# Lung and Heart–Lung Transplantation

# LUNG BIOLOGY IN HEALTH AND DISEASE

*Executive Editor*

**Claude Lenfant**

*Former Director, National Heart, Lung, and Blood Institute*
*National Institutes of Health*
*Bethesda, Maryland*

1. Immunologic and Infectious Reactions in the Lung, *edited by C. H. Kirkpatrick and H. Y. Reynolds*
2. The Biochemical Basis of Pulmonary Function, *edited by R. G. Crystal*
3. Bioengineering Aspects of the Lung, *edited by J. B. West*
4. Metabolic Functions of the Lung, *edited by Y. S. Bakhle and J. R. Vane*
5. Respiratory Defense Mechanisms (in two parts), *edited by J. D. Brain, D. F. Proctor, and L. M. Reid*
6. Development of the Lung, *edited by W. A. Hodson*
7. Lung Water and Solute Exchange, *edited by N. C. Staub*
8. Extrapulmonary Manifestations of Respiratory Disease, *edited by E. D. Robin*
9. Chronic Obstructive Pulmonary Disease, *edited by T. L. Petty*
10. Pathogenesis and Therapy of Lung Cancer, *edited by C. C. Harris*
11. Genetic Determinants of Pulmonary Disease, *edited by S. D. Litwin*
12. The Lung in the Transition Between Health and Disease, *edited by P. T. Macklem and S. Permutt*
13. Evolution of Respiratory Processes: A Comparative Approach, *edited by S. C. Wood and C. Lenfant*
14. Pulmonary Vascular Diseases, *edited by K. M. Moser*
15. Physiology and Pharmacology of the Airways, *edited by J. A. Nadel*
16. Diagnostic Techniques in Pulmonary Disease (in two parts), *edited by M. A. Sackner*
17. Regulation of Breathing (in two parts), *edited by T. F. Hornbein*
18. Occupational Lung Diseases: Research Approaches and Methods, *edited by H. Weill and M. Turner-Warwick*
19. Immunopharmacology of the Lung, *edited by H. H. Newball*
20. Sarcoidosis and Other Granulomatous Diseases of the Lung, *edited by B. L. Fanburg*

21. Sleep and Breathing, *edited by N. A. Saunders and C. E. Sullivan*
22. *Pneumocystis carinii* Pneumonia: Pathogenesis, Diagnosis, and Treatment, *edited by L. S. Young*
23. Pulmonary Nuclear Medicine: Techniques in Diagnosis of Lung Disease, *edited by H. L. Atkins*
24. Acute Respiratory Failure, *edited by W. M. Zapol and K. J. Falke*
25. Gas Mixing and Distribution in the Lung, *edited by L. A. Engel and M. Paiva*
26. High-Frequency Ventilation in Intensive Care and During Surgery, *edited by G. Carlon and W. S. Howland*
27. Pulmonary Development: Transition from Intrauterine to Extrauterine Life, *edited by G. H. Nelson*
28. Chronic Obstructive Pulmonary Disease: Second Edition, *edited by T. L. Petty*
29. The Thorax (in two parts), *edited by C. Roussos and P. T. Macklem*
30. The Pleura in Health and Disease, *edited by J. Chrétien, J. Bignon, and A. Hirsch*
31. Drug Therapy for Asthma: Research and Clinical Practice, *edited by J. W. Jenne and S. Murphy*
32. Pulmonary Endothelium in Health and Disease, *edited by U. S. Ryan*
33. The Airways: Neural Control in Health and Disease, *edited by M. A. Kaliner and P. J. Barnes*
34. Pathophysiology and Treatment of Inhalation Injuries, *edited by J. Loke*
35. Respiratory Function of the Upper Airway, *edited by O. P. Mathew and G. Sant'Ambrogio*
36. Chronic Obstructive Pulmonary Disease: A Behavioral Perspective, *edited by A. J. McSweeny and I. Grant*
37. Biology of Lung Cancer: Diagnosis and Treatment, *edited by S. T. Rosen, J. L. Mulshine, F. Cuttitta, and P. G. Abrams*
38. Pulmonary Vascular Physiology and Pathophysiology, *edited by E. K. Weir and J. T. Reeves*
39. Comparative Pulmonary Physiology: Current Concepts, *edited by S. C. Wood*
40. Respiratory Physiology: An Analytical Approach, *edited by H. K. Chang and M. Paiva*
41. Lung Cell Biology, *edited by D. Massaro*
42. Heart–Lung Interactions in Health and Disease, *edited by S. M. Scharf and S. S. Cassidy*
43. Clinical Epidemiology of Chronic Obstructive Pulmonary Disease, *edited by M. J. Hensley and N. A. Saunders*
44. Surgical Pathology of Lung Neoplasms, *edited by A. M. Marchevsky*
45. The Lung in Rheumatic Diseases, *edited by G. W. Cannon and G. A. Zimmerman*

46. Diagnostic Imaging of the Lung, *edited by C. E. Putman*
47. Models of Lung Disease: Microscopy and Structural Methods, *edited by J. Gil*
48. Electron Microscopy of the Lung, *edited by D. E. Schraufnagel*
49. Asthma: Its Pathology and Treatment, *edited by M. A. Kaliner, P. J. Barnes, and C. G. A. Persson*
50. Acute Respiratory Failure: Second Edition, *edited by W. M. Zapol and F. Lemaire*
51. Lung Disease in the Tropics, *edited by O. P. Sharma*
52. Exercise: Pulmonary Physiology and Pathophysiology, *edited by B. J. Whipp and K. Wasserman*
53. Developmental Neurobiology of Breathing, *edited by G. G. Haddad and J. P. Farber*
54. Mediators of Pulmonary Inflammation, *edited by M. A. Bray and W. H. Anderson*
55. The Airway Epithelium, *edited by S. G. Farmer and D. Hay*
56. Physiological Adaptations in Vertebrates: Respiration, Circulation, and Metabolism, *edited by S. C. Wood, R. E. Weber, A. R. Hargens, and R. W. Millard*
57. The Bronchial Circulation, *edited by J. Butler*
58. Lung Cancer Differentiation: Implications for Diagnosis and Treatment, *edited by S. D. Bernal and P. J. Hesketh*
59. Pulmonary Complications of Systemic Disease, *edited by J. F. Murray*
60. Lung Vascular Injury: Molecular and Cellular Response, *edited by A. Johnson and T. J. Ferro*
61. Cytokines of the Lung, *edited by J. Kelley*
62. The Mast Cell in Health and Disease, *edited by M. A. Kaliner and D. D. Metcalfe*
63. Pulmonary Disease in the Elderly Patient, *edited by D. A. Mahler*
64. Cystic Fibrosis, *edited by P. B. Davis*
65. Signal Transduction in Lung Cells, *edited by J. S. Brody, D. M. Center, and V. A. Tkachuk*
66. Tuberculosis: A Comprehensive International Approach, *edited by L. B. Reichman and E. S. Hershfield*
67. Pharmacology of the Respiratory Tract: Experimental and Clinical Research, *edited by K. F. Chung and P. J. Barnes*
68. Prevention of Respiratory Diseases, *edited by A. Hirsch, M. Goldberg, J.-P. Martin, and R. Masse*
69. *Pneumocystis carinii* Pneumonia: Second Edition, *edited by P. D. Walzer*
70. Fluid and Solute Transport in the Airspaces of the Lungs, *edited by R. M. Effros and H. K. Chang*
71. Sleep and Breathing: Second Edition, *edited by N. A. Saunders and C. E. Sullivan*
72. Airway Secretion: Physiological Bases for the Control of Mucous Hypersecretion, *edited by T. Takishima and S. Shimura*

73. Sarcoidosis and Other Granulomatous Disorders, *edited by D. G. James*
74. Epidemiology of Lung Cancer, *edited by J. M. Samet*
75. Pulmonary Embolism, *edited by M. Morpurgo*
76. Sports and Exercise Medicine, *edited by S. C. Wood and R. C. Roach*
77. Endotoxin and the Lungs, *edited by K. L. Brigham*
78. The Mesothelial Cell and Mesothelioma, *edited by M.-C. Jaurand and J. Bignon*
79. Regulation of Breathing: Second Edition, *edited by J. A. Dempsey and A. I. Pack*
80. Pulmonary Fibrosis, *edited by S. Hin. Phan and R. S. Thrall*
81. Long-Term Oxygen Therapy: Scientific Basis and Clinical Application, *edited by W. J. O'Donohue, Jr.*
82. Ventral Brainstem Mechanisms and Control of Respiration and Blood Pressure, *edited by C. O. Trouth, R. M. Millis, H. F. Kiwull-Schöne, and M. E. Schläfke*
83. A History of Breathing Physiology, *edited by D. F. Proctor*
84. Surfactant Therapy for Lung Disease, *edited by B. Robertson and H. W. Taeusch*
85. The Thorax: Second Edition, Revised and Expanded (in three parts), *edited by C. Roussos*
86. Severe Asthma: Pathogenesis and Clinical Management, *edited by S. J. Szefler and D. Y. M. Leung*
87. *Mycobacterium avium*–Complex Infection: Progress in Research and Treatment, *edited by J. A. Korvick and C. A. Benson*
88. Alpha 1–Antitrypsin Deficiency: Biology • Pathogenesis • Clinical Manifestations • Therapy, *edited by R. G. Crystal*
89. Adhesion Molecules and the Lung, *edited by P. A. Ward and J. C. Fantone*
90. Respiratory Sensation, *edited by L. Adams and A. Guz*
91. Pulmonary Rehabilitation, *edited by A. P. Fishman*
92. Acute Respiratory Failure in Chronic Obstructive Pulmonary Disease, *edited by J.-P. Derenne, W. A. Whitelaw, and T. Similowski*
93. Environmental Impact on the Airways: From Injury to Repair, *edited by J. Chrétien and D. Dusser*
94. Inhalation Aerosols: Physical and Biological Basis for Therapy, *edited by A. J. Hickey*
95. Tissue Oxygen Deprivation: From Molecular to Integrated Function, *edited by G. G. Haddad and G. Lister*
96. The Genetics of Asthma, *edited by S. B. Liggett and D. A. Meyers*
97. Inhaled Glucocorticoids in Asthma: Mechanisms and Clinical Actions, *edited by R. P. Schleimer, W. W. Busse, and P. M. O'Byrne*
98. Nitric Oxide and the Lung, *edited by W. M. Zapol and K. D. Bloch*

99. Primary Pulmonary Hypertension, *edited by L. J. Rubin and S. Rich*

100. Lung Growth and Development, *edited by J. A. McDonald*

101. Parasitic Lung Diseases, *edited by A. A. F. Mahmoud*

102. Lung Macrophages and Dendritic Cells in Health and Disease, *edited by M. F. Lipscomb and S. W. Russell*

103. Pulmonary and Cardiac Imaging, *edited by C. Chiles and C. E. Putman*

104. Gene Therapy for Diseases of the Lung, *edited by K. L. Brigham*

105. Oxygen, Gene Expression, and Cellular Function, *edited by L. Biadasz Clerch and D. J. Massaro*

106. Beta$_2$-Agonists in Asthma Treatment, *edited by R. Pauwels and P. M. O'Byrne*

107. Inhalation Delivery of Therapeutic Peptides and Proteins, *edited by A. L. Adjei and P. K. Gupta*

108. Asthma in the Elderly, *edited by R. A. Barbee and J. W. Bloom*

109. Treatment of the Hospitalized Cystic Fibrosis Patient, *edited by D. M. Orenstein and R. C. Stern*

110. Asthma and Immunological Diseases in Pregnancy and Early Infancy, *edited by M. Schatz, R. S. Zeiger, and H. N. Claman*

111. Dyspnea, *edited by D. A. Mahler*

112. Proinflammatory and Antiinflammatory Peptides, *edited by S. I. Said*

113. Self-Management of Asthma, *edited by H. Kotses and A. Harver*

114. Eicosanoids, Aspirin, and Asthma, *edited by A. Szczeklik, R. J. Gryglewski, and J. R. Vane*

115. Fatal Asthma, *edited by A. L. Sheffer*

116. Pulmonary Edema, *edited by M. A. Matthay and D. H. Ingbar*

117. Inflammatory Mechanisms in Asthma, *edited by S. T. Holgate and W. W. Busse*

118. Physiological Basis of Ventilatory Support, *edited by J. J. Marini and A. S. Slutsky*

119. Human Immunodeficiency Virus and the Lung, *edited by M. J. Rosen and J. M. Beck*

120. Five-Lipoxygenase Products in Asthma, *edited by J. M. Drazen, S.-E. Dahlén, and T. H. Lee*

121. Complexity in Structure and Function of the Lung, *edited by M. P. Hlastala and H. T. Robertson*

122. Biology of Lung Cancer, *edited by M. A. Kane and P. A. Bunn, Jr.*

123. Rhinitis: Mechanisms and Management, *edited by R. M. Naclerio, S. R. Durham, and N. Mygind*

124. Lung Tumors: Fundamental Biology and Clinical Management, *edited by C. Brambilla and E. Brambilla*

125. Interleukin-5: From Molecule to Drug Target for Asthma, *edited by C. J. Sanderson*

126. Pediatric Asthma, *edited by S. Murphy and H. W. Kelly*

127. Viral Infections of the Respiratory Tract, *edited by R. Dolin and P. F. Wright*

128. Air Pollutants and the Respiratory Tract, *edited by D. L. Swift and W. M. Foster*

129. Gastroesophageal Reflux Disease and Airway Disease, *edited by M. R. Stein*

130. Exercise-Induced Asthma, *edited by E. R. McFadden, Jr.*

131. LAM and Other Diseases Characterized by Smooth Muscle Proliferation, *edited by J. Moss*

132. The Lung at Depth, *edited by C. E. G. Lundgren and J. N. Miller*

133. Regulation of Sleep and Circadian Rhythms, *edited by F. W. Turek and P. C. Zee*

134. Anticholinergic Agents in the Upper and Lower Airways, *edited by S. L. Spector*

135. Control of Breathing in Health and Disease, *edited by M. D. Altose and Y. Kawakami*

136. Immunotherapy in Asthma, *edited by J. Bousquet and H. Yssel*

137. Chronic Lung Disease in Early Infancy, *edited by R. D. Bland and J. J. Coalson*

138. Asthma's Impact on Society: The Social and Economic Burden, *edited by K. B. Weiss, A. S. Buist, and S. D. Sullivan*

139. New and Exploratory Therapeutic Agents for Asthma, *edited by M. Yeadon and Z. Diamant*

140. Multimodality Treatment of Lung Cancer, *edited by A. T. Skarin*

141. Cytokines in Pulmonary Disease: Infection and Inflammation, *edited by S. Nelson and T. R. Martin*

142. Diagnostic Pulmonary Pathology, *edited by P. T. Cagle*

143. Particle–Lung Interactions, *edited by P. Gehr and J. Heyder*

144. Tuberculosis: A Comprehensive International Approach, Second Edition, Revised and Expanded, *edited by L. B. Reichman and E. S. Hershfield*

145. Combination Therapy for Asthma and Chronic Obstructive Pulmonary Disease, *edited by R. J. Martin and M. Kraft*

146. Sleep Apnea: Implications in Cardiovascular and Cerebrovascular Disease, *edited by T. D. Bradley and J. S. Floras*

147. Sleep and Breathing in Children: A Developmental Approach, *edited by G. M. Loughlin, J. L. Carroll, and C. L. Marcus*

148. Pulmonary and Peripheral Gas Exchange in Health and Disease, *edited by J. Roca, R. Rodriguez-Roisen, and P. D. Wagner*

149. Lung Surfactants: Basic Science and Clinical Applications, *R. H. Notter*

150. Nosocomial Pneumonia, *edited by W. R. Jarvis*

151. Fetal Origins of Cardiovascular and Lung Disease, *edited by David J. P. Barker*

152. Long-Term Mechanical Ventilation, *edited by N. S. Hill*
153. Environmental Asthma, *edited by R. K. Bush*
154. Asthma and Respiratory Infections, *edited by D. P. Skoner*
155. Airway Remodeling, *edited by P. H. Howarth, J. W. Wilson, J. Bousquet, S. Rak, and R. A. Pauwels*
156. Genetic Models in Cardiorespiratory Biology, *edited by G. G. Haddad and T. Xu*
157. Respiratory-Circulatory Interactions in Health and Disease, *edited by S. M. Scharf, M. R. Pinsky, and S. Magder*
158. Ventilator Management Strategies for Critical Care, *edited by N. S. Hill and M. M. Levy*
159. Severe Asthma: Pathogenesis and Clinical Management, Second Edition, Revised and Expanded, *edited by S. J. Szefler and D. Y. M. Leung*
160. Gravity and the Lung: Lessons from Microgravity, *edited by G. K. Prisk, M. Paiva, and J. B. West*
161. High Altitude: An Exploration of Human Adaptation, *edited by T. F. Hornbein and R. B. Schoene*
162. Drug Delivery to the Lung, *edited by H. Bisgaard, C. O'Callaghan, and G. C. Smaldone*
163. Inhaled Steroids in Asthma: Optimizing Effects in the Airways, *edited by R. P. Schleimer, P. M. O'Byrne, S. J. Szefler, and R. Brattsand*
164. IgE and Anti-IgE Therapy in Asthma and Allergic Disease, *edited by R. B. Fick, Jr., and P. M. Jardieu*
165. Clinical Management of Chronic Obstructive Pulmonary Disease, *edited by T. Similowski, W. A. Whitelaw, and J.-P. Derenne*
166. Sleep Apnea: Pathogenesis, Diagnosis, and Treatment, *edited by A. I. Pack*
167. Biotherapeutic Approaches to Asthma, *edited by J. Agosti and A. L. Sheffer*
168. Proteoglycans in Lung Disease, *edited by H. G. Garg, P. J. Roughley, and C. A. Hales*
169. Gene Therapy in Lung Disease, *edited by S. M. Albelda*
170. Disease Markers in Exhaled Breath, *edited by N. Marczin, S. A. Kharitonov, M. H. Yacoub, and P. J. Barnes*
171. Sleep-Related Breathing Disorders: Experimental Models and Therapeutic Potential, *edited by D. W. Carley and M. Radulovacki*
172. Chemokines in the Lung, *edited by R. M. Strieter, S. L. Kunkel, and T. J. Standiford*
173. Respiratory Control and Disorders in the Newborn, *edited by O. P. Mathew*
174. The Immunological Basis of Asthma, *edited by B. N. Lambrecht, H. C. Hoogsteden, and Z. Diamant*
175. Oxygen Sensing: Responses and Adaptation to Hypoxia, *edited by S. Lahiri, G. L. Semenza, and N. R. Prabhakar*

176. Non-Neoplastic Advanced Lung Disease, *edited by J. R. Maurer*

177. Therapeutic Targets in Airway Inflammation, *edited by N. T. Eissa and D. P. Huston*

178. Respiratory Infections in Allergy and Asthma, *edited by S. L. Johnston and N. G. Papadopoulos*

179. Acute Respiratory Distress Syndrome, *edited by M. A. Matthay*

180. Venous Thromboembolism, *edited by J. E. Dalen*

181. Upper and Lower Respiratory Disease, *edited by J. Corren, A. Togias, and J. Bousquet*

182. Pharmacotherapy in Chronic Obstructive Pulmonary Disease, *edited by B. R. Celli*

183. Acute Exacerbations of Chronic Obstructive Pulmonary Disease, *edited by N. M. Siafakas, N. R. Anthonisen, and D. Georgopoulos*

184. Lung Volume Reduction Surgery for Emphysema, *edited by H. E. Fessler, J. J. Reilly, Jr., and D. J. Sugarbaker*

185. Idiopathic Pulmonary Fibrosis, *edited by J. P. Lynch III*

186. Pleural Disease, *edited by D. Bouros*

187. Oxygen/Nitrogen Radicals: Lung Injury and Disease, *edited by V. Vallyathan, V. Castranova, and X. Shi*

188. Therapy for Mucus-Clearance Disorders, *edited by B. K. Rubin and C. P. van der Schans*

189. Interventional Pulmonary Medicine, *edited by J. F. Beamis, Jr., P. N. Mathur, and A. C. Mehta*

190. Lung Development and Regeneration, *edited by D. J. Massaro, G. Massaro, and P. Chambon*

191. Long-Term Intervention in Chronic Obstructive Pulmonary Disease, *edited by R. Pauwels, D. S. Postma, and S. T. Weiss*

192. Sleep Deprivation: Basic Science, Physiology, and Behavior, *edited by Clete A. Kushida*

193. Sleep Deprivation: Clinical Issues, Pharmacology, and Sleep Loss Effects, *edited by Clete A. Kushida*

194. Pneumocystis Pneumonia: Third Edition, Revised and Expanded, *edited by P. D. Walzer and M. Cushion*

195. Asthma Prevention, *edited by William W. Busse and Robert F. Lemanske, Jr.*

196. Lung Injury: Mechanisms, Pathophysiology, and Therapy, *edited by Robert H. Notter, Jacob Finkelstein, and Bruce Holm*

197. Ion Channels in the Pulmonary Vasculature, *edited by Jason X.-J. Yuan*

198. Chronic Obstuctive Pulmonary Disease: Cellular and Molecular Mechanisms, *edited by Peter J. Barnes*

199. Pediatric Nasal and Sinus Disorders, *edited by Tania Sih and Peter A. R. Clement*

200. Functional Lung Imaging, *edited by David Lipson and Edwin van Beek*

201. Lung Surfactant Function and Disorder, *edited by Kaushik Nag*

202. Pharmacology and Pathophysiology of the Control of Breathing, *edited by Denham S. Ward, Albert Dahan and Luc J. Teppema*

203. Molecular Imaging of the Lungs, *edited by Daniel Schuster and Timothy Blackwell*

204. Air Pollutants and the Respiratory Tract: Second Edition, *edited by W. Michael Foster and Daniel L. Costa*

205. Acute and Chronic Cough, *edited by Anthony E. Redington and Alyn H. Morice*

206. Severe Pneumonia, *edited by Michael S. Niederman*

207. Monitoring Asthma, *edited by Peter G. Gibson*

208. Dyspnea: Mechanisms, Measurement, and Management, Second Edition, *edited by Donald A. Mahler and Denis E. O'Donnell*

209. Childhood Asthma, *edited by Stanley J. Szefler and Søren Pedersen*

210. Sarcoidosis, *edited by Robert Baughman*

211. Tropical Lung Disease, Second Edition, *edited by Om Sharma*

212. Pharmacotherapy of Asthma, *edited by James T. Li*

213. Practical Pulmonary and Critical Care Medicine: Respiratory Failure, *edited by Zab Mosenifar and Guy W. Soo Hoo*

214. Practical Pulmonary and Critical Care Medicine: Disease Management, *edited by Zab Mosenifar and Guy W. Soo Hoo*

215. Ventilator-Induced Lung Injury, *edited by Didier Dreyfuss, Georges Saumon, and Rolf D. Hubmayr*

216. Bronchial Vascular Remodeling In Asthma and COPD, *edited by Aili Lazaar*

217. Lung and Heart–Lung Transplantation, *edited by Joseph P. Lynch III and David J. Ross*

*The opinions expressed in these volumes do not necessarily represent the views of the National Institutes of Health.*

# Lung and Heart–Lung Transplantation

Edited by

## Joseph P. Lynch III
*David Geffen School of Medicine at UCLA*
*University of California*
*Los Angeles, California, U.S.A.*

## David J. Ross
*David Geffen School of Medicine at UCLA*
*University of California*
*Los Angeles, California, U.S.A.*

Taylor & Francis
Taylor & Francis Group
New York   London

Taylor & Francis is an imprint of the
Taylor & Francis Group, an informa business

Published in 2006 by
Taylor & Francis Group
270 Madison Avenue
New York, NY 10016

© 2006 by Taylor & Francis Group, LLC

No claim to original U.S. Government works
Printed in the United States of America on acid-free paper
10 9 8 7 6 5 4 3 2 1

International Standard Book Number-10: 0-8493-3717-8 (Hardcover)
International Standard Book Number-13: 978-0-8493-3717-8 (Hardcover)

**Library of Congress Cataloging-in-Publication Data**

Catalog record is available from the Library of Congress

# informa

Taylor & Francis Group
is the Academic Division of Informa plc.

Visit the Taylor & Francis Web site at
http://www.taylorandfrancis.com

# Introduction

Since the middle of the last century, we have witnessed extraordinary advances in medicine and surgery. Organ transplantation has been the beneficiary of our increased knowledge in fundamental biological processes and in clinical medicine as well.

However, as is often the case, an examination of the more distant past shows that today's discoveries and advances rest on the pioneering work of preceding scientists, not to say luminaries! For example, the foundations of organ transplantation were truly established by the work of Alexis Carrel on cell and tissue culture in the early years of the 20th century. Undoubtedly, Carrel foresaw the potential of his work when in 1905 he and Charles Guthrie of the University of Chicago performed the very first experimental heart transplant.

The journey of lung transplantation began later, at the end of the first half of the 20th century, when Vladimir P. Deminkhov of the former Soviet Union performed the first lung transplant in a dog in early 1947. Later the same year, he transplanted a lower lung lobe into a dog and the dog actually survived one week.

It took another sixteen years to see the very first single-lung transplant performed by James D. Hardy at the University of Mississippi in a 60-year-old man. The patient died eight days later of heart failure. This first case literally opened the door on a surge of interest in lung transplantation. The interest was huge but the progress was slow because of complications, primarily infection and rejection, or technical difficulties, primarily bronchial anastomosis failure. It is reported that in the next 15 years, to 1978, only 39 human lung transplants had been done. It is truly admirable that the interest did not subside; on the contrary, many teams of surgeons and investigators were established worldwide and the work continued.

Recently, the International Society for Heart–Lung Transplantation indicated that 1767 lung transplants had been reported to them in the year 2002. The society cautioned, however, that the reported number may, in fact, be many less than the number of procedures performed. Indeed, the editors of this volume indicate that in the last 25 years "20,000 lung transplants, and 3000 heart–lung transplants have been performed worldwide." This surely underscores the remarkable journey of this procedure.

However, we cannot ignore the risks and complications of lung transplantation. The problems and the fears that developed very early remain major obstacles to further, or more rapid, use of lung transplantation in pulmonary medicine. At the same time, the list of conditions that could benefit from the procedure has lengthened and the actuarial survival rates are increasing.

Should all this overcast the future of lung transplantation? The loud response from this monograph is absolutely not!

This volume, offered by the series of monographs Lung Biology in Health and Disease, presents a comprehensive view of lung transplantation. It reports a multinational experience of basic and clinical scientists who, in fact, have led the journey of lung transplantation. Just about when the series presented its first volume, in 1976, only 39 cases of lung transplantation had been attempted. Today, the experience is about 25,000 combined cases, and the experience is all in this volume.

The editors of this volume, *Lung and Heart–Lung Transplantation*, Drs. Joseph P. Lynch III and David J. Ross, are bringing to the readership the work of 75 authors, all experts in their field, and the multinational experience of six countries. I am extremely grateful to them for this contribution and the opportunity to present it to our readership.

*Claude Lenfant, MD*
*Gaithersburg, Maryland, U.S.A.*

# Preface

*Lung and Heart–Lung Transplantation* provides a comprehensive and state-of-the-art review of clinical and investigative aspects of lung (and heart–lung) transplantation. In this book, international experts from diverse programs representing multiple countries (Australia, Belgium, Canada, Germany, United Kingdom, and United States) and disciplines (surgery, medicine, and immunology) have compiled a superb synthesis of a vast array of information gleaned over the past three decades. Since the first successful heart–lung transplant at Stanford University in 1981, more than 20,000 lung transplants and 3000 heart–lung transplants have been performed worldwide. Over the 25 years spanning the seminal transplant, extensive refinements in surgical techniques, advances in medical knowledge, availability of newer immunosuppressive regimens, and liberal use of antimicrobial prophylactic strategies led to improved prognosis. Unfortunately, despite improvements in survival, chronic allograft rejection remains a vexing and potentially lethal complication, affecting more than half of all lung transplant recipients during the course of the disease. Substantial insights into the pathogenesis of acute and chronic lung allograft rejection have been gleaned from animal models as well as research studies in human lung transplant recipients, but effective treatment for chronic allograft rejection is still lacking. However, a greater understanding of the mechanisms of allograft rejection may stimulate development of newer and more effective strategies to prevent and treat this complication.

This book provides a superlative review of past successes (and failures) associated with lung transplantation, but also provides insight into the latest advances and evolving concepts of lung transplantation. In Chapter 1, Dr. Rutherford and colleagues present a fascinating historical overview of lung transplants and heart–lung transplants, and review cumulative data from the International Registry on outcomes associated with these surgeries worldwide. In Chapter 2, Drs. Cobbold and Waldmann discuss the role of regulatory T cells and dendritic cells in transplantation (rejection and tolerance). In Chapter 3, Dr. Meyer expands on basic immune mechanisms that are operative in allogeneic recognition, rejection, and tolerance. These two basic science chapters provide a framework for understanding the pitfalls inherent in clinical lung transplantation and insights into future strategies to limit or prevent allograft rejection.

Chapters 4 through 9 delineate the indications for lung transplantation for specific disease states [e.g., chronic obstructive pulmonary disease, cystic fibrosis, pulmonary hypertension (primary and secondary forms), interstitial lung diseases, pulmonary Langerhans cell histiocytosis and lymphangioleiomyomatosis, and end-stage lung or pulmonary vascular/cardiac disorders in children]. Each of these chapters reviews the past and current results of lung transplantation in those specific patient cohorts, and also discusses available medical therapies (before or in lieu of lung transplantation) and factors unique to each disease that influence the decision to refer for lung transplantation. Specific parameters or criteria (e.g., physiologic, radiographic, clinical) that guide the decision to refer for lung transplantation are developed for each disease state. For example, in Chapter 4, Drs. Kotloff and Martinez provide an elegant and comprehensive review of both medical and surgical (i.e., lung volume reduction surgery and transplant) treatment options for chronic obstructive pulmonary disease. They discuss in depth various medical therapies (i.e., bronchodilators, corticosteroids, oxygen, pulmonary rehabilitation) and prognostic factors to take into account to assess the suitability of lung transplantation. The role of lung volume reduction surgery and selection criteria for this surgery are discussed in depth. In Chapter 5, Drs. Coakley and Yankaskas discuss complications commonly observed in cystic fibrosis (e.g., differing pharmacokinetics, intestinal dysmotility, and other gastrointestinal complications, diabetes mellitus, chronic sinusitis, and specific infectious complications with cystic fibrosis such as pan-resistant *Pseudomonas aeruginosa*, *Burkholderia cepacea*, *Aspergillus*, and atypical mycobacteria). In Chapter 6, Dr. Saggar and colleagues delineate the specific problems inherent with primary or secondary forms of pulmonary arterial hypertension (e.g., early pulmonary edema following transplantation and the impact of adverse right ventricular function) and controversies regarding single or bilateral lung transplantation for this disease. Chapters 7 and 8 review specific interstitial lung disorders including idiopathic pulmonary fibrosis, nonspecific interstitial pneumonia, connective tissue disease–associated pulmonary fibrosis, sarcoidosis, pulmonary Langerhans cell histiocytosis, and lymphangioleiomyomatosis. For each of these disorders, medical therapies are discussed in detail and criteria are developed for lung transplant candidates. In Chapter 9, Drs. Mallory and Elidemir describe the experience of lung-transplant and heart–lung transplant pediatric patients with diverse end-stage pulmonary or pulmonary vascular/cardiac disorders. Limited availability of donor organs is a major limiting factor and is responsible for prolonged waiting times among patients listed for lung transplantation. Given the potential for death while awaiting lung transplantation, living lobar lung transplantation was adopted as an alternative to cadaveric lung transplantation and may be lifesaving in patients with terminal respiratory illnesses. In Chapter 10, Drs. Bowdish and Barr review the indications for living lobar lung transplantation, criteria for donor and recipient selection, technique, and outcomes of this operation. Given the shortage of donor organs, combined heart–lung transplantation, a technique utilized in the 1980s for end-stage pulmonary vascular disease (particularly for pulmonary arterial hypertension and complex congenital cardiac defects) has been utilized less often in recent years. In Chapter 11, Drs. Moffatt-Bruce and Reitz discuss the indications for heart–lung transplantation, outcomes, and specific complications associated with this operation and also review medical and surgical alternatives (e.g., atrial septostomy, pulmonary thromboendarterectomy, lung transplantation with repair of cardiac defects) that may obviate the need for heart–lung transplantation. The limited lung donor pool and prolonged waiting times for lung transplants have necessitated changes in strategies for organ procurement and allocation as well as improved lung preservation techniques. Chapters 12 through 14 discuss the systems of organ allocation in the United States, Europe, and Australia, including major and complex changes in organ allocation in the United States introduced in 2005. In Chapter 15, Drs. D'Ovidio and Keshavjee articulate novel techniques to enhance lung preservation and expand the donor pool. Chapter 16, by Drs. Schnickel and Ardehali, expands on this concept to advocate more liberal use of donor organs (including use of "nonstandard" lungs). Immunosuppressive therapy is a double-edged sword, as excessive immunosuppression increases the risk for infectious and neoplastic complications while inadequate immunosuppression places the allograft(s) at risk. Chapters 17 and 18 discuss in detail the various immunosuppressive agents currently available, including corticosteroids, antimetabolites, cytotoxic agents, calcineurin inhibitors, and monoclonal or polyclonal antibodies directed against T cells, B cells, or specific receptors. The mechanisms of action, efficacy, monitoring strategies, and complications of each of these agents are discussed in detail. In Chapter 19, Dr. McCurry and colleagues review novel and future approaches to immunosuppression with a focus on inhaled cyclosporine and Campath-1H.

Potentially serious complications of lung transplantation include primary graft dysfunction, complications at the bronchial anastomotic site(s), infections, chronic and acute allograft rejection, cardiovascular and metabolic derangements, and neoplasia. In Chapter 20, Dr. Mulligan discusses primary graft dysfunction, risk factors, management, and outcomes associated with primary graft dysfunction. In Chapter 21, Drs. Angel and

Susanto discuss complications that may arise at the bronchial anastomotic site and potential therapeutic interventions. Chapters 22 through 28 describe the myriad opportunistic infections that may complicate solid organ transplantation. In Chapter 22, Dr. Zamora discusses in detail the incidence and impact of viral infections on lung transplant recipients; their relationship to allograft rejection; and prophylactic, preemptive, and treatment strategies for a host of viral infections. He also discusses the emergence of novel and community-acquired viruses, resistant strains, and strategies for the recognition, prevention, and treatment of viral infections. The incidence, spectrum, diagnostic modalities, clinical impact, and treatment of fungal infections among solid organ transplant recipients are discussed in Chapters 23 through 25. In Chapter 23, Dr. Kubak provides an in-depth discussion of coccidiodomycosis; in Chapter 24, Dr. Kauffman discusses the endemic mycoses, histoplasmosis and blastomycosis, with emphasis on evolving newer therapies. In Chapter 25, Drs. Husain and Silveira emphasize that infections due to *Aspergillus* spp are common among lung transplant recipients (particularly at the bronchial anastomoses) compared to other solid organ transplant recipients and outline prophylactic and treatment strategies for this potentially lethal pathogen. They also discuss *Cryptococcus, Fusarium,* Zygomycetes, and dermatiaceous molds, many of which are resistant to many of the commonly utilized antifungal agents. Other opportunistic pathogens complicating solid organ transplant recipients are discussed in Chapter 26 (bacteria, *Nocardia* spp, and *Pneumocystic jirovecii*), Chapter 27 (*Legionella* spp), and Chapter 28 (nontuberculous mycobacteria and *Mycobacterium tuberculosis*).

Rejection of the allograft(s) remains the Achilles heel of lung transplantation and the major obstacle to long-term survival. Chapters 29 through 32 discuss in depth the epidemiology, pathogenesis, risk factors, and clinical features of acute rejection (Chapter 29), histopathological features of acute and chronic rejection as well as opportunistic infections (Chapter 30), and chronic rejection (Chapters 31 and 32). The basic immunological mechanism operative in chronic and acute allograft rejection (including roles of cytokines, chemokines, HLA matching, gastrointestinal reflux, etc.) are discussed in detail. The role of specific diagnostic or monitoring techniques (e.g., pulmonary function tests, bronchoscopy, imaging procedures, etc.) to identify complications of lung transplantation is reviewed in detail in Chapters 33 and 34. Monitoring of pulmonary physiology is an integral component of follow-up to assure adequate function of the lung allograft(s) and to identify complications that may develop (particularly episodes of rejection or infection). In Chapter 33, Dr. Estenne presents a comprehensive review of physiological responses (normal and abnormal) that may be observed in lung transplant recipients, including effects of lung denervation, sternotomy or thoracotomy, immunosuppressive medications, impaired mucociliary clearance, muscle weakness, and allograft rejection. He details physiological and imaging studies that may be useful to follow lung transplant recipients longitudinally. In Chapter 34, Drs. Suh, Myers, and Goldin elegantly describe the role of radiographic imaging to detect various complications (e.g., mechanical, traumatic, or ischemia-reperfusion injury; infections; acute or chronic rejection; pulmonary embolism; malignancy; drug-induced injury) at various time points following lung transplantation. Finally, Chapters 35 through 37 discuss late complications that may occur following lung transplantation. In Chapter 35, Drs. Patel, Kobashigawa, and Hamilton discuss cardiac, lipid, and atherosclerotic complications among lung transplant recipients. In Chapter 36, Dr. Maurer addresses osteoporosis and metabolic bone disease among lung transplant recipients. Finally, in Chapter 37 Dr. Weigt and colleagues discuss the spectrum of posttransplant lymphoproliferative disorders, including pathogenesis, risk factors, histopathological types, clinical features, diagnosis (including immunohistochemical stains) and treatment.

In summary, this book combines the insights and experience of the best international experts in lung transplantation and provides a global and state-of-the-art perspective of the current and future role of lung transplantation worldwide. The book will be of great interest not only to pulmonologists, transplant physicians, surgeons, nurses, and medical personnel with an interest in transplantation, but also to basic scientists with an interest in transplant immunology.

*Joseph P. Lynch III*
*David J. Ross*

# Contributors

**Luis F. Angel**   Division of Pulmonary and Critical Care and Cardiothoracic Surgery, Departments of Medicine and Surgery, University of Texas Health Science Center at San Antonio, San Antonio, Texas, U.S.A.

**Abbas Ardehali**   Division of Cardiothoracic Surgery, David Geffen School of Medicine at UCLA, Los Angeles, California, U.S.A.

**Robert Aris**   Division of Pulmonary and Critical Care Medicine and Cystic Fibrosis/Pulmonary Research and Treatment Center, University of North Carolina at Chapel Hill, Chapel Hill, North Carolina, U.S.A.

**Mark L. Barr**   Department of Cardiothoracic Surgery, University of Southern California and Childrens Hospital Los Angeles, Los Angeles, California, U.S.A.

**John A. Belperio**   Division of Pulmonary and Critical Care Medicine, Department of Medicine, David Geffen School of Medicine at UCLA, Los Angeles, California, U.S.A.

**Sangeeta M. Bhorade**   Division of Pulmonary and Critical Care Medicine, Department of Internal Medicine, Loyola University Medical Center, Maywood, Illinois, U.S.A.

**Michael E. Bowdish**   Department of Cardiothoracic Surgery, University of Southern California Keck School of Medicine, Los Angeles, California, U.S.A.

**Rami Bustami** Scientific Registry of Transplant Recipients (SRTR), University Renal Research and Education Association (URREA), University of Michigan, Ann Arbor, Michigan, U.S.A.

**Nina M. Clark** Section of Infectious Diseases, Department of Internal Medicine, University of Illinois at Chicago, Chicago, Illinois, U.S.A.

**Raymond D. Coakley** Cystic Fibrosis/Pulmonary Research and Treatment Center, University of North Carolina at Chapel Hill, Chapel Hill, North Carolina, U.S.A.

**Stephen P. Cobbold** Therapeutic Immunology Group, Sir William Dunn School of Pathology, University of Oxford, Oxford, U.K.

**Matthew A. Coke** United Network for Organ Sharing (UNOS), Richmond, Virginia, U.S.A.

**Paul A. Corris** Department of Cardiopulmonary Transplantation, Freeman Hospital, Newcastle upon Tyne, Tyne and Wear, U.K.

**Frank D'Ovidio** Toronto Lung Transplant Program, University of Toronto, Toronto, Canada

**Brian P. Dickover** Division of Pulmonary and Critical Care Medicine, Department of Internal Medicine, Loyola University Medical Center, Maywood, Illinois, U.S.A.

**Stephen Dummer** Department of Infectious Diseases, Vanderbilt University Medical Center, Nashville, Tennessee, U.S.A.

**Lieven J. Dupont** Department of Respiratory Medicine and Lung Transplantation Unit, University Hospital Gasthuisberg, Leuven, Belgium

**Leah B. Edwards** United Network for Organ Sharing (UNOS), Richmond, Virginia, U.S.A.

**Thomas M. Egan** Division of Cardiothoracic Surgery, Department of Surgery, University of North Carolina at Chapel Hill, Chapel Hill, North Carolina, U.S.A.

**Okan Elidemir** Department of Pediatrics, Baylor College of Medicine, Houston, Texas, U.S.A.

**Marc Estenne**   Chest Service and Thoracic Transplantation Unit, Erasme University Hospital, Brussels School of Medicine, Brussels, Belgium

**John L. Faul**   Division of Pulmonary and Critical Care Medicine, Vera Moulton Wall Center for Pulmonary Vascular Disease, Stanford University, Stanford, California, U.S.A.

**Michael C. Fishbein**   Department of Pathology and Laboratory Medicine, David Geffen School of Medicine at UCLA, Los Angeles, California, U.S.A.

**Andrew J. Fisher**   Department of Cardiopulmonary Transplantation, Freeman Hospital, Newcastle upon Tyne, Tyne and Wear, U.K.

**Edward R. Garrity, Jr.**   Division of Pulmonary and Critical Care Medicine, Department of Internal Medicine, Loyola University Medical Center, Maywood, Illinois, U.S.A.

**Jonathan G. Goldin**   Department of Radiological Sciences, David Geffen School of Medicine at UCLA, Los Angeles, California, U.S.A.

**Michele Hamilton**   Division of Cardiology, David Geffen School of Medicine at UCLA, Center for Health Sciences, Los Angeles, California, U.S.A.

**David N. Howell**   Department of Pathology, Duke University and Durham Veterans Affairs Medical Centers, Durham, North Carolina, U.S.A.

**Shahid Husain**   Department of Medicine, University of Pittsburgh, Pittsburgh, Pennsylvania, U.S.A.

**Aldo Iacono**   Division of Pulmonary Medicine, Department of Medicine, University of Maryland, Baltimore, Maryland, U.S.A.

**Carol A. Kauffman**   Division of Infectious Diseases, Veterans Affairs Ann Arbor Healthcare System, University of Michigan Medical School, Ann Arbor, Michigan, U.S.A.

**Shaf Keshavjee**   Toronto Lung Transplant Program, University of Toronto, Toronto, Canada

**Jon A. Kobashigawa**   Division of Cardiology, David Geffen School of Medicine at UCLA, Center for Health Sciences, Los Angeles, California, U.S.A.

**Robert M. Kotloff**   Pulmonary, Allergy, and Critical Care Division, Department of Medicine, University of Pennsylvania, Philadelphia, Pennsylvania, U.S.A.

**Bernard M. Kubak**   Division of Infectious Diseases, Department of Medicine, David Geffen School of Medicine at UCLA, Los Angeles, California, U.S.A.

**Lucy R. Langer**   Division of Hematology and Oncology, Department of Internal Medicine, David Geffen School of Medicine at UCLA, Los Angeles, California, U.S.A.

**Robert D. Levy**   University of British Columbia, Vancouver, British Columbia, Canada

**James L. Lordan**   Department of Cardiopulmonary Transplantation, Freeman Hospital, Newcastle upon Tyne, Tyne and Wear, U.K.

**Brandon S. Lu**   Division of Pulmonary and Critical Care Medicine, Department of Internal Medicine, Loyola University Medical Center, Maywood, Illinois, U.S.A.

**Joseph P. Lynch III**   Division of Pulmonary and Critical Care Medicine and Hospitalists, Department of Internal Medicine, David Geffen School of Medicine at UCLA, Los Angeles, California, U.S.A.

**George B. Mallory**   Department of Pediatrics, Baylor College of Medicine, Houston, Texas, U.S.A.

**Fernando J. Martinez**   Department of Internal Medicine, University of Michigan Health System, Ann Arbor, Michigan, U.S.A.

**Janet R. Maurer**   Health Dialog Services Corporation, Phoenix, Arizona, U.S.A.

**Kenneth R. McCurry**   Division of Cardiothoracic Surgery, Department of Surgery, University of Pittsburgh School of Medicine, Pittsburgh, Pennsylvania, U.S.A.

**Keith C. Meyer**   Section of Allergy, Pulmonary, and Critical Care Medicine, University of Wisconsin School of Medicine and Public Health, Madison, Wisconsin, U.S.A.

**Susan D. Moffatt-Bruce**   Department of Cardiothoracic Surgery, Stanford University Medical School, Stanford, California, U.S.A.

**Michael S. Mulligan** Division of Cardiothoracic Surgery, Department of Surgery, University of Washington, Seattle, Washington, U.S.A.

**Susan Murray** Scientific Registry of Transplant Recipients (SRTR), University of Michigan, Ann Arbor, Michigan, U.S.A.

**Tikvah Myers** Department of Radiological Sciences, David Geffen School of Medicine at UCLA, Los Angeles, California, U.S.A.

**Steven Nathan** Lung Transplant Program, Inova Heart and Vascular Institute, Falls Church, Virginia, U.S.A.

**Jonathan B. Orens** Division of Pulmonary and Critical Care Medicine, Department of Medicine, The Johns Hopkins University School of Medicine, Baltimore, Maryland, U.S.A.

**Scott M. Palmer** Division of Pulmonary and Critical Care Medicine, Department of Medicine, Duke University Medical Center, Durham, North Carolina, U.S.A.

**Jignesh K. Patel** Division of Cardiology, David Geffen School of Medicine at UCLA, Center for Health Sciences, Los Angeles, California, U.S.A.

**Hermann Reichenspurner** Department of Cardiovascular Surgery, University Heart Center, University of Hamburg, Hamburg, Germany

**Bruce A. Reitz** Department of Cardiothoracic Surgery, Stanford University Medical School, Stanford, California, U.S.A.

**David J. Ross** Division of Pulmonary and Critical Care Medicine and Hospitalists, Department of Internal Medicine, David Geffen School of Medicine at UCLA, Los Angeles, California, U.S.A.

**Robert M. Rutherford** Department of Cardiopulmonary Transplantation, Freeman Hospital, Newcastle upon Tyne, Tyne and Wear, U.K.

**Rajan Saggar** Division of Pulmonary and Critical Care Medicine and Hospitalists, Department of Internal Medicine, David Geffen School of Medicine at UCLA, Los Angeles, California, U.S.A.

**Rajeev Saggar** Division of Pulmonary and Critical Care Medicine, Department of Medicine, University of California at Irvine, Irvine, California, U.S.A.

**Gabriel T. Schnickel**   Division of Cardiothoracic Surgery, David Geffen School of Medicine at UCLA, Los Angeles, California, U.S.A.

**Tempie H. Shearon**   Scientific Registry of Transplant Recipients (SRTR), University of Michigan, Ann Arbor, Michigan, U.S.A.

**Fernanda P. Silveira**   Department of Medicine, University of Pittsburgh, Pittsburgh, Pennsylvania, U.S.A.

**Gregory I. Snell**   Department of Allergy, Immunology, and Respiratory Medicine, The Alfred Hospital, Monash University Clinical School, Melbourne, Victoria, Australia

**Sean Studer**   University of Pittsburgh School of Medicine, Pittsburgh, Pennsylvania, U.S.A.

**Robert D. Suh**   Department of Radiological Sciences, David Geffen School of Medicine at UCLA, Los Angeles, California, U.S.A.

**Irawan Susanto**   Division of Pulmonary and Critical Care and Hospitalists, Department of Medicine, David Geffen School of Medicine at UCLA, University of California, Los Angeles, California, U.S.A.

**Lora D. Thomas**   Department of Infectious Diseases, Vanderbilt University Medical Center, Nashville, Tennessee, U.S.A.

**Hendrik Treede**   Department of Cardiovascular Surgery, University Heart Center, University of Hamburg, Hamburg, Germany

**Geert M. Verleden**   Department of Respiratory Medicine and Lung Transplantation Unit, University Hospital Gasthuisberg, Leuven, Belgium

**Herman Waldmann**   Therapeutic Immunology Group, Sir William Dunn School of Pathology, University of Oxford, Oxford, U.K.

**S. Samuel Weigt**   Division of Pulmonary and Critical Care Medicine and Hospitalists, Department of Internal Medicine, David Geffen School of Medicine at UCLA, Los Angeles, California, U.S.A.

**Trevor J. Williams**   Department of Allergy, Immunology, and Respiratory Medicine, The Alfred Hospital, Monash University Clinical School, Melbourne, Victoria, Australia

**James R. Yankaskas**  Cystic Fibrosis/Pulmonary Research and Treatment Center, University of North Carolina at Chapel Hill, Chapel Hill, North Carolina, U.S.A.

**Martin R. Zamora**  Division of Pulmonary Sciences and Critical Care Medicine, University of Colorado Health Sciences Center, Denver, Colorado, U.S.A.

**Adriana Zeevi**  Department of Pathology, University of Pittsburgh and The Starzl Transplant Institute, Pittsburgh, Pennsylvania, U.S.A.

# Contents

*Introduction*   Claude Lenfant  . . . .   *iii*
*Preface*  . . . .   *v*
*Contributors*  . . . .   *xi*

**PART I: CLINICAL ASPECTS (OVERVIEW AND CURRENT DATA)**

1. **Historical Overview of Lung and Heart–Lung Transplantation** . . . . . . . . . . . . . . . . . . . . . . . . . . . . . . . *1*
   *Robert M. Rutherford, James L. Lordan, Andrew J. Fisher, and Paul A. Corris*
   Introduction . . . .  1
   Heart–Lung Transplantation . . . .  2
   Unilateral Lung Transplantation . . . .  4
   Double-Lung Transplantation . . . .  7
   Single Sequential Lung Transplantation . . . .  8
   The ISHLT Registry . . . .  10
   Adult Lung Transplantation . . . .  11
   Adult Heart–Lung Transplantation . . . .  14
   Pediatric Lung Transplantation . . . .  15
   References . . . .  16

## PART II: IMMUNOLOGY OF TRANSPLANTATION—BASIC SCIENCE

2. **Basic Immunological Concepts in Lung Transplantation: The Role of Regulatory T Cells and Dendritic Cells** . . . . . *21*
Stephen P. Cobbold and Herman Waldmann
Introduction . . . . 21
Reprogramming the Immune System for
   Tolerance . . . . 23
Nonoptimal T-Cell Signaling Induces Tolerance and
   Regulatory T Cells . . . . 24
Heterogeneity of Regulatory T Cells . . . . 26
Coreceptor Blockade for Transplantation
   Tolerance . . . . 28
Costimulation Blockade for Tolerance
   Induction . . . . 30
Monoclonal CD3 Antibodies . . . . 31
Antigen Presenting Cells as Modulators of
   Immune Responses . . . . 32
Immune Regulation and Induced Immune
   Privilege . . . . 33
Conclusions . . . . 35
References . . . . 35

3. **Allogeneic Recognition and Immune Tolerance in Lung Transplantation** . . . . . . . . . . . . . . . . . . . . . . . *47*
Keith C. Meyer
Introduction . . . . 47
The Immune System and Self vs. Nonself . . . . 48
Critical Events in Lung Transplantation and Lung
   Allograft Rejection . . . . 49
Determinants of Graft Tolerance: Alloimmunity,
   Autoimmunity, and Regulation . . . . 51
Summary . . . . 55
References . . . . 56

## PART III: CLINICAL ASPECTS

4. **Lung Transplantation for Chronic Obstructive Pulmonary Disease** . . . . . . . . . . . . . . . . . . . . . . . . . . . *61*
Robert M. Kotloff and Fernando J. Martinez
Introduction . . . . 61

Natural History/Predictive Indices . . . . 62
Medical Management . . . . 67
Lung Volume Reduction as an Alternative or Bridge to
    Transplantation . . . . 85
Timing of Referral and Listing for Lung
    Transplantation . . . . 91
Choice of Procedure . . . . 93
Outcomes . . . . 96
Special Considerations Following
    Transplantation . . . . 96
References . . . . 99

5. **Lung Transplant in Cystic Fibrosis** . . . . . . . . . . . . . . . . *121*
   *Raymond D. Coakley and James R. Yankaskas*
   Introduction . . . . 121
   Lung Transplant History and Current
       Challenges . . . . 122
   Referral Criteria for Lung Transplantation and
       Predictors of Short-Term Mortality in
       CF Patients . . . . 123
   A New Allocation Algorithm for Donor Lung
       Allocation in Potential Lung Transplant
       Candidates . . . . 125
   Infectious Contraindications . . . . 126
   Noninfectious Contraindications . . . . 128
   Posttransplant Complications and
       Management . . . . 129
   CF-Related Diabetes . . . . 133
   Summary . . . . 138
   References . . . . 139

6. **Pulmonary Arterial Hypertension and Lung
   Transplantation** . . . . . . . . . . . . . . . . . . . . . . . . . . . . . . *147*
   *Rajan Saggar, David J. Ross, Joseph P. Lynch III,
   and John L. Faul*
   Introduction . . . . 147
   The Biology of Pulmonary Vascular
       Disease . . . . 149
   The Medical Management of PAH . . . . 150
   Conclusions . . . . 157
   References . . . . 158

7.  **Lung Transplantation for Interstitial Lung Disorders** . . . .  *165*
    *Steven Nathan, Rajan Saggar, and Joseph P. Lynch III*
    Introduction . . . .  165
    Idiopathic Pulmonary Fibrosis . . . .  166
    Nonspecific Interstitial Pneumonia . . . .  177
    CVD-Associated PF . . . .  180
    Sarcoidosis . . . .  183
    References . . . .  189

8.  **Pulmonary Langerhans Cell Histiocytosis and**
    **Lymphangioleiomyomatosis**  . . . . . . . . . . . . . . . . . . . .  *205*
    *Joseph P. Lynch III, S. Samuel Weigt,*
    *and Michael C. Fishbein*
    Pulmonary Langerhans Cell Histiocytosis . . . .  205
    Lymphangioleiomyomatosis . . . .  213
    References . . . .  224

9.  **Pediatric Lung Transplantation** . . . . . . . . . . . . . . . . . .  *233*
    *George B. Mallory and Okan Elidemir*
    Introduction . . . .  233
    Indications . . . .  236
    Contraindications and Psychosocial
        Considerations . . . .  238
    Anesthetic and Operative Considerations . . . .  240
    Postoperative Care . . . .  241
    Issues Particular to Pediatric Patients . . . .  245
    Gastrointestinal Function . . . .  248
    Survival . . . .  250
    Conclusion . . . .  251
    References . . . .  251

10. **Living Lobar Lung Transplantation** . . . . . . . . . . . . . . . .  *255*
    *Michael E. Bowdish and Mark L. Barr*
    Introduction . . . .  255
    Indications for Lobar Lung Transplantation and
        Donor Selection . . . .  256
    Operative Technique . . . .  257
    Results . . . .  259
    Recommendations and Future Directions . . . .  264
    References . . . .  266

11. **Heart–Lung Transplantation: Is It a Viable Option in the 21st Century?** .......................... *269*
Susan D. Moffatt-Bruce and Bruce A. Reitz
Introduction .... 269
Historical Overview .... 270
Indications for Heart–Lung Transplantation .... 270
Alternatives to Heart–Lung Transplantation .... 273
Postoperative Complications .... 275
Economic Evaluation of Heart–Lung
Transplantation .... 276
Results of Heart–Lung Transplantation .... 276
Conclusions .... 279
References .... 280

**PART IV: ORGAN ALLOCATION AND DONOR AVAILABILITY**

12. **Lung Allocation in the United States** .............. *285*
Thomas M. Egan, Leah B. Edwards, Matthew A. Coke,
Susan Murray, Tempie H. Shearon, and Rami Bustami
Introduction .... 285
Current Algorithm .... 286
Impetus for Change .... 287
Initial Analyses .... 288
Other Issues to Resolve .... 290
The Lung Allocation Score: How the Algorithm Orders
Candidates .... 294
Determining the Lung Allocation Score .... 297
Initial Feedback .... 298
Lung Review Board .... 299
Summary .... 299
References .... 299

13. **Organ Allocation and Donor Availability—The European Experience** .......................... *301*
Hendrik Treede and Hermann Reichenspurner
Introduction .... 301
Eurotransplant .... 303
Listing and Delisting Policies .... 305
Future European Cooperation Strategies .... 306

14. **Allocation of Donor Organs for Lung Transplantation:**
    **The Australian Experience** ...................... *307*
    *Trevor J. Williams and Gregory I. Snell*
    Introduction .... 307
    The Australian Health Care System .... 308
    Organ Donation in Australia .... 309
    Multiorgan Donors in Australia .... 311
    Lung Transplantation in Australia .... 312
    Outcomes of Lung Transplantation in
      Australia .... 318
    Conclusion .... 321
    References .... 322

15. **Lung Preservation Techniques** .................... *325*
    *Frank D'Ovidio and Shaf Keshavjee*
    Introduction .... 325
    Preservation Solutions .... 326
    Conditions of Administration of the
      Flush Solution .... 329
    Storage of the Lung .... 330
    Non–Heart Beating Donor .... 332
    Therapies Under Investigation .... 334
    References .... 339

16. **Operative Techniques Utilized in Lung**
    **Transplantation and Strategies to Increase**
    **the Donor Pool** ............................. *349*
    *Gabriel T. Schnickel and Abbas Ardehali*
    Introduction .... 349
    Living Lobar Lung Transplantation .... 350
    Non–Heart Beating Donors .... 351
    Nonstandard Donor Lungs .... 353
    Criteria for Standard Donor Lungs .... 353
    Problems with Nonstandard Donor Lungs .... 355
    Primary Graft Dysfunction .... 355
    Infectious Complications .... 356
    Long-Term Allograft Function .... 357
    Experience with Nonstandard Lungs .... 357
    References .... 359

## PART V: IMMUNOSUPPRESSION—ACTION, EFFICACY, DRUG INTERACTIONS, AND TOXICITIES

17. **Immunosuppressive Drugs: Cyclosporine, Tacrolimus, Sirolimus, Azathioprine, Mycophenolate Mofetil, and Corticosteroids** .................... *363*
    *Brandon S. Lu, Edward R. Garrity, Jr.,*
    *and Sangeeta M. Bhorade*
    Introduction . . . . 363
    Calcineurin Inhibitors . . . . 363
    Antimetabolites . . . . 373
    Other Drugs . . . . 379
    Conclusion . . . . 384
    References . . . . 385

18. **Lympholytic Agents (Polyclonal Antilymphocyte Antibodies, Anti-CD3 Monoclonal Antibodies, Anti-CD25 Monoclonal Antibodies)** ....................... *401*
    *Brian P. Dickover, Sangeeta M. Bhorade, and*
    *Edward R. Garrity, Jr.*
    Introduction . . . . 401
    Polyclonal Antilymphocyte Antibodies . . . . 403
    Anti-CD3 Monoclonal Antibodies . . . . 407
    Anti-CD25 Monoclonal Antibodies . . . . 409
    Future Directions . . . . 412
    Conclusion . . . . 413
    References . . . . 413

19. **Novel and Future Approaches to Immunosuppression** ......................... *421*
    *Kenneth R. McCurry, Aldo Iacono,*
    *and Adriana Zeevi*
    Introduction . . . . 421
    Inhalation Cyclosporine . . . . 423
    Use of Inhalation Cyclosporine in Humans . . . . 424
    Campath-1H . . . . 427
    Future Immunosuppression and Therapies . . . . 432
    References . . . . 432

## PART VI: COMPLICATIONS IN LUNG TRANSPLANTATION

20. **Primary Graft Dysfunction Following Lung Transplantation:**
    **Pathogenesis and Impact on Early and Late Outcomes** .... *437*
    *Michael S. Mulligan*
    Introduction .... 437
    Definition and Diagnosis .... 437
    Scientific Principles .... 439
    Donor-Related Risk Factors .... 444
    Recipient-Related Factors .... 447
    Management of PGD .... 452
    Extracorporeal Membrane Oxygenation .... 454
    Outcomes of PGD .... 455
    References .... 456

21. **Airway Complications in Lung Transplantation** ........ *465*
    *Luis F. Angel and Irawan Susanto*
    Introduction .... 465
    Anatomic Considerations and Surgical
       Techniques .... 465
    Airway Complications .... 468
    Interventional Bronchoscopy for the Management
       of Airway Complications .... 477
    Conclusion .... 481
    References .... 481

## PART VII: INFECTIOUS COMPLICATIONS

22. **Viral Infections Complicating Lung and Solid**
    **Organ Transplantation** ........................ *485*
    *Martin R. Zamora*
    Introduction .... 485
    The Herpesviruses .... 486
    Community-Acquired Respiratory Viruses .... 506
    Parvovirus B19 .... 511
    New and Emerging Viruses .... 512
    References .... 514

23. **Coccidioidomycosis After Solid Organ Transplantation** .... *527*
    *Bernard M. Kubak*
    Introduction .... 527
    Mycology .... 528

Epidemiology and Geographic Occurrence . . . . 530
Incidence . . . . 530
Immunology . . . . 532
Pretransplant Evaluation . . . . 532
Clinical Disease . . . . 534
Diagnosis . . . . 536
Treatment of Coccidioidomycosis . . . . 539
Prevention . . . . 542
References . . . . 543

24. **Histoplasmosis and Blastomycosis After Solid Organ Transplantation** . . . . . . . . . . . . . . . . . . . . . . . . . *549*
*Carol A. Kauffman*
Introduction . . . . 549
Histoplasmosis . . . . 549
Blastomycosis . . . . 552
Conclusions . . . . 553
References . . . . 554

25. **Invasive Fungal Infections Complicating Lung and Solid Organ Transplantation: Aspergillosis, Cryptococcosis, and Molds** . . . . . . . . . . . . . . . . . . . . . . *557*
*Shahid Husain and Fernanda P. Silveira*
*Aspergillus* . . . . 557
*Cryptococcus* . . . . 570
Other Mold Infections . . . . 572
References . . . . 575

26. **Bacterial Infections and Pneumocystis Infections** . . . . . . . *587*
*Lora D. Thomas and Stephen Dummer*
Introduction . . . . 587
Bacterial Infections . . . . 588
*Pneumocystis jirovecii* . . . . 599
References . . . . 602

27. ***Legionella* in Solid Organ Transplantation** . . . . . . . . . . . *607*
*Nina M. Clark*
Introduction . . . . 607
Microbiology and Pathogenesis . . . . 608
Epidemiology . . . . 609
Clinical Features . . . . 610

Diagnosis . . . . 611
Treatment and Outcomes . . . . 612
Prevention . . . . 613
Conclusions . . . . 614
References . . . . 614

**28. Mycobacterial Infections Complicating Organ
Transplantation** . . . . . . . . . . . . . . . . . . . . . . . . . . . . . . *623*
*Rajeev Saggar, Bernard M. Kubak, David J. Ross,
and Joseph P. Lynch III*
Mycobacteriosis . . . . 623
*Mycobacterium tuberculosis* . . . . 624
Nontuberculosis Mycobacteriosis . . . . 631
References . . . . 642

**PART VIII: LUNG ALLOGRAFT REJECTION**

**29. Acute Allograft Rejection** . . . . . . . . . . . . . . . . . . . . . . . *661*
*Jonathan B. Orens, Sean Studer, and Robert D. Levy*
Introduction . . . . 661
Incidence of ACR . . . . 662
Diagnosis of ACR . . . . 662
Noninvasive Markers of ACR . . . . 669
References . . . . 676

**30. Pathology of the Lung Transplant** . . . . . . . . . . . . . . . . . *683*
*David N. Howell and Scott M. Palmer*
Introduction . . . . 683
Ischemia–Reperfusion Lung Injury . . . . 687
Infection . . . . 689
Rejection . . . . 697
Tumors and Tumor-Like Conditions . . . . 709
Recurrent Primary Disease . . . . 712
Summary . . . . 714
References . . . . 714

**PART IX: CHRONIC ALLOGRAFT REJECTION**

**31. Obliterative Bronchiolitis** . . . . . . . . . . . . . . . . . . . . . . . *723*
*Geert M. Verleden and Lieven J. Dupont*
Introduction . . . . 723
Incidence and Prevalence of OB/BOS . . . . 723

Clinical Presentation . . . . 724
Histology of Chronic Rejection . . . . 726
Risk Factors for Chronic Rejection . . . . 727
Diagnosis . . . . 731
Treatment of OB/BOS . . . . 734
References . . . . 742

**32. The Role for Alloimmune and Nonalloimmune Injury
and Cytokine Responses in the Pathogenesis of Bronchiolitis
Obliterans Syndrome** . . . . . . . . . . . . . . . . . . . . . . . . **753**
*Robert Aris, John A. Belperio, and Scott M. Palmer*
Introduction . . . . 753
The Role of HLA Mismatches in the
Pathogenesis of BOS . . . . 754
The Role of Gastroesophageal Reflux in the
Pathogenesis of BOS . . . . 758
The Role of Cytokines During the
Pathogenesis of BOS . . . . 760
The Role of the IL-1 Cytokine Family During
the Pathogenesis of BOS . . . . 761
The Role of TNF-α During the Pathogenesis
of BOS . . . . 761
The Role of IL-12 During the Pathogenesis
of BOS . . . . 763
The Role of IFN-γ in the Pathogenesis
of BOS . . . . 764
The Role of IL-10 During the Pathogenesis
of BOS . . . . 764
The Role of IL-6 During the Pathogenesis
of BOS . . . . 766
The Role of TGF-β During the Pathogenesis
of BOS . . . . 766
The Role of Growth Factors During the Pathogenesis
of BOS . . . . 767
The Role of Chemokine Receptor/Chemokines During
the Pathogenesis of BOS . . . . 768
The Role of Receptor/CC Chemokines During
the Pathogenesis of BOS . . . . 769
The Role of Receptor/CXC Chemokines During
the Pathogenesis of BOS . . . . 772

Conclusion . . . . 772
References . . . . 773

**33. Pulmonary Physiology Posttransplant** . . . . . . . . . . . . . . *789*
*Marc Estenne*
Introduction . . . . 789
Effects of Pulmonary Denervation . . . . 790
Pulmonary Function and Gas Exchange . . . . 793
Functional Imaging of the Graft . . . . 800
Chest Wall and Respiratory Muscles . . . . 800
Bronchial Hyperreactivity . . . . 804
Exercise Physiology . . . . 805
Limb Muscle Function . . . . 806
Conclusion . . . . 811
References . . . . 811

**34. Imaging of the Posttransplant Lung** . . . . . . . . . . . . . . . *823*
*Robert D. Suh, Tikvah Myers, and Jonathan G. Goldin*
Introduction . . . . 823
Immediate (Within 24 Hours) . . . . 824
Early (24 Hours to 1 Week) . . . . 830
Intermediate (First 2 Months) . . . . 834
Primary Late (2–4 Months) . . . . 841
Secondary Late (>4 Months) . . . . 849
Any Stage . . . . 861
Future Directions in Imaging . . . . 865
Conclusion . . . . 869
References . . . . 869


**PART X: LONG-TERM COMPLICATIONS OF LUNG
TRANSPLANTATION (AND IMMUNE THERAPY)**

**35. Cardiac, Lipid, and Atherosclerotic Complications Among
    Lung and Heart–Lung Recipients** . . . . . . . . . . . . . . . . . *881*
*Jignesh K. Patel, Jon A. Kobashigawa,
and Michele Hamilton*
Introduction . . . . 881
Preoperative Cardiovascular Evaluation . . . . 882
Early Posttransplant Cardiovascular
    Complications . . . . 886

Lung Transplant vs. Heart–Lung Transplant . . . . 886
Hyperlipidemia . . . . 888
Hypertension . . . . 889
Drugs and Transplant Vasculopathy . . . . 890
Summary . . . . 892
References . . . . 892

**36. Metabolic Bone Disease in Lung
Transplant Recipients** . . . . . . . . . . . . . . . . . . . . . . . . *895*
*Janet R. Maurer*
Introduction . . . . 895
Risk Factors . . . . 895
Management . . . . 897
References . . . . 898

**37. Lymphoproliferative Disorders Complicating Solid
Organ Transplantation** . . . . . . . . . . . . . . . . . . . . . . . . *901*
*S. Samuel Weigt, Joseph P. Lynch III, Lucy R. Langer,
and Michael C. Fishbein*
Introduction . . . . 901
Classification of PTLD . . . . 902
Pathogenesis . . . . 905
Risk Factors for PTLD . . . . 906
Incidence of PTLD . . . . 910
Clinical Manifestations of PTLD in Lung
   Transplantation . . . . 911
Radiographic Imaging . . . . 914
Diagnosis . . . . 914
Risk Reduction or Prevention of PTLD . . . . 916
Treatment of PTLD . . . . 916
References . . . . 921

*Index*   . . . . *935*

# 1

# Historical Overview of Lung and Heart–Lung Transplantation

**Robert M. Rutherford, James L. Lordan, Andrew J. Fisher, and Paul A. Corris**

*Department of Cardiopulmonary Transplantation, Freeman Hospital, Newcastle upon Tyne, Tyne and Wear, U.K.*

## INTRODUCTION

For a remarkable medical success story one has to look no further than the latter part of the 20th century and the emergence of heart–lung and lung transplantation for advanced cardiopulmonary disease. Following the first successful heart–lung transplantations at Stanford, California, U.S.A., in 1981 (1), until the end of 2002, over 20,000 heart–lung and lung transplantation procedures have now been performed worldwide and there are over 100 active transplantation centers (2).

The reason for the explosion in utility of these radical procedures is clear. Heart–lung and lung transplantation significantly improve quality of life (3–6) and survival (7) in carefully selected recipients with end-stage heart and lung disease compared to continued best medical treatment or other surgical approaches.

Our enviable remit is to describe for the reader this journey from experimental therapy to established treatment and the important landmarks passed along the way. The evolution of worldwide heart–lung and lung transplantation activity to the present day will also be discussed as well as expected outcomes following heart–lung and lung transplantation in the 21st century.

## HEART–LUNG TRANSPLANTATION

The surgical techniques for modern solid-organ transplantation can be traced back to vascular experiments performed by Alexis Carrel at the University of Chicago in the early 1900s in animal models (8). During these procedures he demonstrated the successful anastomoses of arteries and veins and utilizing this skill later performed allotransplantation of the heart and lungs from young animals into the neck of adults. In further experiments in the late 1940s, employing a canine model, the Russian surgeon V.P. Demikhov performed numerous heart–lung bloc transplantations without hypothermia or cardiopulmonary bypass (8). These experiments demonstrated that dogs tolerate complete cardiopulmonary denervation very poorly with immediate development of bradypnea followed shortly by respiratory failure and death. The longest surviving dog following this procedure was six days; however, the technical feasibility of transplanting the heart and lungs had been proven.

Two papers published in 1953 provided further interesting observations. Neptune et al. performed three heart–lung allotransplantations in dogs, employing hypothermia with maintenance of circulation up to six hours (9). Marcus et al., utilizing a novel model, performed heterotopic allotransplantation of the heart and lungs into the abdomen of eight animals (10). The trachea of the donor bloc was externalized through the abdominal wall and mechanically oxygenated. The native heart and lungs of the recipients were left in situ but ventilated with nitrogen. These experiments demonstrated that the circulation could be maintained for 75 minutes following death of the host animal heart (10).

The further development of heart–lung transplantation was inextricably linked with advances in cardiac surgery. Development of the artifical pump and oxygenator facilitated tremendous advances in open-heart surgery. Utilizing this technology, Webb and Howard performed heart–lung allotransplantations in dogs with survival up to 22 hours before the inevitable death by respiratory failure (11). Interestingly, in experiments in three dogs involving autotransplantation of the heart alone, spontaneous respirations resumed immediately. In 1958, Blanco et al., also employing a pump oxygenator, performed eight orthoptic heart–lung transplantations with a maximal survival of 4.5 hours (12).

In 1961, Lower et al. achieved return to spontaneous respiration in six dogs following heart–lung transplantation, with two animals surviving over four days before succumbing from respiratory insufficiency (13). In contrast, staged reimplantation of the lungs alone in dogs could result in normal respiratory function (14). It was not known, however, what effect denervation of the lungs would have in humans. An important study by Haglin et al. in 1963, comparing single-lung autotransplantation in baboons and dogs, demonstrated a much superior tolerance of later native lung pneumonectomy, and hence bilateral denervation, in the former (15). This observation was advanced further in a very elegant study by Nakae et al., who performed heart–lung autotransplantation in dogs, cats, and monkeys. Employing stepwise division of the great vessels, trachea, and mediastinum, they demonstrated that relatively normal spontaneous respirations were witnessed following mediastinal denervation in monkeys but not in cats and dogs (16).

Toward the end of the 1960s there were three recorded attempts at heart–lung transplantation in humans, in one infant and two adult recipients (17–19). The latter two patients survived for 8 and 23 days, respectively, and demonstrated the ability to breathe spontaneously, suggesting that humans could tolerate denervation. It was clear, however, that further experience in primates was a prerequisite before any further experimental procedures in humans. Castaneda et al. provided further evidence of the physiological response to mediastinal denervation in primates by performing heart–lung autotransplants in baboons (20). Encouragingly, a small number survived several years and on follow-up demonstrated normal cardiopulmonary physiology. Successful autotransplantation on cardiopulmonary bypass in cynomolgus and rhesus monkeys, employing innovative surgical techniques, with prolonged survival was also demonstrated by the Stanford group in the late 1970s (21).

Around this time a new immunosuppressant drug called cyclosporine with potent antilymphocyte properties was being developed that appeared to offer real hope of attenuation of allograft rejection (22). Having refined their surgical technique and postoperative care, the availability of this drug provided a unique opportunity for the Stanford group to embark on a study involving heart–lung allotransplantation in monkeys. The excitement surrounding cyclosporin turned out to be well founded, and this drug was shown to significantly abrogate allograft rejection without severe toxicity. A number of the animals survived beyond one year and, indeed, on prolonged follow-up several survived more than five years (23). The success of this study provided the catalyst for a clinical trial of heart–lung transplantation in humans.

This primate model also provided crucial experience in the diagnosis, surveillance, and treatment of acute allograft rejection and other complications of transplantation. The phenomenon of the "reimplantation response" was recognized, consisting of early postoperative graft failure due to pulmonary edema, which had been previously described in dogs following unilateral lung transplantation. The etiology of this condition was unclear but did not appear to be an acute rejection injury as it had also been previously witnessed in autotransplantation of the heart and lungs in primates.

## Heart–Lung Transplantation in the Cyclosporine Era

In March 1981, the first heart–lung transplantation of the "cyclosporine era" took place at the Stanford University School of Medicine following approval by the local institutional review board (24). The recipient was a 45-year-old lady with primary pulmonary hypertension (PPH) with a 5-year history of severe progressive symptoms. The donor was a 15-year-old boy, matched for size and blood group, who had sustained a severe head injury. The patient was extubated at 36 hours, and a one-week endomyocardial biopsy revealed no evidence of rejection. The second and fourth post-transplant weeks were characterized, however, by episodes of acute rejection requiring augmentation of immunosuppression. The patient was well enough to leave hospital toward the end of the third postoperative month and at 10 months had achieved a functional level comparable to her premorbid state. This patient was to subsequently survive more than five years following transplantation.

In March 1982, the Stanford group described the outcome of this first and two subsequent heart–lung transplantations for pulmonary vascular disease in humans (1). Their second patient, a 30-year-old man with Eisenmenger's syndrome secondary to atrial and ventricular septal defects, was still alive at 8 months post-transplantation with an excellent functional level. Their third patient, a 29-year-old lady, with transposition of the great vessels and atrial and ventricular septal defects, died on the fourth postoperative day after prolonged cardiopulmonary bypass and ensuing multi-organ failure.

## UNILATERAL LUNG TRANSPLANTATION

Interest in isolated lung transplantation dates back to 1947, when Demikhov performed orthoptic lobar allotransplantations in animals (25). In 1950, Henri Metras published his experience of unilateral lung allotransplantation in dogs, some of whom survived to 20 days (26). The surgical techniques developed by Metras were truly visionary and, indeed, his pioneering work largely forms the basis of present-day lung transplantation. Metras was the first advocate of transplanting the donor pulmonary veins on an atrial cuff and suturing this cuff directly to the recipient's left atrial appendage. He also described a technique of harvesting and anastomosing the left bronchial artery as a means of protecting the bronchial anastomosis from ischemic injury.

Further experiments in the early 1950s demonstrated that dogs could occasionally survive for a short period of time on the function of a unilateral lung allotransplantation following ligation of the pulmonary artery of the contralateral native lung. In 1951, Juvenelle et al. described the first long-term survivor of pulmonary autotransplantation in a canine model (27). In the latter part of the 1950s and early 1960s, a group led by Dr. James Hardy at the University of Mississippi performed over 400 auto and allo lung transplantations in dogs (28). They confirmed the technical feasibility of lung transplantation and also demonstrated that allograft rejection could be significantly delayed from an average of seven to eight days without treatment to around 30 days by treatment with azathioprine. They also found that direct anastomosis of the pulmonary veins led to frequent venous thrombosis, which could be circumvented by adopting the technique espoused by Metras.

Following their extensive experience in a canine model, Dr. Hardy and his collaborators performed the first lung transplantation in a human in June 1963 (29). The recipient was a 58-year-old man with squamous cell carcinoma of the left main bronchus, poor functional status, respiratory failure, and chronic renal impairment. At surgery, tumor deposits were identified in the mediastinum and sepsis in the left lung; however, the decision was made to proceed to left lung transplantation.

On the first postoperative day, the arterial oxygen saturation normalized and a pulmonary angiogram confirmed good perfusion of the graft. In fact, the function of the graft was well maintained until the unfortunate death of the patient on the 18th posttransplant day due to progressive renal failure. Immunosuppression consisted initially of azathioprine, substituted by prednisolone 30 to 60 mg daily in the second week. Post-mortem examination revealed patency of the vascular anastomosis, a small dehiscence in the bronchial anastomosis, and no evidence of cellular rejection in the transplanted lung.

Although not characterized by prolonged survival, this procedure demonstrated the technical feasibility of lung transplantation in human and the ability of the graft to function. The available immunosuppression also appeared to modulate allograft rejection. This experimental procedure stimulated worldwide interest in lung transplantation, and over the next seven years, 23 further single-lung transplantations were performed (19). The outcome of these procedures, however, was universally poor with the majority of patients surviving only a few days or weeks. One patient survived a total of 10 months but did not leave hospital until the ninth postoperative month (30). Understandably, enthusiasm for lung transplantation waned, although a further 17 procedures were conducted over the next decade with unfortunately similar results.

On analysis of these early single-lung transplantations, the majority of deaths were due to respiratory failure in the first two weeks as a result of infection, acute rejection, or a combination of the two. Of the small minority of patients surviving beyond this time period, the most common cause of death was problems involving the bronchial anastomosis. While inadequate immunosuppressive therapy clearly played a role in these poor outcomes, patient selection also clearly contributed. A number of these recipients would not have been considered potential transplant candidates in the modern era as many were acutely ill at the time of transplantation with ventilator dependence, bilateral pulmonary sepsis, and failure of other organ systems.

Contrary to the situation with heart–lung transplantation, the technical challenges of single-lung transplantation had also not been satisfactorily solved prior to the availability of cyclosporine. In particular, healing of the bronchial anastomosis could not be confidently expected in animal models, whereas healing of the tracheal anastomosis in primates following heart–lung transplantation was rarely a problem due to good coronary artery to bronchial artery anastomoses. In the early 1980s, Dr. Joel Cooper's group in Toronto embarked on an important series of studies on bronchial healing in dogs, which were to significantly influence the future development of lung transplantation.

Employing an autotransplantation model, half of the canines were treated with prednisolone and azathioprine following transplantation and the remainder received no treatment. Significantly greater anastamotic complications were witnessed in the treated group (31). Further experiments demonstrated that the adverse effects on healing were entirely due to corticosteroids and substitution of cyclosporine for prednisolone produced healing rates similar to those in untreated animals (32). Another important advance was the use of an omental pedicle brought up into the chest and wrapped around the anastomosis (33,34). This rapidly restored bronchial circulation via collateral vessels from the omentum and improved healing rates further. The omentum also provided a further physical barrier in the event of anastamotic dehiscence.

## Single-Lung Transplantation in the Cyclosporine Era

The success of the Toronto research program, and the contemporaneous success of the Stanford group with heart–lung transplantation employing cyclosporine, persuaded the Toronto group to resume a human unilateral lung transplantation program. They reasoned that for selected patients, this technique could offer not only satisfactory lung function but also a more favorable risk–benefit ratio and more economical use of precious donor organs compared to heart–lung transplantation. In patients with normal or recoverable cardiac function, retention of the native heart would avoid the complications of cardiac denervation and accelerated graft coronary artery atherosclerosis. Patients they deemed not suitable for unilateral lung transplantation included patients with irreversible cardiac failure associated with increased pulmonary vascular resistance and patients with bilateral pulmonary sepsis. There was also concern about performing unilateral transplantation in patients with chronic obstructive pulmonary disease (COPD) due to the risk of hyperinflation of the more compliant remaining native lung.

In November 1983, the Toronto group performed the first single-lung transplantation of the cyclosporine era (35). The recipient was a 53-year-old man with progressive idiopathic pulmonary fibrosis (IPF) and an anticipated life expectancy of less than one year. Corticosteroid therapy had been discontinued prior to the procedure. A right lung transplant was performed employing a cuff of donor left atrium for attachment of the pulmonary veins and an omental wrap for the anastomosis. Immunosuppression initially comprised cyclosporine and azathioprine, but the patient suffered two episodes of acute rejection in the first 16 days, both requiring mechanical ventilation and pulses of methylprednisolone. Anastamotic complications were not encountered, and the patient was discharged at six weeks and returned to work at three months. At 26 months the patient continued to work and was described "in good health" at over four years from surgery.

Patients with pulmonary fibrosis were deemed ideal candidates for unilateral lung transplantation due to a typical absence of sepsis and a favorable compliance and vascular resistance profile of the graft over the remaining native lung. They performed their second transplant one year later in a 35-year-old lady who also had progressive IPF. In the first two post-transplant weeks, acute rejection necessitated intermittent mechanical ventilation. There was also stricture formation of the donor bronchus requiring several bronchoscopic dilatations. The patient was discharged at 6 weeks and after 14 months of follow-up was having an unrestricted normal lifestyle.

A critical milestone in the utility of single-lung transplantation, however, was the demonstration by Mal et al. in 1989 of its applicability to patients with COPD (36). They described performing single-lung transplantations in two patients without significant dynamic hyperinflation of the native lung. The growth of single-lung transplantation for COPD since then has been truly remarkable and is now the most commonly performed lung transplant procedure (2). Dynamic hyperinflation of the native lung, however, can represent a significant threat to the graft and life, particularly if the donor lung is undersized or if there is early postoperative allograft dysfunction leading to a further compliance mismatch. Techniques involving differential ventilation of each lung have been developed to manage such situations (37).

To date, single-lung transplantation has also been utilized successfully for a number of other nonsuppurative interstitial lung diseases and also for repeat lung transplantation. A small number of patients with PPH and congenital heart disease (CHD) have also been treated with isolated lung transplantation with good outcomes reported by the Washington University Group (38). However, heart–lung transplantation and, less commonly, single sequential lung transplantation remain the preferred treatments for these conditions.

## DOUBLE-LUNG TRANSPLANTATION

Following the initial success of heart–lung transplantation for pulmonary hypertension, indications for this procedure swiftly grew to include primary pulmonary pathology such as cystic fibrosis (CF), IPF, COPD, bronchiectasis, and other interstitial lung diseases. As stated previously, there was concern regarding the organ burden that this procedure demanded and the adverse effects of cardiac transplantation in patients with predominantly pulmonary disease. In response, several groups developed the "domino" procedure for this category of patients with the recipient native heart made available for transplantation into another recipient.

In the mid-1980s the Toronto group started looking at the potential of "en bloc" double-lung transplantation for patients with adequate cardiac function with a view to retention of the native heart. The Stanford group's initial experimentation in dogs (39) and, later, monkeys (40) suggested that double-lung implantation was technically feasible, employing anastomosis for the trachea, the common pulmonary artery, and the donor left atrial cuff (containing the four pulmonary veins). Unlike the situation with heart–lung transplantation, however, the coronary artery to bronchial artery collateral circulation would be interrupted, which may have negative implications for healing of the tracheal anastomosis.

From November 1986 to October 1987, the Toronto group performed six double-lung transplantations in patients with obstructive lung disease [three alpha-1-antitrypsin deficiency (A1-AT), one familial emphysema, one postviral bronchiolitis obliterans, one histiocytosis X] (41). A median sternotomy was employed with the recipient on cardiopulmonary bypass. An omental wrap was utilized for the tracheal anastomosis as per the technique for single-lung transplantation. Ischemic airway complications developed in three patients, necessitating later insertion of a stent for bronchial stricture in one patient, and in two patients, following sponta- neous healing of partial anastamotic dehiscences, a tracheal stricture devel- oped in one also requiring a stent. All recipients had returned to a normal lifestyle at 9 to 19 months' follow-up.

These early airway healing problems proved a forerunner of things to come. It quickly became apparent that ischemic airway complications were wit- nessed more frequently with this procedure than with heart–lung or single-lung transplantation leading to increased mortality (42). Moreover, the surgery was technically more difficult than heart–lung transplantation, and the extensive mediastinal dissection involved not infrequently led to denervation of the native heart, thus negating one of the proposed benefits of this surgical approach.

## SINGLE SEQUENTIAL LUNG TRANSPLANTATION

In 1989, the single sequential lung transplantation was introduced as a solu- tion to the problems of double-lung transplantation (43). This procedure is performed through a transverse thoracosternotomy ("clam-shell") incision thus providing excellent access to the pleural space, which is advantageous for division of pleural adhesions. Each lung is sequentially implanted utiliz- ing the technique of a single-lung transplantation with a separate bronchial, pulmonary artery, and left atrial anastomosis. The proposed advantages include better airway healing due to the more distal bronchial anastomosis and reduced disruption of the heart and mediastinum. Importantly, cardio- pulmonary bypass can also be avoided in the majority, unless the recipient has marked pulmonary hypertension where bypass is mandatory.

Avoidance of bypass is possible by removing the most diseased native lung first while maintaining the recipient on one-lung anesthesia via the remaining native lung. Following successful implantation of the first graft, one-lung anesthesia is then directed to this graft allowing explantation of the second native lung and insertion of the second allograft. Significant cardiopulmonary instability during the procedure, however, necessitates conversion to cardiopulmonary bypass in about one-quarter of patients.

Single sequential lung transplantation has rapidly become established as the procedure of choice for bilateral suppurative lung disease. The Washington University group reviewed their airway complication rate following 110 single-lung and 119 single sequential lung transplantations from 1988 to 1994 (44). Of the 348 bronchial anastomoses, significant complications were witnessed in only 9.5%, of which two-thirds were managed effectively with endobronchial therapy. There were five deaths (2.2%) associated with airway complications with only one death in the last 100 patients transplanted.

Strategies to promote airway healing continued to be evaluated, including use of internal mammary artery pedicles (45) and intercostal muscle flaps (45,46) as bronchial wraps. However, further work demonstrated that successful healing could be achieved without recourse to wrapping (47,48) and that use of steroids did not increase the airway complication rate (47). Telescoping of the bronchial anastomosis was also advocated in the early 1990s; however, later studies demonstrated that this predisposed to an increase in stenotic lesions (49). Excellent results have been reported by the Freeman Hospital Group (Newcastle upon Tyne, U.K.) (50), with airway complications of < 2%, by fashioning a short donor bronchus and utilizing an end-to-end anastomosis with a continuous suture through the membranous bronchus and interrupted figure-of-eight sutures through the cartilaginous bronchus. The anastomosis is then protected with peribronchial tissue to prevent fistula formation into the adjacent pulmonary artery.

Interestingly, several groups persisted with en bloc double-lung transplantation with bronchial artery revascularization utilizing a saphenous vein or internal mammary artery graft. This appears to be associated with a lower tracheal anastomosis complication rate (51,52). Bronchial artery revascularization has also been employed for single-lung transplantation and there is a continued debate as to the potential benefits in reducing the future risk of developing obliterative bronchiolitis.

## Living Lobar Lung Transplantation

The success of lung and heart–lung transplantation has outstripped the supply of donor organs available, resulting in a plateau in the number of procedures performed with inevitably increased waiting times and deaths on the waiting list. At the end of 2002, there were just over 3750 patients in the United States on the waiting list (53). In response, attention has focused on the use of "marginal donors" (54), non–heart-beating donors (55), and living lobar lung transplantation (56). The latter was introduced in 1993 in the University of Southern California (56) and involves the transplantation of a right and left lower lobe from two healthy donors into a smaller recipient judged too unwell to wait for cadaveric transplantation. This is clearly a controversial therapy where two donors are put at risk to aid one potentially very sick recipient.

The Southern California Group have accrued, by far, the most experience with this technique and recently published their 10-year outcome data (57). Between 1993 and 2003, 128 living lobar lung transplantations were performed in 123 recipients, of whom, roughly two-thirds were adults. The majority (84%) of the patients had CF and were extremely unwell with 75% of the adult and 51% of the pediatric population hospitalized prior to transplantation and 17.9% ventilator dependent. The one-, three-, and five-year survival data, however, were comparable with the most recent International Society for Heart and Lung Transplantation (ISHLT) bilateral lung cadaveric transplantation outcomes at 70%, 54%, and 45%, respectively, supporting the continued use of this approach.

Patients on ventilators preoperatively, however, and those undergoing retransplantation had significantly poorer outcomes, and the authors cautioned against employing this technique in these patients. The same group also recently published their donor complication rate, and importantly, there were no deaths, although 19.8% suffered more than one complication including 3.2% who required reoperation (58).

## Non–Heart-Beating Donors

At present, nearly all transplanted lungs are obtained from brain-dead donors who have an intact circulation. It has been proposed, however, that the lung may be relatively unique in its ability to "survive" for a period of time following the death of the host and that these organs may be potentially suitable for lung transplantation. Evidence for this has been provided in several animal models (55). This may have huge future ramifications for lung transplantation if lungs from patients who die from trauma and sudden cardiac events enter the donor pool. Clinical experience with this approach, to date, is limited, with published reports involving only a small number of recipients (59,60); however, encouragingly, two of these patients have survived more than four years (60).

## THE ISHLT REGISTRY

In 1983, an ISHLT registry was established to record the activity and outcomes of heart and lung transplantation worldwide. The prompt formation of this registry demonstrated remarkable foresight, as the yearly number of transplantations performed at individual centers is relatively small and inter-center experiences and casemix may be very different, making conclusions and comparison different. A collective pooling of data, however, provides a robust picture of the number, indication, and type of heart and lung transplantation procedures performed, survival outcomes, and complications. To date, the ISHLT has published 21 annual reports detailing such information, which, taken together, map the global evolution of heart and lung transplantation and provide essential comparative data for individual centers and regions.

## ADULT LUNG TRANSPLANTATION[a]

The number of lung transplantations performed annually has increased almost fourfold since 1990, with 1655 procedures performed in 2002. Interestingly, the number of centers around the world reporting adult lung transplantation peaked in 1996 at 128, and since then, there has been a slow decline to 104 centers in 2002. This may represent under-reporting; however, lung transplantation activity has continued to increase by 21% over this time period. This reduction in center volume may, therefore, also reflect a concentration of lung transplantation services. Over 60% of all adult lung transplantations between January 1998 and June 2003, were performed at only 31 centers, where the center average was 20 or more procedures per year. This rationalization of services may be appropriate as the risk of death in the first posttransplant year is significantly lower in centers performing more than 20 lung transplantations per year.

COPD predominates as the main indication for lung transplantation from January 1995 to June 2003 (Fig. 1), and the increase in the number of patients with COPD and CF transplanted over the last decade has paralleled the general increase in lung transplantation activity. However, the largest proportional increase in activity has been witnessed in IPF, which is now the second most common indication for lung transplantation. As a result, 50% of those now transplanted are in the 50- to 64-year age group. Interestingly the number of lung transplantations performed for PPH has declined over the last 10 years, probably reflecting the more efficacious therapies now available for this condition.

The number of single-lung transplantations performed annually has not altered over the last eight years at around 770 procedures per year with 53% performed for COPD, 24% for IPF, and 8.5% for A1-AT. However, the number of bilateral lung procedures has increased significantly in the last few years and now predominates with 861 operations reported in 2002. The bilateral procedure is mandatory for suppurative lung disease and, although not commonly performed, is now preferred to single-lung transplantation for PPH and CHD.

From January 1995 to June 2003, single-lung transplantation has been performed more than twice as often as bilateral lung transplantation for COPD and IPF. However, the proportion of bilateral procedures performed for COPD and IPF is increasing at 23% and 9.7%, respectively, compared to 15.6% and 5.8% in the 1996 ISHLT registry report (61). This probably

---

[a] Reproduced with permission from the ISHLT (2).

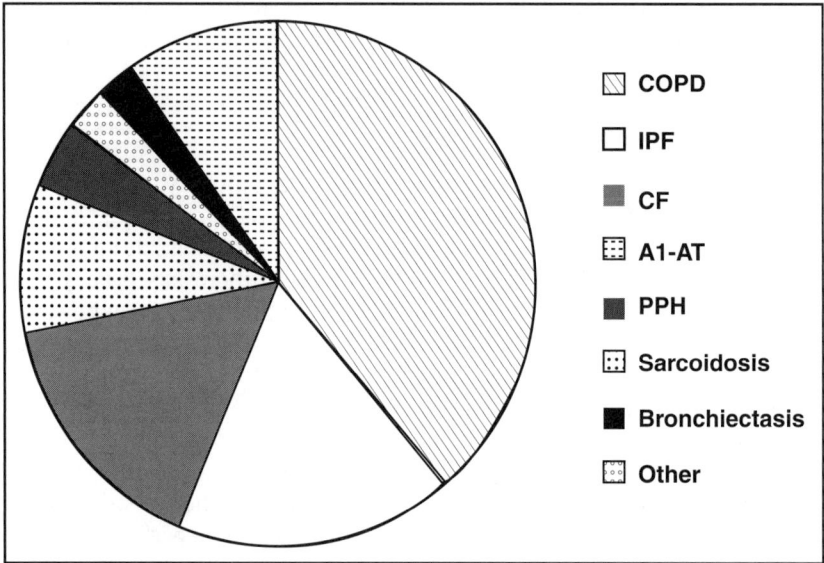

**Figure 1** Indications for adult lung transplantation (January 1995 to June 2003). *Abbreviations*: COPD, chronic obstructive pulmonary disease; IPF, idiopathic pulmonary fibrosis; CF, cystic fibrosis; A1-AT, alpha-1-antitrypsin deficiency; PPH, primary pulmonary hypertension. *Source*: From Ref. 2.

reflects the apparent survival, functional, and quality-of-life benefits of the bilateral procedure.

## Survival After Adult Lung Transplantation

The mortality following lung transplantation is highest in the first year followed by a steady, slower rate of attrition. Registry data from January 1990 to June 2002 note an actuarial survival of 84% at 3 months, 74% at 1 year, 47% at 5 years, and 24% at 10 years (Fig. 2). The time to 50% survival following lung transplantation is 4.4 years. In those patients surviving the first post-transplant year, the time to 50% survival is 6.9 years.

Comparing three five-year eras, 1988–1992, 1993–1997, and 1998–2002, however, survival has significantly improved from one era to the next. This improvement has largely been due to a reduction in mortality in the first post-transplant year, suggesting advances in surgery, perioperative care, immunosuppression, and the prophylaxis and treatment of infection. One-year survival in the most recent era was 77%, compared to 67% in the earliest era, with survival curves paralleling thereafter.

Survival following bilateral lung transplantation from January 1990 to June 2002 has been superior to that following single-lung transplantation, but only after the first posttransplant year, with a time to 50% survival of

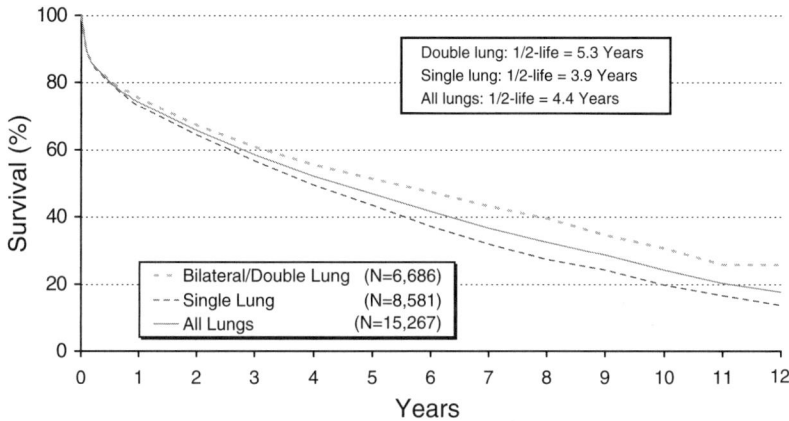

**Figure 2** Lung transplantation—Kaplan–Meier survival for adult recipients (January 1990 to June 2002). *Source*: From Ref. 2.

5.3 and 3.9 years, respectively (Fig. 2). The indications for single- and bilateral lung transplantation, however, differ, and single-lung recipients tend to be older. When 10-year survival is compared for the underlying condition, patients with COPD ($P < 0.001$) and A1-AT deficiency ($P = 0.02$) had a significant survival advantage for the bilateral procedure, although the figures were not adjusted for age.

Analysis of survival by diagnosis reveals that COPD patients enjoy the lowest mortality in the first year but the second lowest 10-year survival at 18.2%. IPF patients also have the lowest survival rates beyond the second year, confirming the poorer long-term prognosis in those transplanted over the age of 50. Conversely, younger patients with CF have excellent 1-year survival (78.6%) and the highest 5- and 10-year survival at 52.9% and 34.1%, respectively. Patients with PPH and sarcoidosis have the lowest 1-year survival and medium 5-year survival, but 10-year survival for sarcoidosis is significantly better at 29.8% versus 20.3% for PPH.

Graft failure and noncytomegalovirus (non-CMV) infections account for over half the deaths in the first post-transplant year, with cardiovascular complications also a significant cause of death in the first month at 11.5%. Even at one year, bronchiolitis obliterans syndrome (BOS) exerts a significant death toll at 5.5% and is the single largest cause of death thereafter at around 30%. Mortality from CMV infection is highest in the first year at 4.2% and declines sharply thereafter. Non-CMV infection also contributes significantly to late mortality and even after five years accounts for 17.3% of deaths. Graft failure also contributes to late mortality, although it is probable that some of these cases have BOS. The proportion of deaths due to post-transplant lymphopoliferative disease (PTLD) and other malignancies increases steadily with time from transplantation and accounts for a significant 12.7% of deaths after five years.

Risk factors for death within one year of transplantation include retransplantation [odds ratio (OR) 2.42], a diagnosis of PPH (OR 2.24) and sarcoidosis (OR 2.29), and, to a lesser extent, A1-AT (OR 1.67) and IPF (OR 1.60). Pretransplant requirement for inotropic or ventilator support confers an increased OR of death at one year of 2.26 and 2.21, respectively. A history of malignancy (OR 1.61) or diabetes mellitus (OR 1.34) at transplantation or CMV mismatch (donor CMV +ve; recipient CMV −ve) also carries an increased risk of death in the first year. Continuous variables that influence mortality at 1 year include patient age (increased risk of death at >50 years of age) and transplant center volume under 20 per year.

Risk factors for death within five years also include ventilator support pretransplantation (OR 2.24), retransplantation (OR 1.98), a diagnosis of IPF (OR 1.30), and recipient age of >50 years. A donor age of >30 years is also associated with increased 5-year mortality. Interestingly, donor death by anoxia is associated with a significantly reduced risk of death at one year (OR 0.73), which is even more marked at five years (OR 0.58). For reasons unexplained, recipients with a thoracotomy prior to transplantation also have a reduced five-year mortality (OR 0.66).

## ADULT HEART–LUNG TRANSPLANTATION

The number of centers reporting heart–lung transplantation climbed steadily through the 1980s and reached a peak in 1994 at 63. In 2002, however, only 37 centers reported this procedure, and unlike the situation with lung transplantation, a dramatic reduction in the utility of this operation has also been witnessed, falling from 240 procedures in 1989 to 71 in 2002. This is clearly partly explained by the success of single sequential lung transplantation, particularly for CF, and improved drug therapy for PPH. Burgeoning programs for isolated heart and lung transplantation may have also further reduced organ availability for this procedure.

From January 1982 to June 2003, CHD (32.1%) and PPH (24.3%) have accounted for the majority of heart–lung transplantations, with CF accounting for a further 15.7%. In recent years, the proportion performed for CHD and PPH has been even higher with the success of isolated lung transplantation.

### Survival After Adult Heart–Lung Transplantation

Survival data from January 1982 to June 2002 demonstrate that heart–lung transplantation is characterized by a high early mortality with an actuarial survival rate of 70% at three months and 62% at one year (Fig. 3). The time to 50% survival is 2.8 years; however, in those surviving the first year, the time to 50% survival improves dramatically to 8.3 years. Five-year survival

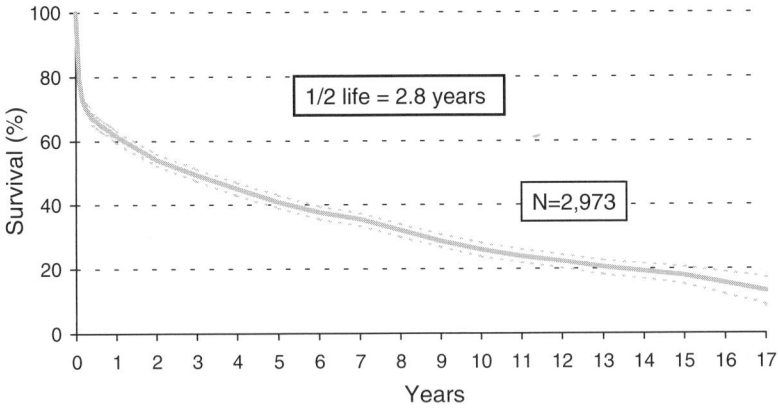

**Figure 3** Overall heart–lung transplantation—Kaplan–Meier survival (January 1982 to June 2002). *Source*: From Ref. 2.

is 41% and 10-year survival is actually slightly higher than for isolated lung transplantation at 26%. Data from January 1990 to June 2002 demonstrate that survival for PPH and Eisenmenger's syndrome is significantly better than for other forms of CHD.

Graft failure and non-CMV infection together account for nearly two-thirds of deaths in the first year. The proportion of deaths in the first month attributable to technical complications, however, is more than double that of lung transplantation at 19.3%. After the first year, the main single cause of death is BOS, although graft failure accounts for 24.4% of deaths after five years. As with lung transplantation, it is not clear what proportion of these patients had BOS.

Compared to lung transplantation, the proportion of deaths after three years due to cardiovascular complications is two to three times greater, which may be due to vasculopathy of the donor heart. The proportion of deaths due to PTLD and other malignancies is highest at one to three years after transplantation at 10.5%, decreasing to 7.3% after five years.

## PEDIATRIC LUNG TRANSPLANTATION[b]

To date, the ISHLT have issued seven annual reports detailing pediatric lung transplantation activity. The number of centers reporting procedures peaked in the mid to late 1990s and has leveled off at about 25 centers from 1999 to 2002. This mirrors the annual number of procedures performed,

---

[b] Reproduced with permission from the ISHLT (62).

which has fallen by nearly 25% in the last few years to about 60 per year. The indications for transplantation vary considerably according to age group.

From January 1991 to June 2003, for those aged <1 year, pulmonary vascular diseases predominate with 46.9% due to CHD, 14.3% due to PPH, and 12.2% for other pulmonary vascular diseases. In children aged 1 to 10 years, CF predominates, accounting for 35.9% of the procedures. Pulmonary vascular diseases still account for more than a quarter of the cases, particularly PPH (13.6%) and CHD (10.9%). IPF also accounts for 7.1% of the cases.

In adolescents (age 11–17 years), CF accounts for two-thirds of lung transplantations, PPH 10%, CHD 6%, and IPF and obliterative bronchiolitis 4%. The number of procedures performed for PPH has decreased considerably over the last few years.

## Survival After Pediatric Lung Transplantation

As with adult lung transplantation the attrition rate is highest in the first year at about 25%. The time to 50% survival is lower than for adults at 3.7 years, but time to 50% survival in those surviving the first year is very similar at 6.7 years, and 10-year survival exceeds that of adults at <40%. There is no significant difference in survival according to recipient age, but there does appear to be a survival advantage for bilateral over single-lung transplantation.

Graft failure and non-CMV infection account for up to 60% of deaths in the first post-transplant year, with technical and cardiovascular complications also accounting for 13.3% of deaths each in the first month. BOS is the leading single cause of late death accounting for 45% of deaths after three years, with non-CMV infection contributing a further 20%. PTLD is also a significant cause of death after five years.

## REFERENCES

1. Reitz BA, Wallwork JL, Hunt SA, et al. Heart–lung transplantation: successful therapy for patients with pulmonary vascular disease. N Engl J Med 1982; 306:557–564.
2. Trulock EP, Edwards LB, Taylor DO, Boucek MM, Keck BM, Hertz MI. The Registry of the International Society for Heart and Lung Transplantation: Twenty-first official adult lung and heart–lung transplant report—2004. J Heart Lung Transplant 2004; 23:804–815.
3. Gross CR, Savik K, Bolman RM III, Hertz MI. Long-term health status and quality of life outcomes of lung transplant recipients. Chest 1995; 108: 1587–1593.
4. Lanuza DM, Lefaiver C, McCabe M, Farcas GA, Garrity E. Prospective study of functional status and quality of life before and after lung transplantation. Chest 2000; 118:115–122.

5. Anyanwu AC, McGuire A, Rodgers CA, Murday AJ. Assessment of quality of life in lung transplantation using a simple generic tool. Thorax 2001; 56:218–222.
6. Van den Berg JW, Geertsma A, van der Bij W, et al. Psychological functioning and quality of life in lung transplant candidates and recipients. Chest 2000; 118:408–416.
7. Charman SC, Sharples LD, McNeil KD, Wallwork J. Assessment of survival benefit after lung transplantation by patient diagnosis. J Heart Lung Transplant 2002; 21:226–232.
8. Reitz BA. Heart–lung transplantation. In: Baumgartner WA, Reitz BA, Achuff SC, eds. Heart and Heart–Lung Transplantation. Philadelphia, PA: W.B. Saunders Company, 1990; 319–346.
9. Neptune WB, Cookson BA, Bailey CP, Appler R, Rajkowski F. Complete homologous heart transplantation. Arch Surg 1953; 66:174–178.
10. Marcus E, Wong SNT, Luisada AA. Homologous heart grafts. Arch Surg 1953; 66:179–191.
11. Webb WR, Howard HS. Cardiopulmonary transplantation. Surg Forum 1957; 8:313–317.
12. Blanco G, Adam A, Rodrigues-Perez D, Fernandez A. Complete homotransplantation of canine heart and lungs. Arch Surg 1958; 76:20–23.
13. Lower RR, Stofer RC, Hurley EJ, Shumway NE. Complete homograft replacement of the heart and both lungs. Surgery 1961; 50:842–845.
14. Lempert N, Blumenstock DA. Survival of dogs after bilateral reimplantation of the lungs. Surg Forum 1964; 15:179–181.
15. Haglin J, Telander RL, Muzzall RE, Kiser JC, Strobel CJ. Comparison of lung autotransplantation in the primate and dog. Surg Forum 1963; 14:196–198.
16. Nakae S, Webb WR, Theodorides T, Sugg WL. Respiratory function following cardiopulmonary denervation in dog, cat and monkey. Surg Gynecol Obstet 1967; 125:1285–1292.
17. Cooley DA, Bloodwell RD, Hallman GL, Nora JJ, Harrison GM, Leachman RD. Organ transplantation for advanced cardiopulmonary disease. Ann Thorac Surg 1969; 8:30–46.
18. Lillehei CW. Discussion of Wildevuur C.R.H., Benfield J.R. A review of 23 human lung transplantations by 20 surgeons. Ann Thorac Surg 1970; 9:489–515.
19. Losman JG, Campbell CD, Replogle RL, Barnard CN. Joint transplantation of the heart and lungs. Past experience and present potentials. J Cardiovasc Surg 1982; 23:440–452.
20. Castaneda AR, Arnar O, Schmidt-Habelman P, Moller JH, Zamora R. Cardiopulmonary autotransplantation in primates. J Cardiovasc Surg 1972; 13: 523–531.
21. Reitz BA, Burton NA, Jamieson JW, et al. Heart and lung transplantation: autotransplantation and allotransplantation in primates with extended survival. J Thorac Cardiovasc Surg 1980; 80:360–372.
22. Borel JF, Feurer C, Magnee C, Stahelin H. Effects of the new anti-lymphocyte peptide cyclosporin A in animals. Immunology 1977; 32:1017–1025.
23. Harjula A, Baldwin JC, Tazelaar HD, Jamieson SW, Reitz BA, Shumway NE. Minimal lung pathology in long-term primate survivors of heart–lung transplantation. Transplantation 1987; 44:852–854.

24. Reitz BA. Heart–lung transplantation. In: Wallwork J, ed. Heart and Heart–Lung Transplantation. Philadelphia, PA: W.B. Saunders Company, 1989; 437–448.
25. Blumenstock DA, Lewis C. The first transplantation of the lung in a human revisted. Ann Thorac Surg 1993; 56:1423–1424.
26. Metras H. Note preliminaire sur la greffe totale du poumon chez le chien. Proc Acad Sci 1950; 231:1176–1177.
27. Juvenelle AA, Citret C, Wiles CE Jr, Stewart JD. Pneumonectomy with reimplantation of the lung in dog for physiologic study. J Thorac Surg 1951; 21:111–115.
28. Hardy JD, Webb WR, Walker GR. Reimplantation and homotransplantations of lung: laboratory studies and clinical potential. Ann Surg 1963; 157: 707–713.
29. Hardy JD, Webb WR, Dalton ML Jr, Walker GR Jr. Lung homotransplantation in man. Report of the initial case. J Am Med Assoc 1963; 186:1065–1074.
30. Derom F, Barbier F, Ringnoir S, et al. Ten-month survival after lung homotransplantation in man. J Thorac Cardiovasc Surg 1971; 61:835–846.
31. Lima O, Cooper JD, Peters WJ, et al. Effects of methylprednisolone and azathioprine on bronchial healing following lung autotransplantation. J Thorac Cardiovasc Surg 1981; 82:211–215.
32. Goldberg M, Lima O, Morgan E, et al. A comparison between cyclosporin A and methylprednisolone plus azathioprine on bronchial healing following canine lung autotransplantation. J Thorac Cardiovasc Surg 1983; 85:821–826.
33. Morgan E, Lima O, Goldberg M, Ayabe H, Ferdman A, Cooper JD. Improved bronchial healing in canine left lung reimplantation using omental pedicle wrap. J Thorac Cardiovasc Surg 1983; 85:134–139.
34. Dubois P, Choiniere L, Cooper JD. Bronchial omentopexy in canine lung allotransplantation. Ann Thorac Surg 1984; 38:211–214.
35. The Toronto Lung Transplant Group. Unilateral lung transplantation for pulmonary fibrosis. N Engl J Med 1986; 314:1140–1145.
36. Mal H, Andreassian B, Pamela F, et al. Unilateral lung transplantation in end-stage pulmonary emphysema. Am Rev Respir Dis 1989; 140:797–802.
37. Smiley RM, Navedo AT, Kirby T, Schulman LL. Postoperative independent lung ventilation in a single-lung transplant recipient. Anesthesiology 1991; 74:1144–1148.
38. Pasque MK, Trulock EP, Cooper JD, et al. Single lung transplantation for pulmonary hypertension: single institution experience in 34 patients. Circulation 1995; 92:2252–2258.
39. Dark JH, Patterson GA, Al-Jilaihawi AN, Hsu H, Egan T, Cooper JD. Experimental en bloc double-lung transplantation. Ann Thorac Surg 1986; 42: 394–398.
40. Patterson GA, Cooper JD, Dark JH, Jones MT, and the Toronto Lung Transplant Group. Experimental and clinical double lung transplantation. J Thorac Cardiovasc Surg 1988; 95:70–74.
41. Cooper JD, Patterson GA, Grossman R, Maurer J. Double-lung transplant for advanced chronic obstructive lung disease. Am Rev Respir Dis 1989; 139: 303–307.

42. Patterson GA, Todd TR, Cooper JD, Pearson FG, Winton TL, Maurer J. Airway complications after double-lung transplantation. Toronto Lung Transplant Group. J Thorac Cardiovasc Surg 1990; 99:14–20.
43. Pasque MK, Cooper JD, Kaiser LR, Haydock DA, Triantafillou A, Trulock EP. Improved technique for bilateral lung transplantation: rationale and initial clinical experience. Ann Thorac Surg 1990; 49:785–791.
44. Date H, Trulock EP, Arcidi JM, Sundaresan S, Cooper JD, Patterson GA. Improved airway healing after lung transplantation. An analysis of 348 bronchial anastamosis. J Thorac Cardiovasc Surg 1995; 110:1424–1432.
45. Turrentine MW, Kesler KA, Wright CD, et al. Effect of omental, intercostal and internal mammary artery pedicle wraps on bronchial healing. Ann Thorac Surg 1990; 49:574–578.
46. Rendina EA, Venuta F, Ricci P, et al. Protection and revascularisation of bronchial anastamoses by the intercostal pedicle wrap. J Thorac Cardiovasc Surg 1994; 107:1251–1254.
47. Wilson IC, Hasan A, Healey M, et al. Healing of the bronchus in pulmonary transplantation. Eur J Cardiothorac Surg 1996; 10:521–526.
48. Auteri JS, Jeevanandam V, Sanchez JA, Marboe CC, Kirby TJ, Smith CR. Normal bronchial healing without bronchial wrapping in canine lung transplantation. Ann Thorac Surg 1992; 53:80–83.
49. Anderson MB, Kriett JM, Harrell J, et al. Techniques for bronchial anastamosis. J Heart Lung Transplant 1995; 14:1090–1094.
50. Jeyakanthan M, Abid Q, Pillay T, Clark SC, Dark JH, Schueler S. Single centre experience with bronchial healing after lung transplantation: a review of 555 anastamoses. J Heart Lung Transplant 2005; 24(suppl):S56–S57.
51. Baudet EM, Dromer C, Dubrez J, et al. Intermediate-term results after en bloc double-lung transplantation with bronchial arterial revascularization. J Thorac Cardiovasc Surg 1996; 12:1292–1299.
52. Norgaard MA, Efsen F, Andersen CB, Svendsen UG, Pettersson G. Medium-term patency and anatomic changes after direct bronchial artery revascularization in lung and heart–lung transplantation with the internal thoracic artery conduit. J Thorac Cardiovasc Surg 1997; 114:326–331.
53. Pierson RN III, Barr ML, McCullough KP, et al. Thoracic organ transplantation. Am J Transplant 2004; 4(suppl 9):93–105.
54. de Perrot M, Snell GI, Babcock WD, et al. Strategies to optimize the use of currently available lung donors. J Heart Lung Transplant 2004; 23:1127–1134.
55. Egan TM. Non-heart beating donors in thoracic transplantation. J Heart Lung Transplant 2004; 23:3–10.
56. Starnes VA, Bowdish ME, Woo MS, et al. A decade of living lobar lung transplantation: recipient outcomes. J Thorac Cardiovasc Surg 2004; 127:114–122.
57. Starnes VA, Barr ML, Cohen RG. Lobar transplantation. Indications, technique and outcome. J Thorac Cardiovasc Surg 1994; 108:403–410.
58. Bowdish ME, Barr ML, Schenkel FA, et al. A decade of living lobar transplantation: perioperative complications after 253 donor lobectomies. Am J Transplant 2004; 4:1283–1288.
59. Steen S, Sjoberg T, Pierre L, Liao Q, Eriksson L, Algotsson L. Transplantation of lungs from a non-heart beating donor. Lancet 2001; 357:825–829.

60. Love RB, D'Allesandro AM, Cornwell RA, Meyer KM. Ten year experience with human lung transplantation from non-heart beating donors. J Heart Lung Transplant 2005; 22(suppl):S87.
61. Hosenpud JD, Novick RJ, Bennett LE, Keck BM, Fiol B, Daily OP. The Registry of the International Society for Heart and Lung Transplantation: thirteenth official report—1996. J Heart Lung Transplant 1996; 15:655–674.
62. Boucek MM, Edwards LB, Keck BM, Trulock EP, Taylor DO, Hertz MI. The Registry of the International Society for Heart and Lung Transplantation: seventh official pediatric report—2004. J Heart Lung Transplant 2004; 23: 933–947.

# 2

# Basic Immunological Concepts in Lung Transplantation: The Role of Regulatory T Cells and Dendritic Cells

**Stephen P. Cobbold and Herman Waldmann**

*Therapeutic Immunology Group, Sir William Dunn School of Pathology, University of Oxford, Oxford, U.K.*

## INTRODUCTION

Transplantation of the lungs represents an interesting immunological paradox as the mucosal interface maintains a relatively immunoprivileged environment to avoid hyperactivity to inhaled antigens or allergens. Despite this, lung allografts seem particularly immunogenic in that even with the most aggressive immunosuppression a high proportion undergo rejection when compared to renal or cardiac allografts. In this review, we summarize the current progress in the development of strategies aimed at inducing immunological tolerance and our understanding of the role and complexity of the regulatory T (Treg) cells that maintain such tolerance. We also consider the role that dendritic cells play in eliciting either graft rejection or tolerance, and how they may be manipulated to provide tolerogenic signals. Finally, we look at how the grafted tissue may upregulate protective genes under the influence of Treg cells, and examine the extent to which conventional immunosuppressive agents interfere with any one of these components of tolerance as a plausible mechanism to explain chronic rejection.

## Immunobiology of Lung Graft Rejection

Lung transplantation is now considered a viable option for patients with end-stage lung diseases such as cystic fibrosis (CF) and chronic obstructive pulmonary disease (COPD). While in one year actuarial survival rates are reasonable at 73.5% (1), they fall below 50% at five years, primarily due to a form of chronic rejection termed the bronchiolitis obliterans syndrome (BOS), which can be shown to be related in severity to the degree of human leukocyte antigen mismatch between donor and recipient (1). While the immunobiology of this rejection is, in principle, the same as that which applies to all organ allografts, it does seem that the transplantation of mucosal tissues, such as the lungs or intestines, is more likely to lead to rejection than that of other solid organs such as the kidney or heart. This is perhaps the opposite of what one might have intuitively predicted, as mucosal tissues are often thought biased to present foreign antigens or allergens for tolerance. To understand why these mucosal tissues seem to be so highly immunogenic, and how we may be able to override this to induce immune tolerance, we need to understand the competing mechanisms of immune activation compared to regulation, and the role of different antigen-presenting cells in the local microenvironment in controlling and directing the immune response.

The graft rejection response in all tissues is initiated by specialized antigen-presenting cells, known as dendritic cells. These are derived from the bone marrow and circulate throughout the body acting as sentinels of infection and inflammation. The normal role of dendritic cells is to sense pathogens via innate signals generated by a range of receptors, such as the Toll-like receptors, that recognize a range of conserved molecules on infectious organisms (2). Such recognition triggers the activation, migration, and maturation of the dendritic cells to enable efficient presentation of antigenic peptides to T cells in the draining lymph nodes. During maturation, the dendritic cells increase the expression of the major histocompatibility complex MHC–bound peptide complexes on their surface and upregulate important costimulatory molecules such as CD40, CD80, and CD86 required for full activation of the T cells, which subsequently proliferate, differentiate, and provide help for other components of immunity such as B cells and macrophages. In the case of an organ graft, a very similar cascade following dendritic cell activation is primarily initiated by proinflammatory signals associated with brain death of the donor, namely hypoxia, cold ischemia, and subsequent reperfusion injury (3). The activated and maturing donor-derived dendritic cells then present both major and minor histocompatibility antigens as targets for driving acute allograft rejection by alloreactive T cells.

This initial interaction between naive T cells and activated dendritic cells is now known to be critical in tailoring the direction of differentiation of the T cells, thus eliciting effector systems appropriate to the nature of the initiating source of antigen. Intracellular pathogens tend to trigger the production of interleukin 12 (IL-12) and the subsequent generation of a Th1 response, macrophage activation, and cellular immunity, while helminths and extracellular antigens tend to promote Th2 differentiation via IL-4 and IL-13 together with help for antibody production and eosinophil activation. Dendritic cells also constitutively migrate to lymph nodes to present both self and "non-harmful" foreign antigens to T cells for tolerance (4), enabling the generation and maintenance of Treg cells, to which we shall return in detail later.

The early migration of donor-type, graft-derived, dendritic cells is primarily thought to stimulate an acute rejection response through the direct presentation of donor alloantigens. In the longer term, however, indirect antigen presentation by recolonizing and migrating recipient dendritic cells and macrophages becomes more relevant to the competing processes of chronic graft rejection and immune regulation. Recipient dendritic cells will present donor graft–derived peptides in the context of recipient-type MHC molecules, so the focus of the immune response in chronic rejection moves away from direct recognition of foreign MHC molecules to self-MHC–restricted presentation of donor-derived peptides including non-MHC (minor) histocompatibility antigens. There is also a risk that normal tissue antigens may be presented in an inflammatory environment, allowing escape from self-tolerance, and there is considerable evidence that an autoreactivity to type V collagen may be a component in the chronic rejection of lungs (5,6) and that inducing oral tolerance to collagen can ameliorate this response in a rat model (7).

## REPROGRAMMING THE IMMUNE SYSTEM FOR TOLERANCE

### Therapeutic Monoclonal Antibodies Against T Cells

The immune system acquires tolerance to self antigens early in life, principally through a process that deletes self-reactive T cell clones as they develop in the thymus. This means that in order to impose therapeutic tolerance in the adult to the alloantigens of grafted tissues, it is necessary either to ablate the entire immune system and attempt to recapitulate development with presentation of the donor graft antigens in the thymus via a fresh source of hemopoietic stem cells or to find a means to reprogram the peripheral T cell repertoire in situ. The development of monoclonal and humanized antibodies that can deplete or modulate T cell function in vivo has made both these routes to tolerance a practical possibility. Monoclonal antibodies that could deplete either CD4$^+$ or CD8$^+$ T cells in mice (8) were found able to suppress the rejection of allogeneic skin or bone marrow grafts (9). While T cell depletion strategies of immunosuppression are still practically useful in clinical bone marrow (10) and organ transplantation to this day (11), it was the discovery that a brief treatment with non-depleting CD4 antibodies could induce a permanent state of antigen-specific tolerance in mice (12) that has provided a potential route to true therapeutic reprogramming of the adult immune system.

The discovery that induction of tolerance was possible in mice given a foreign protein, such as human IgG, under the cover of monoclonal anti-CD4 antibody (13), led to many attempts to use such antibodies clinically as potential immunosuppressive agents in organ transplantation and auto-immunity. All of these early attempts failed to induce any evidence of immune reprogramming, mainly because we did not understand enough about the mechanisms of action and pharmacokinetics of the anti-CD4 anti-bodies used. For example, we now know that blocking antibodies should be used at sufficient doses to maintain saturation of the CD4 expressed on T cells for at least three weeks (in mice) without eliciting any depletion of the $CD4^+$ T cells (14), and this requires that there is no induction of any neutralizing antiglobulin response. We also now know that successful repro-gramming for tolerance depends on the sufficient generation of antigen-specific Treg cells (15) to control any emerging effector cells, and that con-comitant treatment with many conventional immunosuppressive drugs can inhibit Treg cell development (16,17). More recently, it has been shown that a humanized, non-depleting aglycosyl anti-CD4 antibody can be used, at doses equivalent to those used in mice, to induce tolerance to equine IgG in baboons (18), demonstrating that the general principle of immune repro-gramming by coreceptor blockade is feasible in larger primates.

With time, it has become clear that many other antibody specificities are also capable, when used either alone or in combinations, of reprogramming the immune system (19). While non-depleting CD4 antibody used alone is sufficient to achieve tolerance to long-lived protein antigens, such as foreign IgG, it was found to be essential to combine this with anti-CD8 antibodies to achieve reliable tolerance to skin grafts (12). Other antibody specificities that have been shown to induce tolerance to organ or tissue grafts include CD 154 (CD40L), which is often used in combination with CTLA4-Ig (20), CD11a plus ICAM-1 (21), CD2 (22), CD45RB (22), and non-mitogenic CD3 anti-bodies (23). The observation that so many different antibody specificities are able to promote tolerance induction suggests that the mechanism may not be related to the individual functions of the target molecules on the T cell or antigen-presenting cell surface, but to a default response of T cells when they are subjected to nonoptimal signaling in the immune synapse (24).

## NONOPTIMAL T-CELL SIGNALING INDUCES TOLERANCE AND REGULATORY T CELLS

Three types of experiment have demonstrated that nonoptimal or chronic stimulation with antigen can induce tolerance and regulatory T cells.

The first modifies the interaction between the T cell receptor (TCR) and the antigen peptide being presented by the MHC molecule, through the use of variant antigen peptides with conservative amino acid substitutions at TCR contact sites (25). These altered peptide ligands (APLs) are selected to act as either weak agonists or antagonists when compared to the original agonist peptide. APLs of autoantigens have been demonstrated to modulate autoimmune disease induction in mouse models (26,27), and variants of the male transplantation antigen DBY peptide presented by H-2E$^k$ can induce tolerance to male skin grafts in TCR transgenic recipients (28). In the latter case, the APL was found to induce some deletion of antigen-reactive T cells, and also both *foxP3*-positive CD4$^+$CD25$^+$ Treg cells and Tr1-like cells producing IL-10. APLs of myelin basic protein have been tested in clinical trials as a treatment for multiple sclerosis but so far with little success and possibly even some exacerbation of the disease (29).

A second example of chronic antigen stimulation is when TCR transgenic antimale (DBY) T cells were adoptively transferred into male recombinase activating gene (RAG) knockout recipients (30). Surprisingly, none of the male recipients of male-specific T cells developed any long-term signs of graft versus host disease and it was found that all the T cells had become profoundly anergic when tested for proliferation in vitro. In addition, the T cells were able to completely suppress the proliferation and IL-2 secretion of naive T cells in a conventional in vitro suppression assay. These anergic and Treg cells were CD4$^+$CTLA4$^+$ but negative for *foxP3*, CD25, and IL-10 production.

Finally, administering antigen peptide continuously to either TCR transgenic or normal mice subcutaneously via an osmotic pump also leads to tolerance induction (31). Dominant tolerance could be induced in normal mice to the intact antigen by administration of a single peptide epitope and this was dependent on the generation of CD4$^+$CD25$^+$ Treg cells, which appeared indistinguishable from natural CD4$^+$CD25$^+$ Treg cells.

Tolerance can therefore be generated by chronic or nonoptimal antigen stimulation, and the outcome is dependent on the generation of Treg cells. Surprisingly, however, different phenotypes of Treg cells seem to be involved, even when the same transgenic TCR is considered. We also need to consider how anergic or apparently unresponsive T cells can have suppressive properties, at least in the in vitro assays. This phenomenon was originally observed in the tolerance of Vβ6 T cells to the MLS-1a antigen after transplantation of spleen or bone marrow (32) and the "civil service model" of passive competition for antigen presentation and cytokines was proposed (19). A number of experiments have been published to suggest that anergic T cells can compete for both antigen presentation and IL-2 (33,34), and that they also can down-modulate antigen-presenting cell function (35,36) in common with other types of Treg cells.

## HETEROGENEITY OF REGULATORY T CELLS

### "Natural" Treg Cells

It seems that there are many different types of T cells with regulatory capacity (Fig. 1), and it is not yet clear how or whether these are related to each other in terms of their origin, the signals that generate them, and their mechanisms of action. The so-called "natural" Treg cells are generally identified by the coexpression of CD4 and CD25 (37,38) and are thought to be generated primarily in the thymus (39). These natural Tregs seem to be biased toward recognition of agonistic, high-avidity self peptides (40), although it is not yet clear if

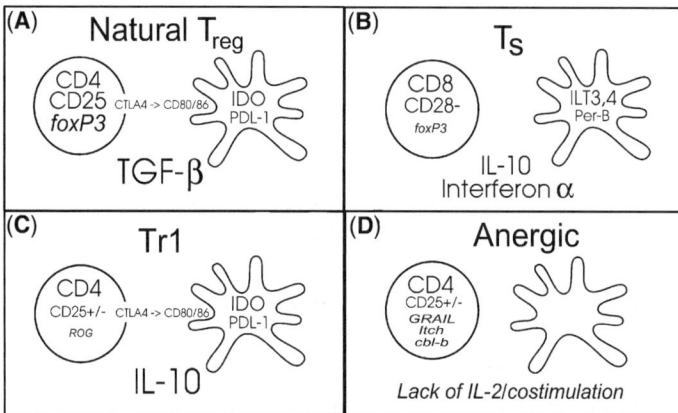

**Figure 1** Different types of Treg cells. The left side of the four panels depicts the four main types of Treg cells that have been characterized so far together with an indication of their interaction with APCs on the right. (**A**) Natural Treg cells are CD4$^+$CD25$^+$*foxP3*$^+$ cells that are associated with TGF-β for their generation and some of their functions. They can down-modulate APC by CTLA4 cross-linking of CD80/86 molecules, the induction of IDO, and the catabolism of tryptophan. Down-modulated APCs also express programmed cell death ligand-1 (PDL-1), which can control the expansion of CD8$^+$ effector T cells. Th3 cells that make predominantly TGF-β may be similar to these Treg cells. (**B**) The CD8$^+$CD28$^-$*foxP3*$^+$ suppressor T cell is associated with an IL-10–and interferon-α–rich environment and is able, at least in the human system, to modulate the dendritic APC to express the molecules ILT3, ILT4, and PIR-B, which present to further T cells to induce anergy and CD4$^+$CD25$^+$ Treg cells. (**C**) Tr1 cells are dependent on IL-10 for their generation and some of their suppressive functions. They can also modulate the APC via CTLA4, CD80/86, and IDO. (**D**) Anergic T cells are associated with T-cell activation in the absence of costimulation and are hyporesponsive to antigen due to the induction of the E3-ubiquitin ligases gene related to anergy in lymphocytes (GRAIL), *Itch*, and *cbl-b*, which cause degradation of the T-cell receptor signaling pathway. Anergic cells may suppress by competing for IL-2 and costimulation. *Abbreviations*: APC, antigen-presenting cell; Treg, regulatory T cells; TGF, transforming growth factor; IDO, indoleamine 2,3-dioxygenase; IL, interleukin.

this is as a result of positive selection or as a resistance to clonal deletion (41,42). These natural Treg cells remain CD62L high (43), populate the peripheral lymphoid system, and are thought to be involved in controlling lymphocyte homeostasis (44) and innate immunity (45). It has been demonstrated that the transcription factor *foxP3* is essential for the generation of these Tregs and that humans or mice that lack *foxP3* function develop an autoimmune pathology involving uncontrolled T cell proliferation in the gut and endocrine tissues (46,47). Viral transduction of the *foxP3* gene into naive T cells converts them both phenotypically and functionally into Treg cells (48–50).

While the natural mechanism in the thymus for specifying the differentiation of thymocytes into Treg cells remains unclear, it now seems that exposing naive, peripheral T cells to transforming growth factor β (TGF-β) during their activation by antigen can also induce foxP3 and regulatory function (51–54). This is intriguing because in, for example, the mouse models of autoimmune colitis, tolerance induced by Treg cells can be broken by the administration of neutralizing antibodies to TGF-β, suggesting that this cytokine plays a role in the activity of Treg cells as well as their induction (55). Most recently, it has been shown that non-depleting CD4 antibodies that induce transplantion tolerance are able to induce *foxP3* expression during exposure to graft antigens, and this is also TGF-β dependent (56). While the source of active TGF-β in these systems remains to be defined, it is of interest to note that a subset of differentiated CD4$^+$ memory T cells, termed Th3 cells (57,58), have also been shown to act as Treg cells in, for example, tolerance to alloantigens presented to the immune system via the anterior chamber of the eye (59). While there is considerable evidence that natural Treg cells can play a role in transplantation tolerance, particularly in adoptive transfer models (60,61), it is becoming clear that other Treg cells, in some cases lacking either CD25 or *foxP3*, are also involved (30,62).

## Treg Type 1 Cells

The Treg type 1 (Tr1) cell represents one example of such an additional type of Treg cell. It is defined and distinguished from natural Treg cells primarily because it is dependent for both its generation and much of its suppressive function on the cytokine IL-10 (63,64). Tr1 cells do not express the *foxP3* gene (65), although they may express some of the other surface markers associated with Treg cells such as CD25, CTLA4, GITR, and CD103 (66,67). The overall pattern of gene expression of Tr1 cells seems to be quite similar to that of Th2 cells, although resting Tr1 cells seem to lack a number of Th2-associated genes such as *GATA-3*, *Egr-1*, *ST2L*, and IL-4. Only very few genes such as the repressor of GATA (*ROG*) (67) and leukemia inhibitory factor (*LIF*) (68) seem to be overexpressed specifically in Tr1 cells. After strong activation with either mature dendritic cells or CD3 cross-linking,

Tr1 cells can express IL-4 and IL-5 cytokines, and appear genetically even more similar to Th2 cells (66), suggesting that the Tr1 cell is perhaps an anergic or partially differentiated Th2 cell. The main functional difference is that while Th2 cells are perfectly capable of rejecting skin grafts rapidly after adoptive transfer to T cell–depleted or RAG-deficient recipients, Tr1 cells fail to reject such grafts and will then go on to suppress rejection by either Th2 or Th1 cells (65,67).

### Other Treg Cell Subsets

There are also other types of Treg cells besides the natural Treg, Th3, and Tr1 populations. These include subpopulations of *foxP3*$^+$ Th1, Th2 cells implicated in the control of airway hyperreactivity (69), CD8$^+$ T cells that express the *foxP3* gene (70,71), as well as more distantly related cells such as natural killer T (NKT) cells, CD4$^-$CD8$^-$, and γδ T cells. NKT cells are defined by a restricted expression of certain αβ TCR rearrangements, are thought to recognize glycosylated antigens in the context of nonclassical MHC molecules, and have been particularly implicated in the regulation of autoimmunity in the nonobese diabetic (NOD) mouse model of type I diabetes (72,73) by acting early in the response to produce cytokines such as IL-4 and IL-13, which deviate the later T cell response from Th1 to Th2. While the main role of NKT cells in the lungs may be to protect against mycobacterial and similar infections (74), there is also some evidence for a regulatory role (75). In many ways, γδ T cells in the lungs may have a similar specificity and role as NKT cells (76). In contrast, *foxP3*-expressing CD8$^+$ Treg cells have been mainly described in human in vitro systems (70,71), although cells with this phenotype can be found in cardiac graft recipients (70), and most recently they have been identified in a rat model of heart transplantation (77). This particular subset of Treg cells are induced by antigen presentation on immature dendritic cells, particularly in the presence of IL-10 and interferon-α (78), and can act to upregulate the inhibitory receptors ILT3, ILT4, and PIR-B (77) on further cohorts of dendritic and endothelial cells (70). It seems, therefore, that any of the CD4$^+$, CD8$^+$, and related T cell subsets can generate cells with either regulatory or effector cell activity depending on the context of antigen presentation.

### CORECEPTOR BLOCKADE FOR TRANSPLANTATION TOLERANCE

Experiments with combinations of depleting CD4 and CD8 antibodies soon showed that either subset could rapidly reject bone marrow or skin allografts (79), and that many autoimmune diseases also involve both CD4$^+$ and CD8$^+$ T cells once established (80,81). Therefore, a number of ways to additionally target the CD8$^+$ component of the response have evolved, including giving donor-specific transfusions (DST) (82) or bone marrow to enhance the deletion of $CD8^+$ T cells while they are blocked from $CD4^+$ help (83), using initial T cell or lymphocyte depletion, or by adding CD8 antibodies to deplete or block the $CD8^+$ T cells (84). Such approaches were found to allow the induction of indefinite graft survival and tolerance to skin, heart, or bone marrow, even across fully MHC-mismatched donors (as defined by the acceptance of a second donor-type graft but rejection of a third-party graft indicating the absence of nonspecific immunosuppression). It is worth noting that tolerance could even be induced in primed recipients by giving initial CD4 plus CD8–depleting antibodies and then continuing with nondepleting CD4 plus CD8 blockade for a further period of three weeks (85). This contrasts with the resistance of memory responses to the induction of tolerance by costimulation blockade (e.g., antibodies to CD40L or CTLA4-Ig fusion protein) (86).

The first really powerful evidence of immune regulation was observed in the mouse models of skin graft tolerance induced by nondepleting CD4 and CD8 antibodies as two related phenomena. The first was that of linked suppression (87), where A-type mice tolerant of B-type skin grafts would reject C-type third-party grafts, demonstrating specificity, but would often accept (BxC) $F_1$ skin. This indicated that regulatory processes targeted to B antigens could override rejection of C antigens if they were expressed on the same tissue or antigen-presenting cell. It was further demonstrated that the regulatory and tolerant phenotype could be transferred from one population of $CD4^+$ T cells to another via the process termed infectious tolerance (88). The tolerant and regulatory state of the immune system was therefore self-sustaining in the continued presence of antigen, with any new T cells generated by the thymus (or artificially introduced from outside) also becoming tolerant. This whole process has generally been called dominant tolerance. Much of the recent work in this area has been to determine which Treg cell and antigen-presenting cell populations play an important role in generating and maintaining dominant tolerance and how different therapeutic manipulations can generate or break the tolerant state.

Previous experiments had suggested that such CD4 treatment in vitro could make T cells anergic to restimulation (89,90), but there had been no clear indication of any mechanism or direct link to regulation. A major step forward has been the discovery that CD4 blockade during T cell activation by cognate antigen can induce the expression of the regulatory master gene *foxP3* (56), both in vitro and in vivo, and that in both cases this is dependent on the presence of active TGF-β. As indicated previously, TGF-β has been strongly implicated in both the differentiation and the suppressive function of natural $CD4^+CD25^+$ Treg cells (91–93), although some of the details, such as whether Tregs themselves are required to express TGF-β, remain controversial (94–98). Furthermore, the addition of active TGF-β1 or TGF-β2 can induce *foxP3* during activation by antigen or CD3 plus

CD28 stimulation in vitro of naive $CD4^+CD25^-$ T cells, and such cultures generate Treg cells that are active both in standard suppression of proliferation assays and after adoptive transfer in autoimmune models in vivo (51,53). Although these observations have now been confirmed by many groups, there is as yet no published evidence for a direct link between TGF-β signaling through the mothers against decapentaplegic peptide homologue (SMAD) pathway and the control elements of the *foxP3* promoter, although there are data to suggest that downregulation of the SMAD7 inhibitor of TGF-β signaling may be involved (52). In addition, although the induction of tolerance by coreceptor blockade in vivo is blocked by neutralizing TGF-β, it has generally not been possible to break established tolerance in this way, indicating that the actions of TGF-β alone are not sufficient to explain the state of dominant and infectious tolerance.

TGF-β has also been implicated in the differentiation of Tr1 regulatory cells (64), and as has already been discussed, Tr1 cells have been shown capable of suppressing both Th1- and Th2- mediated skin graft rejection (65). The tolerant state induced by the combination of partial CD4 depletion and donor-specific transfusion (DST) also seems to depend on both IL-10 and CTLA-4 (99), which may be indicative of Tr1 activity. Furthermore, in the DBY-specific transgenic TCR model of tolerance induction by anti-CD4 there is evidence that RNA transcripts for both *foxP3* (as a marker for $CD4^+CD25^+$ Treg) and *ROG* (as a marker for Tr1 activity) are highly enriched in tolerated male skin grafts (56). It seems likely that the most robust form of transplantation tolerance induced by coreceptor blockade is maintained by a combination of $CD4^+CD25^+$ Treg and Tr1 cells. It remains to be determined whether other types of regulatory populations may also play a role in this situation.

## COSTIMULATION BLOCKADE FOR TOLERANCE INDUCTION

While coreceptor blockade is a potent and robust method of inducing transplantation tolerance in mice, it has never been tested in the clinical setting. Costimulation blockade, using reagents that target either the CD40L (CD154) or CD28 pathways (100–102), has enjoyed a much higher profile, not only in the mouse but also in preclinical primate studies (103–107) and experimental human therapies (108–110). Trials with CTLA4-Ig (or LEA29Y, which has a higher affinity for CD80/CD86) treatment in autoimmune diseases are still ongoing (111), but blocking this pathway has often not been effective in rodent models of established disease (112). Similarly, it is now recognized that costimulation blockade is not effective in a primed immune system or after T cells have been allowed to expand homeostatically (86). Preclinical trials in primates demonstrated that costimulation blockade with monoclonal antibodies to CD154 was able to induce indefinite survival of allogeneic renal allografts (105). Clinical trials with current generation antibodies to CD154 have, however, found an unexpectedly high rate of thrombo-embolic complications (113), as the target antigen is also expressed on platelets (114), and this effectively blocks their current use as a practical therapy.

In an experimental setting there is still considerable use of costimulation blockade–induced tolerance as a means to identify mechanisms of tolerance and immune regulation. While antibodies to CD154 alone can be effective at maintaining long-term graft survival in weaker rejection systems, the antibodies are usually combined with anti-CD8 (84), CTLA4-Ig, or a DST (20) that seems to provide a more robust tolerance induction and generation of Treg cells. Once tolerance has been established by one of these methods, it seems that all the phenomena of linked suppression and infectious tolerance as described earlier are once again observed (84,115). The induction of $CD4^+CD25^+$ Treg cells has been described in both transplantation and autoimmunity models (102).

In the case of anti-CD154 plus a DST, it seems there is an increase in activation-induced T cell death and effective clonal deletion of $CD8^+$ T cells that are otherwise resistant to costimulation blockade alone (116,117). The effects on $CD4^+$ T cells are also still somewhat controversial as it seems that the MR1 hamster anti-mouse CD154 generally used is capable of either blocking costimulation (118) or depleting activated CD154-expressing T cells (119), possibly depending on the dose and timing of antibody administration. If it is working primarily by depleting T cells that are activated by specific antigen (120), in a process more related to clonal deletion rather than the induction of Treg cells, it may still be useful as an adjunct to conventional immunosuppressive agents in the same way that the clinically licensed anti-CD25 antibodies (e.g., daclizumab, basiliximab) are used in human transplantation (121–124). Monoclonal antibodies that deplete either $CD25^+$ or $CD4^+$ T cells in mice, however, while immunosuppressive, have generally been found to deplete Treg cells (125,126) and thereby inhibit the induction of dominant tolerance. It may therefore be important to avoid depletion by anti-CD154 when it is used in tolerogenic protocols by genetically eliminating the function of the Ig-Fc.

## MONOCLONAL CD3 ANTIBODIES

A major commercial barrier to the clinical exploitation of either coreceptor or costimulation blockade is that both systems require combinations of more than one novel reagent to be truly effective. Such combinations can really be developed only if the individual components have been proven safe and effective in the clinic, and as we have seen this is not yet the case for CD4, CD8, CD154, or CTLA4-Ig. One monoclonal antibody that has, however, been approved for use as an immunosuppressive agent in transplantation is OKT3, which recognizes the CD3ε chain of the TCR (127). While this particular antibody has shown no specific evidence of tolerogenic activity, and is generally considered to have too toxic side effects due to mitogenic T cell activation for wider application, the ability to target all T cells in a single agent is appealing. In addition, in experiments using a diphtheria toxin immunoconjugate of a CD3 antibody to deplete three logs of T cells in vivo, it was found to induce long-term survival of renal allografts in rhesus monkeys (128). This observation renewed the clinical interest in pan–T cell or lymphocyte depletion (e.g., with CAMPATH1) as an adjunct to reducing the use of conventional immunosuppressive drugs (129) to induce operational or "prope" tolerance (130).

More recently, second-generation, nonmitogenic antibodies to CD3 have been developed (131–133), and these have less tendency to cause the toxic cytokine release syndrome (134). A non–Fc binding and humanized variant of OKT3 (OKT3γ1Ala-Ala) (135) has been tested in patients with psoriatic arthritis to some effect (136), and more impressively, it was claimed (phase I only) to reduce the need for insulin 12 months after a brief treatment of newly diagnosed type I diabetics (137). Nonmitogenic anti-CD3 antibodies have previously been shown to be effective in treating diabetes even after the onset of symptoms in the NOD mouse model (23), and this has been shown to be due to the TGF-β–dependent function of *foxP3*-positive $CD4^+CD25^+CD62L^+$ Treg cells (138,139). This suggests that under appropriate conditions nonmitogenic anti-CD3 antibodies may be as effective as, and generate a state of tolerance similar to that obtained by, coreceptor or costimulatory blockade.

## ANTIGEN PRESENTING CELLS AS MODULATORS OF IMMUNE RESPONSES

As mentioned previously, tolerance induced by coreceptor or costimulatory blockade induces Treg cells that are antigen specific but that are additionally able to suppress third-party antigens expressed by the same tissue or antigen-presenting cell (87). One likely explanation for this phenomenon of linked suppression is that Treg cells can either suppress or reverse the maturation of dendritic cells such that antigen is presented in a tolerogenic context similar to that of self antigen in the absence of inflammatory stimuli (4). In support of this hypothesis a number of groups have reported that anergic and Treg cells are able to inhibit the upregulation of costimulatory ligands on the surface of antigen-presenting cells normally associated with their maturation (35,140,141). Dendritic cells can also be modulated by treatment with cytokines such as TGF-β (142,143) and IL-10 (144–146) or with analogs of vitamin D3 (147,148), all of which suppress their ability to induce full immune stimulation and can give rise to tolerance via Treg cells. While it was initially thought that the common mechanism of action of such agents was to prevent maturation of the dendritic cells, gene expression studies have revealed a more complex pattern of changes indicating that presentation for tolerance is more likely a specific alternative differentiation pathway (65,149) only in part involving the upregulation of inhibitory ligands such as PDL-1 (150,151) and anti-inflammatory agents such as arginase, hemoxygenase 1, and indoleamine 2,3-dioxygenase (IDO) (65,149).

## IMMUNE REGULATION AND INDUCED IMMUNE PRIVILEGE

IDO is an enzyme that catabolizes tryptophan. It has been shown that $CD8^+$ T cells in particular require a source of this amino acid to proliferate and survive (152). The kynurenine metabolites of tryptophan also seem to be toxic to T cells (153). This means that IDO activity by either dendritic cells or macrophages generates a local environment that is nonpermissive for normal T cell responses to antigen. This mechanism seems to be important in pregnancy to avoid rejection of the semiallogeneic fetus (154) and appears to be regulated via the expression of CTLA4 on the natural $CD4^+CD25^+$ Treg cells (155), which activates the IDO in antigen-presenting cells through ligation of CD80 and CD86 (155). Tr1 cells have also been shown to express surface CTLA4 and these can also act to suppress $CD8^+$ T cell responses via the IDO pathway (156). While CTLA4-Ig has also been considered as a means to achieve blockade of the CD28 costimulatory pathway by competing for CD80/CD86 ligands, it now turns out that it also may have an alternative mechanism of action through induction of IDO in the antigen-presenting cell, particularly in certain subsets of dendritic cells (157).

IDO also seems to be constitutively expressed in the interstitial dendritic cells of normal lungs (158) and can be induced on bronchial epithelial cells by interferon-$\gamma$ (159). Because IDO is an intracellular enzyme, for cells to be able to deplete extracellular tryptophan they must also be capable of transporting the amino acid across their surface membrane. This requires expression of the system L transporter comprising a CD98 heavy chain expressed with a number of different light chains that provide a range of amino acid transporters with varying selectivity and affinity (160,161). In epithelial cells these transporters are differentially expressed on the apical and basal surfaces and can provide polarized transport and depletion of L-tryptophan from the luminal spaces (159). IDO catabolism of external tryptophan by dendritic cells and macrophages is also blocked by inhibitors of the L system transporters, such as 2-aminobicyclo-(2,2,1)-heptane-2-carboxylic acid (161), implying that L system transport is also required in these cells. The lungs, therefore, have both a constitutive and an inducible mechanism of controlling T cell activation via tryptophan depletion (Fig. 2).

IDO may represent only one of a number of examples where Treg cells are able to modulate the activity of antigen-presenting cells, and this is probably an important component of the phenomena of linked suppression and infectious tolerance. Treg cells may induce target tissues to protect themselves from immune attack, in effect generating a local, induced state of

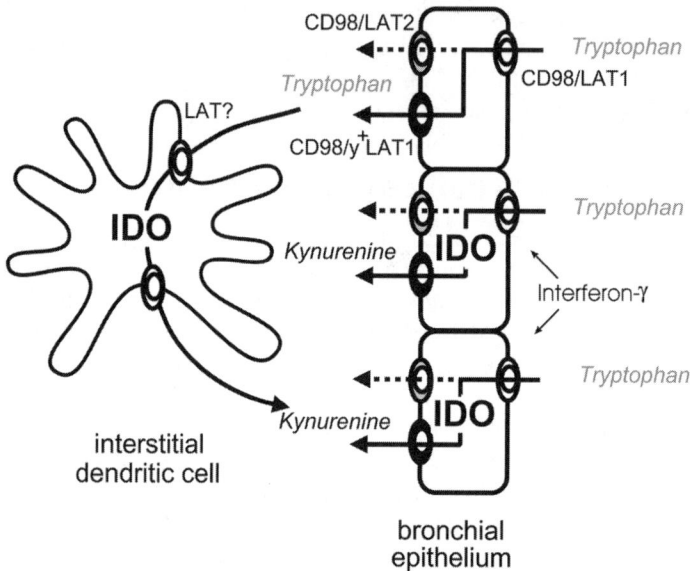

**Figure 2** Tryptophan depletion by bronchial epithelium and interstitial dendritic cells. Interstitial dendritic cells in the lung express IDO constitutively, while in bronchial epithelium it is induced by interferon-γ. Epithelial cells also express different isoforms of the system L amino acid transporter comprising CD98 plus either LAT-1 or LAT-2 on their apical and basolateral faces, together with a high-affinity receptor (CD98/y+) that polarizes the transport of tryptophan as shown. Epithelial cells expressing IDO can catabolize the tryptophan to kynurenine, which is then secreted by the basal amino acid transporter. Any intact tryptophan that is transported across the epithelium can then be acquired and catablized by the interstitial dendritic cells expressing both the transporter and IDO. This leads to an immunosuppressive environment as T cells are unable to proliferate in the absence of tryptophan. *Abbreviation*: IDO, indoleamine 2,3-dioxygenase.

immune privilege (162). Examples of gene products that have been implicated in such protection are FasL (163), PDL-1 (164–167), and hemoxygenase (168), and it is possible that antibodies or other agents that provoke this protection response in tissues may find a role in future tolerogenic therapies. One final word of caution, however, is that many immunosuppressive agents in common use or under development may inhibit the signaling pathways required to induce such tissue self-protection, either directly, perhaps by inhibiting protective responses of the tissue to inflammatory stimuli [e.g., by general inhibition of the nuclear factor κB pathway (169,170)], or indirectly by blocking the T cell activation required to generate Treg cell differentiation [e.g., steroids and calcineurin inhibitors (17,171–173)]. It is perhaps interesting to speculate whether the particular problem of chronic rejection in lung transplantation may even, in part, be a consequence of the extended use of immunosuppressive agents that block the induction of T cell tolerance and tissue self-protection, leading to a continued inflammation driven by activated macrophages and eventual breaking of tolerance even to self antigens giving rise to an autoimmune component (6).

## CONCLUSIONS

The major limitation to therapeutic lung transplantation is the bronchiolitis obliterans syndrome, which is primarily thought to be a form of chronic graft rejection that is either not controlled by current immunosuppressive drugs or may potentially be a result of such drugs blocking the induction of tolerance. Experimental studies, primarily in rodent models, have demonstrated that the immune system can be reprogrammed to a lifelong state of tolerance to various allografts in the absence of any immunosuppression or chronic rejection. Such tolerance is induced and maintained by a population of Treg cells that is heterogenous and still remains to be fully characterized, although common themes, such as the involvement of TGF-$\beta$, the induction of *fox*P3, and the modulation of antigen presentation by tolerogenic dendritic cells, are beginning to emerge. Immunosuppression reduction and tolerogenic strategies are just beginning to show some promise in the clinic for the treatment of autoimmune diseases and in renal transplantation, and it seems likely that these will also play an important role in the future of lung transplantation.

## REFERENCES

1. Chalerraskulrat W, Neuringer LP, Schmitz JL, et al. Human leukocyte antigen mismatches predispose to the severity of bronchiolitis obliterans syndrome after lung transplantation. Chest 2003; 123:1825–1831.
2. Goldstein DR. Toll-like receptors and other links between innate and acquired alloimmunity. Curr Opin Immunol 2004; 16:538–544.
3. Chalasani G, Li Q, Konieczny BT, et al. The allograft defines the type of rejection (acute versus chronic) in the face of an established effector immune response. J Immunol 2004; 172:7813–7820.
4. Huang FP, MacPherson GG. Continuing education of the immune system—dendritic cells, immune regulation and tolerance. Curr Mol Med 2001; 1:457–468.
5. Haque MA, Mizobuchi T, Yasufuku K, et al. Evidence for immune responses to a self-antigen in lung transplantation: role of type V collagen-specific T cells in the pathogenesis of lung allograft rejection. J Immunol 2002; 169:1542–1549.
6. Sumpter TL, Wilkes DS. Role of autoimmunity in organ allograft rejection: a focus on immunity to type V collagen in the pathogenesis of lung transplant rejection. Am J Physiol Lung Cell Mol Physiol 2004; 286:L1129–L1139.
7. Yasufuku K, Heidler KM, Woods KA, et al. Prevention of bronchiolitis obliterans in rat lung allografts by type V collagen-induced oral tolerance. Transplantation 2002; 73:500–505.

8. Cobbold SP, Jayasuriya A, Nash A, Prospero TD, Waldmann H. Therapy with monoclonal antibodies by elimination of T-cell subsets in vivo. Nature 1984; 312:548–551.

9. Cobbold SP, Martin G, Qin S, Waldmann H. Monoclonal antibodies to promote marrow engraftment and tissue graft tolerance. Nature 1986; 323:164–166.

10. Hale G, Cobbold S, Novitzky N, et al. CAMPATH-1 antibodies in stem-cell transplantation. Cytotherapy 2001; 3:145–164.

11. Calne R, Moffatt SD, Friend PJ, et al. Proper tolerance with induction using Campath 1H and low-dose cyclosporin monotherapy in 31 cadaveric renal allograft recipients. Nippon Geka Gakkai Zasshi 2000; 101:301–306.

12. Qin SX, Wise M, Cobbold SP, et al. Induction of tolerance in peripheral T cells with monoclonal antibodies. Eur J Immunol 1990; 20:2737–2745.

13. Benjamin RJ, Cobbold SP, Clark MR, Waldmann H. Tolerance to rat monoclonal antibodies. Implications for serotherapy. J Exp Med 1986; 163: 1539–1552.

14. Scully R, Qin S, Cobbold S, Waldmann H. Mechanisms in CD4 antibody-mediated transplantation tolerance: kinetics of induction, antigen dependency and role of regulatory T cells. Eur J Immunol 1994; 24:2383–2392.

15. Chen ZK, Cobbold SP, Waldmann H, Metcalfe S. Amplification of natural regulatory immune mechanisms for transplantation tolerance. Transplantation 1996; 62:1200–1206.

16. Kirk AD, Burkly LC, Batty DS, et al. Treatment with humanized monoclonal antibody against CD154 prevents acute renal allograft rejection in nonhuman primates. Nat Med 1999; 5:686–693.

17. Smiley ST, Csizmadia V, Gao W, Turka LA, Hancock WW. Differential effects of cyclosporine A, methylprednisolone, mycophenolate, and rapamycin on CD154 induction and requirement for NFkappaB: implications for tolerance induction. Transplantation 2000; 70:415–419.

18. Winsor-Hines D, Merrill C, O'Mahony M, et al. Induction of immunological tolerance/hyporesponsiveness in baboons with a nondepleting CD4 antibody. J Immunol 2004; 173:4715–4723.

19. Waldmann H, Cobbold S. Regulating the immune response to transplants, a role for CD4+ regulatory cells? Immunity 2001; 14:399–406.

20. Zheng XX, Markees TG, Hancock WW, et al. CTLA4 signals are required to optimally induce allograft tolerance with combined donor-specific transfusion and anti-CD154 monoclonal antibody treatment. J Immunol 1999; 162:4983–4990.

21. Ohta Y, Gotoh M, Ohzato H, et al. Direct antigen presentation through binding of donor intercellular adhesion molecule-1 to recipient lymphocyte function-associated antigen-1 molecules in xenograft rejection. Transplantation 1998; 65:1094–1100.

22. Sido B, Otto G, Zirnmermann R, Muller P, Meuer S, Dengler TJ. Prolonged allograft survival by the inhibition of costimulatory CD2 signals but not by modulation of CD48 (CD2 ligand) in the rat. Transpl Int 1996; 9(suppl 1): S323–S327.

23. Chatenoud L. CD3-specific antibody-induced active tolerance: from bench to bedside. Nat Rev Immunol 2003; 3:123–132.

24. Dustin MX. Stop and go traffic to tune T cell responses. Immunity 2004; 21:305–314.
25. Chen YZ, Matsushita S, Nishimura Y. Response of a human T cell clone to a large panel of altered peptide ligands carrying single residue substitutions in an antigenic peptide: characterization and frequencies of TCR agonism and TCR antagonism with or without partial activation. J Immunol 1996; 157:3783–3790.
26. Paas-Rozner M, Sela M, Mozes E. A dual altered peptide ligand down-regulates myasthenogenic T cell responses by up-regulating CD25- and CTLA-4-expressing CD4+ T cells. Proc Natl Acad Sci USA 2003; 100:6676–6681.
27. Nicholson LB, Greer JM, Sobel RA, Lees MB, Kuchroo VK. An altered peptide ligand mediates immune deviation and prevents autoimmune encephalomyelitis. Immunity 1995; 3:397–405.
28. Chen TC, Waldmann H, Fairchild PJ. Induction of dominant transplantation tolerance by an altered peptide ligand of the male antigen Dby. J Clin Invest 2004; 113:1754–1762.
29. Bielekova B, Goodwin B, Richert N, et al. Encephalitogenic potential of the myelin basic protein peptide (amino acids 83–99) in multiple sclerosis: results of a phase II clinical trial with an altered peptide ligand. Nat Med 2000; 6:1167–1175.
30. Chen TC, Cobbold SP, Fairchild PJ, Waldmann H. Generation of anergic and regulatory T cells following prolonged exposure to a harnless antigen. J Immunol 2004; 172:5900–5907.
31. Apostolou I, von Boehmer H. In vivo instruction of suppressor commitment in naive T cells. J Exp Med 2004; 199:1401–1408.
32. Qin SX, Cobbold S, Benjamin R, Waldmann H. Induction of classical transplantation tolerance in the adult. J Exp Med 1989; 169:779–794.
33. Lombardi G, Sidhu S, Batchelor R, Lechler R. Anergic T cells as suppressor cells in vitro. Science 1994; 264:1587–1589.
34. Barthlott T, Kassiotis G, Stockinger B. T cell regulation as a side effect of homeostasis and competition. J Exp Med 2003; 197:451–460.
35. Lechler R, Chai JG, Marelli-Berg F, Lombardi G. T-cell anergy and peripheral T-cell tolerance. Philos Trans R Soc Lond B Biol Sci 2001; 356: 625–637.
36. Taams LS, Wauben MH. Anergic T cells as active regulators of the immune response. Hum Immunol 2000; 61:633–639.
37. Sakaguchi S, Sakaguchi N, Asano M, Itoh M, Toda M. Immunologic self-tolerance maintained by activated T cells expressing IL-2 receptor alpha-chains (CD25). Breakdown of a single mechanism of self-tolerance causes various autoimmune diseases. J Immunol 1995; 155:1151–1164.
38. Thornton AM, Shevach EM. CD4+CD25+ immunoregulatory T cells suppress polyclonal T cell activation in vitro by inhibiting interleukin 2 production. J Exp Med 1998; 188:287–296.
39. Sakaguchi S, Sakaguchi N, Shimizu J, et al. Immunologic tolerance maintained by CD25+ CD4+ regulatory T cells: their common role in controlling autoimmunity, tumor immunity, and transplantation tolerance. Immunol Rev 2001; 182: 18–32.

40. Jordan MS, Boesteanu A, Reed AJ, et al. Thymic selection of CD4+CD25+ regulatory T cells induced by an agonist self-peptide. Nat Immunol 2001; 2:301–306.

41. Lerman MA, Larkin J III, Cozzo C, Jordan MS, Caton AJ. CD4+ CD25+ regulatory T cell repertoire formation in response to varying expression of a neo-self-antigen. J Immunol 2004; 173:236–244.

42. van Santen HM, Benoist C, Mathis D. Number of T reg cells that differentiate does not increase upon encounter of agonist ligand on thymic epithelial cells. J Exp Med 2004; 200:1221–1230.

43. Chatenoud L, Salomon B, Bluestone JA. Suppressor T cells—they're back and critical for regulation of autoiinmunity! Immunol Rev 2001; 182:149–163.

44. Annacker O, Pimenta-Araujo R, Burlen-Defranoux O, Barbosa TC, Cumano A, Bandeira A. CD25+ CD4+ T cells regulate the expansion of peripheral CD4 T cells through the production of IL-10. J Immunol 2001; 166: 3008–3018.

45. Maloy KJ, Salaun L, Cahill R, Dougan G, Saunders NJ, Powrie F. CD4+CD25+ T(R) cells suppress innate immune pathology through cytokine-dependent mechanisms. J Exp Med 2003; 197:111–119.

46. Brunkow ME, Jeffery EW, Hjerrild KA, et al. Disruption of a new forkhead/winged-helix protein, scurfin, results in the fatal lymphoproliferative disorder of the scurfy mouse. Nat Genet 2001; 27:68–73.

47. Bennett CL, Christie I, Ramsdell F, et al. The immune dysregulation, polyendocrinopathy, enteropathy, X-linked syndrome (IPEX) is caused by mutations of FOXP3. Nat Genet 2001; 27:20–21.

48. Hori S, Nomura T, Sakaguchi S. Control of regulatory T cell development by the transcription factor foxp3. Science 2003; 299:1057–1061.

49. Khattri R, Cox T, Yasayko SA, Ramsdell F. An essential role for Scurfin in CD4+CD25+ T regulatory cells. Nat Immunol 2003; 4:337–342.

50. Fontenot ID, Gavin MA, Rudensky AY. Foxp3 programs the development and function of CD4+ CD25+ regulatory T cells. Nat Immunol 2003; 4:330–336.

51. Chen W, Jin W, Hardegen N, et al. Conversion of peripheral CD4+CD25− naive T cells to CD4+CD25+ regulatory T cells by TGF-b induction of transcription factor FoxP3. J Exp Med 2003; 198:1875–1886.

52. Fantini MC, Becker C, Monteleone G, Pallone F, Galle PR, Neurath MF. Cutting edge: TGF-beta induces a regulatory phenotype in CD4+CD25− T cells through Foxp3 induction and down-regulation of Smad7. J Immunol 2004; 172:5149–5153.

53. Fu S, Zhang N, Yopp AC, et al. TGF-beta induces Foxp3 + T-regulatory cells from CD4+ CD25− precursors. Am J Transplant 2004; 4:1614–1627.

54. Park HB, Paik DJ, Jang E, Hong S, Youn J. Acquisition of anergic and suppressive activities in transforming growth factor-beta-costimulated CD4+CD25− T cells. Int Immunol 2004; 16:1203–1213.

55. Powrie F, Carlino J, Leach MW, Mauze S, Coffinan RL. A critical role for transforming growth factor-beta but not interleukin 4 in the suppression of T helper type 1-mediated colitis by CD45RB(low) CD4+ T cells. J Exp Med 1996; 183:2669–2674.

56. Cobbold SP, Castejon R, Adams E, et al. Induction of foxP3+ regulatory T cells in the periphery of T cell receptor transgenic mice tolerized to transplants. J Immunol 2004; 172:6003–6010.
57. Fukaura H, Kent SC, Pietrusewicz MJ, Khoury SJ, Werner HL, Hafler DA. Induction of circulating myelin basic protein and proteolipid protein-specific transforming growth factor-beta 1-secreting Th3 T cells by oral administration of myelin in multiple sclerosis patients. J Clin Invest 1996; 98:70–77.
58. Werner HL. Oral tolerance: immune mechanisms and the generation of Th3-type TGF-beta-secreting regulatory cells. Microbes Infect 2001; 3:947–954.
59. Kosiewicz MM, Alard P, Streilein JW. Alterations in cytokine production following intraocular injection of soluble protein antigen: impairment in IFN-gamma and induction of TGF-beta and IL-4 production. J Immunol 1998; 161:5382–5390.
60. Graca L, Le Moine A, Lin CY, Fairchild PJ, Cobbold SP, Waldmann H. Donor-specific transplantation tolerance: the paradoxical behavior of CD4+CD25+ T cells. Proc Natl Acad Sci USA 2004; 101:10122–10126.
61. Wood KJ, Sakaguchi S. Regulatory T cells in transplantation tolerance. Nat Rev Immunol 2003; 3:199–210.
62. Graca L, Thompson S, Lin CY, Adams E, Cobbold SP, Waldmann H. Both CD4(+)CD25(+) and CD4(+)CD25(−) regulatory cells mediate dominant transplantation tolerance. J Immunol 2002; 168:5558–5565.
63. Groux H, O'Garra A, Bigler M, et al. A CD4+ T-cell subset inhibits antigen-specific T-cell responses and prevents colitis. Nature 1997; 389:737–742.
64. Roncarolo MG, Bacchetta R, Bordignon C, Narula S, Levings MK. Type 1 T regulatory cells. Immunol Rev 2001; 182:68–79.
65. Cobbold SP, Nolan KN, Graca L, et al. Regulatory T cells and dendritic cells in transplantation tolerance: molecular markers and mechanisms. Immunol Rev 2003; 196:109–124.
66. Cobbold S, Adams E, Graca L, Waldmann H. Serial analysis of gene expression provides new insights into regulatory T cells. Semm Immunol 2003; 15:209–214.
67. Zelenika D, Adams E, Humm S, et al. Regulatory T cells overexpress a subset of Th2 gene transcripts. J Immunol 2002; 168:1069–1079.
68. Metcalfe SM, Muthukumarana PA, Thompson HL, Haendel MA, Lyons GE. Leukaemia inhibitory factor (LIF) is functionally linked to axotxophin and both LIF and axotrophin are linked to regulatory immune tolerance. FEBS Lett 2005; 579:609–614.
69. Stock P, Akbari O, Berry G, Freeman GJ, Dekruyff RH, Umetsu DT. Induction of T helper type 1-like regulatory cells that express Foxp3 and protect against airway hyper-reactivity. Nat Immunol 2004; 5:1149–1156.
70. Manavalan JS, Kim-Schulze S, Scotto L, et al. Alloantigen specific CD8+CD28–FOXP3+ T suppressor cells induce ILT3+ ILT4+ tolerogenic endothelial cells, inhibiting alloreactivity. Int Immunol 2004; 16:1055–1068.
71. Cosmi L, Liotta F, Lazzeri E, et al. Human CD8+CD25+ thymocytes sharing phenotypic and functional features with CD4+CD25+ regulatory thymocytes. Blood 2003; 102:4107–4144.

72. Sharif S, Arreaza GA, Zucker P, Delovitch TL. Regulatory natural killer T cells protect against spontaneous and recurrent type 1 diabetes. Ann NY Acad Sci 2002; 958:77–88.

73. Ikehara Y, Yasunami Y, Kodama S, et al. CD4(+) Valphal4 natural killer T cells are essential for acceptance of rat islet xenografts in mice. J Clin Invest 2000; 105:1761–1767.

74. Dieli F, Taniguchi M, Kronenberg M, et al. An anti-inflammatory role for V alpha 14 NK T cells in Mycobacteriurn bovis bacillus Calmette–Guerin-infected mice. J Immunol 2003; 171:1961–1968.

75. Park JM, Terabe M, van den Broeke LT, Donaldson DD, Berzofsky JA. Unmasking immunosurveillance against a syngeneic colon cancer by elimination of CD4+ NKT regulatory cells and IL-13. Int J Cancer 2005; 114:80–87.

76. Uezu K, Kawakami K, Miyagi K, et al. Accumulation of gammadelta T cells in the lungs and their regulatory roles in Thl response and host defense against pulmonary infection with Cryptococcus neoformans. J Immunol 2004; 172: 7629–7634.

77. Liu J, Liu Z, Witkowski P, et al. Rat CD8+ FOXP3+ T suppressor cells mediate tolerance to allogeneic heart transplants, inducing PIR-B in APC and rendering the graft invulnerable to rejection. Transpl Immunol 2004; 13:239–247.

78. Manavalan JS, Rossi PC, Vlad G, et al. High expression of ILT3 and ILT4 is a general feature of tolerogenic dendritic cells. Transpl Immunol 2003; 11: 245–258.

79. Cobbold S, Waldmann H. Skin allograft rejection by L3/T4+ and Lyt-2+ T cell subsets. Transplantation 1986; 41:634–639.

80. Kantwerk G, Cobbold S, Waldmann H, Kolb H. L3T4 and Lyt-2 T cells are both involved in the generation of low-dose streptozotocin-induced diabetes in mice. Clin Exp Immunol 1987; 70:585–592.

81. Hayward AR, Cobbold SP, Waldmann H, Cooke A, Simpson E. Delay in onset of insulitis in NOD mice following a single injection of CD 4 and CD 8 antibodies. J Autoimmim 1988; 1:91–96.

82. Pearson TC, Madsen JC, Morris PJ, Wood KJ. The induction of transplantation tolerance using donor antigen and CD4 monoclonal antibody. Transplant Proc 1990; 22:1955–1956.

83. Seung E, Mordes JP, Rossini AA, Greiner DL. Hematopoietic chimerism and central tolerance created by peripheral-tolerance induction without myeloablative conditioning. J Clin Invest 2003; 112:795–808.

84. Honey K, Cobbold SP, Waldmann H. CD40 ligand blockade induces CD4 ÷ T cell tolerance and linked suppression. J Immunol 1999; 163:4805–4810.

85. Cobbold SP, Martin G, Waldmann H. The induction of skin graft tolerance in major histocompatibility complex-mismatched or primed recipients: primed T cells can be tolerized in the periphery with anti-CD4 and anti-CD8 antibodies. Eur J Immunol 1990; 20:2747–2755.

86. Wu Z, Bensinger SJ, Zhang J, et al. Homeostatic proliferation is a barrier to transplantation tolerance. Nat Med 2004; 10:87–92.

87. Davies JD, Leong LY, Mellor A, Cobbold SP, Waldmann H. T cell suppression in transplantation tolerance through linked recognition. J Immunol 1996; 156:3602–3607.

88. Qin S, Cobbold SP, Pope H, et al. "Infectious" transplantation tolerance. Science 1993; 259:974–977.
89. Vincent C, Fournel S, Wijdenes J, Revillard JP. Specific hyporesponsiveness of alloreactive peripheral T cells induced by CD4 antibodies. Eur J Immumol 1995; 25:816–822.
90. Woods M, Guy R, Waldmann H, Glennie M, Alexander DR. A humanised therapeutic CD4 mAb inhibits TCR-induced IL-2, IL-4, and IL-10 secretion and expression of CD25, CD40L, and CD69. Cell Immunol 1998; 185:101–113.
91. Chen W, Wahl SM. TGF-beta: the missing link in CD4(+)CD25(+) regulatory T cell-mediated immunosuppression. Cytokine Growth Factor Rev 2003; 14: 85–89.
92. Yamagiwa S, Gray JD, Hashimoto S, Horwitz DA. A role for TGF-beta in the generation and expansion of CD4+CD25+ regulatory T cells from human peripheral blood. J Immunol 2001; 166:7282–7289.
93. Nakamura K, Kitani A, Strober W. Cell contact-dependent immunosuppression by CD4(+)CD25(+) regulatory T cells is mediated by cell surface-bound transforming growth factor beta. J Exp Med 2001; 194:629–644.
94. Nakamura K, Kitani A, Fuss I, et al. TGF-beta 1 plays an important role in the mechanism of CD4+CD25+ regulatory T cell activity in both humans and mice. J Immunol 2004; 172:834–842.
95. Wahl SM, Swisher J, McCartney-Francis N, Chen W. TGF-beta: the perpetrator of immune suppression by regulatory T cells and suicidal T cells. J Leukoc Biol 2004; 76:15–24.
96. Gregg RK, Jain R, Schoenleber SJ, et al. A sudden decline in active membrane-bound TGF-{beta} impairs both T regulatory cell function and protection against autoimmune diabetes. J Immunol 2004; 173:7308–7316.
97. Tang Q, Boden EK, Henriksen KJ, Bour-Jordan H, Bi M, Bluestone JA. Distinct roles of CTLA-4 and TGF-beta in CD4+CD25+ regulatory T cell function. Eur J Immunol 2004; 34:2996–3005.
98. Piccirillo CA, Letterio JJ, Thornton AM, et al. CD4(+)CD25(+) Regulatory T Cells Can Mediate Suppressor Function in the Absence of Transforming Growth Factor beta1 Production and Responsiveness. J Exp Med 2002; 196:237–246.
99. Kingsley CI, Karim M, Bushell AR, Wood KJ. CD25+CD4+ regulatory T cells prevent graft rejection: CTLA-4- and EL-10-dependent irnmunoregulation of alloresponses. J Immunol 2002; 168:1080–1086.
100. Pearson TC, Alexander DZ, Winn KJ, Linsley PS, Lowry RP, Larsen CP. Transplantation tolerance induced by CTLA4-Ig. Transplantation 1994; 57:1701–1706.
101. Larsen CP, Alexander DZ, Hollenbaugh D, et al. CD40-gp39 interactions play a critical role during allograft rejection. Suppression of allograft rejection by blockade of the CD40-gp39 pathway. Transplantation 1996; 61:4–9.
102. Salomon B, Bluestone JA. Complexities of CD28/B7: CTLA-4 costimulatory pathways in autoimmunity and transplantation. Annu Rev Immunol 2001; 19:225–252.
103. Blair PJ, Riley JL, Harlan DM, et al. CD40 ligand (CD154) triggers a short-term CD4(+) T cell activation response that results in secretion of immuno-modulatory cytokines and apoptosis. J Exp Med 2000; 191:651–660.

104. Krieger NR, Yuh D, McIntyre WB, et al. Prolongation of cardiac graft survival with anti-CD4Ig plus hCTLA4Ig in primates. J Surg Res 1998; 76:174–178.
105. Kirk AD, Harlan DM, Armstrong NN, et al. CTLA4-Ig and anti-CD40 ligand prevent renal allograft rejection in primates. Proc Natl Acad Sci USA 1997; 94:8789–8794.
106. Ossevoort MA, Ringers J, Boon L, et al. Blocking of costimulation prevents kidney graft rejection in rhesus monkeys. Transplant Proc 1998; 30: 2165–2166.
107. Kirk AD, Tadaki DK, Celniker A, et al. Induction therapy with monoclonal antibodies specific for CD80 and CD86 delays the onset of acute renal allograft rejection in non-human primates. Transplantation 2001; 72:377–384.
108. Elster EA, Hale DA, Mannon RB, Cendales LC, Swanson SJ, Kirk AD. The road to tolerance: renal transplant tolerance induction in nonhuman primate studies and clinical trials. Transpl Immunol 2004; 13:87–99.
109. Kalunian KC, Davis JC Jr, Merrill JT, Totoritis MC, Wofsy D. Treatment of systemic lupus erythematosus by inhibition of T cell costimulation with anti-CD154: a randomized, double-blind, placebo-controlled trial. Arthritis Rheum 2002; 46:3251–3258.
110. Goronzy JJ, Weyand CM. T-cell regulation in rheumatoid arthritis. Curr Opin Rheumatol 2004; 16:212–217.
111. Moreland LW, Alten R, Van den Bosch F, et al. Costimulatory blockade in patients with rheumatoid arthritis: a pilot, dose-finding, double-blind, placebo-controlled clinical trial evaluating CTLA-4Ig and LEA29Y eighty-five days after the first infusion. Arthritis Rheum 2002; 46:1470–1479.
112. Rossini AA, Mordes JP, Greiner DL, Stoff JS. Islet cell transplantation tolerance. Transplantation 2001; 72:S43–S46.
113. Kawai T, Andrews D, Colvin RB, Sachs DH, Cosimi AB. Thromboembolic complications after treatment with monoclonal antibody against CD40 ligand. Nat Med 2000; 6:114.
114. Sidiropoulos PI, Boumpas DT. Lessons learned from anti-CD40L treatment in systemic lupus erythematosus patients. Lupus 2004; 13:391–397.
115. Graca L, Honey K, Adams E, Cobbold SP, Waldmann H. Cutting edge: anti-CD154 therapeutic antibodies induce infectious transplantation tolerance. J Immunol 2000; 165:4783–4786.
116. Jones TR, Ha J, Williams MA, et al. The role of the IL-2 pathway in costimulation blockade-resistant rejection of allografts. J Immunol 2002; 168: 1123–1130.
117. Iwakoshi NN, Mordes JP, Markees TG, Phillips NE, Rossini AA, Greiner DJ. Treatment of allograft recipients with donor-specific transfusion and anti-CD154 antibody leads to deletion of alloreactive CD8+ T cells and prolonged graft survival in a CTLA4-dependent manner. J Immunol 2000; 164:512–521.
118. Nagelkerken L, Haspels I, van Rijs W, et al. FcR interactions do not play a major role in inhibition of experimental autoimmune encephalomyelitis by anti-CD154 monoclonal antibodies. J Immunol 2004; 173:993–999.
119. Monk NJ, Hargreaves RE, Marsh JE, et al. Fc-dependent depletion of activated T cells occurs through CD40L-specific antibody rather than costimulation blockade. Nat Med 2003; 9:1275–1280.

120. Hargreaves RE, Monk NJ, Jurcevic S. Selective depletion of activated T cells: the CD40L-specific antibody experience. Trends Mol Med 2004; 10:130–135.
121. Waldmann TA, O'Shea J. The use of antibodies against the IL-2 receptor in transplantation. Curr Opin Immunol 1998; 10:507–512.
122. Adu D, Cockwell P, Ives NJ, Shaw J, Wheatley K. Interleukin-2 receptor monoclonal antibodies in renal transplantation: meta-analysis of randomised trials. Br Med J 2003; 326:789.
123. Bumgardner GL, Hardie I, Johnson RW, et al. Results of 3-year phase III clinical trials with daclizumab prophylaxis for prevention of acute rejection after renal transplantation. Transplantation 2001; 72:839–845.
124. Sollinger H, Kaplan B, Pescovitz MD, et al. Basiliximab versus antithymocyte globulin for prevention of acute renal allograft rejection. Transplantation 2001; 72:1915–1919.
125. Dubois B, Chapat L, Goubier A, Papiernik M, Nicolas JF, Kaiserlian D. Innate CD4+CD25+ regulatory T cells are required for oral tolerance and control CD8+ T cells mediating skin inflammation. Blood 2003; 102:3295–3301.
126. Onizuka S, Tawara I, Shimizu J, Sakaguchi S, Fujita T, Nakayama E. Tumor rejection by in vivo administration of anti-CD25 (interleukin-2 receptor alpha) monoclonal antibody. Cancer Res 1999; 59:3128–3133.
127. Smith SL. Ten years of Orthoclone OKT3 (muromonab-CD3): a review. J Transpl Coord 1996; 6:109–119; quiz 120–121.
128. Armstrong N, Buckley P, Oberley T, et al. Analysis of primate renal allografts after T-cell depletion with anti-CD3-CRM9. Transplantation 1998; 66:5–13.
129. Knechtle SJ, Fernandez LA, Pirsch JD, et al. Campath-1H in renal transplantation: The University of Wisconsin experience. Surgery 2004; 136:754–760.
130. Calne R, Friend P, Moffatt S, et al. Proper tolerance, perioperative campath 1H, and low-dose cyclosporin monotherapy in renal allograft recipients. Lancet 1998; 351:1701–1702.
131. Meijer RT, Surachno S, Yong SL, et al. Treatment of acute kidney allograft rejection with a non-mitogenic CD3 antibody. Clin Exp Immunol 2003; 133:485–492.
132. Plain KM, Chen J, Merten S, He XY, Hall BM. Induction of specific tolerance to allografts in rats by therapy with non-mitogenic, non-depleting anti-CD3 monoclonal antibody: association with TH2 cytokines not anergy. Transplantation 1999; 67:605–613.
133. Bolt S, Routledge E, Lloyd I, et al. The generation of a humanized, non-mitogenic CD3 monoclonal antibody which retains in vitro immunosuppressive properties. Eur J Immunol 1993; 23:403–411.
134. Vossen AC, Tibbe GJ, Kroos MJ, van de Winkel JG, Benner R, Savelkoul HF. Fc receptor binding of anti-CD3 monoclonal antibodies is not essential for immunosuppression, but triggers cytokine-related side effects. Eur J Immunol 1995; 25:1492–1496.
135. Herold KC, Burton JB, Francois F, Poumian-Ruiz E, Glandt M, Bluestone JA. Activation of human T cells by FcR nonbinding anti-CD3 mAb, hOKT3gamma1(Ala-Ala). J Clin Invest 2003; 111:409–418.
136. Utset TO, Auger JA, Peace D, et al. Modified anti-CD3 therapy in psoriatic arthritis: a phase I/II clinical trial. J Rheumatol 2002; 29:1907–1913.

137. Herold KC, Hagopian W, Auger JA, et al. Anti-CD3 monoclonal antibody in new-onset type 1 diabetes mellitus. N Engl J Med 2002; 346:1692–1698.

138. Belghith M, Bluestone JA, Barriot S, Megret J, Bach JF, Chatenoud L. TGF-beta-dependent mechanisms mediate restoration of self-tolerance induced by antibodies to CD3 in overt autoimmune diabetes. Nat Med 2003; 9:1202–1208.

139. You S, Slehoffer G, Barriot S, Bach JF, Chatenoud L. Unique role of CD4+CD62L+ regulatory T cells in the control of autoimmune diabetes in T cell receptor transgenic mice. Proc Natl Acad Sci USA 2004; 101(suppl 2):14580–14585.

140. Cederbom L, Hall H, Ivars F. CD4+CD25+ regulatory T cells down-regulate co-stimulatory molecules on antigen-presenting cells. Eur J Immunol 2000; 30:1538–1543.

141. Misra N, Bayry J, Lacroix-Desmazes S, Kazatchkine MD, Kaveri SV. Cutting edge: human CD4+CD25+ T cells restrain the maturation and antigen-presenting function of dendritic cells. J Immunol 2004; 172:4676–4680.

142. Lipscomb MF, Pollard AM, Yates JL. A role for TGF-beta in the suppression by murine bronchoalveolar cells of lung dendritic cell initiated immune responses. Reg Immunol 1993; 5:151–157.

143. Strobl H, Knapp W. TGF-beta1 regulation of dendritic cells. Microbes Infect 1999; 1:1283–1290.

144. Steinbrink K, Jonuleit H, Muller G, Schiller G, Knop J, Enk AH. Interleukin-10-treated human dendritic cells induce a melanoma-antigen-specific anergy in CD8(+) T cells resulting in a failure to lyse tumor cells. Blood 1999; 93:1634–1642.

145. Ding L, Shevach EM. IL-10 inhibits mitogen-induced T cell proliferation by selectively inhibiting macrophage costimulatory function. J Immunol 1992; 148:3133–3139.

146. Kubsch S, Graulich E, Knop J, Steinbrink K. Suppressor activity of anergic T cells induced by IL-10-treated human dendritic cells: association with IL-2- and CTLA-4-dependent G1 arrest of the cell cycle regulated by p27Kipl. Eur J Immunol 2003; 33:1988–1997.

147. Gregori S, Casorati M, Amuchastegui S, Smiroldo S, Davalli AM, Adorini L. Regulatory T cells induced by 1 alpha,25-dihydroxyvitamin D3 and mycophenolate mofetil treatment mediate transplantation tolerance. J Immunol 2001; 167:1945–1953.

148. Adorini L, Penna G, Giarratana N, Uskokovic M. Tolerogenic dendritic cells induced by vitamin D receptor ligands enhance regulatory T cells inhibiting allograft rejection and autoimmune diseases. J Cell Biochem 2003; 88:227–233.

149. Nolan KF, Strong V, Soler D, et al. IL-10-conditioned dendritic cells, decommissioned for recruitment of adaptive immunity, elicit innate inflammatory gene products in response to danger signals. J Immunol 2004; 172:2201–2209.

150. Latchman YE, Liang SC, Wu Y, et al. PD-L1-deficient mice show that PD-L1 on T cells, antigen-presenting cells, and host tissues negatively regulates T cells. Proc Natl Acad Sci USA 2004; 101:10691–10696.

151. Probst HC, McCoy K, Okazaki T, Honjo T, van den Broek M. Resting dendritic cells induce peripheral CD8+ T cell tolerance through PD-1 and CTLA-4. Nat Immunol 2005; 6:280–286.

152. Lee GK, Park HJ, Macleod M, Chandler P, Munn DH, Mellor AL. Tryptophan deprivation sensitizes activated T cells to apoptosis prior to cell division. Immunology 2002; 107:452–460.
153. Terness P, Bauer TM, Rose L, et al. Inhibition of allogeneic T cell proliferation by indoleamine 2,3-dioxygenase-expressing dendritic cells: mediation of suppression by tryptophan metabolites. J Exp Med 2002; 196:447–457.
154. Munn DH, Zhou M, Attwood JT, et al. Prevention of allogeneic fetal rejection by tryptophan catabolism. Science 1998; 281:1191–1193.
155. Aluvihare VR, Kallikourdis M, Betz AG. Regulatory T cells mediate maternal tolerance to the fetus. Nat Immunol 2004; 5:266–271.
156. Mellor AL, Chandler P, Baban B, et al. Specific subsets of murine dendritic cells acquire potent T cell regulatory functions following CTLA4-mediated induction of indoleamine 2,3 dioxygenase. Int Immunol 2004; 16:1391–1401.
157. Mellor AL, Baban B, Chandler P, et al. Cutting edge: induced indoleamine 2,3 dioxygenase expression in dendritic cell subsets suppresses T cell clonal expansion. J Immunol 2003; 171:1652–1655.
158. Swanson KA, Zheng Y, Heidler KM, Mizobuchi T, Wilkes DS. CD11c+ cells modulate pulmonary immune responses by production of indoleamine 2,3-dioxygenase. Am J Respir Cell Mol Biol 2004; 30:311–318.
159. Zegarra-Moran O, Folli C, Manzari B, Ravazzolo R, Varesio L, Galietta LJ. Double mechanism for apical tryptophan depletion in polarized human bronchial epithelium. J Immunol 2004; 173:542–549.
160. Kudo Y, Boyd CA. The physiology of immune evasion during pregnancy; the critical role of placental tryptophan metabolism and transport. Pflugers Arch 2001; 442:639–641.
161. Kudo Y, Boyd CA. The role of L-tryptophan transport in L-tryptophan degradation by indoleamine 2,3-dioxygenase in human placental explants. J Physiol 2001; 531:417–423.
162. Ferguson TA, Green DR, Griffith TS. Cell death and immune privilege. Int Rev Immunol 2002; 21:153–172.
163. Green DR, Ferguson TA. The role of Fas ligand in immune privilege. Nat Rev Mol Cell Biol 2001; 2:917–924.
164. Aramaki O, Shirasugi N, Takayama T, et al. Programmed death-1-programmed death-Ll interaction is essential for induction of regulatory cells by intratracheal delivery of alloantigen. Transplantation 2004; 77:6–12.
165. Gao W, Demirci G, Li XC. Negative T cell costimulation and islet tolerance. Diabetes Metab Res Rev 2003; 19:179–185.
166. Dong H, Chen L. B7-H1 pathway and its role in the evasion of tumor immunity. J Mol Med 2003; 81:281–287.
167. Nishimura H, Honjo T. PD-1: an inhibitory immunoreceptor involved in peripheral tolerance. Trends Immunol 2001; 22:265–268.
168. Ke B, Ritter T, Kato H, et al. Regulatory cells potentiate the efficacy of IL-4 gene transfer by up-regulating Th2-dependent expression of protective molecules in the infectious tolerance pathway in transplant recipients. J Immunol 2000; 164:5739–5745.
169. Yoshimura S, Bondeson J, Brennan FM, Foxwell BM, Feldmann M. Role of NFkappaB in antigen presentation and development of regulatory T cells

elucidated by treatment of dendritic cells with the proteasome inhibitor PSI. Eur J Immunol 2001; 31:1883–1893.

170.  Farivar AS, Mackinnon-Patterson B, Woolley S, et al. FR167653 reduces obliterative airway disease in rats. J Heart Lung Transplant 2004; 23:985–992.

171.  Nomoto K, Eto M, Yanaga K, Nishimura Y, Maeda T. Interference with cyclophosphamide-induced skin allograft tolerance by cyclosporin A. J Immunol 1992; 149:2668–2674.

172.  Watson CJ, Cobbold SP, Davies HS, et al. Immunosuppression of canine renal allograft recipients by CD4 and CD8 monoclonal antibodies. Tissue Antigens 1994; 43:155–162.

173.  Li Y, Li XC, Zheng XX, Wells AD, Turka LA, Strom TB. Blocking both signal 1 and signal 2 of T-cell activation prevents apoptosis of alloreactive T cells and induction of peripheral allograft tolerance. Nat Med 1999; 5:1298–1302.

3

# Allogeneic Recognition and Immune Tolerance in Lung Transplantation

**Keith C. Meyer**

*Section of Allergy, Pulmonary, and Critical Care Medicine, University of Wisconsin School of Medicine and Public Health, Madison, Wisconsin, U.S.A.*

## INTRODUCTION

The mammalian immune system evolved to protect individuals from various biological threats, which range from viruses and bacteria to multicellular parasites and neoplastic cells, by recognizing antigenic determinants that are distinct from self-expressed molecular moieties. Cells and tissues from individuals of the same species express a plethora of genetically determined major and minor antigens that differentiate self from nonself, and immune cells can be stimulated when exposed to nonself antigens from other individuals of the same species unless they are genetically identical, monozygotic twins. Although the immune system did not evolve to recognize and react to transplanted tissues, the ability that it has developed to resist infections and neoplasms by recognizing self versus nonself or "abnormal self" plays a key role in rejecting transplanted tissues and organs.

Animal studies and human transplantation have demonstrated that tolerance of nonself tissue is linked to the degree of similarity among both major and minor antigens expressed on cell surfaces and appears to be particularly determined by the family of proteins that comprise the major histocompatibility complex (MHC). More recent investigations have identified regulatory aspects of the immune system, such as regulatory lymphocytes, that serve to limit reactions to both self and nonself antigens. This chapter will examine current knowledge of allogeneic immune responses and immune regulation, how these responses pertain to lung allograft rejection, and the mechanisms by which stable immune tolerance may be achieved.

## THE IMMUNE SYSTEM AND SELF VS. NONSELF

Exposure to allogeneic cells or tissues will trigger both cellular and humoral immune responses, and successful transplantation that does not require the prolonged use of immunosuppressive drugs is only possible for syngeneic individuals. Such allorecognition of genetically encoded glycoprotein polymorphisms among members of the same species by the immune system constitutes the major hurdle to long-term graft survival in clinical organ transplantation.

The family of glycoproteins that comprises the major determinants of self versus nonself are the MHC antigens that are encoded on chromosome 6p in humans and chromosome 17 in mice. The most important of these extremely polymorphic surface recognition receptors, which are defined as human leukocyte antigens (HLA), are class I (HLA-A, -B, and -C) and class II (HLA-DP, -DQ, and -DR) molecules. Nucleated cells constitutively express low levels of MHC-I and little or no MHC-II antigens, but numerous stimuli can upregulate MHC expression (1). Although mismatched HLA antigens can cause rapid tissue rejection, minor histocompatibility antigens have also been characterized and can cause rejection that proceeds at a slower rate (2–4).

Because innate immunity does not require previous sensitization to respond to a stimulus, it is the first limb of the immune system to respond to foreign tissue and can simultaneously induce adaptive immune responses. Inflammatory components of the innate immune response that may play a role in transplant rejection include endothelial activation, bioactive lipid mediator production, chemokine and cytokine release, neutrophil sequestration and activation, complement activation, and costimulatory molecule production. However, severe combined immunodeficiency mice with intact innate immunity can tolerate allogeneic tissues indefinitely yet promptly reject allografts when reconstituted with T cells despite having displayed long-term allograft acceptance prior to T-cell reconstitution (5).

In contrast to innate immunity, the adaptive immune response is characterized by the recognition of specific antigens by T cells and involves sensitization to specific peptides. This requires the activation of naive host lymphocytes and the generation of antigen-specific T cell repertoires via clonal expansion and differentiation that culminates in the development of effector and memory T cells. Immunoregulatory lymphocytes are simultaneously generated that serve to control and limit adaptive immune responses. Antigen-presenting cells (APCs)—dendritic cells, activated B cells, and macrophages—play a key role in the generation of adaptive alloimmune responses. Dendritic cells are particularly efficient T cell stimulators. They capture and process the antigen while expressing costimulatory molecules and present peptides (derived from processed antigens and bound to MHC molecules) to T cells after migrating to nearby secondary lymphoid tissues (6).

Although naive T cells could recognize alloantigens in grafted tissue, a recent investigation has shown that the conversion of a naive T cell to an alloreactive cell occurs in secondary lymphoid organs, where naive T cells that are normally present in secondary lymphoid organs detect alloantigens presented by APCs (7). Both direct and indirect allorecognition pathways lead to the sensitization and generation of allospecific T cells (8). T cells can be activated via an indirect allorecognition pathway whereby they interact with preprocessed allopeptides (derived from donor APCs and taken up by recipient APCs) bound to self-MHC that have been redistributed onto the surface of recipient APCs (9). Direct allorecognition occurs when donor APCs that bear nonspecific peptides bound to allo-MHC molecules activate recipient T cells (10). A third mechanism of allorecognition (a "hybrid" pathway) involves elements of both the direct and indirect pathways (11,12). By examining various models that have been developed to explain the generation of recipient alloreactive effector T cells, four subsets of recipient T cells that are sensitized to allograft antigens have been recognized (8,13,14). These include (i) CD4+ T cells that directly recognize donor MHC-II, (ii) CD4+ T cells that are indirectly sensitized via donor peptides bound to self-MHC-II on recipient APCs, (iii) CD8+ T cells directly sensitized to donor MHC-I peptides, and (iv) CD8+ T cells sensitized via cross-presentation by recipient APCs associated with MHC-I peptides. These models indicate that both CD4+ and CD8+ T cells play a role in host rejection responses to implanted foreign tissue.

## CRITICAL EVENTS IN LUNG TRANSPLANTATION AND LUNG ALLOGRAFT REJECTION

To minimize ischemia time and preservation injury, HLA matching is generally not performed for lung transplantation due to the limitations of time and distance. Donor lungs are matched with recipients on the basis of blood group and chest dimensions, and rejection of the transplanted lung must be prevented by pharmacological immunosuppression, which is based on chronic administration of calcineurin inhibitors.

Prior to removal, the lungs of a brain-dead donor may sustain considerable injury, and nonimmunological events can cause injury that can significantly impair posttransplant allograft function (15). Warm and cold ischemia at the time of organ harvest can also damage the lung, and ischemia–reperfusion injury, which occurs to some degree in all recipients, can be severe. Such reperfusion injury can cause inflammatory changes that are not directly related to alloantigenic stimulation, and allograft damage may enhance exposure of alloantigens to recipient APCs and lymphocytes.

In addition to perioperative injury, the transplanted lung is at risk of both rejection and infection. Occasionally, hyperacute rejection can occur if the recipient already has circulating antibodies directed against antigens on the graft and is characterized by acute endothelial cell damage and dramatic disruption of allograft perfusion (16,17). Such preformed antibodies can be generated in response to pregnancy, previous blood transfusions, or previous transplants. Therefore, panel reactivity testing is performed prior to transplant to identify individuals with preformed antibodies (panel reactive antibodies) that may cause hyperacute rejection (17,18). Acute lung rejection is characterized by the appearance of lymphocytic infiltrates around small vessels in the graft (19) and is likely a combination of antigen-specific responses plus nonspecific inflammatory responses. Complement activation has been demonstrated in both hyperacute and acute rejection, and it appears to play a pivotal role in hyperacute rejection (20).

Although acute lung rejection is characterized by perivascular and/or peribronchial infiltration by activated lymphocytes into the lung allograft, such lymphocyte infiltration may not be present on lung biopsy despite a clinical situation that is consistent with lung rejection and not explained by other processes despite the appearance of fever and deteriorating lung function. A possible explanation for this clinical situation is a humoral antibody response that is directed against graft components and leads to complement deposition and graft injury that is not accompanied by lymphocyte infiltrates. Magro et al. (21) have shown that such episodes of lung rejection ("pauci-inflammatory capillary injury syndrome") correlate with septal capillary injury and deposits of antiendothelial antibodies (plus complement components) that did not appear to be MHC class I or II specific antibodies. They speculate that non-HLA endothelial cell antigens stimulate a humoral rejection response that may play an important role in both acute and chronic lung allograft rejection (21,22).

The major factor that limits long-term survival and quality of life following lung transplantation is bronchiolitis obliterans syndrome (BOS), which still occurs in more than half of all lung transplant recipients who survive at five years following transplantation despite improvements in surgical and organ preservation techniques, management of infections and reperfusion injury, and immunosuppression regimens (23). Some risk factors that have been linked to the development of BOS include acute rejection, HLA mismatching, and cytomegalovirus (CMV) infection. Although alloimmune responses to the transplanted lung are thought to be the major cause of BOS, alloimmune-independent factors, such as inhaled irritants, airway ischemia, viral infections, and gastroesophageal reflux disease (GERD), may also play an important role (Table 1). Furthermore, although much emphasis is placed on T cell–mediated rejection, especially in acute rejection, it

**Table 1**  Potential Causes of Bronchiolitis
Obliterans Syndrome

---

*Alloimmune dependent*
Episodes of acute rejection
Degree of HLA mismatching
Lymphocytic bronchitis/bronchiolitis
Anti-HLA alloantibodies
Anti-endothelial cell antibodies
*Alloimmune independent*
Airway ischemia
CMV infection/pneumonitis
Non-CMV viral infection
Bacterial infection
GERD
Medical noncompliance
Advanced donor age
Induction of autoimmunity (e.g., collagen V)

---

*Abbreviations*: HLA, human leukocyte antigen; CMV, cytomegalovirus; GERD, gastroesophageal reflux disease.

should be recognized that B cell responses and humoral rejection appear to
play a particularly important role in chronic graft rejection (24).

## DETERMINANTS OF GRAFT TOLERANCE: ALLOIMMUNITY, AUTOIMMUNITY, AND REGULATION

Immune tolerance to self-antigens and many exogenous antigens is required to
avoid or limit inflammation and prevent significant autoinjury, and transplantation has provided an excellent means of "dissecting" the immune system and
understanding immune responses and their regulation. Activation of T and B
cells appears to require two signals (25). The first is the engagement of the antigen receptor, and the second is the engagement of costimulatory receptors.
Engagement of the antigen receptor without activation of costimulatory
receptors (interaction of CD28 on naive CD4+ cells with B7.1 or B7.2 on
APCs for T cells, interaction of CD40L on activated CD4+ cells with its
CD40 ligand on B cell surfaces for B cells) results in anergy or tolerized lymphocytes. However, true anergy has been difficult to demonstrate in animal
models, and regulatory mechanisms that prevent lymphocyte activation may
account for tolerance observed in animal models of MHC mismatching (26).

Various retrospective analyses of organ allograft survival have linked
HLA phenotypes of donor and recipient, especially HLA-DR antigens, to
alloimmune responses and graft survival (27). However, graft survival for
some donor–recipient mismatches has not been shown to differ versus

completely HLA-identical allografts (28), and some donor–recipient mismatches appear to be more immunogenic than others (27,29). Retrospective analyses of lung transplantation have correlated HLA mismatch with survival rates (30,31) and with the incidence and severity of BOS (8,32). However, Quantz et al. (31) in their multicenter study of 3549 patients found very few lung transplants performed that had two or less HLA mismatches. Although an increased number of HLA mismatches correlated significantly with decreased survival, the effect of HLA mismatch on survival appeared to be small, and HLA mismatching did not correlate with the development of BOS (31). Other investigators have identified the development of anti-HLA antibodies as a risk factor for decreased survival and the development of BOS in smaller cohorts of patients (33–35). These studies indicate a role for alloimmunity in lung allograft rejection, but other factors may also govern graft tolerance versus rejection.

Although much research in organ transplantation has focused on alloimmunity and HLA-mismatching as a cause of graft rejection, relatively little has been done to explore the role of autoimmune responses that may be initiated by transplantation, although some attention has recently been focused on similarities between autoimmune diseases and the responses to transplanted organs (36,37). Tissue remodeling following reperfusion injury, infection-induced graft inflammation, or episodes of acute rejection may expose self-antigens that are normally sequestered and tolerated by the host, inducing immune recognition and graft rejection that are not due to HLA mismatch and allogeneic immune responses. Sumpter and Wilkes (38) have suggested that an autoimmune response to an extracellular matrix component, collagen V, may play an important role in acute and chronic lung allograft rejection and may explain, in part, why chronic rejection and long-term graft survival are worse for lung transplantation than any other organ. They have shown that in a murine model of lung rejection, perivascular and peribronchiolar lymphocytic infiltrates and IgG2a antibody deposition appear and correlate with the location of collagen V in the normal lung (39). Additionally, this group has shown that collagen V–specific T cells appear in rat lungs during acute and chronic rejection responses (40), and that lung allograft rejection can be significantly blunted in their rat lung transplant model if the animals are orally tolerized by administration of collagen V prior to transplant (41).

Considerable numbers of APCs and other passenger leukocytes, which are capable of migration and residing in donor tissues, are passively transferred with allograft implantation, and persistence of passenger leukocytes in the transplanted lung has been correlated with better outcome following lung transplantation (42). Although migration of passenger APCs from transplanted organs to regional host lymphoid tissue appears to be important in initiating and propagating alloimmune rejection responses, donor cells may help induce organ tolerance. This concept is supported by the observations of Pham et al. (43) that infusion of donor bone marrow at the time of lung transplantation increases donor cell chimerism, induces donor-specific hyporeactivity, and reduces the incidence of BOS. Although these data are preliminary, they suggest that donor bone marrow–derived cells may play an important role in immune tolerance of allografts, although the precise function of donor versus recipient leukocytes in regulating rejection responses is not yet known.

Regulatory T lymphocytes can control and limit harmful immune responses, while allowing protective responses against pathogens to occur as required. Although there are numerous mechanisms by which autoreactive lymphocytes are purged during immune system development, some may escape to the periphery (e.g., the respiratory and oral mucosa), and if not kept in check by regulatory T cells or other mechanisms, they can cause an autoimmune disease, such as lupus erythematosus (44,45). CD4+/CD25+ regulatory cells, which can be found in naive mice, appear to play a key role in maintaining peripheral tolerance to self-antigens (44–46), and CD4+/CD25+ regulatory T cells have been recently characterized in humans (47,48). Depletion of CD4+/CD25+ regulatory cells via thymectomy in neonatal mice causes systemic autoimmunity, and depletion of regulatory T cells in adult, wild-type mice reverses peripheral tolerance and causes autoimmune disease to appear as well (44). Although T regulatory cells have been identified as CD4+/CD25+, a CD4+/CD25– T cell subset has been associated with tolerance to skin grafts in mice (49). CD8+ regulatory T cells have also been identified and linked to attenuated immune responses (50,51), although they may function to limit inflammation and destruction of organs, such as a liver that is chronically infected with hepatitis C and would otherwise be destroyed if an equilibrium between host and pathogen could not be established and maintained (52).

Regulatory T cell subsets have been examined fairly extensively, and two basic types of T regulatory cells have been described (53,54). Natural T regulatory cells are derived from the thymus and suppress T-cell activation via an antigen-independent, contact-driven mechanism. The second type, adaptive T regulatory cells, is generated from thymically derived regulatory T cells or from CD4+ helper T cells in response to peripheral antigen stimulation. Regulatory T cells with different phenotypes have now been identified in many experimental models of transplantation (55,56).

Regulatory T cells appear to suppress T-cell responses via an antigen-specific mechanism that is driven by specific cytokines, which include interleukin-2 (IL-2), IL-4, and IL-10 combined with secretion of transforming growth factor-beta (TGF-β) (57–61). Although regulatory T cells have been shown to inhibit donor-specific rejection, they do not appear to affect rejection of third-party grafts (49,62,63). TGF-β, which has potent immunosuppressive properties, may be particularly important for the generation of regulatory T cells and maintenance of peripheral tolerance (61,64–66), and it has been shown to be systemically upregulated in rats that become tolerant to their lung allografts (67). Similarly, IL-10 is produced by lung dendritic cells and promotes the differentiation of antigen-specific regulatory T cells (68). Systemic IL-10 induces in vivo expansion of regulatory T cell populations (69), and IL-10 produced by regulatory T cells can abrogate CD4+ T cell responses to alloantigens (70). Differentiation of T cells to a regulatory phenotype is also influenced by expression of LAG-3. LAG-3 is a CD4-linked molecule that binds MHC class II molecules and reduces proliferation of CD4+ T cells that express LAG-3 and allows these cells to suppress effector T cells (71). In addition to the recently recognized role of regulatory T cells in maintaining immune tolerance, other mechanisms for the maintenance of peripheral tolerance have recently been described, such as the expression of an inhibitory Fc receptor (FcγRIIB) on B cells, which can prevent spontaneous lupus-like autoimmunity from developing in mice (72,73).

Much of the variability in the incidence and severity of acute and chronic rejection among organ allograft recipients may well be due to the ability of their regulatory T cells to prevent alloimmune (e.g., acute rejection) and autoimmune (e.g., BOS in lung transplantation) responses. Recent data support a role for regulatory T cells in preventing lung allograft rejection. Meloni et al. (74) found that recipients who were clinically stable and doing well had increased CD4+/CD25+ T cells in peripheral blood versus patients with BOS. Induction of oral tolerance to lung allografts in rats by feeding with collagen V has been shown to be mediated by TGF-β–producing T cells (40,41). This tolerance to collagen V appears to be mediated by CD4+CD45RChigh regulatory cells that can mediate tolerance when adoptively transferred; these cells are permissive to TGF-β–mediated signaling and do not express SMAD7 (75). Another recently published investigation indirectly supports the regulatory immune mechanisms that may prevent allograft rejection by promoting the development and persistence of regulatory T lymphocytes. Zheng and colleagues (76) examined IL-10 production phenotypes in human lung allograft recipients and found that there were significantly less persistent rejectors in the group with a high IL-10 production phenotype in comparison to those with a low or intermediate phenotype, supporting an important role for IL-10 in suppressing rejection responses in lung allograft recipients.

Many approaches may prove helpful for preventing lung allograft rejection (Table 2). Whether rejection of lung allografts occurs via alloimmune responses to nonself antigens in the context of MHC molecules, autoimmune responses to a self-antigen, such as collagen V, or a combination of alloimmune and autoimmune responses, the most important determinant of allograft survival and sustained function may be suppression of rejection responses by regulatory components of the immune system. Indeed, the use of calcineurin inhibitors to block development of CD4+ lymphocyte–mediated alloimmune rejection responses may have the untoward effect of

**Table 2**   Measures to Optimize the Induction and
Maintenance of Lung Allograft Tolerance

| |
| --- |
| Prevent or limit graft preservation injury |
| Prevent or limit reperfusion injury |
| Prevent or suppress viral and bacterial infection |
| HLA matching |
| Suppress allogeneic immune responses |
| Enhance regulatory T-cell function |
|    Donor leukocyte transfer (e.g., bone marrow cells) |
|    Induce tolerance (e.g., oral administration of collagen V) |
|    Limit use of calcineurin inhibitors |

*Abbreviation*: HLA, human leukocyte antigen.

blocking the development of regulatory T cells that can mediate allograft tolerance. Cyclosporin and tacrolimus block IL-2 expression, which is required for optimal proliferation and function of regulatory T cells (77), and the administration of cyclosporine A to mice appears capable of suppressing peripheral tolerance and inducing systemic autoimmunity (78–80).

## SUMMARY

Rejection of lung allografts by a recipient's immune system has been perceived as mediated by effector T lymphocytes that recognize foreign antigens, especially nonself MHC molecules. Suppression of this alloimmune response to transplanted tissue with immunosuppressive agents, such as the calcineurin inhibitors, has allowed long-term graft acceptance and sustained function for many lung transplant recipients. However, tolerance of organ allografts may be achieved and maintained by regulatory mechanisms that are just now being more widely recognized and understood. Regulatory T cells clearly play an important role in preventing the rejection of grafted allogeneic tissues. They are not only capable of preventing alloimmune rejection responses, but they may also suppress autoimmune responses associated with transplantation (e.g., loss of tolerance to a self-antigen, such as collagen V in lung transplants). Strategies that promote the proliferation and persistence of regulatory T cells in lung allograft recipients may prove more beneficial than the use of relatively nonselective immunosuppression for long-term allograft acceptance. Such strategies may be as simple and nontoxic as inducing tolerance via the gastrointestinal tract by giving candidates oral tolerogenic antigens, such as collagen V, prior to lung transplantation. A better understanding of tolerance mechanisms and how they can be exploited clinically is likely to lead to considerably better outcomes following lung transplantation.

## REFERENCES

1. Gould DS, Auchincloss H Jr. Direct and indirect recognition: the role of MHC antigens in graft rejection. Immunol Today 1999; 20:77–82.
2. Roopenian D, Choi EY, Brown A. The immunogenomics of minor histocompatibility antigens. Immunol Rev 2002; 190:86–94.
3. Perreault C, Roy DC, Fortin C. Immunodominant minor histocompatibility antigens: the major ones. Immunol Today 1998; 19:69–74.
4. Malarkannan S, Pooler LM. Minor histocompatibility antigens: molecular barriers for sucessful tissue transplantation. In: Wilkes DS, Burlingham WJ, eds. Immunobiology of Organ Transplantation. New York: Kluwer Academic/Plenum, 2004:71–105.
5. Bingaman AW, Ha J, Waitze SY, et al. Vigorous allograft rejection in the absence of danger. J Immunol 2000; 164:3065–3071.
6. Liu YJ. Dendritic cell subsets and lineages, and their functions in innate and adaptive immunity. Cell 2001; 106:259–262.
7. Lakkis FG, Arakelov A, Konieczny BT, Inoue Y. Immunologic "ignorance" of vascularized organ transplants in the absence of secondary lymphoid tissue. Nat Med 2000; 6:686–688.
8. Chalermskulrat W, Neuringer IP, Schmitz JL, et al. Human leukocyte antigen mismatches predispose to the severity of bronchiolitis obliterans syndrome after lung transplantation. Chest 2003; 123:1825–1831.
9. Fangmann J, Dalchau R, Fabre JW. Rejection of skin allografts by indirect allorecognition of donor class I major histocompatibility complex peptides. J Exp Med 1992; 175:1521–1529.
10. Lechler RI, Lombardi G, Batchelor JR, Reinsmoen N, Bach FH. The molecular basis of alloreactivity. Immunol Today 1990; 11:83–88.
11. Frasca L, Amendola A, Hornick P, et al. Role of donor and recipient antigen-presenting cells in priming and maintaining T cells with indirect allospecificity. Transplantation 1998; 66:1238–1243.
12. Burlingham WJ, Torrealba J. Immunologic tolerance as taught by allografts. In: Wilkes DS, Burlingham WJ, eds. Immunobiology of Organ Transplantation. New York: Kluwer Academic/Plenum, 2004:139–158.
13. Kishimoto K, Sandner S, Imitola J, et al. Th1 cytokines, programmed cell death, and alloreactive T cell clone size in transplant tolerance. J Clin Invest 2002; 109:1471–1479.
14. Valujskikh A, Lantz O, Celli S, Matzinger P, Heeger PS. Cross-primed CD8(+) T cells mediate graft rejection via a distinct effector pathway. Nat Immunol 2002; 3:844–851.
15. Meyer KC. The role of neutrophils in transplantation. In: Wilkes DS, Burlingham WJ, eds. Immunobiology of Organ Transplantation. New York: Kluwer Academic/Plenum, 2004:493–507.
16. Kissmeyer-Nielsen F, Olsen S, Petersen VP, Fjeldborg O. Hyperacute rejection of kidney allografts, associated with pre-existing humoral antibodies against donor cells. Lancet 1966; 2:662–665.
17. Patel R, Terasaki PI. Significance of the positive crossmatch test in kidney transplantation. N Engl J Med 1969; 280:735–739.

18. Koka P, Cecka JM. Sensitization and crossmatching in renal transplantation. Clin Transpl 1989; 379–390.
19. Yousem SA, Berry GJ, Cagle PT, et al. Revision of the 1990 working formulation for the classification of pulmonary allograft rejection: Lung Rejection Study Group. J Heart Lung Transplant 1996; 15:1–15.
20. Baldwin WM III, Ota H, Wasowska BA, et al. Complement system in allorecognition and rejection of organ transplants. In: Wilkes DS, Burlingham WJ, eds. Immunobiology of Organ Transplantation. New York: Kluwer Academic/ Plenum, 2004:139–158.
21. Magro CM, Klinger DM, Adams PW, et al. Evidence that humoral allograft rejection in lung transplant patients is not histocompatibility antigen-related. Am J Transplant 2003; 3:1264–1272.
22. Magro CM, Ross P Jr, Kelsey M, Waldman WJ, Pope-Harman A. Association of humoral immunity and bronchiolitis obliterans syndrome. Am J Transplant 2003; 3:1155–1166.
23. Estenne M, Hertz MI. Bronchiolitis obliterans after human lung transplantation. Am J Respir Crit Care Med 2002; 166:440–444.
24. Michaels PJ, Fishbein MC, Colvin RB. Humoral rejection of human organ transplants. Springer Semin Immunopathol 2003; 25:119–140.
25. Field EH, Wood KJ. Regulatory T cells: professional supressor cells. In: Wilkes DS, Burlingham WJ, eds. Immunobiology of Organ Transplantation. New York: Kluwer Academic/Plenum, 2004:313–327.
26. Kruisbeek AM, Amsen D. Mechanisms underlying T-cell tolerance. Curr Opin Immunol 1996; 8:233–244.
27. Claas FHJ. HLA immunogenetics and transplantation. In: Wilkes DS, Burlingham WJ, eds. Immunobiology of Organ Transplantation. New York: Kluwer Academic/Plenum, 2004:45–52.
28. Maruya E, Takemoto S, Terasaki PI. HLA matching: identification of permissible HLA mismatches. Clin Transpl 1993: 511–520.
29. Hendriks GF, D'Amaro J, Persijn GG, et al. Excellent outcome after transplantation of renal allografts from HLA-DRw6-positive donors even in HLA-DR mismatches. Lancet 1983; 2:187–189.
30. Smits JM, Vanhaecke J, Haverich A, et al. Three-year survival rates for all consecutive heart-only and lung-only transplants performed in Eurotransplant, 1997–1999. Clin Transpl 2003; 89–100.
31. Quantz MA, Bennett LE, Meyer DM, Novick RJ. Does human leukocyte antigen matching influence the outcome of lung transplantation? An analysis of 3,549 lung transplantations. J Heart Lung Transplant 2000; 19:473–479.
32. van den Berg JW, Hepkema BG, Geertsma A, et al. Long-term outcome of lung transplantation is predicted by the number of HLA-DR mismatches. Transplantation 2001; 71:368–373.
33. Reinsmoen NL, Nelson K, Zeevi A. Anti-HLA antibody analysis and crossmatching in heart and lung transplantation. Transpl Immunol 2004; 13:63–71.
34. Lu KC, Jaramillo A, Mendeloff EN, et al. Concomitant allorecognition of mismatched donor HLA class I- and class II-derived peptides in pediatric lung transplant recipients with bronchiolitis obliterans syndrome. J Heart Lung Transplant 2003; 22:35–43.

35. Palmer SM, Davis RD, Hadjiliadis D, et al. Development of an antibody specific to major histocompatibility antigens detectable by flow cytometry after lung transplant is associated with bronchiolitis obliterans syndrome. Transplantation 2002; 74:799–804.

36. Wrenshall L. Role of the microenvironment in immune responses to transplantation. Springer Semin Immunopathol 2003; 25:199–213.

37. Matthews JB, Ramos E, Bluestone JA. Clinical trials of transplant tolerance: slow but steady progress. Am J Transplant 2003; 3:794–803.

38. Sumpter TL, Wilkes DS. Role of autoimmunity in organ allograft rejection: a focus on immunity to type V collagen in the pathogenesis of lung transplant rejection. Am J Physiol Lung Cell Mol Physiol 2004; 286:L1129–L1139.

39. Wilkes DS, Heidler KM, Bowen LK, et al. Allogeneic bronchoalveolar lavage cells induce the histology of acute lung allograft rejection, and deposition of IgG2a in recipient murine lungs. J Immunol 1995; 155:2775–2783.

40. Haque MA, Mizobuchi T, Yasufuku K, et al. Evidence for immune responses to a self-antigen in lung transplantation: role of type V collagen-specific T cells in the pathogenesis of lung allograft rejection. J Immunol 2002; 169:1542–1549.

41. Yasufuku K, Heidler KM, O'Donnell PW, et al. Oral tolerance induction by type V collagen downregulates lung allograft rejection. Am J Respir Cell Mol Biol 2001; 25:26–34.

42. O'Connell PJ, Mba-Jonas A, Leverson GE, et al. Stable lung allograft outcome correlates with the presence of intragraft donor-derived leukocytes. Transplantation 1998; 66:1167–1174.

43. Pham SM, Rao AS, Zeevi A, et al. Effects of donor bone marrow infusion in clinical lung transplantation. Ann Thorac Surg 2000; 69:345–350.

44. Asano M, Toda M, Sakaguchi N, Sakaguchi S. Autoimmune disease as a consequence of developmental abnormality of a T cell subpopulation. J Exp Med 1996; 184:387–396.

45. Sakaguchi S, Sakaguchi N, Asano M, Itoh M, Toda M. Immunologic self-tolerance maintained by activated T cells expressing IL-2 receptor alpha-chains (CD25). Breakdown of a single mechanism of self-tolerance causes various autoimmune diseases. J Immunol 1995; 155:1151–1164.

46. Suri-Payer E, Amar AZ, Thornton AM, Shevach EM. CD4+CD25+ T cells inhibit both the induction and effector function of autoreactive T cells and represent a unique lineage of immunoregulatory cells. J Immunol 1998; 160:1212–1218.

47. Dieckmann D, Plottner H, Berchtold S, Berger T, Schuler G. Ex vivo isolation and characterization of CD4(+)CD25(+) T cells with regulatory properties from human blood. J Exp Med 2001; 193:1303–1310.

48. Jonuleit H, Schmitt E, Stassen M, Tuettenberg A, Knop J, Enk AH. Identification and functional characterization of human CD4(+)CD25(+) T cells with regulatory properties isolated from peripheral blood. J Exp Med 2001; 193:1285–1294.

49. Graca L, Thompson S, Lin CY, Adams E, Cobbold SP, Waldmann H. Both CD4(+)CD25(+) and CD4(+)CD25(−) regulatory cells mediate dominant transplantation tolerance. J Immunol 2002; 168:5558–5565.

50. Gaur A, Ruberti G, Haspel R, Mayer JP, Fathman CG. Requirement for CD8+ cells in T cell receptor peptide-induced clonal unresponsiveness. Science 1993; 259:91–94.
51. Koh DR, Fung-Leung WP, Ho A, Gray D, Acha-Orbea H, Mak TW. Less mortality but more relapses in experimental allergic encephalomyelitis in CD8–/– mice. Science 1992; 256:1210–1213.
52. Accapezzato D, Francavilla V, Paroli M, et al. Hepatic expansion of a virus-specific regulatory CD8(+) T cell population in chronic hepatitis C virus infection. J Clin Invest 2004; 113:963–972.
53. Bluestone JA, Abbas AK. Natural versus adaptive regulatory T cells. Nat Rev Immunol 2003; 3:253–257.
54. Piccirillo CA, Shevach EM. Naturally-occurring CD4+CD25+ immunoregulatory T cells: central players in the arena of peripheral tolerance. Semin Immunol 2004; 16:81–88.
55. McHugh RS, Shevach EM. The role of suppressor T cells in regulation of immune responses. J Allergy Clin Immunol 2002; 110:693–702.
56. Waldmann H, Cobbold S. Regulating the immune response to transplants: a role for CD4+ regulatory cells? Immunity 2001; 14:399–406.
57. Furtado GC, Curotto de Lafaille MA, Kutchukhidze N, Lafaille JJ. Interleukin 2 signaling is required for CD4(+) regulatory T cell function. J Exp Med 2002; 196:851–857.
58. Suzuki H, Kundig TM, Furlonger C, et al. Deregulated T cell activation and autoimmunity in mice lacking interleukin-2 receptor beta. Science 1995; 268:1472–1476.
59. Bushell A, Niimi M, Morris PJ, Wood KJ. Evidence for immune regulation in the induction of transplantation tolerance: a conditional but limited role for IL-4. J Immunol 1999; 162:1359–1366.
60. Hara M, Kingsley CI, Niimi M, et al. IL-10 is required for regulatory T cells to mediate tolerance to alloantigens in vivo. J Immunol 2001; 166:3789–3796.
61. Gorelik L, Flavell RA. Abrogation of TGF beta signaling in T cells leads to spontaneous T cell differentiation and autoimmune disease. Immunity 2000; 12:171–181.
62. Graca L, Cobbold SP, Waldmann H. Identification of regulatory T cells in tolerated allografts. J Exp Med 2002; 195:1641–1646.
63. van Maurik A, Herber M, Wood KJ, Jones ND. Cutting edge: CD4+CD25+ alloantigen-specific immunoregulatory cells that can prevent CD8+ T cell-mediated graft rejection: implications for anti-CD154 immunotherapy. J Immunol 2002; 169:5401–5404.
64. Gorelik L, Flavell RA. Transforming growth factor-beta in T-cell biology. Nat Rev Immunol 2002; 2:46–53.
65. Nakamura K, Kitani A, Strober W. Cell contact-dependent immunosuppression by CD4(+)CD25(+) regulatory T cells is mediated by cell surface-bound transforming growth factor beta. J Exp Med 2001; 194:629–644.
66. Monteleone G, Kumberova A, Croft NM, McKenzie C, Steer HW, MacDonald TT. Blocking Smad7 restores TGF-beta1 signaling in chronic inflammatory bowel disease. J Clin Invest 2001; 108:601–609.

67. Yasufuku K, Heidler KM, Woods KA, et al. Prevention of bronchiolitis obliterans in rat lung allografts by type V collagen-induced oral tolerance. Transplantation 2002; 73:500–505.

68. Akbari O, DeKruyff RH, Umetsu DT. Pulmonary dendritic cells producing IL-10 mediate tolerance induced by respiratory exposure to antigen. Nat Immunol 2001; 2:725–731.

69. Goudy KS, Burkhardt BR, Wasserfall C, et al. Systemic overexpression of IL-10 induces CD4+CD25+ cell populations in vivo and ameliorates type 1 diabetes in nonobese diabetic mice in a dose-dependent fashion. J Immunol 2003; 171:2270–2278.

70. Groux H. Type 1 T-regulatory cells: their role in the control of immune responses. Transplantation 2003; 75:8S–12S.

71. Huang CT, Workman CJ, Flies D, et al. Role of LAG-3 in regulatory T cells. Immunity 2004; 21:503–513.

72. Bolland S, Ravetch JV. Spontaneous autoimmune disease in Fc(gamma)RIIB-deficient mice results from strain-specific epistasis. Immunity 2000; 13:277–285.

73. McGaha TL, Sorrentino B, Ravetch JV. Restoration of tolerance in lupus by targeted inhibitory receptor expression. Science 2005; 307:590–593.

74. Meloni F, Vitulo P, Bianco AM, et al. Regulatory CD4+CD25+ T cells in the peripheral blood of lung transplant recipients: correlation with transplant outcome. Transplantation 2004; 77:762–766.

75. Mizobuchi T, Yasufuku K, Zheng Y, et al. Differential expression of Smad7 transcripts identifies the CD4+CD45RChigh regulatory T cells that mediate type V collagen-induced tolerance to lung allografts. J Immunol 2003; 171: 1140–1147.

76. Zheng HX, Burckart GJ, McCurry K, et al. Interleukin-10 production genotype protects against acute persistent rejection after lung transplantation. J Heart Lung Transplant 2004; 23:541–546.

77. Thornton AM, Shevach EM. CD4+CD25+ immunoregulatory T cells suppress polyclonal T cell activation in vitro by inhibiting interleukin 2 production. J Exp Med 1998; 188:287–296.

78. Huss R. In vitro determination of self-reactivity in the early postcyclosporine period. Transpl Immunol 1993; 1:228–234.

79. Sakaguchi S, Sakaguchi N. Thymus and autoimmunity. Transplantation of the thymus from cyclosporin A-treated mice causes organ-specific autoimmune disease in athymic nude mice. J Exp Med 1988; 167:1479–1485.

80. Sakaguchi S, Sakaguchi N. Organ-specific autoimmune disease induced in mice by elimination of T cell subsets. V. Neonatal administration of cyclosporin A causes autoimmune disease. J Immunol 1989; 142:471–480.

# 4

# Lung Transplantation for Chronic Obstructive Pulmonary Disease

**Robert M. Kotloff**

*Pulmonary, Allergy, and Critical Care Division, Department of Medicine, University of Pennsylvania, Philadelphia, Pennsylvania, U.S.A.*

**Fernando J. Martinez**

*Department of Internal Medicine, University of Michigan Health System, Ann Arbor, Michigan, U.S.A.*

## INTRODUCTION

Chronic obstructive pulmonary disease (COPD) is defined as a progressive respiratory disease characterized by airflow limitation that is not fully reversible (1,2). This definition includes several distinct pathophysiologic conditions including chronic bronchitis and emphysema. Chronic bronchitis is defined clinically by the presence of a daily, productive cough for more than three months with a duration of more than two successive years; emphysema is pathologically defined by an enlargement of air spaces (3,4); abnormalities of small airways are frequently seen (5,6). Importantly, most patients have features of all three of these pathologic conditions (4).

Lung transplantation represents one of the many therapeutic options for patients with severe COPD. Given the potential toxicity of this therapeutic intervention, an accurate assessment of prognosis is important as is maximization of more conservative therapy. This chapter presents a detailed description of prognostic factors in COPD and the latest concepts regarding pharmacological and nonpharmacological therapy within the context of lung transplantation.

## NATURAL HISTORY/PREDICTIVE INDICES

Accurate prognostication in patients with COPD remains difficult. This is particularly relevant in determining eligibility for lung transplantation in patients with severe chronic airflow obstruction. In an effort to standardize listing criteria, representatives from the International Society for Heart and Lung Transplantation (ISHLT), the American Society of Transplant Physicians, the American Thoracic Society, and the European Respiratory Society enumerated general health guidelines and disease-specific guidelines for identifying patients at risk from their underlying disease (7). These criteria are currently under revision, a process that will be particularly relevant for COPD patients, as studies of outcome in COPD have confirmed widely varying survival rates.

### Features Influencing COPD Survival

Pulmonary Function

**Spirometry:**   Over the past several decades many authors have examined the natural history of COPD in an attempt to identify prognostic factors, as reviewed by numerous authors (8–10). The vast majority of these studies have identified pulmonary function as the single best predictor of survival, although careful comparison of individual studies is limited by varying selection criteria, treatment regimens (including oxygen therapy), and definitions of underlying disease.

Most studies have confirmed that forced expiratory volume in one second ($FEV_1$) is a strong predictor of survival (8,10). In a sentinel study, Burrows and colleagues confirmed that indices of ventilatory capacity were the most predictive of long-term survival in 200 patients with an initial $FEV_1$ <60% predicted (11). Longer-term follow-up of the same patients plus an additional 100 patients confirmed that postbronchodilator $FEV_1$ % predicted was the best predictor of long-term survival (12). In the Intermittent Positive Pressure Breathing Trial (IPPB), where a wide spectrum of COPD patients without hypoxemia were recruited, baseline prebronchodilator $FEV_1$ and patient age were the best predictors of mortality (13,14). Importantly, although the percentage rise in $FEV_1$ after bronchodilator administration was positively related to survival, this was not noted when the postbronchodilator $FEV_1$ was substituted for prebronchodilator $FEV_1$. The importance of bronchodilator reversibility was prospectively tested in 1586 subjects with asthma ($n = 491$) or COPD ($n = 1095$) (15); the latter exhibited a mean $FEV_1$ of 38.5% predicted, which increased to 49.2% predicted after bronchodilators and steroid therapy. The extent of bronchoreversibility did not improve the ability to predict survival when the best $FEV_1$ % predicted was included in the model. These data confirm the importance of best achieved $FEV_1$ % predicted as a mortality predictor in COPD (16).

Several authors have attempted to identify the threshold $FEV_1$ % predicted at which mortality rises. The IPPB investigators suggested that survival was worst in patients with a postbronchodilator $FEV_1$ less than 30% predicted. A similar threshold was established by another group of investigators who examined a smaller group of patients (mean age of 60 years) being treated with long-term oxygen therapy (LTOT) (17). A threshold post-bronchodilator $FEV_1$ less than 30% predicted seems a reasonable threshold to identify COPD patients at increased risk of mortality. A decreasing $FEV_1$ during follow-up has also been suggested to identify a group of COPD patients at particular risk of mortality (18–20).

**Diffusing capacity:** An impaired diffusing capacity has been suggestive of a decreased survival in some studies (12,21–23). In the early series of Burrows and colleagues, a decreased diffusing capacity of the lung for carbon monoxide (DLCO) was weakly predictive of mortality in univariate but not multivariate analysis (11). In contrast, Boushy et al. noted that those patients with a DLCO $<3$ ml/min/mmHg exhibited a significantly higher mortality (22). This finding has been confirmed by some (23), but not by all (13). As such, a decreased DLCO may be an additional predictor of mortality in patients with severe chronic airflow obstruction, although a clear threshold value for individual patients is difficult to establish.

**Arterial blood gases:** Several groups have suggested that a low $PaO_2$ is associated with decreased survival in COPD (8,24). In addition, oxygen therapy in hypoxemic patients has been demonstrated to improve survival in large, multicenter controlled trials (25); the beneficial effect may not appear to carry over to individuals with only moderate hypoxemia (26). The varying survival characteristics of different COPD cohorts has been attributed, in part, to the negative effects of hypoxemia, particularly in early studies where LTOT was not routinely employed (8,13). This argument has been supported by analyses suggesting that long-term survival in patients with a $PaO_2 >60$ mmHg was not different from those patients with more severe hypoxemia treated with LTOT (27,28). Furthermore, some have suggested that an improved outcome in patients with COPD occurs in those who are adherent to therapy (including oxygen administration) versus those who are not compliant (16). As such, hypoxemia is likely a weak predictor of mortality, particularly in those with more severe baseline hypoxemia, although much of the detrimental impact can be minimized by the use of LTOT.

A strong argument can be made that hypercarbia is an independent predictor of mortality in COPD (8,22,23,29). Interestingly, Aida and colleagues did not confirm a worse survival in patients with an initial

$PaCO_2 \geq 45\,mmHg$ in 4552 COPD patients receiving LTOT (30); during the course of 6–18 months of follow-up in 466 patients, those patients whose $PaCO_2$ rose by $\geq 5\,mmHg$ had a worse prognosis. Although some patients presenting with a $PaCO_2 > 50\,mmHg$ during an exacerbation experience significant mortality during long-term follow-up (11% hospital, 20% 60-day, 43% 1-year, and 49% 2-year) (31), not all investigators have confirmed such a finding (32,33). As such, an elevated resting $PaCO_2$ measured during a time of stability, or a rise in $PaCO_2$ during intermediate follow-up, are associated with a worse survival in patients with COPD.

**Exercise capacity:** Overall impairment in functional status has been associated with impaired survival in COPD. Several investigators have noted worse survival in COPD patients with a lesser exercise capacity (8,34). This has been quantified using a pedometer; in the initial three-week stabilization period prior to randomization in the Nocturnal Oxygen Therapy Trial (NOTT) (35); those patients classified as achieving a "low" walk distance ($<3950\,ft/day$) had a worse survival than those classified as the "high walking group." The walking distance has been demonstrated to provide prognostic information. One group suggested that postrehabilitation 12-minute walk distance was the most significant variable related to prognosis after pulmonary rehabilitation (36). This finding was confirmed in a separate similar study (37). In a large cohort of well-characterized patients, another group confirmed that six-minute walk distance was independently predictive of survival, particularly if distance decreased serially during follow-up (38). Additional study of more complex exercise modality has confirmed the value of exercise capacity as a prognostic variable, particularly the slope of change in $PaO_2$ as a function of the change in oxygen consumption ($VO_2$) (39) and the peak $VO_2$ achieved (40).

## Pathophysiology of Chronic Airflow Limitation

The pathophysiologic basis underlying chronic airflow limitation (CAL) appears to influence to subsequent mortality. COPD represents a heterogenous group of diseases characterized by CAL (1); underlying diseases include chronic bronchitis, emphysema, long standing asthma, bronchiectasis, and obliterative bronchiolitis (3). An aggressive clinical, radiographic, and physiologic evaluation can define the underlying phenotype (3), although clinical and physiologic features can overlap (41). The course and prognosis of different phenotypes can influence survival. Burrows and colleagues studied 117 subjects with CAL ($FEV_1$ 47.1–51.3% predicted) and characterized subjects as "asthmatic bronchitis" if they were atopic and had a minimal smoking history ($<10$ pack years), "typical COPD" if there was no asthma or atopy history along with a $>10$ pack year smoking history, and "mixed" if these features were not met (42). A significant difference in survival was noted favoring patients with asthmatic bronchitis.

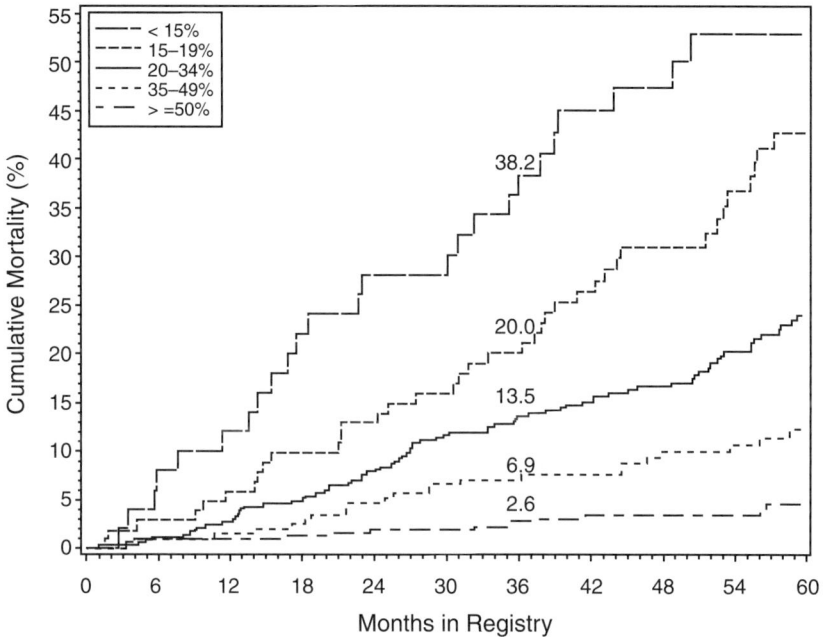

**Figure 1** Kaplan–Meier analysis of mortality, stratified by baseline value of FEV$_1$. percentage of predicted in participants in the National Heart, Lung, and Blood Institute Registry of Individuals with Severe AAT Deficiency. *Abbreviation*: FEV$_1$, forced expiratory volume in one second. *Source*: From Ref. 51.

Confirmation of an emphysematous phenotype is likely associated with a worse survival (11,22). The previously described data suggesting a worse prognosis with lower DLCO could support this. Unfortunately, DLCO is not a foolproof diagnostic study for identifying emphysema (3,41). Computed tomography (CT) diagnosis and quantification of emphysema may provide improved data (43). In fact, increased emphysema volume has proven prognostic in patients with alpha-1 antitrypsin deficiency ($\alpha$l-ATD) (44). As a complement, a self-reported diagnosis of asthma is associated with improved survival (45,46).

The prognosis of $\alpha$l-ATD associated COPD has been examined in great detail. Three-year mortality was 40% in those with an initial FEV$_1$ <30% predicted, compared to 7% when the FEV$_1$ was between 30% and 65% predicted in one early study (47). A separate database analysis demonstrated negligible two-year mortality when the FEV$_1$ was above 35% predicted but mortality increased exponentially below this threshold, reaching 50% when the FEV$_1$ was 15% predicted (48). Other analyses have confirmed the relationship between decreasing initial FEV$_1$ and mortality (Fig. 1) (49–51). It is evident that in emphysema associated with $\alpha$l-ATD prognosis worsens when the FEV$_1$ % predicted falls below 25% to 30% predicted.

Demographic/Clinical Characteristics

Although controversial (52), some investigators have suggested that females with COPD have an improved prognosis compared with males (53,54). In addition, comorbidity strongly influences survival in COPD patients (55). Incalzi et al. described survival in consecutive patients discharged after an acute exacerbation of COPD (56). The most common comorbidities included hypertension (28%), diabetes mellitus (14%), and ischemic heart disease (10%). With a median survival of 3.1 years, death was predicted by chronic renal insufficiency [hazard ratio (HR) 1.79, 95% confidence interval (CI) 1.05–3.02] and electrocardiogram (EKG) evidence of myocardial infarction (HR 1.42, 95% CI 1.02–1.96), in addition to age, $FEV_1$, and EKG signs of right ventricular hypertrophy (HR 1.76, 95% CI 1.30–2.38). These data support the concept that cardiovascular disease is an important comorbid condition in COPD patients (57,58).

The presence of pulmonary hypertension is unusual in COPD (59), although it is more common with worse obstructive disease (60) and appears to be an independent predictor of survival. Incalzi et al. confirmed that an S1, S2, S3 pattern (HR 1.81, 95% CI 1.22–2.69) and right atrial overload (HR 1.58, 95% CI 1.15–2.18) on EKG were associated with increased mortality in COPD patients hospitalized with an acute exacerbation (61). Another group confirmed in multivariate analysis that only age and initial pulmonary artery pressure (PAP) influenced survival in 84 patients with COPD treated with LTOT (62). The cumulative survival was 71% at three years and 48% at five years; those patients with a PAP > 25 mmHg had a 36.3% five-year survival, compared to 62.2% in those with a lower PAP. Although others have not confirmed these findings (17), most studies have confirmed the importance of an increased PAP on survival in COPD patients (63–65). As such, the presence of pulmonary hypertension, independent of $FEV_1$, influences survival in COPD.

The nutritional status has also been demonstrated to strongly influence COPD prognosis (66–69) and posttransplant survival (70). In landmark studies, Schols and colleagues confirmed an independent, negative effect of body mass index (BMI) despite adjustment for age, gender, spirometry, and arterial blood gases in multivariate analyses (67). Furthermore, in a prospective study, a weight gain <2 kg in eight weeks in depleted or non-depleted patients was positively associated with worse survival (67). Importantly, these data have been extended by recent data confirming that midthigh muscle cross-sectional area measured by CT is a more powerful predictor than BMI in a cohort of COPD patients (71). As such, markers of nutritional impairment appear to be potent, independent features negatively affecting prognosis in COPD.

**Multidimensional indices:** Recently, investigators have incorporated the multitude of clinical abnormalities in COPD patients into multidimensional indices that reflect different clinical and physiological

**Table 1** Variables and Point Values of the BODE Index

| | Points on the BODE index | | | |
|---|---|---|---|---|
| Variable | 0 | 1 | 2 | 3 |
| FEV$_1$ (% pred) | ≥65 | 50–64 | 36–49 | ≤35 |
| Six-minute walk distance (m) | ≥350 | 250–349 | 150–249 | ≤149 |
| MMRC dyspnea scale | 0–1 | 2 | 3 | 4 |
| Body mass index | >21 | ≤21 | – | – |

*Abbreviations*: FEV$_1$, forced expiratory volume in one second; MMRC, modified Medical Research Council.
*Source*: From Ref. 69.

dimensions (72,73). The most compelling of these was published by Celli et al., who developed a multidimensional index (BODE) reflecting the body mass index (B), the degree of airflow obstruction (O), dyspnea (D), and the exercise capacity measured by the 6-minute walk test (E) (Table 1) (69). This index was developed in 207 patients and validated in a separate cohort of 625 COPD patients with varying phenotype. Figure 2 illustrates the difference in survival of patients stratified by an FEV$_1$-based system in contrast to the BODE index. It is evident that the quartiles of BODE score are better able to define patient groups with differing survival characteristics. Subsequently, an international group of experts defined candidate variables that were potentially useful and independent in predicting survival in COPD (74). Principal components analysis was performed using 30 variables; six groups remained including pulmonary function (including FEV$_1$), symptoms (including cough and breathlessness), health status, bronchoreversibility, BMI, and dyspnea [modified Medical Research Council (MMRC) scale]. The role of multidimensional indices in identifying patients who may optimally benefit from lung transplantation requires additional study.

## MEDICAL MANAGEMENT

### Goals of Therapy

COPD is generally a progressive disease with increasing severity resulting in increasing symptoms, greater impairment in health-related quality of life (HRQol), more frequent exacerbations, and greater health-care costs (75). As such, management should be comprehensive in nature. The Global Initiative for Chronic Obstructive Lung Disease (GOLD) workshop (2) has recommended an excellent management plan consisting of

- assessing and monitoring disease,
- reducing risk factors,

(A)

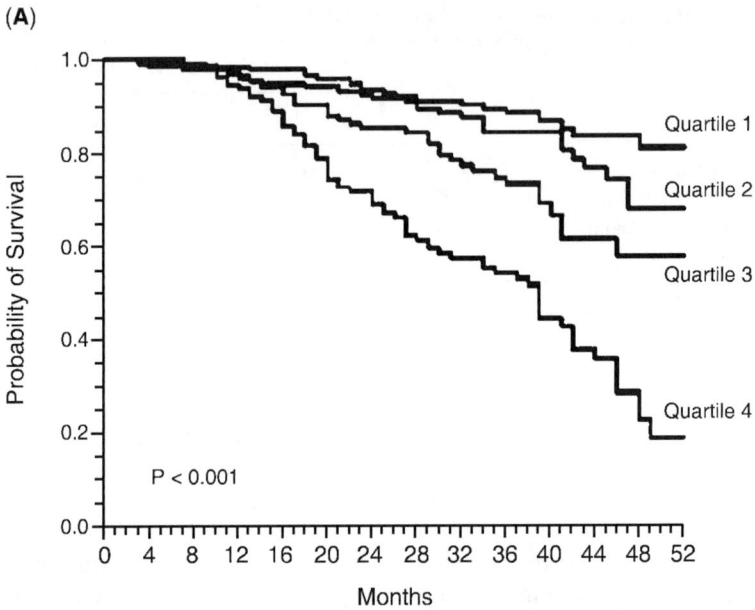

No. at Risk    625      611      574      521      454   322   273   159  80

(B)

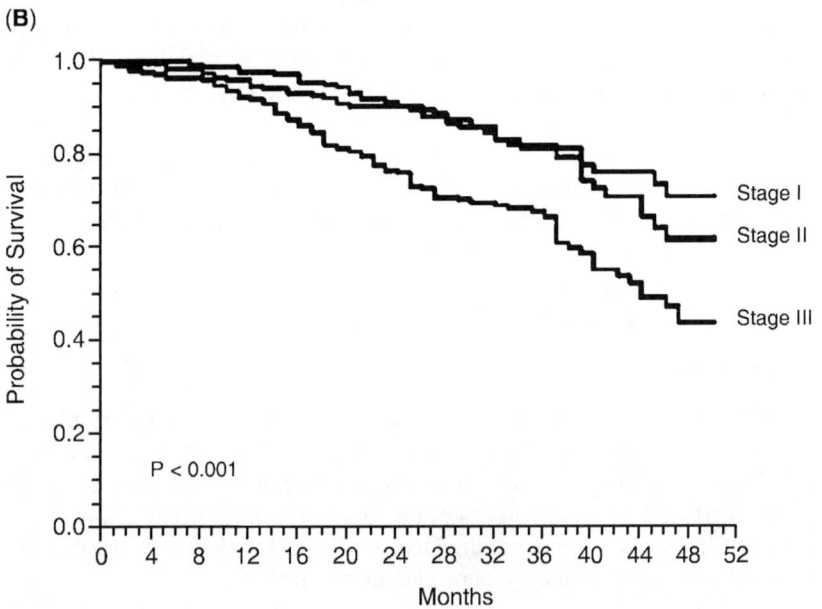

No. at Risk    625      611      574      521      454   322   273   159  80

**Figure 2**   (*Caption on facing page*)

- managing stable disease, and
- managing exacerbations.

Furthermore, effective management was stated to include

- preventing disease progression,
- alleviating symptoms,
- improving exercise tolerance,
- improving health status,
- preventing and treating complications,
- preventing and treating exacerbations, and
- reducing mortality.

The various therapeutic options for the treatment of COPD will be briefly discussed in the context of these recommendations, particularly as they relate to patients with severe CAL, those most likely to be referred for lung transplantation.

### Assessing and Monitoring Disease

**Diagnosis:** The broad definition, as suggested by international guidelines, includes a disease of airflow obstruction that is not fully reversible, an appropriate risk factor, and chronic symptoms (cough, sputum production, dyspnea, chest tightness) (1,2). Given the limitations of the clinical examination (76), confirmation of airflow obstruction is required to assure an accurate diagnosis. Spirometry, an easy to perform and widely available standardized physiologic test has been accepted as the key to confirmation of a COPD diagnosis (77). In addition, spirometric data are able to physiologically stratify the severity of airflow obstruction. In this way, the $FEV_1$ as % predicted has been utilized to define severe, moderate, and mild disease (1,2,78).

The role of high-resolution computed tomography (HRCT) for the diagnosis of mild to moderate disease is evolving (43,79). CT provides excellent visual anatomic detail for detecting, characterizing, and quantitatively determining the severity of emphysema. Furthermore, emphysema severity on CT correlates well with the pathologic severity of emphysema, using either

---

**Figure 2** (*Facing page*) Kaplan–Meier survival curves for the four quartiles of the body mass index, degree of airflow obstruction and dyspnea, and exercise capacity index (BODE score, **A**) and three spirometric stages of disease severity as defined by the American Thoracic Society (**B**). In (**A**), quartile 1 is a score of 0–2, quartile 2 is a score of 3–4, quartile 3 a score of 5–6, and quartile 4 a score of 7–10. Survival differed significantly among the four groups ($P < 0.001$ by the log-rank test). In (**B**), stage I is defined by $FEV_1$ that is $> 50\%$ of the predicted value, stage II by an $FEV_1$ that is 36–50% of the predicted value, and stage III by an $FEV_1$ that is no more than 35% of the predicted value. Survival differed significantly among the three groups ($P < 0.001$ by the log-rank test). *Abbreviation*: $FEV_1$, forced expiratory volume in one second. *Source*: From Ref. 69.

visual scoring systems or quantitative analysis based on Hounsfield unit (HU) threshold measurements (43,79). Similarly, quantitative analysis of emphysema correlates with decreasing DLCO (80) and is useful in identifying emphysema, usually mild, in patients with an isolated decrement in DLCO (81,82). The role of such imaging on subsequent medical therapy in individual patients with milder disease requires further investigation. In the setting of evaluating COPD patients for surgical therapy of COPD, CT has proven quite useful. This includes proven utility in the evaluation of patients for lung volume reduction surgery (LVRS) (83) and lung transplantation (84).

**Monitoring:** As COPD is generally a progressive disorder, serial monitoring is important in optimizing therapeutic interventions (85). Symptomatic monitoring includes quantifying worsening of dyspnea, which strongly influences HRQol in these patients (86–88). Similarly, identifying and treating exacerbations of disease are important interventions, particularly in more advanced disease, as these acute deteriorations in clinical status have a significant effect on pulmonary function and health status (89). The impact of acute episodes on HRQol may take several weeks to recover (90–92). The role of serial physiologic monitoring remains poorly defined although serial spirometric monitoring may provide a diagnostic advantage over a single test (77,93). Radiological follow-up may be important as patients with COPD are at risk of developing other smoking-related illnesses such as bronchogenic carcinoma. As such, the literature advocating routine screening in high-risk patients is evolving rapidly (94). Identifying these is important as there may be important repercussions to the transplant decision-making process (95,96).

Reduce Risk Factors

Cigarette smoking is the most common risk factor for the development of COPD in developed countries (1,2). As such, smoking cessation is a vital component in a comprehensive approach to the COPD patient. This is particularly relevant to lung transplant decision making as active smoking has been considered an absolute contraindication for lung transplantation (95). A detailed description of smoking cessation techniques is beyond the scope of this work, but comprehensive reviews of the topic have been presented (97,98). A comprehensive approach to smoking cessation intervention is ideal and includes counseling. Three counseling modalities have been shown to be effective: practical counseling, social support as part of treatment, and social support arranged outside of treatment (2). Pharmacotherapy has advanced significantly over the past decade, with an aggressive approach to nicotine replacement treatment proven effective; many replacement forms are available (97–99). In addition, the antidepressants buproprion and nortryptilline have been documented to increase long-term quit rates (97,98,100,101).

Not only is smoking cessation imperative to allow listing for lung transplantation, but the importance of smoking cessation has been confirmed by sentinel studies conducted by the Lung Health Study Research Group. This randomized trial of current smokers with borderline to moderate impairment of pulmonary function confirmed that patients who were able to discontinue smoking preserved their lung function over short-term (102) and long-term follow-ups (103). Importantly, this effect was only seen with complete cessation or with a >85% reduction in smoking rate (104). These investigators have confirmed that smoking cessation in this study was associated with improved long-term mortality (HR 1.18, 95% CI 1.02–1.37) compared to usual care (105) and to improved respiratory symptoms (106).

### Medical Management of the Stable Patient with COPD

Medical management of the COPD patient must be multifactorial given the myriad manifestations of the disease (107). This is particularly important for COPD patients with severe disease, those most likely to be evaluated for lung transplantation. Early therapeutic interventions were primarily aimed at improving physiologic derangement. Unfortunately, as COPD is generally defined by lack of complete reversibility, these patients experience a limited spirometric response to bronchodilators. Furthermore, relief in symptoms correlates only weakly with changes in spirometric indices (77,108), although it does correlate more closely with the change in operational lung volumes (109–112). As such, alternative physiologic techniques are now employed when assessing the benefits of specific therapeutic interventions, including bronchodilators (111,113,114). In addition, international expert guidelines have recommended a more comprehensive approach to the treatment of COPD patients (1,2,115). As such, therapeutic goals have been defined, which include preventing disease progression, alleviating symptoms, improving exercise tolerance, improving health status, preventing and treating complications, preventing and treating exacerbations, and reducing mortality (2). Numerous therapeutic approaches have been used clinically in COPD patients. These have generally been incorporated into stepwise approaches as highlighted in Figures 3A and B, which illustrate symptom-based and disease management approaches (1). A separate set of tabular recommendations based on the GOLD guidelines are enumerated in Table 2. In discussing available therapeutic alternatives, we attempt, whenever possible, to present a comprehensive assessment of treatment outcomes, particularly as they apply to COPD patients with advanced disease.

### Bronchodilator Therapy

Bronchodilators have constituted the mainstay of therapy in COPD for many years and remain cornerstones of treatment in all published recommendations (116,117). They improve pulmonary function, exercise capacity,

**(A)**

**(B)**

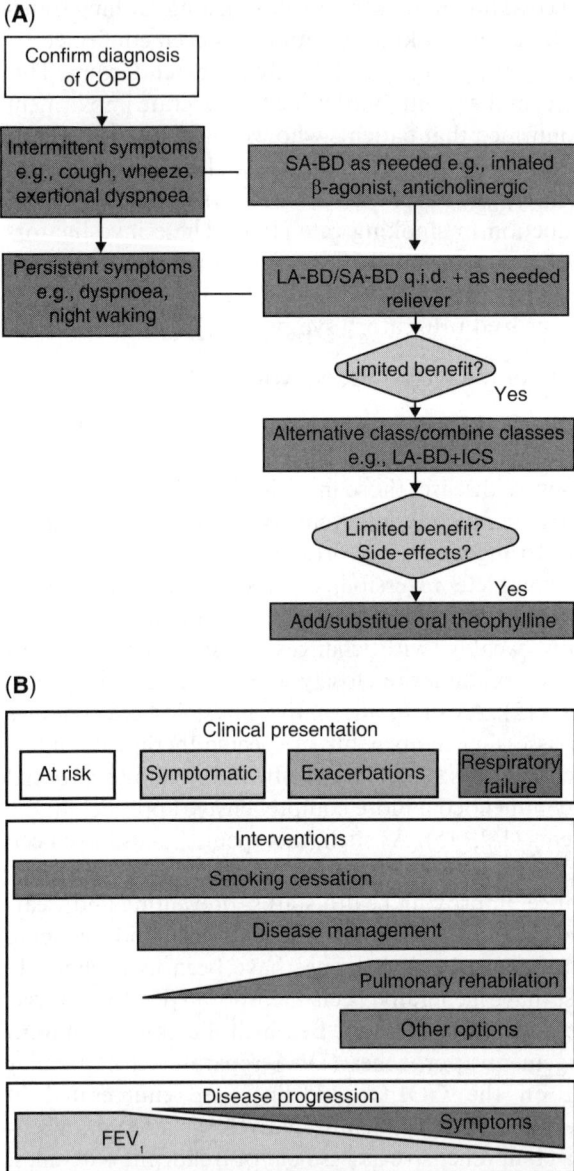

**Figure 3** (**A**) Algorithm for pharmacological management of COPD. Assess effectiveness by treatment response criteria. (**B**) Continuum of care for COPD patient emphasizing a multidisciplinary, comprehensive approach to disease management. *Abbreviations*: COPD, chronic obstructive pulmonary disease; SA-BD, short-acting bronchodilator; LA-BD, long-acting bronchodilator; ICS, inhaled corticosteroid. *Source*: From Ref. 1.

**Table 2** Therapy at Each Stage of Chronic Obstructive Pulmonary Disease as Adapted from the Global Initiative for Chronic Obstructive Lung Disease Guidelines

| Stage | Characteristics | Recommended therapy |
|---|---|---|
| All | – | Avoidance of risk factors<br>Influenza vaccination |
| 0: at risk | Chronic symptoms (cough, sputum)<br>Exposure to risk factors | |
| I: mild COPD | $FEV_1/FVC < 70\%$<br><br>$FEV_1 \geq 80\%$ predicted | Short-acting bronchodilator as needed |
| II: moderate COPD | IIA<br>$FEV_1/FVC$ $< 70\%$ predicted<br>$50\% \leq FEV_1$ $< 80\%$ predicted<br>With or without symptoms | Regular treatment with one or more bronchodilators<br>Pulmonary rehabilitation<br>Inhaled corticosteroids if significant symptoms and lung function response are evident |
| | IIB<br>$FEV_1/FVC < 70\%$<br>$30\% \leq FEV_1$ $< 50\%$ predicted<br>With or without symptoms | Regular treatment with one or more bronchodilators<br>Pulmonary rehabilitation<br>Inhaled corticosteroids if significant symptoms and lung function response are evident or if repeated exacerbations are present |
| II: severe COPD | $FEV_1/FVC < 70\%$<br>$FEV_1 < 30\%$ predicted or<br>Presence of respiratory failure or right heart failure | Regular treatment with one or more bronchodilators<br>Pulmonary rehabilitation<br>Inhaled corticosteroids if significant symptoms and lung function response are evident or if repeated exacerbations are present<br>Treatment of complications<br>Long-term oxygen therapy if respiratory failure is evident<br>Consider surgical therapies |

*Abbreviations*: COPD, chronic obstructive pulmonary disease; $FEV_1$, forced expiratory volume in one second; FVC, forced vital capacity.
*Source*: From Ref. 2.

relieve symptoms, decrease the frequency and severity of exacerbations, improve quality of life, and, potentially, decrease disease progression and mortality (116). Several classes are available for use in the COPD patient.

Anticholinergics

The anticholinergic agents are derived from belladonna and other alkaloid plants that have been used to treat pulmonary disorders for centuries. Over the past several decades, increased knowledge has been accumulated defining the cholinergic pathways in the lung (118). There are multiple muscarinic receptors in the lung, including periganglionic excitatory ($M_1$) and smooth muscle ($M_3$) receptors that stimulate smooth muscle contraction and mucous secretion (118). In contrast, inhibitory postganglionic muscarinic receptors ($M_2$) can downregulate acetylcholine release and thereby limit the magnitude of vagally mediated bronchoconstriction (118); these $M_2$ receptors have recently been shown to be functional in patients with stable COPD (119). Available anticholinergic agents have been quarternary derivatives of anticholinergic compounds that do not cross biologic barriers easily but, unfortunately, block all muscarinic receptors (108). Increased selectivity in antimuscarinic agents has created a class of agents with an excellent therapeutic profile (118). For example, tiotropium exhibits the unique pharmacological property of binding to all muscarinic receptors with varying duration of binding. The slow dissociation from $M_3$ receptors ($t_{1/2}$ of 35 hours compared to 16 minutes for ipratropium) and a faster dissociation from $M_2$ receptors ($t_{1/2}$ of 3.6 hours) creates a functional receptor subtype selectivity of $M_3$ and $M_1$ over $M_2$ receptors (120). These properties and accumulating clinical data have generated increased enthusiasm for their use in COPD patients.

**Short-acting anticholinergics:** Anticholinergics have been demonstrated to yield measurable improvement in airflow, which is at least equal and in many settings better than can be achieved with β-agonists (108,121). Of 38 published studies comparing anticholinergic agents and short acting β-agonists, all but two found the anticholinergic agents to be equal and generally superior to short acting β-agonists (122). In addition, anticholinergic drugs can induce bronchodilation even when β-agonists have failed to improve airflow (123,124). An additional beneficial effect of anticholinergic therapy includes a longer duration of action in comparison to short-acting β-agonists (125). In a systematic review, the long-term effect of anticholinergic therapy was examined in pooled data from seven randomized controlled trials comparing ipratropium bromide and β-agonists (126). After three months of therapy, the mean $FEV_1$ improvement was significantly higher in the ipratropium arm of the studies (mean 28-mL increase) than the β-agonist studies (mean 1-mL decrease, $P < 0.05$). All seven trials demonstrated a decline in the acute effect of β-agonist treatment with prolonged treatment; five of seven studies demonstrated improvement in the acute effect of ipratropium. Unfortunately, long-term ipratropium therapy has not been shown to influence the natural, spirometric progression of COPD (102).

The exercise response after anticholinergic therapy has been reviewed in a systematic analysis (127). The majority of the 17 studies examining steady-state exercise confirmed a response (3/4 single-dose studies and 3/3 maintenance-dose studies). Nine of 12 studies confirmed a positive effect on maximal exercise capacity. Two investigative groups have suggested an increasing effect of higher doses on exercise tolerance (128,129). The mechanism underlying the benefit in maximal exercise tolerance and decrease in exertional dyspnea after inhalation of ipratropium has been suggested to reflect decreasing dynamic hyperinflation (130).

In addition to improving pulmonary function and exercise capacity, inhaled short-acting anticholinergic agents have been demonstrated to improve symptoms. In the pooled studies described by Rennard et al., ipratropium led to significant improvements in dyspnea in ex-smoking patients (126). Similar improvements have been noted in large studies of ipratropium and long-acting β-agonists. In patients with severe COPD ($FEV_1$ 37% predicted), patients treated with either ipratropium or salmeterol experienced similar improvements in transitional dyspnea index scores during 12 weeks of follow-up (131). In a methodologically similar study, improvements in dyspnea after ipratropium administration were modest, only achieving statistical significance from placebo in the first 6 weeks of a 12-week study (132). In contrast, others have not identified improvements in total symptom scores between inhaled ipratropium and placebo (133), potentially reflecting a difference in methodology.

Improving HRQol has been recently described after ipratropium administration. Mahler et al. noted an improvement in the chronic respiratory disease questionnaire (CRDQ) with ipratropium administration for 12 weeks compared with placebo (131). Interestingly, a similar study did not confirm these findings (132), nor did a recent study utilizing the St. George's Respiratory Questionnaire (SGRO) (133). Given the importance of exacerbations on HRQol, the impact of anticholinergic therapy on this outcome has been examined. Three groups failed to identify a beneficial effect of ipratropium use, although the definitions of exacerbations varied widely (131–133). A pharmacoeconomic analysis of two placebo-controlled, three-month-long, randomized studies of ipratropium versus ipratropium plus albuterol or albuterol alone confirmed a significant decrease in exacerbation frequency in the ipratropium arms (134). Corroborating these findings, the same investigative group has reported that the use of ipratropium alone or in combination with a β-agonist resulted in a lower total cost of care for patients with stages I–III COPD (75).

**Long-acting anticholinergics:** The advantageous properties of the more selective anticholinergics such as tiotropium have been widely touted

(135). Numerous studies have examined the effect of tiotropium in COPD patients as reviewed in two systematic reviews (136,137). The prolonged physiologic effect of tiotropium has been confirmed in a study of patients with severe COPD (mean $FEV_1$ 41% predicted) (138). These data confirm that a dose of 18 µg/day, defined as optimal from efficacy and safety analyses (139), provides sustained spirometric improvement. Systematic reviews of the published data suggest that tiotropium not only improves $FEV_1$ in contrast to placebo but also in comparison to ipratropium (137) and, potentially, to salmeterol (140). In contrast to ipratropium, data from post hoc analysis of two one-year tiotropium studies suggest that the longer-acting agent may be able to minimize decrement in $FEV_1$ during one year of follow-up (141). Prospective confirmation of this intriguing finding is being tested in a large, multicenter trial. Given the importance of lung volumes in COPD patients, one group has confirmed beneficial effects of tiotropium on resting lung volumes (142).

Data regarding effects of tiotropium on exercise capacity are more limited. A large, multicenter, placebo-controlled trial has confirmed that tiotropium improves submaximal exercise capacity in patients with moderately severe COPD (mean $FEV_1$ 41% predicted) (114). This effect occurred while leading to decreased dyspnea at similar workloads; improvement in operational lung volumes was closely related to the improved functional status. A separate, novel investigational approach examined the additive value of tiotropium or placebo to pulmonary rehabilitation in a cohort of patients with severe COPD (mean $FFV_1$ 34% predicted) (143). Endurance time improved in both groups after pulmonary rehabilitation, although tiotropium resulted in clear additional functional benefits.

Several investigators have examined the effect of tiotropium on dyspnea. Systematic reviews have confirmed improvement compared to placebo and ipratropium (136,137); the effect was similar to salmeterol (136,137). Similarly, data supporting a beneficial effect of tiotropium on HRQol have been quite consistent. The improvement has been confirmed when tiotropium is contrasted with placebo or ipratropium, although to a similar extent as salmeterol (136,137). There are similarly robust data confirming a decrease in exacerbation rate with tiotropium (136,137). These include studies confirming decrease in hospitalization rates (137).

On the bases of these data, investigators have suggested a pharmacological algorithm to therapy in COPD patients emphasizing the early use of bronchodilators, including an anticholinergic agent (Fig. 4) (117).

### β-Adrenergic Agonists

Although there is little sympathetic innervation of airway smooth muscle, sympathomimetics have been documented to be efficacious in COPD (108). Detailed discussions of the effects of short- and long-acting β-agonists have

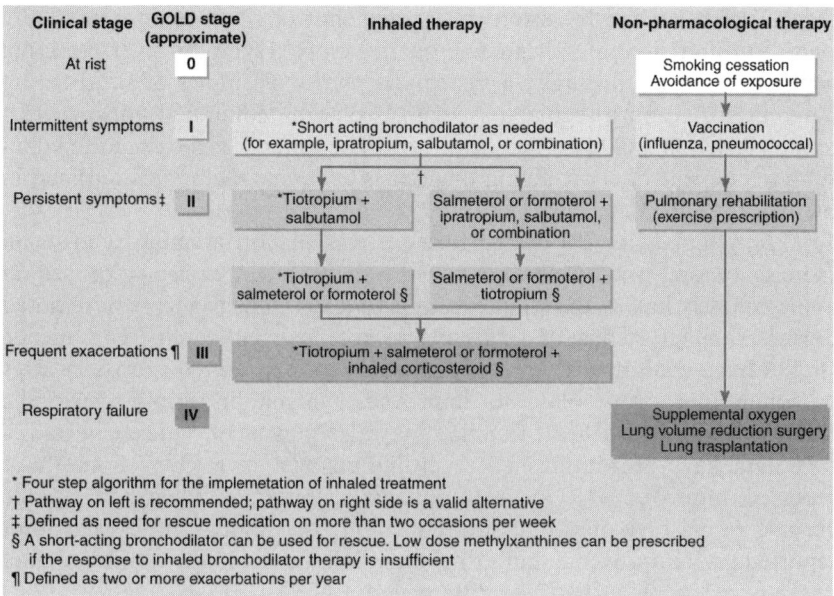

| Clinical stage | GOLD stage (approximate) | Inhaled therapy | | Non-pharmacological therapy |
|---|---|---|---|---|
| At rist | 0 | | | Smoking cessation Avoidance of exposure |
| Intermittent symptoms | I | \*Short acting bronchodilator as needed (for example, ipratropium, salbutamol, or combination) | | Vaccination (influenza, pneumococcal) |
| Persistent symptoms‡ | II | \*Tiotropium + salbutamol | Salmeterol or formoterol + ipratropium, salbutamol, or combination | Pulmonary rehabilitation (exercise prescription) |
| | | \*Tiotropium + salmeterol or formoterol § | Salmeterol or formoterol + tiotropium § | |
| Frequent exacerbations ¶ | III | \*Tiotropium + salmeterol or formoterol + inhaled corticosteroid § | | |
| Respiratory failure | IV | | | Supplemental oxygen Lung volume reduction surgery Lung trasplantation |

\* Four step algorithm for the implemetation of inhaled treatment
† Pathway on left is recommended; pathway on right side is a valid alternative
‡ Defined as need for rescue medication on more than two occasions per week
§ A short-acting bronchodilator can be used for rescue. Low dose methylxanthines can be prescribed
   if the response to inhaled bronchodilator therapy is insufficient
¶ Defined as two or more exacerbations per year

**Figure 4** Clinical algorithm for the treatment of COPD. Clinical stages are defined symptomatically. GOLD stage refers to the classification of COPD based on spirometry after bronchodilator. *Abbreviation*: COPD, chronic obstructive pulmonary disease. *Source*: From Ref. 117.

been published (121,127,144–146). In addition, alternative mechanisms for these long-acting agents have been detailed (147).

**Short acting β-agonists:** Short-acting β-agonists have been shown to result in bronchodilation, although the magnitude has been highly variable (121). For example, a review of the effects of bronchodilators on exercise capacity described the results reported in 14 such studies demonstrating a change in $FEV_1$ ranging from 93 to 240 ml (127). Some of this variability reflects individual patient variability. For example, one large study demonstrated that more than two-thirds of COPD patients who had a ≤10% increase in $FEV_1$ after an inhaled bronchodilator at baseline demonstrated an increase ≥15% at some time daring the three-year trial (14). An additional source of variability lies in the dose of β-agonist administered. As such, higher doses may result in further increase in $FEV_1$ (121), although this may be seen in a minority of patients (148). The available β-agonists differ in the time of onset, degree of $β_2$-receptor selectivity, and the duration of onset. One investigative group has confirmed the value of short-acting β-agonists as "as needed" medications in contrast to regular use in a randomized, double-blind, placebo-controlled trial of 53 COPD patients (149). Patients in the regular use arm used twice as much albuterol as those in the "as needed" period. Despite this greater short-acting β-agonist use, there were no differences in spirometry, quality of life, symptoms, or 6-minute walk distance. Interestingly, a systematic review of studies of short-acting β-agonists used on a regular basis versus placebo confirmed improvement in lung function and breathlessness (150). The totality of the published data support the role of short-acting β-agonists as rescue therapy as outlined in the recent GOLD guidelines (Table 2) (2).

A systematic review described the effects of short-acting β-agonists on exercise capacity in 14 studies (127). Steady-state exercise improved in approximately half of the studies, although lesser improvements were noted during maximal exercise testing. As was noted for anticholinergics agents, studies have confirmed that improvements noted in exercise capacity after β-agonist inhalation relate to improved dynamic hyperinflation (151). Improvement in right heart function may also play a role (152). Contradictory data have been published regarding changes in HRQol. Some have reported improved HRQol with inhaled salbutamol [measured by the chronic respiratory questionnaire (CRQ)] (153), although others have not reported such improvement after nebulized albuterol (154). Additional data are required to reconcile these differences.

**Long-acting β-agonists:** β-agonists with a prolonged duration of action have become clinically available. The clinical effects have been the subject of detailed reviews (121,144–146). These agents result in significant bronchodilation in COPD patients (144). Although the onset of action of salmeterol appears to be somewhat shorter than with other inhaled β-agonists or inhaled anticholinergic agents, its duration of action has been longer than the comparators, with the exception of inhaled formoterol, which is similar (145). These data must be interpreted with caution as significant interpatient variability has been reported. For example, in a single-blind crossover study of salbutamol (200 µg), salmeterol (50 µg), formoterol (24 µg), or placebo in 16 COPD patients (mean $FEV_1$ 39.3% predicted), a similar time of onset to improvement of $FEV_1$ by 15% was noted among the β-agonists (155). Interestingly, the onset of action was more rapid with inhaled formoterol in nine patients while it was more rapid in five patients after inhaled salmeterol. In fact, formoterol has been shown to result in a similar onset of bronchodilation to salbutamol (156,157). The potency of salmeterol and formoterol seems to be similar (144), although one recent study has suggested that salmeterol demonstrates greater potency than formoterol in patients with severe COPD (mean $FEV_1$ 21.5% predicted) (158) while another suggested similar results in a less severely ill population (mean $FEV_1$ 35.4% predicted) (159). As such, some have suggested that formoterol is more active in mild to moderate COPD while salmeterol is more active in patients with severe disease (144). Importantly, treatment with salmeterol does not preclude a further bronchodilator response to salbutamol (160,161).

Several large studies have examined the role of long-acting β-agonists during long-term treatment. The pivotal studies of salmeterol compared with ipratropium confirmed a similar peak improvement in $FEV_1$ between both bronchodilators, although the duration of effect was longer with salmeterol (131,132). Similar findings were noted by investigators who compared two doses of formoterol with ipratropium and placebo (133). Both doses of formoterol exhibited a greater area under the curve for $FEV_1$ response than placebo and ipratropium. The effects of salmeterol on $FEV_1$ have been maintained over 24 weeks of therapy (162), although others have argued that tolerance may be seen with this duration of therapy (163). Overall, the spirometric response to long-acting β-agonists is equivalent to ipratropium in patients with chronic obstruction that is not acutely reversible to short acting β-agonists in the pulmonary function laboratory (164). Similarly, salmeterol and formoterol increase inspiratory capacity in patients with poor acute reversibility (165).

An improvement in symptoms is a consistent finding in studies of long-acting β-agonists. Both Mahler et al. (131) and Rennard et al. (132) confirmed an improvement in dyspnea with both salmeterol and ipratropium. Similarly, Dahl and colleagues noted an improvement in global symptom scores with both formoterol doses compared to placebo (133). Despite improvement in symptoms, improvement in maximal exercise capacity is less evident (127). One group has suggested an improved distance walked with salmeterol and ipratropium compared to placebo while the time to recovery of $SaO_2$ after exercise was improved with both bronchodilators (166). A separate group has noted a greater inspiratory capacity (IC) during submaximal exercise with salmeterol versus ipratropium six hours after dosing, although the IC was similar one hour after dosing; dyspnea ratings were similar with both bronchodilators (167). An additional investigative group has confirmed an increase in maximal exercise capacity and endurance time with salmeterol therapy. The increase in peak oxygen uptake correlated with increased tidal volume (113).

Numerous investigators have examined the effect of long-acting β-agonists on HRQol in COPD patients. A systematic review has confirmed an improvement in St. George's respiratory questionnaire (SGRQ) although below the minimal clinically important difference (136). Several groups have examined the effect of long-acting β-agonists on exacerbations. Although the effect has been inconsistent (168), a systematic review of the literature has suggested a significant decrement in exacerbation rate relative risk (RR) 0.79, 95% CI 0.69–0.90 (136). In general, these agents appear to be quite safe (116). A large analysis involving three cohort studies (12,294 patients treated with nedocromil, 15,407 with salmeterol, and 8098 with bambuterol) suggested an increased risk of adverse cardiac side effects with an oral β-agonist (bambuterol) but not inhaled salmeterol (169). A smaller study of 12 COPD patients with preexisting cardiac arrhythmias and hypoxemia ($PaO_2 < 60\,mmHg$)

examined the effect of formoterol 12 μg bid, formoterol 24 μg bid, salmeterol 50 μg bid, and placebo (170). A higher heart rate and more frequent supraventricular or ventricular premature beats were noted with higher-dose formoterol than lower-dose formoterol or salmeterol. As such, long-acting β-agonists seem to have favorable side-effect profiles.

**Combination of inhaled bronchodilators:**   Given the different mode of action of anticholinergic and β-agonist agents, the combination of these two classes has been explored by several investigative groups. It is apparent that the combination of ipratropium and short-acting β-agonists results in an increased physiologic response than either agent administered separately (171–183). Other investigators have not confirmed these findings (184–186), with some suggesting that the combination does not provide benefit over maximal doses of either agent alone (184), particularly higher doses of β-agonists (187). Interestingly, some investigators have suggested that beneficial effects of combination therapy are realized when the anticholinergics agent is administered before the β-agonist (188–190).

Some have examined the combination of anticholinergic agents and long-acting β-agonists, with contradictory results. Although one group has suggested that the combination of salmeterol and ipratropium was not more effective than salmeterol alone (191), another group has suggested that the combination of formoterol plus ipratropium was more effective than ipratropium alone but did not provide additional bronchodilation to formoterol alone (192). Some have suggested that the effect of combination therapy may depend on the dose of bronchodilator administered (193) and the timing of bronchodilator administration (194). Long-term studies of these combinations are scarce. Van Noord et al. noted that the combination of ipratropium and salmeterol produced a greater peak in $FEV_1$ (12%) than salmeterol alone (195). Salmeterol has been combined with tiotropium in a randomized, double-blind, crossover six-week study (196). Importantly, the combination of tiotropium and formoterol administered once daily led to the greatest improvement (Fig. 5).

Limited data have been published examining the effect of combined bronchodilator therapy on exercise capacity (127). Improvement in submaximal or maximal exercise has been inconsistent. Additional improvement in symptoms with combination therapy has been marginal in some (154) but significant in other (173,197) studies. During short-term treatment the combination of formoterol/ipratropium provided better symptomatic relief than salbutamol/ipratropium (197). Interestingly, a differential improvement in symptoms was not consistently seen during 12 weeks of therapy with salmeterol alone versus salmeterol plus ipratropium (195). These investigators noted a decrease in exacerbation rate between the placebo (36%), salmeterol (23%), and salmeterol plus ipratropium (13%) treated groups. The differences proved significant only in the patients treated with combination bronchodilation. In a separate publication these investigators noted a

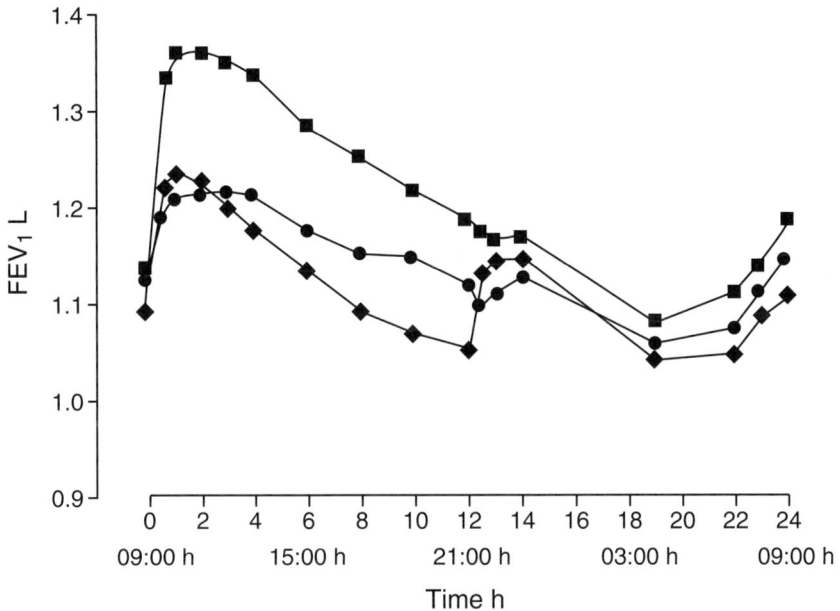

**Figure 5** Mean $FEV_1$ (adjusted for period, center, and patient within the center) before and 24 hours after the inhalation of tiotropium once a day (●), formoterol twice a day (◆), and tiotropium plus formoterol once a day (■) at the end of a six-week treatment period. *Abbreviation*: $FEV_1$, forced expiratory volume in one second. *Source*: From Ref. 196.

clinically significant difference in mean symptom scores of the SGRQ with salmeterol and combination therapy compared with placebo (198). Similarly, the proportion of patients experiencing a clinically meaningful improvement in the CRQ was greater with combination than with salmeterol monotherapy or placebo (198). These data support the use of combinations of bronchodilators in symptomatic patients with COPD.

Methylxanthines

Methylxanthines have been used to treat respiratory disorders for many decades (108), although the use of theophylline has decreased over the past decade (199). This change in practice pattern reflects the controversy regarding theophylline benefits (121,200), the availability of alternative bronchodilator regimens (see above) (144), and theophylline's narrow therapeutic spectrum (121). Investigative groups have confirmed that theophylline is a weak bronchodilator in patients with COPD, with improvement in $FEV_1$ ranging from 10% to 21% (200). A limited number of studies have compared various β-agonists and theophylline, administered alone or in combination. In general, the mean increase in $FEV_1$ has been similar; when administered in combination, statistically significant additive effects have been observed (200,201). Data comparing theophylline and long-acting β-agonists are scarce. In general, the β-agonists seem to be more active in the short term, although the difference becomes less marked with prolonged therapy (144). The bronchodilatory effect of theophylline is most often achieved with prolonged administration (200). Salmeterol and theophylline have been demonstrated to result in similar spirometric improvements by several groups (202,203); the combination has been demonstrated to result in additional bronchodilation (203). Importantly, in the latter study 150/1185 screened patients were unable to tolerate theophylline during a wash-in period and 30 additional patients were unable to achieve therapeutic theophylline levels (203). As such, theophylline may provide additional bronchodilation but is unlikely to be an effective initial bronchodilator.

Theophylline has been demonstrated to have additional beneficial effects including improving mucociliary clearance, respiratory muscle function, cardiovascular function, and respiratory drive (121,200). These additional effects may aid in explaining benefits in addition to spirometric changes that have been described with theophylline. For example, despite modest bronchodilation theophylline has been suggested to improve symptoms (203,204), exercise tolerance (127), and HRQol (203). In combination with salmeterol, fewer exacerbations were noted than in patients treated with theophylline alone or salmeterol alone (203). It should be noted that theophylline therapy may not improve the cost-effectiveness of care. In a pharmacoeconomic analysis, Hilleman and colleagues noted that theophylline therapy alone was associated with greater treatment costs ($1946) in patients with milder COPD than ipratropiurn alone ($1362) or β-agonists alone ($1542) (75). As such, theophylline therapy is not likely the ideal bronchodilator, particularly in patients with milder disease.

The role of methylxanthines in COPD will likely be expanded by the new generation of phosphodiesterase receptor inhibitors. These enzymes have direct bronchodilating effects as well as an anti-inflammatory effect (205). Two agents have been extensively studied in COPD patients. Cilomilast has been confirmed to result in a modest improvement in $FEV_1$ compared with placebo (206). Importantly, in patients with moderate COPD ($FEV_1$ 58% predicted) 12 weeks of cilomilast led to decreased inflammation on bronchial biopsies (207). A different agent, roflumilast, has been shown to result in modest bronchodilation, improvement in HRQol, and to decrease exacerbation rate compared with placebo (208). This same agent has been shown to ameliorate the development of emphysema in a murine model of COPD (209). Additional data are required to better define the role of such novel agents in the management of patients with severe COPD.

## Corticosteroids

The role of corticosteroid therapy remains controversial in COPD (210,211) although data are becoming more congruent (212,213). The role of inflammation has been accepted and described by numerous authors (214,215); these changes have been particularly evident in patients with severe COPD (6,216). It appears that neutrophilic and lymphocytic inflammation have been described in the central airways of COPD patients while a more intense lymphocytic inflammatory process (particularly CD8+ lymphocytes) is present in the peripheral airways and parenchyma (217). Given the presence of inflammation in COPD patients and the known benefit of steroids in asthmatics (218), inhaled corticosteroids have been frequently used in clinical practice to treat patients with COPD.

Physiologic end-points after short-term steroid therapy have been examined by numerous groups. Conflicting reports have been described with oral steroid therapy. In a meta-analysis of controlled trials performed through 1989, which defined response as an increase in $FEV_1$ of 20%, only 10% of the subjects exhibited response more frequently after taking oral steroids than with placebo (219). It has been difficult to define the patient population that is most likely to experience these benefits (220–223). Long-term data with oral steroids are scarce. Two retrospective studies noted a favorable effect of prednisolone on $FEV_1$ over a 20-year period (224). In a randomized study of elderly patients with "steroid-dependent" COPD, discontinuation of oral steroids did not result in a significant change in spirometric or other functional indices (225). Given the potential risks of oral steroid therapy (226), further data are required to adequately assess the risk and benefits of such therapy.

In an effort to improve the risk profile, the role of inhaled steroids have been investigated in COPD patients (212,213). Several large randomized studies of inhaled steroids with long duration of follow-up have been published in the last several years. Although the studies were methodologically quite different, the studies demonstrated little (227) to no (228) change in the rate of decline in $FEV_1$ over the course of follow-up. Interestingly, several groups have confirmed a decrement in pulmonary function after discontinuation of inhaled steroid therapy (229,230). Nevertheless, it is unlikely that inhaled corticosteroids alter deterioration in pulmonary function to any great extent.

Although the effect of inhaled steroids on pulmonary function is modest, a survival benefit has been suggested in prospective (210), retrospective, population-based (231–233), and single center (234) studies. Improved respiratory symptoms have been reported (235,236). Similarly, chronic inhaled steroid use has been suggested to minimize decrease in HRQol compared to placebo (237); this effect has been felt to relate, in part, to amelioration of the exacerbation rate (described later) (238). The modulation of exacerbation frequency is an important benefit of steroid therapy (239). This effect seems to be most prominent in patients with more severe disease (136). Additional insight has been provided by an observational study utilizing the Ontario version of the Canadian Institute for Health Information hospital discharge database (240). These investigators examined outcome in all 22,260 patients aged more than 65 years who were discharged from the hospital with a principal diagnosis of COPD; admission data were linked to subsequent inhaled steroid prescriptions and subsequent death or rehospitalization for COPD during year after the index hospitalization. After adjustment for age, gender, other medications, and comorbidity, the group receiving inhaled steroids after hospital discharge experienced an improved COPD hospitalization-free survival. The totality of these data suggests that inhaled steroids have a role in patients with more severe disease as judged by more severely impaired pulmonary function, frequent exacerbations, or COPD-related hospitalization.

## Combined Inhaled Corticosteroids and Long-Acting Bronchodilators

The combination of inhaled corticosteroids and long-acting bronchodilators have been increasingly examined in COPD patients (213,241). In general, the result of adding a long-acting β-agonist has been additive, although in patients with more severe airflow obstruction the changes are more impressive (242–246). The combination of these agents has generally been associated with improved spirometry, reduced exertional breathlessness, reduced exacerbation frequency, and a beneficial effect on health status. Interestingly, the impact on pulmonary function can be seen within the first few days of therapy (247). Population-based studies have suggested a decreased risk of hospitalization and mortality in COPD patients treated with combination products (248,249). In patients with severe disease being evaluated for lung transplantation, combination therapy should be strongly considered.

## Long-Term Oxygen Therapy

One of the few therapeutic interventions that can positively affect survival in patients with COPD is the appropriate delivery of long-term oxygen therapy (250). Several randomized trials have documented an improved survival in patients with oxygen (25). It appears that continuous therapy is appropriate in patients who meet criteria for advanced hypoxemia, although a plausible mechanism for the improvement in survival is not clear (25). The role of oxygen therapy in patients with less severe hypoxemia remains unclear. In studies of patients with milder daytime hypoxemia (26,251,252), oxygen therapy has not resulted in significant benefits, although all studies were limited by low power. Further data are required to better define the role of $O_2$ therapy with milder hypoxemia, including exercise-induced desaturation.

## Pulmonary Rehabilitation

Pulmonary rehabilitation has been shown to improve exercise capacity and decrease exertional breathlessness. Meta-analyses have clearly confirmed benefits in exercise capacity and health status (253–255). These beneficial effects have been noted in patients with milder and those with more severe COPD (254). The improvement in perception of dyspnea and in 6-minute walk distance from an outpatient trial of pulmonary rehabilitation was found to diminish but persists up to two years following a comprehensive six-month program of pulmonary rehabilitation followed by maintenance rehabilitation of six months duration (256). The rehabilitation arm of the study were found to have statistically significant lower frequency of exacerbations ($3.7 \pm 2.2$) as compared to controls ($6.9 \pm 3.9$) (256). Other recent studies have confirmed the benefit of similar long-term maintenance from pulmonary rehabilitation programs (256–259). Importantly, a maintenance program of telephone contacts and intermittent supervised session has been documented to better maintain benefits (260).

COPD patients with chronic respiratory impairment who, despite optimal medical management, are persistently symptomatic, have reduced exercise tolerance, or experience a restriction in activities are felt to be candidates for pulmonary rehabilitation (261). Severity of symptoms, disability, and handicap, not the severity of the physiologic impairment, should be the primary characteristics that determine the need for pulmonary rehabilitation (262). Clearly, comprehensive pulmonary rehabilitation is a useful adjunctive therapy in situations where medical therapy for COPD has been maximized. As such, it should be a routine part of the overall comprehensive care of patients with COPD undergoing evaluation for lung transplantation; this approach likely has beneficial effects on post-transplant functional outcome (263).

## LUNG VOLUME REDUCTION AS AN ALTERNATIVE OR BRIDGE TO TRANSPLANTATION

Given the importance of hyperinflation to dyspnea (109,264) and mortality (265) in COPD, numerous innovative approaches have taken to reducing lung volume with invasive procedures. These approaches include bronchoscopic and surgical lung volume reduction.

### Lung Volume Reduction Surgery

Over the past 50 years, numerous surgical approaches to ameliorate symptoms in COPD patients have been studied (266). The most successful has been LVRS. An exhaustive description of the surgical techniques for LVRS is outside the scope of this chapter. The surgical approach to LVRS has included median sternotomy (267), standard thoracotomy, and video-assisted thoracoscopic surgery (VATS) (268). Laser ablation has fallen out of favor as postoperative improvements were similar to stapled, unilateral LVRS but with a higher complication rate (269). In general, comparative studies have confirmed greater improvement with bilateral than unilateral procedures (270,271). In the recently completed National Emphysema Treatment Trial (NETT), bilateral VATS and MS exhibited similar morbidity and mortality, although the overall length of stay was longer for MS (10 days vs. 9 days, $P = 0.01$) (272). By 30 days after surgery, 70.5% of MS patients and 80.9% of VATS patients were living independently.

Since the early report of Cooper and colleagues (273), numerous reports of LVRS have been published, with summaries reviewed by several authors (274,275). Although the initial report of Cooper and colleagues documented an 82% improvement in $FEV_1$ 6.4 months after bilateral LVRS via MS (273), subsequent studies confirmed lesser, although significant, mean improvements in spirometry (275). The most compelling are the results of the NETT that confirmed a modest improvement in $FEV_1$ for patients treated surgically compared to a decrement in medically treated patients (276).

In general, bilateral procedures have been associated with greater short-term improvement (270,277). Several investigative groups have suggested similar physiologic response from bilateral LVRS performed via VATS or MS, although morbidity and mortality results vary (275). The most compelling data come from the NETT, where similar functional benefits between bilateral LVRS performed using MS or VATS were noted (272).

Significant variance has been reported around the mean improvement in $FEV_1$ (278–280). These data confirm that a significant proportion of patients experience little improvement in $FEV_1$, even in the short-term. Although data are limited, lung volumes have generally decreased during short-term follow-up (275), while changes in $DL_{CO}$ have been modest (275). Much less long-term follow-up data have been published (275). One group has reported a higher rate of drop in $FEV_1$ in patients experiencing the greatest improvement in the initial six months after surgery (those treated with bilateral stapling) (281). The lowest rate of drop was noted in those with the least initial improvement (those treated unilaterally). Another investigative group has reported a gradual decrement in $FEV_1$ over the course of three years after bilateral LVRS (282), while one has noted that a majority of patients still exhibited spirometric improvement three and five years after bilateral LVRS (283).

Most investigators have described consistent improvement in walk distance (275). Similarly, numerous groups have reported short-term increases in maximal work load, $VO_2$, $V_E$, and VT, with little change in respiratory rate and a decrease in work of breathing (275). The NETT confirmed an increase in maximal achieved wattage during oxygen supplemented cycle ergometry in surgical patients, while lesser improvement was noted in patients that continued aggressive medical management (276). Dolmage and colleagues recently reported an improved peak $VO_2$ and power with greater minute ventilation and tidal volume in a randomized controlled trial of LVRS (19/39 randomized to surgery) (284). Importantly, these individuals confirmed an improvement in operational lung volumes with LVRS (284), the physiologic change that correlates best with improved breathlessness after surgery (285). Long-term exercise data are scanty. One group has reported a higher 6-minute walk distance in six patients 18 months after surgery compared with preoperative values (286); a separate group described maintenance of improvement in 6-minute walk distance despite spirometric decrement over three years after bilateral surgery (282). The NETT investigative group noted that surgical patients, in contrast to medically treated patients, were more likely to maintain improved maximal wattage during oxygen-supplemented cardiopulmonary exercise testing up to two years after surgery (276).

Several groups have demonstrated short-term improvement in dyspnea after LVRS (275,276,282). Data regarding improved breathlessness during long-term follow-up are limited. Appleton and colleagues reported a sustained improvement in MMRC scores and in baseline dyspnea index during a mean of 51 months after bilateral LVRS (287), while Yusen and colleagues reported improved MRC scores in 52% and 40% of patients three or five years after bilateral LVRS, respectively (283).

Improvement in health status following LVRS has been reviewed extensively (288). These changes have been reported in the short-term with generic instruments (275,289) and disease-specific instruments (275,276,290). In randomized trials, clinically significant improvement in SGRQ scores was seen favoring surgical compared to medically treated patients (276). These investigators also reported improvement in SF-36 subscores during this period of follow-up. Similarly, the NETT reported that surgical patients compared to medically treated patients were more likely to experience clinically significant improvement in the SGRQ up to two years after surgery (276).

Given the heterogeneity in response, much has been written regarding identifying which patients should and which should not be considered for surgery. As LVRS is a palliative procedure for a COPD patient with an emphysematous phenotype, the clinical evaluation aims to identify patients with emphysema. As such, the presence of frequent respiratory infections and chronic, copious sputum production may identify patients with primary airway disease who are less favorable LVRS candidates (3).

Pulmonary function testing has proven instrumental in identifying optimal candidates for surgery. A lower limit of $FEV_1$ that identifies individuals at prohibitive risk has not been agreed upon (275,291). Patients with airflow obstruction from structural emphysema appear to be the ones who benefit most from LVRS. As such, a relationship between low inspiratory resistance, a measure of primarily airway disease, and lesser short-term improvements in $FEV_1$ has been reported (292). This measurement provides additional information compared to emphysema distribution as defined by perfusion scintigraphy (293). Finally, one group has recently confirmed that greater histopathological abnormalities of the smaller airways are associated with poorer short-term response to LVRS (294).

A very low $DL_{CO}$ likely increases risk (275). The NETT identified two subgroups of patients at particularly high risk of surgical mortality after bilateral LVRS (276); patients with a postbronchodilator $FEV_1 \leq 20\%$ predicted and a $DL_{CO} \leq 20\%$ predicted exhibited a much higher mortality with LVRS than with medical management [odds ratio (OR) 2.98, 95% CI 1.3–7.7]. Impaired outcome and higher mortality has been suggested in patients with hypercapnia (275); others have not confirmed this finding (275,295). The most definitive data come from the NETT, where baseline $PaCO_2$ was not associated with impaired outcome despite over 30% of randomized patients exhibiting baseline hypercapnia (276).

Preoperative exercise capacity has been documented to be a predictor of outcome (275,291). The NETT investigators noted that a threshold of 40% of the baseline maximal achieved workload during oxygen supplemented cycle ergometry identified a clear breakpoint in mortality for the overall study group. This threshold corresponded to a work load of 25 W for females and 40 W for males (276). These thresholds, in conjunction with computed tomography data, allowed a clear separation of non–high risk patients into four distinct categories (Fig. 6 and Table 3).

Thoracic imaging is crucially important in the evaluation of potential LVRS patients (296). CT is likely an ideal imaging technique in these patients (297,298). Emphysema heterogeneity appears to be of particular importance (275,296). The importance of visual grading of emphysema distribution was provided by NETT investigators (276). Radiologists at 17 participating clinical centers classified HRCT scans as exhibiting predominantly upper lobe or non–upper lobe emphysema based on visual scoring of disproportionate disease between nonanatomic thirds divided equally from apex to the base (299). Using this method, in conjunction with the maximal achieved workload during oxygen-supplemented maximal cycle ergometry, NETT investigators published two sentinel studies. Earlier work identified an increased risk of surgical mortality in patients with severe obstruction ($FEV_1 < 20\%$ predicted) and diffuse emphysema on HRCT (RR 5.96, 95% CI 2.2–20.1) (276). Patients with upper-lobe predominant emphysema and a low postrehabilitation exercise capacity exhibited a decreased risk of mortality (RR 0.47, $P = 0.005$) after LVRS. Patients with non–upper lobe predominant emphysema and a high postrehabilitation exercise capacity exhibited an increased risk of death during follow-up after LVRS (RR 2.06, $P = 0.02$) (Table 3). Patients with upper lobe predominant emphysema and a high postrehabilitation exercise capacity or patients with non–upper lobe predominant emphysema and a low postrehabilitation exercise capacity did not exhibit a survival advantage or disadvantage (276). Patients with

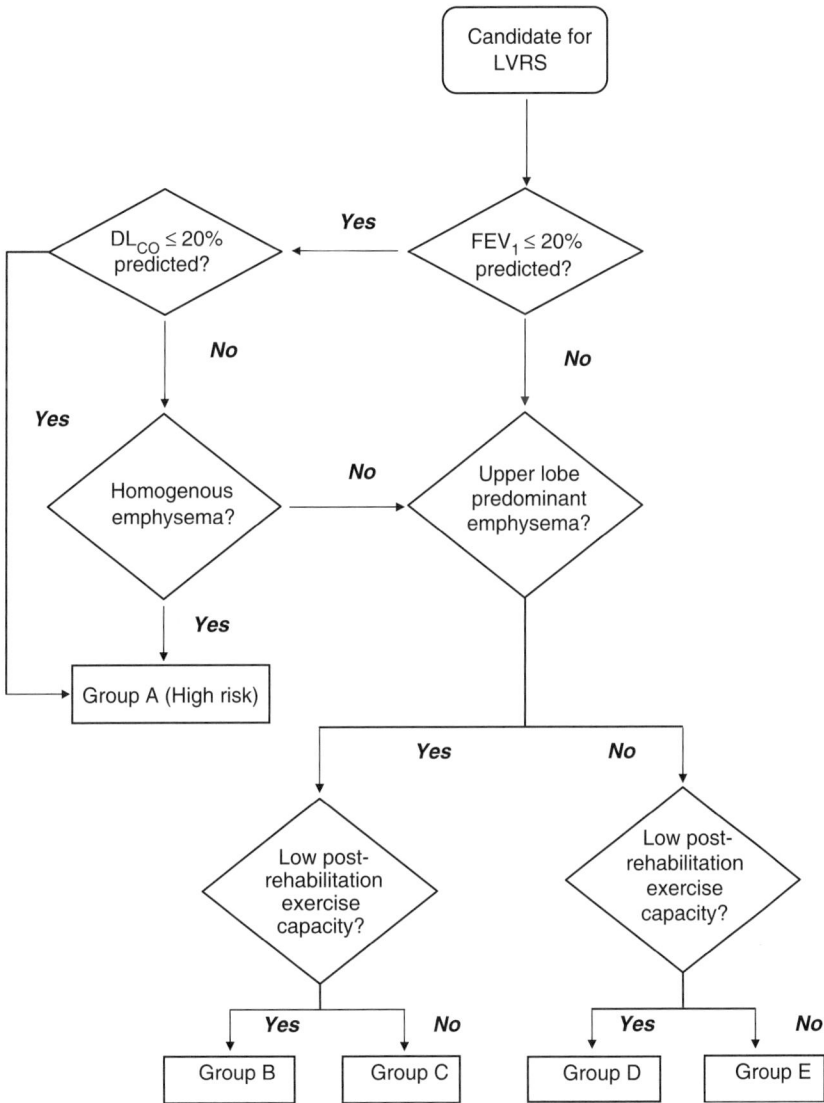

**Figure 6** Diagnostic algorithm for patients being considered for LVRS based on data from the NETT. *Abbreviations*: LVRS, lung volume reduction surgery; NETT, National Emphysema Treatment Trial. *Source*: From Refs. 276 and 340.

upper-lobe predominant emphysema undergoing LVRS were more likely to improve their exercise capacity compared to medically treated patients (Table 3). Figure 6 and Table 3 illustrate an approach to the evaluation of patients based on NETT data.

**Table 3** Results of Bilateral Lung Volume Reduction Surgery Compared to Medical Therapy in Patients with Severe Emphysema[a]

| Patients | 90-day mortality | | | Total mortality | | | |
|---|---|---|---|---|---|---|---|
| | LVRS | Medical therapy | P value | LVRS | Medical therapy | Risk ratio[b] | P value |
| Group A | 20/70 (28.6) | 0/70 (0) | <0.001 | 42/70 | 30/70 | 1.82 | 0.06 |
| Group B | 4/139 (2.9) | 5/151 (3.3) | 1.00 | 26/139 | 51/151 | 0.47 | 0.005 |
| Group C | 6/206 (2.9) | 2/213 (0.9) | 0.17 | 34/206 | 39/213 | 0.98 | 0.70 |
| Group D | 7/84 (8.3) | 0/65 (0) | 0.02 | 28/84 | 26/65 | 0.81 | 0.49 |
| Group E | 11/109 (10.1) | 1/111 (0.9) | 0.003 | 27/109 | 14/111 | 2.06 | 0.02 |

| Patients | Improvement in exercise capacity[c] | | | | Improvement in health-related quality of life[d] | | | |
|---|---|---|---|---|---|---|---|---|
| | LVRS | Medical therapy | Odds ratio | P value | LVRS | Medical therapy | Odds ratio | P value |
| Group A | 4/58 (7) | 1/48 (2) | 3.48 | 0.37 | 6/58 (10) | 0/48 (0) | – | 0.03 |
| Group B | 25/84 (30) | 0/92 (0) | – | <0.001 | 40/84 (48) | 9/92 (10) | 8.38 | <0.001 |
| Group C | 17/115 (15) | 4/138 (3) | 5.81 | 0.001 | 47/115 (41) | 15/138 (11) | 5.67 | <0.001 |
| Group D | 6/49 (12) | 3/41 (7) | 1.77 | 0.50 | 18/49 (37) | 3/41 (7) | 7.35 | 0.001 |
| Group E | 2/65 (3) | 2/59 (3) | 0.90 | 1.00 | 10/65 (15) | 7/59 (12) | 1.35 | 0.61 |

Values in parentheses indicate percentage. Groups A–E refer to the patients as defined in Figure 6.

Risk ratio for total mortality in surgically versus medically treated patients during a mean follow-up of 29.2 months.

Increase in the maximal workload of more than 10 W from the patient's post-rehabilitation baseline value (24 months after randomization).

Improvement in the health-related quality of life was defined as a decrease in the score on the St. George's Respiratory Questionnaire of more than eight points (on a 100-point scale) from the patient's post-rehabilitation baseline score (24 months after randomization).

*Abbreviation:* LVRS, lung volume reduction surgery.

*Source:* Adapted from Refs. 276 and 340.

## Bronchoscopic Lung Volume Reduction

Novel techniques that allow selective lung volume reduction via a broncho-scopic approach have recently become available (300). These techniques gen-erally result in localized areas of atelectasis and lung volume reduction. The techniques utilized include those where a one-way valve is placed into hyper-inflated, emphysematous segments, an approach tested in small case series with inconsistent benefits (301–303). Most recently, improvement in dynamic hyperinflation in highly selected patients treated with bronchoscopic place-ment of valves has been documented (303). Additional data are required to better define the therapeutic role of such techniques in emphysema patients.

## Impact of LVRS on Subsequent Lung Transplantation

LVRS should be considered as a palliative (and in some instances, life-extending) surgical option for the subset of patients with advanced, upper-lobe predominant emphysema who meet criteria for this procedure. For patients with an $FEV_1$ in the range of 25% to 40% of predicted, LVRS is the exclusive surgical consideration since this degree of airflow obstruction is above the threshold for which lung transplantation is typically offered. For those patients with an $FEV_1$ below 25% who meet criteria for both sur-gical procedures, there is the option of offering LVRS first, reserving trans-plantation for failure to respond to LVRS or to subsequent functional decline after a period of sustained improvement. Successful LVRS can post-pone the need for transplantation for up to several years, and the associated improvement in functional and nutritional status can optimize the patient's suitability as a transplant candidate (304–306). On the other hand, prior performance of LVRS can lead to formation of pleural adhesions that can render subsequent pneumonectomy at the time of transplantation somewhat more difficult. It may be necessary to leave residual native lung tissue and visceral pleura behind, particularly to protect the recurrent laryngeal and phrenic nerves (305). One clinical series of 15 patients who underwent lung transplantation following LVRS documented an increased transfusion requirement, related to perioperative pleural bleeding, compared to a matched cohort without antecedent LVRS. Nonetheless, no significant difference was noted in survival rates or long-term pulmonary function between the two groups (304). In sum, performance of LVRS does not preclude subsequent lung transplantation and, in experienced surgical hands, should not contribute to excessive post-transplantation morbidity or mortality.

## TIMING OF REFERRAL AND LISTING FOR LUNG TRANSPLANTATION

As is evident from the preceding discussion, it is inherently difficult to make definitive statements about mortality risk in patients with COPD and αl-ATD. Even in the advanced stages of disease, long-term survival is possible. As a result, determining the point in a patient's course at which the risk of death from COPD exceeds that associated with transplantation is problematic. Acknowledging that the precise point cannot be accurately defined from available literature, a consensus statement generated by an international panel of experts in the field recommended that transplantation be considered for COPD patients once the $FEV_1$ has fallen below 25% of predicted (307). Additional factors that were suggested as guidelines included a $PaCO_2$ exceeding 55 mmHg and pulmonary hypertension, especially with evidence of cor pulmonale. While these characteristics clearly define patients with far advanced COPD, they do not necessarily identify a group at imminent risk of death for whom lung transplant would therefore be a life-extending procedure (10). Indeed, studies that have compared survival of COPD patients on the waiting list with post-transplantation survival have yielded conflicting results, with one study from the United States suggesting that transplantation does not confer a survival advantage (308) while two European studies came to the opposite conclusion (309,310). In light of these uncertainties, some have advocated that lung transplant should be viewed as a life-enhancing rather than life-extending procedure for COPD patients. From this perspective, transplantation should be offered to patients with far advanced disease (defined by the parameters given earlier) who have been maximally treated with pharmacologic therapy and rehabilitation (described earlier), and who are willing to accept the considerable risks of transplantation in the hope of realizing dramatic improvement in quality of life even if the absolute number of years lived is the same. Figure 7 provides a potential approach to decision making in the patient with COPD referred for transplantation.

Decisions about the timing of referral for transplantation in the United States have been affected by recent changes in the lung allocation policy. The previous policy prioritized patients on the basis of time accrued on the waiting list. With waiting times approximating two years or more at many of the larger centers, early referral of patients was advocated so that they could be listed and begin to accrue time. Those patients who remained "too healthy" at the time they became senior on the list could be removed from the active waiting list rather than transplanted. The new lung allocation policy, introduced in May 2005, allocates lungs on the basis of "net transplant benefit," the difference between predicted one-year survival with and without transplantation (311). These survival predictions are generated with a statistical model that employs 12 clinical parameters, the most important of which is the underlying diagnosis. Patients with the greatest predicted net transplant benefit receive the highest priority. Since waiting time is not a factor, there is no longer any rationale for referring and listing patients prior to the time that they are deemed to be ready for transplantation. For the COPD population, there is an additional and potentially more

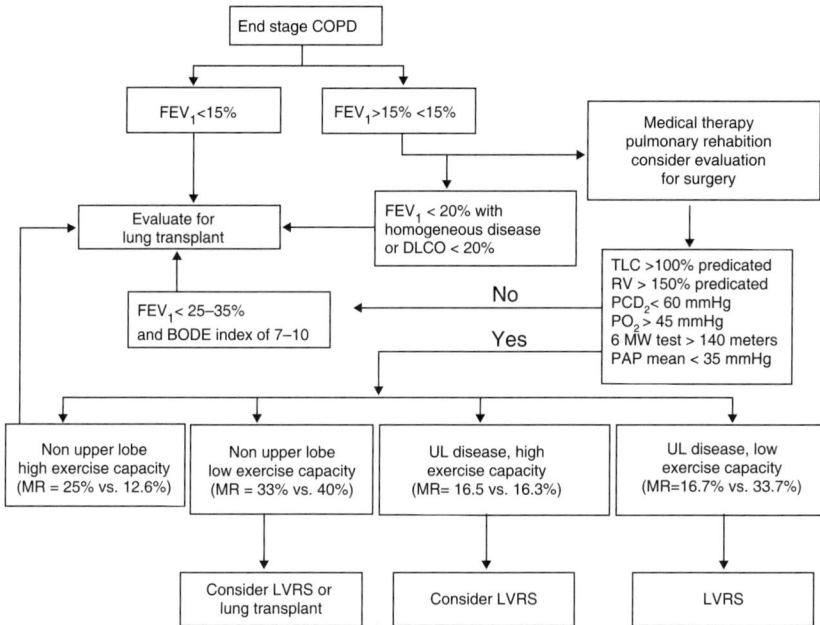

**Figure 7** Potential algorithm of surgical options for COPD patients. Comparisons of LVRS versus medical therapy in each of the four groups were made with a median follow-up period of 29 months. *Abbreviations*: COPD, chronic obstructive pulmonary disease; LVRS, lung volume reduction surgery; TLC, total lung capacity; RV, residual volume; 6MW test, six-minute walk test; UL, upper lobe predominant emphysema on CT; non–upper lobe, non–upper lobe predominant emphysema distribution on CT; MR, mortality rates. *Source*: From Ref. 96.

ominous implication to the new system. Using the restrictive definition of net transplant benefit that is at the core of the new system, it is unlikely that COPD patients will receive high lung allocation scores. This likely will lead to protracted waiting times, particularly at centers that have a large number of patients with idiopathic pulmonary fibrosis and cystic fibrosis, patient populations that will receive priority under the new system.

## CHOICE OF PROCEDURE

Whether COPD patients are best served by single lung transplantation (SLT) or bilateral lung transplantation (BLT) is a controversy that dates back to the early days of human lung transplantation and continues to the present day. To date, SLT has been the most commonly performed procedure in this patient population, accounting for ~70% of procedures (312). Among patients with αl-ATD, however, utilization patterns are more evenly distributed between the two procedures (312), reflecting the bias of some programs to offer what is perceived to be the functionally superior albeit more rigorous BLT procedure to this younger patient population. Factors relevant to the debate on which procedure to employ include physiologic considerations, functional outcomes, survival benefit, and donor organ availability.

Initial attempts to perform SLT for COPD resulted in severe ventilation/perfusion derangements. In two well-documented cases published in 1970, ventilation was preferentially directed toward the native lung, leading to progressive hyperinflation and crowding of the allograft (313). Conversely, the poorly ventilated allografts received the preponderance of blood flow, resulting in shunt physiology and hypoxemia. Based on this experience, it was prematurely concluded that ventilation/perfusion mismatch was the natural and unavoidable consequence of placing an allograft with normal compliance and vascular resistance in parallel with an emphysematous lung (313,314). SLT was thus deemed to be physiologically unsuitable for treatment of COPD, and replacement of both lungs via heart–lung or bilateral techniques emerged as the procedure of choice. This bias persisted until the late 1980s when advances in the field of lung transplantation emboldened a number of investigators to reattempt SLT for COPD, this time with successful outcomes (315,316). It is now clear that in the absence of allograft dysfunction, ventilation and perfusion are preferentially directed toward the allograft in a balanced fashion. Progressive hyperinflation of the native lung does occasionally pose a problem, typically under the influence of positive pressure ventilation, but this complication is fortunately rather uncommon (discussed subsequently).

Functional outcomes following SLT and BLT have been extensively investigated (315–320). Both procedures lead to dramatic improvement in the $FEV_1$, but the magnitude of improvement is far greater following BLT (Fig. 8). Similarly, BLT is associated with superior exercise performance as assessed by 6-minute walk test distance (Fig. 8), but this may in part reflect age-related and not procedure-related influences since BLT recipients tend to be a younger patient population. When peak exercise performance is examined, using the age-adjusted parameter of % predicted maximum oxygen consumption, BLT recipients achieve only slightly higher levels of exercise (317,321). Curiously, peak exercise performance is suboptimal in both groups, with maximum oxygen consumption falling in the range of 40% to 60% of predicted. In neither group is this exercise limitation attributable to ventilatory constraints. Rather, peripheral muscle dysfunction, due to chronic deconditioning, muscle weakness, and calcineurin inhibitor-induced myopathy, has been implicated (322,323).

Both single-center and international registry data have suggested that BLT is associated with superior survival compared to SLT (319,324). Direct comparison between these groups is confounded by the fact that BLT recipients are generally younger. A recent study involving analysis of over 2200 lung transplant recipients with COPD addressed this issue by controlling for

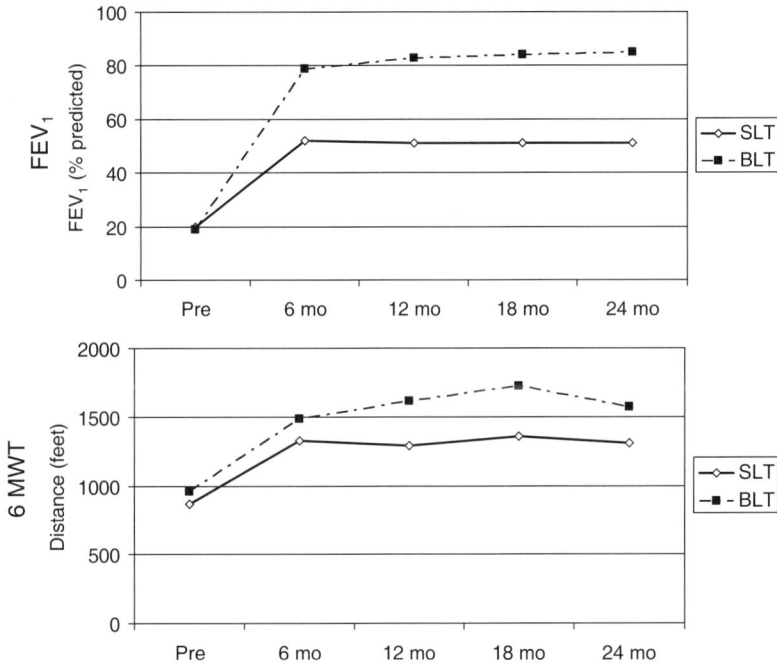

**Figure 8** Functional outcomes following SLT and BLT. These figures demonstrate the magnitude of improvement in $FEV_1$ (*upper panel*) and 6MWT (*lower panel*) distance following SLT ($n = 83$ patients) and BLT ($n = 45$ patients). Data points represent mean values at each time point. *Abbreviations*: SLT, single lung transplantation; BLT, bilateral lung transplantation; $FEV_1$, forced expiratory volume in one second; 6MWT, six-minute walk test. *Source*: Data derived from the University of Pennsylvania Lung Transplant database.

recipient age (325). The analysis confirmed that BLT is associated with superior long-term survival in recipients <60 years of age. It is postulated that the survival advantage offered by BLT relates to the greater degree of improvement in lung function and thus the greater reserve available to handle functional decline that accompanies chronic rejection. For patients >60 years, there was a trend toward poorer survival associated with BLT, which appeared to be due to an excessive perioperative mortality rate. While this suggests that older patients may not be well suited to handle the more rigorous bilateral procedure, the small number of BLT recipients >60 years included in the analysis ($n = 27$) limits firm conclusions.

The final consideration in weighing the pros and cons of the two procedures is organ availability. In the context of an extremely scarce donor pool, SLT would appear to provide a more efficient use of limited resources. However, transplant centers that advocate for BLT argue that transplantation of two lungs permits greater use of marginal organs that would otherwise be deemed unsuitable if used as single allografts (319). Whether this greater willingness to employ marginal donors would truly counterbalance the increased consumption of organs that would accompany a widespread shift from SLT to BLT remains uncertain.

In sum, the technical ease and efficient use of the limited donor pool are the major assets of SLT. This procedure is well suited for older and frailer patients who might not be able to tolerate the rigors of the more extensive bilateral procedure. With functional outcomes permitting resumption of a normal lifestyle in all but the most vigorous patients, SLT is certainly an acceptable procedure. However, the superior long-term survival achieved with BLT in those <60 years provides a compelling argument for the preferential use of BLT in "younger" recipients. Such a practice would have to be coupled with a more liberal use of marginal organs and other strategies to expand the limited donor pool in order to prevent further disparity in meeting the needs of an ever-increasing number of candidates awaiting transplantation.

## OUTCOMES

Recipients with underlying COPD enjoy the highest one-year post-transplant survival of any patient population, approximating 85% (324,326). This reflects the relative technical ease of the surgical procedure in a group of patients who typically do not have extensive pleural or mediastinal adhesions, septic lung disease, or significant pulmonary hypertension. Beyond the first year, COPD recipients are subject to the same life-threatening complications that afflict all lung transplant recipients, resulting in intermediate and long-term survival rates that are similar to other patient populations. Median survival for the COPD recipient population is ~5 years, and 10-year survival is achieved by only 20% to 25% of patients (324). As discussed before, intermediate-term survival rates are better following BLT compared with SLT for patients <60 years of age. For example, in a large cohort of patients between the ages of 50 and 60 years, five-year survival was 61% for BLT recipients and only 40% for SLT (325).

## SPECIAL CONSIDERATIONS FOLLOWING TRANSPLANTATION

The various complications that can compromise the outcome of lung transplantation for all recipients are discussed in detail elsewhere in this book. This section will address several issues of particular relevance to patients with underlying COPD.

### Native Lung Hyperinflation

As discussed before, initial concerns about preferential ventilation and hyperinflation of the highly compliant native lung following SLT for COPD have subsequently proven to be overstated. Nonetheless, native lung hyperinflation can occasionally complicate the immediate postoperative period or develop more insidiously months to years later. The incidence of clinically significant acute native lung hyperinflation has been reported to be 15 % to 30% among COPD patients undergoing SLT (327,328). Although risk factors have not been well defined, the combination of positive pressure ventilation and significant allograft edema serves to magnify the compliance differential between the two lungs and may predispose to this complication. The hemodynamic consequences of marked overdistention and air trapping of the native lung are identical to those seen in association with tension pneumothorax: impaired venous return, diminished cardiac output, and hypotension. Marked contralateral shift of the mediastinum leads to extrinsic compression of the allograft, resulting in atelectasis and impaired gas exchange. The risk of acute hyperinflation can be minimized by early extubation of the patient, which in uncomplicated cases can often be performed at the completion of the surgical procedure. For patients who cannot be extubated and who develop severe respiratory or hemodynamic consequences of acute hyperinflation, replacement of the standard endotracheal tube with a double lumen tube permits initiation of independent lung ventilation (329,330). In this way, the native lung can be ventilated with a low respiratory rate and prolonged expiratory time to facilitate more complete emptying.

Beyond the perioperative period, some SLT recipients with COPD demonstrate exaggerated or progressive native lung hyperinflation associated with suboptimal or deteriorating pulmonary function. In cases where the allograft is intrinsically normal but crowded by the native lung, surgical volume reduction of the native lung can lead to significant and sustained improvement in pulmonary function (331,332). It is important to recognize that native lung hyperinflation may at times be the consequence, rather than the cause, of allograft dysfunction. In this regard, development of bronchiolitis obliterans within the allograft can occasionally result in secondary hyperinflation of the native lung, presumably due to a combination of volume loss and diminished ventilation of the diseased allograft. In this setting, the results of surgical volume reduction of the native lung have been disappointing (333). The distinction between the two clinical situations in which native lung hyperinflation is encountered is obviously critical but often difficult. Demonstration of air trapping or bronchiectasis within the allograft by high-resolution CT suggests the presence of bronchiolitis obliterans and argues against consideration of surgical volume reduction.

## Bronchogenic Carcinoma

Patients with COPD, as well as those with underlying pulmonary fibrosis, are at risk for developing lung cancer involving the native lung. Several published series have documented an overall prevalence of bronchogenic carcinoma of

2.0% to 3.7% among lung transplant recipients with underlying COPD (334,335). The traditional risk factors of cigarette smoking and airflow obstruction account for the particular vulnerability of this recipient population. Data are conflicting as to whether factors related to transplantation (e.g., immunosuppression) confer additional risk for developing lung cancer or whether the prevalence is comparable to that of the general population with similar risk factors (334).

In the majority of cases, bronchogenic carcinoma is encountered in the remaining native lung following SLT. Occasionally, lung cancer that was previously unsuspected may be incidentally found in the explanted lung at the time of transplantation, placing the recipient at risk for subsequent recurrence (334,336). Whether developing de novo or recurring after transplant pneumonectomy, lung cancers in the transplant recipient often demonstrate rapid progression over a short period of time, leading to initial suspicion of an infectious rather than neoplastic process. In one series, the survival rate one year after diagnosis of lung cancer was only 33% (334). This aggressive behavior may reflect loss of antitumor immune surveillance in the immunosuppressed host or may be due to a more specific effect of cyclosporine in promoting tumor growth.

### Special Considerations in α1-ATD Recipients

Lung transplantation effectively treats the pulmonary manifestations of αl-ATD, but the underlying antiprotease-deficient state persists. This raises the question of whether these patients are at risk for recurrent protease-mediated injury to the allograft and, in turn, whether αl-antitrypsin replacement therapy is warranted in the posttransplant period. As the development of emphysema in non-smoking αl-ATD patients evolves over many decades, far exceeding the currently anticipated life expectancy of transplant recipients, it is not clear that enzyme replacement would prolong life or preserve graft function. However, two studies examining antiprotease defenses in αl-ATD patients following transplantation suggest that the allograft may in fact be vulnerable to protease injury during times of increased neutrophil burden in the lower respiratory tract (337,338). Both studies demonstrated that levels of αl-antitrypsin in bronchoalveolar lavage fluid recovered from αl-ATD transplant recipients were extremely low when compared to normal controls. Despite this, antiprotease levels were sufficient to prevent unopposed neutrophil elastase activity in healthy, stable patients. However, unopposed elastase activity was documented in 43% and 59% of patients, respectively, in the two studies, occurring during periods of allograft inflammation due to ischemia–reperfusion injury, lower respiratory tract infection, and bronchiolitis obliterans.

Recently, recurrence of emphysema in the allograft was documented 11 years after transplantation for αl-ATD (339). The patient had resumed smoking following transplantation and this was presumed to play a central role in accelerating the recurrence of disease. Bronchoalveolar lavage fluid obtained after disease recurrence demonstrated free elastase activity, suggesting that the endogenous antiprotease defenses had been overwhelmed.

These studies provide a possible rationale for the selective use of enzyme replacement therapy at times when increased neutrophil burden in the lower respiratory tract is expected, such as with bacterial respiratory tract infections, acute lung injury, and bronchiolitis obliterans. However, unless it becomes clear that recurrence of emphysema is a common phenomenon among long-term survivors, such a strategy cannot be advocated. As the one case report of recurrent disease illustrates, absolute avoidance of cigarette smoking in the post-transplant period is critical in αl-ATD patients.

## REFERENCES

1. Celli BR, MacNee W, et al. ATS/ERS Task Force. Standards for the diagnosis and treatment of patients with COPD: a summary of the ATS/ERS position paper. Eur Respir J 2004; 23:932–946.
2. Pauwels RA, Buist AS, Calverley PMA, Jenkins CR, Hurd SS. Committee GOLD Scientific. Global strategy for the diagnosis, management, and prevention of chronic obstructive pulmonary disease. NHLBI/WHO Global Initiative for Chronic Obstructive Lung Disease (GOLD) Workshop Summary. Am J Respir Crit Care 2001; 163:1256–1276.
3. Flaherty KR, Kazerooni EA, Martinez FJ. Differential diagnosis of chronic airflow obstruction. J Asthma 2000; 37:201–223.
4. Barnes PJ. Chronic obstructive pulmonary disease. N Eng J Med 2000; 343:269–280.
5. Jeffery PK. Remodeling in asthma and chronic obstructive lung disease. Am J Respir Crit Care 2001; 164:S28–S38.
6. Hogg JC, Chu F, Utokaparch S, et al. The nature of small-airway obstruction in chronic obstructive pulmonary disease. N Engl J Med 2004; 350:350.
7. American Thoracic Society. International guidelines for the selection of lung transplant candidates. Am J Respir Crit Care Med 1998; 158:335–339.
8. Hodgkin JE. Prognosis in chronic obstructive pulmonary disease. Clin Chest Med 1990; 11:555–569.
9. Nishimura K, Tsukino M. Clinical course and prognosis of patients with chronic obstructive pulmonary disease. Curr Op Pulm Med 2000; 6:127–132.
10. Martinez FJ, Kotloff R. Prognostication in chronic obstructive pulmonary disease: implications for lung transplantation. Sem Respir Crit Care Med 2001; 22:489–498.
11. Burrows B, Earle RH. Prediction of survival in patients with chronic airways obstruction. Am Rev Respir Dis 1969; 99:865–871.
12. Traver GA, Cline MG, Burrows B. Predictors of mortality in chronic obstructive pulmonary disease. A 15-year follow-up study. Am Rev Respir Dis 1979; 119:895–902.

13. Anthonisen NR. Prognosis in chronic obstructive pulmonary disease: results from multicenter clinical trials. Am Rev Respir Dis 1989; 140:S95–S99.

14. Anthonisen NR, Wright EC, IPPB Trial Group. Bronchodilator response in chronic obstructive pulmonary disease. Am Rev Respir Dis 1986; 133:814–819.

15. Hansen EF, Pharaneth K, Laursen LC, Kok-Jensen A, Dirksen A. Reversible and irreversible airflow obstruction as predictor of overall mortality in asthma and chronic obstructive pulmonary disease. Am J Respir Crit Care Med 1999; 159:1267–1271.

16. Piccioni P, Caria E, Bignamini E, et al. Predictors of survival in a group of patients with chronic airflow obstruction. J Clin Epidemiol 1998; 51:547–555.

17. Cooper CB, Waterhouse J, Howard P. Twelve year clinical study of patients with hypoxic cor pulmonale given long term domiciliary oxygen therapy. Thorax 1987; 42:105–110.

18. Diener CF, Burrows B. Further observations on the course and prognosis of chronic obstructive lung disease. Am Rev Respir Dis 1975; 111:719–724.

19. Postma DS, Burema J, Gimeno F, et al. Prognosis in severe chronic obstructive pulmonary disease. Am Rev Respir Dis 1979; 119:357–367.

20. Postma DS, DeVries K, Koeter GH, et al. Independent influence of reversibility of air-flow obstruction and non-specific hyperreactivity on the long-term course of lung function in chronic air-flow obstruction. Am Rev Respir Dis 1979; 134:276–280.

21. Bates DV, Knott JMS, Christie RV. Respiratory function in emphysema in relation to prognosis. Q J Med 1956; 25:137–157.

22. Boushy SF, Thompson HK Jr, North LB, Beale AR, Snow TR. Prognosis in chronic obstructive pulmonary disease. Am Rev Respir Dis 1973; 108: 1373–1383.

23. Kanner RE, Renzetti AD Jr, Stanish WM, Barkman HW Jr, Klauber MR. Predictors of survival in subjects with chronic airflow limitation. Am J Med 1983; 74:249–255.

24. Chailleux E, Fauroux B, Binet G, Dautzenberg B, Polu JM. Predictors of survival in patients receiving domiciliary oxygen therapy or mechanical ventilatory. A 10-year analysis of ANTADIR observatory. Chest 1996; 109:741–749.

25. Crockett AJ, Cranston JM, Moss JR, Alpers JH. A review of long-term oxygen therapy for chronic obstructive pulmonary disease. Resp Med 2001; 95:437–443.

26. Gorecka D, Gorzelak K, Sliwinski P, Tobiasz M, Zielinski J. Effect of long term oxygen therapy on survival in patients with chronic obstructive pulmonary disease with moderate hypoxemia. Thorax 1997; 52:674–679.

27. Veale D, Chailleux E, Taytard A, Cardinaud JP. Characteristics and survival of patients prescribed long-term oxygen therapy outside of prescription guidelines. Eur Respir J 1998; 12:780–784.

28. Cranston JM, Nguyen AM, Crockett AJ. The relative survival of COPD patients on long-term oxygen therapy in Australia: A comparative study. Resp 2004; 9:237–242.

29. Foucher P, Baudouin N, Merati M, et al. Relative survival analysis of 252 patients with COPD receiving long-term oxygen therapy. Chest 1998; 113: 1580–1587.

30. Aida A, Miyamoto K, Nishimura M, Aiba M, Kira S, Kawakami Y. Japan Respiratory Failure Research Group. Prognostic value of hypercapnia in patients with chronic respiratory failure during long-term oxygen therapy. Am J Respir Crit Care Med 1998; 158:188–193.

31. Connors AF Jr, Dawson NV, Thomas C, et al. Investigators for the SUPPORT. Outcomes following acute exacerbation of severe chronic obstructive lung disease. Am J Respir Crit Care Med 1996; 154:959–967.

32. Costello R, Deegan P, Fitzpatrick M, McNicholas WT. Reversible hypercapnia in chronic obstructive pulmonary disease: a distinct pattern of respiratory failure with a favorable prognosis. Am J Med 1997; 103:239–244.

33. Saryal S, Celik G, Karabiyikoglu G. Distinctive features and long-term survival of reversible and chronic hypercapnic patients with COPD. Monaldi Arch Chest Dis 1999; 54:212–216.

34. Strom K. Oral corticosteroid treatment during long-term oxygena therapy in chronic obstructive pulmonary disease: a risk factor for hospitalization and mortality in women. Respir Med 1998; 92:50–56.

35. Petty TL, Bliss PL. Ambulatory oxygen therapy, exercise, and survival with advanced chronic obstructivce pulmonary disease (The Nocturnal Oxygen Therapy Trial revisited). Respir Care 2000; 45:204–213.

36. Gerardi DA, Lovett L, Benoit-Connors ML, Reardon JZ, ZuWallack RL. Variables related to increased mortality following out-patient pulmonary rehabilitation. Eur Respir J 1996; 9:431–435.

37. Bowen JB, Votto JJ, Thrall RS, et al. Functional status and survival following pulmonary rehabilitation. Chest 2000; 118:697–703.

38. Pinto-Plata VM, Cote C, Cabral H, Taylor J, Celli BR. The 6-min walk distance: change over time and value as a predictor of survival in severe COPD. Eur Respir J 2004; 23:28–33.

39. Hiraga T, Maekura R, Okuda Y, et al. Prognostic predictors for survival in patients with COPD using cardiopulmonary exercise testing. Clin Physiol Funct Imaging 2003; 23:324–331.

40. Oga T, Nishimura K, Tsukino M, Sato S, Hajiro T. Analysis of the factors related to mortality in chronic obstructive pulmonary disease: role of exercise capacity and health stauts. Am J Resp Crit Care Med 2003; 167:544–549.

41. Gelb AF, Zamel N, Hogg JC, Muller NL, Schein MJ. Pseudophysiologic emphysema resulting from severe small-airways disease. Am J Respir Crit Care Med 1998; 158:815–819.

42. Burrows B. The course and prognosis of different types of chronic airflow limitation in a general population sample from Arizona: comparison with the Chicago "COPD" Series. Am Rev Respir Dis 1989; 140:S92–S94.

43. Goldin JG. Quantitative CT of emphysema and the airways. J Thorac Imag 2004; 19:235–240.

44. Dawkins PA, Dowson LJ, Guest PJ, Stockley RA. Predictors of mortality in alpha1-antitrypsin deficiency. Thorax 2003; 58:1020–1026.

45. Keistinen T, Tuuponen T, Kivela SL. Survival experience of the population needing hospital treatment for asthma or COPD at age 50–54. Respir Med 1998; 92:568–572.

46. Vestbo J, Prescott E, Lange P, Schnohr P, Jensen G. Vital prognosis after hospitalization for COPD: a study of a random population sample. Respir Med 1998; 92:772–776.
47. Wu MC, Eriksson E. Lung function, smoking and survival in severe alpha-1 antitrypsin deficiency PiZZ. J Clin Epidemiol 1988; 41:1157–1165.
48. Seersholm N, Dirksen A, Kok-Jensen A. Airways obstruction and two year survival in patients with severe alpha$_1$-antitrypsin deficiency. Eur Respir J 1994; 7:1985–1987.
49. Seersholm N, Kok-Jensen A. Survival in relation to lung function and smoking cessation in patients with severe hereditary alpha-1-antitrypsin deficiency. Am J Respir Crit Care Med 1995; 151:369–373.
50. The alpha-1-Antitrypsin Deficiency Registry Study Group. Survival and FEV$_1$ decline in individuals with severe deficiency of a$_1$-antitrypsin. Am J Respir Crit Care Med 1998; 158:49–59.
51. Stoller JK, Tomashefki J Jr, Crystal RG, et al. For the a1-Antitrypsin Deficiency Registry Study Group. Mortality in individuals with severe deficiency of a1-antitrypsin. Findings from the National Heart, Lung, and Blood Institute Registry. Chest 2005; 127:1196–1204.
52. Ringbaek TJ, Seersholm N, Viskum K. Standardised mortality rates in females and males with COPD and asthma. Eur Respir J 2005; 25:891–895.
53. Miyamoto K, Aida A, Nishimura M, Aiba M, Kira S, Kawakami Y. Japan The Respiratory Failure Research Group. Gender effect on prognosis of patients receiving long-term home oxygen therapy. Am J Respir Crit Care Med 1995; 152:972–976.
54. Sunyer J, Anto JM, McFarlane D, et al. Sex differences in mortality of people who visited emergency rooms for asthma and chronic obstructive pulmonary disease. Am J Respir Crit Care 1998; 158:851–856.
55. Rennard SI. Clinical approach to patients with chronic obstructive pulmonary disease and cardiovascular disease. Proc Am Thorac Soc 2005; 2:94–100.
56. Incalzi RA, Fuso L, DeRosa M, et al. Co-morbidity contributes to predict mortality of patients with chronic obstructive pulmonary disease. Eur Respir J 1997; 10:2794–2800.
57. Hunninghake DB. Cardiovascular disease in chronic obstructive pulmonary disease. Proc Am Thorac Soc 2005; 2:44–49.
58. Sin DD, Man SFP. Chronic obstructive pulmonary disease as a risk factor for cardiovascular morbidity and mortality. Proc Am Thorac Soc 2005; 2:8–11.
59. Wright JL, Levy RD, Churg A. Pulmonary hypertension in chronic obstructive pulmonary disease: current theories of pathogenesis and their implications for treatment. Thorax 2005; 60:605–609.
60. Higenbottam T. Pulmonary hypertension and chronic obstrucive pulmonary disease. A case for treatment. Proc Am Thorac Soc 2005; 2:12–19.
61. Incalzi RA, Fuso L, De Rosa M, et al. Electrocardiographic signis of chronic cor pulmonale: a negative prognostic finding in chronic obstructive pulmonary disease. Circulation 1999; 99:1600–1605.
62. Oswald-Mammosser M, Weitzenblum E, Quoix E, et al. Prognostic factors in COPD patients receiving long-term oxygen therapy. Importance of pulmonary artery pressure. Chest 1995; 107:1193–1198.

63. Skwarsky K, MacNee W, Wraith PK, et al. Predictors of survival in patients with chronic obstructive pulmonary disease treated with long term oxygen therapy. Chest 1991; 100:1522–1527.
64. Keller A, Ragaz A, Borer P. Predictors of early mortality in patients with long-term oxygen home therapy. Respiration 1985; 48:216–221.
65. Wurternberger G, Zielinski J, Sliwinksy P, et al. Survival in chronic obstructive pulmonary disease after diagnosis of pulmonary hypertension related to long-term oxygen therapy. Lung 1990; 168(suppl):762–769.
66. Gray-Donald K, Gibbons L, Shapiro SH, MacKlem PT, Martin JG. Nutritional status and mortality in chronic obstructive pulmonary disease. Am J Respir Crit Care Med 1996; 153:961–966.
67. Schols AMWJ, Slangen J, Volovics L, Wouters EFM. Weight loss is a reversible factor in the prognosis of chronic obstructive pulmonary disease. Am J Respir Crit Care Med 1998; 157:1791–1797.
68. Landbo C, Prescott E, Lange P, Vestbo J, Almdal TP. Prognostic value of nutritional status in chronic obstructive pulmonary disease. Am J Respir Crit Care Med 1999; 160:1856–1861.
69. Celli BR, Cote CG, Marin JM, et al. The body-mass index, airflow obstruction, dyspnea, and exercise capacity index in chronic obstructive pulmonary disease. N Eng J Med 2004; 350:1005–1012.
70. Madill J, Gutierrez C, Grossman J, et al. Program Toronto Lung Transplant. Nutritional assessment of the lung transplant patient: body mass index as a predictor of 90-day mortality following transplantation. J Heart Lung Trans 2001; 20:288–296.
71. Marquis K, Debigare R, Lacasse Y, et al. Midthigh muscle cross-sectional area is a better predictor of mortality than body mass index inpatients with chronic obstructive pulmonary disease. Am J Respir Crit Care Med 2002; 166:809–813.
72. Wegner RE, Jorres RA, Kirsten DK, Magnussen H. Factor analysis of exercise capacity, dyspnoea ratings and lung function in patients with severe COPD. Eur Respir J 1994; 7:725–729.
73. Mahler DA, Harver A. A factor analysis of dyspnea ratings, respiratory muscle strength, and lung function in patients with chronic obstructive pulmonary disease. Am Rev Respir Dis 1992; 145:467–470.
74. Celli BR, Calverley PMA, Rennard SI, et al. Proposal for a multidimensional staging system for chronic obstructive pulmonary disease. Respir Med 2005; 99:1546–1554.
75. Hilleman DE, Dewan N, Malesker M, Friedman M. Pharmacoeconomic evaluation of COPD. Chest 2000; 118:1278–1285.
76. Holleman DR Jr, Simel DL. Does the clinical examination predict airflow limitation? JAMA 1995; 273:313–319.
77. Ferguson GT, Enright PL, Buist AS, Higgins MW. Office spirometry for Lung Health Assessment in Adults. A consensus statement from the National Lung Health Education Program. Chest 2000; 117:1146–1161.
78. Pearson MG, Bellamy D, Calverley PMA, et al. BTS guidelines for the management of chronic obstructive pulmonary disease. Thorax 1997; 52(suppl 5): S1–S28.

79. Kazerooni EA, Whyte RI, Flint A, Martinez FJ. Imaging of emphysema and lung volume reduction surgery. RadioGraphics 1997; 17:1023–1036.

80. Baldi S, Miniati M, Bellina CR, et al. Relationship between extent of pulmonary emphysema by high-resolution computed tomography and lung elastic recoil in patients with chronic obstructive pulmonary disease. Am J Respir Crit Care Med 2001; 164:585–589.

81. Klein JS, Gamsu G, Webb WR, Golden JA, Muller NL. High-resolution CT diagnosis of emphysema in symptomatic patients with normal chest radiographs and isolated low diffusing capacity. Radiology 1992; 182:817–821.

82. Spaggiari E, Zompatori M, Verduri A, et al. Early smoking-induced lung lesions in asymptomatic subjects. Correlations between high resolution dynamic CT and pulmonary function testing. Radiol Med (Torino) 2005; 109:27–39.

83. Flaherty KR, Martinez FJ. The role of computed tomography in emphysema and lung volume reduction surgery. In: Lipson D, van Beek E, eds. Functional Lung Imaging Lung Biology in Health and Disease. Boca Raton: Taylor & Francis, LLC, 2005:431–451.

84. Kotloff RM, Lipson DA. Lung transplantation: radiographic considerations. In: Lipson D, van Beek E, eds. Functional Lung Imaging Lung Biology in Health and Disease. Boca Raton: Taylor & Francis, LLC, 2005:593–620.

85. Celli BR. The importance of spirometry in COPD and asthma. Effect on approach to management. Chest 2000; 117:S15–S19.

86. Jones PW. Health status measurement in chronic obstructive pulmonary disease. Thorax 2001; 56:880–887.

87. Hajiro T, Nishimura K, Tsukino M, Ikeda A, Oga T. Stages of disease severity and factors that affect the health status of patients with chronic obstructive pulmonary disease. Respir Med 2000; 94:841–846.

88. Mahler DA, Tomlinson D, Olmstead EM, Tosteson ANA, O'Connor GT. Changes in dyspnea, health status, and lung function in chronic airway disease. Am J Respir Crit Care Med 1995; 151:61–65.

89. Miravitlles M, Ferrer M, Pont A, et al. For the IMPAC Study Group. Effect of exacerbations on quality of life in patients with chronic obstructive pulmonary diseasee: a 2 year follow-up study. Thorax 2004; 59:387–395.

90. Aaron SD, Vandemheen KL, Clinch JJ, et al. Measurement of short-term changes in dyspnea and disease-specific quality of life following an acute COPD exacerbation. Chest 2002; 121:688–696.

91. Spencer S, Jones PW. For the GLOBE Study Group. Time course of recovery of health status following an infective exacerbation of chronic bronchitis. Thorax 2003; 58:589–593.

92. Seemungal TAR, Donaldson GC, Bhowmik A, Jeffries DJ, Wedzicha JA. Time course and recovery of exacerbations in patients with chronic obstructive pulmonary disease. Am J Respir Crit Care Med 2000; 161:1608–1613.

93. Hankinson JL, Wagner GR. Medical screening using periodic spirometry for detection of chronic lung disease. Occup Med 1993; 8:353–361.

94. Kazerooni EA. Lung cancer screening. In: Fishman E, Jeffrey R, eds. Multidector CT: Principles, Techniques & Clinical Applications. Philadelphia: Lippincott, Williams & Wilkins, 2004:61–76.

95. Glanville AR, Estenne M. Indications, patient selection and timing of referral for lung transplantation. Eur Respir J 2003; 22:845–852.
96. Nathan SD. Lung transplantation. Disease-specific considerations for referral. Chest 2005; 127:1006–1016.
97. The tobacco use and dependence clinical practice guideline panel staff, and consortium representatives. A clinical practice guideline for treating tobacco use and dependence. JAMA 2000; 282:3244–3254.
98. Lancaster T, Stead L, Silagy C, Sowden A. Effectiveness of interventions to help people stop smoking: findings from the Cochrane Library. BMJ 2000; 321:355–358.
99. Henningfield JE. Nicotine medications for smoking cessation. N Eng J Med 1995; 333:1196–1203.
100. Jorenby DE, Leischow SJ, Nides MA, et al. A controlled trial of sustained-release bupropion, a nicotine patch, or both for smoking cessation. N Eng J Med 1999; 340:685–691.
101. Tashkin DP, Kanner R, Bailey W, et al. Smoking cessation in patients with chronic obstructive pulmonary disease: a double-blind, placebo-controlled, randomised trial. Lancet 2001; 357:1571–1575.
102. Anthonisen NR, Connett JE, Kiley JP, et al. For the Lung Health Study Group. The effects of smoking intervention and the use of an inhaled anticholinergic bronchodilator on the rate of decline in $FEV_1$: the Lung Health Study. JAMA 1994; 272:1497–1505.
103. Anthonisen NR, Connett JE, Murray RP. For the Lung Health Study Research Group. Smoking and lung function of Lung Health Study participants after 11 years. Am J Respir Crit Care Med 2002; 166:675–679.
104. Simmons MS, Connett JE, Nides MA, et al. Smoking reduction and the rate of decline in $FEV_1$: results from the Lung Health Study. Eur Respir J 2005; 25:1011–1017.
105. Anthonisen NR, Skeans MA, Wise RM, Manfreda J, Kanner RE, Connett JE. For the Lung Health Study Research Group. The effects of a smoking cessation intervention on 14.5-year mortality. A randomized clinical trial. Ann Int Med 2005; 142:233–239.
106. Kanner RE, Connett JE, Williams DE, Buist AS, For the Lung Health Study Research Group. Effects of randomized assignment to a smoking cessation intervention and changes in smoking habits on respiratory symptoms in smokers with early chronic obstructive pulmonary disease: The Lung Health Study. Am J Med 1999; 106:410–416.
107. Agusti AGN. COPD, a multicomponent disease: implicationis for management. Respir Med 2005; 99:670–682.
108. Ferguson GT. Update on pharmacologic therapy for chronic obstructive pulmonary disease. Clin Chest Med 2000; 21.
109. O'Donnell DE, Revill SM, Webb KA. Dynamic hyperinflation and exercise intolerance in chronic obstructive pulmonary disease. Am J Respir Crit Care 2001; 164:770–777.
110. O'Donnell DE, Lam M, Webb KA. Measurement of symptoms, lung hyperinflation, and endurance during exercise in chronic obstructive pulmonary disease. Am J Respir Crit Care 1998; 158:1557–1565.

111. O'Donnell DE. Assessment of bronchodilator efficacy in symptomatic COPD. Is spirometry useful? Chest 2000; 117:S42–S47.
112. Diaz O, Villafranca C, Ghezzo H, et al. Role of inspiratory capacity on exercise tolerance in COPD patients with and without tidal expiratory flow limitation at rest. Eur Resp J 2000; 16:269–275.
113. O'Donnell DE, Voduc N, Fitzpatrick M, Webb KA. Effect of salmeterol on the ventilatory response to exercise in chronic obstructive pulmonary disease. Eur Respir J 2004; 24:86–94.
114. O'Donnell DE, Fluge T, Gerken F, et al. Effects of tiotropium on lung hyperinflation, dyspnoea and exercise tolerance in COPD. Eur Respir J 2004; 23:832–840.
115. O'Donnell DE, Aaron S, Bourbeau J, et al. Canadian Thoracic Society recommendations for management of chronic obstructive pulmonary disease-2003. Can Respir J 2003; 10 (suppl A).
116. Weder MM, Donohue JF. Role of bronchodilators in chronic obstructive pulmonary disease. Semin Respir Crit Care Med 2005; 26:221–234.
117. Cooper CB, Tashkin DP. Recent developments in inhaled therapy in stable chronic obstructive pulmonary disease. BMJ 2005; 330:640–644.
118. Barnes PJ. The role of anticholinergics in chronic obstructive pulmonary disease. Am J Med 2004; 117(12A):S24–S32.
119. On LS, Boonyongsunchai P, Webb S, Davies L, Calverley PMA, Costello RW. Function of pulmonary neuronal $M_2$ muscarinic receptors in stable chronic obstructive pulmonary disease. Am J Respir Crit Care 2001; 163:1320–1325.
120. Disse B. Antimuscarinic treatment for lung diseases. From research to clinical practice. Life Sciences 2001; 68:257–264.
121. Cazzola M, Spina D, Matera MG. The use of bronchodilators in stable chronic obstructive pulmonary disease. Pulm Pharmacol Therapeut 1997; 10:129–144.
122. Chapman KR. Clinical implications of anticholinergic bronchodilator therapy in COPD. Res Clin Forums 1991; 13:43–50.
123. Klock LE, Miller TD, Morris AH, et al. A comparative study of atropine sulfate and isoproterenol hydrochloride in chronic bronchitis. Am Rev Respir Dis 1975; 112:371–376.
124. Marini JJ, Lakshminarayan S. The effect of atropine inhalation in "irreversible" chronic bronchitis. Chest 1980; 77:591–596.
125. Braun SR, McKenzie WN, Copeland C, Knight L, Ellersieck M. A comparison of the effect of ipratropium and albuterol in the treatment of chronic obstructive pulmonary disease. Arch Intern Med 1989; 149:544–547.
126. Rennard SI, Serby CW, Ghafouri M, Johnson PA, Friedman M. Extended therapy with ipratropium is associated with improved lung function in patients with COPD. A retrospective analysis of data from seven clinical trials. Chest 1996; 110:62–70.
127. Liesker JJW, Wijkstra PJ, Hacken NHTT, Koeter GH, Postma DS, Kerstjens HAM. A systematic review of the effects of bronchodilators on exercise capacity in patients with COPD. Chest 2002; 121:597–608.
128. Ikeda A, Nishimura K, Koyama H, Tsukino M, Mishima M, Izumi T. Dose response study of ipratropium bromide aerosol on maximum exercise performance in stable patients with chronic obstructive pulmonary disease. Thorax 1996; 51:48–53.

129. Tsukino M, Nishimura K, Ikeda A, et al. Effects of theophylline and ipratropium bromide on exercise performance in patients with stable chronic obstructive pulmonary disease. Thorax 1998; 53:269–273.
130. O'Donnell DE, Lam M, Webb KA. Spirometric correlates of improvement in exercise performance after anticholinergic therapy in chronic obstructive pulmonary disease. Am J Respir Crit Care 1999; 160:542–549.
131. Mahler DA, Donohue JF, Barbee RA, et al. Efficacy of salmeterol xinafoate in the treatment of COPD. Chest 1999; 115:957–965.
132. Rennard SI, Anderson W, ZuWallack R, et al. Use of a long-acting inhaled $\beta_2$-adrenergic agonist, salmeterol xinafoate, in patients with chronic obstructive pulmonary disease. Am J Respir Crit Care 2001; 163:1087–1092.
133. Dahl R, Greefhorst LAPM, Nowak D, et al. Inhaled formoterol dry powder versus ipratropium bromide in chronic obstructive pulmonary disease. Am J Respir Crit Care 2001; 164:778–784.
134. Friedman M, Serby CW, Menjoge SS, Wilson JD, Hilleman DE, Witek TJ Jr. Pharmacoeconomic evaluation of a combination of ipratropium plus albuterol compared with ipratropium alone and albuterol alone in COPD. Chest 1999; 115:635–641.
135. Koumis T, Samuel S. Tiotropium bromide: a new long-acting bronchodilator for the treatment of chronic obstructive pulmonary disease. Clin Ther 2005; 27:377–392.
136. Sin DD, McAlister FA, Man SFP, Anthonisen NR. Contemporary management of chronic obstructive pulmonary disease. Scientific review. JAMA 2003; 290:2301–2312.
137. Barr RG, Bourbeau J, Camargo CA, Ram FSF. Inhaled tiotropium for stable chronic obstructive pulmonary disease. Cochrane Database Syst Rev 2005; 18(2):CD002876.
138. Calverley PMA, Lee A, Towse L, Van Noord J, Witek TJ, Kelsen S. Effect of tiotropium bromide on circadian variation in airflow limitation in chronic obstructive pulmonary disease. Thorax 2003; 58:855–860.
139. Littner MR, Ilowite JS, Tashkin DP, et al. Long-acting bronchodilation with once-daily dosing of tiotropium (Spiriva) in stable chronic obstructive pulmonary disease. Am J Respir Crit Care 2000; 161:1136–1142.
140. Brusasco V, Hodder R, Miravitlles M, Korducki L, Towse L, Kesten S. Health outcomes following treatment for six months with once daily tiotropium compared with twice daily salmeterol in patients with COPD. Thorax 2003; 58:399–404.
141. Anzueto A, Tashkin D, Menjoge S, Kesten S. One-year analysis of longitudinal changes in spirometry in patients with COPD receiving tiotropium. Pulm Pharmacol Therapeut 2005; 18:75–81.
142. Celli B, ZuWallack R, Wang S, Kesten S. Improvement in resting inspiratory capacity and hyperinflation with tiotropium in COPD patients with increased static lung volumes. Chest 2003; 124:1743–1748.
143. Casaburi R, Kukafka D, Cooper CC, Witek TJ Jr, Kesten S. Improvement in exercise tolerance with the combination of tiotropium and pulmonary rehabilitation in patients with COPD. Chest 2005; 127:809–817.

144. Cazzola M, Donner CF. Long-acting $\beta_2$-agonists in the management of stable chronic obstructive pulmonary disease. Drugs 2000; 60:307–320.

145. Jarvis B, Markham A. Inhaled salmeterol. A review of its efficacy in chronic obstructive pulmonary disease. Drugs and Aging 2001; 18:441–472.

146. Bartow RA, Brogden RN. Formoterol. An update of its pharmacological properties and therapeutic efficacy in the management of asthma. Drugs 1998; 55:303–322.

147. Johnson M, Rennard SI. Alternative mechanisms for long-acting $\beta_2$-adrenergic agonists in COPD. Chest 2001; 120:258–270.

148. Jaeschke R, Guyatt GH, Cook D, et al. The effect of increasing doses of beta-agonists on airflow in patients with chronic airflow limitation. Resp Med 1993; 87:433–438.

149. Cook D, Guyatt GH, Wong E, et al. Regular versus as-needed short-acting inhaled $\beta$-agonist therapy for chronic obstructive pulmonary disease. Am J Respir Crit Care 2001; 163:85–90.

150. Ram FSF, Sestini P. Regular inhaled short acting $\beta_2$ agonists for the management of stable chronic obstructive pulmonary disease: Cochrane systematic review and meta-analysis. Thorax 2003; 58:580–584.

151. Belman MJ, Botnick WC, Shin JW. Inhaled bronchodilators reduce dynamic hyperinflation during exercise in patients with chronic obstructive pulmonary disease. Am J Respir Crit Care Med 1996; 153:967–975.

152. Saito S, Miyamoto K, Nishimura M, et al. Effects of Inhaled bronchodilators on pulmonary hemodynamics at rest and during exercise in patients with COPD. Chest 1999; 115:376–382.

153. Guyatt GH, Townsend ER, Pugsley SO, et al. Bronchodilators in chronic airflow limitation. Effects on airway function, exercise capacity, and quality of life. Am Rev Respir Dis 1987; 135:1069–1074.

154. The COMBIVENT Inhalation Solution Study Group. Routine nebulized ipratropium and albuterol together are better than either alone in COPD. Chest 1997; 112:1514–1521.

155. Cazzola M, Santangelo G, Piccolo A, et al. Effect of salmeterol and formoterol in patients with chronic obstructive pulmonary disease. Pulm Pharmacol 1994; 7:103–107.

156. Benhamou D, Cuvelier A, Muir JF, et al. Rapid onset of bronchodilation in COPD: a placebo-controlled study comparing formoterol (Foradil® Aerolizer™) with salbutamol (Ventodisk™). Resp Med 2001; 95:817–821.

157. Cazzola M, Centanni S, Regorda C, et al. Onset of action of single doses of formoterol administered via turbuhaler in patients with stable COPD. Pulm Pharmacol Therapeut 2001; 14:41–45.

158. Cazzola M, Matera MG, Santangelo G, Vinciguerra A, Rossi F, D'Amato G. Salmeterol and formoterol in partially reversible severe chronic obstructive pulmonary disease: a dose-response study. Respir Med 1995; 89:357–362.

159. Celik G, Kayacan O, Beder S, Durmaz G. Formoterol and salmeterol in partially reversible chronic obstructive pulmonary disease: a crossover, placebo-controlled comparison of onset and duration of action. Respiration 1999; 66:434–439.

160. Cazzola M, Di Perna F, Noschese P, et al. Effects of formoterol, salmeterol or oxitropium bromide on airway responses to salbutamol in COPD. Eur Respir J 1998; 11:1337–1341.
161. Cazzola Mario, Di Lorenzo Gabriele, Di Perna Felice, Calderaro Francesco, Testi Renato, Centanni Stefano. Additive Effects of Salmeterol and Fluticasone or Theophylline in COPD. Chest 2000; 118:1576–1581.
162. Hanania NA, Kalberg C, Yates J, Emmett A, Horstman D, Knobil K. The bronchodilator response to salmeterol is maintained with regular, long-term use in patients with COPD. Pulm Pharmacol Therapeut 2005; 18:19–22.
163. Donohue JF, Menjoge S, Kesten S. Tolerance to bronchodilating effects of salmeterol in COPD. Respir Med 2003; 97:1014–1020.
164. Husereau D, Shukla V, Boucher M, Mensinkai S, Dales R. Long acting b2-agonists for stable chronic obstructive pulmonary disease with poor reversibioity: a systematic review of randomised controlled trials. BMC Pulm Med 2004; 4:1–11.
165. Bouros D, Kottakis J, Le Gros V, Overend T, Della Cioppa G, Siafakas N. Effects of formoterol and salmeterol on resting inspiratory capacity in COPD patients with poor $FEV_1$ reversibility. Curr Med Res Opinion 2004; 20:581–586.
166. Patakas D, Andreadis D, Mavrofridis E, Argyropoulou P. Comparison of the effects of salmeterol and ipratropium on exercise performance and breathlessness in patients with stable chronic obstructive pulmonary disease. Resp Med 1998; 92:1116–1121.
167. Ayers ML, Mejia R, Ward J, Lentine T, Mahler DA. Effectiveness of salmeterol versus ipratropium bromide on exertional dyspnea in COPD. Eur Resp J 2001; 17:1132–1137.
168. Tashkin DP, Cooper CB. The role of long-acting bronchodilators in the management of stable COPD. Chest 2004; 125:249–259.
169. Martin RM, Dunn NR, Freemantle SN, Mann RD. Risk of non-fatal cardiac failure and ischaemic heart disease with long acting $\beta_2$-agonists. Thorax 1998; 53:558–562.
170. Cazzola M, Imperatore F, Salzillo A, et al. Cardiac effects of formoterol and salmeterol in patients suffering from COPD with preexisting cardiac arrhythmias and hypoxemia. Chest 1998; 114:411–415.
171. COMBIVENT Inhalation Aerosol Study Group. In chronic obstructive pulmonary disease, a combination of ipratropium and albuterol is more effective than either agent alone: an 85-day multicenter trial. Chest 1994; 105: 1411–1419.
172. Ikeda A, Nishimura K, Koyama H, Izumi T. Bronchodilating effects of combined therapy with clinical dosages of ipratropium bromide and salbutamol for stable COPD: comparison with ipratropium bromide alone. Chest 1995; 107:401–405.
173. Campbell S. For COPD a combination of ipratropium bromide and albuterol sulfate is more effective than albuterol base. Arch Intern Med 1999; 159:156–160.
174. Dorinsky PM, Reisner C, Ferguson GT, Menjoge SS, Serby CW, Witek Jr TJ. The combination of ipratropium and albuterol optimizes pulmonary function reversibility testing in patients with COPD. Chest 1999; 115:966–971.

175. Casali L, Grassi C, Rampulla C, et al. Clinical pharmacology of a combination of a bronchodilators. Int J Clin Pharmacol Biopharm 1979; 7:277–280.
176. Lees AW, Allan GW, Smith J. Nebulised ipratropium bromide and salbutamol in chronic bronchitis. Br J Clin Pract 1980; 3:240–242.
177. Leitch AG, Hopkin JM, Ellis DA, et al. The effect of aerosol ipratropium bromide and salbutamol on exercise tolerance in chronic bronchitis. Thorax 1978; 33:711–713.
178. Petrie GR, Palmer KNV. Comparison of aerosol ipratropium bromide and salbutamol in chronic bronchitis and asthma. BMJ 1975; 1:430–432.
179. Lightbody IM, Ingram CG, Legge JS, et al. Ipratropium bromide, salbutamol and prednisolone in bronchial asthma and chronic bronchitis. Br J Dis Chest 1978; 72:181–186.
180. Wesseling G, Mostert R, Wouters EFM. A comparison of effects of anticholinergic and $\beta_2$-agonist and combination therapy on respiratory impedance in COPD. Chest 1992; 101:166–173.
181. Marlin GE. Studies of ipratopium bromide and fenoterol administered by metered-dose inhaler and aerosolized solution. Respiration 1986; 50(suppl 2): 290–293.
182. Serra G, Giacopelli A. Controlled clinical study of a long-term treatment of chronic obstructive lung disease using a combination of fenoterol and ipratropium bromide in aerosol form. Respiration 1986; 50(suppl 2):249–253.
183. Morton O. Response to Duovent of chronic reversible airways obstruction a controlled trial in general practice. Postgrad Med J 1984; 60(suppl 1):32–35.
184. Easton PA, Jadue C, Dhingra S, Anthonisen NR. A comparison of the bronchodilating effects of a beta-2 adrenergic agent (albuterol) and an anticholinergic agent (ipratropium bromide), given by aerosol alone or in sequence. N Engl J Med 1986; 315:735–739.
185. Lloberes P, Ramis L, Montserrat JM, et al. Effect of three different bronchodilators during an exacerbation of chronic obstructive pulmonary disease. Eur Respir J 1988; 1:536–539.
186. Le Doux EJ, Morris JF, Temple WP, et al. Standard and double dose ipratropium bromide and combined ipratropium bromide and inhaled metaproterenol in COPD. Chest 1989; 95:1013–1016.
187. Ullah MI, Newman GB, Saunders KB. Influence of age on response to ipratropium and salbutamol in asthma. Thorax 1981; 36:52309.
188. Rebuck AS, Chapman KR, Abboud RT, et al. Nebulized anticholinergic and sympathomimetic treatment of asthma and chronic obstructive airway disease in the emergency room. Am J Med 1987; 82:59–64.
189. Lakshminarayan S. Iprartopium bromide in chronic bronchitis/emphysema: a review of the literature. Am J Med 1986; 81(suppl 5A):76–80.
190. Newhnham DM, Dhillon DP, Winter JH, et al. Bronchodilator reversibility to low and high doses of terbutaline and ipratropium bromide in patients with chronic obstructive pulmonary disease. Thorax 1993; 48:1151–1155.
191. Matera MG, Caputi M, Cazzola M. A combination with clinical recommended dosages of salmeterol and ipratropium is not more effecive than salmeterol alone in patients with chronic obstructive pulmonary disease. Respir Med 1996; 90:497–499.

192. Sichletidis L, Kottakis J, Marcou S, Constantinidis, TC, Antoniades, A. Bronchodilatory responses to formoterol, ipratropium, and their combination in patients with stable COPD. Int J Clin Pract 1999; 53:185–188.

193. Cazzola M, Di Perna F, Centanni S, et al. Influence of higher than conventional doses of oxitropium bromide on formoterol-induced bronchodilation in COPD. Resp Med 1999; 93:909–911.

194. Cazzola M, Di Perna F, Califano C, Vinciguerra A, D'Amato M. Incremental benefit of adding oxitropium bromide to formoterol in patients with stable COPD. Pulm Pharmacol Therapeut 1999; 12:267–271.

195. Van Noord JA, de Munck DRAJ, Bantje THA, Hop WCJ, Akveld MLM, Bommer AM. Long-term treatment of chronic obstructive pulmonary disease with salmeterol and the additive effect of ipratropium. Eur Resp J 2000; 15:878–885.

196. van Noord JA, Aumann JL, Janssens E, et al. Comparison of tiotropium once daily, formoterl twice daily and both combined once daily in patients with COPD. Eur Respir J 2005; 26:214–222.

197. D'Urzo AD, De Salvo MC, Ramirez-Rivera A, et al. In patients with COPD, treatment with a combination of formoterol and ipratropium is more effective than a combination of salbutamol and ipratropium: A 3-week, randomized, double-blind, within-patient, multicenter study. Chest 2001; 119: 1347–1356.

198. Rutten-van Molken M, Roos B, Van Noord JA. An empirical comparison of the St George's Respiratory Questionnaire (SGRQ) and the Chronic Respiratory Disease Questionnaire (CRQ) in a clinical trial setting. Thorax 1999; 54:995–1003.

199. Van Andel AE, Reisner C, Menjoge SS, Witek TJ. Analysis of inhaled corticosteroid and oral theophylline use among patients with stable COPD from 1987 to 1995. Chest 1999; 115:703–707.

200. vas Fragoso CA, Miller MA. Review of the clinical efficacy of theophylline in the treatment of chronic obstructivce pulmonary disease. Am Rev Respir Dis 1993; 147:S40–S47.

201. Nishimura K, Koyama H, Ikeda A, Izumi T. Is oral theophylline effective in combination with both inhaled anticholinergic agent and inhaled beta-2-agonist in the treatment of stable COPD. Chest 1993; 104:179–184.

202. Taccola M, Bancalari L, Ghignoni G, Paggiaro PL. Salmeterol versus slow-release theophylline in patients with reversible obstructive pulmonary disease. Monaldi Arch Chest Dis 1999; 54:302–306.

203. ZuWallack RL, Mahler DA, Reilly D, et al. Salmeterol plus theophylline combination therapy in the treatment of COPD. Chest 2001; 119:1661–1670.

204. Nishimura K, Koyama H, Ikeda A, Suguira N, Kawakatsu K, Izumi T. The additive effect of theophylline on a high-dose combination of inhaled salbutamol and ipratropium in stable COPD. Chest 1995; 107:718–723.

205. Lipworth BJ. Phosphodiesterase-4 inhibitors for asthma and chronic obstructive pulmonary disease. Lancet 2005; 365:167–175.

206. Compton CH, Gubb J, Nieman R, et al. Cilomilast, a selective phosphodiesterase-4 inhibitor for treatment of patients with chronic obstructive pulmonary disease: a randomised, dose-ranging study. Lancet 2001; 358:265–270.

207. Gamble E, Grootendorst DC, Brightling CE, et al. Antiinflammatory effects of the phosphodiesterase-4 inhibitor Cilomilast (Ariflo) in chronic obstructive pulmonary disease. Am J Respir Crit Care Med 2003; 168:976–982.
208. Rabe KF, Bateman ED, O'Donnell DE, Witte S, Bredenbroker D, Bethke TD. Roflumilast-an oral anti-inflammatory treatment for chronic obstructive pulmonary disease: a randomised controlled trial. Lancet 2005; 366:563–571.
209. Martorana PA, Beume R, Lucattelli M, Wollin L, Lungarella G. Roflumilast fully prevents emphysema in mice chronically exposed to cigarette smoke. Am J Respir Crit Care Med 2005; In Press. Published on June 16, 2005 as doi:10.1164/rccm.200411–1549OC.
210. Burge S. Should inhaled corticosteroids be used in the long term treatment of chronic obstructive pulmonary disease. Drugs 2001; 61:1535–1544.
211. Borron W, deBoisblanc BP. Steroid therapy for chronic obstructive pulmonary disease. Curr Opin Pulm Med 1998; 4:61–65.
212. Man SFP, Sin DD. Inhaled corticosteroids in chronic obstructive pulmonary disease. Is there a clinical benefit? Drugs 2005; 65:579–591.
213. Calverley PMA. The role of corticosteroids in chronic obstructive pulmonary disease. Semin Respir Crit Care Med 2005; 26:235–245.
214. Barnes PJ, Shapiro SD, Pauwels RA. Chronic obstructive pulmonary disease: molecular and cellular mechanisms. Eur Respir J 2003; 22:672–688.
215. Sutherland ER, Martin RJ. Airway inflammation in chronic obstructive pulmonary disease: comparisons with asthma. J Allergy Clin Immunol 2003; 112:819–827.
216. Grumelli S, Corry DB, Song LZ, et al. An immune basis for lung parenchymal destruction in chronic obstructive pulmonary disease and emphysema. PLOS Med 2004; 1:75–83.
217. Saetta MP, Turato G, Maestrelli P, Mapp CE, Fabbri LM. Cellular and structural bases of chronic obstructive pulmonary disease. Am J Respir Crit Care 2001; 163:1304–1309.
218. Barnes PJ, Pedersen S, Busse WW. Efficacy and safety of inhaled corticosteroids. New developments. Am J Respir Crit Care Med 1998; 157: 1S–53.
219. Callahan CM, Dittus RS, Katz BP. Oral corticosteroid therapy for patients with stable chronic obstructive pulmonary disease. A meta-analysis. Ann Intern Med 1991; 114:216–223.
220. Chanez P, Vignola AM, O'Shaugnessy T, et al. Corticosteroid reversibility in COPD is related to features of asthma. Am Rev Respir Crit Care Med 1997; 155:1529–1534.
221. Pizzichini E, Pizzichini M, Gibson P, et al. Sputum eosinophilia predicts benefit from prednisone in smokers with chronic obstructive bronchitis. Am J Respir Crit Care Med 1998; 158:1511–1517.
222. Brightling CE, Monteiro W, Ward R, et al. Sputum eosinophilia and short-term response to prednisolone in chronic obstructive pulmonary disease: a randomised controlled trial. Lancet 2000; 356:1480–1485.
223. Fujimoto K, Kubo K, Yamamoto H, Yamaguchi S, Matsuzawa Y. Eosinophilic inflammation in the airway is related to glucocorticoid reversibility in patients with pulmonary emphysema. Chest 1999; 115:697–702.

224. Postma DS, Steenhuis EJ, van der Weele LT, Sluiter HJ. Severe chronic airflow obstruction: can corticosteroids slow down obstruction? Eur J Respir Dis 1985; 67:56–64.
225. Rice KL, Rubins JB, Lebahn F, et al. Withdrawal of chronic systemic corticosteroids in patients with COPD. A randomized trial. Am J Respir Crit Care 2000; 162:174–178.
226. McEvoy CE, Niewoehner DE. Adverse effects of corticosteroid therapy for COPD. A critical review. Chest 1997; 111:732–743.
227. Sutherland ER, Allmers H, Ayas NT, Venn AJ, Martin AJ. Inhaled corticosteroids reduce the progression of airflow limitation in chronic obstructive pulmonary disease: a meta-analysis. Thorax 2003; 58:937–941.
228. Highland KB, Strange C, Heffner JE. Long-term effects of inhaled corticosteroids on $FEV_1$ in patients with chronic obstructive pulmonary disease. Ann Int Med 2003; 138:969–973.
229. O'Brien A, Russo-Magno P, Karki A, et al. Effects of withdrawal of inhaled steroids in men with severe irreversible airflow obstruction. Am J Respir Crit Care 2001; 164:365–371.
230. Wouters EF, Postma DS, Fokkens B, et al. For the COSMIC (COPD and Seretide: a Multi-Center Intervention and Characterization) Study Group. Withdrawal of fluticasone proprionate from combined salmeterol/fluticasone treatment in patients with COPD causes immediate and sustained disease deterioration: a randomised controlled trial. Thorax 2005; 60:480–487.
231. Sin DD, Tu JV. Inhaled corticosteroids and the risk of mortality and readmission in elderly patients with chronic obstructive pulmonary disease. Am J Respir Crit Care Med 2001; 164:580–584.
232. Sin DD, Man SFP. Inhaled corticosteroids and survival in chronic obstructive pulmonary disease: does the dose matter? Eur J Respir 2003; 21:260–266.
233. Kiri VA, Pride NB, Soriano JB, Vestbo J. Inhaled corticosteroids in chronic obstructive pulmonary disease: results from two observational designs free of immortal bias. Am J Respir Crit Care Med 2005; 172:460–464.
234. Tkacova R, Toth S, Sin DD. Inhaled corticosteroids and survival in COPD patients receiving long-term home oxygen therapy. Respir Med 2005 (Epub ahead of print).
235. Paggiaro PL, Dahle R, Bakran I, Frith L, Hollingworth K, Efthimiou. Group International COPD Study. Multicentre randomised placebo-controlled trial of inhaled fluticasone propionate in patients with chronic obstructive pulmonary disease. Lancet 1998; 351:773–780.
236. Group The Lung Health Study Research. Effect of inhaled triamcinolone on the decline in pulmonary function in chronic obstructive pulmonary disease. N Eng J Med 2000; 343:1902–1909.
237. Spencer S, Calverley PMA, Sherwood BP, Jones PW. Health status deterioration in patients with chronic obstructive pulmonary disease. Am J Respir Crit Care Med 2001; 163:122–128.
238. Spencer S, Calverley PMA, Burge PS, Jones PW. Impact of preventing exacerbations on deterioration of health status in COPD. Eur Respir J 2004; 23: 698–702.

239. Alseedi A, Sin DD, McAlister FA. The effects of inhaled corticosteroids in chronic obstructive pulmonary disease: a systemic review of randomized placebo-controlled trials. Am J Med 2002; 113:59–65.
240. Sin DD, Tu JV. Inhaled corticosteroids and the risk of mortality and readmission in elderly patients with chronic obstructive pulmonary disease. Am J Respir Crit Care 2001; 164:580–584.
241. Sin DD, Johnson M, Gan WQ, Man SF. Combination therapy of inhaled corticosteroids and long-acting beta2-adrenergics in management of patients with chronic obstructive pulmonary disease. Curr Pharm Des 2004; 10:3547–3560.
242. Mahler DA, Wire P, Horstman D, et al. Effectiveness of fluticasone propionate and salmeterol combination delivered via the diskus device in the treatment of chronic obstructive pulmonary disease. Am J Respir Crit Care Med 2002; 166:1084–1091.
243. Calverley P, Pauwels R, Vestbo J, et al. Group. for the TRISTAN (Trial of inhaled steroids and long-acting B2 agoists) study. Combined salmeterol and fluticasone in the treatment of chronic obstructive pulmonary disease: a randomised controlled trial. Lancet 2003; 361:449–456.
244. Szafranski W, Cukier A, Ramirez A, et al. Efficacy and safety of budesonide/ formoterol in the management of chronic obstructive pulmonary disease. Eur Respir J 2003; 21:74–81.
245. Calverley PM, Boonsawat W, Cseke Z, Zhong N, Peterson S, Olsson H. Maintenance therapy with budesonide and formoterol in chronic obstructive pulmonary disease. Eur Respir J 2003; 22:912–919.
246. Hanania NA, Darken P, Horstman D, et al. The efficacy and safety of fluticasone proprionate (250 μg)/salmeterol (50 μg) combined in the diskus inhaler for the treatment of COPD. Chest 2003; 124:834–843.
247. Vestbo J, Pauwels R, Anderson JA, Jones P, Calverley P. On behalf of the TRISTAN study group. Early onset of effect of salmeterol and fluticasone proprionate in chronicc obstructive pulmonary disease. Thorax 2005; 60:301–304.
248. Soriano JB, Vestbo J, Pride NB, Kiri V, Maden C, Maier WC. Survival in COPD patients after regular use of fluticasone propionate and salmeterol in general practice. Eur J Respir 2002; 20:819–825.
249. Soriano JB, Kiri VA, Pride NB, Vestbo J. Inhaled corticosteroids with/without long-acting beta-agonists reduce the risk of reshospitalization and death in COPD patients. Am J Respir Med 2003; 2:67–74.
250. Tarpy SP, Celli BR. Long-term oxygen therapy. N Eng J Med 1995; 333:710–714.
251. Fletcher EC, Lukett RA, Goodnight-White S, Miller CC, Qian W, Costarangos-Galarza C. A double-blind trial of nocturnal supplemental oxygen for sleep desaturation in patients with chronic obstructive pulmonary disease and a daytime $PaO_2$ above 60 mm Hg. Am Rev Respir Dis 1992; 145:1070–1076.
252. Chaouat A, Weitzenblum E, Kessler R, et al. A randomized trial of nocturnal oxygen therapy in chronic obstructive pulmonary disease patients. Eur J Respir 1999; 14:1002–1008.
253. Lacasse Y, Wong E, Guyatt GH, King D, Cook DJ, Goldstein RS. Meta-analysis of respiratory rehabilitation in chronic obstructive pulmonary disease. Lancet 1996; 348:1115–1119.

254. Salman GF, Mosier MC, Beasley BW, Calkins DR. Rehabilitation for patients with chronic obstructive pulmonary disease. Meta-analysis of randomized controlled trials. J Gen Intern Med 2003; 18:213–221.

255. Cambach W, Wagenaar R, Koelman T, van Keimpema A, Kemper H. The long-term effects of pulmonary rehabilitation in patients with asthma and chronic obstructive pulmonary disease: a research synthesis. Archives of Physical Medicine and Rehabilitation 1999; 80:103–111.

256. Guell R, Casan P, Belda J, et al. Long-term effects of outpatient rehabilitation of COPD. A randomized trial. Chest 2000; 117:976–983.

257. Griffiths TL, Campbell IA, Lewis-Jenkins V, et al. Results at 1 year of outpatient multidisciplinary pulmonary rehabilitation: a randomised controlled trial. Lancet 2000; 355:362–368.

258. Troosters T, Gosselink R, Decramer M. Short-and Long-term effects of outpatient rehabilitation in patients with chronic obstructive pulmonary disease: a randomized trial. Am J Med 2000; 109:207–212.

259. Foglio K, Bianchi L, Bruletti G, Battista L, Pagani M, Ambrosino N. Long-term effectiveness of pulmonary rehabilitation in patients with chronic airway obstruction. Eur J Resp 1999; 13:125–132.

260. Ries AL, Kaplan RM, Myers R, Prewitt LM. Maintenance after pulmonary rehabilitation in chronic lung disease. A randomized trial. Am J Respir Crit Care Med 2003; 167:880–888.

261. Morgan MDL, Calverley PMA, Clark CJ, et al. Pulmonary rehabilitation. Thorax 2001; 56:827–834.

262. Bourjeily G, Rochester CL. Exercise training in chronic obstructive pulmonary disease. Clin Chest Med 2000; 214.

263. Stiebelleher L, Quittan M, End A, et al. Aerobic endurance training program improves exercise performance in lung transplant recipients. Chest 1998; 113:906–912.

264. O'Donnell DE. Dyspnea in advanced chronic obstructive pulmonary disease. J Heart Lung Transplant 1998; 17:544–554.

265. Casanova C, Cote C, de Torres JP, et al. Inspiratory-to-total lung capacity ratio predicts mortality in patients with chronic obstructive pulmonary disease. Am J Respir Crit Care Med 2005; 171:591–597.

266. Meyers BF, Patterson GA. Chronic obstructive pulmonary disease. 10: bullectomy, lung volume reduction surgery, and transplantation for patients with chronic obstructive pulmonary disease. Thorax 2003; 58:634–638.

267. Cooper JD, Patterson GA. Lung volume reduction surgery for severe emphysema. Sem Thorac Cardiovasc Surg 1996; 8:52–60.

268. Brenner M, Yusen R, McKenna R Jr, et al. Lung volume reduction surgery for emphysema. Chest 1996; 110:205–218.

269. McKenna RJ, Brenner M, Gelb AF, et al. A randomized, prospective trial of stapled lung reduction versus laser bullectomy for diffuse emphysema. J Thorac Cardiovasc Surg 1996; 111:317–322.

270. McKenna RJ Jr, Brenner M, Fischel RJ, Gelb AF. Should lung volume reduction for emphysema be unilateral or bilateral. J Thorac Cardiovasc Surg 1996; 112:1331–1338.

271. Argenziano M, Thorashow B, Jellen PA, et al. Functional comparison of unilateral versus bilateral lung volume reduction surgery. Ann Thorac Surg 1997; 64:321–327.
272. National Emphysema Treatment Trial Research Group. Safety and efficacy of median sternotomy versus video-assisted thoracic surgery for lung volume reduction surgery. J Thor Cardiovas Surg 2004; 127:1350–1360.
273. Cooper JD, Trulock EP, Triantafillou AN, et al. Bilateral pneumectomy (volume reduction) for chronic obstructive pulmonary disease. J Thorac Cardiovasc Surg 1995; 109:106–116.
274. Benditt JO. Surgical therapies for chronic obstructive pulmonary disease. Respir Care 2004; 49:53–61.
275. Flaherty KR, Martinez FJ. Lung volume reduction surgery for emphysema. Clin Chest Med 2000; 21:819–848.
276. National Emphysema Treatment Trial Research Group. A randomized trial comparing lung-volume-reduction surgery with medical therapy for severe emphysema. N Engl J Med 2003; 348:2059–2073.
277. Lowdermilk GA, Keenan RJ, Landreneau RJ, et al. Comparison of clinical results for unilateral and bilateral thoracoscopic lung volume reduction. Ann Thorac Surg 2000; 69:1670–1674.
278. Keller CA, Ruppel G, Hibbett A, Osterloh J, Naunheim KS. Thoracoscopic lung volume reduction surgery reduces dyspnea and improves exercise capacity in patients with emphysema. Am J Respir Crit Care Med 1997; 156:60–67.
279. Kotloff RM, Tino G, Bavaria JE, et al. Bilateral lung volume reduction surgery for advanced emphysema. A comparison of median sternotomy and thoracoscopic approaches. Chest 1996; 110:1399–1406.
280. Yusen RD, Trulock EP, Pohl MS, Biggar DG. The Washington University Emphysema Surgery Group. Results of lung volume reduction surgery in patients with emphysema. Semin Thorac Cardiovasc Surg 1996; 8:99–109.
281. Brenner M, McKenna RJ Jr, Gelb AF, Fischel RJ, Wilson AF. Rate of $FEV_1$ change following lung volume reduction surgery. Chest 1998; 113:652–659.
282. Flaherty KR, Kazerooni EA, Curtis JL, et al. Short-term and long-term outcomes after bilateral lung volume reduction surgery. Prediction by Quantitative CT. Chest 2001; 119:1337–1346.
283. Yusen RD, Lefrak SS, Gierada DS, et al. A prospective evaluation of lung volume reduction surgery in 200 consecutive patients. Chest 2003; 123: 1026–1037.
284. Dolmage TE, Waddell TK, Maltais F, et al. The influence of lung volume reduction surgery on exercise in patients with COPD. Eur Respir J 2004; 23: 269–274.
285. Martinez FJ, de Oca MM, Whyte RI, Stetz J, Gay SE, Celli BR. Lung-volume reduction improves dyspnea, dynamic hyperinflation, and respiratory muscle function. Am J Respir Crit Care Med 1997; 155:1984–1990.
286. Cordova F, O'Brien G, Furukawa S, Kuzma AM, Travaline J, Criner GJ. Stability of improvement in exercise performance and quality of life following bilateral lung volume reduction surgery in severe COPD. Chest 1997; 112: 907–915.

287. Appleton S, Adams R, Porter S, Peacock M, Ruffin R. Sustained improvements in dyspnea and pulmonary function 3 to 5 years after lung volume reduction surgery. Chest 2003; 123:1838–1846.

288. Yusen RD, Morrow LE, Brown KL. Health-related quality of life after lung volume reduction surgery. Sem Thorac Cardiovasc Surg 2002; 14:403–412.

289. Moy ML, Ingenito EP, Mentzer SJ, Evans RB, Reilly JJ Jr. Health-related quality of life improves following pulmonary rehabiliation and lung volume reduction surgery. Chest 1999; 115:383–389.

290. Goldstein RS, Todd TRJ, Guyatt GH, et al. Influence of lung volume reduction surgery (LVRS) on health related quality of life in patients with chronic obstructive pulmonary disease. Thorax 2003; 58:405–410.

291. Naunheim KS, Hazelrigg SR, Kaiser LR, et al. Risk analysis for thoracoscopic lung volume reduction: a multi-institutional experience. Eur J Cardiothorac Surg 2000; 17:673–679.

292. Ingenito EP, Evans RB, Loring SH, et al. Relation between preoperative inspiratory lung resistance and the outcome of lung-volume-reduction surgery for emphysema. N Engl J Med 1998; 338:1181–1185.

293. Ingenito EP, Loring SH, Moy ML, et al. Comparison of physiological and radiological screening for lung volume reduction surgery. Am J Respir Crit Care Med 2001; 163:1068–1073.

294. Kim V, Criner FJ, Abdallah HY, Gaughan JP, Furukawa SS, Solomides CC. Small airway morphometry and improvement in pulmonary function after lung volume reduction surgery. Am J Respir Crit Care Med 2005; 171: 40–47.

295. Mitsui K, Kurokawa Y, Kaiwa Y, et al. Thoracoscopic lung volume reduction surgery for pulmonary emphysema patients with severe hypercapnia. Jpn J Thorac Cardiovasc Surg 2001; 49:481–488.

296. Gierada DS. Radiologic assessment of emphysema for lung volume reduction surgery. Sem Thorac Cardiovasc Surg 2002; 14:381–390.

297. Kazerooni EA. Radiologic evaluation of emphysema for lung volume reduction surgery. Clin Chest Med 1999; 20:845–861.

298. Goldin JG. Quantitative CT of the lung. Radiol Clin North Am 2002; 40: 45–58.

299. Sciurba FC. Preoperative predictors of outcome following lung volume reduction surgery. Thorax 2002; 57(suppl II):ii47–ii52.

300. Maxfied RA. New and emerging minimally invasive techniques for lung volume reduction. Chest 2004; 125:777–783.

301. Toma TP, Hopkinson NS, Hillier J, et al. Bronchoscopic volume reduction with valve implants in patients with severe emphysema. Lancet 2002; 361: 931–933.

302. Snell GI, Holsworth L, Borrill ZL, et al. The potential for bronchoscopic lung volume reduction using bronchial prostheses. A pilot study. Chest 2003; 124:1073–1080.

303. Hopkinson NS, Toma TP, Hansell DM, et al. Effect of bronchoscopic lung volume reduction on dynamic hyperinflation and exercise in emphysema. Am J Respir Crit Care Med 2005; 171:453–460.

304. Burns KE, Keenan RJ, Grgurich WF, Manzetti JD, Zenati MA. Outcomes of lung volume reduction surgery followed by lung transplantation: a matched cohort study. Ann Thorac Surg 2002; 73:1587–1593.

305. Meyers BF, Yusen RD, Guthrie TJ, et al. Outcome of bilateral lung volume reduction in patients with emphysema potentially eligible for lung transplantation. J Thorac Cardiovasc Surg 2001; 122:10–17.

306. Senbaklavaci O, Wisser W, Ozpeker C, et al. Successful lung volume reduction surgery brings patients into better condition for later lung transplantation. Eur J Cardiothorac Surg 2002; 22:363–367.

307. Maurer JR, Frost AE, Glaville AR, Estenne M, Higenbottam T, Glanville, AR. International guidelines for the selection of lung transplant candidates. Am J Respir Crit Care Med 1998; 158:335–339.

308. Hosenpud JD, Bennett LE, Keck BM, Edwards EB, Novick RJ. Effect of diagnosis on survival benefit of lung transplantation for end-stage lung disease. Lancet 1998; 351:24–27.

309. Charman SC, Sharples LD, McNeil KD, Wallwork J. Assessment of survival benefit after lung transplantation by patient diagnosis. J Heart Lung Trans 2002; 21:226–232.

310. Demeester JD, Smits JMA, Persijn GG, Haverich A. Listing for lung transplantation: life expectancy and transplant effect, stratified by type of end-stage lung disease, the Eurotransplant Experience. J Heart Lung Trans 2001; 20: 518–524.

311. Egan TM, Kotloff RM. Pro/Con debate: lung allocation should be based on medical urgency and transplant survival and not on waiting time. Chest 2005; 128:407–415.

312. Trulock EP, Edwards LB, Taylor DO, Boucek MM, Keck BM, Hertz MI. The Registry of the International Society for Heart and Lung Transplantation: twenty-first official adult lung and heart-lung transplant report–2004. J Heart Lung Transplant 2004; 23:804–815.

313. Stevens PM, Johnson PC, Bell RL, Beall AC, Jenkins DE. Regional ventilation and perfusion after lung transplantation in patients with emphysema. N Eng J Med 1970; 282:245–249.

314. Bates DV. The other lung. N Engl J Med 1970; 282:277–279.

315. Levine SM, Anzueto A, Peters JI, et al. Medium term functional results of single-lung transplantation for endstage obstructive lung disease. Am J Respir Crit Care Med 1994; 150:398–402.

316. Mal H, Sleiman C, Jebrak G, et al. Functional results of single-lung transplantation for chronic obstructive lung disease. Am J Respir Crit Care Med 1994; 149:1476–1481.

317. Levy RD, Ernst P, Levine SM, et al. Exercise performance after lung transplantation. J Heart Lung Transplant 1993; 12:27–33.

318. Pochettino A, Kotloff RM, Rosengard BR, et al. Bilateral versus single lung transplantation for chronic obstructive pulmonary disease: Intermediate-term results. Ann Thorac Surg 2000; 70:1813–1819.

319. Sundaresan RS, Shiraishi Y, Trulock EP, et al. Single or bilateral lung transplantation for emphysema? J Thoracic Cardiovas Surg 1996; 112: 1485–1495.

320. Williams TJ, Patterson GA, McClean PA, Zamel N, Maurer JR. Maximal exercise testing in single and double lung transplant recipients. Am Rev Respir Dis 1992; 145:101–105.
321. Schwaiblmair M, Reichenspurner H, Muller C, et al. Munich Lung Transplant Group. Cardiopulmonary exercise testing before and after lung and heart-lung transplantation. Am J Respir Crit Care Med 1999; 159:1277–1283.
322. Pantoja JG, Andrade FH, Stoki DS, Frost AE, Eschenbacher WL, Reid MB. Respiratory and limb muscle function in lung allograft recipients. Am J Respir Crit Care Med 1999; 160:1205–1211.
323. Tirdel GB, Girgis R, Fishman RS, Theodore J. Metabolic myopathy as a cause of the exercise limitation in lung transplant recipients. J Heart Lung Transplant 1998; 17:1231–1237.
324. Registry of the International Society for Heart and Lung Transplantation-2004. http://www.ishlt.org/registries/heartLungRegistry.asp. Accessed: July 1, 2005.
325. Meyer DM, Bennett LE, Novick RJ, Hosenpud JD. Single versus bilateral, sequential lung transplantation for end-stage emphysema: influence of recipient age on survival and secondary end-points. J Heart Lung Transplant 2001; 20:935–941.
326. UNOS. 2004. 2004 Annual Report of the U.S. Organ Procurement and Transplantation Network and the Scientific Registry of Transplant Recipients: Transplant Data 1994–2003.
327. Weill D, Torres F, Hodges TN, Olmos JJ, Zamora MR. Acute native lung hyperinflation is not associated with poor outcomes after single lung transplant for emphysema. J Heart Lung Transplant 1999; 18:1080–1087.
328. Yonan NA, el-Gamel A, Egan J, Kakadellis J, Rahman A, Deiraniya AK. Single lung transplantation for emphysema: predictors for native lung hyperinflation. J Heart Lung Transplant 1998; 17:192–201.
329. Gavazzeni V, Iapichino G, Mascheroni D, et al. Prolonged independent lung respiratory treatment after single lung transplantation in pulmonary emphysema. Chest 1993; 103:96–100.
330. Popple C, Higgins TL, McCarthy P, Baldyga A, Mehta A. Unilateral auto-PEEP in the recipient of a single lung transplant. Chest 1993; 103:297–299.
331. Anderson MB, Kriett JM, Kapelanski DP, Perricone A, Smith CM, Jamieson SW. Volume reduction surgery in the native lung after single lung transplantation for emphysema. J Heart Lung Transplant 1997; 16:752–757.
332. Venuta F, De Giacomo T, Rendina EA, et al. Thoracoscopic volume reduction of the native lung after single lung transplantation for emphysema. Am J Respir Crit Care Med 1998; 157:292–293.
333. Schulman LL, O'Hair DP, Cantu E, McGregor C, Ginsberg ME. Salvage by volume reduction of chronic allograft rejection in emphysema. J Heart Lung Transplant 1999; 18:107–112.
334. Arcasoy SM, Hersh C, Christie JD, et al. Bronchogenic carcinoma complicating lung transplantation. J Heart Lung Transplant 2001; 20:1044–1053.
335. Collins J, Kazerooni EA, Lacomis J, et al. Bronchogenic carcinoma after lung transplantation: frequency, clinical characteristics, and imaging findings. Radiology 2002; 224:131–138.

336. de Perrot M, Fischer S, Waddell TK, et al. Management of lung transplant recipients with bronchogenic carcinoma in the native lung. J Heart Lung Transplant 2003; 22:87–89.
337. King MB, Campbell EJ, Gray BH, Hertz MI. The proteinase-antiproteinase balance in alpha-1-proteinase inhibitor-deficient lung transplant recipients. Am J Respir Crit Care Med 1994; 149:966–971.
338. Meyer KC, Nunley DR, Dauber JH, et al. Neutrophils, unopposed neutrophil elastase, and alpha1-antiprotease defenses following human lung transplantation. Am J Respir Crit Care Med 2001; 164:97–102.
339. Mal H, Guignabert C, Thabut G, et al. Recurrence of pulmonary emphysema in an alpha-1 proteinase inhibitor-deficient lung transplant recipient. Am J Respir Crit Care Med 2004; 170:811–814.
340. Martinez FJ, Flaherty KR, Iannettoni MD. Patient selection for lung volume reduction surgery. Chest Surg Clin N Am 2003; 13:669–685.

# 5

# Lung Transplant in Cystic Fibrosis

**Raymond D. Coakley and James R. Yankaskas**

*Cystic Fibrosis/Pulmonary Research and Treatment Center, University of North Carolina at Chapel Hill, Chapel Hill, North Carolina, U.S.A.*

## INTRODUCTION

Cystic fibrosis (CF) is the most common fatal inherited disease among whites, affecting more than 30,000 patients in North America (1,2). CF is similarly prevalent in Europe (3) and other parts of the world, including Israel, Australia, and parts of South America (1,2).

Although CF affects multiple organs of epithelial origin, the bulk of the morbidity and mortality in the condition is due to lung disease. CF is caused by mutations in the gene that encodes the CF transmembrane conductance regulator (CFTR) protein. Lack of functional CFTR expression results in abnormal movement of electrolytes and liquid across the plasma membranes of epithelial cells. In the lung, this appears to promote depletion of airway surface liquid, dehydration of the mucus layer that lines airways, and stagnation of the excessively viscous mucus (4). As a result, lungs become chronically infected and inflamed. Characteristically, bronchiectasis develops, with progressive respiratory failure ensuing in 90% of affected individuals (5). In this context, CF has become a dominant indication for lung transplantation.

Improvements in patient care have led to a dramatic increase in the median survival of CF patients over the past 30 years from ~16 years in 1970 to >35 years in 2004 (6), and further improvements in CF patients' survival are projected (7). However, current therapeutic modalities are not curative, and merely slow the development of lung disease, deferring the age at which respiratory failure develops. Thus, we predict that bilateral lung transplantation will remain the ultimate life-preserving option for most patients.

Since the first report of successful application of lung transplantation in CF patients (8), refinements in surgical technique and perioperative medical management have resulted in increasingly successful outcomes. In fact, CF is currently among the most common indications for lung transplantation, and the survival benefit derived by CF patients exceeds that of other patient groups (9). Nonetheless, significant morbidity and mortality are associated with transplantation, which substitutes respiratory failure with chronic immunosuppression and its consequences. Further, CF patients present specific challenges for the transplant team, both before and after surgery.

In this chapter, we review the history of lung transplantation in CF, consider evolving issues relating to indication, timing of transplantation, donor organ allocation, and discuss the management of the CF patient pre– and post–lung transplantation. Finally, we will consider outcomes of the procedure in the CF population.

## LUNG TRANSPLANT HISTORY AND CURRENT CHALLENGES

The first heart–lung transplant for CF was performed in 1983, and lung transplantation has become an effective form of therapy (10). Technical developments led to effective en bloc double-lung transplantation (8) and then to bilateral sequential double-lung transplantation (the current procedure of choice in North America). By 2003, more than 1560 heart–lung or double-lung transplants for CF had been performed in the United States.

The small number of usable donor lungs and the variability in CF clinical course make the timing of transplant referral and allocation of donor organs difficult. These problems are discussed in the following section. Chronic airway infections with common and rare microbes, and multiorgan involvement with CF, pose some clinical problems that are unique to CF individuals. First, existing airway infections and altered antibiotic pharmacokinetics require the knowledge and use of antibiotics and doses tailored to CF bacteriology and drug metabolism in the immediate posttransplant period. Second, the infection with multidrug-resistant *Pseudomonas* species or with *Burkholderia* species alters transplant candidacy and posttransplant treatment at most lung transplant centers. Third, the effects of airway nontuberculous Mycobacteria (NTM) (e.g., *Mycobacterium avium complex* and *Mycobacterium abscessus*) and fungi (e.g., *Aspergillus* spp.) on transplant management and outcomes are not known. Fourth, CF lung transplant recipients may be more susceptible to renal failure, CF-related diabetes mellitus (DM), and osteoporosis. Fifth, the risks and best screening strategies for posttransplant cancer have not been defined.

## REFERRAL CRITERIA FOR LUNG TRANSPLANTATION AND PREDICTORS OF SHORT-TERM MORTALITY IN CF PATIENTS

Although the survival benefit of lung transplantation in CF patients is well documented (9), the decision to transplant is by no means straightforward. Formidable challenges with regard to patient selection, optimal timing of surgery, and equitable allocation of scarce donor organs must be faced. Benefits of transplantation must be weighed against significant accompanying risk, and, given the frustratingly unpredictable rates of clinical decline in CF patients, timing the procedure is challenging. Furthermore, the needs of CF patients must be balanced against those of other patient groups.

Generally accepted criteria for lung transplant referral are discussed elsewhere in this book, and have been modified for CF patients. Following collective consideration by the American Society for Transplant Physicians, American Thoracic Society, European Respiratory Society, and the International Society for Heart and Lung Transplantation, modified guidelines for CF patients were set out in the "International Guidelines for the Selection of Lung Transplant Candidates" (11). At their core is a progressive impairment of pulmonary function manifested by forced expiratory volume in one second ($FEV_1$) of <30% predicted. Other factors that may affect the determination in individual cases include more rapid progressive respiratory deterioration in patients, with $FEV_1$ >30% predicted. This rapid deterioration is characterized by increasing hospitalizations, an unusually rapid fall in $FEV_1$, massive hemoptysis, and increasing cachexia despite optimal medical management. A patient with a $PaCO_2$ of >50 mmHg or a $PaO_2$ of <55 mm Hg while breathing room air, and females whose conditions are deteriorating rapidly, may also be appropriately considered.

The decision to refer a CF patient for transplantation should be based on a firm conviction that the patient will live longer as a result of the procedure. However, this has been less easy to establish than in some other conditions [such as primary pulmonary hypertension (PPH) and idiopathic pulmonary fibrosis (IPF)] in which the clinical course is more predictable. For this reason, the most accurate specific predictors of short-term mortality in CF patients have been sought. The best-characterized and most widely exploited parameter of clinical deterioration is an $FEV_1$ <30% predicted. Kerem et al. reported that $FEV_1$ was the most significant predictor of two-year mortality (~50%) in 673 CF patients (12). In patients older than 18 years, the sensitivity of $FEV_1$ <30% as a predictor of death within two years was 42% with a specificity of 95%. The associated negative predictive value was 97%, suggesting that transplantation could be deferred if a patient's $FEV_1$ remained above this level. An $FEV_1$ <20% was associated with an even lower predicted survival of 20%. Liou and colleagues subsequently studied a larger cohort of ~5800 patients. They confirmed that

$FEV_1$ predicted benefit from lung transplantation, though they suggested that it was more accurately anticipated by a sophisticated multivariate model designed to identify patients with a predicted five-year survival of 30% or less (13,14). A subsequent study by Mayer-Hamblett and colleagues, the largest published to date, including >14,000 CF patients enrolled in the Cystic Fibrosis Foundation Patient Registry, identified age, height, $FEV_1$, respiratory microbiology, number of hospitalizations for pulmonary exacerbation, and number of home intravenous (IV) antibiotic courses as predictors of two-year mortality (15). Disappointingly, however, a model based on these parameters was not demonstrably superior to $FEV_1$ alone as a predicator of short-term mortality. Although both their model and their $FEV_1$ had excellent negative predictive values (98% and 97%, respectively), they had relatively poor positive predictive values (33% and 28%, respectively). This is disappointing, since $FEV_1$ has obvious limitations as a selection criterion when applied to individual CF patients, as physicians readily appreciate when confronted with the tremendous clinical variability observed from case to case in CF.

It must be noted that the parameters analyzed in these models did not include all those that might better predict mortality. However, though other factors have been associated with poor short-term outcomes, results in various studies have been variable, and in many cases studies were limited by accrual of data from single centers and limited sample size.

In the study by Kerem et al., $PaCO_2 > 55$ mmHg (7.3 kPa), $PaO_2$ <50 mmHg (6.65 kPa), age <18 years, and female gender were adverse prognostic indicators (12). Hypercapnia has also been identified as a negative prognostic indicator in other studies. Stanchina and colleagues demonstrated that hypercapnia and severe unilateral lung perfusion abnormalities were primary risk factors for death in CF patients on a lung transplant waiting list (16). Venuta et al. demonstrated that mortality in CF patients awaiting lung transplantation was increased in the presence of hypercapnia. In this study, elevated mean pulmonary arterial pressure, resting tachycardia, and increased cardiac index were also risk factors of earlier death (17,18).

Other potentially useful parameters include measures of exercise performance. In a recent study, elevated breathing reserve index (minute ventilation/maximal voluntary ventilation) was an independent predictor of mortality (as was $FEV_1$ and $PaCO_2$) (19). In a study of 167 CF patients awaiting lung transplantation, a multivariate Cox proportional hazards model identified a shorter 6-minute walk distance as well as higher systolic pulmonary artery pressure and DM as significant risk factors for death on the waiting list (20). Other studies also confirm that pulmonary arterial pressure is a discriminating clinical variable. Both Fraser et al. and Venuto et al. reported its prognostic significance in CF patients as estimated with Doppler echocardiography (18,21). However, given the technical difficulties of echocardiography in very ill patients, direct measurements of pulmonary artery pressure made during catheterization studies are likely to be more accurate and instructive. Finally, wasting has also been suggested to be a negative prognostic indicator in these patients (22).

## A NEW ALLOCATION ALGORITHM FOR DONOR LUNG ALLOCATION IN POTENTIAL LUNG TRANSPLANT CANDIDATES

In the face of challenging medical and ethical issues surrounding transplantation, and given the limited donor pool, the United States initially adopted a straightforward donor organ allocation scheme based primarily on an $FEV_1$ of <30% predicted, suggesting an anticipated survival of two to three years, the anticipated upper end of the current waiting time for lung allocation (23). At this point, patients are generally symptomatic from a respiratory standpoint during daily activities [New York Heart Association (NYHA) class III or IV]. Until recently, potential transplant recipients were grouped by geographical location and ABO blood group, and organs were offered to those with most accrued "waiting time," the single most influential determinant in organ allocation (though physical size is also taken into account, insofar as it influences the feasibility of graft placement). This allocation system does not discriminate between CF patients and other lung transplant candidates.

This system benefited from simplicity and, in particular, allowed CF patients to accrue time, even occasionally becoming inactive on the list if their clinical status was stable by the time they were likely to receive offers of donor organs, due to their seniority on the waiting list. In doing so, patients were in some cases able to "store" their waiting list time pending changes in clinical status. Under this system, however, organ allocation was less likely for patients with more rapidly progressive disease, a population less likely to accrue sufficient time before death intervenes. Furthermore, a significant limitation of the initially adopted system is that it failed to favor organ allocation in patients with a greater likelihood of survival benefit from transplantation. With this regard, it is noteworthy that CF patients accounted for only 16% of patients awaiting lung transplantation in the United States in 2002, whereas 39% of those awaiting the procedure had emphysema, a patient group in which survival benefit has been far less readily demonstrable than in CF.

The need for a more sophisticated system of organ allocation has been fueled by a precipitous increase in the number of patients listed for lung transplantation (300% increase between 1992 and 2002), while the number of transplants performed increased to a lesser extent (from 667 to 1041) over a similar period, reflecting donor organ scarcity. Though the number of active registrants increased in part due to earlier referral for the procedure, and the number of those awaiting lung transplant has stabilized in recent years, attrition of those patients already on the list is still a key concern.

Given the scarcity of organs from suitable brain-dead donors, patients with the highest risk of imminent death as well as those with the greatest chance of survival benefit after transplantation should be given the first priority to receive donor offers. In this light, an alternative allocation system was developed and implemented in the United States in 2005. It is described in detail elsewhere in this text and only details pertinent to CF are discussed here.

Under this new schema, prioritization for organ allocation is based on an allocation score that balances predicted risk of short-term death ("waitlist urgency measure") with predicted survival benefit after transplantation ("transplant benefit score"). A raw allocation score is calculated on the basis of transplant benefit score (measured in days) minus waitlist urgency measure (measured in days), and the raw allocation score is normalized to a continuous allocation score from 1 to 100 to determine the "lung allocation score." A higher score reflects greater likelihood of organ allocation. The clinical parameters used to calculate these scores are individualized for different patient groups. CF and immunodeficiency disorders, such as immunoglobulin deficiency, comprise a single group. In CF, patient parameters used to calculate the waitlist urgency measure include forced vital capacity (FVC), pulmonary artery systolic pressure, supplemental oxygen requirement at rest, age, body mass index, presence of insulin-dependent diabetes, functional status (NYHA class), 6-minute walk distance, and ventilator use. In CF patients, parameters used to calculate transplant benefit score include ventilator use, age, creatinine, and functional status (NYHA class). The transplant benefit score will reflect a greater actuarial survival in CF patients, and, crucially, the diagnosis will increase their likelihood of being allocated organs. All clinical data will have to be updated on a regular basis, except right heart catheterization, which will be repeated only at the discretion of the physician when deterioration is suspected and updated information is necessary to more optimally represent a patient's need for transplantation. It is anticipated that other physiological parameters will be repeated at regular intervals, and also if the patient's clinical status changes, so that this data may be used to update the lung allocation score.

Likely, these parameters will be optimized as time passes and better prospective data become available. FVC was selected since it was found to be strongly predictive of death of patients already on the lung transplant waiting list. However, these patients have already been selected for an $FEV_1 < 30\%$. Thus, the predictive value of FVC in all CF patients is less well defined, and $FEV_1 < 30\%$ should still be a key referral indication.

## INFECTIOUS CONTRAINDICATIONS

The required posttransplant immunosuppression regimen precludes lung transplantation for patients with HIV, hepatitis B (with expression of hepatitis B surface antigen), and active *Mycobacterium tuberculosis* infections. Other organisms can cause significant morbidity and mortality after transplantation (24). Some infections (e.g., *Burkholderia cenocepacia*) are clearly associated with lower survival rates. The choice of whether to transplant CF patients with certain infections differs across the country, and the approaches to patients with such infections are likely to evolve with time and experience.

### *Pseudomonas aeruginosa*

About 80% of CF patients develop chronic *Pseudomonas* infections, and the antibiotic resistance of these bacteria often increases with repeated courses of antibiotic treatment. Multiply antibiotic-resistant (MAR) *P. aeruginosa* are defined by resistance to all antibiotics in two of the following classes: (i) β-lactams (including imipenem and aztreonam), (ii) aminoglycosides, and (iii) fluoroquinolones. Aris et al. found no differences in perioperative complications or two-year survival in 27 CF lung transplant recipients with MAR bacteria compared to 39 recipients with susceptible *Pseudomonas* (25). The six patients in that study with *Burkholderia* had 50% one- and two-year survival, in contrast to 90% and 76% survival rates for those with MAR *Pseudomonas*. In a five-year predicted survival model based on analysis of 845 CF lung transplant recipients, Liou et al. did not find *Pseudomonas* infection to predict worse outcome (26). Few transplant centers exclude *P. aeruginosa*–infected CF patients on the basis of in vitro antibiotic susceptibility tests.

### *Burkholderia* Species

*Burkholderia* is a genus of plant pathogens that rarely infect normal humans, but was recognized as a CF pathogen in 1984 (27). A rapidly fatal course may occur with Burkholderia infection, but the clinical courses are widely variable (28). The nine DNA-defined genomovars in the genus now have species definitions (29). *Burkholderia* are isolated from about 3% of CF patients reported to the U.S. CF Foundation, and *B. cenocepacia* (genomovar III) and *Burkholderia multivorans* (genomovar II) are the most frequent species. Several centers have reported worse posttransplant survival for such patients (30). These survival statistics and the limited supply of donor organs have led many centers to exclude *Burkholderia*-infected CF patients. The significant successes at some centers (25,31) and the possibility that complications are species-specific (32), or that better treatments may be developed, have preserved lung transplant options for such patients at some centers (33).

### Nontuberculous Mycobacteria

NTM, especially *M. avium complex* and *M. abscessus*, are isolated from about 13% of CF patients in the United States (34). It can be difficult to distinguish colonization from disease in such patients, and many do well without anti-NTM antibiotics (35). Mycobacterial burden (assessed by the frequency of acid-fast bacillus smear and culture-positive samples), high-resolution chest

CT scan changes, and the responses to airway clearance and antibacteria therapy treatment may help to distinguish NTM colonization and disease. Post-transplant empyema (36) and death have been reported (37). There is no consensus about the best management of NTM-infected CF patients or the effects of NTM on lung transplant candidacy and outcomes.

### Aspergillus

*Aspergillus* is a genus of ubiquitous fungi that may infect both CF and post-transplant airways. In a consecutive case series, the University of Wisconsin center reported that 17 of 32 (53%) CF transplant recipients had *Aspergillus fumigatus* in their respiratory secretions before transplantation, and that 59% of these had persistent *A. fumigatus* after transplantation. Four of those with pretransplant isolates developed tracheo-bronchial aspergillosis, and one died. These rates were higher than those in lung transplant recipients without CF. The authors recommended early surveillance in such patients (38). A survey of 37 U.S. lung transplant centers found a wide range of surveillance, prophylaxis, and treatment practices, reflecting the lack of controlled trials on this issue (39).

### NONINFECTIOUS CONTRAINDICATIONS

There are few absolute noninfectious contraindications for CF lung transplantation. Significant psychological or social dysfunction is a strong contraindication if it would compromise adherence to the posttransplant care regimen and reduce the likelihood of long-term survival (10). Dysfunction in other organs (e.g., heart, liver, and kidneys) is a relative contraindication, which is comparable to lung transplantation for other indications. Several pulmonary complications that are common in CF merit specific consideration.

### Pneumothorax

Pneumothorax occurs with increasing frequency in older CF patients, and is currently reported at 0.7% per year in CF adults (6). Management of large pneumothoraces often requires tube drainage (40). Optimal choice of chemical agent for pleurodesis in CF patients has not been definitively established, but more recently favored agents are generally effective in CF. Conservative management is recommended, but prior pneumothorax and even pleurodesis do not significantly affect CF lung transplant outcomes (41).

### Massive Hemoptysis

Massive hemoptysis due to chronic airway inflammation and bronchial artery hypertrophy is common in CF, occurring at an annual rate of 0.9% per year and in 4.1% of patients overall (42). Standard treatment with antibiotics, cough suppression, and correction of coagulopathies is often effective. Bronchial artery embolization provides more definitive hemostasis, and does not affect transplant candidacy or outcomes (43).

## Respiratory Failure and Mechanical Ventilation

Respiratory failure is the most common cause of death in CF. A 1978 review of the outcomes of mechanical ventilation for severe CF respiratory disease demonstrated poor outcomes and recommended palliative care in most cases (44). Noninvasive ventilation with nasal or face masks avoids many complications of endotracheal tubes (such as impaired cough) and has sustained CF patients awaiting lung transplantation (45,46). Mechanical ventilation has been used successfully for CF patients awaiting lung transplantation. The University of North Carolina reported 42 CF patients who required intensive care unit (ICU) care for respiratory failure. Of these, 37 (88%) required tracheal intubation and mechanical ventilation. Twenty-three (55%) survived to ICU discharge. Seventeen (40%) received lung transplants, and 14 were alive one year later. Without lung transplantation, three (7%) were alive one year after ICU discharge (47). The authors noted that a few patients with prolonged intubation did well, but that long-term positive pressure ventilation was usually associated with poor outcomes. Initial evaluation for lung transplantation after intubation was impractical.

## Preoperative Management

CF lung transplant candidates have severe pulmonary disease and often require more intense medical care in the months preceding surgery. Effective airway clearance, nutrition, and physical conditioning are particularly important. The techniques are described in review articles and consensus statements (48–50). Knowledge of local transplant candidacy practices is important because some transplant centers have limits on systemic corticosteroid doses or other criteria. Some CF physicians choose antibiotics conservatively in order to reserve drugs with good effectiveness for use during the posttransplant period, when immunosuppression levels are the highest.

## POSTTRANSPLANT COMPLICATIONS AND MANAGEMENT

Postoperative medical complications and management of lung transplant patients are described in detail elsewhere in this book. Therefore, these discussions will be limited to postoperative medical issues specific to CF patients.

## Drug Pharmacokinetics in CF Patients

Pharmacokinetics are altered in CF patients before and after transplantation and differ from other patient groups. This can complicate postoperative management. Achieving satisfactory levels of immunosuppressive drugs can be challenging because of variable absorption after oral ingestion in CF patients. Patients with CF have lower bioavailability of cyclosporine than other transplant patients and greater intersubject variability of pharmacokinetic parameters (51,52). This should be considered when dosing and monitoring are planned. In patients requiring very high doses of calcineurin inhibitor to achieve therapeutic levels, concomitant administration of "azole" class antifungals (such as itraconazole), diltiazem, or clarithromycin has been used successfully to slow down clearance of calcineurin inhibitors and allow lower doses while achieving satisfactory serum levels (53,54). To circumvent altered oral drug absorption in CF patients, alternative routes of drug administration (such as the sublingual route) have been explored (55). Tobramycin pharmacokinetics are altered after transplantation in CF patients. Clearance is decreased, while volume of distribution and serum half-life are increased (56). This should be taken into account when dosing patients in the postoperative period. Although oral ganciclovir has limited bioavailability, its pharmacokinetics in CF patients appear to be satisfactory when compared to other patient groups (57).

## Immunosuppression

Immunosuppressive regimens in CF patients are conventionally similar to those used in non-CF patients. We have used cyclosporine and azathioprine in conjunction with a corticosteroid taper in our CF population and have frequently substituted or added tacrolimus and mycophenolate when medical complications related to these agents are encountered or chronic rejection develops (58). In patients infected with *B. cepacia*, our practice has been to use standard immunosuppression regimens, but consider accelerated corticosteroid tapers and more conservative steroid pulses for acute rejection on a case by case basis, while the patients continue with prolonged (3–4 months) courses of three to four drug antibiotic regimens. Induction regimens, including OKT3 (murine monoclonal antibodies), rabbit antithymocyte globulin, and monoclonal antibodies directed against the interleukin-2 receptor, have been used in ~40% of lung transplant patients (9). However, their specific impact in CF patients is uncharacterized, as are the effects of simolimus and other novel immunosuppressants in the context of CF.

## Intestinal Complications

Gastrointestinal (GI) complications are common in CF (59) and are prone to worsen after transplantation. Among the most important are the intestinal dysmotility and gastroesophageal reflux disease (GERD).

### Intestinal Dysmotility

Immunosuppressive and analgesic agents can exacerbate intestinal dysmotility in CF patients (60). In a retrospective review of 80 CF patients who underwent lung transplantation, Gilljam et al. reported GI issues to be frequent (61). Distal intestinal obstruction syndrome (DIOS) was diagnosed in 20% of patients. Two-thirds had a single episode, mainly in the early postoperative period. One-third of these patients had recurrent episodes. DIOS was generally responsive to medical treatment, though surgery was performed in 2/15 patients. DIOS has potentially catastrophic sequelae and should be anticipated in the early posttransplantation period. Management of DIOS is similar pre- and postoperatively, employing intestinal lavage (62). However, prophylaxis in at-risk patients with osmotically active laxatives (Golytely or lactulose) is prudent.

Gastroesophageal Reflux Disease

GERD is common in CF, affecting between 25% and 50% of patients (63,64). Among CF patients who experience GERD, it has been suggested that esophagitis will develop in as many as 50%. Though GERD may be a consequence of chronic lung disease in CF (due to the associated abnormal abdomino-thoracic pressure gradients and attendant therapies, such as β-agonists that reduce lower esophageal sphincter tone) (59), it does not abate after transplantation, and, on the contrary, appears to worsen, possibly due to esophageal dysmotility, delayed gastric emptying, or inadvertent partial or total surgical vagotomy. In one prospective trial, lung transplantation was found to almost double the number of patients in whom abnormal esophageal acid contact time was detected (65). This is worrisome, as there is a speculative link between GERD and the development of bronchiolitis obliterans syndrome (BOS) in posttransplant patients, and the presence of GERD has been correlated with decreased $FEV_1$ after transplantation (66). Medical staff should have a low threshold for initiating a diagnostic workup, even when prominent symptoms are lacking. Management of GERD in CF patients after transplant is not different in CF patients compared to other patient groups, though there is a case for more aggressive surgical intervention early in potential transplant candidates.

Other potential GI complications in CF patients include cholecystitis, mucocele of the appendix, peptic ulcer disease, and colonic carcinoma (61). Gastric bezoar can complicate as many as 11% of CF patients after transplant (66a). The risk of GI neoplasia in CF transplant patients is discussed below.

## Malabsorption and Malnutrition

Most CF transplant candidates manifest pancreatic exocrine insufficiency and exhibit increased resting energy expenditure. Malnutrition is an important risk factor in transplantation (67), and malabsorption persists after transplantation, so patients should continue taking pancreatic enzyme supplements and supplemental fat-soluble vitamins postoperatively. Resting energy requirements are expected to decline in the absence of persistent inflammation/infection after transplant, and patients are likely to gain weight while receiving corticosteroids. Indeed, some improvements in nutritional indices have been reported in CF patients after transplant (68). Nonetheless, since they may be severely malnourished at the time of surgery, parenteral/enteral nutrition is important and regular nutritional evaluation and intervention are recommended.

## Hepatobiliary Disease

Patients with CF are predisposed to hepatobiliary disease, including hepatic cholestasis, cirrhosis, cholelithiasis, and common bile duct stenosis. Any of these problems may become clinically significant after transplant. Prevalence estimates of clinically significant liver disease/cirrhosis in CF vary from 1% to 9% (6,60,70). Importantly, a high proportion of CF patients (24–30%) have transiently abnormal liver function tests or hepatomegaly even in the absence of cirrhosis (70–72). This should be taken into account when abnormal liver function tests and hepatomegaly are detected in CF patients after transplant. Treatment with the hydrophilic bile acid ursodeoxycholic acid improves bile flow and biochemical indices of liver injury in CF (73), and can be used after transplantation. Though >90% of cirrhosis cases in CF are diagnosed before the age of 14 (70), the development of clinically apparent cirrhosis after lung transplant is not frequent. However, limited data suggest that 72% of CF adults have focal biliary cirrhosis (74); therefore, since a significant proportion of lung transplant patients consume alcohol (75), abstinence should be encouraged in CF patients.

## Infectious Complications

Specific infection control guidelines for CF patients have been published (76). These should be rigorously enforced both before and after transplantation, given the high prevalence of multidrug-resistant organisms in CF patients and the risks of exposure to these organisms in other patient groups.

The specific issues in relation to preoperative infections with multidrug-resistant microorganisms in CF have already been discussed. We conventionally treat CF patients for two to three weeks with broad-spectrum antibiotics in the perioperative period, based on up-to-date bacterial culture and sensitivity results. In patients with *B. cepacia* complex, more prolonged (3–4 months) antibiotic therapy is employed.

After transplantation, CF patients become vulnerable to the same opportunistic infections that affect other patient groups, and these are considered elsewhere in the book. However, *A. fumigatus* is a special case, since high rates of preoperative colonization might predispose CF patients to serious postoperative tracheobronchial aspergillosis in the postoperative period. With this regard, an increased need for early surveillance for *A. fumigatus* has been suggested (38).

## Rhinosinusoidal Disease

Chronic bacterial rhinosinusitis occurs in most CF patients, and sinus infection with multidrug-resistant organisms persists after transplantation. This might have serious consequences in the immunosuppressed host. In 37 CF patients who underwent sinus surgery after lung transplantation, Holzmann et al. demonstrated correlations between (both positive and negative) sinus and bronchoalveolar lavage cultures, and reported that those patients in whom sinus surgery was successful had a lower incidence of tracheobronchitis and pneumonia (77).

## Hypertension

Patients with CF do not appear to be predisposed to develop hypertension. In fact, before transplantation, hypertension is uncommon and blood pressure may even be lower in CF patients (78). Patients may develop hypertension after transplantation as a consequence of corticosteroid therapy, immuno-suppression-associated vascular disease, and renal dysfunction. The incidence of hypertension after lung transplantation is very high ($\sim$50% in the first year and $\sim$85% after that) (79). The management of posttransplant hypertension is similar pre- and posttransplant and is described elsewhere in the text.

## Renal Insufficiency

Although intrinsic renal dysfunction is not a feature of CF, except for an attenuated capacity to excrete sodium chloride, medullary nephrocalcinosis is identified in almost 90% of CF patients at autopsy (80), and renal dysfunction is common in CF patients after transplant. This reflects both cumulative preoperative exposure to potentially nephrotoxic agents and a high incidence of diabetes prior to and after transplantation, as well as treatment with nephrotoxic agents, diabetes, infection, and dehydration in the post-transplant period (81). Thus, it is not surprising that CF patients may have even more rapid rates of glomerular filtration rate decline than other patient groups after lung transplantation (82). Renal-protective management strategies after transplantation include selection of renal-sparing antibiotics where feasible, exploitation of nebulized antibiotics, once daily dosing of amino-glycosides where systemic therapy is essential, avoidance of nonsteroidal anti-inflammatory drugs, careful monitoring and control of diabetes, and monitoring and normalization of electrolytes, including phosphate and oxa-late. In addition, the identification of satisfactory newer immunosuppression protocols may have renal-sparing effects.

## CF-RELATED DIABETES

Although CF-related diabetes (CFRD) occurs in $\sim$6% of all CF patients (83), the incidence increases steeply with advancing age. As many as 35% of patients aged 20–30 years and 43% of patients aged >30 years were affected in one series (84). The incidence of DM in all lung transplant patients during the first year is ~18% (79), which suggests that CF transplant patients have a much higher incidence of DM than other patient groups. Since diabetes is a risk factor of accelerated decline in pulmonary status (85), an even higher proportion of CF patients who are candidates for lung transplantation will be expected to have CFRD. Diabetes is not a contraindication for lung transplantation, unless end-organ damage is present, though its presence is associated with reduced posttransplant survival (9).

The principles of CFRD management pre- and posttransplant are similar and are described in detail elsewhere (83). However, glycemic control is more difficult to achieve after transplant because of concomitant immuno-suppressive/corticosteroid therapy. Subjects with CF are rarely ketosis prone and phenotypically lie between type 1 and type 2 DM. Unfortunately, immunosuppressive regimens add to the risk of vascular end-organ damage after transplant, and, for this reason, we strongly favor early insulin therapy in all CF transplant patients with abnormal glucose control, even though a subset of patients may have tolerable glucose control with oral hypoglycemic drugs before transplant. The risk of new-onset DM appears to be higher with tacrolimus than cyclosporine therapy in solid organ transplant recipients, although tacrolimus may have favorable effects in terms of reduced severity of coronary artery vasculopathy, hyperlipidemia, and hypertension (86).

There are case reports of lung and islet transplantation, with reduction of insulin requirement and normalization of C-peptide levels for several years (87,88).

## Neurologic Complications

Neurologic complications after lung transplantation are common and include severe headache, seizure, infection, and stroke (89). Calcineurin inhibitor toxicity is common, affecting between 10% and 28% of patients who receive cyclosporine-based immunosuppression (90), and has been reported after transplant in CF (91). Risk factors include hypomagnesemia, hypertension, high doses of corticosteroids, and low serum cholesterol. Clinical improvement may be associated with dose reduction or discontinuation of the implicated agent and even substitution with an alternative calcineurin inhibitor (92).

## Posttransplant Lymphoproliferative Disorder and Neoplastic Disorders

Posttransplant lymphoproliferative disorder (PTLD) is a serious and potentially fatal neoplastic complication of the immunosuppressive regimens required for graft protection after lung transplantation. Potent depression of T-cell number and function appears to underlie the neoplastic proliferation of B-cells seen in the condition (93). Primary EBV infection is the major risk factor (94). CF patients, who are younger and less likely to have been previously exposed to EBV, are therefore at special risk (95). In one series, of 14 EBV seronegative CF patients who underwent lung transplantation, 12 seroconverted and 5 developed PTLD (96). Intensive acyclovir prophylaxis may be protective and confer lower risk (97).

Other neoplastic complications occur with increased frequency after lung transplantation (92), but the risk in CF patients has not been shown to be elevated, except for the GI tract. Digestive tract cancers (small bowel, colon, and biliary tract) appear to occur more commonly in CF patients (98,99). In fact, this phenomenon appears to be further accentuated in CF patients after transplant (100), emphasizing the importance of appropriate screening measures in this patient group.

## Bone Disease

Risk factors for bone loss prior to transplant in CF patients include chronic illness, malnutrition, reduced lean body mass and physical activity, delayed puberty and gonadal failure, corticosteroid exposure, and vitamin D/K deficiency. Immunosuppressive therapy carries a very significant additional risk of subsequent bone loss. The combination contributes to an extremely high incidence of osteoporosis in CF transplant patients (101–103). After transplantation, CF patients have a very high incidence of pathologic fracture, ranging from 37% to 42% (104), and it has been suggested that osteonecrosis is particularly prevalent in CF patients after lung transplant (105). Therapy after transplant mirrors that required by CF patients prior to transplant (106), but more frequently requires intensification. Nutritional and vitamin supplementation, as well as antiresorptive and anabolic therapies, have roles in treating osteoporosis in CF transplant patients (107). Since CF patients receiving conventional care (i.e., two daily combination vitamin A, D, E, and K tablets) may still exhibit vitamin D deficiency, more aggressive supplementation is required based on close monitoring of serum 25-hydroxyvitamin D levels. Close attention to adequate supplementation of calcium and vitamin K is also advised. Hormone replacement therapy, where indicated, is recommended to maintain bone mass density (BMD) in patients with CF and delayed puberty/gonadal failure after transplant. Bisphosphonates, including pamidronic acid, etidronic acid, and alendronic acid, reduce bone resorption by inhibiting the recruitment and function of osteoclasts and may be efficacious in glucocorticoid-induced osteoporosis. Pamidronic acid has been shown to be beneficial in improving BMD in CF patients before and after transplantation (108,109). Bone pain, which can complicate IV pamidronate therapy, is less clinically significant in patients on corticosteroids, and therefore the pamidronate may be better tolerated after transplant (108,109). Teriparatide is the first U.S.

FDA-approved anabolic growth agent for bone, and has been shown to increase BMD and decrease fracture incidence in postmenopausal women (107), and may be useful in transplant patients. Calcitonin may also be beneficial in these patients.

### BOS and Graft Rejection

BOS occurs in CF patients, but they have not been shown to be at increased risk of this serious complication. In all patients with BOS, the airways become bronchiectatic and are frequently colonized with *P. aeruginosa*. In CF patients, sinus infection is a likely early source. The management of BOS in CF patients is not different in CF patients compared to other patient groups and is described elsewhere in this book. In a limited open-label, uncontrolled pilot trial of azithromycin therapy for BOS, two of five patients who demonstrated improved lung function with therapy had CF. One non-CF patient failed to respond (110). This suggests that macrolides, which are indicated in CF patients infected with *P. aeruginosa* pretransplantation, may also benefit these patients after surgery. The incidence of BOS in CF patients may be modified by cytokine gene polymorphisms. Interestingly, polymorphisms in the TGFβ gene are associated with accelerated decline in lung function in CF patients prior to transplant as well as the occurrence of BOS afterward (111,112).

### Outcomes of Lung Transplantation in CF Patients

By the end of 2004, 12,357 lung transplants had been preformed in the United States, according to the United Organ Procurement Network Web site (113). Between January 1995 and July 2003, 1746 transplants were performed in CF patients (16% of all lung transplants), making them the third largest cohort of patients to undergo the procedure in the United States, after chronic obstructive pulmonary disease (COPD)/emphysema (39%) and IPF (17%). CF is the most frequent indication for double-lung transplantation, as a large proportion of IPF and emphysema patients receive single lungs.

Retrospective analyses confirmed survival benefit of lung transplantation in CF patients. Several authors have calculated the time of survival benefit after lung transplantation (i.e., the time point at which total survival after transplant equals that while remaining on the waiting list). This figure was 260 days in Charman's single-center analysis of 174 CF patients, and 182 days in Hosenpud's multicenter analysis of 664 CF patients (114,115).

Vricella et al. reported a single-center experience of 64 patients transplanted for CF between 1988 and 2000. Their actuarial survival was 93.2%, 61.8%, and 48.1% at 1, 5, and 10 years, respectively (116). Forty-seven CF patients transplanted in Denmark had even better survival (89%, 80%, and 70% at 1, 3, and 8 years, respectively).

**Table 1** Relative Survival Benefit Following Lung Transplant by Diagnosis

| Year | α-1 (N = 1356) | CF (N = 1923) | COPD (N = 4955) | IPF (N = 2119) | PPH (N = 737) | Sarcoidosis (N = 317) |
|---|---|---|---|---|---|---|
| 1 | 74.7 | 78.6 | 79.9 | 67.5 | 64.8 | 66.7 |
| 3 | 60.0 | 63.0 | 62.4 | 51.6 | 54.4 | 52.8 |
| 5 | 50.2 | 52.9 | 46.8 | 40.0 | 45.2 | 44.9 |
| 7 | 40.2 | 44.9 | 33.7 | 28.3 | 37.3 | 40.4 |
| 10 | 26.0 | 34.1 | 18.2 | 17.5 | 20.3 | 29.8 |

*Note*: Survival comparisons—CF versus COPD: $P=0.0001$; CF versus IPF: $P<0.0001$; CF versus PPH: $P<0.0001$; CF versus sarcoidosis: $P=0.0014$.
*Abbreviations*: CF, cystic fibrosis; COPD, chronic obstructive pulmonary disease; IPF, idiopathic pulmonary fibrosis; PPH, primary pulmonary hypertension.
*Source*: From Ref. 9.

The outcomes of lung transplantation in CF patients, compared to patients with other diagnoses, are excellent. Data reported from the Heart Lung Transplant Registry of the International Society for Heart Lung Transplantation indicate the survival of patients transplanted for CF exceeds that of other diagnoses at all time points (Table 1) (9). This difference reflects, at least in part, the younger age of CF transplant patients, since recipient age is an important predictor of postoperative survival. The odds ratio for one-year mortality rose steeply after the age of 40. However, other factors may contribute, including the experience CF patients have with complex medical regimens.

Certain preoperative factors pertinent to CF patients have been shown to adversely affect one-year mortality after lung transplantation. These include mechanical ventilator or inotrope dependence at the time of initial transplantation, repeat transplantation, panel reactive antibody >10%, donor or recipient history of diabetes, cytomegalovirus status (donor positive/recipient negative), female donor and female recipient, anoxia as a cause of donor death, and recipient hospitalization immediately prior to transplant (9). Total number of human leukocyte antigen (HLA) mismatches, increasing donor age, and infection requiring IV antibiotics were additional risk factors for five-year mortality. In contrast, other recipient factors ($PaCO_2$, chronic steroid use, transfusions, and recent infection requiring IV drug therapy), donor factors (clinical infection, history of hypertension, history of cancer), and factors relating to the transplant (procedure type, ABO compatibility, HLA mismatch, year of transplant, height ratio) did not influence one-year outcomes (9).

CF patients with *B. cepacia* represent a special group, and are transplanted at a limited number of institutions. Egan et al. reported long-term lung transplant outcomes of 123 CF patients, 22 of whom were colonized with *B. cepacia*, at a single center between 1990 and 2001. The actuarial survival at 1, 5, and 10 years was 81%, 59%, and 38%, respectively (33). Although survival was reduced in the patients colonized with *B. cepacia* (one and five year survival of 60% and 36%, respectively), it was not dissimilar to that reported elsewhere for PPH, IPF, and sarcoidosis (Table 1), arguing that this is a defensible use of donor resources. In this analysis, survival was not affected by being on a ventilator immediately prior to transplantation. Survival of five patients who underwent retransplantation for BOS was 60% at one year. A report of the 10-year experience from the Toronto Lung Transplant Program indicated 10-year actuarial survival for CF patients with and without *B. cepacia* infection of 52% and 15%, respectively (117).

The documented beneficial outcomes of transplantation in CF patients extend beyond survival. Although it has been well established that lung transplantation improves quality of life (QOL) (118–120), this effect may be more prominent in CF patients. Durst et al. reported positive psychological outcomes in adolescent CF patients who underwent lung transplantation (121). Vermeulen et al., comparing CF and non-CF patients, demonstrated greater changes in QOL indices after transplantation in the CF recipients (122).

Data on return to work (RTW) after lung transplantation are less readily available than for patients who underwent transplantation of other organs. More than 80% of all patients alive after lung transplantation have no activity limitation (9). Among all transplant patients, 20% to 30% work full time between one and seven years after the procedure (9). Cicutto reported a 37% employment rate in 117 patients after lung transplantation, most of whom had CF or COPD (123). Since younger age was a predictor of RTW, rates for CF patients are likely to be higher. This is consistent with the findings of a study of 99 lung transplant patients by Paris et al., which documented a 37% employment rate for those who are physically able. This is comparable to other types of solid organ transplant recipients, and interestingly, statistically higher RTW rates for CF patients versus patients transplanted for other reasons were reported (124).

## SUMMARY

Respiratory failure will occur in most CF patients, regardless of their genotype or age at diagnosis. The progression of lung disease is slower in many CF patients who are diagnosed as adults, but survival is still difficult to predict. Despite substantial risks and costs, lung transplantation is an effective treatment. CF patients have survival at least as good as patients who receive transplants for other underlying diseases, and many CF patients resume work.

Many transplant-related medical issues are similar for patients with CF and other diseases. The multisystem involvement of CF and its infectious complications produce some transplant and CF related problems that require knowledge of both areas. The importance and benefits of having good working relationships between the lung transplant and the CF care teams in caring for these patients cannot be overemphasized.

## REFERENCES

1. Boucher RC, Knowles MR, Yankaskas JR. Cystic fibrosis. In: Murray and Nadel's Textbook of Respiratory Medicine. Amsterdam: Elsevier, 2005: 1217–1251.
2. FitzSimmons SC. The changing epidemiology of cystic fibrosis. J Pediatr 1993; 122(1):1–9.
3. Gradient of distribution in Europe of the major CF mutation and of its associated haplotype. European Working Group on CF Genetics (EWGCFG). Hum Genet 1990; 85(4):436–445.
4. Boucher RC. New concepts of the pathogenesis of cystic fibrosis lung disease. Eur Respir J 2004; 23(1):146–158.
5. Fiel SB. Clinical management of pulmonary disease in cystic fibrosis. Lancet 1993; 341(8852):1070–1074.
6. Cystic Fibrosis Foundation Patient Registry 2004 Annual Data Report. Bethesda, MD: Cystic Fibrosis Foundation, 2005.
7. Elborn JS, Shale DJ, Britton JR. Cystic fibrosis: current survival and population estimates to the year 2000. Thorax 1991; 46(12):881–885.
8. Ramirez JC, Patterson GA, Winton TL, de Hoyos AL, Miller JD, Maurer JR. Bilateral lung transplantation for cystic fibrosis. The Toronto Lung Transplant Group. J Thorac Cardiovasc Surg 1992; 103(2):287–294.
9. Trulock EP, Edwards LB, Taylor DO, Boucek MM, Keck BM, Hertz MI. The Registry of the International Society for Heart and Lung Transplantation: twenty-first official adult lung and heart-lung transplant report—2004. J Heart Lung Transplant 2004; 23(7):804–815.
10. Yankaskas JR, Mallory GB Jr. Lung transplantation in cystic fibrosis: Consensus Conference Statement. Chest 1998; 113:217–226.
11. International guidelines for the selection of lung transplant candidates. The American Society for Transplant Physicians (ASTP)/American Thoracic Society (ATS)/European Respiratory Society (ERS)/International Society for Heart and Lung Transplantation (ISHLT). Am J Respir Crit Care Med 1998; 158(1):335–339.
12. Kerem E, Reisman J, Corey M, Canny GJ, Levison H. Prediction of mortality in patients with cystic fibrosis. N Engl J Med 1992; 326(18):1187–1191.
13. Liou TG, Adler FR, FitzSimmons SC, Cahill BC, Hibbs JR, Marshall BC. Predictive 5-year survivorship model of cystic fibrosis. Am J Epidemiol 2001; 153(4):345–352.
14. Liou TG, Adler FR, Cahill BC, et al. Survival effect of lung transplantation among patients with cystic fibrosis. J Am Med Assoc 2001; 286(21):2683–2689.
15. Mayer-Hamblett N, Rosenfeld M, Emerson J, Goss CH, Aitken ML. Developing cystic fibrosis lung transplant referral criteria using predictors of 2-year mortality. Am J Respir Crit Care Med 2002; 166(12, Pt 1):1550–1555.

16. Stanchina ML, Tantisira KG, Aquino SL, Wain JC, Ginns LC. Association of lung perfusion disparity and mortality in patients with cystic fibrosis awaiting lung transplantation. J Heart Lung Transplant 2002; 21(2):217–225.

17. Venuta F, Rendina EA, De Giacomo T, et al. Timing and priorities for cystic fibrosis patients candidates to lung transplantation. Eur J Pharm Sci 1998; 8(5):274–277.

18. Venuta F, Rendina EA, Rocca GD, et al. Pulmonary hemodynamics contribute to indicate priority for lung transplantation in patients with cystic fibrosis. J Thorac Cardiovasc Surg 2000; 119(4, Pt 1):682–689.

19. Tantisira KG, Systrom DM, Ginns LC. An elevated breathing reserve index at the lactate threshold is a predictor of mortality in patients with cystic fibrosis awaiting lung transplantation. Am J Respir Crit Care Med 2002; 165(12):1629–1633.

20. Vizza CD, Yusen RD, Lynch JP, Fedele F, Alexander PG, Trulock EP. Outcome of patients with cystic fibrosis awaiting lung transplantation. Am J Respir Crit Care Med 2000; 162(3, Pt 1):819–825.

21. Fraser KL, Tullis DE, Sasson Z, Hyland RH, Thornley KS, Hanly PJ. Pulmonary hypertension and cardiac function in adult cystic fibrosis: role of hypoxemia. Chest 1999; 115(5):1321–1328.

22. Sharma R, Florea VG, Bolger AP, et al. Wasting as an independent predictor of mortality in patients with cystic fibrosis. Thorax 2001; 56(10):746–750.

23. Arcasoy SM, Kotloff RM. Lung transplantation. N Engl J Med 1999; 340(14):1081–1091.

24. Flume PA, Egan TM, Paradowski LJ, Detterbeck FC, Thompson JT, Yankaskas JR. Infectious complications of lung transplantation. Impact of cystic fibrosis. Am J Respir Crit Care Med 1994; 149(6):1601–1607.

25. Aris RM, Gilligan PH, Neuringer IP, Gott KK, Rea J, Yankaskas JR. The effects of panresistant bacteria in cystic fibrosis patients on lung transplant outcome. Am J Respir Crit Care Med 1997; 155:1699–1704.

26. Liou TG, Adler FR, Huang D. Use of lung transplantation survival models to refine patient selection in cystic fibrosis. Am J Respir Crit Care Med 2005; 171(9):1053–1059.

27. Isles A, MacLusky I, Corey M, et al. *Pseudomonas cepacia* infection in cystic fibrosis: an emerging problem. J Pediatr 1984; 104:206–210.

28. Frangolias DD, Mahenthiralingam E, Rae S, et al. Burkholderia cepacia in cystic fibrosis. Variable disease course. Am J Respir Crit Care Med 1999; 160(5, Pt 1):1572–1577.

29. Reik R, Spilker T, LiPuma JJ. Distribution of Burkholderia cepacia complex species among isolates recovered from persons with or without cystic fibrosis. J Clin Microbiol 2005; 43(6):2926–2928.

30. De Soyza A, Corris PA. Lung transplantation and the Burkholderia cepacia complex. J Heart Lung Transplant 2003; 22(9):954–958.

31. Chaparro C, Maurer J, Gutierrez C, et al. Infection with Burkholderia cepacia in cystic fibrosis: outcome following lung transplantation. Am J Respir Crit Care Med 2001; 163(1):43–48.

32. Aris RM, Routh JC, LiPuma JJ, Heath DG, Gilligan PH. Lung transplant- ation for cystic fibrosis patients with Burkholderia cepacia complex. Survival

linked to genomovar type. Am J Respir Crit Care Med 2001; 164(11): 2102–2106.

33. Egan TM, Detterbeck FC, Mill MR, et al. Long term results of lung transplantation for cystic fibrosis. Eur J Cardiothorac Surg 2002; 22(4):602–609.
34. Olivier KN, Weber DJ, Wallace RJ Jr, et al. Nontuberculous mycobacteria in cystic fibrosis: I. Multicenter prevalence study of a potential pathogen in a susceptible population. Am J Respir Crit Care Med 2003; 167(6):828–834.
35. Olivier KN, Weber DJ, Lee JH, et al. Nontuberculous mycobacteria: II. Nested cohort study of impact on cystic fibrosis lung disease. Am J Respir Crit Care Med 2003; 167(6):835–840.
36. Fairhurst RM, Kubak BM, Shpiner RB, Levine MS, Pegues DA, Ardehali A. Mycobacterium abscessus empyema in a lung transplant recipient. J Heart Lung Transplant 2002; 21(3):391–394.
37. Sanguinetti M, Ardito F, Fiscarelli E, et al. Fatal pulmonary infection due to multidrug-resistant Mycobacterium abscessus in a patient with cystic fibrosis. J Clin Microbiol 2001; 39(2):816–819.
38. Helmi M, Love RB, Welter D, Cornwell RD, Meyer KC. Aspergillus infection in lung transplant recipients with cystic fibrosis: risk factors and outcomes comparison to other types of transplant recipients. Chest 2003; 123(3): 800–808.
39. Dummer JS, Lazariashvilli N, Barnes J, Ninan M, Milstone AP. A survey of anti-fungal management in lung transplantation. J Heart Lung Transplant 2004; 23(12):1376–1381.
40. Schidlow DV, Taussig LM, Knowles MR. Cystic Fibrosis Foundation Consensus Conference Report on pulmonary complications of cystic fibrosis. Pediatr Pulmonol 1993; 15:187–198.
41. Curtis HJ, Bourke SJ, Dark JH, Corris PA. Lung transplantation outcome in cystic fibrosis patients with previous pneumothorax. J Heart Lung Transplant 2005; 24(7):865–869.
42. Flume PA, Yankaskas JR, Ebeling M, Hulsey T, Clark LL. Massive hemoptysis in cystic fibrosis. Chest 2005; 128(2):729–738.
43. Brinson GM, Noone PG, Mauro MA, et al. Bronchial artery embolization for the treatment of hemoptysis in patients with cystic fibrosis. Am J Respir Crit Care Med 1998; 157:1951–1958.
44. Davis PB, di Sant'Agnese PA. Assisted ventilation for patients with cystic fibrosis. J Am Med Assoc 1978; 239(18):1851–1854.
45. Hodson ME, Madden BP, Steven MH, Tsang VT, Yacoub MH. Non-invasive mechanical ventilation for cystic fibrosis patients—a potential bridge to transplantation. Eur Respir J 1991; 4(5):524–527.
46. Piper AJ, Parker S, Torzillo PJ, Sullivan CE, Bye PTP. Nocturnal nasal IPPV stabilizes patients with cystic fibrosis and hypercapnic respiratory failure. Chest 1992; 102(3):846–850.
47. Sood N, Paradowski LJ, Yankaskas JR. Outcomes of intensive care unit care in adults with cystic fibrosis. Am J Respir Crit Care Med 2001; 163(2): 335–338.
48. Davis PB, Drumm M, Konstan MW. Cystic fibrosis. Am J Respir Crit Care Med 1996; 154(5):1229–1256.

49. Gibson RL, Burns JL, Ramsey BW. Pathophysiology and management of pulmonary infections in cystic fibrosis. Am J Respir Crit Care Med 2003; 168(8):918–951.

50. Yankaskas JR, Marshall BC, Sufian B, Simon RH, Rodman D. Cystic fibrosis adult care—Consensus Conference Report. Chest 2004; 125:S1–S39.

51. Knoop C, Vervier I, Thiry P, et al. Cyclosporine pharmacokinetics and dose monitoring after lung transplantation: comparison between cystic fibrosis and other conditions. Transplantation 2003; 76(4):683–688.

52. Rousseau A, Monchaud C, Debord J, et al. Bayesian forecasting of oral cyclosporin pharmacokinetics in stable lung transplant recipients with and without cystic fibrosis. Ther Drug Monit 2003; 25(1):28–35.

53. McLachlan AJ, Tett SE. Effect of metabolic inhibitors on cyclosporine pharmacokinetics using a population approach. Ther Drug Monit 1998; 20(4): 390–395.

54. Knower MT, Labella-Walker K, McFadden PM, Kantrow SP, Valentine VG. Clarithromycin for safe and cost-effective reduction of cyclosporine doses in lung allograft recipients. South Med J 2000; 93(11):1087–1093.

55. Reams BD, Palmer SM. Sublingual tacrolimus for immunosuppression in lung transplantation: a potentially important therapeutic option in cystic fibrosis. Am J Respir Med 2002; 1(2):91–98.

56. Dupuis RE, Sredzienski ES. Tobramycin pharmacokinetics in patients with cystic fibrosis preceding and following lung transplantation. Ther Drug Monit 1999; 21(2):161–165.

57. Snell GI, Kotsimbos TC, Levvey BJ, et al. Pharmacokinetic assessment of oral ganciclovir in lung transplant recipients with cystic fibrosis. J Antimicrob Chemother 2000; 45(4):511–516.

58. Yankaskas JR, Aris R. Outpatient care of the cystic fibrosis patient after lung transplantation. Curr Opin Pulm Med 2000; 6(6):551–557.

59. Gaskin KJ. Intestines. In: Yankaskas JR, Knowles MR, eds. Cystic Fibrosis in Adults. Philadelphia: Lippincott-Raven Publishers, 1999:325–342.

60. Lubetkin EI, Lipson DA, Palevsky HI, et al. GI complications after orthotopic lung transplantation. Am J Gastroenterol 1996; 91(11):2382–2390.

61. Gilljam M, Chaparro C, Tullis E, Chan C, Keshavjee S, Hutcheon M. GI complications after lung transplantation in patients with cystic fibrosis. Chest 2003; 123(1):37–41.

62. Cleghorn GJ, Stringer DA, Forstner GG, Durie PR. Treatment of distal intestinal obstruction syndrome in cystic fibrosis with a balanced intestinal lavage solution. Lancet 1986; 1(8471):8–11.

63. Scott RB, O'Loughlin EV, Gall DG. Gastrooesophageal reflux in patients with cystic fibrosis. J Pediatr 1985; 106(2):223–227.

64. Brodzicki J, Trawinska-Bartnicka M, Korzon M. Frequency, consequences and pharmacological treatment of gastroesophageal reflux in children with cystic fibrosis. Med Sci Monit 2002; 8(7):CR529–CR537.

65. Young LR, Hadjiliadis D, Davis RD, Palmer SM. Lung transplantation exacerbates gastroesophageal reflux disease. Chest 2003; 124(5):1689–1693.

66. Hadjiliadis D, Duane DR, Steele MP, et al. Gastroesophageal reflux disease in lung transplant recipients. Clin Transplant 2003; 17(4):363–368.

66a. Dellon E, Morgan D, Mohanty S, Davis K, Aris R. High incidence of gastric bezoars in cystic fibrosis patients after lung transplantation. Transplantation 2006. In press.

67. Sharples L, Hathaway T, Dennis C, Caine N, Higenbottam T, Wallwork J. Prognosis of patients with cystic fibrosis awaiting heart and lung transplantation. J Heart Lung Transplant 1993; 12(4):669–674.

68. Stephenson A, Brotherwood M, Robert R, et al. Increased vitamin A and E levels in adult cystic fibrosis patients after lung transplantation. Transplantation 2005; 79(5):613–615.

69. Scott-Jupp R, Lama M, Tanner MS. Prevalence of liver disease in cystic fibrosis. Arch Dis Child 1991; 66(6):698–701.

70. Feigelson J, Anagnostopoulos C, Poquet M, Pecau Y, Munck A, Navarro J. Liver cirrhosis in cystic fibrosis—therapeutic implications and long term follow up. Arch Dis Child 1993; 68(5):653–657.

71. Nagel RA, Westaby D, Javaid A, et al. Liver disease and bile duct abnormalities in adults with cystic fibrosis. Lancet 1989; 2(8677):1422–1425.

72. Gaskin KJ, Waters DL, Howman-Giles R, et al. Liver disease and common-bile-duct stenosis in cystic fibrosis. N Engl J Med 1988; 318(6):340–346.

73. Colombo C, Castellani MR, Balistreri WF, Seregni E, Assaisso ML, Giunta A. Scintigraphic documentation of an improvement in hepatobiliary excretory function after treatment with ursodeoxycholic acid in patients with cystic fibrosis and associated liver disease. Hepatology 1992; 15(4):677–684.

74. Vawter GF, Shwachman H. Cystic fibrosis in adults: an autopsy study. Pathol Annu 1979; 14(Pt 2):357–382.

75. Evon DM, Burker EJ, Sedway JA, Cicale R, Davis K, Egan T. Tobacco and alcohol use in lung transplant candidates and recipients. Clin Transplant 2005; 19(2):207–214.

76. Saiman L, Siegel J. Infection control recommendations for patients with cystic fibrosis: microbiology, important pathogens, and infection control practices to prevent patient-to-patient transmission. Am J Infect Control 2003; 31(3, Suppl): S1–S62.

77. Holzmann D, Speich R, Kaufmann T, et al. Effects of sinus surgery in patients with cystic fibrosis after lung transplantation: a 10-year experience. Transplantation 2004; 77(1):134–136.

78. Super M, Irtiza-Ali A, Roberts SA, et al. Blood pressure and the cystic fibrosis gene: evidence for lower pressure rises with age in female carriers. Hypertension 2004; 44(6):878–883.

79. Hertz MI, Taylor DO, Trulock EP, et al. The registry of the international society for heart and lung transplantation: nineteenth official report—2002. J Heart Lung Transplant 2002; 21(9):950–970.

80. Katz SM, Krueger LJ, Falkner B. Microscopic nephrocalcinosis in cystic fibrosis. N Engl J Med 1988; 319(5):263–266.

81. Schindler R, Radke C, Paul K, Frei U. Renal problems after lung transplantation of cystic fibrosis patients. Nephrol Dial Transplant 2001; 16(7):1324–1328.

82. Broekroelofs J, Navis GJ, Stegeman CA, et al. Long-term renal outcome after lung transplantation is predicted by the 1-month postoperative renal function loss. Transplantation 2000; 69(8):1624–1628.

83. Moran A, Hardin D, Rodman D, et al. Diagnosis, screening and management of cystic fibrosis related diabetes mellitus: a consensus conference report. Diabetes Res Clin Pract 1999; 45(1):61–73.

84. Moran A, Doherty L, Wang X, Thomas W. Abnormal glucose metabolism in cystic fibrosis. J Pediatr 1998; 133(1):10–17.

85. Rosenecker J, Hofler R, Steinkamp G, et al. Diabetes mellitus in patients with cystic fibrosis: the impact of diabetes mellitus on pulmonary function and clinical outcome. Eur J Morphol 2001; 6(8):345–350.

86. Heisel O, Heisel R, Balshaw R, Keown P. New onset diabetes mellitus in patients receiving calcineurin inhibitors: a systematic review and meta-analysis. Am J Transplant 2004; 4(4):583–595.

87. Tschopp JM, Brutsche MH, Frey JG, et al. End-stage cystic fibrosis: improved diabetes control 2 years after successful isolated pancreatic cell and double-lung transplantation. Chest 1997; 112(6):1685–1687.

88. Cretin N, Buhler L, Fournier B, et al. Results of human islet allotransplantation in cystic fibrosis and type I diabetic patients. Transplant Proc 1998; 30(2):315–316.

89. Goldstein LS, Haug MT III, Perl J, et al. Central nervous system complications after lung transplantation. J Heart Lung Transplant 1998; 17(2):185–191.

90. Walker RW, Brochstein JA. Neurologic complications of immunosuppressive agents. Neurol Clin 1988; 6(2):261–278.

91. Lischke R, Simonek J, Stolz AJ, et al. Cyclosporine-related neurotoxicity in a patient after bilateral lung transplantation for cystic fibrosis. Transplant Proc 2004; 36(9):2837–2839.

92. Kotloff RM, Ahya VN. Medical complications of lung transplantation. Eur Respir J 2004; 23(2):334–342.

93. Armitage JM, Kormos RL, Stuart RS, et al. Posttransplant lymphoproliferative disease in thoracic organ transplant patients: ten years of cyclosporine-based immunosuppression. J Heart Lung Transplant 1991; 10(6):877–887.

94. Randhawa PS, Jaffe R, Demetris AJ, et al. Expression of Epstein-Barr virus-encoded small RNA (by the EBER-1 gene) in liver specimens from transplant recipients with posttransplantation lymphoproliferative disease. N Engl J Med 1992; 327(24):1710–1714.

95. Cohen AH, Sweet SC, Mendeloff E, et al. High incidence of posttransplant lymphoproliferative disease in pediatric patients with cystic fibrosis. Am J Respir Crit Care Med 2000; 161(4 Pt 1):1252–1255.

96. Aris RM, Maia DM, Neuringer IP, et al. Posttransplantation lymphoproliferative disorder in the Epstein–Barr virus-naive lung transplant recipient. Am J Respir Crit Care Med 1996; 154(6, Pt 1):1712–1717.

97. Levine SM, Angel L, Anzueto A, et al. A low incidence of posttransplant lymphoproliferative disorder in 109 lung transplant recipients. Chest 1999; 116(5):1273–1277.

98. Lloyd-Still JD. Cystic fibrosis, Crohn's disease, biliary abnormalities, and cancer. J Pediatr Gastroenterol Nutr 1990; 11(4):434–437.

99. Neglia JP, FitzSimmons SC, Maisonneuve P, et al. The risk of cancer among patients with cystic fibrosis. Cystic Fibrosis and Cancer Study Group. N Engl J Med 1995; 332(8):494–499.

100. Maisonneuve P, FitzSimmons SC, Neglia JP, Campbell PW III, Lowenfels AB. Cancer risk in nontransplanted and transplanted cystic fibrosis patients: a 10-year study. J Natl Cancer Inst 2003; 95(5):381–387.
101. Aris RM, Neuringer IP, Weiner MA, Egan TM, Ontjes D. Severe osteoporosis before and after lung transplantation. Chest 1996; 109(5):1176–1183.
102. Rodino MA, Shane E. Osteoporosis after organ transplantation. Am J Med 1998; 104(5):459–469.
103. Aris RM, Renner JB, Winders AD, et al. Increased rate of fractures and severe kyphosis: sequelae of living into adulthood with cystic fibrosis. Ann Intern Med 1998; 128(3):186–193.
104. Parfitt AM. Risk of vertebral fracture after lung transplantation in cystic fibrosis. Aust N Z J Med 1997; 27(6):707.
105. Schoch OD, Speich R, Schmid C, et al. Osteonecrosis after lung transplantation: cystic fibrosis as a potential risk factor. Transplantation 2000; 69(8): 1629–1632.
106. Aris RM, Merkel PA, Bachrach LK, et al. Guide to bone health and disease in cystic fibrosis. J Clin Endocrinol Metab 2005; 90(3):1888–1896.
107. Hecker TM, Aris RM. Management of osteoporosis in adults with cystic fibrosis. Drugs 2004; 64(2):133–147.
108. Brenckmann C, Papaioannou A. Bisphosphonates for osteoporosis in people with cystic fibrosis. Cochrane Database Syst Rev 2001; 4:CD002010.
109. Aris RM, Lester GE, Renner JB, et al. Efficacy of pamidronate for osteoporosis in patients with cystic fibrosis following lung transplantation. Am J Respir Crit Care Med 2000; 162(3, Pt 1):941–946.
110. Verleden GM, Dupont LJ. Azithromycin therapy for patients with bronchiolitis obliterans syndrome after lung transplantation. Transplantation 2004; 77(9):1465–1467.
111. Knowles MR, Konstan M, Schluchter M, et al. CF gene modifiers: comparing variation between unrelated individuals with different pulmonary phenotypes (abstract). Pediatr Pulmonol 2004; Suppl 27:139.
112. Holweg CT, Weimar W, Uitterlinden AG, Baan CC. Clinical impact of cytokine gene polymorphisms in heart and lung transplantation. J Heart Lung Transplant 2004; 23(9):1017–1026.
113. http://www.optn.org.
114. Charman SC, Sharples LD, McNeil KD, Wallwork J. Assessment of survival benefit after lung transplantation by patient diagnosis. J Heart Lung Transplant 2002; 21(2):226–232.
115. Hosenpud JD, Bennett LE, Keck BM, Edwards EB, Novick RJ. Effect of diagnosis on survival benefit of lung transplantation for end-stage lung disease. Lancet 1998; 351(9095):24–27.
116. Vricella LA, Karamichalis JM, Ahmad S, Robbins RC, Whyte RI, Reitz BA. Lung and heart–lung transplantation in patients with end-stage cystic fibrosis: the Stanford experience. Ann Thorac Surg 2002; 74(1):13–17.
117. de Perrot M, Chaparro C, McRae K, et al. Twenty-year experience of lung transplantation at a single center: Influence of recipient diagnosis on long-term survival. J Thorac Cardiovasc Surg 2004; 127(5):1493–1501.

118.  Lanuza DM, Lefaiver C, Mc CM, Farcas GA, Garrity E Jr. Prospective study
      of functional status and quality of life before and after lung transplantation.
      Chest 2000; 118(1):115–122.
119.  TenVergert EM, Essink-Bot ML, Geertsma A, van Enckevort PJ, de Boer WJ,
      van der BW. The effect of lung transplantation on health-related quality of
      life: a longitudinal study. Chest 1998; 113(2):358–364.
120.  Kugler C, Strueber M, Tegtbur U, Niedermeyer J, Haverich A. Quality of life
      1 year after lung transplantation. Prog Transplant 2004; 14(4):331–336.
121.  Durst CL, Horn MV, MacLaughlin EF, Bowman CM, Starnes VA, Woo MS.
      Psychosocial responses of adolescent cystic fibrosis patients to lung transplan-
      tation. Pediatr Transplant 2001; 5(1):27–31.
122.  Vermeulen KM, van der BW, Erasmus ME, Duiverman EJ, Koeter GH,
      TenVergert EM. Improved quality of life after lung transplantation in indivi-
      duals with cystic fibrosis. Pediatr Pulmonol 2004; 37(5):419–426.
123.  Cicutto L, Braidy C, Moloney S, Hutcheon M, Holness DL, Downey GP.
      Factors affecting attainment of paid employment after lung transplantation.
      J Heart Lung Transplant 2004; 23(4):481–486.
124.  Paris W, Diercks M, Bright J, et al. Return to work after lung transplantation.
      J Heart Lung Transplant 1998; 17(4):430–436.

# 6

# Pulmonary Arterial Hypertension and Lung Transplantation

**Rajan Saggar, David J. Ross, and Joseph P. Lynch III**
*Division of Pulmonary and Critical Care Medicine and Hospitalists, Department of Internal Medicine, David Geffen School of Medicine at UCLA, Los Angeles, California, U.S.A.*

**John L. Faul**
*Division of Pulmonary and Critical Care Medicine, Vera Moulton Wall Center for Pulmonary Vascular Disease, Stanford University, Stanford, California, U.S.A.*

## INTRODUCTION

Heart–lung transplantation (HLT) was developed in the 1980s as a cure for adults with severe pulmonary vascular disease, specifically idiopathic pulmonary hypertension and complex cyanotic congenital heart disease (1). Indeed, 22 of the first 23 HLTs performed at Stanford University between 1982 and 1985 were for patients with end-stage pulmonary vascular disease and resulted in a 60% three-year survival. HLT and lung transplantation (LT) remain important therapies for idiopathic pulmonary arterial hypertension (IPAH) (formerly termed primary pulmonary hypertension), but recent advances in medical therapy make transplantation unnecessary in a significant proportion of patients with PAH. By the early 1990s, the advent of continuous prostacyclin therapies, initially introduced as a bridge therapy to transplantation, resulted in significant improvements in survival outcomes (2,3). These benefits were comparable to those of HLT, and many patients who were thought to be destined for HLT were subsequently removed from the transplant list. In the new millennium, the increasing use of newer and more effective medical strategies for PAH should further delay progression of disease in many patients to the extent that many will no longer require transplantation (4–6). We will therefore premise our discussion of the role of LT as a surgical cure and therapy for IPAH with comments on the current medical strategies for IPAH.

When considering a patient for transplantation there are three major considerations. First, what is the etiology? Second, what is the natural history of the patients disease with current medical therapy? Third, what comorbid conditions might preclude a successful transplantation?

## Diagnosis and Classification Systems

PAH is defined by the presence of a mean pulmonary arterial pressure (PAP) of 25 mmHg or greater at rest, or a mean PAP of $\geq$30 mmHg during exercise. We further classify PAH according to the revised World Health Organization classification system (Table 1). This classification system allows patients to be placed in groups with candidacy for therapy (for instance, some medications in the United States have limited indications for use in patients in Group 1). The classification system also helps to determine patient prognosis and candidacy for transplantation.

**Table 1** World Health Organization Working Classification System for Pulmonary Arterial Hypertension (Venice 2003)

---

Group 1: PAH
  IPAH
  FPAH
  APAH
    Collagen vascular disease
    Congenital systemic-to-pulmonary shunts
    Portal hypertension
  Associated with significant venous or capillary involvement
    PVOD
    PCH
  Persistent pulmonary hypertension of the newborn
Group 2: Pulmonary hypertension with left heart failure
Group 3: Pulmonary hypertension with lung diseases and/or hypoxemia
Group 4 Pulmonary hypertension due to chronic thrombotic and/or embolic
  diseases
Group 5: Miscellaneous

---

*Abbreviations*: PAH, pulmonary arterial hypertension; IPAH, idiopathic pulmonary arterial hypertension; FPAH, familial pulmonary arterial hypertension; APAH, associated with pulmonary arterial hypertension; PVOD, pulmonary veno-occlusive disease; PCH, pulmonary capillary hemangiomatosis.
*Source*: From Ref. 7.

## Factors that Affect Prognosis in PAH

Even within Group 1, prognosis is highly dependent on the etiology of PAH. Eisenmenger's syndrome has a good prognosis, while PAH associated with human immunodeficiency virus infection or collagen vascular disease has a generally poor prognosis (8,9). Furthermore, children with IPAH have a more aggressive course and a worse prognosis (10). In IPAH, prognosis is best suggested by the New York Heart Association (NYHA) functional class, although right atrial pressure, mean PAP, and cardiac output by cardiac catheterization also provide important information (3,11,12). Conventional indicators that patients are candidates for transplantation include advanced NYHA functional class (III/IV despite optimum medical therapy), a cardiac index $<2\,\text{L}/\text{min}/\text{m}^2$, a right atrial pressure $>15\,\text{mmHg}$, and a mean PAP $>55\,\text{mmHg}$.

## THE BIOLOGY OF PULMONARY VASCULAR DISEASE

The precise cause of the progressive obliteration in the pulmonary vascular tree in IPAH is thought to depend on a combination of several factors. Most importantly, there are genetic factors that lead to dysregulation of bone morphogenetic signaling. The first series of genetic mutations associated with human familial PAH (FPAH) were described in the gene that encodes bone morphogenetic protein receptor type 2. Further mutations in the gene for BMPR2 have been demonstrated not only in other families with FPAH, but also in approximately 25% of patients with sporadic, diet-pill–associated disease (13–17). The genetic abnormality is found on the long arm of chromosome 2 and is transmitted in an autosomal dominant fashion, but with reduced (15%) penetrance. The inheritance does not explain the strong predilection for PAH to develop in women. Mutations in a separate gene, *Alk 1*, have also been associated with a familial form of PAH seen in families with hereditary hemorrhagic telangiectasia (HHT) (18,19). These families do not demonstrate mutations in the gene for BMPR2. The penetrance of disease in these families is low, suggesting that a combination of factors might be required to develop severe disease. Additional factors that have been implicated include (i) a loss of pulmonary arterial bed (due to intraluminal thrombosis or lung disease); (ii) vasoconstriction due to an excess of vasoconstrictive compounds (e.g., endothelin, serotonin) and/or a deficiency of endogenous pulmonary arterial vasodilators (e.g., prostacyclin and nitric oxide); and (iii) vascular remodeling due to a disordered accumulation of pulmonary arterial endothelial cells and smooth muscle cells that lead to luminal narrowing (18). Current effective therapies directed at these processes include anticoagulants, endothelin receptor antagonists, phosphodiesterase inhibitors, prostacyclin analogs, and nitric oxide.

The pathology of severe PAH is characterized by a progressive luminal narrowing due to intimal thickening, onion-skin formation, and plexiform lesions (20,21). While prior classification systems emphasized the pathology to describe subtypes of disease, current guidelines emphasize clinical aspects of the disease since these clinical markers help to guide patient management and prognosis.

## THE MEDICAL MANAGEMENT OF PAH

In addition to therapies aimed at reversing or attenuating pulmonary vascular disease, patient management in PAH involves the management of heart failure. Most patients receive high-dose diuretics and digoxin, although there are no controlled studies of whether their use in pulmonary hypertension leads to improved prognosis.

### The Natural History of Untreated PAH

The natural history of PAH depends on the etiology, the age of the patient, the use of medical therapies, and the presence or absence of right heart failure (22). The National Institutes of Health registry dating from the 1980s determined a 50% five year mortality for patients with untreated IPAH (22). It appears that FPAH has a course that progresses more rapidly and occurs earlier in each successive generation (17,23). Generally, children have a more rapid progression of disease. In a prospective follow-up study of 194 patients in the Patient Registry for the Characterization of Primary Pulmonary Hypertension supported by the National Heart, Lung, and Blood Institute, the estimated median survival was 2.8 years (95% CI, 1.9–3.7 years). Survival rates at one year were 68% (CI, 61–75%); at three years, 48% (CI, 41–55%); and at five years, 34% (CI, 24–44%). In that study, the variables associated with poor survival included an NYHA functional class of III or IV, the presence of Raynaud's phenomenon, an elevated mean right atrial pressure, an elevated mean PAP, a low cardiac index, and a low diffusing capacity for carbon monoxide ($DL_{co}$) (22).

### Natural History of Treated PAH

The outcomes for patients receiving medical therapy for PAH have been closely studied over the past 10 years. In addition to many short-duration (three months) randomized controlled studies (Table 2), there are long-term (>2 years), open-label studies that report subject mortality and progression of disease (31). In both settings, the patient's functional class, etiology, and therapy significantly influence prognosis.

Although rarely used nowadays, there are some data that suggest a benefit with calcium-channel blockers in patients with PAH (3,32,33). In our experience, only a small subset (<5%) of IPAH patients respond to an acute challenge with calcium-channel blockers (34). "Responders" are patients who experience a ≥20% decrease in mean pulmonary-artery pressure (mPAP)

**Table 2** Randomized Controlled Trials in Primary Pulmonary Hypertension

| Therapy | $N$ | Duration (weeks) | End point | References |
|---------|-----|------------------|-----------|-----------|
| Epoprostenol | 81 | 12 | 6-minute walk distance | (24) |
| Trepostinil | 470 | 12 | 6-minute walk distance | (25) |
| Iloprost | 203 | 12 | 6-minute walk distance | (26) |
| Beraprost | 130 | 12 | 6-minute walk distance | (27) |
| Bosentan | 32 | 12 | 6-minute walk distance | (28) |
| Bosentan | 213 | 12 | 6-minute walk distance | (29) |
| Sitaxsetan | 178 | 12 | $VO_{2max}$ | (30) |

and pulmonary vascular resistance (PVR) with calcium-channel blockers. In these subjects, long-term therapy leads to sustained hemodynamic improvement and prolonged survival (35). In a trial designed to assess the efficacy of calcium-channel blockers in idiopathic PAH, Rich et al. found that patients taking coumadin had better survival (50% at five years compared to 25% in those who did not receive coumadin) (36). However, anticoagulants were recommended on the basis of nonuniformity of pulmonary blood flow on lung scan, which could have led to subgroup bias with some patients with thromboembolic disease having a better prognosis when treated with coumadin (36). In support of the concept that coumadin might improve outcome, one retrospective, single-center study found that 78 IPAH patients given coumadin had better survival than 37 patients not receiving anticoagulant (37).

The most important advance in the management of patients with IPAH during the 1990s was the introduction of epoprostenol. Chronic intravenous epoprostenol therapy leads to an improvement in both exercise tolerance and hemodynamic measures, and survival in IPAH (2,24). Barst et al. reported one-, three-, and five-year survival with epoprostenol of 87%, 63%, and 54% compared with 77%, 41%, and 27% in historical controls, respectively (24). However, epoprostenol is not equally effective across all patient groups. For example, in patients who receive epoprostenol, those with fenfluramine-induced PAH had a poorer survival rate (50% at one year) than patients with IPAH (88% at one year). There appears to be a different prognosis even when the groups are corrected for PVR and functional class: those with diet-pill–induced disease had an 18% five-year survival versus 39% in IPAH (38). This difference suggests referral for a transplantation evaluation as soon as the diagnosis of diet-pill–associated PAH is made. Similarly, while epoprostenol is also effective for the treatment of PAH from scleroderma, it does not confer a survival advantage (39). Smaller series suggest that it may help patients with PAH from congenital heart disease (40).

In addition to epoprostenol, other prostanoid analogs appear to show benefit. In a retrospective, nonrandomized trial, beraprost given to IPAH patients maintained improvement in exercise tolerance and hemodynamic profile along with a survival benefit at one, two, and three years compared with controls (41). Hoeper et al. documented improvement in exercise capacity and hemodynamics at one year in IPAH patients who received inhaled iloprost (42). However, administration of iloprost required six to eight inhalations daily, given every two to three hours while the patient was awake. Treprostinil is another prostanoid analog that can be administered by continuous subcutaneous or intravenous infusions and leads to improved 6-minute walk distance, dyspnea, and hemodynamic profile (27). The benefits seen with treprostinil have been demonstrated to persist up to 18 months. Since many of these new agents significantly improve exercise tolerance and hemodynamic measures, they should be considered for IPAH patients as a possible alternative to transplantation.

Endothelin receptor antagonists have been developed to treat PAH, and currently both dual receptor antagonists and selective endothelin receptor antagonists are commonly prescribed. They are active orally and lead to improved exercise endurance, hemodynamics, and functional class over the short term. Long-term studies that examine survival up to 36 months demonstrate Kaplan–Meier survival estimates of 96% at 12 months and 89% at 24 months, compared to a predicted survival of 69% and 57%, respectively. At one and three years, 85% and 70% of patients, respectively, remained alive and on bosentan monotherapy (29).

Using animal models, there are several other classes of drugs that appear to attenuate or reverse PAH, including elastase inhibitors (43), statins (44), and arginine (45). However, long-term data on their impact on patient survival are currently lacking. Oral sildenafil, in particular, might prove a useful therapy since it appears both to have a potent vasodilator effect and to reverse established disease in animal models. Sildenafil might also have superior efficacy over epoprostenol in patients with restrictive lung disease (46).

IPAH patients with a patent foramen ovale appear to have improved survival compared to those without this feature (47). Atrial septostomy (i.e., the creation of a small perforation in the atrial septum) has therefore been used for patients with end-stage right heart failure and leads to less episodes of syncope and better exercise performance (48). The creation of a right-to-left shunt (a surgical atrial septostomy) can cause reductions in arterial saturation. This downside is outweighed by the benefits of a lower mean right atrial pressure and increases in left ventricular preload, which help to "unload" the right ventricle and improve cardiac output.

## LT for IPAH

The overall performance of LT for all indications has increased 52% since 1993. In contrast, lung transplant for IPAH have actually declined by

15% (49). This unique trend reflects the advent of prostacyclin therapy and newer oral therapy with endothelin receptor antagonists and sildenafil.

LT for pulmonary vascular disease has been closely studied ever since the first report in 1982 (1). In the 2004 annual reports, the Organ Procurement and Transplant Network (OPTN)/Scientific Registry of Transplant Recipients (SRTR) (OPTN/SRTR data as of May 3, 2004) and the International Society of Heart and Lung Transplantation (ISHLT) registry (49) reported 74% and 65% one-year patient survival rates, respectively, after deceased donor lung transplants for IPAH. These results are the lowest survival rates of all lung transplant indications. Interestingly, the increased mortality is most prevalent in the first three months and is thought to be strongly influenced by intra- or perioperative factors. If patients survive at least three months, the ISHLT registry reports an 89% one-year survival for IPAH lung transplant recipients, a rate comparable to other lung allograft recipients such as those with chronic obstructive pulmonary disease (COPD) and cystic fibrosis. More importantly, this trend continues for up to 10 years (49), supporting the concept that a perioperative survival disadvantage exists among IPAH lung transplant recipients. Some workers have also suggested that some IPAH patients are at an increased risk for the early development of bronchiolitis obliterans syndrome (BOS), compared to non-IPAH lung transplant recipients (50).

## Surgical Procedure of Choice

The appropriate surgical procedure for patients with IPAH and secondary PAH (mostly Eisenmenger's syndrome, chronic thromboembolic disease, and parenchymal lung disease) has been the subject of long-standing debate. Initially, HLT was considered the procedure of choice (51). In the early 1990s, a shift occurred favoring LT. This change was based on observations that pulmonary hemodynamics and right ventricular function normalized quickly after LT, and these effects persisted at three months or even as long as four years after single-lung transplantation (SLT) for IPAH (52–55). SLT might be benefical over bilateral lung transplantation (BLT) for IPAH and secondary PAH because of the improved operative risk profile [relative ease of SLT, simultaneous repair of simple intracardiac defects (56–58), shorter cardiopulmonary bypass (CPB) and ischemic times, and similar postoperative right ventricular functional and hemodynamic recovery] and improved donor availability, without compromising postoperative graft/patient morbidity and mortality. Also, it is possible that SLT allows for pathologic regression of IPAH in the native lung as a consequence of the marked hemodynamic changes post transplantation (59).

The Pittsburgh group compared recipients of SLT versus BLT with either underlying IPAH or secondary PAH and found identical functional status and postoperative recovery (hemodynamics, duration of mechanical ventilation, ICU/hospital stay, and incidence of acute/chronic rejection) (60). However, they reported that SLT recipients had a significantly lower $PaO_2/FiO_2$ at one hour and higher mPAP at 12 and 24 hours. Bando et al. concluded that despite a significantly shortened CPB duration in their cohort, SLT recipients with underlying PAH (idiopathic or secondary) had significantly less functional recovery (less reduction in mPAP and increase in cardiac index) and higher graft mortality compared with BLT and HLT recipients (61). A similar nonsignificant trend ($P = 0.07$) was seen in the percentage of mPAP reduction in an IPAH cohort, with SLT recipients faring worse than BLT (62).

Some centers favor BLT because of the physiologically increased functional reserve, making patients less prone to respiratory insufficiency with subsequent insult (i.e., acute cellular rejection) (63,64). The Hopkins experience evaluated 15 patients with IPAH (all of whom received CPB) and found BLT to have a highly significant survival advantage compared to SLT, at all time points up to four years (62). The most recent ISHLT registry 2004 report suggests a nonsignificant trend ($P = 0.3$) toward increased survival favoring BLT compared to SLT in patients with underlying IPAH (49).

The surgical procedure of choice for patients with underlying IPAH and secondary PAH remains unclear since retrospective data support all three modalities. The ultimate decision regarding type of procedure appears to be center specific and depends on historical experience, donor availability, the degree of preoperative cardiac dysfunction, and the complexity of underlying congenital heart disease in the cases of Eisenmenger's physiology.

### IPAH/Secondary PAH and Ischemia Reperfusion Lung Injury

The relatively high mortality in PAH patients who receive lung transplants occurs in the early postoperative period (49) (within 30 days of LT) and is largely attributable to primary graft failure (PGF) ($\sim$30%) and non–cytomegalovirus infections ($\sim$23%) (49). PGF represents the fraction of patients without clear evidence of infection, rejection, or technical complications as a cause of respiratory failure and mortality. PGF is the extreme of a clinical spectrum of early posttransplant lung injury termed ischemia reperfusion lung injury (IRLI) (also pulmonary reimplantation response, reperfusion/reimplantation edema, and allograft dysfunction).

IRLI typically occurs within 72 hours after LT and is a syndrome characterized by noncardiogenic pulmonary edema, hypoxemia, and diffuse alveolar damage (65). Since the definition can be somewhat nebulous, the analysis of risk factors contributing to IRLI becomes complex. Radiographically, lung infiltrates compatible with IRLI post LT have been reported in 97% of patients, making this feature of the definition somewhat unreliable (66). There are also reports to support risk factors for IRLI, including several perioperative factors, e.g., preservation/reperfusion technique (38,67–69), graft ischemia time (70–73), use of CPB (74–78), use of induction chemotherapy (79), and recipient characteristics [e.g., allosensitization (80), preoperative PAH, right ventricular dysfunction (77), among others].

It remains controversial whether the diagnosis of IPAH before transplantation (IPAH or secondary PAH) is a risk factor for IRLI/PGF. Animal studies using SLT in rats for chemical-induced PAH demonstrate a preferential flow of blood to the allograft, which was fatal in cases of severe preoperative PAH, presumably because of increased IRLI (81,82). A retrospective review in humans comparing SLT for PAH and emphysema confirmed significantly increased allograft blood flow in the PAH patients (83,84). However, despite highly significant differences in pre- and postoperative systolic PAP between the two groups, the incidence and severity of IRLI based on chest X-ray (CXR) scores and $PaO_2/FiO_2$ ratio at 24 hours were not statistically different. The CXR score at 24 hours predicted intensive care unit length of stay (ICU-LOS) of $\geq 7$ days for both groups; however, the threshold score of the patients with PAH was significantly lower. The authors concluded that perioperative PAH and increased allograft blood flow do not directly lead to post-LT IRLI. The reason why this PAH cohort was significantly more susceptible to increased ICU-LOS possibly relates to a limited compensatory pulmonary vascular reserve in the face of IRLI. This conclusion obviated the question regarding a possible advantage to BLT in patients with underlying PAH. No comment was made regarding the use of CPB; however, CPB was likely used in a greater percentage of patients with underlying PAH and possibly contributed to the conclusions.

The Australian group compared BLT for PAH versus all other non-PAH indications and found significantly decreased $PaO_2/HO_2$ ratio in the first 24 hours and increased postoperative blood loss, without any differences in reoperation rate, time on mechanical ventilation, tracheostomy rate, ICU or hospital length of stay, or hospital mortality (85). Importantly, CPB was used in all PAH patients and only in 5% of the non-PAH cohort, possibly accounting for the noted differences.

The analysis of risk factors contributing to IRLI/PGF is difficult since the retrospective studies to date do not follow a standard definition (71,78, 86–88). Preoperative PAH (88) and right ventricle dysfunction (moderate to severe right ventricle hypokinesis) (86) have been reported as risk factors for IRLI; however, some studies do not support this finding (78) and others simply did not pursue this specific analysis (71,87). Similarly, there are studies to both support (86–88) and refute (71,78) the correlation between IRLI/PGF and increased mortality. Using $PaO_2/FiO_2$ as the determinant of IRLI/PGF grading (grades 0–3), recently defined by ISHLT consensus, there is significant discriminant validity for mortality at 30 days, especially when evaluated at 72 hours (89). Furthermore, IRLI/PGF might increase the risk of late BOS, further affecting mortality after LT (90).

## Morbidity and Mortality Associated with LT for IPAH/Secondary PAH

Several authors report a relatively high early intra- or postoperative morbidity and mortality in patients who receive LT for pulmonary vascular disease (91,92). The ISHLT registry identifies IPAH as a risk factor for one-year mortality (OR 2.24; $P < 0.0001$) and recipient PVR as a continuous risk factor for 1- and 5-year mortality ($P = 0.01$ and $P = 0.002$, respectively) (49). The Washington University study cohort (including adults and children with either IPAH or PAH secondary to a congenital heart defect) found 10% to 26% of patients having either reoperation (the majority with bleeding), urgent reintubation, tracheostomy, cardiac arrest, sepsis, or postoperative extracorporeal membrane oxygenation (ECMO) (93). The hospital mortality for the IPAH subgroup was 10% (data not analyzed by surgical procedure type), significantly less than the 23% reported for LT for PAH secondary to a congenital heart defect. Of note, preoperative mPAP was not a risk factor predictive of hospital mortality.

Extrapolating ISHLT registry data, there is an approximate "background" mortality of ~7.3% in the first 30 days after LT for all indications (data for January 1992 through June 2003) (49). The reported recipient mortality in hospital or at 30 days after either SLT or BLT for IPAH/secondary PAH is between 5% and 19% (54,60–62,93,94).

Is it the presence of PAH, the degree of PAH (e.g., preoperative mPAP), or the type of PAH (IPAH vs. secondary PAH) that accounts for the increased early morbidity and mortality in this cohort of patients? All available studies are retrospective with few patients and have several confounding and uncontrolled factors, including CPB requirements, surgical procedure type, preoperative management (IPAH patients often were treated with prostacyclin and coumadin), functional status assessment at the time of LT (e.g., NYHA functional class/6-minute walk), among others, making it difficult to answer this question.

The Hopkins group attempted to address these issues in one retrospective study and found similar actuarial four-year survival between IPAH and secondary PAH patients (62). However, within the IPAH group, the BLT subgroup had significantly improved survival at all time points up to four years; no significant survival differences were seen in the secondary PAH subgroups even with further analysis taking into account an mPAP threshold of 40 mmHg. When all patients with mPAP > 40 mmHg were combined (all required CPB), either IPAH or secondary PAH, there was a trend to a survival advantage for BLT recipients at all time points.

The Denver group found no survival advantage for BLT when comparing patients with and without secondary PAH (excluding Eisenmenger's syndrome) (95). Interestingly, only a single patient required CPB for intraoperative hemorrhage and no patients had preoperative severe PAH, i.e., mPAP > 40 mmHg, making the results difficult to extrapolate to all patients with secondary PAH.

### Special Considerations with LT and Pulmonary Vascular Disease

The effect of LT for pulmonary vascular disease can allow for almost immediate improvement in right ventricular function (55), but how is the left ventricle affected? The concept of transient left ventricular failure was first described in 1993 (96) and reported again as a possible complication of LT for PAH (97). Presumably, this phenomenon results from the increased preload for the left ventricle after LT normalizes the PVR.

IPAH is not generally considered a recurrent or de novo disease after LT. However, several interesting case reports have emerged. Anastomotic pulmonary hypertension secondary to narrowing of the pulmonary artery (98), recurrent pulmonary veno-occlusive disease after HLT (99), and de novo pulmonary capillary hemangiomatosis after BLT (100) have all been reported.

The Minnesota group has reported IPAH as an independent risk factor for obliterative bronchiolitis (OB) with an odds ratio of 2.7 versus non-IPAH patients (50). The Australian group found no difference in rates of BOS among BLT recipients comparing an IPAH/Eisenmenger's syndrome cohort to all other indications (85). Furthermore, there is probably no difference in freedom from BOS between IPAH and PAH secondary to Eisenmenger's syndrome (93). Most retrospective studies have not found a correlation between the type of procedure (i.e., HLT, SLT, or BLT) and the subsequent development of BOS for LT recipients with underlying PAH (60,62); one study did find a significant decrease in freedom from BOS in SLT versus BLT recipients with underlying pulmonary vascular disease (Eisenmenger's syndrome and IPAH) (93).

LT for pulmonary vascular disease in the setting of a systemic connective tissue disease is controversial and traditionally considered a significant risk for graft failure. LT for PAH associated with systemic disorders (with the exception of sarcoidosis) is mostly performed on patients with underlying connective tissue disease, such as progressive systemic sclerosis (PSSc), rheumatoid arthritis, and systemic lupus erythematosus. Several centers have reported experiences comparable to those obtained in patients who undergo LT for isolated pulmonary disease (101–105). Unfortunately, we have personally seen cases of "renal crisis" requiring sustained hemodialysis after LT for PSSc (105).

### CONCLUSIONS

LT remains an important cure for patients with end-stage PAH. However, several important points need to be emphasized. First, we predict that fewer patients will progress to LT since the medical management of PAH continues to improve and a wider spectrum of effective therapies are evolving for this patient population. Second, technical advances in both pediatric cardiac surgery and cardiac diagnostics will ensure that the prevalence of unrepaired congenital heart defects will continue to decline. It is notable that many patients who underwent HLT for Eisenmenger's complex were born before the era of heart bypass surgery. Third, the outcomes for PAH patients soon after LT remain poorer than for other patient populations, but we look forward to improved outcomes in the near future. Currently, potential candidates need to understand the risks and benefits of LT for PAH.

## REFERENCES

1. Reitz BA, Wallwork JL, Hunt SA, et al. Heart-lung transplantation: successful therapy for patients with pulmonary vascular disease. N Engl J Med 1982; 306(10):557–564.
2. Magnani B, Galie N. Prostacyclin in primary pulmonary hypertension. Eur Heart J 1996; 17(l):18–24.
3. McLaughlin VV. Medical management of primary pulmonary hypertension. Expert Opin Pharmacother 2002; 3(2):159–165.
4. Paramothayan NS, Lasserson TJ, Wells AU, Walters EH. Prostacyclin for pulmonary hypertension in adults. Cochrane Database Syst Rev 2005; 2:CD002994.
5. Cohen H, Chahine C, Hui A, Mukherji R. Bosentan therapy for pulmonary arterial hypertension. Am J Health Syst Pharm 2004; 61(11):1107–1119.
6. Budev MM, Minai OA, Arroliga AC. Overview of treprostinil sodium for the treatment of pulmonary arterial hypertension. Drugs Today (Barc) 2004; 40(3):225–234.
7. Simonneau G, Galie N, Rubin LJ, et al. Clinical classification of pulmonary hypertension. J Am Coll Cardiol 2004; 43(12 suppl S):5S–12S.
8. Pellicelli AM, D'Ambrosio C, Vizza CD, et al. HIV-related pulmonary hypertension. From pathogenesis to clinical aspects. Acta Cardiol 2004; 59(3):323–330.
9. Velasquez EM, Glancy DL. Cardiovascular disease in patients infected with the human immunodeficiency virus. J La State Med Soc 2003; 155(6):314–324.
10. Yung D, Widlitz AC, Rosenzweig EB, Kerstein D, Maislin G, Barst RJ. Outcomes in children with idiopathic pulmonary arterial hypertension. Circulation 2004; 110(6):660–665.
11. Reichart B, Gulbins H, Meiser BM, Kur F, Briegel J, Reichenspurner H. Improved results after heart-lung transplantation: a 17-year experience. Transplantation 2003; 75(l):127–132.
12. Bennett LE, Keck BM, Hertz MI, Trulock EP, Taylor DO. Worldwide thoracic organ transplantation: a report from the UNOS/ISHLT international registry for thoracic organ transplantation. Clin Transpl 2001:25–40.
13. Deng Z, Haghighi F, Helleby L, et al. Fine mapping of PPH1, a gene for familial primary pulmonary hypertension, to a 3-cM region on chromosome 2q33. Am J Respir Crit Care Med 2000; 161(3 Pt 1):l055–1059.

14. Gottmann U, van der Woude FJ, Braun C. Endothelin receptor antagonists: a new therapeutic option for improving the outcome after solid organ transplantation? Curr Vase Pharmacol 2003; 1(3):281–299.

15. Lane KB, Machado RD, Pauciulo MW, et al. Heterozygous germline mutations in BMPR2, encoding a TGF-beta receptor, cause familial primary pulmonary hypertension. The International PPH Consortium. Nat Genet 2000; 26(l):81–84.

16. Loyd JE. Genetics and pulmonary hypertension. Chest 2002; 122(suppl 6):284S–286S.

17. Morse JH, Jones AC, Barst RJ, Hodge SE, Wilhelmsen KC, Nygaard TG. Mapping of familial primary pulmonary hypertension locus (PPH1) to chromosome 2q31-q32. Circulation 1997; 95(12):2603–2606.

18. Morrell NW, Yang X, Upton PD, et al. Altered growth responses of pulmonary artery smooth muscle cells from patients with primary pulmonary hypertension to transforming growth factor-beta(l) and bone morphogenetic proteins. Circulation 2001; 104(7):790–795.

19. Abdalla SA, Gallione CJ, Barst RJ, et al. Primary pulmonary hypertension in families with hereditary haemorrhagic telangiectasia. Eur Respir J 2004; 23(3):373–377.

20. Heath D, Edwards JE. The pathology of hypertensive pulmonary vascular disease; a description of six grades of structural changes in the pulmonary arteries with special reference to congenital cardiac septal defects. Circulation 1958; 18(4 Pt l):533–547.

21. Voelkel NF, Tuder RM. Severe pulmonary hypertensive diseases: a perspective. Eur Respir J 1999; 14(6):1246–1250.

22. D'Alonzo GE, Barst RJ, Ayres SM, et al. Survival in patients with primary pulmonary hypertension. Results from a national prospective registry. Ann Intern Med 1991; 115(5):343–349.

23. Morse JH. Genetic studies of pulmonary arterial hypertension. Lupus 2003; 12(3):209–212.

24. Barst RJ, Rubin LJ, Long WA, et al. A comparison of continuous intravenous epoprostenol (prostacyclin) with conventional therapy for primary pulmonary hypertension. The Primary Pulmonary Hypertension Study Group. N Engl J Med 1996; 334(5):296–302.

25. Simonneau G, Barst RJ, Galie N, et al. Continuous subcutaneous infusion of treprostinil, a prostacyclin analogue, in patients with pulmonary arterial hypertension: a double-blind, randomized, placebo-controlled trial. Am J Respir Crit Care Med 2002; l65(6):800–804.

26. Olschewski H, Simonneau G, Galie N, et al. Inhaled iloprost for severe pulmonary hypertension. N Engl J Med 2002; 347(5):322–329.

27. Galie N, Humbert M, Vachiery JL, et al. Effects of beraprost sodium, an oral prostacyclin analogue, in patients with pulmonary arterial hypertension: a randomized, double-blind, placebo-controlled trial. J Am Coll Cardiol 2002; 39(9):1496–1502.

28. Channick RN, Simonneau G, Sitbon O, et al. Effects of the dual endothelin-receptor antagonist bosentan in patients with pulmonary hypertension: a randomised placebo-controlled study. Lancet 2001; 358(9288):1119–1123.

29. McLaughlin VV, Sitbon O, Badesch DB, et al. Survival with first-line bosentan in patients with primary pulmonary hypertension. Eur Respir J 2005; 25(2):244–249.

30. Barst RJ, Langleben D, Frost A, et al. Sitaxsentan therapy for pulmonary arterial hypertension. Am J Respir Crit Care Med 2004; 169(4):441–447.

31. Sitbon O, Badesch DB, Channick RN, et al. Effects of the dual endothelin receptor antagonist bosentan in patients with pulmonary arterial hypertension: a 1-year follow-up study. Chest 2003; 124(l):247–254.

32. Rubin LJ, Moser K. Long-term effects of nitrendipine on hemodynamics and oxygen transport in patients with cor pulmonale. Chest 1986; 89(l):141–145.

33. Rubin LJ, Nicod P, Hillis LD, Firth BG. Treatment of primary pulmonary hypertension with nifedipine. A hemodynamic and scintigraphic evaluation. Ann Intern Med 1983; 99(4):433–438.

34. Rich S, Kaufmann E. High dose titration of calcium channel blocking agents for primary pulmonary hypertension: guidelines for short-term drug testing. J Am Coll Cardiol 1991; 18(5):1323–1327.

35. Rich S, Brundage BH, Levy PS. The effect of vasodilator therapy on the clinical outcome of patients with primary pulmonary hypertension. Circulation 1985; 71(6):1191–1196.

36. Rich S, Kaufmann E, Levy PS. The effect of high doses of calcium-channel blockers on survival in primary pulmonary hypertension. N Engl J Med 1992; 327(2):76–81.

37. Cohen M, Edwards WD, Fuster V. Regression in thromboembolic type of primary pulmonary hypertension during 2 1/2 years of antithrombotic therapy. J Am Coll Cardiol 1986; 7(1):172–175.

38. Ardehali A, Laks H, Russell H, et al. Modified reperfusion and ischemia-reperfusion injury in human lung transplantation. J Thorac Cardiovasc Surg 2003; 126(6):1929–1934.

39. Badesch DB, Tapson VF, McGoon MD, et al. Continuous intravenous epoprostenol for pulmonary hypertension due to the scleroderma spectrum of disease. A randomized, controlled trial. Ann Intern Med 2000; 132(6):425–434.

40. Rosenzweig EB, Kerstein D, Barst RJ. Long-term prostacyclin for pulmonary hypertension with associated congenital heart defects. Circulation 1999; 99(14): 1858–1865.

41. Nagaya N, Uematsu M, Okano Y, et al. Effect of orally active prostacyclin analogue on survival of outpatients with primary pulmonary hypertension. J Am Coll Cardiol 1999; 34(4):1188–1192.

42. Hoeper MM, Schwarze M, Ehlerding S, et al. Long-term treatment of primary pulmonary hypertension with aerosolized iloprost, a prostacyclin analogue. N Engl Med 2000; 342(25):1866–1870.

43. Cowan KN, Heilbut A, Humpl T, Lam C, Ito S, Rabinovitch M. Complete reversal of fatal pulmonary hypertension in rats by a serine elastase inhibitor. Nat Med 2000; 6(6):698–702.

44. Nishimura T, Vaszar LT, Faul JL, et al. Simvastatin rescues rats from fatal pulmonary hypertension by inducing apoptosis of neointimal smooth muscle cells. Circulation 2003; 108(13):1640–1645.

45. Mitani Y, Maruyama K, Sakurai M. Prolonged administration of L-arginine ameliorates chronic pulmonary hypertension and pulmonary vascular remodeling in rats. Circulation 1997; 96(2):689–697.
46. Ghofrani HA, Wiedemann R, Rose F, et al. Combination therapy with oral sildenafil and inhaled iloprost for severe pulmonary hypertension. Ann Intern Med 2002; 136(7):515–522.
47. Glanville AR, Burke CM, Theodore J, Robin ED. Primary pulmonary hypertension. Length of survival in patients referred for heart-lung transplantation. Chest 1987; 91(5):675–681.
48. Sandoval J, Gaspar J, Pulido T, et al. Graded balloon dilation atrial septostomy in severe primary pulmonary hypertension. A therapeutic alternative for patients nonresponsive to vasodilator treatment. J Am Coll Cardiol 1998; 32(2):297–304.
49. Trulock EP, Edwards LB, Taylor DO, Boucek MM, Keck BM, Hertz MI. The Registry of the International Society for Heart and Lung Transplantation: twenty-first official adult heart transplant report—2004. J Heart Lung Transplant 2004; 23(7):804–815.
50. Kshettry VR, Kroshus TJ, Savik K, Hertz MI, Bolman RM. Primary pulmonary hypertension as a risk factor for the development of obliterative bronchiolitis in lung allograft recipients. Chest 1996; 110(3):704–709.
51. Griffith BP, Hardesty RL, Trento A, et al. Heart-lung transplantation: lessons learned and future hopes. Ann Thorac Surg 1987; 43(1):6–16.
52. Pasque MK, Trulock EP, Kaiser LR, Cooper JD. Single-lung transplantation for pulmonary hypertension. Three-month hemodynamic follow-up. Circulation 1991; 84(6):2275–2279.
53. Pasque MK, Kaiser LR, Dresler CM, Trulock E, Triantafillou AN, Cooper JD. Single lung transplantation for pulmonary hypertension. Technical aspects and immediate hemodynamic results. J Thorac Cardiovasc Surg 1992; 103(3): 475–481; discussion 481–482.
54. Pasque MK, Trulock EP, Cooper JD, et al. Single lung transplantation for pulmonary hypertension. Single institution experience in 34 patients. Circulation 1995; 92(8):2252–2258.
55. Katz WE, Gasior TA, Quinlan JJ, et al. Immediate effects of lung transplantation on right ventricular morphology and function in patients with variable degrees of pulmonary hypertension. J Am Coll Cardiol 1996; 27(2):384–391.
56. Fremes SE, Patterson GA, Williams WG, Goldman BS, Todd TR, Maurer J. Single lung transplantation and closure of patent ductus arteriosus for Eisenmenger's syndrome. Toronto Lung Transplant Group. J Thorac Cardiovasc Surg 1990; 100(1):1–5.
57. Kreitmann B, Metras D, Badier M. Unilateral lung transplantation for Eisenmenger's syndrome. J Thorac Cardiovasc Surg 1992; 104(2):529–530.
58. Lupinetti FM, Boiling SF, Bove EL, et al. Selective lung or heart-lung transplantation for pulmonary hypertension associated with congenital cardiac anomalies. Ann Thorac Surg 1994; 57(6):1545–1548; discussion 1549.
59. Levy NT, Liapis H, Eisenberg PR, Botney MD, Trulock EP. Pathologic regression of primary pulmonary hypertension in left native lung following

right single-lung transplantation. J Heart Lung Transplant 2001; 20(3): 381–384.

60. Gammie JS, Keenan RJ, Pham SM, et al. Single- versus double-lung transplantation for pulmonary hypertension. J Thorac Cardiovasc Surg 1998; 115(2):397–402; discussion 402–403.

61. Bando K, Armitage JM, Paradis IL, et al. Indications for and results of single, bilateral, and heart-lung transplantation for pulmonary hypertension. J Thorac Cardiovasc Surg 1994; 108(6):1056–1065.

62. Conte JV, Borja MJ, Patel CB, Yang SC, Jhaveri RM, Orens JB. Lung transplantation for primary and secondary pulmonary hypertension. Ann Thorac Surg 2001; 72(5):1673–1079; discussion 1679–1680.

63. Levine SM, Jenkinson SG, Bryan CL, et al. Ventilation-perfusion inequalities during graft rejection in patients undergoing single lung transplantation for primary pulmonary hypertension. Chest 1992; 101(2):401–405.

64. Birsan T, Zuckermann Z, Aitermiou O, et al. Bilateral lung transplantation for pulmonary hypertension. Transplant Proc 1997; 29(7):2892–2894.

65. de Perrot M, Liu M, Waddell TK, Keshavjee S. Ischemia-reperfusion-induced lung injury. Am J Respir Crit Care Med 2003; 167(4):490–511.

66. Anderson DC, Glazer HS, Semenkovich JW, et al. Lung transplant edema: chest radiography after lung transplantation—the first 10 days. Radiology 1995; 195(1):275–281.

67. Keshavjee SH, Yamazaki F, Cardoso PF, McRitchie DI, Patterson GA, Cooper JD. A method for safe twelve-hour pulmonary preservation. J Thome Cardiovasc Surg 1989; 98(4):529–534.

68. Steen S, Kimblad PO, Sjoberg T, Lindberg L, Ingemansson R, Massa G. Safe lung preservation for twenty-four hours with Perfadex. Ann Thome Surg 1994; 57(2):450–457.

69. Sundaresan S, Lima O, Date H, et al. Lung preservation with low-potassium dextran flush in a primate bilateral transplant model. Ann Thome Surg 1993; 56(5):1129–1135.

70. Thabut G, Mai H, Cerrina J, et al. Graft ischemic time and outcome of lung transplantation: a multicenter analysis. Am J Respir Crit Care Med 2005; 171(7):786–791.

71. Sleiman C, Mai H, Fournier M, et al. Pulmonary reimplantation response in single-lung transplantation. Eur Respir J 1995; 8(l):5–9.

72. Ware LB, Golden JA, Finkbeiner WE, Matthay MA. Alveolar epithelial fluid transport capacity in reperfusion lung injury after lung transplantation. Am J Respir Crit Care Med 1999; 159(3):980–988.

73. Prop J, Ehrie MG, Crapo ID, Nieuwenhuis P, Wildevuur CR. Reimplantation response in isografted rat lungs. Analysis of causal factors. J Thorac Cardiovasc Surg 1984; 87(5):702–711.

74. Gammie JS, Cheul Lee J, Pham SM, et al. Cardiopulmonary bypass is associated with early allograft dysfunction but not death after double-lung transplantation. J Thorac Cardiovasc Surg 1998; 115(5):990–997.

75. Wan S, LeClerc JL, Vincent JL. Cytokine responses to cardiopulmonary bypass: lessons learned from cardiac transplantation. Ann Thorac Surg 1997; 63(1):269–276.

76. AebaR, Griffith BP, Kormos RL, et al. Effect of cardiopulmonary bypass on early graft dysfunction in clinical lung transplantation. Ann Thorac Surg 1994; 57(3):715–722.

77. Chatila WM, Criner GJ. Complications of long-term mechanical ventilation. Respir Care Clin N Am 2002; S(4):631–647.

78. Khan SU, Salloum J, O'Donovan PB, et al. Acute pulmonary edema after lung transplantation: the pulmonary reimplantation response. Chest 1999; 116(1):187–194.

79. Palmer SM, Miralles AP, Lawrence CM, Gaynor JW, Davis RD, Tapson VF. Rabbit antithymocyte globulin decreases acute rejection after lung transplantation: results of a randomized, prospective study. Chest 1999; 116(l):127–133.

80. Lau CL, Palmer SM, Posther KE, et al. Influence of panel-reactive antibodies on posttransplant outcomes in lung transplant recipients. Ann Thorac Surg 2000; 69(5):1520–1524.

81. Kawaguchi AT, Kawashima Y, Mizuta T, et al. Single lung transplantation in rats with fatal pulmonary hypertension. J Thorac Cardiovasc Surg 1992; 104(3):825–829.

82. Kawaguchi AT, Mizuta T, Matsuda H, et al. Single lung transplantation in rats with chemically induced pulmonary hypertension. J Thorac Cardiovasc Surg 1992; 103(3):483–489.

83. Boujoukos AJ, Martich GD, Vega JD, Keenan RJ, Griffith BP. Reperfusion injury in single-lung transplant recipients with pulmonary hypertension and emphysema. J Heart Lung Transplant 1997; 16(4):439–448.

84. Bando K, Keenan RJ, Paradis TJL, et al. Impact of pulmonary hypertension on outcome after single-lung transplantation. Ann Thorac Surg 1994; 58(5): 1336–1342.

85. Ueno T, Smith JA, Snell GI, et al. Bilateral sequential single lung transplantation for pulmonary hypertension and Eisenmenger's syndrome. Ann Thorac Surg 2000; 69(2):381–387.

86. Chatila WM, Furukawa S, Gaughan JP, Criner GJ. Respiratory failure after lung transplantation. Chest 2003; 123(l):165–173.

87. Thabut G, Vinatier I, Stern JB, et al. Primary graft failure following lung transplantation: predictive factors of mortality. Chest 2002; 121(6):1876–1882.

88. King RC, Binns OA, Rodriguez F, et al. Reperfusion injury significantly impacts clinical outcome after pulmonary transplantation. Ann Thorac Surg 2000; 69(6):l681–1685.

89. Christie TD, Carby M, Bag R, Corris P, Hertz M, Weill D. Report of the ISHLT working group on primary lung-graft dysfunction part II: a consensus statement of the international society for heart and lung transplantation. J Heart Lung Transplant 2005; 24:1454–1460.

90. Fiser SM, Tribble CG, Long SM, et al. Ischemia-reperfusion injury after lung transplantation increases risk of late bronchiolitis obliterans syndrome. Ann Thorac Surg 2002; 73(4):1041–1047; discussion 1047–1048.

91. Mikhail G, al-Kattan K, Banner N, et al. Long-term results of heart-lung transplantation for pulmonary hypertension. Transplant Proc 1997; 29(l–2): 633.

92. Bridges ND, Mallory GB Jr, Huddleston CB, Canter CE, Sweet SC, Spray TL. Lung transplantation in children and young adults with cardiovascular disease. Ann Thorac Surg 1995; 59(4):813–820; discussion 820–821.
93. Mendeloff EN, Meyers BF, Sundt TM, et al. Lung transplantation for pulmonary vascular disease. Ann Thorac Surg 2002; 73(l):209–217; discussion 217–219.
94. Davis RD Jr, Trulock EP, Manley J, et al. Differences in early results after single-lung transplantation. Washington University Lung Transplant Group. Ann Thorac Surg 1994; 58(5):1327–1334; discussion 1334–1335.
95. Huerd SS, Hodges TN, Grover FL, et al. Secondary pulmonary hypertension does not adversely affect outcome after single lung transplantation. J Thorac Cardiovasc Surg 2000; 119(3):458–465.
96. Chapelier A, Vouhe P, Macchiarini P, et al. Comparative outcome of heart-lung and lung transplantation for pulmonary hypertension. J Thorac Cardiovasc Surg 1993; 106(2):299–307.
97. Birsan T, Kranz A, Mares P, et al. Transient left ventricular failure following bilateral lung transplantation for pulmonary hypertension. J Heart Lung Transplant 1999; 18(4):304–309.
98. Soriano CM, Gaine SP, Conte JV, Fairman RP, White C, Rubin LJ. Anastomotic pulmonary hypertension after lung transplantation for primary pulmonary hypertension: report of surgical correction. Chest 1999; 116(2):564–566.
99. Izbicki G, Shitrit D, Schechtman I, et al. Recurrence of pulmonary veno-occlusive disease after heart–lung transplantation. J Heart Lung Transplant 2005; 24(5):635–637.
100. de Perrot M, Waddell TK, Chamberlain D, Hutcheon M, Keshavjee S. De novo pulmonary capillary hemangiomatosis occurring rapidly after bilateral lung transplantation. J Heart Lung Transplant 2003; 22(6):698–700.
101. Rosas V, Conte JV, Yang SC, et al. Lung transplantation and systemic sclerosis. Ann Transplant 2000; 5(3):38–43.
102. Pigula FA, Griffith BP, Zenati MA, Dauber JH, Yousem SA, Keenan RJ. Lung transplantation for respiratory failure resulting from systemic disease. Ann Thorac Surg 1997; 64(6):1630–1634.
103. Yeatman M, McNeil K, Smith JA, et al. Lung transplantation in patients with systemic diseases: an eleven-year experience at Papworth Hospital. J Heart Lung Transplant 1996; 15(2):l44–149.
104. Levine SM, Anzueto A, Peters JL Calhoon JH, Jenkinson SG, Bryan CL. Single lung transplantation in patients with systemic disease. Chest 1994; 105(3):837–841.
105. Saggar R, Ardehali A, Beygui R, et al. Connective Tissue Disease and Lung Transplantation. (Abst. 252967), presented at American Transplant Congress, Seattle, WA 2005.

# 7

# Lung Transplantation for Interstitial Lung Disorders

**Steven Nathan**

*Lung Transplant Program, Inova Heart and Vascular Institute, Falls Church, Virginia, U.S.A.*

**Rajan Saggar and Joseph P. Lynch III**

*Division of Pulmonary and Critical Care Medicine and Hospitalists, Department of Internal Medicine, David Geffen School of Medicine at UCLA, Los Angeles, California, U.S.A.*

## INTRODUCTION

End-stage lung disease due to myriad interstitial lung diseases (ILDs) accounts for approximately 20% of lung transplants (LTs) performed worldwide (1). Data from the International Society of Heart and Lung Transplantation (ISHLT) Registry from January 1995 to June 2004 cited idiopathic pulmonary fibrosis (IPF) as the second most frequent diagnosis leading to LT, comprising 17% of all LTs (1). Sarcoidosis and collagen vascular disease–associated pulmonary fibrosis (CVD-PF) accounted for 2.5% and 0.5% of LTs performed in that time frame, respectively (1). The prognoses of these diverse ILDs differ, and criteria for listing patients with these disorders have not been validated. When to list patients for LT is a difficult decision, since predicting life expectancy in individual patients is imperfect at best. Further, waiting times for organ procurement are unpredictable, but may be prolonged. Unfortunately, death rates while awaiting LT are highest in patients with IPF compared to other disorders. Early listing of patients with IPF is critical to improve outcome. Given the rarity of ILDs, appropriate timing for listing for LT has not been well established. In this chapter, we first discuss IPF because there is the greatest amount of experience and published data relating to this disorder. We later discuss the role of LT for patients with CVD-PF and sarcoidosis.

## IDIOPATHIC PULMONARY FIBROSIS

IPF is a specific form of chronic fibrosing interstitial pneumonitis affecting older adults associated with the histopathological pattern of usual interstitial pneumonia (UIP) (2–4). The term cryptogenic fibrosing alveolitis (CFA) is synonymous with IPF (4,5). The course of IPF/CFA is characterized by inexorable progression, with worsening respiratory insufficiency, restrictive lung disease, and hypoxemia (2). The disease is usually fatal within three to five years of diagnosis (mean survival ranging from 2.8 to 4 years) (6–15). Ten-year survival is less than 15% (6–15). Medical therapy has not been shown to affect outcome (discussed in detail later), and LT is the best therapeutic option for severe, progressive IPF. Because of the poor prognosis of IPF, and the lack of effective therapy, international guidelines published in 1998 (16) advised that patients with IPF be referred early for LT (discussed in detail later).

### Results of Lung Transplantation for IPF

Data from the ISHLT Registry from January 1995 to June 2004 indicate that 2257 of 13,007 (17%) LTs in adults were performed for IPF (1). IPF comprised 24% of all single-lung transplants (SLTs) and 10.0% of bilateral sequential lung transplants (BSLTs) in that time frame. The ISHLT Registry cited one-, three-, and five-year survival rates of 68%, 52%, and 50%, respectively, among IPF patients following LT (17). Initial studies from single centers noted similar mortality rates with SLT or BSLT in patients with PF (18,19). However, a recent review of 821 patients who received LTs for IPF (636 SLT, 185 BSLT) in the United States between 1994 and 2000 reported significantly better early (one month) and late (three year) survival rates with SLT compared to BSLT (20). Among recipients aged 30 to 49 years, early survival rates were 91% (SLT) versus 77% (BSLT); late survival rates were 64% (SLT) versus 46% (BSLT). Survival was also significantly better with SLT in patients aged 50 to 59 years. Early survival rates were 89.5% versus 81.7%, and late 54% versus 47%, respectively. No differences in survival were noted between SLT and BSLT among patients 60 to 69 years of age. When post-transplant survival was reanalyzed contingent upon survival to one month, survival by procedure type (SLT vs. BSLT) was similar. The increased mortality with BSLT at one month was independent of age or presence of pulmonary arterial hypertension (PAH) in the recipient. The reason for increased mortality with BSLT is not clear, but likely reflects an increase in surgical problems or graft failure in the early transplant period with BSLT.

### Definition of IPF and Other Idiopathic Interstitial Pneumonias

IPF is the most common of the idiopathic interstitial pneumonias (IIPs), comprising 47% to 71% of cases (6–8,21,22). Clinical and radiographic features of IPF overlap extensively with nonspecific interstitial pneumonia (NSIP) (23), which we discuss in detail later in this chapter. Other IIPs [e.g., respiratory bronchiolitis interstitial lung disease (RB-ILD) (24–26), desquamative interstitial pneumonia (DIP) (25,27,28), acute interstitial pneumonia (AIP) (29–32), lymphocytic interstitial pneumonia (LIP) (33,34), or cryptogenic organizing pneumonia (COP) (35–37)] rarely require LT and are not discussed further here.

### Epidemiology and Prevalence of IPF

IPF is rare, with an estimated prevalence of 6 to 20 cases per 100,000 (4,38–40). IPF is more common in males, older adults, and current or former smokers (4,39). The prevalence increases dramatically in older adults. In one study from New Mexico, the prevalence of IPF among adults from age 35 to 44 years was 2.7 per 100,000 but exceeded 175 per 100,000 for individuals >75 years of age (39). The etiology of IPF is not known, but environmental factors may play a contributory role (41–44). Gastroesophageal reflux was implicated as a risk factor for IPF in one study (45), but this relationship is controversial. Familial IPF accounts for 0.5% to 3% of cases (4,46,47).

### Clinical Features

Cardinal features of IPF include dry cough, exertional dyspnea, end-inspiratory velcro rales, diffuse parenchymal infiltrates on chest radiographs, honeycomb cysts on high-resolution computed tomographic (HRCT) scans, a restrictive defect on pulmonary function tests (PFTs), and impaired oxygenation (2,4,38). Physical examination reveals crackles in >80% of patients and clubbing in 25% to 50% (2,4). Extrapulmonary involvement does not occur (4,38). The clinical course of IPF/UIP is heterogenous, but most patients die of progressive respiratory insufficiency within months to years of onset (4,38).

### Histopathology

UIP is the histopathological pattern observed in IPF, but UIP can be observed in other diseases (e.g., CVDs; asbestosis; and diverse occupational, environmental, or drug exposures) (4,48). The salient histopathological features of UIP include temporal and geographic heterogeneity, alternating zones of normal and abnormal lung, predilection for peripheral (subpleural) and basilar regions, fibroblastic foci (aggregates of proliferating fibro-blasts and myofibroblasts), excessive collagen and extracellular matrix, and honeycomb change (2,3). Additional features include smooth muscle hyper-trophy, metaplasia and hyperplasia of type II pneumocytes, destroyed and disrupted alveolar architecture, traction bronchiectasis and bronchioloecta-sis, and pulmonary hypertensive changes (3).

## Treatment of IPF

Treatment options for IPF are limited, and are of unproven efficacy. Histori-cally, corticosteroids (CS) and/or immunosuppressive or cytotoxic agents were used in an attempt to ablate any inflammatory component (2,9,38,49). However, prospective, randomized studies assessing these agents are lacking. Surveys in the 1990s found that 39% to 66% of patients with IPF were treated with CS while immunosuppressive or cytotoxic agents were employed in only 2% to 17% (11,21,49). Early studies cited response rates of 10% to 30% with CS (alone or combined with immunosuppressive agents) (5,50–53), but complete or sustained remissions were rare. More importantly, most "responders" likely had IIPs other than UIP (e.g., NSIP, RB-ILD, COP, etc) (48). In more recent studies, response rates to CS among patients with UIP were low (0–17%) (2,21,54,55). Similarly, early prospective studies cited favorable responses to azathioprine (AZA) plus prednisone (53,56), but these studies comprised a limited number of patients and likely included patients with IIPs other than UIP. Further, impact on survival was not demonstrated. Cyclo-sphosphamide (CP) (either oral or intravenous pulse) has been used to treat IPF, but results are unimpressive (11,49,57–59). Toxicities associated with CP are substantial (60), and we do not advocate this agent for IPF. Oral colchicine was ineffective in retrospective (11) and prospective, randomized trials (61,62). Importantly, several large retrospective studies found no survival benefit with any form of therapy (11,49,63,64).

In 2000, an international consensus statement on IPF published by the American Thoracic Society (ATS) and European Respiratory Society (ERS) concluded that "no data exist that adequately document any of the current treatment approaches improves survival or the quality of life for patients with IPF" (4). Given the potential toxicities associated with CS, the ATS/ERS statement advised that high-dose CS should not be used to treat IPF. However, since anecdotal responses to CS or immunosuppressive agents were occasionally noted in patients with IPF/UIP, these experts acknowledged that patients with severe or progressive disease should be offered treatment (4). In this context, treatment with oral CP or AZA (plus low-dose CS) was recommended. It should be emphasized that these recom-mendations reflected expert consensus, but have not been validated in clinical trials. Despite the lack of evidence affirming efficacy, we believe a 6-month trial of AZA is reasonable for patients with IPF desiring therapy.

Additional agents evaluated in preliminary studies include *N*-acetyl cysteine (NAC) (40,65,66), pirfenidone (5-methyl-1-phenyl-2-[1*H*]-pyridone) (67,68), and recombinant interferon-gamma-1b (rIFN-γ-1b) (69,70). Although these studies show promise, an impact on survival has not been established. NAC has antioxidant properties and attenuates fibrosis in animal models (40). Oral NAC (600 mg t.i.d. for 5 days) augmented glutathione levels in bronchoalveolar lavage (BAL) in IPF patients (65). In a prospective open-label trial, 18 patients with IPF treated with oral NAC for 12 weeks exhibited slight improvement in PFTs (66). A phase III multicenter, international trial (IFIGENIA) study evaluating the efficacy of NAC in IPF has recently been completed. Both patient cohorts received AZA and low-dose prednisone in addition to NAC or placebo. Preliminary results suggested that treatment with NAC slowed down the rate of decline in forced vital capacity (FVC) and diffusing capacity for carbon monoxide (DL$_{CO}$) compared with controls (70a). A recent prospective trial in Japan randomized 107 patients with IPF to pirfenidone ($n = 72$) or placebo ($n = 35$) (68). No difference was noted in the primary end point [lowest O$_2$ saturation during a 6-minute walk test (6MWT)] between groups, but positive treatment effects were noted in secondary end points at nine months. These changes were small, and of uncertain clinical significance. Pirfenidone is not commercially available, but a randomized, placebo-controlled trial evaluating this agent is planned in the United States in 2006.

The most studied of these novel agents is rIFN-γ-1b (70). A double-blind, placebo-controlled multicenter trial randomized 330 patients with CS-recalcitrant IPF to rIFN-γ-1b plus prednisone (7.5 mg/day) or placebo (69). Analysis at a median of 58 weeks found no differences in any of the primary or secondary end points between rIFN-γ-1b– and placebo-treated cohorts. However, there was a trend ($P = 0.08$) toward lower mortality in the rIFN-γ-1b group (10% vs. 17%, respectively). Further, post hoc subgroup analysis of patients with FVC $>$ 62% predicted at entry suggested a survival benefit with rIFN-γ-1b ($P = 0.04$) (69). These data are promising, but additional data are required to determine the efficacy (if any) of rIFN-γ-1b. An additional study is currently under way (the INSPIRE trial) in which 800 patients with mild to moderate IPF will be randomized in a 2:1 ratio to rIFN-γ-1b or placebo. Given the expense of rIFN-γ-1b ($>$\$50,000 annually), widespread use of this agent should be deferred pending the outcome of this ongoing study. Additional novel therapies with potential antifibrotic properties have theoretical value, but have not been tested in IPF (discussed in detail elsewhere) (40,71–73).

## When Should Patients with IPF Be Referred for Lung Transplantation?

Based on the current lack of proven medical therapies, and the high mortality associated with IPF, it is unwise to defer referral for LT pending an assessment of response to therapy. Median survival for patients with IPF is approximately three years from the time of diagnosis (6,11,49,74). However, reports on mortality can be biased in a number of ways. Lead-time bias may be present if patient outcomes are reported from the time of referral or diagnosis at large referral centers. One study cited a mean survival of 35 months from the time of diagnosis as compared to 81 months from the time of onset of symptoms (63). Other studies citing median survival of 4.3 and 5.8 years included only patients in whom PFTs were available over a six-month time frame and therefore were biased by patients having to survive six months to be evaluated (15,75). Nonetheless, numerous studies have noted that responses to therapy are achieved in <15% of patients with IPF (2,4), and historically, IPF patients had the highest mortality while on the LT waiting list (76). Therefore, it is prudent to refer patients to an LT center at the time of diagnosis of IPF (provided no contraindications exist). The decision as to when to list for LT is best made by the local transplant team, who are more familiar with the organ allocation system, local waiting times, and other factors that might affect pre- and post-transplant survival. This principle is underscored by data showing that patients with IPF who died while on the list were diagnosed on average nearly two years prior to referral (77). Early referral also allows for the proper preparation of the patient. This might include optimizing the patient's physical status through pulmonary rehabilitation and other time-dependent measures such as weight loss and reduction of steroid dose. Sufficient time is needed for appropriate education and psychological preparation, factors that are integral to the overall success of LT.

International guidelines endorsed by the ISHLT were published in 1998 (16). These guidelines recommended that patients with IPF be referred early for LT. In the absence of specific contraindications, the guidelines advocated referring patients for LT evaluation when any of the following indications were present: symptoms, failure to improve or stabilize following CS or immunosuppressive therapy, and progressive or new abnormalities on PFTs (16). The committee noted that the disease should be considered "advanced" when the FVC fell below 60% to 70% of the predicted values or the $DL_{CO}$ corrected for alveolar volume fell below 50% to 60% predicted. They also stated that serial PFTs were important to gauge the evolution of the disease.

The decision to list for LT is determined by a risk analysis of the likelihood of mortality during the projected wait period versus the likely mortality following LT. Despite this, the risk assessment of mortality frequently favors listing owing to the unpredictability and poor prognosis associated with IPF.

## What Factors Are Predictive of Mortality in IPF?

For reasons that are not clear, the male gender has been associated with higher mortality in several (11,78,79), but not all (63), studies. Interestingly, three studies noted improved survival among cigarette smokers with UIP compared to those who have never smoked (12,63,78), but others found no such effect (49,54,79). The "protective effect" of cigarette smoking may relate to the inhibitory effects of cigarette smoke on cytokine release or fibroblast proliferation (80). Advanced age has been associated with increased mortality in several studies (4,11,23,74,81,82). Age has a profound effect on survival. In one study, median survival rates were 63 months for patients between 50 and 60 years of age compared to 116 months for patients <50 years of age (23). The improved survival in younger patients in this study may reflect a differing natural history of disease in younger patients or fewer comorbidities. When to list patients for LT requires a careful assessment of risk factors for mortality. Given the high mortality associated with LT, deferring listing is appropriate for selected patients (e.g., patients with moderate disease and an indolent course). In the sections that follow, we discuss specific risk factors for mortality that should be taken into account when deciding who should be listed for LT. The decision about when to list for LT is dependent on the local organ allocation system and projected waiting times.

## Prognostic Value of Histological Features

Among patients with IIPs, the histological pattern UIP on surgical lung biopsy (SLBx) is the single most important factor predicting mortality (6,14). All studies have noted increased mortality with UIP compared to NSIP (7,8,15,21,54,74,81,83). However, even among patients with UIP, additional histological factors may influence prognosis. Two studies found that increasing fibroblastic foci correlated with mortality (12,83), but others (15) found no such correlation.

## Pulmonary Functional Parameters as Predictors of Mortality

Physiological parameters are essential to assess the severity of the disease and the rate of progression (74,84). A retrospective study of 487 patients with UIP found that older age, male gender, lower $DL_{CO}$, and worsening lung function were associated with higher mortality (11). Numerous studies in IPF cited higher mortality rates when $DL_{CO}$ or lung volumes were severely impaired (10,49,74,81), but correlations between physiologic aberrations and mortality are inexact. The cutoff points predicting outcomes are variable. Several studies cited higher mortality rates with FVC < 60–67% predicted or when $DL_{CO}$ falls below 30% to 45% predicted (10,69,84–87). Changes in total lung capacity (TLC) are less predictive of prognosis (84,88). However, given the heterogenous pace of the disease (both UIP and NSIP), the value of any pulmonary functional parameter in predicting outcomes is limited (74,77).

Rate of change in physiological parameters provides more useful prognostic information than parameters at a single point in time. Serial change in FVC was an independent predictor of mortality in several studies (15,74,75). Not surprisingly, improvement or stability of FVC or $DL_{CO}$ has been associated with an improved prognosis. Conversely, deterioration in VC ( > 10% decrease) or $DL_{CO}$ ( > 15% decrease) at three months (89), six months (14,74,75,81), or later time points (74,75,86,90) predicts a worse survival. A retrospective study of 129 patients (UIP in 80; NSIP in 29) found that change in FVC was the best physiologic predictor of mortality in patients with UIP ($P = 0.05$) (14). By multivariate analysis (controlling for histologic diagnosis), a > 10% decrease in FVC at six months remained an independent risk factor for mortality [hazard ration (HR) 2.47, $P = 0.006$] (14). Changes in TLC or $DL_{CO}$ did not provide further prognostic information. The rIFN-$\gamma$-1b multicenter study found that a 10% decline in the FVC was associated with a 2.4-fold increased risk of death (70). Another study evaluated 315 patients from that cohort; higher $DL_{CO}$ was associated with lower mortality (87). One study of 81 patients with UIP noted that changes in FVC at six and 12 months provided more accurate prognostic information than baseline values alone (75). Six-month changes in FVC, forced expiratory volume in 1 second ($FEV_1$), $DL_{CO}$, TLC, $paO_2$, $O_2$ saturation, and alveolar–arterial (A–a) $O_2$ gradient were predictive of survival even after adjusting for baseline values. Five-year survival (stratified by smoking history) ranged from 18% to 22% among patients exhibiting >10% decline in FVC as compared to 42% to 46% among patients with stable FVC and 64% to 68% among patients with >10% increase in FVC. British investigators evaluated a cohort of patients with fibrotic IIP (i.e., UIP or fibrotic NSIP) (74). Increasing age ($P = 0.03$) and lower $DL_{CO}$ ($P = 0.001$) or FVC ($P < 0.0005$) levels were independently linked to mortality. After six months of follow-up, serial PFT trends [$DL_{CO}$, FVC, $FEV_1$, and composite physiologic index (CPI) scores] and the histopathological pattern independently correlated with survival. At 12 months, serial PFTs trends (particularly $DL_{CO}$ and CPI) were the major prognostic determinants. The histological pattern provided no additional prognostic information when PFT trends were clear-cut or when functional impairment was severe. Jegal et al. examined prognostic factors in 179 patients with fibrotic IIPs (UIP in 131; NSIP in 48) (81). Five-year survival was better for fibrotic NSIP (76%) compared to UIP (44%), $P = 0.007$. For all patients, three variables at the time of presentation had important prognostic value (by multivariate analysis): pathology pattern, age, and $DL_{CO}$. However, after six months of follow-up, only changes in FVC, initial $DL_{CO}$, and age were independent prognostic factors. The histological pattern no longer provided additional prognostic information. These various studies affirm that serial PFTs are important to gauge the pace and evolution of the disease. Declines in FVC or $DL_{CO}$ over time are associated with a high mortality, and should prompt listing for LT. However, stability does not guarantee a good prognosis. In the IFN-γ-1b trial, 43% of the deaths occurred in patients with stable PFTs (70).

## Oxygenation

Hypoxemia (at rest or exercise) is an independent predictor of mortality in fibrotic IIPs (both UIP and fibrotic NSIP). The impact of resting hypoxemia was underscored in a series of 48 patients with IIPs awaiting LT (77). Initial FVC, $FEV_1$, or TLC did not differ between patients who were alive ($n = 28$) or died ($n = 20$) while awaiting LT. However, resting hypoxemia was associated with higher mortality. Among patients with room air $PaO_2$ < 50 mmHg at rest, none survived beyond 15 months. Desaturation with exercise is a more sensitive index of gas exchange abnormalities. Cardiopulmonary exercise testing (CPET) has prognostic value, but the 6MWT (91,92) is easier to perform, noninvasive, and more reproducible than CPET or static PFTs (93). In one study of 105 patients with IIPs (UIP, $n = 83$; NSIP, $n = 22$), desaturation ($\leq 88\%$ $O_2$ saturation) during 6MWT was an independent predictor of mortality (both UIP and NSIP) (HR 4.47, $P =$ 0.005) (91). Not surprisingly, patients with UIP who desaturated exhibited significantly lower values of FVC, $DL_{CO}$, and resting $O_2$ saturation compared to patients with UIP who did not desaturate. Four-year mortality rate of UIP patients who desaturated was 65.5% compared to 31% for patients who did not. For NSIP patients, four-year mortality was 34.4% versus 0% for patients who did not desaturate. For all patients, a decrease in saturation of 4% or more ($\Delta$ saturation $\geq 4\%$) was a significant predictor of mortality (HR 13.6, $P = 0.001$). Another study of 41 patients with IPF found that exercise-induced hypoxemia by CPET correlated strongly with mortality (94). Hallstrand et al. prospectively followed 28 patients with progressive IPF for a median of 5.4 years (range 4.3–6.2) to determine the relationship between parameters of the timed walk test (maximum 6 minutes) and mortality (92). By multivariate analysis, only $\Delta SO_2$, walk velocity, and $DL_{CO}$ were associated with mortality. In summary, although disparate results have been noted, arterial desaturation (at rest or exercise) is associated with a poor prognosis, and should prompt consideration for LT.

## HRCT Scans as Predictors of Mortality

The extent and pattern of aberrations on HRCT have prognostic significance. The extent of fibrosis on CT (CT-fib) correlates with functional impairment (87,95) and mortality (10,78,87,90). Both global qualitative and semiquantitative scoring systems may predict prognosis. In a prospective study of 39 patients with IPF, the CT-fib assessed by a semiquantitative scoring system correlated with poor response to therapy and increased mortality (90). In that study, CT-fib scores $\geq 2$ (which corresponds to honeycomb change) predicted subsequent mortality within three years with 80%

sensitivity and 82% specificity. HRCT was a better predictor of survival than PFTs or clinical/radiographic/physiologic (CRP) scores (discussed later). Using a similar system, British investigators assessed risk factors for two-year mortality in a cohort of 115 patients with UIP awaiting LT (10). By multivariate analysis, only CT-fib scores and $DL_{CO}$ % predicted were independent predictors of mortality. The risk of death increased by 106% for each unit increase in CT-fib score and 4% for every 1% decrease in $DL_{CO}$ % predicted. Receiving operating curve (ROC) analysis gave the best fit (predictive value) using a combination of CT-fib and $DL_{CO}$ scores. The area under the ROC curve was remarkably similar to that in the earlier study (90). Another study assessed the prognostic value of CT fibrotic scores in a cohort of 168 patients with IIPs (UIP 106, NSIP 33, other 29) (78). A CT-fib score $\geq 2$ in any lobe was highly predictive of UIP (sensitivity 90%, specificity 86%) and was associated with increased mortality (relative risk of 3.35, $P = 0.02$). Others have shown that CT patterns that are "typical" of IPF were associated with greater fibrosis on lung biopsy and a higher mortality compared to "atypical" CT scans (55). Flaherty et al. confirmed that CT scans characteristic of UIP (i.e., considered as "probable or definite UIP" by experienced radiologists) predicted a worse survival (96). In that study, 96 patients with IIPs were evaluated (UIP in 73, NSIP in 23). Among patients with biopsy-proven UIP, mortality was higher when CT features were characteristic ("definite or probable UIP") compared to those with nondiagnostic CT scans ($P = 0.04$). Median survival rates were 2.08 years for patients with UIP by histology and CT compared with 5.76 years for patients with histologic UIP but atypical CT. These data suggest that CT features typical or characteristic of UIP reflect advanced disease. A recent study of 315 IPF patients enrolled in the rIFN-γ-1b protocol identified three independent predictors of mortality by multivariate analysis (87). Greater CT-fib correlated with increased risk of death, whereas higher $DL_{CO}$ and treatment assigned to rIFN-γ-1b were associated with reduced risk of death.

## Composite Scoring Systems

Several models that incorporate CRP criteria have been developed to provide better predictors of survival (10,23,74,97). In an early study, Watters et al. developed a composite score incorporating clinical (dyspnea), radiographic (chest X rays), and physiological parameters (i.e., the CRP score) as a means to more objectively monitor the course of IPF (97). The latest iteration of the CRP scoring system incorporates multiple factors, including age, smoking history, clubbing, changes on chest X-ray (extent of profusion of interstitial opacities and/or pulmonary hypertension), % predicted TLC, and $PaO_2$ at the end of maximal exercise (23). This modified CRP score predicted five-year survival with remarkable accuracy. This quantitative CRP scoring system is invaluable for research investigations, but is cumbersome and impractical for use in clinical settings (98). British investigators developed a CPI that incorporates CT and physiologic parameters to assess outcomes in patients with IPF (74). The CPI evaluates disease extent by CT and selected functional variables (i.e., % predicted FVC, $FEV_1$, and $DL_{CO}$). Exercise components were not included. Multivariate analysis of a cohort of IPF patients identified several variables that correlated with mortality, including greater extent of disease on CT; greater functional impairment (FVC, $FEV_1$, $DL_{CO}$, $PaO_2$, A–a $O_2$ gradient); and higher CPI score. Importantly, CPI was the most powerful predictor of mortality, and correlated better with survival than CT or any pulmonary functional parameter (74). Further, CPI score was a better predictor of outcome than the physiological component of the original (97) or modified (23) CRP score. The CPI is promising, but may not be easily adapted into clinical practice settings. Another model derived specifically from IPF patients awaiting LT found that a DLco <39% predicted together with an HRCT-fibrosis score of 2.25 yielded a sensitivity and specificity for death within the next two years of 82% and 84%, respectively (10). Use of these or other models requires further prospective validation in other potential LT candidates (98).

**Impact of PAH on Prognosis**

Secondary PAH has been reported in 28% to 84% of patients with advanced IPF (82,99–101). Nadrous et al. analyzed 88 patients with IPF who had estimates of systolic pulmonary artery pressure (sPAP) by echocardiography (82). Importantly, 84% had elevated sPAP, including 27 (31%) with sPAP > 50 mmHg. sPAP correlated inversely with $DL_{CO}$ and $paO_2$, and was an independent predictor of mortality. Median survival was significantly worse among patients with sPAP ≥ 50 mmHg (0.7 years) compared to patients with sPAP ≤ 35 mmHg (4.8 years) or sPAP between 36 and 50 mmHg (4.1 years). Other parameters associated with worse survival by univariate analysis included male gender, lower $DL_{CO}$, use of oxygen, history of coronary artery disease, and worse New York Heart Association class. These data suggest that PAH is common among patients with IPF (particularly those with low $DL_{CO}$ or $PaO_2$). Screening for PAH is reasonable since it has prognostic value and may have implications for management. Although data are limited, favorable responses to sildenafil (102) and inhaled prostacyclin and iloprost (103) have been noted in IPF patients with PAH. Awareness of the prognostic importance of PAH should prompt the use of Doppler echocardiography (DE) to estimate sPAP in any patient with end-stage lung disease or requiring supplemental oxygen. Assessment of right ventricular (RV) size and function is helpful to identify patients who may be candidates for right heart catheterization (RHC). However, DE has only modest predictive value for PAH (99,104). Abnormal RV findings are not reliable, and considerably overdiagnose PAH (99,104). Further, in a study of 374 LT candidates with end-stage lung disease, estimates of sPAP by DE and RHC were discordant by >10 mmHg in 52% of patients (99). However, among 120 patients with end-stage lung disease and no RV abnormalities on DE, only 4% had PAH by RHC (99). Accordingly, RHC is reasonable among patients with abnormal DE but is usually not required when DE is normal. We believe that RHC should be done in any patient with end-stage lung disease who is being considered for LT. Reduced 6MWT distance and elevated brain natriuretic peptide (BNP) levels are surrogate markers of PAH in patients with PF (100). In a recent study, 39 patients with PF and severe restrictive disease (FVC < 55% predicted) (including 28 with UIP) underwent RHC, measurement of plasma BNP levels, and 6MWT (100). Among patients with IPF, elevated BNP concentrations correlated with increased PAP and pulmonary vascular resistance and correlated inversely with 6MWT distance. Importantly, PFTs did not discriminate between patients with normal and elevated PAP. These data suggest that plasma BNP concentrations are an excellent noninvasive marker to screen for PAH in patients with PF. Secondary PAH is not a contraindication to LT, but its presence may influence the operative and perioperative management of these patients. Some studies cited increased mortality among SLT recipients with elevated PAP (preoperative PAP > 30 mmHg) (105), while others did not (106). Recently, a large study found that PAH in IPF patients was associated with increased mortality following LT (either SLT or BSLT) (107). The ISHLT Registry evaluated 830 patients with IPF transplanted between 1995 and 2002: 77% had SLT, and 23% had BSLT (107). By multivariate analysis, mean PAP and BSLT were independent risk factors for 90-day mortality after adjustment for potential confounders. Further, there was a linear relationship between PAP and 90-day mortality among SLTs. Only 8.3% of patients with SLT had mean PAP > 40 mmHg, so the conclusions are limited.

In summary, the decision of when to list IPF patients for LT is complex, and requires careful assessment of CRP and hemodynamic parameters (Table 1).

**Table 1**  Indications for Lung Transplantation for IPF/UIP

---

Severe impairment in pulmonary function tests
  FVC < 65% predicted
  $DL_{CO}$ < 40% predicted
Declining PFTs
Need for supplemental oxygen
Pulmonary arterial hypertension (sPAP > 50 mmHg)
Severe fibrosis or honeycomb change on HRCT scans

---

*Abbreviations*: FVC, forced vital capacity; $DL_{CO}$, diffusing capacity for carbon monoxide; PFT, defect on pulmonary function test; sPAP, systolic pulmonary artery pressure; HRCT, high-resolution computed tomography.

## Disease-Specific Considerations

Patients with IPF are at increased risk for various comorbid conditions (e.g., coronary artery disease, pulmonary embolism, and bronchogenic carcinoma). In a large meta-analysis of mortality among studies of IPF published from 1964 to 1983, 24% of deaths were ascribed to cardiac causes (108). Other causes of death included bronchogenic carcinoma (10%), pulmonary infections (3%), and pulmonary emboli (3%). This meta-analysis likely represented a heterogenous group of IIPs and may not apply only to IPF/UIP by today's current definition (4). Nonetheless, this study emphasizes that not all deaths are directly attributable to IPF and that potential comorbid conditions need to be carefully assessed during the LT workup. Recent studies confirm that the incidence of coronary artery disease is increased in patients with IPF (109). Further, a higher propensity for pulmonary emboli has been noted in IPF (110). One possible mechanism might relate to microvascular injury, which occurs as part of the pathogenic sequence in IPF (111). A high incidence of antiphopholipid antibodies has also been noted in IPF (111). Lung cancer has been noted in 5% to 13% of patients with IPF (2,64,108,112), but a direct causative link remains controversial (113). CS therapy instituted for IPF may be associated with significant complications including glucose intolerance (89). Interestingly, a higher incidence of diabetes mellitus has been noted in steroid-naive IPF patients (114). The propensity for these potential comorbid conditions is important not only in the pretransplant evaluation phase, but also in the post-transplant period when some of these entities may be manifest.

## NONSPECIFIC INTERSTITIAL PNEUMONIA

### Introduction

The histopathologic designation of NSIP was first applied in 1994 by Katzenstein and Fiorelli (115) to describe cases of IIPs that do not fit the histopathological critera for other categories of IIP (i.e., UIP, DIP, RBILD, AIP, LIP, COP). In that sentinel report, Katzenstein and Fiorelli emphasized that the term NSIP referred to immunocompetent patients with a clinical syndrome resembling IPF, but with a distinctly better prognosis. An international ATS/ERS consensus statement on the classification of IIPs published in 2002 (48) recognized NSIP as a distinct histopathological pattern found in response to occupational exposures, CVDs, or as an idiopathic form. The relationship between NSIP and UIP remains uncertain.

### Histopathology

NSIP is an inflammatory and/or fibrotic process involving the lung interstitium but lacks the requisite features of other IIPs (4,115). The NSIP pattern encompasses a broad spectrum, with varying degrees of alveolar wall inflammation and fibrosis (7,8,21). In striking contrast to UIP, a cardinal feature of NSIP is temporal uniformity (4,115). Other IIPs (e.g., DIP, RBILD, AIP, LIP) exhibit temporal uniformity, but these disorders differ from NSIP in other important respects (discussed elsewhere) (4,48).

## Clinical Features

Clinical features of NSIP overlap with UIP. Both disorders exhibit basilar crackles, cough, dyspnea, restrictive ventilatory defects, and impaired oxygenation (2,23,81). However, patients with NSIP tend to be younger (55,78,81). More importantly, the course of NSIP is more subacute, evolving over weeks to months (23,81), whereas UIP is more indolent (2). BAL cell profiles in NSIP often reveal lymphocytosis (21,55,81), but this is not uniform (54). HRCT scans typically reveal ground-glass opacities (GGO) or consolidation, with no or minimal honeycomb change (78,81,116–118). However, bibasilar and subpleural predominance, reticular abnormalities, traction bronchiectasis and bronchiolectasis, and architectural distortion are found in most patients with NSIP (similar to UIP) (117,118). CT features of CVD-associated NSIP are similar to idiopathic NSIP (119,120).

## Course and Prognosis

The prognosis of NSIP and responsiveness to therapy are much better than for UIP (2,8,21,23,54,81,121). However, prospective studies are lacking. Early retrospective studies cited >80% survival with cellular NSIP, but follow-up was relatively short (two to five years) (6,8,21,54,55,78,121). With longer follow-up, prognosis is distinctly worse. British investigators cited mortality of 61% in a cohort of 28 patients with idiopathic NSIP (mean survival was 52 months) (54). A subsequent retrospective study from the same center cited median survival rates of 56 months for fibrotic NSIP and 33 months for UIP (74). Among 43 patients with NSIP, 5- and 10-year survival rates were only 46% and 39%, respectively (74). Korean investigators cited 5-year survival rates of 56% among 48 patients with fibrotic NSIP and 34% among 131 patients with UIP (81). Further, the impact of therapy for NSIP is difficult to ascertain. Early studies suggested favorable responses to CS (alone or combined with immunosuppressive agents) in 60% to 83% of patients (8,21,121,122), but subsequent studies were less sanguine (response rates of 25–40%) (54,55,78).

## What Is the Relationship Between NSIP and UIP?

Controversy exists as to whether NSIP is a separate disease entity or a continuum of disease related to IPF/UIP (7,22,74). Histologically, NSIP lesions display temporal homogeneity, whereas UIP is temporally heterogenous (115). Further, neither fibroblastic foci nor honeycombing, cardinal features of UIP (3), is prominent in NSIP (23,115). However, histological features of NSIP and UIP overlap, and distinguishing fibrotic NSIP from UIP is difficult (54,78). Importantly, both NSIP and UIP may coexist in individual patients. Review of SLBx from patients with IIPs observed both NSIP and UIP (i.e., discordant UIP) in 13% to 26% of patients (22,123). If the two histopathological patterns coexist, UIP becomes the default diagnosis, as such cases have a prognosis that most closely approximates that of UIP (96). Katzenstein et al. examined whole-lung explants from 21 patients undergoing LT for ILD (124). Antemortem SLBx demonstrated UIP pattern in 15 patients, nonclassifiable pattern in 5, and NSIP in 1 patient. A histological review of whole-lung explants showed a predominant pattern of UIP in 20 patients (95%) and NSIP in one (5%) patient. However, areas resembling NSIP were observed in the background of otherwise typical UIP in 12 of 15 SLBx (80%) and in 16 of 20 (80%) explant specimens. These various studies support the concept that NSIP and UIP are part of a spectrum of fibrotic disorders. NSIP and UIP may represent different points in the progression of a single disease or may represent distinct (albeit overlapping) processes. The spectrum of NSIP is broad, and encompasses an inflammatory (cellular) variant (8,21) as well a fibrotic variant (74,81,83). In the original description of NSIP, it was subdivided into three histological patterns: group I, cellular infiltrate with minimal or no fibrosis; group II, mixed cellularity and fibrosis; group III, dense fibrosis (115). Subsequent studies support segregating NSIP into cellular (group I) and fibrotic (groups II or III) subtypes because these histological variants differ in prognosis (21,22,54,74,78,121). Cellular NSIP comprises only one-quarter to one-third of patients with NSIP, and has a good prognosis (five-year survival rates >80%) (8,21,22,54,78). Prognosis with fibrotic NSIP is distinctly worse, with five-year survival rates of 39% to 60% (54,74,81). It is possible that cellular NSIP represents an early phase that may progress to fibrotic NSIP and ultimately UIP. If so, the survival advantage of NSIP may simply represent lead-time bias. This concept is supported by recent studies (14,74).

## When Should Patients with NSIP Be Referred for LT?

ISHLT guidelines for selecting LT candidates discussed IPF and "systemic disease with PF" but did not specifically address NSIP (16). However, fibrotic NSIP is potentially fatal (54,74,81,91), and LT is the best option for a subset of NSIP patients with deteriorating PFTs and oxygen dependency. As was previously discussed, deteriorating PFTs (74,81) or hypoxemia (91) are surrogate markers for mortality in patients with IIP, and deteriorating FVC, $DL_{CO}$, or oxygenation outweigh the importance of histological pattern after the first 6 to 12 months of follow-up (74,81). Our approach is to aggressively treat NSIP with a combination of CS and AZA for a minimum of three to six months. Responders are continued on medical therapy, and LT is deferred. However, patients failing therapy and exhibiting a deteriorating course are listed for LT (criteria similar to those in Table 1).

### Results of Lung Transplantation for NSIP

Data regarding LT for NSIP are lacking since the ISHLT Registry does not include NSIP as a separate diagnosis.

### CVD-ASSOCIATED PF

### Introduction

PF may complicate each of the CVDs, but limited data are available regarding the role of LT. Most centers are reluctant to perform LT in patients with CVD, in part due to concern about extrapulmonary complications. However, the 1998 ISHLT consensus statement stated that LT is a legitimate option for patients with CVD (or other systemic disorders), provided patients had failed an adequate course of medical therapy and the systemic disease was quiescent (16). Candidates should be considered on an individual basis, and extrapulmonary organ involvement that could negatively impact long-term prognosis needs to be taken into account.

### Lung Transplantation for CVD-PF

Both SLT and BLT have been performed for CVD-PF, but data are limited. The ISHLT Registry noted that only 65 patients with CVD had LTs (SLT in 34, BSLT in 31) between January 1995 and June 2004 (representing 0.5% of LTs performed during that time frame) (1).

### Clinical Features and Natural History of CVD-PF

CRP features of CVD-PF overlap with those of IPF, but the course of CVD-PF is much more indolent (125). Survival is much better in patients with CVD-PF compared to IPF, even when matched for initial severity of disease (126).

### Progressive Systemic Sclerosis

Pulmonary complications of progressive systemic sclerosis (PSSc) include fibrosing alveolitis (FA), pulmonary hypertension, recurrent aspiration pneumonia (among patients with esophageal dysfunction), and rarely, bronchiolitis obliterans [with or without organizing pneumonia (OP)], pulmonary hemorrhage, bronchoalveolar cell carcinoma, opportunistic infections, or complications of drug therapy (125). Chronic ILD (also termed fibrosing alveolitis) complicates PSSc in >80% of patients, and is the most common cause of death from PSSc (125). Antibodies to topoisomerase I (anti-Scl-70) occur in 20–40% of patients with PSSc, and are often associated with chronic ILD (125,127). Autoantibodies against histones (128) or endothelial cells (129) are associated with an increased frequency of FA. Neither the duration of the PSSc nor the extent of extrapulmonary involvement correlated with the extent of FA as assessed by CT (125). The clinical course of FA complicating PSSc is heterogenous, but a gradual decline over many years is typical (125). Pulmonary dysfunction and exercise impairment are less severe in PSSc-FA than in IPF, even when patients are matched for extent and pattern of disease on CT and other demographic factors (age, smoking history, sex) (95). Coarse reticular patterns or honeycombing on CT correlated with increased fibrosis and a more rapid rate of deterioration (130). Pulmonary hypertension (131) or $DL_{CO} < 40\%$ predicted (132) have been associated with an increased mortality. Factors associated with a deteriorating course include peripheral vascular involvement, digital pitting or ulcerations, severe Raynaud's phenomenon, and history of smoking (131,132). Historically, the approach to PSSc-associated FA has been nihilistic. However, some patients manifest active alveolitis, which may be amenable to therapy. Favorable responses have been noted with CS and immunosuppressive agents. Cyclophosphamide (oral or pulse) has been most often utilized, with benefit in some patients (125,133–135). Rates of response are likely highest in patients with active alveolitis or early disease.

## Rheumatoid Arthritis

Pulmonary complications of rheumatoid arthritis (RA) are protean and include pleural effusions, FA, obliterative bronchiolitis (with or without OP), lymphocytic infiltration of small airways, Caplan's syndrome, rheumatoid pulmonary nodules, bronchiectasis, pulmonary hypertension, opportunistic infections, or complications of therapy (125). Aberrations on HRCT scans were noted in 29% to 52% of patients with RA, even in the absence of pulmonary symptoms (136–138). The presence of FA in RA does not correlate with the extent, duration, or activity of the articular or systemic components (125). Risk factors for RA-FA include male gender, age >60 years, history of smoking, high titers of circulating rheumatoid factor, variant α-1-antitrypsin phenotypes, and human leukocyte antigen B40 (125). The course of FA complicating RA is usually indolent, but 1% to 4% of patients with RA develop severe, disabling FA (125). Optimal therapy for rheumatoid lung disease is not known, as controlled therapeutic trials have not been done. However, treatment regimens employed for RA include CS, immunosuppressive or cytotoxic agents, or anti–tumor necrosis factor-α (TNF-α) inhibitors. Lung transplantation is reserved for patients with severe, progressive PF refractory to medical therapy.

## Polymyositis and Dermatomyositis

Pulmonary complications of polymyositis (PM) or dermatomyositis (DM) include respiratory failure due to severe neuromuscular weakness, aspiration pneumonia due to weakness of the pharyngeal musculature, diaphragmatic paresis or dysfunction, FA, bronchiolitis obliterans (with or without OP), and opportunistic infections (125). Chronic ILD complicates PM/DM in 3% to 10% of patients, and can be the presenting feature (125,139). Although surgical lung biopsies are rarely performed for ILD complicating PM and DM, NSIP is the most common pattern, comprising 45–82% of cases (139–142). Other histological patterns include COP, UIP, diffuse alveolar damage, and LIP (139–142). The severity of FA does not correlate with the course of the muscle disease, muscle enzymes, or systemic features (125). Serological autoantibodies to the enzyme histidyl-tRNA-synthetase (anti-Jo1, anti-PL7, and anti-PL12) or KJ are present in a majority of patients with PM or DM with FA, but in < 20% of patients with PM or DM without FA (125,143). These autoantibodies are rarely present in other CVDs (125,144). CS and/or immunosuppressive agents are the cornerstone of therapy for myopathic and systemic manifestations of PM or DM, and favorable responses have been noted with these agents for FA, but data are sparse (125,145,146). Therapy is most likely to be efficacious in patients with active alveolitis before irreversible fibrosis has occurred.

## Systemic Lupus Erythematosus

Pulmonary complications of systemic lupus erythematosus (SLE) are protean and include pleuritis, acute lupus pneumonitis, FA, alveolar hemorrhage (capillaritis), pulmonary embolism (due to circulating anticardiolipin antibodies), bronchiolitis obliterans (with or without OP), pulmonary vasculitis, diaphragmatic dysfunction, opportunistic infections, or drug toxicity from immunosuppressive therapy (144,147). Clinically significant FA complicates SLE in 3% to 13% of patients, but is rarely severe (144,147). However, progressive, severe FA may occur in a subset of patients with SLE in the context of overlap syndrome (147). CS and/or immunosuppressive or cytotoxic agents may be efficacious (144,147), but therapeutic trials are lacking.

## Overlap Syndrome and Mixed Connective Tissue Disease

Overlap syndrome is characterized by clinical manifestations overlapping with two or more of the five major CVDs (e.g., PSSc, RA, PM, DM, or SLE) (125). Features of two or more CVDs may occur concurrently, or the disease may evolve from one CVD to another (125). Mixed connective tissue disease (MCTD) displays overlapping features of SLE, PSSc, or PM/DM (125,148). High-titer circulating antibodies (anti-RNP) to a ribonuclease-sensitive extractable nuclear antigen and a speckled antinuclear antibody are present; antibodies to Sm are absent (148,149). Pulmonary manifestations occur in up to 85% of patients with MCTD (125,148,149). Of these, FA (149) and PAH (150) are the most common. FA develops in 25% to 85% of patients with MCTD during the course of the disease (148,149). The clinical expression of FA complicating MCTD is variable (125). Treatment is similar to FA complicating other CVDs.

## Sjogren's Syndrome

Sjogren's syndrome (SS) is characterized by lymphocytic infiltration and destruction of exocrine glands and symptoms of xerostomia and/or xeropthalmia (sicca syndrome) (151). SS may occur as a primary syndrome or as a secondary syndrome in the context of a specific autoimmune disorder (e.g., RA, SLE, PM/DM, PSSc) (125). Pulmonary manifestations of SS are protean and include FA, LIP, lymphoproliferative disorders (pseudolymphoma and lymphoma), xerotrachea, OP, pleural effusions, or fibrosis (125,151–153). FA complicating SS is indistinguishable from FA complicating other CVDs. The reported incidence of FA in SS ranges from 9% to 55%, depending on variations in diagnostic testing and populations studied (151–156). Clinical or serological features fail to identify patients with SS most likely to develop pulmonary disease (151,153,157). The course of FA complicating SS is variable. Favorable responses to CS and immunosuppressive or cytotoxic agents have been noted (156–158), but controlled studies are lacking.

## SARCOIDOSIS

### Introduction

Sarcoidosis is a granulomatous disorder of uncertain etiology with variable clinical expression and clinical course (159–162). Spontaneous remissions (SRs) occur in nearly two thirds of patients but a chronic or progressive course is noted in 10% to 30% (160,163–167). Chronic pulmonary sarcoidosis may result in debilitating respiratory failure (160,168). Fatality rates ascribed to sarcoidosis range from 2% to 5% (160,165,166,169,170), but the rates are lower (< 1%) in nonreferral settings (163,164,171,172). Lung transplantation is a viable option for patients with severe fibrocystic pulmonary sarcoidosis failing medical therapy (173).

### Results of Lung Transplantation for Sarcoidosis

Both single and bilateral LTs have been performed for end-stage pulmonary sarcoidosis (76). Data from the ISHLT Registry noted that 323 patients with sarcoidosis had LTs between January 1995 and June 2004 (representing 2.5% of LTs performed within that time frame (1).

## Clinical Features and Prognosis of Sarcoidosis

Fever, erythema nodosum, polyarthritis, and bilateral hilar lymphadenopathy (BHL) (Lofgren's syndrome) are common early features of sarcoidosis, and predict an excellent prognosis (SRs in >85%) (160–162,174). By contrast, bone involvement, lupus pernio (disfiguring cutaneous lesions), black race, chronic hypercalcemia, and chronic pulmonary sarcoidosis are associated with a worse prognosis (161,165,175).

## Radiographic Classification Scheme: Influence on Prognosis

Chest radiographs are abnormal in >90% of patients with sarcoidosis (160–162). The most characteristic finding is BHL, with or without concomitant right paratracheal node enlargement (160,162). Parenchymal infiltrates are present in 25–55% of patients with sarcoidosis (160,162). These infiltrates have a predilection for mid and upper lung zones (160). The radiographic staging system developed more than four decades ago continues to be useful prognostically. This schema applies the following criteria on chest radiographs: stage 0, normal; stage I, BHL without parenchymal infiltrates; stage II, BHL with parenchymal infiltrates; stage III, parenchymal infiltrates without BHL; stage IV, extensive destruction, architecture distortion, and irreversible fibrosis (162). SRs occur in 60% to 90% of patients with stage I disease, 40% to 70% with stage II disease, and 10% to 20% with stage III disease (160–163,166,171). Serious sequelae are rare with stage I sarcoidosis, but may be appreciable in later stages. Virtually all fatalities due to pulmonary sarcoidosis are in patients with radiographic II, III, or IV disease (160). The course of the disease is usually dictated within the first two years of onset. SRs occur in up to 40% within the first six months (162,176,177); >80% of SRs occur within the first two years (166). Persistence of radiographic infiltrates beyond two years suggests a chronic or progressive course (166). In some patients, multiple exacerbations of the disease over the years result in progressive destruction of lung parenchyma and debilitating respiratory insufficiency (160,165).

## HRCT in Sarcoidosis

Typical features of parenchymal involvement in sarcoidosis on HRCT scans include parenchymal opacities or nodules in the mid or upper lung zones, patchy involvement, distribution along bronchovascular bundles, focal or confluent alveolar opacities with consolidation, GGO, thickened intra- or interlobular septae, fibrosis, distortion, and cysts (178,179). Distortion, cysts, bullae, or traction bronchiectasis reflect fibrosis and predict unresponsiveness to therapy (178,179). By contrast, focal alveolar opacities, GGO, or nodules are often associated with an inflammatory component and predict a higher rate of response to therapy (178,180).

## Influence of Pulmonary Function on Prognosis

Physiological parameters at the onset do not predict long-term outcome in patients with sarcoidosis (181–184). However, serial studies are important to follow the course of the disease and assess response to therapy. Vital capacity (VC) improves more frequently than $DL_{CO}$ (184–186), TLC (187), or arterial oxygenation (188). Changes in VC and $DL_{CO}$ are usually concordant; discordant changes occur in fewer than 5% of patients (167,188). Spirometry and flow-volume loops are the most useful and cost-effective parameters to follow the course of the disease (184). Additional studies such as $DL_{CO}$, TLC, or gas exchange have a role in selected patients. Criteria for assessing "response" or improvement have not been validated. Most investigators define a change in FVC > 10–15% or $DL_{CO}$ > 20% as significant (188,189). Responses to therapy are usually evident within 6 to 12 weeks of initiation of therapy (184,190).

## Treatment of Sarcoidosis

Treatment of sarcoidosis is controversial. CS are the cornerstone of therapy for severe or progressive sarcoidosis (pulmonary or extrapulmonary), and often produce dramatic resolution of disease (159,175,176,191,192). The long-term benefit of CS therapy is less clear, as relapses may occur upon taper or cessation of therapy (175,193,194). Alternative therapeutic modalities (particularly immunosuppressive or cytotoxic agents) are reserved for patients failing, experiencing adverse effects, or at risk of adverse effects from CS (159,191,195–201). Alternative therapeutic modalities include methotrexate (202,203), AZA (196,197,204), lenflunamide (201), cyclophosphamide (205), antimalarials (chloroquine or hydroxychloroquine) (198,206,207), and anti-TNF inhibitors (199,200,208–211). A discussion of medical therapy for sarcoidosis is beyond the scope of this chapter, and is not addressed here.

## Which Patients Should Be Considered for LT?

Given the potential for spontaneous resolution in patients with sarcoidosis, LT should be reserved for patients with chronic, progressive disease who have failed medical therapy. Typically, this includes patients with radiographic stage IV disease, characterized by advanced fibrotic changes, honeycombing, hilar retraction, bullae, cysts, and emphysema (160,162,212). HRCT scans should be done in patients with stage II or III disease to discriminate active inflammation (alveolitis) from fibrosis. Nodules, GGO, consolidation, or alveolar opacities suggest granulomatous inflammation, which may reverse with therapy (178,180,213–215). By contrast, honeycomb change, cysts, coarse broad bands, distortion, or traction bronchiectasis indicate irreversible fibrosis (216–219). Patients with severe pulmonary

**Table 2**  Indications for Lung Transplantation for Sarcoidosis

---

Severe impairment in pulmonary function tests
  FVC  < 45% predicted
  $FEV_1$  < 40% predicted
  $DL_{CO}$  < 40% predicted
Declining PFTs
Need for supplemental oxygen
Pulmonary arterial hypertension (sPAP  > 50 mmHg)
Severe fibrosis or honeycomb change on HRCT scans
Failure to respond to medical therapy

---

*Abbreviations*: FVC, forced vital capacity; $FEV_1$, forced expiratory volume in one second; $DL_{CO}$, diffusing capacity for carbon monoxide; PFT, defect on pulmonary function test; sPAP, systolic pulmonary artery pressure; HRCT, high-resolution computed tomography.

dysfunction but with CT features suggesting active inflammation should be aggressively treated medically before resorting to LT. Conversely, medical therapy is of no value and potentially toxic in patients with severe architectural distortion, honeycomb change, and fibrosis (178,212,220). These patients should be referred promptly for LT, provided the symptoms and the extent of pulmonary dysfunction warrant it. Indications and contraindications for LT for sarcoidosis are generally similar to other indications (Table 2) (221). However, LT would not be an appropriate use of resources for patients with severe extrapulmonary sarcoidosis that is disabling or life-threatening (159). Additionally, mycetomas, which may be observed in end-stage pulmonary sarcoidosis (178,212,220), have been associated with a worse prognosis post LT (222), and are considered by many centers to be a contraindication to LT.

### Predicting Mortality in Patients with Sarcoidosis

Mortality rates among sarcoid patients awaiting LT are high (27–53%) (76,223,224). This high attrition rate on the waiting list likely reflects late diagnosis of advanced disease and delayed referral for LT (173). Deciding when to refer patients with sarcoidosis for LT is difficult, as models predicting mortality in sarcoidosis are lacking. Importantly, algorithms or parameters predicting mortality for IPF and other types of ILDs may not apply to sarcoidosis. Severe restrictive lung disease is associated with increased mortality among sarcoid patients (168), but no clear cutoff point for any pulmonary functional parameter predicts outcome. Typically, patients with sarcoidosis referred for LT have severe impairment in PFTs (mean % predicted FVC < 44%; mean % predicted $FEV_1$ < 38%) (76,224). A large retrospective review of the United Network for Organ Sharing (UNOS) database from 1995 to 2000 identified 405 patients with sarcoidosis listed for LT in the United States; 111 (27.4%) died while awaiting LT (224).

Surprisingly, PFTs did not correlate with mortality. Mean % predicted FVC among survivors was 43.1% compared to 41.3% among nonsurvivors ($P = 0.14$). Mean % predicted $FEV_1$ values were similar among survivors (35.8%) compared to nonsurvivors (36.7 %; $P = 0.48$). Three factors were associated with increased mortality while on the transplant list: (i) the presence of PAH, (ii) the amount of supplemental oxygen needed, and (iii) African American race (224). The mean PAP of survivors was 31.7 mmHg, compared to 41.4 mmHg among nonsurvivors ($P < 0.01$). Mean supplemental oxygen requirements were 2.2 versus 2.9 L/min among survivors and nonsurvivors, respectively ($P < 0.01$). Another single-center study of 43 patients with sarcoidosis awaiting LT found that mean $PAP \geq 35$ mmHg, cardiac index $\leq 2$ L/min/m$^2$, and right atrial pressure (RAP) $\geq 15$ mmHg were associated with a higher risk of death (223). By multivariate analysis, mean RAP $> 15$ mmHg was the only independent prognostic variable [5.2-fold odds ratio (OR) for mortality].

In conclusion, PAH is an ominous sign in sarcoidosis, and warrants referral for LT as well as consideration for aggressive medical therapy. Importantly, PAH is common in advanced sarcoidosis (225,226). The mechanism for PAH has not been elucidated, and may reflect several factors including hypoxemic vasoconstriction, primary involvement or destruction of the pulmonary vasculature, cardiac dysfunction, and distortion or loss of lung parenchyma (225). The UNOS database identified 363 patients with sarcoidosis listed for LT in the United States between January 1995 and December 2002 who had undergone RHC (225). This represented 72.5% of all listed sarcoid patients; clinical variables were similar among patients with or without RHC. Pulmonary hypertension (defined as mean PAP > 25 mmHg) was present in 74% of patients; severe PAH (defined as mean PAP > 40 mmHg) was noted in 36%. Importantly, PFTs did not differ between those with or without PAH. However, supplemental $O_2$ requirements were higher in those with PAH (2.7 L/min) compared to those without PAH (1.6 L/min). In addition, PAH doubled the risk of patients being disabled due to disease (OR, 2.08). By multivariate analysis, only two variables were associated with PAH: $O_2$ requirements and pulmonary capillary wedge pressure. Patients with severe PAH were nearly seven times more likely to require supplemental $O_2$. Although vasodilators, prostaglandins, or endothelin-receptor antagonists have not been extensively studied in sarcoidosis, these agents may have a role as a bridge to transplantation in patients with severe PAH or right heart failure (227).

In summary, sarcoid patients with PAH or requiring supplemental $O_2$ should be referred promptly to transplant centers, as these findings are associated with increased mortality with medical therapy alone. Although we recognize the limitations of DE in assessing sPAP (99), we believe DE should be performed in patients with severe pulmonary sarcoidosis, particularly those requiring supplemental oxygen. When DE is abnormal, performing a confirmatory RHC is reasonable to assess the extent of PAP and the responsiveness to vasodilators. To our knowledge, the prognostic value of other noninvasive tests (e.g., 6MWT and serum BNP) has not been studied in sarcoidosis. Despite the lack of discriminatory ability of standard PFT parameters, referral for LT is reasonable when the FVC falls below 50% predicted and/or $FEV_1$ falls below 40% predicted.

## Results of LT for Sarcoidosis

Data from the ISHLT Registry indicate that 2.3% of SLTs (157 of 6731) and 2.6% of BLTs (166 of 6276) were performed for patients with sarcoidosis from 1995 to 2004 (1). There are no data attesting to the benefit of one procedure over the other. However, bilateral bronchiectasis or aspergillomas may necessitate BLT. There is no evidence that PAH mandates BLT, but this is the preference of some programs.

Short- and late-term mortality rates following LT for sarcoidosis were slightly higher compared to LT performed for other diseases (17,76). The ISHLT Registry cited one-, three-, and five-year survival rates of 67%, 53%, and 45% among sarcoid patients receiving LT (17). By comparison, one-, three-, and five-year survival rates for other indications are, respectively, as follows: chronic obstructive pulmonary disease (80%, 62%, and 47%); IPF (68%, 52%, and 50%); cystic fibrosis (79%, 63%, and 53%); alpha-1-antitrypsin deficiency (75%, 60%, and 50%); and primary pulmonary hypertension (65%, 54%, and 45%) (17). A retrospective review of UNOS data from 1995 to 2000 cited 30-day survival post LT of 83% among 133 patients with sarcoidosis compared to 91% among LT recipients for other conditions ($P = 0.002$) (228). In that study, graft failure was the most common cause of death in sarcoid patients, whereas infection was the leading cause of death among nonsarcoid LT recipients. The adjusted OR for mortality among sarcoid patients was 1.45 (95% confidence interval, 0.84–2.48), but this was not statistically significant ($P = 0.18$). After controlling for both health insurance and other conditions that may affect survival after LT, patients with sarcoidosis were no more likely to die than persons undergoing LT for other conditions (228). Significant predictors of mortality included combined heart–lung transplant, need for mechanical ventilation, treatment in an intensive care unit at time of LT, pre-LT $FEV_1$, need for supplemental oxygen, and donor age. Race influenced mortality. African American recipients were nearly 50% more likely to die (adjusted OR, 1.49; $P = 0.045$). Interestingly, recipients receiving organs from African Americans had nearly 50% higher risk for mortality (adjusted OR, 1.44; $P = 0.008$). The impact of race was independent of health insurance status. Previous studies cited worse outcomes among African Americans receiving renal (229) or hepatic transplants (230); this may reflect greater major histocompatibility polymorphisms or immunologic hyper-responsiveness among African Americans.

Recurrent non-necrotizing granulomata have been noted in the lung allografts in more than one-third of sarcoid patients (231–233), but are not usually associated with symptoms (233). However, a few cases of clinically significant recurrence have been noted (234,235).

## REFERENCES

1. Trulock EP, Edwards LB, Taylor DO, Boucek MM, Keck BM, Hertz MI. Registry of the International Society for Heart and Lung Transplantation: Twenty-Second Official Adult Lung and Heart–Lung Transplant Report— 2005. J Heart Lung Transplant 2005; 24(8):956–967.
2. Lynch III JP, Wurfel M, Flaherty K, et al. Usual interstitial pneumonia. Semin Respir Crit Care Med 2001; 22:357–387.
3. Katzenstein AL, Myers JL. Idiopathic pulmonary fibrosis: clinical relevance of pathologic classification. Am J Respir Crit Care Med 1998; 157(4, Pt 1): 1301–1315.
4. American Thoracic Society. Idiopathic pulmonary fibrosis: diagnosis and treatment. International consensus statement. American Thoracic Society (ATS), and the European Respiratory Society (ERS). Am J Respir Crit Care Med 2000; 161(2, Pt 1):646–664.
5. Turner-Warwick M, Burrows B, Johnson A. Cryptogenic fibrosing alveolitis: response to corticosteroid treatment and its effect on survival. Thorax 1980; 35:593–599.
6. Bjoraker JA, Ryu JH, Edwin MK, et al. Prognostic significance of histopathologic subsets in idiopathic pulmonary fibrosis. Am J Respir Crit Care Med 1998; 157(1):199–203.
7. Nicholson AG, Wells AU. Nonspecific interstitial pneumonia—nobody said it's perfect. Am J Respir Crit Care Med 2001; 164(9):1553–1554.
8. Travis WD, Matsui K, Moss J, Ferrans VJ. Idiopathic nonspecific interstitial pneumonia: prognostic significance of cellular and fibrosing patterns: survival comparison with usual interstitial pneumonia and desquamative interstitial pneumonia. Am J Surg Pathol 2000; 24(1):19–33.
9. Mapel DW, Samet JM, Coultas DB. Corticosteroids and the treatment of idiopathic pulmonary fibrosis. Past, present, and future. Chest 1996; 110(4): 1058–1067.
10. Mogulkoc N, Brutsche MH, Bishop PW, Greaves SM, Horrocks AW, Egan JJ. Pulmonary function in idiopathic pulmonary fibrosis and referral for lung transplantation. Am J Respir Crit Care Med 2001; 164(1):103–108.
11. Douglas WW, Ryu JH, Schroeder DR. Idiopathic pulmonary fibrosis: impact of oxygen and colchicine, prednisone, or no therapy on survival. Am J Respir Crit Care Med 2000; 161:1172–1178.
12. King TE Jr, Schwarz MI, Brown K, et al. Idiopathic pulmonary fibrosis: relationship between histopathologic features and mortality. Am J Respir Crit Care Med 2001; 164(6):1025–1032.
13. Wells AU, Desai SR, Rubens MB, et al. Idiopathic pulmonary fibrosis: a composite physiologic index derived from disease extent observed by computed tomography. Am J Respir Crit Care Med 2003; 167(7):962–969.

14. Flaherty KR, Mumford JA, Murray S, et al. Prognostic implications of physiologic and radiographic changes in idiopathic interstitial pneumonia. Am J Respir Crit Care Med 2003; 168(5):543–548.
15. Flaherty KR, Colby TV, Travis WD, et al. Fibroblastic foci in usual interstitial pneumonia: idiopathic versus collagen vascular disease. Am J Respir Crit Care Med 2003; 167(10):1410–1415.
16. The American Society for Transplant Physicians (ASTP)/American Thoracic Society (ATS)/European Respiratory Society (ERS)/International Society for Heart and Lung Transplantation (ISHLT). International guidelines for the selection of lung transplant candidates. Am J Respir Crit Care Med 1998; 158(1):335–339.
17. Trulock EP, Edwards LB, Taylor DO, Boucek MM, Keck BM, Hertz MI. The registry of the International Society for Heat and Lung Transplantation: Twenty-First Official Adult Heart Transplant Report—2004. J Heart Lung Transplant 2004; 23(7):804–815.
18. Charman SC, Sharples LD, McNeil KD, Wallwork J. Assessment of survival benefit after lung transplantation by patient diagnosis. J Heart Lung Transplant 2002; 21(2):226–232.
19. Meyers BF, Lynch JP, Trulock EP, Guthrie T, Cooper JD, Patterson GA. Single versus bilateral lung transplantation for idiopathic pulmonary fibrosis: a ten-year institutional experience. J Thorac Cardiovasc Surg 2000; 120(1): 99–107.
20. Meyer DM, Edwards LB, Torres F, Jessen ME, Novick RJ. Impact of recipient age and procedure type on survival after lung transplantation for pulmonary fibrosis. Ann Thorac Surg 2005; 79(3):950–957; discussion 7–8.
21. Nagai S, Kitaichi M, Itoh H, Nishimura K, Izumi T, Colby T. Idiopathic nonspecific interstitial pneumonia/fibrosis: comparison with idiopathic pulmonary fibrosis and BOOP. Eur Respir J 1998; 12:1010–1019.
22. Flaherty KR, Travis WD, Colby TV, et al. Histopathologic variability in usual and nonspecific interstitial pneumonias. Am J Respir Crit Care Med 2001; 164(9):1722–1727.
23. Flaherty KR, Martinez FJ, Travis W, Lynch JP III. Nonspecific interstitial pneumonia (NSIP). Semin Respir Crit Care Med 2001; 22(4):423–434.
24. Yousem SA, Colby TV, Gaensler EA. Respiratory bronchiolitis-associated interstitial lung disease and its relationship to desquamative interstitial pneumonia. Mayo Clin Proc 1989; 64(11):1373–1380.
25. Ryu JH, Colby TV, Hartman TE, Vassallo R. Smoking-related interstitial lung diseases: a concise review. Eur Respir J 2001; 17(1):122–132.
26. Moon J, du Bois RM, Colby TV, Hansell DM, Nicholson AG. Clinical significance of respiratory bronchiolitis on open lung biopsy and its relationship to smoking related interstitial lung disease. Thorax 1999; 54(11):1009–1014.
27. Hartman TE, Primack SL, Swensen SJ, Hansell D, McGuinness G, Muller NL. Desquamative interstitial pneumonia: thin-section CT findings in 22 patients. Radiology 1993; 187(3):787–790.
28. Hartman TE, Primack SL, Kang EY, et al. Disease progression in usual interstitial pneumonia compared with desquamative interstitial pneumonia. Assessment with serial CT. Chest 1996; 110(2):378–382.

29. Ichikado K, Suga M, Muller NL, et al. Acute interstitial pneumonia: comparison of high-resolution computed tomography findings between survivors and nonsurvivors. Am J Respir Crit Care Med 2002; 165(11):1551–1556.
30. Johkoh T, Muller NL, Taniguchi H, et al. Acute interstitial pneumonia: thin-section CT findings in 36 patients. Radiology 1999; 211(3):859–863.
31. Vourlekis JS, Brown KK, Cool CD, et al. Acute interstitial pneumonitis. Case series and review of the literature. Medicine (Baltimore) 2000; 79(6):369–378.
32. Bouros D, Nicholson AC, Polychronopoulos V, du Bois RM. Acute interstitial pneumonia. Eur Respir J 2000; 15(2):412–418.
33. Johkoh T, Muller NL, Pickford HA, et al. Lymphocytic interstitial pneumonia: thin-section CT findings in 22 patients. Radiology 1999; 212(2):567–572.
34. McGuinness G, Scholes JV, Jagirdar JS, et al. Unusual lymphoproliferative disorders in nine adults with HIV or AIDS: CT and pathologic findings. Radiology 1995; 197(1):59–65.
35. Alasaly K, Muller N, Ostrow DN, Champion P, FitzGerald JM. Cryptogenic organizing pneumonia. A report of 25 cases and a review of the literature. Medicine (Baltimore) 1995; 74(4):201–211.
36. Lee KS, Kullnig P, Hartman TE, Muller NL. Cryptogenic organizing pneumonia: CT findings in 43 patients. Am J Roentgenol 1994; 162(3):543–546.
37. Cordier JF. Organising pneumonia. Thorax 2000; 55(4):318–328.
38. Gross TJ, Hunninghake GW. Idiopathic pulmonary fibrosis. N Engl J Med 2001; 345(7):517–525.
39. Coultas DB, Zumwalt RE, Black WC, Sobonya RE. The epidemiology of interstitial lung diseases. Am J Respir Crit Care Med 1994; 150(4):967–972.
40. Thannickal V, Flaherty K, Hyzy R, Lynch JP III. Emerging drugs for idiopathic pulmonary fibrosis. Expert Opin Emerg Drugs 2005; 10(4):707–727.
41. Baumgartner KB, Samet JM, Coultas DB, et al. Occupational and environmental risk factors for idiopathic pulmonary fibrosis: a multicenter case–control study. Collaborating Centers. Am J Epidemiol 2000; 152(4):307–315.
42. Iwai K, Mori T, Yamada N, Yamaguchi M, Hosoda Y. Idiopathic pulmonary fibrosis. Epidemiologic approaches to occupational exposure. Am J Respir Crit Care Med 1994; 150(3):670–675.
43. Mullen J, Hodgson MJ, DeGraff CA, Godar T. Case–control study of idiopathic pulmonary fibrosis and environmental exposures. J Occup Environ Med 1998; 40(4):363–367.
44. Harris JM, Cullinan P, McDonald JC. Occupational distribution and geographic clustering of deaths certified to be cryptogenic fibrosing alveolitis in England and Wales. Chest 2001; 119(2):428–433.
45. Tobin RW, Pope CE II, Pellegrini CA, Emond MJ, Sillery J, Raghu G. Increased prevalence of gastroesophageal reflux in patients with idiopathic pulmonary fibrosis. Am J Respir Crit Care Med 1998; 158(6):1804–1808.
46. Marshall RP, Puddicombe A, Cookson WO, Laurent GJ. Adult familial cryptogenic fibrosing alveolitis in the United Kingdom. Thorax 2000; 55(2):143–146.
47. Whyte M, Hubbard R, Meliconi R, et al. Increased risk of fibrosing alveolitis associated with interleukin-1 receptor antagonist and tumor necrosis factor-alpha gene polymorphisms. Am J Respir Crit Care Med 2000; 162(2, Pt 1):755–758.

48. American Thoracic Society/European Respiratory Society International - Multidisciplinary Consensus Classification of the Idiopathic Interstitial Pneumonias. This joint statement of the American Thoracic Society (ATS), and the European Respiratory Society (ERS) was adopted by the ATS board of directors, June 2001 and by the ERS Executive Committee, June 2001. Am J Respir Crit Care Med 2002; 165(2):277–304.

49. Hubbard R, Johnston I, Britton J. Survival in patients with cryptogenic fibrosing alveolitis. A population-based cohort study. Chest 1998; 113:396–400.

50. Watters LC, Schwarz MI, Cherniack RM, et al. Idiopathic pulmonary fibrosis. pretreatment bronchoalveolar lavage cellular constituents and their relationships with lung histopathology and clinical response to therapy. Am Rev Respir Dis 1987; 135(3):696–704.

51. Tukiainen P, Taskineu E, Holsti P, et al. Prognosis of cryptogenic fibrosing alveolitis. Thorax 1983; 38:349–355.

52. Turner-Warwick M, Haslam PL. The value of serial bronchoalveolar lavages in assessing the clinical progress of patients with cryptogenic fibrosing alveolitis. Am Rev Respir Dis 1987; 135(1):26–34.

53. Winterbauer RH, Hammar SP, Hallman KO, et al. Diffuse interstitial pneumonitis. Clinicopathologic correlations in 20 patients treated with prednisone/azathioprine. Am J Med 1978; 65(4):661–672.

54. Nicholson AG, Colby TV, du Bois RM, Hansell DM, Wells AU. The prognostic significance of the histologic pattern of interstitial pneumonia in patients presenting with the clinical entity of cryptogenic fibrosing alveolitis. Am J Respir Crit Care Med 2000; 162(6):2213–2217.

55. Daniil ZD, Gilchrist FC, Nicholson AG, et al. A histologic pattern of nonspecific interstitial pneumonia is associated with a better prognosis than usual interstitial pneumonia in patients with cryptogenic fibrosing alveolitis. Am J Respir Crit Care Med 1999; 160(3):899–905.

56. Raghu G, Depaso WJ, Cain K, et al. Azathioprine combined with prednisone in the treatment of idiopathic pulmonary fibrosis: a prospective double-blind, randomized, placebo-controlled clinical trial. Am Rev Respir Dis 1991; 144(2):291–296.

57. Kolb M, Kirschner J, Riedel W, Wirtz H, Schmidt M. Cyclophosphamide pulse therapy in idiopathic pulmonary fibrosis. Eur Respir J 1998; 12:1409–1414.

58. Zisman DA, Lynch JP III, Toews GB, Kazerooni EA, Flint A, Martinez FJ. Cyclophosphamide in the treatment of idiopathic pulmonary fibrosis: a prospective study in patients who failed to respond to corticosteroids. Chest 2000; 117(6):1619–1626.

59. Johnson MA, Kwan S, Snell NJ, Nunn AJ, Darbyshire JH, Turner-Warwick M. Randomised controlled trial comparing prednisolone alone with cyclophosphamide and low dose prednisolone in combination in cryptogenic fibrosing alveolitis. Thorax 1989; 44(4):280–288.

60. Lynch JP III, McCune WJ. Immunosuppressive and cytotoxic pharmacotherapy for pulmonary disorders. Am J Respir Crit Care Med 1997; 155(2):395–420.

61. Selman M, Carrillo G, Salas J, et al. Colchicine, D-penicillamine, and prednisone in the treatment of idiopathic pulmonary fibrosis. A controlled clinical trial. Chest 1998; 114:507–512.

62. Douglas WW, Ryu JH, Swensen SJ, et al. Colchicine versus prednisone in the treatment of idiopathic pulmonary fibrosis. A randomized prospective study. Members of the lung study group. Am J Respir Crit Care Med 1998; 158(1): 220–225.

63. King TE Jr, Tooze JA, Schwarz MI, Brown KR, Cherniack RM. Predicting survival in idiopathic pulmonary fibrosis: scoring system and survival model. Am J Respir Crit Care Med 2001; 164(7):1171–1181.

64. Nagai S, Kitaichi M, Hamada K, et al. Hospital-based historical cohort study of 234 histologically proven Japanese patients with IPF. Sarcoidosis Vasc Diffuse Lung Dis 1999; 16(2):209–214.

65. Meyer A, Buhl R, Magnussen H. The effect of oral *N*-acetylcysteine on lung glutathione levels in idiopathic pulmonary fibrosis. Eur Respir J 1994; 7(3): 431–436.

66. Behr J, Maier K, Degenkolb B, Krombach F, Vogelmeier C. Antioxidative and clinical effects of high-dose *N*-acetylcysteine in fibrosing alveolitis. Adjunctive therapy to maintenance immunosuppression. Am J Respir Crit Care Med 1997; 156(6):1897–1901.

67. Raghu G, Johnson WC, Lockhart D, Mageto Y. Treatment of idiopathic pulmonary fibrosis with a new antifibrotic agent, pirfenidone: results of a prospective, open-label phase II study. Am J Respir Crit Care Med 1999; 159(4, Pt 1): 1061–1069.

68. Azuma A, Nukiwa T, Tsuboi E, et al. Double-blind, placebo-controlled trial of pirfenidone in patients with idiopathic pulmonary fibrosis. Am J Respir Crit Care Med 2005; 171(9):1040–1047.

69. Raghu G, Brown KK, Bradford WZ, et al. A placebo-controlled trial of interferon gamma-1b in patients with idiopathic pulmonary fibrosis. N Engl J Med 2004; 350(2):125–133.

70. King TE Jr, Safrin S, Starko KM, et al. Analyses of efficacy end points in a controlled trial of interferon-gamma1b for idiopathic pulmonary fibrosis. Chest 2005; 127(1):171–177.

70a. Demendts M, Behr J, Buhl R, et al. High-dose acetylcysteine in idiopathic pulmonary fibrosis. N Eng J Med 2005; 353:2229–2242.

71. Selman M, Thannickal VJ, Pardo A, Zisman DA, Martinez FJ, Lynch JP III. Idiopathic pulmonary fibrosis: pathogenesis and therapeutic approaches. Drugs 2004; 64(4):405–430.

72. Thannickal VJ, Toews GB, White ES, Lynch JP III, Martinez FJ. Mechanisms of pulmonary fibrosis. Annu Rev Med 2004; 55:395–417.

73. Thannickal VJ, Flaherty KR, Martinez FJ, Lynch JP III. Idiopathic pulmonary fibrosis: emerging concepts on pharmacotherapy. Expert Opin Pharmacother 2004; 5(8):1671–1686.

74. Latsi PI, du Bois RM, Nicholson AG, et al. Fibrotic idiopathic interstitial pneumonia: the prognostic value of longitudinal functional trends. Am J Respir Crit Care Med 2003; 168(5):531–537.

75. Collard HR, King TE Jr, Bartelson BB, Vourlekis JS, Schwarz MI, Brown KK. Changes in clinical and physiologic variables predict survival in idiopathic pulmonary fibrosis. Am J Respir Crit Care Med 2003; 168(5):538–542.

76. Shorr AF, Davies DB, Nathan SD. Outcomes for patients with sarcoidosis awaiting lung transplantation. Chest 2002; 122(1):233–238.

77. Timmer SJ, Karamzadeh AM, Yung GL, Kriett J, Jamieson SW, Smith CM. Predicting survival of lung transplantation candidates with idiopathic interstitial pneumonia: does PaO(2) predict survival? Chest 2002; 122(3):779–784.

78. Flaherty KR, Toews GB, Travis WD, et al. Clinical significance of histological classification of idiopathic interstitial pneumonia. Eur Respir J 2002; 19(2):275–283.

79. Schwartz DA, Helmers RA, Galvin JR, et al. Determinants of survival in idiopathic pulmonary fibrosis. Am J Respir Crit Care Med 1994; 149(2, Pt 1): 450–454.

80. Nakamura Y, Romberger DJ, Tate L, et al. Cigarette smoke inhibits lung fibroblast proliferation and chemotaxis. Am J Respir Crit Care Med 1995; 151(5): 1497–1503.

81. Jegal Y, Kim DS, Shim TS, et al. Physiology is a stronger predictor of survival than pathology in fibrotic interstitial pneumonia. Am J Respir Crit Care Med 2005; 171(6):639–644.

82. Nadrous HF, Pellikka PA, Krowka MJ, et al. Pulmonary hypertension in patients with idiopathic pulmonary fibrosis. Chest 2005; 128(4):2393–2399.

83. Nicholson AG, Fulford LG, Colby TV, du Bois RM, Hansell DM, Wells AU. The relationship between individual histologic features and disease progression in idiopathic pulmonary fibrosis. Am J Respir Crit Care Med 2002; 166(2):173–177.

84. Flaherty KR, Martinez FJ. The role of pulmonary function testing in pulmonary fibrosis. Curr Opin Pulm Med 2000; 6(5):404–410.

85. Erbes R, Schaberg T, Loddenkemper R. Lung function tests in patients with idiopathic pulmonary fibrosis. Are they helpful for predicting outcome? Chest 1997; 111(1):51–57.

86. Hanson D, Winterbauer RH, Kirtland SH, Wu R. Changes in pulmonary function test results after 1 year of therapy as predictors of survival in patients with idiopathic pulmonary fibrosis. Chest 1995; 108(2):305–310.

87. Lynch DA, Godwin JD, Safrin S, et al. High-resolution computed tomography in idiopathic pulmonary fibrosis: diagnosis and prognosis. Am J Respir Crit Care Med 2005; 172(4):488–493.

88. Dunn TL, Watters LC, Hendrix C, Cherniack RM, Schwarz MI, King TE Jr. Gas exchange at a given degree of volume restriction is different in sarcoidosis and idiopathic pulmonary fibrosis. Am J Med 1988; 85(2):221–224.

89. Flaherty KR, Toews GB, Lynch JP III, et al. Steroids in idiopathic pulmonary fibrosis: a prospective assessment of adverse reactions, response to therapy, and survival. Am J Med 2001; 110(4):278–282.

90. Gay SE, Kazerooni EA, Toews GB, et al. Idiopathic pulmonary fibrosis: predicting response to therapy and survival. Am J Respir Crit Care Med 1998; 157(4, Pt 1):1063–1072.

91. Lama VN, Flaherty KR, Toews GB, et al. Prognostic value of desaturation during a 6-minute walk test in idiopathic interstitial pneumonia. Am J Respir Crit Care Med 2003; 168(9):1084–1090.

92. Hallstrand TS, Boitano LJ, Johnson WC, Spada CA, Hayes JG, Raghu G. The timed walk test as a measure of severity and survival in idiopathic pulmonary fibrosis. Eur Respir J 2005; 25(1):96–103.

93. Eaton T, Young P, Milne D, Wells AU. Six-minute walk, maximal exercise tests: reproducibility in fibrotic interstitial pneumonia. Am J Respir Crit Care Med 2005; 171(10):1150–1157.

94. Miki K, Maekura R, Hiraga T, et al. Impairments and prognostic factors for survival in patients with idiopathic pulmonary fibrosis. Respir Med 2003; 97(5):482–490.

95. Wells AU, Hansell DM, Rubens MB, Cailes JB, Black CM, du Bois RM. Functional impairment in lone cryptogenic fibrosing alveolitis and fibrosing alveolitis associated with systemic sclerosis: a comparison. Am J Respir Crit Care Med 1997; 155(5):1657–1664.

96. Flaherty KR, Thwaite EL, Kazerooni EA, et al. Radiological versus histological diagnosis in UIP and NSIP: survival implications. Thorax 2003; 58(2): 143–148.

97. Watters LC, King TE, Schwarz MI, Waldron JA, Stanford RE, Cherniack RM. A clinical, radiographic, and physiologic scoring system for the longitudinal assessment of patients with idiopathic pulmonary fibrosis. Am Rev Respir Dis 1986; 133(1):97–103.

98. Perez A, Rogers RM, Dauber JH. The prognosis of idiopathic pulmonary fibrosis. Am J Respir Cell Mol Biol 2003; 29(3, Suppl):S19–S26.

99. Arcasoy SM, Christie JD, Ferrari VA, et al. Echocardiographic assessment of pulmonary hypertension in patients with advanced lung disease. Am J Respir Crit Care Med 2003; 167(5):735–740.

100. Leuchte HH, Neurohr C, Baumgartner R, et al. Brain natriuretic peptide and exercise capacity in lung fibrosis and pulmonary hypertension. Am J Respir Crit Care Med 2004; 170(4):360–365.

101. Harari S, Simonneau G, De Juli E, et al. Prognostic value of pulmonary hypertension in patients with chronic interstitial lung disease referred for lung or heart-lung transplantation. J Heart Lung Transplant 1997; 16(4):460–463.

102. Ghofrani HA, Wiedemann R, Rose F, et al. Sildenafil for treatment of lung fibrosis and pulmonary hypertension: a randomised controlled trial. Lancet 2002; 360(9337):895–900.

103. Olschewski H, Ghofrani HA, Walmrath D, et al. Inhaled prostacyclin and iloprost in severe pulmonary hypertension secondary to lung fibrosis. Am J Respir Crit Care Med 1999; 160(2):600–607.

104. Homma A, Anzueto A, Peters JI, et al. Pulmonary artery systolic pressures estimated by echocardiogram vs. cardiac catheterization in patients awaiting lung transplantation. J Heart Lung Transplant 2001; 20(8):833–839.

105. Bando K, Keenan RJ, Paradis IL, et al. Impact of pulmonary hypertension on outcome after single-lung transplantation. Ann Thorac Surg 1994; 58(5): 1336–1342.

106. Huerd SS, Hodges TN, Grover FL, et al. Secondary pulmonary hypertension does not adversely affect outcome after single lung transplantation. J Thorac Cardiovasc Surg 2000; 119(3):458–465.

107. Whelan TP, Dunitz JM, Kelly RF, et al. Effect of preoperative pulmonary artery pressure on early survival after lung transplantation for idiopathic pulmonary fibrosis. J Heart Lung Transplant 2005; 24(9):1269–1274.

108. Panos RJ, Mortenson RL, Niccoli SA, King TE Jr. Clinical deterioration in patients with idiopathic pulmonary fibrosis: causes and assessment. Am J Med 1990; 88(4):396–404.

109. Kizer JR, Zisman DA, Blumenthal NP, et al. Association between pulmonary fibrosis and coronary artery disease. Arch Intern Med 2004; 164(5):551–556.

110. Nathan SD, Barnett SD, Urban BA, Nowalk C, Moran BR, Burton N. Pulmonary embolism in idiopathic pulmonary fibrosis transplant recipients. Chest 2003; 123(5):1758–1763.

111. Magro CM, Allen J, Pope-Harman A, et al. The role of microvascular injury in the evolution of idiopathic pulmonary fibrosis. Am J Clin Pathol 2003; 119(4):556–567.

112. Hubbard R, Venn A, Lewis S, Britton J. Lung cancer and cryptogenic fibrosing alveolitis. A population-based cohort study. Am J Respir Crit Care Med 2000; 161(1):5–8.

113. Samet JM. Does idiopathic pulmonary fibrosis increase lung cancer risk? Am J Respir Crit Care Med 2000; 161(1):1–2.

114. Enomoto T, Usuki J, Azuma A, Nakagawa T, Kudoh S. Diabetes mellitus may increase risk for idiopathic pulmonary fibrosis. Chest 2003; 123(6):2007–2011.

115. Katzenstein AL, Fiorelli RF. Nonspecific interstitial pneumonia/fibrosis. Histologic features and clinical significance. Am J Surg Pathol 1994; 18(2):136–147.

116. Kim TS, Lee KS, Chung MP, et al. Nonspecific interstitial pneumonia with fibrosis: high-resolution CT and pathologic findings. Am J Roentgenol 1998; 171(6):1645–1650.

117. Hartman TE, Swensen SJ, Hansell DM, et al. Nonspecific interstitial pneumonia: variable appearance at high-resolution chest CT. Radiology 2000; 217(3):701–705.

118. MacDonald SL, Rubens MB, Hansell DM, et al. Nonspecific interstitial pneumonia and usual interstitial pneumonia: comparative appearances at and diagnostic accuracy of thin-section CT. Radiology 2001; 221(3):600–605.

119. Nishiyama O, Kondoh Y, Taniguchi H, et al. Serial high resolution CT findings in nonspecific interstitial pneumonia/fibrosis. J Comput Assist Tomogr 2000; 24(1):41–46.

120. Kim DS, Yoo B, Lee JS, et al. The major histopathologic pattern of pulmonary fibrosis in scleroderma is nonspecific interstitial pneumonia. Sarcoidosis Vasc Diffuse Lung Dis 2002; 19(2):121–127.

121. Cottin V, Donsbeck AV, Revel D, Loire R, Cordier JF. Nonspecific interstitial pneumonia. Individualization of a clinicopathologic entity in a series of 12 patients. Am J Respir Crit Care Med 1998; 158(4):1286–1293.

122. Park JS, Lee KS, Kim JS, et al. Nonspecific interstitial pneumonia with fibrosis: radiographic and CT findings in seven patients. Radiology 1995; 195(3):645–648.

123. Monaghan H, Wells AU, Colby TV, du Bois RM, Hansell DM, Nicholson AG. Prognostic implications of histologic patterns in multiple surgical lung biopsies from patients with idiopathic interstitial pneumonias. Chest 2004; 125(2):522–526.

124. Katzenstein AL, Zisman DA, Litzky LA, Nguyen BT, Kotloff RM. Usual interstitial pneumonia: histologic study of biopsy and explant specimens. Am J Surg Pathol 2002; 26(12):1567–1577.

125. Lynch JP III, Orens J, Kazerooni EA. Collagen vascular diseases. In: Sperber M, ed. Diffuse Lung Diseases: A Comprehensive Clinical–Radiological Overview. London: Springer-Verlag, 1999:325–355.

126. Wells AU, Cullinan P, Hansell DM, et al. Fibrosing alveolitis associated with systemic sclerosis has a better prognosis than lone cryptogenic fibrosing alveolitis. Am J Respir Crit Care Med 1994; 149(6):1583–1590.

127. Manoussakis MN, Constantopoulos SH, Gharavi AE, Moutsopoulos HM. Pulmonary involvement in systemic sclerosis. Association with anti-Scl 70 antibody and digital pitting. Chest 1987; 92(3):509–513.

128. Sato S, Ihn H, Kikuchi K, Takehara K. Antihistone antibodies in systemic sclerosis. Association with pulmonary fibrosis. Arthritis Rheum 1994; 37(3): 391–394.

129. Salojin KV, Le Tonqueze M, Saraux A, et al. Antiendothelial cell antibodies: useful markers of systemic sclerosis. Am J Med 1997; 102(2):178–185.

130. Chan TY, Hansell DM, Rubens MB, du Bois RM, Wells AU. Cryptogenic fibrosing alveolitis and the fibrosing alveolitis of systemic sclerosis: morphological differences on computed tomographic scans. Thorax 1997; 52(3): 265–270.

131. Groen H, Wichers G, ter Borg EJ, van der Mark TW, Wouda AA, Kallenberg CG. Pulmonary diffusing capacity disturbances are related to nailfold capillary changes in patients with Raynaud's phenomenon with and without an underlying connective tissue disease. Am J Med 1990; 89(1):34–41.

132. Peters-Golden M, Wise RA, Schneider P, Hochberg M, Stevens MB, Wigley F. Clinical and demographic predictors of loss of pulmonary function in systemic sclerosis. Medicine (Baltimore) 1984; 63(4):221–231.

133. Akesson A, Scheja A, Lundin A, Wollheim FA. Improved pulmonary function in systemic sclerosis after treatment with cyclophosphamide. Arthritis Rheum 1994; 37(5):729–735.

134. Steen VD, Lanz JK Jr, Conte C, Owens GR, Medsger TA Jr. Therapy for severe interstitial lung disease in systemic sclerosis. A retrospective study. Arthritis Rheum 1994; 37(9):1290–1296.

135. Davas EM, Peppas C, Maragou M, Alvanou E, Hondros D, Dantis PC. Intravenous cyclophosphamide pulse therapy for the treatment of lung disease associated with scleroderma. Clin Rheumatol 1999; 18(6):455–461.

136. Gabbay E, Tarala R, Will R, et al. Interstitial lung disease in recent onset rheumatoid arthritis. Am J Respir Crit Care Med 1997; 156(2, Pt 1):528–535.

137. Fujii M, Adachi S, Shimizu T, Hirota S, Sako M, Kono M. Interstitial lung disease in rheumatoid arthritis: assessment with high-resolution computed tomography. J Thorac Imaging 1993; 8(1):54–62.

138. McDonagh J, Greaves M, Wright AR, Heycock C, Owen JP, Kelly C. High resolution computed tomography of the lungs in patients with rheumatoid arthritis and interstitial lung disease. Br J Rheumatol 1994; 33(2):118–122.

139. Marie I, Hatron PY, Hachulla E, Wallaert B, Michon-Pasturel U, Devulder B. Pulmonary involvement in polymyositis and in dermatomyositis. J Rheumatol 1998; 25(7):1336–1343.

140. Marie I, Hachulla E, Hatron PY, et al. Polymyositis and dermatomyositis: short term and longterm outcome, and predictive factors of prognosis. J Rheumatol 2001; 28(10):2230–2237.

141. Tazelaar HD, Viggiano RW, Pickersgill J, Colby TV. Interstitial lung disease in polymyositis and dermatomyositis. Clinical features and prognosis as correlated with histologic findings. Am Rev Respir Dis 1990; 141(3):727–733.

142. Douglas WW, Tazelaar HD, Hartman TE, et al. Polymyositis-dermatomyositis-associated interstitial lung disease. Am J Respir Crit Care Med 2001; 164(7):1182–1185.

143. Marguerie C, Bunn CC, Beynon HL, et al. Polymyositis, pulmonary fibrosis and autoantibodies to aminoacyl-tRNA synthetase enzymes. Q J Med 1990; 77(282):1019–1038.

144. Orens JB, Martinez FJ, Lynch JP III. Pleuropulmonary manifestations of systemic lupus erythematosus. Rheum Dis Clin North Am 1994; 20(1):159–193.

145. Schnabel A, Reuter M, Gross WL. Intravenous pulse cyclophosphamide in the treatment of interstitial lung disease due to collagen vascular diseases. Arthritis Rheum 1998; 41(7):1215–1220.

146. Nawata Y, Kurasawa K, Takabayashi K, et al. Corticosteroid resistant interstitial pneumonitis in dermatomyositis/polymyositis: prediction and treatment with cyclosporine. J Rheumatol 1999; 26(7):1527–1533.

147. Keane MP, Lynch JP III. Pleuropulmonary manifestations of systemic lupus erythematosus. Thorax 2000; 55(2):159–166.

148. Lazaro MA, Maldonado Cocco JA, Catoggio LJ, Babini SM, Messina OD, Garcia Morteo O. Clinical and serologic characteristics of patients with overlap syndrome: is mixed connective tissue disease a distinct clinical entity? Medicine (Baltimore) 1989; 68(1):58–65.

149. Sullivan WD, Hurst DJ, Harmon CE, et al. A prospective evaluation emphasizing pulmonary involvement in patients with mixed connective tissue disease. Medicine (Baltimore) 1984; 63(2):92–107.

150. Jolliet P, Thorens JB, Chevrolet JC. Pulmonary vascular reactivity in severe pulmonary hypertension associated with mixed connective tissue disease. Thorax 1995; 50(1):96–97.

151. Constantopoulos SH, Papadimitriou CS, Moutsopoulos HM. Respiratory manifestations in primary Sjogren's syndrome. A clinical, functional, and histologic study. Chest 1985; 88(2):226–229.

152. Papathanasiou MP, Constantopoulos SH, Tsampoulas C, Drosos AA, Moutsopoulos HM. Reappraisal of respiratory abnormalities in primary and secondary Sjogren's syndrome. A controlled study. Chest 1986; 90(3):370–374.

153. Dalavanga YA, Constantopoulos SH, Galanopoulou V, Zerva L, Moutsopoulos HM. Alveolitis correlates with clinical pulmonary involvement in primary Sjogren's syndrome. Chest 1991; 99(6):1394–1397.

154. Kadota J, Kusano S, Kawakami K, Morikawa T, Kohno S. Usual interstitial pneumonia associated with primary Sjogren's syndrome. Chest 1995; 108(6): 1756–1758.
155. Kelly C, Gardiner P, Pal B, Griffiths I. Lung function in primary Sjogren's syndrome: a cross sectional and longitudinal study. Thorax 1991; 46(3): 180–183.
156. Tsuzaka K, Ogasawara T, Tojo T, et al. Relationship between autoantibodies and clinical parameters in Sjogren's syndrome. Scand J Rheumatol 1993; 22(1):1–9.
157. Deheinzelin D, Capelozzi VL, Kairalla RA, Barbas Filho JV, Saldiva PH, de Carvalho CR. Interstitial lung disease in primary Sjogren's syndrome. Clinical-pathological evaluation and response to treatment. Am J Respir Crit Care Med 1996; 154(3, Pt 1):794–799.
158. Ogasawara H, Sekiya M, Murashima A, et al. Very low-dose cyclosporin treatment of steroid-resistant interstitial pneumonitis associated with Sjogren's syndrome. Clin Rheumatol 1998; 17(2):160–162.
159. Lynch J III, Baughman R, Sharma O. Extrapulmonary sarcoidosis. Semin Respir Infect 1998; 13:229–254.
160. Lynch JP III, Kazerooni EA, Gay SE. Pulmonary sarcoidosis. Clin Chest Med 1997; 18(4):755–785.
161. Newman LS, Rose CS, Maier LA. Sarcoidosis. N Engl J Med 1997; 336(17): 1224–1234.
162. Statement on sarcoidosis. Joint statement of the American Thoracic Society (ATS), the European Respiratory Society (ERS) and the World Association of Sarcoidosis and Other Granulomatous Disorders (WASOG) adopted by the ATS board of directors and by the ERS executive committee, February 1999. Am J Respir Crit Care Med 1999; 160(2):736–755.
163. Hillerdal G, Nou E, Osterman K, Schmekel B. Sarcoidosis: epidemiology and prognosis. A 15-year European study. Am Rev Respir Dis 1984; 130(1):29–32.
164. Henke CE, Henke G, Elveback LR, Beard CM, Ballard DJ, Kurland LT. The epidemiology of sarcoidosis in Rochester, Minnesota: a population-based study of incidence and survival. Am J Epidemiol 1986; 123(5):840–845.
165. Neville E, Walker A, James DG. Prognostic factors predicting the outcome of sarcoidosis: an analysis of 818 patients. Q J Med 1983; 208:525–533.
166. Romer FK. Presentation of sarcoidosis and outcome of pulmonary changes. Dan Med Bull 1982; 29(1):27–32.
167. Judson MA, Baughman RP, Thompson BW, et al. Two year prognosis of sarcoidosis: the ACCESS experience. Sarcoidosis Vasc Diffuse Lung Dis 2003; 20(3):204–211.
168. Baughman RP, Winget DB, Bowen EH, Lower EE. Predicting respiratory failure in sarcoidosis patients. Sarcoidosis Vasc Diffuse Lung Dis 1997; 14(2): 154–158.
169. Huang CT, Heurich AE, Sutton AL, Lyons HA. Mortality in sarcoidosis. A changing pattern of the causes of death. Eur J Respir Dis 1981; 62(4):231–238.
170. Perry A, Vuitch F. Causes of death in patients with sarcoidosis. A morphologic study of 38 autopsies with clinicopathologic correlations. Arch Pathol Lab Med 1995; 119(2):167–172.

171. Reich JM, Johnson RE. Course and prognosis of sarcoidosis in a nonreferral setting. Analysis of 86 patients observed for 10 years. Am J Med 1985; 78(1):61–67.

172. Reich JM. Mortality of intrathoracic sarcoidosis in referral vs population-based settings: influence of stage, ethnicity, and corticosteroid therapy. Chest 2002; 121(1):32–39.

173. Judson MA. Lung transplantation for pulmonary sarcoidosis. Eur Respir J 1998; 11(3):738–744.

174. Mana J, Gomez-Vaquero C, Montero A, et al. Lofgren's syndrome revisited: a study of 186 patients. Am J Med 1999; 107(3):240–245.

175. Johns CJ, Michele TM. The clinical management of sarcoidosis. A 50-year experience at the Johns Hopkins Hospital. Medicine (Baltimore) 1999; 78(2): 65–111.

176. Gibson GJ, Prescott RJ, Muers MF, et al. British Thoracic Society sarcoidosis study: effects of long term corticosteroid treatment. Thorax 1996; 51(3): 238–247.

177. Hunninghake GW, Gilbert S, Pueringer R, et al. Outcome of the treatment for sarcoidosis. Am J Respir Crit Care Med 1994; 149(4, Pt 1):893–898.

178. Lynch JP III. Computed tomographic scanning in sarcoidosis. Semin Respir Crit Care Med 2003; 24:393–418.

179. Remy-Jardin M, Giraud F, Remy J, Wattinne L, Wallaert B, Duhamel A. Pulmonary sarcoidosis: role of CT in the evaluation of disease activity and functional impairment and in prognosis assessment. Radiology 1994; 191(3): 675–680.

180. Remy-Jardin M, Giraud F, Remy J, Copin MC, Gosselin B, Duhamel A. Importance of ground-glass attenuation in chronic diffuse infiltrative lung disease: pathologic-CT correlation. Radiology 1993; 189(3):693–698.

181. Finkel R, Teirstein AS, Levine R, Brown LK, Miller A. Pulmonary function tests, serum angiotensin-converting enzyme levels, and clinical findings as prognostic indicators in sarcoidosis. Ann N Y Acad Sci 1986; 465:665–671.

182. Keogh BA, Hunninghake GW, Line BR, Crystal RG. The alveolitis of pulmonary sarcoidosis. Evaluation of natural history and alveolitis-dependent changes in lung function. Am Rev Respir Dis 1983; 128(2):256–265.

183. Lieberman J, Schleissner LA, Nosal A, Sastre A, Mishkin FS. Clinical correlations of serum angiotensin-converting enzyme (ACE) in sarcoidosis. A longitudinal study of serum ACE, 67gallium scans, chest roentgenograms, and pulmonary function. Chest 1983; 84(5):522–528.

184. Alhamad EH, Lynch JP III, Martinez FJ. Pulmonary function tests in interstitial lung disease: what role do they have? Clin Chest Med 2001; 22(4): 715–750, ix.

185. Johns CJ, Macgregor MI, Zachary JB, Ball WC. Extended experience in the long-term corticosteroid treatment of pulmonary sarcoidosis. Ann N Y Acad Sci 1976; 278:722–731.

186. Odlum CM, FitzGerald MX. Evidence that steroids alter the natural history of previously untreated progressive pulmonary sarcoidosis. Sarcoidosis 1986; 3(1):40–46.

187. Bradvik I, Wollmer P, Blom-Bulow B, Albrechtsson U, Jonson B. Lung mechanics and gas exchange in steroid treated pulmonary sarcoidosis. A seven year follow-up. Sarcoidosis 1991; 8(2):105–114.

188. Winterbauer RH, Hutchinson JF. Use of pulmonary function tests in the management of sarcoidosis. Chest 1980; 78(4):640–647.

189. Zaki M, Lyons H, Leilop L, Huang C. Corticosteroid therapy in sarcoidosis. A five-year, controlled follow-up study. NY State J Med 1987; 87:496–499.

190. Goldstein DS, Williams MH. Rate of improvement of pulmonary function in sarcoidosis during treatment with corticosteroids. Thorax 1986; 41(6):473–474.

191. Baughman RP, Sharma OP, Lynch JP III. Sarcoidosis: is therapy effective? Semin Respir Infect 1998; 13(3):255–273.

192. Sharma OP. Pulmonary sarcoidosis and corticosteroids. Am Rev Respir Dis 1993; 147(6, Pt 1):1598–1600.

193. Gottlieb JE, Israel HL, Steiner RM, Triolo J, Patrick H. Outcome in sarcoidosis. The relationship of relapse to corticosteroid therapy. Chest 1997; 111(3): 623–631.

194. Johns CJ, Schonfeld SA, Scott PP, Zachary JB, MacGregor MI. Longitudinal study of chronic sarcoidosis with low-dose maintenance corticosteroid therapy. Outcome and complications. Ann N Y Acad Sci 1986; 465:702–712.

195. O'Leary TJ, Jones G, Yip A, Lohnes D, Cohanim M, Yendt ER. The effects of chloroquine on serum 1,25-dihydroxyvitamin D and calcium metabolism in sarcoidosis. N Engl J Med 1986; 315(12):727–730.

196. Muller-Quernheim J, Kienast K, Held M, Pfeifer S, Costabel U. Treatment of chronic sarcoidosis with an azathioprine/prednisolone regimen. Eur Respir J 1999; 14(5):1117–1122.

197. Lewis SJ, Ainslie GM, Bateman ED. Efficacy of azathioprine as second-line treatment in pulmonary sarcoidosis. Sarcoidosis Vasc Diffuse Lung Dis 1999; 16(1):87–92.

198. Baltzan M, Mehta S, Kirkham TH, Cosio MG. Randomized trial of prolonged chloroquine therapy in advanced pulmonary sarcoidosis. Am J Respir Crit Care Med 1999; 160(1):192–197.

199. Baughman RP, Lower EE. Infliximab for refractory sarcoidosis. Sarcoidosis Vasc Diffuse Lung Dis 2001; 18(1):70–74.

200. Utz JP, Limper AH, Kalra S, et al. Etanercept for the treatment of stage II and III progressive pulmonary sarcoidosis. Chest 2003; 124(1):177–185.

201. Baughman RP, Lower EE. Leflunomide for chronic sarcoidosis. Sarcoidosis Vasc Diffuse Lung Dis 2004; 21(1):43–48.

202. Lower EE, Baughman RP. Prolonged use of methotrexate for sarcoidosis. Arch Intern Med 1995; 155(8):846–851.

203. Baughman RP, Winget DB, Lower EE. Methotrexate is steroid sparing in acute sarcoidosis: results of a double blind, randomized trial. Sarcoidosis Vasc Diffuse Lung Dis 2000; 17:60–66.

204. Pacheco Y, Marechal C, Marechal F, Biot N, Perrin Fayolle M. Azathioprine treatment of chronic pulmonary sarcoidosis. Sarcoidosis 1985; 2(2):107–113.

205. Demeter SL. Myocardial sarcoidosis unresponsive to steroids. Treatment with cyclophosphamide. Chest 1988; 94(1):202–203.

206. Zic JA, Horowitz DH, Arzubiaga C, King LE Jr. Treatment of cutaneous sarcoidosis with chloroquine. Review of the literature. Arch Dermatol 1991; 127(7):1034–1040.

207. Sharma OP. Neurosarcoidosis: a personal perspective based on the study of 37 patients. Chest 1997; 112(1):220–228.

208. Pettersen JA, Zochodne DW, Bell RB, Martin L, Hill MD. Refractory neurosarcoidosis responding to infliximab. Neurology 2002; 59(10):1660–1661.

209. Katz JM, Bruno MK, Winterkorn JM, Nealon N. The pathogenesis and treatment of optic disc swelling in neurosarcoidosis: a unique therapeutic response to infliximab. Arch Neurol 2003; 60(3):426–430.

210. Khanna D, Liebling MR, Louie JS. Etanercept ameliorates sarcoidosis arthritis and skin disease. J Rheumatol 2003; 30(8):1864–1867.

211. Pritchard C, Nadarajah K. Tumour necrosis factor alpha inhibitor treatment for sarcoidosis refractory to conventional treatments: a report of five patients. Ann Rheum Dis 2004; 63(3):318–320.

212. Lynch JP III, Kazerooni E. Sarcoidosis. In: Sperber M, ed. Radiologic Diagnosis of Chest Disease. 2nd edn. London: Springer-Verlag, 2001:193–220.

213. Muller NL, Miller RR. Ground-glass attenuation, nodules, alveolitis, and sarcoid granulomas. Radiology 1993; 189(1):31–32.

214. Drent M, De Vries J, Lenters M, et al. Sarcoidosis: assessment of disease severity using HRCT. Eur Radiol 2003; 13(11):2462–2471.

215. Akira M, Kozuka T, Inoue Y, Sakatani M. Long-term follow-up CT scan evaluation in patients with pulmonary sarcoidosis. Chest 2005; 127(1):185–191.

216. Murdoch J, Muller NL. Pulmonary sarcoidosis: changes on follow-up CT examination. Am J Roentgenol 1992; 159(3):473–477.

217. Brauner MW, Lenoir S, Grenier P, Cluzel P, Battesti JP, Valeyre D. Pulmonary sarcoidosis: CT assessment of lesion reversibility. Radiology 1992; 182(2): 349–354.

218. Abehsera M, Valeyre D, Grenier P, Jaillet H, Battesti JP, Brauner MW. Sarcoidosis with pulmonary fibrosis: CT patterns and correlation with pulmonary function. Am J Roentgenol 2000; 174(6):1751–1757.

219. Hennebicque AS, Nunes H, Brillet PY, Moulahi H, Valeyre D, Brauner MW. CT findings in severe thoracic sarcoidosis. Eur Radiol 2005; 15(1):23–30.

220. Israel HL, Lenchner GS, Atkinson GW. Sarcoidosis and aspergilloma. The role of surgery. Chest 1982; 82(4):430–432.

221. Maurer J, Frost A, Estenne M, Higenbottam T, Glanville A. International guidelines for the selection of lung transplant candidates. J Heart Lung Transplant 1998; 17:703–709.

222. Hadjiliadis D, Sporn TA, Perfect JR, Tapson VF, Davis RD, Palmer SM. Outcome of lung transplantation in patients with mycetomas. Chest 2002; 121(1):128–134.

223. Arcasoy SM, Christie JD, Pochettino A, et al. Characteristics and outcomes of patients with sarcoidosis listed for lung transplantation. Chest 2001; 120(3):873–880.

224. Shorr AF, Davies DB, Nathan SD. Predicting mortality in patients with sarcoidosis awaiting lung transplantation. Chest 2003; 124(3):922–928.

225. Shorr AF, Helman DL, Davies DB, Nathan SD. Pulmonary hypertension in advanced sarcoidosis: epidemiology and clinical characteristics. Eur Respir J 2005; 25(5):783–788.
226. Gluskowski J, Hawrylkiewicz I, Zych D, Zielinski J. Effects of corticosteroid treatment on pulmonary haemodynamics in patients with sarcoidosis. Eur Respir J 1990; 3(4):403–407.
227. Preston IR, Klinger JR, Landzberg MJ, Houtchens J, Nelson D, Hill NS. Vasoresponsiveness of sarcoidosis-associated pulmonary hypertension. Chest 2001; 120(3):866–872.
228. Shorr AF, Helman DL, Davies DB, Nathan SD. Sarcoidosis, race, and short-term outcomes following lung transplantation. Chest 2004; 125(3):990–996.
229. Young CJ, Gaston RS. African Americans and renal transplantation: disproportionate need, limited access, and impaired outcomes. Am J Med Sci 2002; 323(2):94–99.
230. Nair S, Eustace J, Thuluvath PJ. Effect of race on outcome of orthotopic liver transplantation: a cohort study. Lancet 2002; 359(9303):287–293.
231. Nunley DR, Hattler B, Keenan RJ, et al. Lung transplantation for end-stage pulmonary sarcoidosis. Sarcoidosis Vasc Diffuse Lung Dis 1999; 16(1):93–100.
232. Walker S, Mikhail G, Banner N, et al. Medium term results of lung transplantation for end stage pulmonary sarcoidosis. Thorax 1998; 53(4):281–284.
233. Collins J, Hartman MJ, Warner TF, et al. Frequency and CT findings of recurrent disease after lung transplantation. Radiology 2001; 219(2):503–509.
234. Bjortuft O, Foerster A, Boe J, Geiran O. Single lung transplantation as treatment for end-stage pulmonary sarcoidosis: recurrence of sarcoidosis in two different lung allografts in one patient. J Heart Lung Transplant 1994; 13(1, Pt 1):24–29.
235. Martinez FJ, Orens JB, Deeb M, Brunsting LA, Flint A, Lynch JP III. Recurrence of sarcoidosis following bilateral allogeneic lung transplantation. Chest 1994; 106(5):1597–1599.

# 8

# Pulmonary Langerhans Cell Histiocytosis and Lymphangioleiomyomatosis

**Joseph P. Lynch III and S. Samuel Weigt**

*Division of Pulmonary and Critical Care Medicine and Hospitalists, Department of Internal Medicine, David Geffen School of Medicine at UCLA, Los Angeles, California, U.S.A.*

**Michael C. Fishbein**

*Department of Pathology and Laboratory Medicine, David Geffen School of Medicine at UCLA, Los Angeles, California, U.S.A.*

## PULMONARY LANGERHANS CELL HISTIOCYTOSIS

Pulmonary Langerhans cell histiocytosis (PLCH), formerly termed pulmonary eosinophilic granuloma, is a rare disorder that results in progressive respiratory insufficiency in 15% to 30% of cases; fatality rates range from 2% to 27% (1–7). Isolated PLCH is principally a disease of adult smokers (2,8) and is rare in children (6,7,9–11). Fewer than 20% of adults with PLCH manifest extrapulmonary involvement (1–3,5,8,12,13). In contrast, Langerhans cell histiocytosis (LCH) in children typically involves extrapulmonary organs (principally bone, skin, pituitary gland, lymph nodes, and viscera) (6,14,15). In children, pulmonary involvement may be observed with multisystemic LCH (9,15–19). French investigators analyzed 348 cases of LCH from 32 centers over a decade; mean age was 2.5 years (19). Most common sites of involvement included bone (50%), soft tissue without organ dysfunction (39%), and organ dysfunction (11%). In a recent study of 220 children with LCH, 83 (38%) had multisystemic involvement, 36 (16%) had pulmonary involvement, and only 2 (1%) had isolated PLCH (15). In 1999, Howarth et al. reviewed 314 patients (children and adults) with LCH seen at the Mayo Clinic over a 50-year period (18). Most common sites of involvement included bone lesions (60%), multisystemic involvement (31%), PLCH (41%), mucocutaneous (25%), diabetes insipidus (14%), and lymph nodes (7%) (18). Importantly, 83 of 87 patients with *isolated* PLCH were adults. A survey of 274 *adults* with LCH from 13 countries found that 188 patients (69%) had multisystemic disease, 81 (29%) had diabetes insipidus, and 44 (16%) had isolated PLCH (20). German investigators reported on 58 adults with LCH: 42 (72%) had single organ involvement, 16 (28%) had multisystemic involvement, and 23 (40%) had isolated PLCH (21). Histologically, the lesions of PLCH are identical to LCH affecting bone, pituitary gland, skin, or other organs (discussed later) (8,18,22).

## Prevalence and Epidemiology

The prevalence of PLCH is estimated at two to five cases per million persons (8,22). More than 95% of cases of PLCH occur in smokers (1–3,5,8,12,23), suggesting that constituents of cigarette smoke are critical to the pathogenesis. Pulmonary LCH has been almost exclusively reported among Caucasians (2,3,8,22), but no familial or inheritable trait has been identified.

## Clinical Features

The clinical features and natural history of PLCH are variable. Cough or dyspnea are noted in 60% to 75% of patients (1,8,22). Symptoms usually develop insidiously over several weeks or months (22). Ten to 25% of patients are asymptomatic, with incidental findings on chest radiographs (1–3,22). Pneumothorax, due to rupture of pleural cysts, occurs in 6% to 20% of patients, and may be the presenting feature (1–4,22,24). Recurrent pneumothoraces require surgical pleurodesis for control (3,8). At thoracotomy, numerous subpleural cysts and blebs are usually evident. Pulmonary arterial hypertension (PAH) is common in severe PLCH (25) and reflects a proliferative vasculopathy involving muscular arteries and veins. In one study of 21 patients with advanced PLCH referred for lung transplantation, all patients had PAH (mean pulmonary arterial pressure of 59 mmHg) (25). Pulmonary hypertension is disproportionate to the degree of pulmonary functional impairment or hypoxemia (25). Extrapulmonary involvement [particularly osteolytic bone lesions or diabetes insipidus (from involvement of the pituitary)] occurs in 15% to 20% of patients with PLCH (1–3,5,8,13, 22,26,27). Constitutional symptoms (low-grade fever, malaise, weight loss, or anorexia) are present in 15% to 30% of patients (2,3,8).

## Radiographic Features

Chest radiographs in PLCH typically demonstrate diffuse reticular, reticulonodular, or cystic lesions with a predilection for the mid and upper lung zones; the costophrenic angles are spared (2,3,8,22,28). High-resolution computed tomography (HRCT) scans demonstrate numerous thin-walled cysts (>80% of cases) with a proclivity for the upper and mid lung fields; peribronchiolar nodules (typically 1–4 mm in diameter) are evident in 60–80% of patients (Fig. 1C) (8,22,24,29–31). There is no central or peripheral predominance. These cysts are usually round and <10 mm, but may coalesce, exceeding 4 cm (24,30). The cysts and nodules are associated with intervening areas of normal lung tissue (8,12,22,24,30). The nodules represent peribronchiolar granulomas (24,30,31). As the disease progresses,

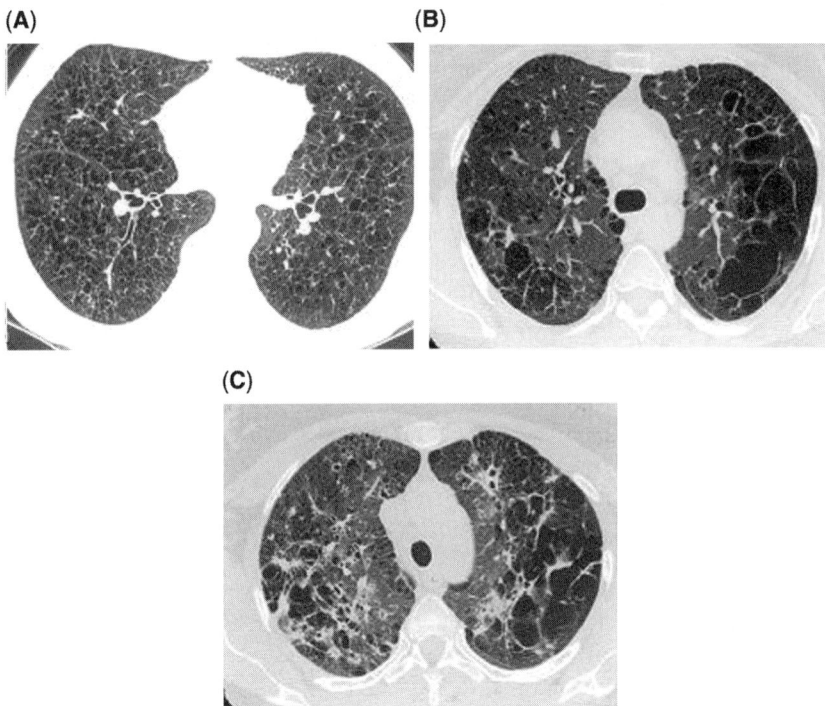

**Figure 1** (**A**) Pulmonary LCH. HRCT from a 56-year-old male with PLCH shows multiple well-defined cystic spaces with walls measuring 1–2 cm in size. A few ill-defined scattered interstitial nodules are also present but subtle. (**B**) Pulmonary LCH. HRCT from another patient demonstrates marked destruction of lung parenchyma by cysts, some of which have coalesced and assumed bizarre shapes. A few faint nodules are visible. (**C**) Pulmonary LCH. HRCT from the same patient demonstrates extensive cystic radiolucencies. Marked peribronchiolar thickening and scattered dense nodules are present, consistent with an active inflammatory component. *Abbreviations*: LCH, Langerhans cell histiocytosis; HRCT, high-resolution computed tomography; PLCH, pulmonary Langerhans cell histiocytosis. *Source*: From Refs. 32 and 33.

the nodules are replaced by cysts, some of which become confluent, leading to bizarre shapes or bullae (22,24,30,32,33). Pleural effusions and hilar adenopathy are rare (22,24,29) but mediastinal lymphadenopathy may be detected by CT scans in up to one-third of patients (8).

## Pulmonary Function Tests

Aberrations in PFTs are noted in >80% of patients with PLCH (1–3,22,26,34). Reductions in vital capacity (VC), total lung capacity (TLC), or diffusing capacity of the lung for carbon monoxide ($DL_{co}$) are typical (1–3,8,24,26,34). Severe reductions in $DL_{co}$ are associated with more extensive cystic disease on chest CT and a worse prognosis (8). Pure obstructive or mixed obstructive–restrictive patterns are present in one-third of patients (1–3,34). Air-trapping (increased residual volume) occurs in nearly half of patients with PLCH, but hyperinflation is uncommon (8,34). Cardiopulmonary exercise tests (CPETs) typically reveal reductions in exercise tolerance, maximal workload, oxygen consumption ($VO_2$ max), and anaerobic threshold, worsening gas exchange, and increases in dead space ($V_D/V_T$) with exercise (34). Aberrations in pulmonary function tests (PFTs) or CPETs do not consistently correlate with radiographic findings. Serial PFTs should be performed to monitor the course of the disease.

## Pathology

Grossly, the lungs in PLCH may show cysts, honeycomb change, and nodules. Histologically, PLCH is characterized by inflammatory, nodular, cystic, and fibrotic lesions distributed in a bronchocentric fashion (Fig. 2A and B) (1,2,5,26,34,35). Eosinophils may be present in the inflammatory nodular lesions (Fig. 2B), but are not universally found. The cardinal feature is aggregates of Langerhans cells (LCs) (belonging to the family of dendritic cells) within nodular lesions, airspaces, and alveolar interstitium (Fig. 2C and D) (1,2,8,36,37). LCs are distinctive, large, ovoid mononuclear phagocytes with a prominently grooved, folded nucleus, inconspicuous nucleoli, and finely dispersed chromatin (1,8,37). LCs express CDla antigen (the common thymocyte antigen) (Fig. 2C) (8,22,38,39), surface markers associated with activation (such as B7) (22), a new cell marker termed Langerin (CD207) (40), and stain for S100 protein (Fig. 2D) (36,37,41). Ultrastructurally, LCs contain the characteristic Birbeck granule that resembles a tennis racket (Fig. 2D, inset). Older lesions, with more fibrosis, minimal or no eosinophils, and rare LCs, are recognizable by the distinct "stellate" pattern of fibrosis (Fig. 2E) (1,2,5,26,34,35).

    Pulmonary LCH occurs in distinct phases. Early in the course of the disease, a cellular granulomatous phase, characterized by proliferation of LCs, dominates (1,2,36). Variable numbers of eosinophils, lymphocytes, plasma cells, fibroblasts, and foci of fibrosis surround or infiltrate these

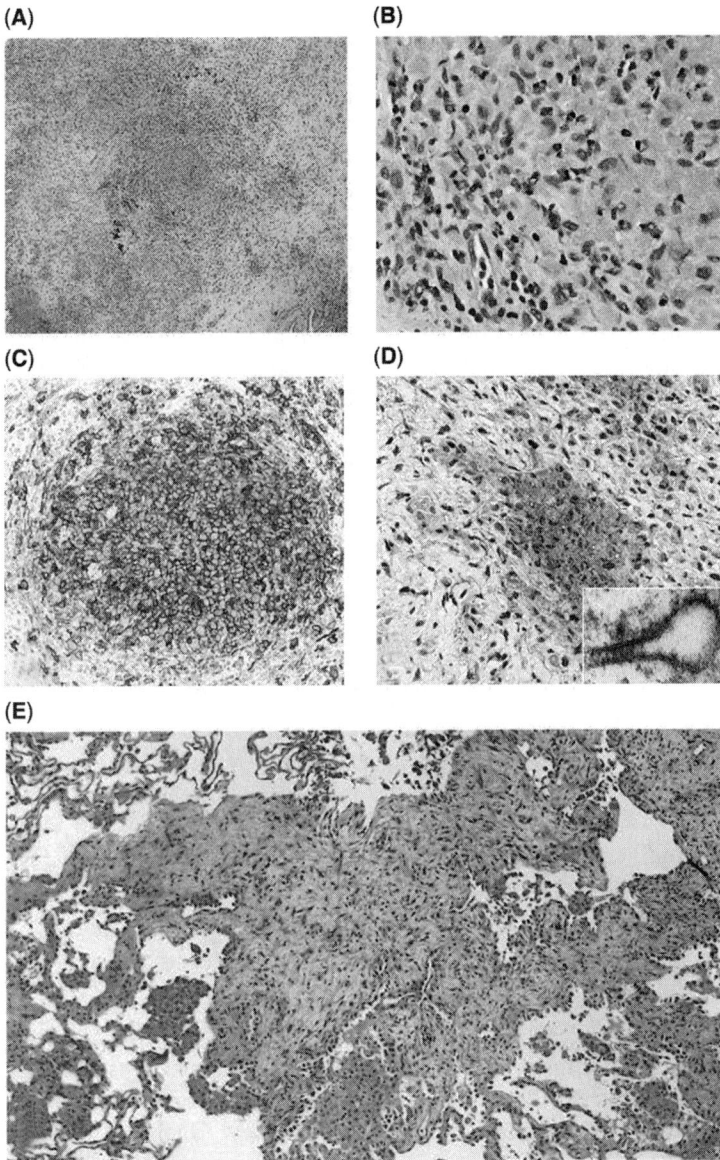

**Figure 2** Langerhans cell histiocytosis. (**A**) Nodular lesion replacing lung paren-chyma (H&E, × 40); (**B**) high magnification showing numerous eosinophils (H&E, × 400); (**C** and **D**) immunohistochemical staining for CDla (**C**) and S100 (**D**) show-ing characteristic nodular aggregates of Langerhans cells (inset shows ultrastructural characteristic Birbeck granule that resembles a tennis racket); and (**E**) stellate scar, thought to reflect old, burnt-out lesion of LCH (H&E, × 100). *Abbreviation*: LCH, Langerhans cell histiocytosis.

granulomatous lesions (1,2,8,36). Early lesions involve bronchioles (22). Cavitation likely represents the lumen of the preexisting bronchiole destroyed by the granulomatous process (22). As the inflammatory process evolves, bronchioles and alveolar walls are destroyed and replaced by fibrotic connective tissue, resulting in dilated, distorted bronchioles and alveolar parenchymal cysts (1,26). In late phases, extensive destruction and fibrosis of the lung parenchyma is evident (2,5). Blebs, subpleural cysts, and interstitial and intraluminal fibrosis may be evident (1). Late or end-stage PLCH may be relatively acellular, with <5% LCs and extensive alveolar and honeycomb cysts (22,36). In this context, distinguishing PLCH from other end-stage chronic fibrotic lung disorders is difficult. The retention of a nodular or stellate configuration is a clue to the diagnosis (Fig. 2E) (1,2) that can be confirmed by immunohistochemistry or electron microscopy.

**Pathogenesis**

The pathogenesis of PLCH in adults likely represents an exaggerated immune response to cigarette smoking initiated or regulated by LCs (1–3,5, 8,26,42). More than 95% of adults with PLCH are smokers (1–3,5,8,26,42). Further, constituents of cigarette smoke serve as T-cell mitogens, stimulate macrophage cytokine production, and recruit LCs to the lung (8,43,44). LCs serve as accessory cells, activating T lymphocytes and recruiting other immune effector cells to the lung (22,45). Bronchial epithelial (44) and bombesin-positive neuroendocrine cells in the airways may contribute to the local recruitment and activation of LCs and stimulate growth of fibroblasts (8,46,47). Interestingly, exposure to cigarette smoke in mice evoked interstitial granulomatous inflammation, with features consistent with PLCH (48). Following cessation of exposure, the density of pulmonary LCs in mice returned to normal levels.

**Course and Prognosis**

The natural history of PLCH has not been well defined, but most patients improve or stabilize within 6 to 12 months of onset of symptoms (1–6,8, 22,24). Data are limited to large retrospective studies, with variable treatment regimens. In 1978, French investigators reported 78 cases of PLCH (3). Among 67 cases with follow-up data, the following outcomes were noted: improved (13%); stable (40%); worse (21 %); and death (25%). The impact of treatment was not clear. The following factors were associated with a worse prognosis: multisystem generalized disease; extensive honeycombing on chest radiographs; severe reductions in $DL_{co}$; extremes of age; and multiple pneumothoraces (3). In 1981, Friedman et al. reviewed 100 cases of "pulmonary eosinophilic granuloma" (PLCH) confirmed by surgical lung biopsy (2). Follow-up was available for only 60 patients (both treated and untreated). Complete resolution of symptoms was noted in 33 patients (55%); 22 (37%) had persistent symptoms; five patients worsened but only one (2%) died (2). In a subsequent study from the Mayo Clinic, 74 of 87 patients (85%) with *isolated* PLCR achieved "disease-free survival" (18). Treatment regimens included prednisone (58%); chemotherapy (10%); surgical excision (7%); and no treatment (25%). Ten patients (11%) with isolated PLCH died; three additional patients developed progressive pulmonary disease. A European study observed 45 patients with PLCH for a median of six years; 12 patients (27%) died or required lung transplantation (26). Median survival from the time of diagnosis was 13 years. Reduced forced expiratory volume in one second ($FEV_1$) to forced vital capacity (FVC) ratio was an independent predictor of mortality by multivariate analysis. A review of 102 cases of PLCH *in adults* from the Mayo Clinic from 1976 to 1998 noted a median survival of 12.5 years; 5- and 10-year survival rates after the diagnosis were 74% and 64%, respectively (49). Only 15 patients (15%) died from respiratory failure. Treatment regimens were varied and included smoking cessation (100%); prednisone alone (39%); prednisone plus chemotherapeutic agents (15%); and lung transplantation (1%) (49). Variables associated with shorter survival included older age, low $FEV_1$, high residual volume (RV), low ratio $FEV_1/FVC$, and reduced $DL_{co}$ (49). Another study from the Mayo Clinic noted that the presence of PAH on echocardiography markedly increased mortality [hazard ratio (HR), 28.8] (50).

## Therapy

Because of the rarity of PLCH, and its highly variable natural history, the role of therapy is controversial (8,22,49). For multisystemic LCH in children, the Histiocyte Society recommends treatment with vinblastine and corticosteroids (51). A variety of chemotherapeutic regimens have been used to treat disseminated LCH including vinca alkaloids, etoposide, cladribine (2-chlorodeoxyadenosine), cyclophosphamide, methotrexate, cyclosporine A, and antithymocyte globulin (15,17,18,51–57). Anecdotal responses were noted with interleukin-2 (IL-2) (58) and etanercept (59) for disseminated LCH in children (55). Most published series of LCH reflected pediatric age groups, but small series in adults with severe, multisystemic LCH cited favorable responses to etoposide (20,60), vinblastine (with or without corticosteroids) (20,52), or cladribine (53). The International Histiocyte Society Registry recently initiated a registry of LCH in adults (20). Overall, 274 adults with LCH were identified from 13 countries; only 44 (16%) had lung involvement. Most commonly used therapies included vinblastine (with or without corticosteroids) in 30% and etoposide in 10%. Only 30% of patients with isolated PLCH were treated. Five-year survival rates following diagnosis were 92% for multisystemic disease and 89% for isolated PLCH (20).

Therapeutic approaches for disseminated LCH may not apply to isolated PLCH in adults, as the pathogenesis of these disorders may differ (8,22). No controlled or prospective therapeutic trials have been performed for PLCH, and efficacy of therapy is unproven. However, given the link between cigarette smoking and PLCH, patients must be urged in the strongest possible terms to discontinue smoking (8,61). Anecdotal responses have been noted with corticosteroids and immunosuppressive and cytotoxic agents (3–5,16,26,42), but effects of therapy may be confounded by the impact of smoking cessation or the potential for spontaneous resolution (22). One uncontrolled study cited radiographic improvement in 12 of 14 patients treated with prednisone for progressive PLCH; the other two patients were stable (42). In another study, the use of corticosteroids was associated with worse survival (26), but this may reflect a selection bias. In the cohort reported from the Mayo Clinic, prednisone (alone or combined with immunosuppressive agents) was prescribed in 54 of 102 patients (53%) (49). Although data were not provided, the authors stated "no specific therapeutic interventions have been shown to prolong survival." A multicenter therapeutic trial is needed to clarify the impact (if any) of therapy (6), but has not yet been done. Given the paucity of data, we reserve therapy for patients with severe, progressive, or debilitating disease. In this context, an empirical trial of corticosteroids for three to six months is reasonable. Prolonged therapy should be continued only in patients manifesting *unequivocal* and *objective* improvement. The role of immunosuppressive or cytotoxic agents for isolated PLCH in adults has not been established. These agents should be reserved for severe, progressive PLCH recalcitrant to corticosteroid therapy and despite cessation of smoking. Vasodilators have a theoretical role to treat pulmonary hypertension in patients with PLCH (25), but data are limited. However, two patients with PLCH treated with intravenous epoprostenol developed acute pulmonary edema (25).

## Lung Transplantation for PLCH

Lung transplantation has been successfully accomplished in patients with severe PLCH refractory to medical therapy (62,63). Data from the International Society for Heart and Lung Transplantation (ISHLT) Registry from January 1995 to June 2004 identified only 39 patients with PLCH among 13,007 lung transplant recipients (0.3%) (64). Criteria for listing patients with PLCH have not been developed. However, we believe patients should be referred for lung transplantation when the following factors are present: (i) severe or progressive respiratory insufficiency despite smoking cessation and medical therapy (e.g., FVC <55% predicted; FEV$_1$ <40% predicted; DL$_{co}$ <40% predicted); (ii) need for supplemental oxygen (at rest or with exertion); (iii) poor and declining quality of life; and (iv) severe exercise limitation and PAH. Prior thoracotomy or pleurodesis do not preclude transplantation. Recurrent PLCH has been noted among lung transplant recipients who resume cigarette smoking. In one series of seven PLCH patients who had lung transplant, the diseases recurred in the lung allografts in two patients within 12 months; both had resumed cigarette smoking (63). In contrast, five patients who did not resume smoking remained well 15 to 90 months following lung transplantation. Recurrence of LCH in lung allografts was cited in two additional case reports (65,66). Patients must be vigorously counseled not to resume smoking following transplantation.

## LYMPHANGIOLEIOMYOMATOSIS

Lymphangioleiomyomatosis (LAM) is a rare disorder exclusively affecting women, characterized by proliferation of atypical smooth muscle and thin-walled cysts within lung, kidney, uterus, or abdominal–pelvic organs (67–74). Pulmonary and abdomino-pelvic lesions identical to LAM may occur in patients with tuberous sclerosis complex (TSC), an autosomal-dominant familial disorder associated with mental retardation and cutaneous manifestations (67,75–80).

### Prevalence and Epidemiology

Lymphangioleiomyomatosis is exceptionally rare (prevalence of 0.4–3 cases per million) (69,81,82). More than 95% of cases are in premenopausal women; the mean age of onset is between 30 and 36 years (67,69–71,73,83).

### Pathology

Grossly, the lungs in LAM may first appear emphysematous. However, as the disease progresses, the entire lung is replaced by cysts (Fig. 3A and B). Histologically, one sees numerous cystic regions, surrounded by a multifocal proliferation of immature-appearing smooth muscle cells. Unlike other forms of interstitial lung disease, there is very little fibrosis in LAM. Smooth muscle cells in pulmonary LAM are similar histologically and by immunohistochemical analysis to angiomyolipomas, which are benign mesenchymal tumors consisting of blood vessels, abnormal smooth muscle, and fat (67,69,84,85). The smooth muscle LAM cells are heterogenous and may exhibit features of large spindle cells, smaller cells with little cytoplasm, or may be "epithelioid" in appearance (Fig. 3C and D) (67,74). LAM cells grow in a haphazard arrangement, unlike normal smooth muscle cells (86). Immunohistochemical stains are positive for muscle-specific actin (Fig. 3E), desmin, and melanoma-related marker (HMB-45) (Fig. 3F) (67,81,84). HMB-45 immunoreactivity is never found in normal smooth muscle (67,81, 84,87). Immunohistochemical staining for estrogen (Fig. 3G) and progesterone (Fig. 3H) receptors may be positive.

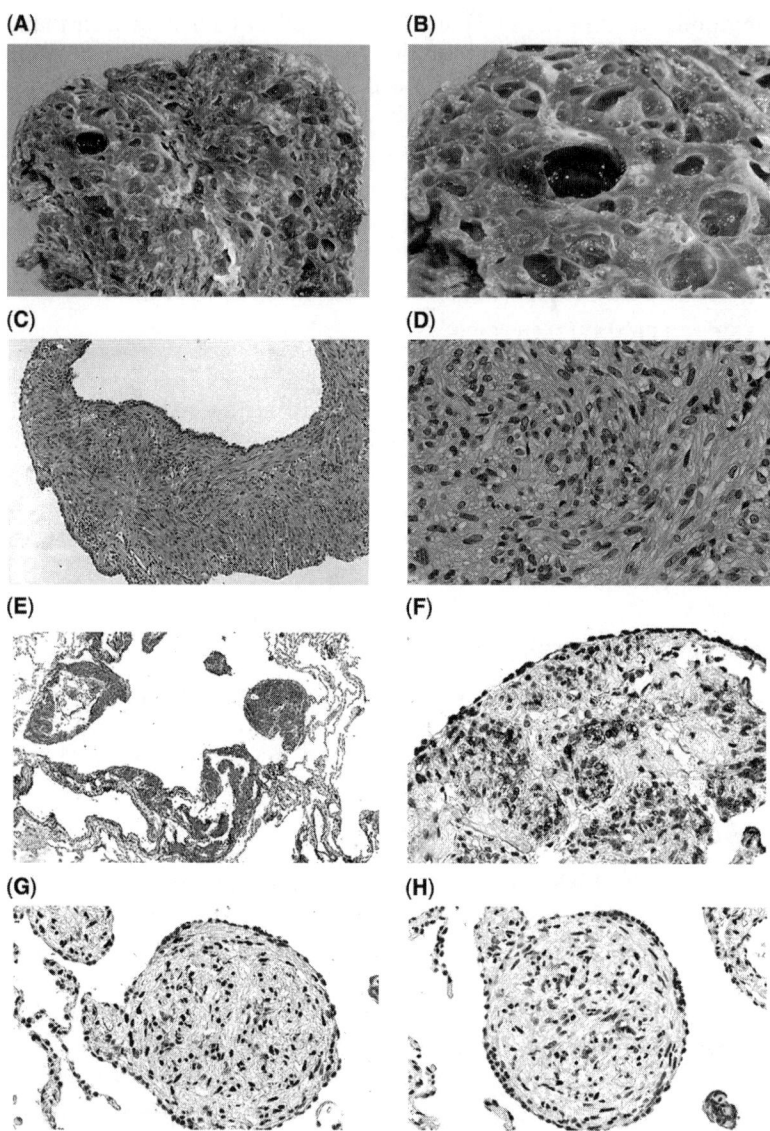

**Figure 3** Pathology of lymphangioleiomyomatosis. (**A** and **B**) Gross photographs showing complete obliteration of lung parenchyma with replacement of normal tissue with multiple cystic lesions. (**C** and **D**) Histologic sections showing cystic spaces surrounded by proliferations of disorganized smooth muscle cells (H&E, × 40 and × 400). (**E–H**) Immunohistochemical stains positive for smooth muscle actin (**E**), HMB45 (**F**), estrogen receptors (**G**), and progesterone receptors (**H**) (ABC immunoperoxidase stain).

## Pathogenesis

The pathogenesis of the smooth-muscle proliferation in LAM is poorly understood, but estrogens likely play a major role (67,81,88). Angiomyolipomas in both LAM and TSC express HMB-45, suggesting a common origin from a progenitor smooth-muscle cell (67,69,81,85). Further, chromosomal abnormalities (13ql4 and 14q24) are noted in TSC, LAM, and uterine leiomyomas (81,89). Both leiomyomas and LAM involve proliferations of smooth muscle in women of childbearing age (81). In TSC, germline mutations in one of two genes (TSC-1 or TSC-2) are present (67,90). A second somatic mutation, termed loss of heterozygosity, results in loss of the gene product from the cell (67,91). Since TSC genes suppress tumor growth (81), this additional mutation allows cellular proliferation and the formation of hamartomas (67). Loss of heterozygosity for TSC-2 (but not TSC-1) has also been noted in angiomyolipomas (with or without LAM) and no evidence for TSC (67,91). It is possible that sequential mutations of the TSC-2 gene may be operative in at least *some* patients with LAM (81,90,92).

### Clinical Manifestations of Pulmonary LAM

Clinical manifestations of pulmonary LAM are due to immature smooth muscle proliferations and cyst formation within airways, blood vessels, lymphatics, and lung parenchyma (71,72,74,83). In pulmonary LAM, innumerable small cysts, representing destroyed airways and alveoli, are interspersed throughout the lung (32,33,83,93,94). The most common symptom of LAM is dyspnea, which usually begins in the third or fourth decade of life and progresses inexorably over years (67,69–73,83). Dyspnea is usually due to airflow obstruction from cystic lesions, but may reflect other specific complications of LAM (e.g., pneumothorax, chylothorax, or alveolar hemorrhage). Rupture of subpleural cysts may give rise to pneumothoraces (67,69,73,83). Further, proliferating smooth muscle may obstruct pulmonary venules (causing focal edema and pulmonary hemorrhage) or lymphatics (leading to chylothorax) (67,69,71,74,83). During the course of the disease, complications of LAM include pneumothorax (50–80%); chylous effusions (7–39%); and focal alveolar hemorrhage (28–40%) (67,69,70,72,73,83).

### Radiographic Features

Chest radiographs in LAM demonstrate a wide spectrum of abnormalities, including pneumothoraces, cystic or reticulonodular shadows, pleural effusions (typically chylous), or hyperinflation (67,69,70,73,83,94). HRCT scans are highly distinctive in LAM (67,70,73,93,94). The cardinal feature is numerous thin-walled cysts (ranging in size from a few millimeters to 6 cm) with normal intervening lung parenchyma (Figs. 4–7) (29,32,33,67,69,70,73, 83,93). The cysts are distributed diffusely without predilection for specific

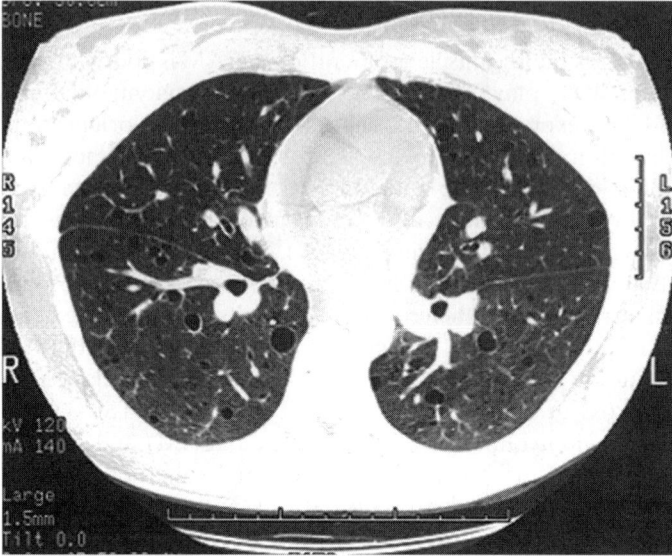

**Figure 4** Lymphangioleiomyomatosis. HRCT from a 28-year-old woman with a history of recurrent pneumothoraces. Multiple well-circumscribed cysts are present bilaterally, with large areas of intervening lung parenchyma. *Abbreviation*: HRCT, high-resolution computed tomography. *Source*: From Ref. 33.

**(A)**                                         **(B)**

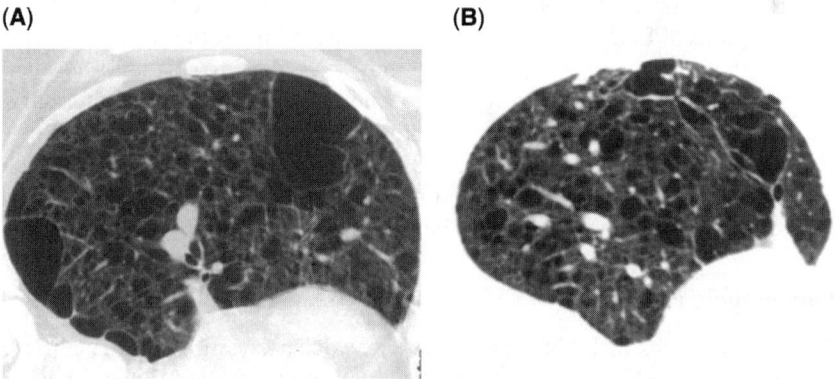

**Figure 5** Lymphangioleiomyomatosis. (**A**) HRCT from a 44-year-old woman demonstrating multiple thin-walled cysts bilaterally. Note the two large lesions, representing confluent cysts. (**B**) HRCT from the same patient demonstrating numerous thin-walled cysts bilaterally. *Abbreviation*: HRCT, high-resolution computed tomography. *Source*: From Ref. 32.

**(A)**     **(B)**

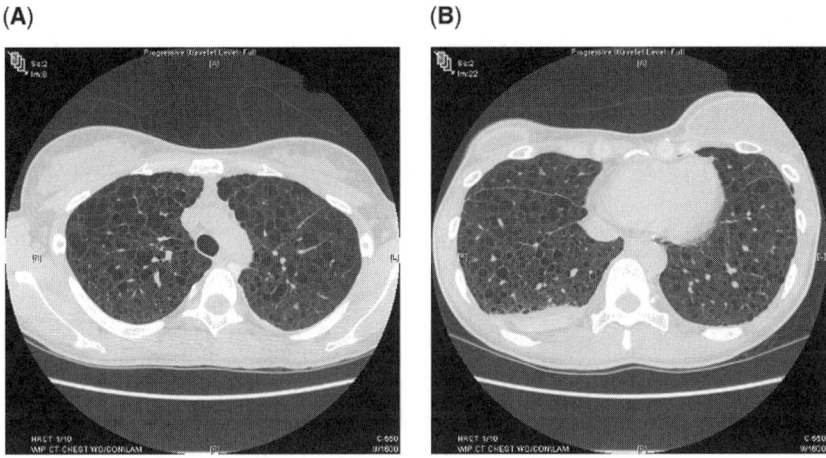

**Figure 6** Lymphangioleiomyomatosis. (**A**) HRCT (upper lobes) from a 32-year-old woman with a history of recurrent pneumothoraces. Multiple well-circumscribed cysts are present bilaterally. (**B**) HRCT (lower lobes) from the same patient showing numerous well-circumscribed cysts bilaterally. A small right chylous effusion is also present. *Abbreviation*: HRCT, high-resolution computed tomography.

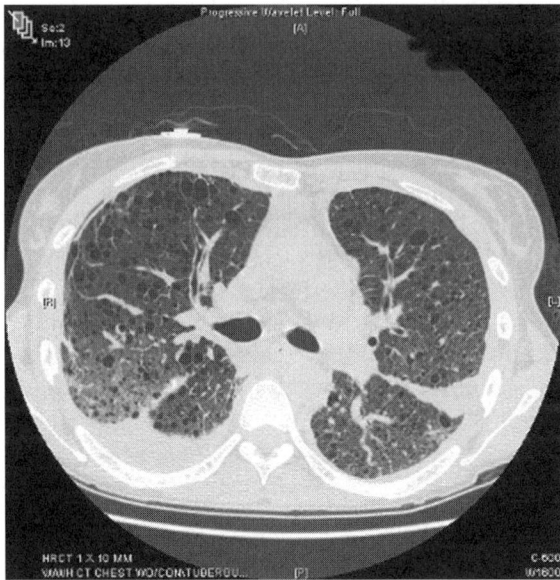

**Figure 7** Lymphangioleiomyomatosis (LAM). HRCT from a 48-year-old woman with LAM and recurrent chylous effusions following surgical (VATS) pleurodesis and ligation of the thoracic duct. Multiple well-circumscribed cysts are present bilaterally; modest bilateral chylous effusions are also present. *Abbreviations*: HRCT, high-resolution computed tomography; VATS, video-assisted thoracoscopic surgery.

regions or lobes (29,93,94). Ground-glass opacities occur in 12% to 59% of cases (69,73), and may reflect foci of alveolar hemorrhage, pulmonary hemosiderosis, or diffuse proliferation of smooth-muscle cells (67,69) (70,74). Cavities, nodules, interstitial fibrosis, or irregular lung–pleural interfaces are not found in LAM (29). Semiquantitative and quantitative analyses of extent of disease by thin-section computed tomography (CT) scan correlate well with physiologic parameters (e.g., $FEV_1$, $DL_{co}$, and gas exchange at rest and exercise) (93,94) and exercise performance (95).

## Pulmonary Function Tests

PFTs in LAM typically demonstrate airflow limitation (often with air-trapping), impaired $DL_{co}$, and hypoxemia; lung volumes are usually normal or increased (67,69,70,72,73,83,96). The rate of progression of airflow obstruction is highly variable, ranging from a few years to more than two decades (67,83). A review of 47 patients with LAM in the United Kingdom cited a mean fall in $FEV_1$ of 118 mL/yr, but there was marked variability between patients (82). In retrospective review of 31 cases of LAM, French investigators noted a mean decline in $FEV_1$ of 106 mL/yr (97). The largest study examined annual rate of decline in lung functional parameters in a cohort of 275 patients with LAM followed for ~4 years in the United States (98). Overall annual rates of decline were 1.7% predicted for $FEV_1$ and 2.4% predicted for $DL_{co}$ (98). Overall, the most significant predictors of functional decline were initial lung function and age. The rate of decline in $FEV_1$ was negatively correlated with the initial $DL_{co}$ and age. That is, rates of decline in $FEV_1$ were lower in older patients and patients with higher $DL_{co}$ and $FEV_1$. Conversely, patients with higher initial $FEV_1$ and $DL_{co}$ (i.e., less severe disease) had more rapid decline in $DL_{co}$. Reduced $DL_{co}$ is also the best predictor of exercise-induced hypoxemia (99). Restrictive defects in LAM reflect the presence of chylous pleural effusions or effects of pleurodesis (100). Impairments in exercise performance and gas exchange correlate with the extent of cystic disease on quantitative CT scanning (94,95,99). Reductions in $FEV_1/FVC$ ratio and increased TLC were associated with a worse prognosis and poor survival (73,96). In contrast to LCH, pulmonary hypertension is uncommon in LAM (62).

## Extrapulmonary Involvement

Lymphangiomyolipomas or cysts may involve abdominal or retroperitoneal lymph nodes, spleen, kidney, periadrenal blood vessels, liver, uterus, and ovaries (67,69,70,85,86,101–103). Renal angiomyolipomas, composed of fat, blood vessels, and smooth muscle (HMB-45-positive), have been noted in 15% to 54% of patients with pulmonary LAM and often antedate the diagnosis of pulmonary LAM (69,70,85,101,103). Uterine leiomyomas were found in 41% of patients with LAM in one study (69). Angiomyolipomas are often incidental findings noted on CT, but growth of these smooth muscle tumors or cysts may cause local pain, bleeding, chylous ascites, or compression of contiguous structures (67,70,85). Angiomyolipomas are hyperechogenic on ultxasonography and reveal fat attenuation on CT (67,70). Ultrasonography or abdominal CT scans are important to diagnose and follow renal, intra-abdominal, or pelvic cystic or angiomyolipomatous lesions (85,102–104). Management of angiomyolipomas or cysts depends upon size, growth rate, and presence or absence of symptoms (67,70,85,105). Asymptomatic patients with lesions <4 cm in greatest dimension can be followed with yearly ultrasonography or CT. Larger lesions require closer follow-up (≤6-month intervals) (67,85). Expanding or symptomatic lesions may require surgical resection or embolization (85,106). Partial or total nephrectomy may be required to manage complications of renal angiolipomas (e.g., hemorrhage and refractory pain) (70,85). The diagnosis of pulmonary LAM can be established without lung biopsy provided chest CT features are characteristic and one or more of the following features are present: renal angiomyolipomas; chronic chylous ascites with abdominal lymphadenopathy; or characteristic histological findings on lymph node biopsy (67–70). Meningiomas were detected in ~2% of patients with LAM or TSC (107). An increased risk of renal cell carcinoma was noted in patients with TSC and angiomyolipoma (62).

## The Course and Prognosis of LAM

The course of LAM is usually indolent, but most patients ultimately die of progressive respiratory failure. However, the prognosis is heterogenous, and the impact of therapy is controversial. Early retrospective reviews cited 5- and 10-year survival rates of only 60% and 20% (71,72). More recent studies noted improved survival, which likely in part reflect earlier diagnosis (particularly with the advent of CT scans). In a cohort of 32 LAM patients from Stanford and the Mayo Clinic, 25 patients (78%) were alive at a mean of 8.5 years after onset of the disease (83). A study from Asia cited survival rates of >70% at five years after the onset of LAM, but only 38% (10 of 26 patients) were alive at 8.5 years (73). A study of 69 LAM patients from France cited survival rates (by Kaplan–Meier analysis) of 91% at 5 years, 79% at 10 years, and 71% after 15 years (69). In a recent study of 57 patients with LAM from the United Kingdom, 10-year survival from onset of symptoms was 91% (108). Over the period of observation, five patients had died and six were alive following a lung transplant.

## Treatment

Optimal therapy of LAM is not known (68). Owing to the rarity of LAM, no randomized or controlled therapeutic studies have been done. Because LAM is exclusively a disease of females, estrogens are believed to be central to the pathogenesis (88). Treatment strategies have focused on reducing estrogens, either by oophorectomy or antiestrogen regimens [e.g., progesterone, tamoxifen, androgens, lynestrenol, luteinizing hormone–releasing hormone (LHRH) antagonists (e.g., goserelin), gonadotropin-releasing hormone (GrRH) agonists (e.g., leuprolide acetate), and somatostatin] (67,69, 70,73,82,83,109,110). Pregnancy or exogenous estrogens are strongly contraindicated (67–69,82). Treatment strategies have shown little or no benefit, but data are limited to retrospective studies. In 1990, Taylor et al. analyzed the effect of diverse therapies among 30 patients with LAM (83). Oophorectomy *alone* was ineffective in all 16 patients (83). Two of 19 patients treated with intramuscular (IM) medroxyprogesterone acetate (MPA) alone stabilized or improved; none of the nine patients treated with tamoxifen improved (83). In 1995, Kitaichi et al. reviewed the impact of antihormonal therapy in 40 patients with LAM (73). Only two patients (5%) improved; nine stabilized; 29 deteriorated. Oophorectomy or progesterone alone was never effective. Urban and coworkers noted no responses in eight patients with LAM treated with a variety of antiestrogen therapies, including oophorectomy, MPA, lynestrenol (a progestin), or tamoxifen (111). Tamoxifen has partial estrogen-agonist activity, which raises concerns about its potential to exacerbate the proliferative process (67). Korean investigators reported 10 patients with LAM who were treated with MPA and/or tamoxifen and had $\geq 12$ months of follow-up (110). The disease worsened in eight; no patient improved. French investigators identified 69 women with LAM from 1973 to 1996, of whom 57 (84%) received various hormonal therapies including progesterone ($n = 46$), tamoxifen ($n = 22$), GrRh agonists ($n = 14$), somatostatin ($n = 6$), and oophorectomy ($n = 5$) (69). Among 34 patients with serial PFTs, $FEV_1$ improved by $\geq 15\%$ in 4 patients (12%), 11 deteriorated, and 19 remained stable. Anecdotal responses were cited with a synthetic analog of LHRH (109), interferon$\alpha$-2b (112), and somatostatin (113), but these agents are of unproven value. One retrospective analysis of 43 patients with LAM in the United Kingdom noted a slower rate of decline of PFTs ($FEV_1$, TLC) among patients treated with progesterone (82), but differences were not statistically significant. A subsequent retrospective study from these investigators analyzed factors influencing disease progression in a cohort of 57 LAM patients, 36 of whom were treated with progesterone (108). There was more rapid progression of dyspnea (MRC grade 3) among those who became pregnant after the onset of symptoms (HR 2.7), patients treated with progesterone (HR 2.2), and cigarette smokers (HR 2.0). These associations were of borderline statistical significance. However, these data do *not* support a beneficial effect of progesterone on lung function. A larger study from the United States followed 275 patients with LAM for ~4 years (98). Overall, 139 patients (50%) were treated with progesterone (67 oral and 72 IM). No benefit in rates of decline in $FEV_1$

and $DL_{co}$ were noted among patients receiving progesterone (either oral or IM) compared to untreated patients (98). Absolute annual declines in $FEV_1$ were 59 mL among patients not treated with progesterone versus 119 mL/yr and 76 mL/yr declines among patients treated with oral or IM progesterone, respectively (98). Absolute annual declines in $DL_{co}$ were 0.57 ml/min/mmHg among patients *not* treated with progesterone versus 0.95 and 0.70 ml/min/mm Hg among patients treated with oral or IM progesterone, respectively (98). In summary, cumulative data from these various clinical series (69,73,82,83,110) suggest that current therapies are of limited efficacy at best. Unfortunately, there are no clear guidelines for optimal therapy.

Given the poor prognosis of untreated LAM, it is reasonable to offer an empirical trial of antiestrogen therapy for symptomatic patients. However, patients should be informed that these therapies have *not been proven to alter the course of the disease.* The decision to treat needs to be individualized, and must take into account the patient's wishes. Progesterone has been used most often [either IM MPA (dose of 400–800 mg/mo) or oral progesterone (10–20 mg/day)] (67,69,70,73,82,83). Pharmacokinetics reveal higher and more sustained levels with the IM route (67), but no studies have evaluated clinical efficacy for various regimens. Antihormonal therapies appear to be more efficacious in ameliorating chylothorax or chylous ascites, but have limited or no effect on modulating the pulmonary parenchymal cystic process (61,70,73,83). Rapamycin, a macrolide with immunosuppressive properties, inhibits hyperphosphylation of ribosomal protein S6, p70S6K activity, and the increased DNA synthesis of LAM cells in vitro (92,114). Whether these in vitro inhibitory effects of rapamycin on smooth muscle cell proliferation in LAM have clinical application is not known, but a randomized, placebo-controlled clinical trial to address this hypothesis is currently underway (personal communication, Francis X. McCormack, M.D., University of Cincinnati, September 2005). Bronchodilators or supplemental oxygen have adjunctive roles in selected patients with pulmonary LAM (67,69,70).

## Management of Chylous Effusions and Pneumothoraces in LAM

Pneumothorax complicates LAM in 50% to 80% of patients and chylothorax in 10% to 39% of patients (67,69,70,72,73,83). Both complications may occur repetitively in individual patients, mandating an aggressive surgical approach to therapy. Thoracostomy tubes may be adequate therapy for pneumothorax or chylothorax in some patients, but recurrences are common. Video-assisted thoracoscopic surgery (VATS) with pleurodesis is warranted for recurrent pneumothoraces or chylothoraces complicating LAM (68–70,115). Unfortunately, pleurodesis (mechanical or chemical) increases morbidity (particularly bleeding) at the time of eventual lung transplantation (69,116). Recurrent chylothorax may result in large, symptomatic pleural effusions, requiring repetitive drainage (Fig. 8). Criteria for diagnosis of chylothorax include pleural fluid triglyceride >110 mg/dL or the presence of chylomicrons in pleural fluid (117). Chylothorax does not correlate with the severity of lung involvement in LAM (115). Mechanisms for chylothorax formation in LAM include (i) leak from the thoracic duct; (ii) oozing from pleural lymphatics or collateral vessels; and (iii) transdiaphragmatic flow of chylous ascites (115). Management of chylous pleural effusions or ascites in patients failing antiestrogen therapy is difficult. Simple thoracentesis, paracentesis, or thoracostomy tubes may provide palliation, but are usually not definitive (115). A low-fat diet, with or without supplementation with medium-chain triglycerides, and total parenteral nutrition (TPN) have been tried, but are usually ineffective (67,69,70,115,118,119). Additional treatment options for chylous effusions include tube thoracostomy (with sclerosing agents) (118,120); thoracotomy with thoracic duct ligation (±mechanical or talc pleurodesis) (68); parietal pleurectomy (72,115); and peritoneal–jugular shunts (115,121). Sclerosing agents used for pleurodesis include nitrogen mustard (120), tetracycline (118), bleomycin (115), and

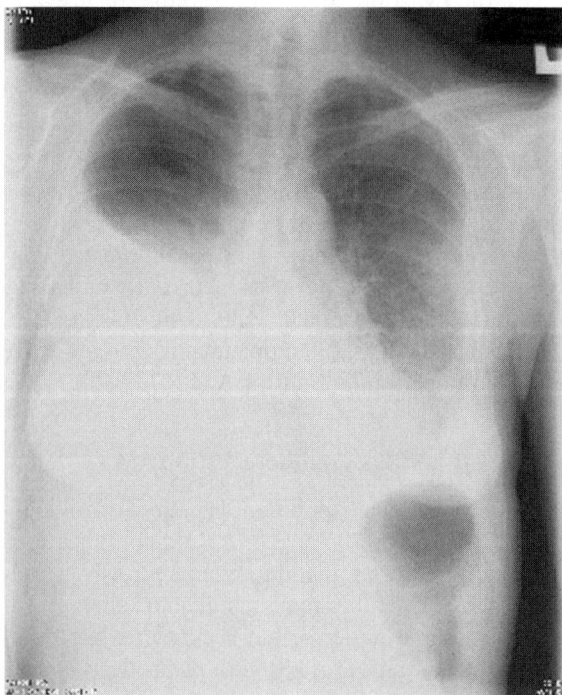

**Figure 8** Lymphangioleiomyomatosis (LAM). Chest radiograph from a 48-year-old woman with LAM and recurrent chylous effusions. A massive right pleural effusion and moderate left pleural effusions are present.

talc (122). In one LAM patient with chylothorax refractory to conventional therapies, intrapleural injection of povidone (INN polyvidone) was efficacious (119). Given the rarity of LAM, optimal management of chylous effusions is controversial. We agree with Ryu et al. (115) that the approach should be individualized, taking into account the severity or persistence of chylothorax, comorbidities, and local expertise. For refractory chylorax, we favor VATS with talc pleurodesis *and* thoracic duct ligation. In cases of unilateral pleurodesis, single-lung transplantation can be performed on the contralateral side (116). However, given the risk of future complications in the native lung (i.e., pneumothorax, chylothorax), we favor bilateral lung transplantation for patients with LAM.

## Lung Transplantation for LAM

Single- or double-lung transplantation has been successful in patients with LAM and end-stage pulmonary insufficiency (62,64,116,123–125). Data from the ISHLT Registry from January 1995 to June 2004 identified 138 patients with LAM among 13,007 lung transplant recipients (1.1%) (64). One review of 34 LAM patients cited one- and two-year survival rates of 69% and 58%, respectively, following lung transplantation (116). A retrospective review of 14 LAM patients who underwent lung transplantation at Washington University cited two- and five-year survival rates of 90% and 69%, respectively (123). We are aware of one patient who received a living-donor lobar lung transplant for end-stage LAM (126). When to list LAM patients for lung transplantation is difficult, as the prognosis is widely heterogenous among patients. Survival is worse in LAM patients with predominantly cystic LAM lesions on surgical lung biopsy (73,96,127), but estimating survival in individual patients is not possible. Guidelines for lung transplantation in LAM include progressive respiratory insufficiency despite medical therapy, a rapidly deteriorating course, $FEV_1/FVC < 50\%$, $TLC > 130\%$, and $FEV_1 < 30\%$, and severe cystic disease on HRCT (81).

LAM-associated complications of transplantation include massive operative hemorrhage due to extensive pleural adhesions (particularly in patients with multiple pneumothoraces or pleurodeses); pneumothorax in the native lung (for single lung transplant recipients); postoperative chylothorax or fistulas requiring thoracic duct ligation or sclerosis (62,116, 123,128). Recurrence of LAM was noted in at least four cases in the donor lung allografts (129–132), but is uncommon [1 of 29 lung transplant recipients in one review (116) and 1 of 14 in another] (123). Recent reports using molecular techniques confirmed that foci of LAM in lung allografts were derived from the recipient (132,133). Previous reports suggesting that recurrent LAM cells were of male (donor) origin (131,133) may have reflected donor-derived endothelial cells or reactive pneumocytes rather than smooth muscle (LAM) cells.

## REFERENCES

1. Colby TV, Lombard C. Histiocytosis X in the lung. Hum Pathol 1983; 14(10):847–856.
2. Friedman PJ, Liebow AA, Sokoloff J. Eosinophilic granuloma of lung. Clinical aspects of primary histiocytosis in the adult. Medicine (Baltimore) 1981; 60(6):385–396.
3. Basset F, Corrin B, Spencer H, et al. Pulmonary histiocytosis X. Am Rev Respir Dis 1978; 118(5):811–820.
4. Selman M, Carillo G, Gaxiola M, Ramos C. Pulmonary histiocytosis X (Eosinophilic granuloma): clinical behavior, pathogenesis, and therapeutic strategies of an unusual interstitial lung disease. Clin Pulm Med 1996; 3:191–198.
5. Travis WD, Borok Z, Roum JH, et al. Pulmonary Langerhans cell granulomatosis (histiocytosis X). A clinicopathologic study of 48 cases. Am J Surg Pathol 1993; 17(10):971–986.
6. McClain KL, Gonzalez JM, Jonkers R, De Juli E, Egeler M. Need for a cooperative study: pulmonary langerhans cell histiocytosis and its management in adults. Med Pediatr Oncol 2002; 39(1):35–39.
7. Ha SY, Helms P, Fletcher M, Broadbent V, Pritchard J. Lung involvement in Langerhans cell histiocytosis: prevalence, clinical features, and outcome. Pediatrics 1992; 89(3):466–469.
8. Vassallo R, Ryu JH, Colby TV, Hartman T, Limper AH. Pulmonary Langerhans-cell histiocytosis. N Engl J Med 2000; 342(26):1969–1978.
9. Smets A, Mortele K, de Praeter G, Francois O, Benoit Y, Kunnen M. Pulmonary and mediastinal lesions in children with Langerhans cell histiocytosis. Pediatr Radiol 1997; 27(11):873–876.
10. Nondahl SR, Finlay JL, Farrell PM, Warner TF, Hong R. A case report and literature review of "primary" pulmonary histiocytosis X of childhood. Med Pediatr Oncol 1986; 14(1):57–62.
11. Bernstrand C, Cederlund K, Sandstedt B, et al. Pulmonary abnormalities at long-term follow-up of patients with Langerhans cell histiocytosis. Med Pediatr Oncol 2001; 36(4):459–468.
12. Soler P, Bergeron A, Kambouchner M, et al. Is high-resolution computed tomography a reliable tool to predict the histopathological activity of pulmonary Langerhans cell histiocytosis? Am J Respir Crit Care Med 2000; 62(1):264–270.
13. Sundar KM, Gosselin MV, Chung HL, Cahill BC. Pulmonary Langerhans cell histiocytosis: emerging concepts in pathobiology, radiology, and clinical evolution of disease. Chest 2003; 123(5):1673–1683.
14. Adler BD, Padley SP, Muller NL, Remy-Jardin M, Remy J. Chronic hypersensitivity pneumonitis: high-resolution CT and radiographic features in 16 patients. Radiology 1992; 185(1):91–95.
15. Braier J, Latella A, Balancini B, et al. Outcome in children with pulmonary Langerhans cell histiocytosis. Pediatr Blood Cancer 2004; 43(7):765–769.
16. Ladisch S, Gadner H. Treatment of Langerhans cell histiocytosis—evolution and current approaches. Br J Cancer Suppl 1994; 23:S41–S46.
17. Braier J, Chantada G, Rosso D, et al. Langerhans cell histiocytosis: retrospective evaluation of 123 patients at a single institution. Pediatr Hematol Oncol 1999; 16(5):377–385.

18. Howarth DM, Gilchrist GS, Mullan BP, Wiseman GA, Edmonson JH, Schomberg PJ. Langerhans cell histiocytosis: diagnosis, natural history, management, and outcome. Cancer 1999; 85(10):2278–2290.
19. The French Langerhans' Cell Histiocytosis Study Group. A multicentre retrospective survey of Langerhans' cell histiocytosis: 348 cases observed between 1983 and 1993. Arch Dis Child 1996; 75(1):17–24.
20. Arico M, Girschikofsky M, Genereau T, et al. Langerhans cell histiocytosis in adults. Report from the International Registry of the Histiocyte Society. Eur J Cancer 2003; 39(16):2341–2348.
21. Gotz G, Fichter J. Langerhans'-cell histiocytosis in 58 adults. Eur J Med Res 2004; 9(11):510–514.
22. Tazi A, Soler P, Hance AJ. Adult pulmonary Langerhans' cell histiocytosis. Thorax 2000; 55(5):405–416.
23. Vassallo R, Jensen EA, Colby TV, et al. The overlap between respiratory bronchiolitis and desquamative interstitial pneumonia in pulmonary Langerhans cell histiocytosis: high-resolution CT, histologic, and functional correlations. Chest 2003; 124(4):1199–1205.
24. Moore AD, Godwin JD, Muller NL, et al. Pulmonary histiocytosis X: comparison of radiographic and CT findings. Radiology 1989; 172(1):249–254.
25. Fartoukh M, Humbert M, Capron F, et al. Severe pulmonary hypertension in histiocytosis X. Am J Respir Crit Care Med 2000; 161(1):216–223.
26. Delobbe A, Durieu J, Duhamel A, Wallaert B. Determinants of survival in pulmonary Langerhans' cell granulomatosis (histiocytosis X). Groupe d'Etude en Pathologie Interstitielle de la Societe de Pathologie Thoracique du Nord. Eur Respir J 1996; 9(10):2002–2006.
27. Lewis JG. Eosinophilic granuloma and its variants with special reference to lung involvement. A report of 12 patients. Q J Med 1964; 33:337–359.
28. Lacronique J, Roth C, Battesti JP, Basset F, Chretien J. Chest radiological features of pulmonary histiocytosis X: a report based on 50 adult cases. Thorax 1982; 37(2):104–109.
29. Koyama M, Johkoh T, Honda O, et al. Chronic cystic lung disease: diagnostic accuracy of high-resolution CT in 92 patients. AJR Am J Roentgenol 2003; 180(3):S27–S35.
30. Brauner MW, Grenier P, Tijani K, Battesti JP, Valeyre D. Pulmonary Langerhans cell histiocytosis: evolution of lesions on CT scans. Radiology 1997; 204(2):497–502.
31. Stern EJ, Webb WR, Golden JA, Gamsu G. Cystic lung disease associated with eosinopbilic granuloma and tuberous sclerosis: air trapping at dynamic ultrafast high-resolution CT. Radiology 1992; 182(2):325–329.
32. Lynch J III, Raghu G. Major pulmonary disease syndromes of unknown etiology. In: Crapo JD, Glassroth, Karlinsky J, King E Jr, eds. Baum's Textbook of Pulmonary Diseases. 7th ed. Lippincott, Williams & Wilkins, Philadelpia, PA: 2004:629–656.
33. Lynch J III, Keane M. Treatment of parenchymal lung diseases. In: Spina D, Page CP, Metzger WJ, O'Connor BJ, eds. Drugs for the Treatment of Respiratory Diseases. Cambridge University Press, Cambridge, UK, 2003: 247–335.

34. Crausman RS, Jennings CA, Tuder RM, Ackerson LM, Irvin CG, King TE Jr. Pulmonary histiocytosis X: pulmonary function and exercise pathophysiology. Am J Respir Crit Care Med 1996; 153(1):426–435.
35. Housini I, Tomashefski JF Jr, Cohen A, Crass J, Kleinerman J. Transbronchial biopsy in patients with pulmonary eosinophilic granuloma. Comparison with findings on open lung biopsy. Arch Pathol Lab Med 1994; 118(5):523–530.
36. Flint A, Lloyd RV, Colby TV, Wilson BW. Pulmonary histiocytosis X. Immunoperoxidase staining for HLA-DR antigen and S100 protein. Arch Pathol Lab Med 1986; 110(10):930–933.
37. Webber D, Tron V, Askin F, Churg A. S-100 staining in the diagnosis of eosinophilic granuloma of lung. Am J Clin Pathol 1985; 84(4):447–453.
38. Chollet S, Soler P, Dournovo P, Richard MS, Ferrans VJ, Basset F. Diagnosis of pulmonary histiocytosis X by immunodetection of Langerhans cells in bronchoalveolar lavage fluid. Am J Pathol 1984; 115(2):225–232.
39. Tazi A, Bonay M, Grandsaigne M, Battesti JP, Hance AJ, Soler P. Surface phenotype of Langerhans cells and lymphocytes in granulomatous lesions from patients with pulmonary histiocytosis X. Am Rev Respir Dis 1993; 147(6, Pt 1):1531–1536.
40. Smetana K Jr, Mericka O, Saeland S, Homolka J, Brabec J, Gabius HJ. Diagnostic relevance of Langerin detection in cells from bronchoalveolar lavage of patients with pulmonary Langerhans cell histiocytosis, sarcoidosis and idiopathic pulmonary fibrosis. Virchows Arch 2004; 444(2):171–174.
41. Soler P, Chollet S, Jacque C, Fukuda Y, Ferrans VJ, Basset F. Immunocytochemical characterization of pulmonary histiocytosis X cells in lung biopsies. Am J Pathol 1985; 118(3):439–451.
42. Schonfeld N, Frank W, Wenig S, et al. Clinical and radiologic features, lung function and therapeutic results in pulmonary histiocytosis X. Respiration 1993; 60(1):38–44.
43. Youkeles LH, Grizzanti JN, Liao Z, Chang CJ, Rosenstreich DL. Decreased tobacco-glycoprotein–induced lymphocyte proliferation in vitro in pulmonary eosinophilic granuloma. Am J Respir Crit Care Med 1995; 151(1):145–150.
44. Tazi A, Bonay M, Bergeron A, Grandsaigne M, Hance AJ, Soler P. Role of granulocyte-macrophage colony stimulating factor (GM-CSF) in the pathogenesis of adult pulmonary histiocytosis X. Thorax 1996; 51(6):611–614.
45. Hance AJ. Pulmonary immune cells in health and disease: dendritic cells and Langerhans' cells. Eur Respir J 1993; 6(8):1213–1220.
46. Aguayo SM. Determinants of susceptibility to cigarette smoke. Potential roles for neuroendocrine cells and neuropeptides in airway inflammation, airway wall remodeling, and chronic airflow obstruction. Am J Respir Crit Care Med 1994; 49(6):1692–1698.
47. Aguayo SM, King TE Jr, Waldron JA Jr, Sherritt KM, Kane MA, Miller YE. Increased pulmonary neuroendocrine cells with bombesin-like immunoreactivity in adult patients with eosinophilic granuloma. J Clin Invest 1990; 86(3):838–844.
48. Zeid NA, Muller HK. Tobacco smoke induced lung granulomas and tumors: association with pulmonary Langerhans cells. Pathology 1995; 27(3): 247–254.

49. Vassallo R, Ryu JH, Schroeder DR, Decker PA, Limper AH. Clinical outcomes of pulmonary Langerhans'-cell histiocytosis in adults. N Engl J Med 2002; 346(7):484–490.
50. Chaowalit N, Pellikka PA, Decker PA, et al. Echocardiographic and clinical characteristics of pulmonary hypertension complicating pulmonary Langerhans cell histiocytosis. Mayo Clin Proc 2004; 79(10):1269–1275.
51. Gadner H, Grois N, Arico M, et al. A randomized trial of treatment for multisystem Langerhans' cell histiocytosis. J Pediatr 2001; 138(5):728–734.
52. Giona F, Caruso R, Testi AM, et al. Langerhans' cell histiocytosis in adults: a clinical and therapeutic analysis of 11 patients from a single institution. Cancer 1997; 80(9):1786–1791.
53. Saven A, Burian C. Cladribine activity in adult Langercans-cell histiocytosis. Blood 1999; 93(12):4125–4130.
54. Zeller B, Storm-Mathisen I, Smevik B, Lie SO. Multisystem Langerhans-cell histiocytosis with life-threatening pulmonary involvement–good response to cyclosporine A. Med Pediatr Oncol 2000; 35(4):438–442.
55. Minkov M, Grois N, Broadbent V, Ceci A, Jakobson A, Ladisch S. Cyclosporine A therapy for multisystem Langerhans cell histiocytosis. Med Pediatr Oncol 1999; 33(5):482–485.
56. Choi SW, Bangaru BS, Wu CD, Finlay JL. Gastrointestinal involvement in disseminated Langerhans cell histiocytosis (LCH) with durable complete response to 2-chlorodeoxyadenosine and high-dose cytarabine. J Pediatr Hematol Oncol 2003; 25(6):503–506.
57. Goh NS, McDonald CE, MacGregor DP, Pretto JJ, Brodie GN. Successful treatment of Langerhans cell histiocytosis with 2-chlorodeoxyadenosine. Respirology 2003; 8(1):91–94.
58. Hirose M, Saito S, Yoshimoto T, Kuroda Y. Interleukin-2 therapy of Langerhans cell histiocytosis. Acta Paediatr 1995; 84(10):1204–1206.
59. Henter JI, Karlen J, Calming U, Bernstrand C, Andersson U, Fadeel B. Successful treatment of Langerhans'-cell histiocytosis with etanercept. N Engl J Med 2001; 345(21):1577–1578.
60. Tsele E, Thomas DM, Chu AC. Treatment of adult Langerhans cell histiocytosis with etoposide. J Am Acad Dermatol 1992; 27(1):61–64.
61. Mogulkoc N, Veral A, Bishop PW, Bayindir U, Pickering CA, Egan JJ. Pulmonary Langerhans' ceil histiocytosis: radiologic resolution following smoking cessation. Chest 1999; 115(5):1452–1455.
62. Boehler A. Lung transplantation for cystic lung diseases: lymphangioleiomyomatosis, histiocytosis X, and sarcoidosis. Semin Respir Crit Care Med 2001; 22:509–516.
63. Etienne B, Bertocchi M, Gamondes JP, et al. Relapsing pulmonary Langerhans cell histiocytosis after lung transplantation. Am J Respir Crit Care Med 1998; 157(1);288–291.
64. Hertz MI, Boucek MM, Deng MC, et al. Scientific Registry of the International Society for Heart and Lung Transplantation: introduction to the 2005 annual reports. J Heart Lung Transplant 2005; 24(8):939–944.
65. Gabbay E, Dark JH, Ashcroft T, et al. Recurrence of Langerhans' cell granulomatosis following lung transplantation. Thorax 1998; 53(4):326–327.

66. Habbib SB, Congelton J, Carr D, Mickey M. Recurrence of Langerhan's cell histiocytosis following bilateral lung transplantation. Thorax 1998; 53:323–325.
67. Johnson S. Rare diseases. 1. Lymphangioleiomyomatosis: clinical features, management and basic mechanisms. Thorax 1999; 54(3):254–264.
68. Johnson SR, Tattersfield AE. Clinical experience of lymphangioleiomyomatosis in the UK. Thorax 2000; 55(12):1052–1057.
69. Urban T, Lazor R, Lacronique J, et al. Pulmonary lymphangioleiomyomatosis. A study of 69 patients. Groupe d'Etudes et de Recherche sur les Maladies "Orphelines" Pulmonaires (GERM"O"P). Medicine (Baltimore) 1999; 78(5): 321–337.
70. Chu SC, Horiba K, Usuki J, et al. Comprehensive evaluation of 35 patients with lymphangioleiomyomatosis. Chest 1999; 115(4):1041–1052.
71. Corrin B, Liebow AA, Friedman PJ. Pulmonary lymphangiomyomatosis. A review. Am J Pathol 1975; 79(2):348–382.
72. Silverstein EF, Ellis K, Wolff M, Jaretzki Ad. Pulmonary lymphangiomyomatosis. AJR Am J Roentgenol Radium Ther Nucl Med 1974; 120(4):832–850.
73. Kitaichi M, Nishimura K, Itoh H, Izumi T. Pulmonary lymphangioleiomyomatosis: a report of 46 patients including a clinicopathologic study of prognostic factors. Am J Respir Crit Care Med 1995; 151(2, Pt 1):527–533.
74. Hayashi T, Fleming MV, Stetier-Stevenson WG, et al. Immunohistochemical study of matrix metalloproteinases (MMPs) and their tissue inhibitors (TIMPs) in pulmonary lymphangioleiomyomatosis (LAM). Hum Pathol 1997; 28(9):1071–1078.
75. Castro M, Shepherd CW, Gomez MR, Lie JT, Ryu JH. Pulmonary tuberous sclerosis. Chest 1995; 107(1):189–195.
76. Peccatori I, Pitingolo F, Battini G, et al. Pulmonary lymphangioleiomyomatosis and tuberous sclerosis complex. Contrib Nephrol 1997; 122:98–101.
77. Bonetti F, Chiodera P. Lymphangioleiomyomatosis and tuberous sclerosis: where is the border? Eur Respir J 1996; 9(3):399–401.
78. Roach ES, Smith M, Huttenlocher P, Bhat M, Alcorn D, Hawley L. Diagnostic criteria: tuberous sclerosis complex. Report of the Diagnostic Criteria Committee of the National Tuberous Sclerosis Association. J Child Neurol 1992; 7(2):221–224.
79. Costello LC, Hartman TE, Ryu JH. High frequency of pulmonary lymphangioleiomyomatosis in women with tuberous sclerosis complex. Mayo Clin Proc 2000; 75(6):591–594.
80. Torres VE, Bjornsson J, King BF, et al. Extrapulmonary lymphangioleiomyomatosis and lymphangiomatous cysts in tuberous sclerosis complex. Mayo Clin Proc 1995; 70(7):641–648.
81. NHLBI. Workshop Summary. Report of workshop on lymphangioleiomyomatosis. National Heart, Lung, and Blood Institute. Am J Respir Crit Care Med 1999; 159(2):679–683.
82. Johnson SR, Tattersfield AE. Decline in lung function in lymphangioleiomyomatosis: relation to menopause and progesterone treatment. Am J Respir Crit Care Med 1999; 160(2):628–633.
83. Taylor JR, Ryu J, Colby TV, Raffin TA. Lymphangioleiomyomatosis. Clinical course in 32 patients. N Engl JMed 1990; 323(18):1254–1260.

84. Chan JK, Tsang WY, Pau MY, Tang MC, Pang SW, Fletcher CD. Lymphangiomyomatosis and angiomyolipoma: closely related entities characterized by hamartomatous proliferation of HMB-45-positive smooth muscle. Histopathology 1993; 22(5):445–455.
85. Bernstein SM, Newell JD Jr, Adamezyk D, Mortenson RL, King TE Jr, Lynch DA. How common are renal angiomyolipomas in patients with pulmonary lymphangiomyomatosis? Am J Respir Crit Care Med 1995; 152(6, Pt 1):2138–2143.
86. Matsui K, Tatsuguchi A, Valencia J, et al. Extrapulmonary lymphangioleiomyomatosis (LAM): clinicopathologic features in 22 cases. Hum Pathol 2000; 31(10):1242–1248.
87. Guinee DG Jr, Feuerstein I, Koss MN, Travis WD. Pulmonary lymphangioleiomyomatosis. Diagnosis based on results of transbronchial biopsy and immunohistochemical studies and correlation with high-resolution computed tomography findings. Arch Pathol Lab Med 1994; 118(8):846–849.
88. Kalassian KG, Doyle R, Kao P, Ruoss S, Raffin TA. Lymphangioleiomyomatosis: new insights. Am J Respir Crit Care Med 1997; 155(4):1183–1186.
89. McCormack FX, Smolarek TA, Menon AG. Lymphangioleiomyomatosis and leiomyoma: possibility of shared genetic origins? In: Moss J, ed. LAM and Other Diseases Characterized by Smooth Muscle Proliferation. New York: Marcel Dekker, 1998:373–386.
90. Carsillo T, Astrinidis A, Henske EP. Mutations in the tuberous sclerosis complex gene TSC2 are a cause of sporadic pulmonary lymphangioleiomyomatosis. Proc Natl Acad Sci USA 2000; 97(11):6085–6090.
91. Smolarek TA, Wessner LL, McCormack FX, Mylet JC, Menon AG, Henske EP. Evidence that lymphangiomyomatosis is caused by TSC2 mutations: chromosome 16p13 loss of heterozygosity in angiomyolipomas and lymph nodes from women with lymphangiomyomatosis. Am J Hum Genet 1998; 62(4):810–815.
92. Goncharova EA, Goncharov DA, Eszterhas A, et al. Tuberin regulates p70 S6 kinase activation and ribosomal protein S6 phosphorylation. A role for the TSC2 tumor suppressor gene in pulmonary lymphangioleiomyomatosis (LAM). J Biol Chem 2002; 277(34):30958–30967.
93. Aberle DR, Hansell DM, Brown K, Tashkin DP. Lymphangiomyomatosis: CT, chest radiographic, and functional correlations. Radiology 1990; 176(2):381–387.
94. Muller NL, Chiles C, Kullnig P. Pulmonary lymphangiomyomatosis: correlation of CT with radiographic and functional findings. Radiology 1990; 175(2): 335–339.
95. Crausman RS, Lynch DA, Mortenson RL, et al. Quantitative CT predicts the severity of physiologic dysfunction in patients with lymphangioleiomyomatosis. Chest 1996; 109(1):131–137.
96. Crausman RS, Jennings CA, Mortenson RL, Ackerson LM, Irvin CG, King TE Jr. Lymphangioleiomyomatosis: the pathophysiology of diminished exercise capacity. Am J Respir Crit Care Med 1996; 153(4, Pt 1):1368–1376.
97. Lazor R, Valeyre D, Lacronique J, Wallaert B, Urbane T, Cordier JF. Low initial KCO predicts rapid FEV1 decline in pulmonary lymphangioleiomyomatosis. Respir Med 2004; 98(6):536–541.

98. Taveira-Dailva AM, Stylianou MP, Hedin CJ, Hathaway O, Moss J. Decline in lung function in patients with lymphangioleiomyomatosis treated with or without progesterone. Chest 2004; 126(6):1867–1874.

99. Taveira-DaSilva AM, Stylianou MP, Hedin CJ, et al. Maximal oxygen uptake and severity of disease in lymphangioleiomyomatosis. Am J Respir Crit Care Med 2003; 168(12):1427–1431.

100. Avila NA, Kelly JA, Dwyer AT, Johnson DL, Jones EC, Moss J. Lymphangioleiomyomatosis: correlation of qualitative and quantitative thin-section CT with pulmonary function tests and assessment of dependence on pleurodesis. Radiology 2002; 223(1):189–197.

101. Maziak DE, Kesten S, Rappaport DC, Maurer J. Extrathoracic angiomyolipomas in lymphangioleiomyomatosis. Eur Respir J 1996; 9(3):402–405.

102. Woodring JH, Howard RS II, Johnson MV. Massive low-attenuation mediastinal, retroperitoneal, and pelvic lymphadenopathy on CT from lymphangioleiomyomatosis. Case report. Clin Imaging 1994; 18(1):7–11.

103. Avila NA, Kelly JA, Chu SC, Dwyer AJ, Moss J. Lymphangioleiomyomatosis: abdominopelvic CT and US findings. Radiology 2000; 216(1):147–153.

104. Lemaitre L, Robert Y, Dubrulle F, et al. Renal angiomyolipoma: growth followed up with CT and/or US. Radiology 1995; 197(3):598–602.

105. Steiner MS, Goldman SM, Fishman EK, Marshall FF. The natural history of renal angiomyolipoma. J Urol ; 150(6):1782–1786.

106. Han YM, Kim JK, Roh BS, et al. Renal angiomyolipoma: selective arterial embolization: effectiveness and changes in angiomyogenic components in long-term follow up. Radiology 1997; 204:65–70.

107. Moss J, DeCastro R, Patronas NJ, Taveira-DaSilva A. Meningiomas as in lymphangioleiomyomatosis. J Am Med Assoc 2001; 286(15):1879–1881.

108. Johnson SR, Whale CI, Hubbard RB, Lewis SA, Tattersfield AE. Survival and disease progression in UK patients with lymphangioleiomyomatosis. Thorax 2004; 59(9):800–803.

109. Rossi GA, Balbi B, Oddera S, Lantero S, Ravazzoni C. Response to treatment with an analog of the luteinizing-hormone-releasing hormone in a patient with pulmonary lymophangioleiomyomatosis. Am Rev Respir Dis 1991; 143(1): 174–176.

110. Oh YM, Mo EK, Jang SH, et al. Pulmonary lymphangioleiomyomatosis in Korea. Thorax 1999; 54(7):618–621.

111. Urban T, Kuttenn F, Gompel A, Marsac J, Lacronique J. Pulmonary lymphangiomyomatosis. Follow-up and long-term outcome with antiestrogen therapy: a report of eight cases. Chest 1992; 102(2):472–476.

112. Klein M, Krieger O, Ruckser R, et al. Treatment of lymphangioleiomyomatosis by ovariectomy, interferon alpha 2b and tamoxifen—a case report. Arch Gynecol Obstet 1992; 252(2):99–102.

113. DeBove P, Murris-Espin M, Buscail L, et al. Somatostatin receptors in pulmonary lymphangioleiomyomatosis: therapeutic relevance. Eur Respir J 1997; 10(Suppl 25):297S.

114. Krymskaya VP. Tumour suppressors hamartin and tuberin: intracellular signalling. Cell Signal 2003; 15(8):729–739.

115. Ryu JH, Doerr CH, Fisher SD, Olson EJ, Sahn SA. Chylothorax in lymphangioleiomyomatosis. Chest 2003; 123(2):623–627.
116. Boehler A, Speich R, Russi EW, Weder W. Lung transplantation for lymphangioleiomyomatosis. N Engl J Med 1996; 335(17):1275–1280.
117. Doerr CH, Miller DL, Ryu JH. Chylothorax. Semin Respir Crit Care Med 2001; 22(6):617–626.
118. Luna CM, Gene R, Jolly EC, et al. Pulmonary lymphangiomyomatosis associated with tuberous sclerosis. Treatment with tamoxifen and tetracycline-pleurodesis. Chest 1985; 88(3):473–475.
119. Dauriat G, Brugiere O, Mai H, et al. Refractory chylothorax after lung transplantation for lymphangioleiomyomatosis successfully cured with instillation of povidone. J Thorac Cardiovasc Surg 2003; 126(3):875–877.
120. Lieberman J, Agliozzo CM. Intrapleural nitrogen mustard for treating chylous effusion of pulmonary lymphangioleiomyomatosis. Cancer 1974; 33(6):1505–1511.
121. Valentine VG, Raffin TA. The management of chylothorax. Chest 1992; 102(2):586–591.
122. Sullivan EJ. Lymphangioleiomyomatosis: a review. Chest 1998; 114(6):1689–1703.
123. Pechet TT, Meyers BF, Guthrie TJ, et al. Lung transplantation for lymphangioleiomyomatosis. J Heart Lung Transplant 2004; 23(3):301–308.
124. Speich R, Nicod LP, Aubert JD, et al. Ten years of lung transplantation in Switzerland: results of the Swiss Lung Transplant Registry. Swiss Med Wkly 2004; 134(1–2):18–23.
125. Trulock EP, Edwards LB, Taylor DO, Boucek MM, Keck BM, Herte MI. The Registry of the International Society for Heart and Lung Transplantation: twenty-first official adult lung and heart-lung transplant report—2004. J Heart Lung Transplant 2004; 23(7):804–815.
126. Chen F, Fukuse T, Hasegawa S, Bando T, et al. Living-donor lobar lung transplantation for pulmonary and abdominopelvic lymphangioleiomyomatosis. Thorac Cardiov Surg 2005; 53:122–127.
127. Matsui K, Beasley MB, Nelson WK, et al. Prognostic significance of pulmonary lymphangioleiomyomatosis histologic score. Am J Surg Pathol 2001; 25(4):479–484.
128. Collins J, Muller NL, Kazerooni EA, McAdams HP, Leung AN, Love RB. Lung transplantation for lymphangioleiomyomatosis: role of imaging in the assessment of complications related to the underlying disease. Radiology 1999; 210(2):325–332.
129. Bittmann I, Dose TB, Muller C, Dienemann H, Vogelmeier C, Lohrs U. Lymphangioleiomyomatosis: recurrence after single lung transplantation. Hum Pathol 1997; 28(12):1420–1423.
130. O'Brien JD, Lium JH, Parosa JF, Deyoung BR, Wick MR, Trulock EP. Lymphangiomyomatosis recurrence in the allograft after single-lung transplantation. Am J Respir Crit Care Med 1995; 151(6):2033–2036.
131. Nine JS, Yousem SA, Paradis IL, Keenan R, Griffith BP. Lymphangioleiomyomatosis: recurrence after lung transplantation. J Heart Lung Transplant 1994; 13(4):714–719.

132. Karbowniczek M, Astrinidis A, Balsara BR, et al. Recurrent lymphangiomyo-matosis after transplantation: genetic analyses reveal a metastatic mechanism. Am J Respir Crit Care Med 2003; 167(7):976–982.
133. Bittmann I, Rolf B, Amann G, Lohrs U. Recurrence of lymphangioleiomyo-matosis after single lung transplantation: new insights into pathogenesis. Hum Pathol 2003; 34(1):95–98.

# 9

# Pediatric Lung Transplantation

**George B. Mallory and Okan Elidemir**
*Department of Pediatrics, Baylor College of Medicine,
Houston, Texas, U.S.A.*

## INTRODUCTION

Modern lung transplantation began with the work of Cooper and colleagues at the University of Toronto in the early 1980s. Although heart–lung transplantation in children had been uncommonly performed in the United States and the United Kingdom in the 1980s (1,2), pediatric lung transplantation evolved through the 1990s, so that small but significant numbers of lung transplants were performed in this age group in select centers in North America and Europe. Published reports from a number of centers indicated success in adopting the surgical techniques, immunosuppression, and post-transplant care to younger patients with outcomes comparable to that seen in adults (3–7). There has been and will continue to be a population of infants, children, and adolescents in need of lung transplantation since chronic pulmonary disease and pulmonary vascular disease are among the 10 most common categories of death in childhood despite the prevalence being far lower than that seen in adults (8).

Recent U.S. data available from the United Network for Organ Sharing (UNOS) show that lung transplantation remains relatively limited within the pediatric age group (Table 1) (9). As of August 2005, 5.3% of U.S. lung transplant candidates were 17 years of age and younger, compared to 7.6% of the heart, 4.2% of the liver, and 1.3% of the kidney transplant waiting list (9). However, when the actual numbers of solid organ transplants performed in

**Table 1**  Pediatric Lung and Other Solid Organ Transplantation
in the United States, 2000–2005

|  | Lung | Heart | Liver | Kidney | Intestine | Heart–Lung |
|---|---|---|---|---|---|---|
| No. of pediatric transplant candidates listed[a] | 177 | 247 | 828 | 814 | 140 | 25 |
| Adult transplant candidate total listed (%)[a] | 5.3 | 8.0 | 4.7 | 1.3 | 75 | 15.6 |
| No. of pediatric cadaveric transplants performed[b] | 237 | 1232 | 1964 | 3694 | 338 | 32 |
| No. of free-standing pediatric transplant centers[a] | 9 | 27 | 21 | 31 | 7 | 8 |

[a]From UNOS Web site for data in August 2005.
[b]UNOS figures for 2000–2004
*Abbreviation*: UNOS, United Network for Organ Sharing.

the United States in 2004 are compared across organs, there are more than
five times as many heart, 10 times as many liver, 14 times as many kidney,
and even one and one-half times as many small intestine transplants performed in the pediatric group than lung transplants (Fig. 1). Most pediatric
lung transplant recipients fall into the 11- to 17-year age group where cystic
fibrosis is the dominant disease leading to lung transplantation with considerably fewer lung transplant recipients in younger categories (Fig. 2). Only 6.7%
of lung transplants in the pediatric age group occur in the first year of life in
contrast to 29% of pediatric heart recipients, 41% of pediatric liver recipients,
and 21% of pediatric small bowel recipients over a five-year period, 2000–
2004 (9).

Over the last decade, the number of heart–lung transplants performed
within the United States has fallen in part because organ blocks became less
available in the United States (9). In 2004, there were only 39 heart–lung
transplants performed in the United States, among which six were in the
pediatric age group (9). Also, isolated lung and heart transplantation has been
applied to clinical scenarios that heretofore led to heart–lung transplantation.

The fact that suitable, healthy lungs are harvested at a much lower rate
from brain-dead patients than other solid organs explains only in part the
low numbers of pediatric lung recipients. We believe that the low number
of dedicated, freestanding pediatric lung transplant centers is a more important explanation for the low numbers of lung transplants done in infants and
children in the United States. Furthermore, there are no pediatric lung

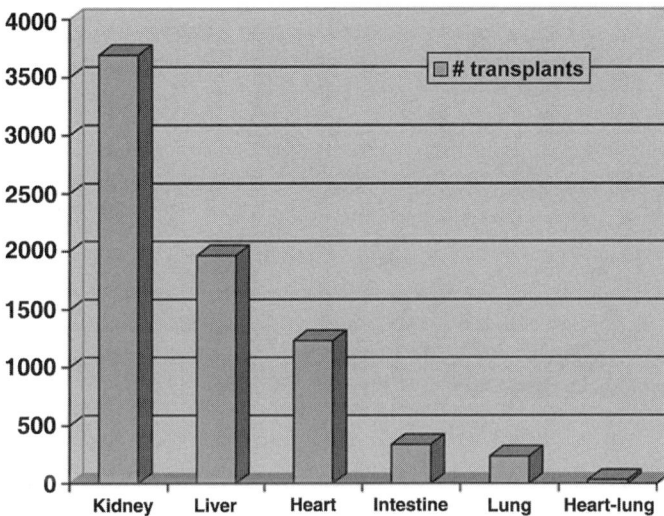

**Figure 1** Number of transplants performed in the United States in the age group of 17 years and younger by organ, 2000–2004. *Source*: From Ref. 9.

transplant centers in Australia, Japan, and, until recently, Canada. In Europe, most pediatric centers appear to focus on adolescents, eschewing infants and young children altogether. For the year 2003, the International Society for Heart and Lung Transplantation (ISHLT) reported 63 total pediatric lung transplants (17 years of age and younger) performed world-wide, of which only 16 were performed outside the United States (9,10). As of August 2005, there were only nine certified pediatric lung transplant centers in the United States but only in three centers—Los Angeles Children's Hospital, St. Louis Children's Hospital, and Texas Children's Hospital—were four or more annual lung transplants performed on average over the past three years (9). The actual peak in worldwide pediatric lung transplantation was reached in 1995 through 1998 with a roughly 20% drop in numbers since that time (10). Thus, the numbers of transplants, patients on the waiting list, and experienced and active centers lag behind adult lung transplantation and other pediatric solid organ transplantation.

There remain a few adult and pediatric lung transplant centers where heart–lung transplantation remains a common operation for end-stage lung disease. While the total number of heart–lung transplant operations have decreased over time since a peak in the mid-1990s, the number performed for intrinsic lung disease and pulmonary vascular disease without congenital heart disease have fallen most dramatically (11). Nevertheless, due to its continuing popularity in some European centers, cystic fibrosis remains the third most common indication for heart–lung transplantation.

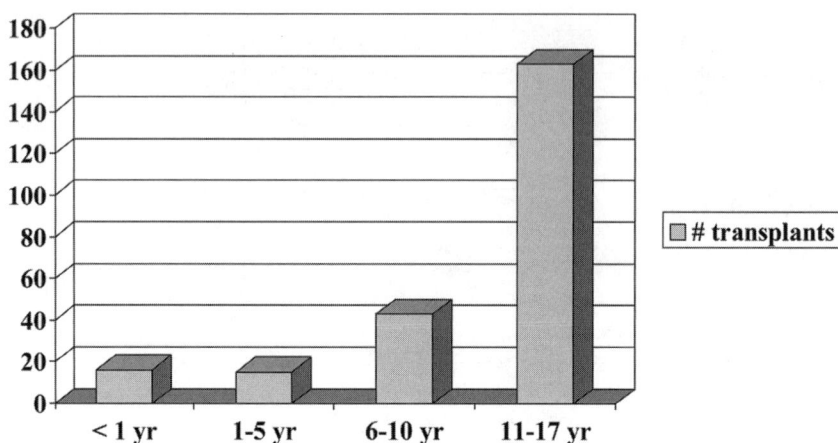

**Figure 2** Age distribution for pediatric lung transplants performed in the United States, 2000–2004. *Source*: From Ref. 9.

## INDICATIONS

The diseases leading to pediatric lung transplantation are distinct from those noted in most adult series (Table 2) (10). The most common indications in infants are disorders related to pulmonary hypertension. The combination of congenital heart disease, congenital pulmonary vascular disease, and idiopathic pulmonary hypertension accounts for 64% of the transplanted infants. Infantile pulmonary alveolar proteinosis, most commonly due to surfactant protein B deficiency, has become the most common indication for infantile lung transplantation in St. Louis (12). In the intermediate age group from 1 to 10 years, cystic fibrosis represents over one-third of the transplanted patients as does the combined category of pulmonary vascular diseases. In the age group from 11 through 17 years, cystic fibrosis represents nearly three-quarters of the total. Among miscellaneous disease entities leading to lung transplantation beyond one year of age, from our own experience, are postviral bronchiolitis obliterans, bronchopulmonary dysplasia, respiratory insufficiency after bone marrow transplantation, and interstitial lung diseases with varying degrees of pulmonary fibrosis. Despite the continuing advances in therapy that have led to an encouraging increase in mean life expectancy, cystic fibrosis is, and will likely remain, the dominant underlying diagnosis leading to lung transplantation in older children and adolescents for the next decade.

The general criteria for lung and heart–lung transplantation in infants and children are similar to those used in adults: individuals at risk of dying from single organ failure and/or who have a poor quality of life despite maximal medical therapy. In infants in whom organ procurement within

**Table 2** Underlying Diagnosis of Pediatric Lung Transplant Recipients Transplanted Worldwide Between 1991 and 2001

| | Diagnostic category | | |
| --- | --- | --- | --- |
| | Age < 1 year | Age 1–10 years | Age 11–17 years |
| Cystic fibrosis (%) | 0 | 36.5 | 72 |
| Primary pulmonary hypertension (%) | 13.7 | 13.2 | 10 |
| Pulmonary vascular disease (%) | 13.7 | 3.0 | 0 |
| Congenital heart disease (%) | 47.1 | 10.7 | 2 |
| Idiopathic pulmonary fibrosis/interstital lung disease (%) | 5.9 | 9.7 | 3 |
| Retransplantation/ graft failure (%) | 5.9 | 9.7 | 6 |
| Other (%) | 13.7 | 17.3 | 7 |

*Source*: From Ref. 10.

days or weeks is often possible and in whom recuperation is often gratifyingly rapid, a candidate on mechanical ventilation and technologic support including nitric oxide inhalation and even extracorporeal membrane oxygenation (ECMO) may sometimes be appropriate for listing and transplantation (13). Depending on location, transplant center, and waiting list, older children are usually considered candidates if death within six months to two years seems likely. For children with rare diseases or atypical courses of more common diseases, prognostication—and the linked listing and timing of transplantation—will depend on careful serial measurements of cardiopulmonary function to ascertain the natural history of the underlying disease process.

With the new distribution algorithm introduced by UNOS in 2005, the impact on the timing of referral of pediatric candidates, the duration of waiting time, and survival to transplantation are uncertain. Patients aged ≥12 years will have a score based on a complex disease-specific equation. Patients ≤11 years will still be listed by date of listing and cumulative waiting time. Donors aged ≤17 years will be preferentially directed to pediatric candidates, but only at the local level before being made available to local adult candidates. The UNOS Thoracic Committee is committed to a prospective evaluation of the system and, at least in theory, to modification of the system if there are not more pediatric organs made available to pediatric recipients, as is currently the case with heart, liver, and kidney transplant recipients.

## CONTRAINDICATIONS AND PSYCHOSOCIAL CONSIDERATIONS

Over time, the medical and surgical contraindications for lung transplantation in children have narrowed down (Table 3). In the current era, most contraindications are relative, and absolute contraindications are rare in the populations at risk. Issues of active infection are generally straightforward. Outcome after lung transplantation in cystic fibrosis patients infected with the most virulent and transmissible form of *Burkholderia cepacia* infection is poor, with an early mortality from infection approaching 50% (14,15). Recent microbiological research on this organism has shown what laboratories have heretofore identified as *B. cepacia* can now be differentiated into distinct species (16). Speciation in reference laboratories can identify *B. cenocepacia*, which appears to be the most virulent and invasive species after transplantation (15), and it remains an absolute contraindication in many transplant centers, including our own. We believe that nontuberculous mycobacteria with in vitro sensitivities to antimicrobial therapy and pulmonary fungal infection or colonization are almost always amenable to therapy provided perioperatively and postoperatively and should not be

**Table 3**  Medical and Surgical Contraindications to Pediatric Lung Transplantation

---

Absolute
   Severe scoliosis or thoracic cage deformity
   Severe tracheomegaly and/or tracheomalacia
   Hepatic[a], renal[a], left ventricular failure[a]
   Severe transpleural systemic to bronchial artery collateral arteries
   *B. cenocepacia* lower respiratory infection (not all centers)
   Active malignancy
   HIV infection
   Active viral infection
   Active mycobacterial infection
   Bacteremia or septicemia
   Irreversible and significant respiratory muscle dysfunction
   Poorly controlled diabetes mellitus
Relative
   Symptomatic osteoporosis or osteopenia
   Pneumonectomy (unless volume-occupying device in place)
   Pan-resistant microorganisms within the respiratory tract
   *Burkholderia multivorans* and similar members of the complex
   Daily systemic corticosteroids
   Severe malnutrition

---

[a]Multiorgan transplantation such as liver–lung, renal–lung, or heart–lung transplantation might be an appropriate option.

considered contraindications to transplantation. Poorly controlled diabetes mellitus is often a manifestation of suboptimal adherence to a prescribed regimen and should be considered a strong contraindication.

Anatomic or surgical contraindications are generally center specific. Chemical pleurodesis increases the operative time in a somewhat unpredictable fashion and always leads to widespread bleeding sites within the parietal pleura. Nevertheless, most transplant surgeons today feel that candidates with pleurodesis are acceptable, if not ideal, candidates. Tracheal dilation (tracheomegaly) and/or collapsibility (tracheomalacia) make the airway anastomosis problematic and could conceivably lead to long-term mechanical ventilation. A tracheostomy alone generally would not be considered a contraindication since early posttransplant decannulation could obviate the problem of a long-term portal of entry for microorganisms into the lower airway. In patients with pulmonary atresia with nonconfluent pulmonary arteries, pulmonary blood flow depends exclusively on bronchial arteries. Especially in the context of previous thoracotomy, there may also be diffuse arterial connections across the pleura. In the early experience at St. Louis Children's Hospital, this particular clinical scenario predisposed to diffuse small arterial bleeding, which led to the early demise of several patients, even with the use of aprotinin (3).

Nonmedical contraindications include financial and psychosocial factors. Although most insurers in the United States cover lung transplantation at the present time, at times, a contractual offer from the insurer may predispose to a magnitude of financial loss to the providers that some institutions may choose not to list. Also, many policies do not provide for travel and living expenses. Community fund-raising may be necessary for many families to afford heavy uncovered costs. In view of the complexities and rigors of life after lung transplantation, patients and families and the transplant team must consider psychosocial issues seriously. It would seem obvious that serious mental health disorders or disability that would obviate cooperation with the administration of medication and/or follow-up testing are strong contraindications to transplantation. Individual or family dysfunction manifest as repeated nonadherence to medical regimens in the past should be considered a contraindication, although it may be appropriate to give an individual patient and family the opportunity to demonstrate a capacity for adherence over a defined period of time. A thorough evaluation of the child and family by a child psychologist, pediatric social worker, and the team of transplant caregivers should be required before accepting or rejecting any individual candidate. Transplant centers depend on the integrity and truthfulness of referring physicians and caregivers in receiving all relevant information about patients and families that bear on past and future health behaviors. In borderline situations, probationary listing of a child with a clear written, signed contract of expectations may be appropriate.

Like their adult counterparts in the United States, pediatric candidates for lung transplantation are listed by ABO blood group, height range, and, as of April 2005, calculated score. The waiting period has been and likely will continue to be highly variable from region to region and center to center. Our own experience in a newly established center in Texas is that the average time from listing until transplantation has been a median of two to three months, under both the previous and the new distribution schemes. Historically, wait time has been significantly longer in established pediatric centers. Since organs will continue to be distributed locally first, there will continue to be disparities in waiting for the conceivable future. The new algorithm does prioritize pediatric organs for pediatric recipients in the local distribution.

Size considerations are clearly more important for pediatric recipients and donors because of the wide variability in size of the thorax and lungs during the span of childhood. Lobar transplantation and downsizing of donor lungs with a surgical stapling device are options for the transplant surgeon in the event that oversized lungs are offered. Although lungs are quite distensible, the use of undersized lungs risks overexpansion of the organ into the noncompliant portion of the lung's intrinsic pressure–volume curve and a disappointing physiologic outcome.

## ANESTHETIC AND OPERATIVE CONSIDERATIONS

The pediatric anesthesiologist plays a critical role in the timely admission of the patient to the operating room. There is often little time after the patient and family are notified for the patient to be admitted and have a limited number of tests in a highly dramatic context. All patients receive initial immunosuppression and intravenous antibiotics. In the operating room, the patent needs to be anesthetized and both arterial and central venous lines are placed. At Texas Children's Hospital, the anesthesiologist inserts a thoracic epidural catheter in most patients after induction of anesthesia, but before surgery, to administer an infusion of local anesthetic and fentanyl. Most transplant recipients in our institution continue to receive thoracic epidural medication for three to six days postoperatively.

Most pediatric transplant surgeons elect cardiopulmonary bypass (CPB) for all lung transplant procedures (17). The disadvantages of CPB are the associated coagulopathy that accompanies heparinization and the capillary leak syndrome, which affects all organs to a variable degree after CPB. The advantages of CPB include the opportunity to deflate the native lungs to permit easier dissection of the lung and hilum, the ability to clamp and cleanse (with instillation of antibiotic) the proximal tracheobronchial airway, and the minimization of ischemic time. Furthermore, with CPB, the newly implanted lungs are ventilated and perfused simultaneously, avoiding the need for the entire cardiac output to perfuse a single lung, while the second lung is being sewn in. Clearly, operative and anesthetic approaches will be specific to each institution.

Although single lung transplantation is a relatively common option in adult lung transplantation, few pediatric recipients have this surgery. Bilateral lung transplantation is the operative approach of choice for most young patients because of growth considerations, for cystic fibrosis patients because cystic fibrosis as a disease with bilateral infection does not allow for single lung procedures, and for the entire pediatric age group because there usually are two lungs available for most small patients. In most centers, heart–lung transplantation is usually reserved for patients with end-stage lung or pulmonary vascular disease who have irreparable congenital heart defects or left ventricular failure. Experience has shown that there is excellent potential for complete reversibility of right ventricular failure in pediatric patients with pulmonary hypertension. The specific incisions and anastomotic techniques utilized in pediatric lung transplantation are not substantially different from those employed in adult lung transplantation and are beyond the scope of this chapter (18).

In 1990, Starnes introduced living donor lung transplantation (LDLT). The recipient undergoes bilateral pneumonectomy and then receives implantation of lower lobes from each of the two healthy adult donors (19). Given the size of the organ in even the shortest adults, LDLT is not a realistic option for children younger than age six years (20). Ideally, the donor should be taller than the recipient so that the donor lobe can readily fill the recipient hemithorax. Because of important ethical concerns, a pulmonary physician and psychologist entirely separate from the transplant team should evaluate all potential donors (20). Donors should be ≥18 years and in excellent health. Altruistic motive and full disclosure of the potential morbidity and mortality of elective lobectomy are mandatory. At the time of LDLT, three simultaneous thoracic operations are carried out—a requirement of resources that many transplant centers cannot mobilize. Although the most recent results achieved by Starnes in adults and children is encouraging, technical considerations have been a problem in other institutions. With no end in sight to the shortage of donors, LDLT will be an option in aggressive programs and for selected patients and families. In many adult programs, one-year survival after deceased donor transplantation exceeds 90%. LDLT, even in Starnes' hands, has never yielded better than 80% one-year survival.

Regardless of the surgical procedure (except for lower numbers with LDLT), operative survival of the lung transplantation operation in children appears to be as high in infants, children, and adolescents as in adults at >95% (3,21).

## POSTOPERATIVE CARE

Immediate postoperative issues include graft function, bleeding, and stabilization of a critically ill patient after a major operation. A thorough physical examination, initial chest radiograph, continuous monitoring of blood pressure, central venous pressures, gas exchange, and assessment of urine output are critical in assessing the integrity of graft and patient on arrival in the intensive care unit. Fluid administration, including the administration of blood products and inotropic agents, is done according to cardiac status and renal function. In our center, we prefer to minimize fluid administration in the first 48 hours after transplantation and use intravenous infusions of prostaglandin El, dopamine, and vasopressin to dilate the pulmonary vascular bed, maintain cardiac output, and support systemic vascular resistance. We employ flexible bronchoscopy first in the operating room prior to reperfusion to inspect the bronchial anastomosis. Then, in the pediatric intensive care unit within the first 6 to 24 hours after surgery, we assess the vascular supply of the bronchial mucosa just distal to the anastomosis and perform bronchoalveolar lavage for the diagnosis of lower respiratory infection. Weaning from ventilatory support should proceed as quickly as the patient wakes up and graft function permits. Because of concerns about the absolute volume of the pulmonary vascular bed and its propensity for capillary leak, LDLT recipients are often kept under neuromuscular blockade, sedation, and relative hypotension for the first 24 to 48 hours prior to the commencement of weaning from ventilatory support.

### Immunosuppression

Immunosuppression is often begun prior to surgery with an oral dose of cyclosporine or tacrolimus and intravenous corticosteroids. Cyclosporine or tacrolimus is resumed promptly after surgery. Beginning on arrival in the intensive care unit, it is our practice to give cyclosporine intravenously as a three-hour infusion twice daily to simulate the pharmacokinetics of an oral dose. Cyclosporine is titrated initially to trough blood levels of 400 ng/mL. We initiate oral dosing after oral function and gastric emptying have been established. Recent insights suggest that it may be more accurate to adjust cyclosporine by using peak or C2 (concentration two hours after an oral dose) to optimize drug dosing. Our recent experience demonstrates that pediatric recipients with trough levels in the above range have C2 values in the 1500–2000 ng/mL range, which is tolerated without apparent injury to the kidney or evident central nervous system toxicity. Some centers have embraced tacrolimus as the calcineurin inhibitor of choice for initial immunosuppression. Initial tacrolimus dosing may be by intravenous drip or oral or nasogastric tube bolus dosing. Tacrolimus trough levels are titrated to 10–15 ng/mL, or slightly higher initially in some programs, on whole-blood samples. In the 1990s, azathioprine was traditionally used as part of a three-drug strategy with dosing at 2.0–3.0 mg/kg/day initially given intravenously. From recently published epidemiologic data, mycophenolate mofetil (MMF) has replaced azathioprine as the second agent in 50% of patients transplanted after 1999 (10). Although pediatric dosing has not been universally established, adult dosing would suggest a pediatric dose of 15–20 mg/kg of MMF twice daily either intravenously or orally. Therapeutic drug monitoring is available for MMF dose titration and seems logical even if empiric studies to assess efficacy are currently lacking. Our patients with cystic fibrosis require 30–50 mg/kg to obtain therapeutic mycophenolate levels. Toxicity has been rare.

Corticosteroid dosing also varies by center. In our program, a dose of intravenous methylprednisolone is given pretransplant and continued in moderate dosing the first three days posttransplant and then weaned to 2 mg/kg/ day. We discharge most patients on a dose of oral prednisone or prednisolone of 1.0 mg/kg/day. Tapering of corticosteroid dosing to 0.25–0.5 mg/kg/day is common by the second to third month posttransplant and should aim for 0.15 mg/kg/day by one year posttransplant and in the long run. In most centers, daily prednisone or prednisolone is continued long term, although some programs do consider alternate day dosing.

## Antimicrobial Strategies

Antibiotic treatment before and after transplantation is not, in the strict sense, prophylaxis. Most donor lungs, if cultured, grow one or more potential pathogens. Cystic fibrosis patients have intrathoracic airways, including the proximal trachea and bronchi, which remain "diseased" and in situ after transplantation, presumably infected microscopically by typical gram-negative organisms. Furthermore, we have routinely performed blood cultures in our patients immediately on arrival in the intensive care unit after transplantation. Twenty percent of cystic fibrosis patients have had positive blood cultures, most commonly growing one of their pretransplant lung pathogens. Therefore, it is our practice to choose an antibiotic regimen before, during, and immediately after lung transplantation geared to the most likely pathogens. At Texas Children's Hospital, the initial antibiotic choice in non–cystic fibrosis patients is limited to a second- or third-generation cephalosporin and vancomycin because of the high prevalence of methicillin-resistant staphylococcus in the community. In cystic fibrosis patients, at least two intravenous antipseudomonal antibiotics are chosen based on the most recent respiratory microbiological specimen. Other agents are chosen if *Pseudomonas aeruginosa* is either not present or not the exclusive pathogen. In fact, we have been impressed by the increasing prevalence of other gram-negative organisms, especially *Achromobacter xylosoxidans* in the last few years. Two antibiotic agents are chosen, as is the usual practice in cystic fibrosis care, to obtain synergism between antibiotics and to lessen the chance of emergence of antibiotic-resistant organisms.

In cystic fibrosis patients with a history of aspergillus infection, allergic bronchopulmonary aspergillosis, or recent sputum cultures positive for

*Aspergillus* species, intravenous antifungal therapy with low-dose amphotericin B or voriconazole is begun. Depending on clinical course and the results of respiratory culture at the time of transplant and the first BAL culture at 24-hours posttransplant, intravenous amphotericin B may be changed within 3 to 10 days to the nebulized route, usually 10 mg in sterile water three times daily, for an additional one to two weeks. After initial parenteral therapy, transition to oral voriconazole is made. We prefer voriconazole to itraconazole due to its broad antifungal coverage and much more reliable enteral absorption.

Lung transplant recipients who have circulating antibody for cytomegalovirus (CMV) before transplantation or who receive an organ from a donor with positive CMV serology are treated with intravenous ganciclovir for the first days posttransplant. Oral valganciclovir is introduced as soon as the oral route has been established and continued for the first five months after transplantation. This regimen permits the diagnosis of CMV infection at the 6-month evaluation. Trimethoprim–sulfamethoxazole is commenced in the first week after transplantation as prophylaxis for *Pneumocystis jiroveci* pneumonia (previously *Pneumocystis carinii*). Some programs continue pneumocystis prophylaxis long term; others discontinue after three months. Oral nystatin is commonly prescribed to reduce the likelihood of clinically significant oral candidiasis. Oral acyclovir is used in some programs routinely as prophylactic treatment for herpes simplex infection, but we have never routinely used it.

### Allograft Rejection

From published intermediate-term results, it appears that young children may have a lower risk of both acute and chronic rejection compared to older children and adults (3,21). Nonetheless, timely surveillance and accurate diagnosis of allograft rejection remains central to the posttransplant care of children in our practice. The standard pediatric flexible bronchoscope has an outer diameter of 3.4 to 3.6 mm and a suction channel of only 1.2 mm. Standard biopsy forceps cannot be used through this diminutive channel. Olympus makes a biopsy forceps (FB-56D) and cytology brushes without (BC-201C-1006) and with protective sheath (BC-203D-2006) for the smaller pediatric scopes.

Although the length of the jaw of the forceps seems quite adequate and the forceps opens efficiently within the distal airway, the dimensions of the jaw yields a cup volume of approximately 0.5 L (compared to 2.0-L volume of standard adult forceps) and leads to diminutive and sometimes histologically inadequate specimens. Alternative techniques have been developed (22). However, for most children of four to six years of age and older, we use a bronchoscope 4.9 mm in outer diameter, which permits standard biopsy forceps. The recent advent of the laryngeal mask considerably facilitates this procedure in smaller and sicker patients.

Standard histopathologic markers of lung graft rejection are used to make the diagnosis of acute vascular rejection. Treatment consists of intravenous methylprednisolone 10 mg/kg for three consecutive days. For recurrent acute rejection, cytolytic therapy with an antilymphocyte preparation, a six week course of once weekly orally methotrexate 0.15 mg/kg and/or a change in the daily immunosuppressant regimen is indicated. There have been no large retrospective comparative studies or prospective randomized studies in pediatric lung transplantation to indicate which pharmacologic program is optimal. It does appear that repeated episodes of acute graft rejection do predispose to chronic rejection.

Bronchiolitis obliterans syndrome (BOS) is an applicable concept for the pediatric lung transplant patient (23). Because of somatic growth after lung transplantation, the definition of BOS relies on change in percentage predicted values of forced expiratory volume in 1 second and/or forced midexpiratory flow rate of 25% to 75% as opposed to a change in absolute numbers. As a general rule, a new diagnosis of BOS would lead to augmentation of immunosuppression similar to what is employed in adults.

## ISSUES PARTICULAR TO PEDIATRIC PATIENTS

In the remainder of the chapter, we will focus on selected topics where there may be unique pediatric issues or problems. There is limited published material on many of these topics so the material should be received as it is written—one center's perspective based on a relatively large clinical experience.

### Somatic Growth

Growth retardation is an issue for all pediatric transplant recipients. Many transplant candidates may have chronic malnutrition and/or stunting of skeletal growth due to the long-standing impact of the underlying disease process. Furthermore, posttransplant care with the long-term use of daily prednisone (which is the rule in most pediatric lung transplant recipients in contradistinction to pediatric heart, liver, and renal transplant recipients) commonly leads to a rate of skeletal growth that remains below the age-adjusted normal range. Augmentation of nutrition and correction of metabolic abnormalities are fundamental posttransplant goals. In some recipients, even when daily prednisone is lowered to 0.1–0.15 mg/kg/day, growth remains suboptimal. The growth response can be impressive and has been reported to be both safe and effective in pediatric renal and liver transplant recipients (24,25). A recent retrospective review of the experience at St. Louis Children's Hospital suggests a higher incidence of BOS in individuals who received growth hormone therapy (26). We believe that a cautious approach to growth hormone therapy after lung transplantation is indicated.

## Nutrition

The delivery of effective nutrition in the immediate posttransplant period may be difficult in some patients. In patients with early graft rejection, the use of higher-dose corticosteroids counteracts the goal of anabolism. In many infants, rather severe gastroesophageal reflux disease (GERD), and in older patients, gastroparesis, can compromise the delivery of adequate calories by the enteral route (27). Older patients with cystic fibrosis are at risk of small bowel obstruction, a variant form of the distal intestinal obstruction syndrome, in the early posttransplant period when inactivity and opiate medication slow down intestinal transit. This complication can compromise transition to oral medication and nutritional rehabilitation and may require surgery (28). We now use enteral lactulose 30 cc twice daily after transplant and have largely prevented this complication.

Because of our belief that GERD can cause unsuspected graft injury, we perform a pH probe study in the second posttransplant month in almost all transplant recipients. If the study demonstrates >10% time with esophageal acidity, we recommend elective laporoscopic Nissen fundoplication. A separate problem arises when infants or young toddlers endure for months without normal oral stimulation; the process of oral retraining can be prolonged and emotionally demanding for the family. A careful and coordinated therapeutic oral motor stimulation and enteral supplemental feeding program needs to be delineated and modified as progress is made.

In older patients and adolescents, most individuals literally and figuratively enjoy nutritional gains after transplantation. A small number of patients may experience a marked increase in weight, quickly putting them into the range of mild to moderate obesity. Others, particularly, in our experience, adolescent females, may have prolonged anorexia with a clinical syndrome with parallels to anorexia nervosa. Aggressive psychosocial intervention, including consideration of anti-depressant medication, is usually needed.

## Neurodevelopmental Issues

Infants who have experienced severe respiratory failure from birth, such as those with surfactant protein B deficiency, or those chronically ill for months prior to transplantation, will likely have neurodevelopmental deficits even after prompt physical recovery after successful lung transplantation. In concert with the common oral motor and behavioral feeding challenges previously mentioned, a broad-based therapeutic program developed by therapists but delivered in large part by families is of major importance. Both the transplant physician and the primary care pediatrician may need to lobby strongly for these services after transplantation. We emphasize that the goal of lung transplantation is to give each individual a chance at a reasonably normal lifestyle, which includes social interactions with peers and a mainstream school environment.

## Seizures

The emergence of generalized seizures in the first months after lung transplantation is common in pediatric lung transplant recipients (29). Most seizures occur in the first several weeks after transplantation and are self-limited although quite frightening to patients and families. Brief hospitalization is usually necessary. Imaging studies, when performed, show what has been called a reversible posterior leukoencephalopathy (30). However, our experience is that the prognosis for the vast majority of these patients is good. We prefer phenytoin as the anticonvulsant of choice since it competitively enhances calcineurin inhibitor hepatic drug clearance less than phenobarbitol and carbamazepine. Most patients take phenytoin for <3 months and have no recurrence of seizures. In the context of uncomplicated self-limited seizures, we do not perform electroencephaolography, lumbar puncture, or imaging studies. Since there is such wide interindividual variability in calcineurin inhibitor absorption and clearance, retrospective studies have been unable to prove a simple link to cyclosporine or tacrolimus blood levels.

## Viral Infections

By natural circumstance of immunity and lifestyle, it is the natural proclivity for children to experience dozens of primary viral infections in the early years of life. From that point of view, they represent an epidemiologic risk group for particularly severe diseases with certain pathogens, most notably the respiratory viruses—respiratory syncytial virus, parainfluenza virus, and adenovirus. On the other hand, some viral infections, such as Epstein–Barr virus and varicella, have milder clinical manifestations in normal children than if primary infection occurs later in life. Because of the higher likelihood of immunologic innocence in chronically ill children, the timely diagnosis and focused treatment of viral infections is especially important in children after lung transplantation more so than in their adult counterparts. Scrupulous attention to preventative measures consisting of active immunization with vaccines and passive immunization of selected infants and very young children with palivizumab (anti-RSV IgG) is imperative. We believe that it is wise to keep these patients out of social situations such as day care in which the likelihood of exposure to community viral pathogens is especially high. Our own preference is to avoid varicella–zoster immune globulin after varicella exposure in healthy lung transplant recipients, since the timely early administration of acyclovir is highly effective in our experience and, just as importantly, confers long-lasting immunity.

### Posttransplant Lymphoproliferative Disease

The incidence of posttransplant lymphoproliferative disease (PTLD) seems to be higher in children than in adults (31), and data suggest that primary Epstein–Barr virus infection after transplantation is a related risk factor (32). In the St. Louis experience, fully 20% of the CF lung transplant recipients developed PTLD (31), with a high morbidity and significant mortality. Because the first response to PTLD has historically included a reduction in immunosuppression, survival after PTLD is complicated by a high incidence of BOS. Clinical scientists have developed the ability to grow clones of recipient Epstein–Barr–specific cytotoxic T lymphocytes for therapeutic use in PTLD (33). The availability of rituximab (anti-CD20 antibody) shows early promising results, which may lead to a significant lowering in morbidity and mortality (34). Unfortunately, relapse after successful rituximab therapy may dampen our initial enthusiasm for this effective new therapy.

### GASTROINTESTINAL FUNCTION

We have already mentioned the apparently high incidence of gastroesophageal reflux disease in infants after lung transplantation. In addition, older patients seem to be at risk of severe gastroparesis after lung transplantation (27). It has been speculated that mediastinal dissection and severing of the vagal connections to the explanted lungs results in a virtual vagotomy affecting upper gastrointestinal function. Gastroparesis may severely complicate the transition from intravenous to enteral immunosuppressant drug administration. Frequent emesis leading to low therapeutic drug levels predisposes to graft rejection. Furthermore, patients with cystic fibrosis are at risk of small bowel obstruction due to the dehydrated nature of their intestinal mucus complicated by the use of opiates and the marked decrease in locomotion in the first days after transplantation. Intestinal obstruction may be refractory to medical measures and may require surgical intervention, which further complicates recovery and the transition to enteral drug administration (28). It was our impression in St. Louis that this complication appeared to be more common and difficult in the pediatric cystic fibrosis population than in the adult population. We therefore make preoperative and early postoperative use of oral cathartic agents routinely in cystic fibrosis lung transplant recipients.

### Lung Function Testing

Spirometry is universally employed after lung transplantation as a mainstay in assessing graft function. Children from the age of four to six years can usually perform spirometry with sensitive coaching. There are new approaches to children somewhat younger that may lead to reproducible flow–volume curves with forced maneuvers in children as young as 2.5 years of age (35). Infants and younger toddlers do not have the developmental capacity for cooperating with voluntary respiratory maneuvers. In many centers, infant pulmonary function laboratories perform modified spirometry under sedation using the rapid thoracoabdominal compression technique. In St. Louis, we found that the regularly scheduled use of this technique was helpful in differentiating those patients with good lung health from those with intrinsic airway abnormalities or evolving BOS (36). Further work with this group of patients is needed before standards and definitions of BOS can be established. In older patients, we procure home spirometers incorporating laptop computers, which has permitted the earlier diagnosis of pulmonary complications after transplantation leading to timely and often less costly interventions. We believe that this modality is cost-effective. We now use a laptop-based system because it permits easy assessment of adherence, facilitates downloads in our pulmonary laboratory, and helps patients and families send us updated lung function data via e-mail with ease.

## Lung Growth

The human lung grows early in life in response to the rhythmic application of physical stretch in a proper nutritional and hormonal milieu. When we launched into infant lung transplantation in the mid-1990s, it was unclear if the process of transplantation, the use of immunosuppressants, or the unavoidable denervation of the lungs might stunt the growth of transplanted lungs. Perhaps an even more cogent concern was the growth potential of mature adult lungs or lobes transplanted into the growing thorax. Although there are no human data to address the latter, two papers have examined lung growth in the younger patient. In St. Louis, we used infant lung function testing to assess airflow as a surrogate for airway caliber and functional residual capacity as a surrogate for alveolar growth in a cohort of infants and young children <3 years of age at the time of transplantation (36). The physiologic data support the contention that transplanted lungs grow. Ro and colleagues at the Children's Hospital of Philadelphia used serial chest CT scans in a young population of broader age range to assess the caliber of the central intrathoracic airways over time (37). Their data also support the hypothesis that the airways of transplanted lungs appear to grow with somatic growth.

## Cosmetic Issues

Adolescence is a period of life during which there is normally a rapid and profound change in self-image. Periods of emotional instability are common. Cyclosporine is an immunosuppressant, which commonly impacts physical appearance, often of major concern to adolescent females. The degree and manifestations of hirsutism vary considerably among individuals but may be successfully managed, at least on the face, with depilatory medications (38). Gingival hypertrophy is also common but may be decreased when the individual pays careful attention to regular dental hygiene. Flare-up in acne vulgaris is common with systemic corticosteroids but may also be seen with the use of cyclosporine (39). Either aggressive attention to these medical problems or change to tacrolimus may be important means to limit non-adherence. The moon facies associated with higher-dose corticosteroids usually recedes during the first year after transplantation as the dose of prednisone is weaned.

## Psychosocial Needs

The care of infants, children, and adolescents is more complex than the care of sentient adults in that the care must be developmentally adjusted and family-based. Because there are so few pediatric lung transplant centers in the world today, the vast majority of pediatric lung candidates will not live in or near the transplant center. Thus, this fact guarantees disruption of the physical integrity of a family and limits the availability of extended family and a reliable assortment of familiar community supports. Relocation to the transplant center to await cadaveric organs is common in the United States due to the time and distance involved in getting to the hospital when an organ is finally located, which brings further imposing financial and emotional costs to caring for terminally ill children. For these reasons, the authors believe that a multidisciplinary team of pediatric caregivers with special orientation to lung transplantation, including a pediatric transplant nurse coordinator, a social worker, a child life specialist, and a child psychologist, are vital to the successful care and treatment of pediatric lung transplant candidates and recipients. Further, the transplant center hospital should foster and access supportive services within the community to help provide a "home away from home."

## SURVIVAL

From the most recent published international data, it appears that average survival for pediatric lung transplantation (half-life of 3.5 years) falls just below that for lung transplant recipients of all ages (half-life of 3.8 years) (10,40). Interestingly, adolescents had the lowest conditional actuarial survival (5.4 years) and infants the longest within the pediatric age spectrum (7.1 years) (10). In the only large series within one medical center where pediatric and adult lung transplant recipients with cystic fibrosis were compared, the pediatric cohort had a slightly higher survival rate at every time point after transplantation (41). Nonetheless, the threat of primary viral infection, the higher incidence of PTLD, and adolescent nonadherence arguably put pediatric lung transplant recipients at greater risk of death after transplantation than their adult counterparts.

Recently, Liou used survival data in a large cohort of cystic fibrosis patients to suggest that, in contrast to adults, lung transplantation did not appear to confer any survival advantage to children and adolescents with cystic fibrosis (42). We believe that his survival model does not and cannot take into account the clinical judgment of referring physicians and transplant pulmonologists who select individuals at higher risk of death from the cohort of patients with similar clinical characteristics to be candidates for transplantation. In that light, Aurora has argued that with attention to certain clinical details, lung transplantation appears to confer a survival advantage to selected pediatric patients with cystic fibrosis (5). We believe that there is every reason to be scrupulous in the selection of younger candidates for lung transplantation and redoubled efforts at improving posttransplant care to improve survival. With improving clinical care for cystic fibrosis, this important area of clinical decision making will be an ever-changing one.

## CONCLUSION

Experience has shown definitively that lung transplantation can be successfully performed in infants, children, and adolescents. While indications are similar to those in adults, the disease entities are often different. The surgical approach differs from the usual approach in adult centers due to the strong preference for bilateral lung transplantation and cardiopulmonary bypass. Postoperative management requires special sensitivity to the issues of primary viral infection, somatic growth, scholastic progress, and functioning within a family environment. At present, the paucity of pediatric lung transplant centers severely limits the options for infants, children, and adolescents with end-stage lung and pulmonary vascular disease.

## REFERENCES

1. Starnes VA, Marshall SE, Lewiston NJ, et al. Heart–lung transplantation in infants, children, and adolescents. J Pediatr Surg 1991; 26(4):434–438.
2. Smyth RL, Scott JP, Whitehead B, et al. Heart–lung transplantation in children. Transplant Proc 1990; 22(4):1470–1471.
3. Sweet SC, Huddleston CB, Spray TL, et al. Pediatric lung transplantation at St. Louis Children's Hospital 1990–1995. Am J Respir Crit Care Med 1997; 155(3):1027–1035.
4. Metras D, Viard L, Kreitmann B, et al. Lung infections in pediatric lung transplantation: experience in 49 cases. Eur J Card Thorac Surg 1999; 15(4):490–494.
5. Aurora P, Whitehead B, Wade A, et al. Lung transplantation and life extension in children with cystic fibrosis. Lancet 1999; 354(9190):1591–1593.
6. Starnes VA, Woo MS, MacLaughlin EF, et al. Comparison of outcomes between living donor and cadaveric lung transplantation in children. Ann Thorac Surg 1999; 68(6):2279–2283.

7. Gaynor JW, Bridges ND, Clark BJ, et al. Update on lung transplantation in children. Curr Opin Pediatr 1998; 10(3):256–261.

8. Hoyert DL, Arias E, Smith BL, et al. Deaths: final data for 1999. Natl Vital Stat Rep 2001; 49(8):1–114.

9. United Network for Organ Sharing (Accessed August 2005 at http://www.unos.org).

10. Boucek MM, Edwards LB, Keck BM, et al. Registry of the International Society for Heart and Lung Transplantation: eighth official pediatric report 2005. J Heart Lung Transplant 2005; 24(8):968–982.

11. Boucek MM, Edwards LB, Keck BM, et al. The Registry of the International Society for Heart and Lung Transplantation: fifth official pediatric report— 2001 to 2002. J Heart Lung Transplant 2002; 21(8):827–840.

12. Hamvas A, Nogee LM, Mallory GB, et al. Lung transplantation for treatment of infants with surfactant protein B deficiency. J Pediatr 1997; 130(2):231–239.

13. Huddleston CB, Sweet SC, Mallory GB, et al. Lung transplantation in very young infants. J Thorac Cardiovasc Surg 1999; 118(5):796–804.

14. Aris RM, Routh JC, LiPuma J, et al. Lung transplantation for cystic fibrosis patients with Burkholderia cepacia complex: survival linked to genomovar type. Am J Respir Crit Care Med 2001; 164(11):2102–2106.

15. Chaparro C, Maurer J, Gutierrez C, et al. Infection with Burkholderia cepacia in cystic fibrosis: outcome following lung transplantation. Am J Resp Crit Care Med 2001; 163(1):43–48.

16. Mahenthiralingam E, Baldwin A, VanDamme P. Burkholderia cepacia complex infection in patients with cystic fibrosis. J Med Microbiol 2002; 51(7):533–538.

17. Spray TL, Mallory GB, Canter CB, et al. Pediatric lung transplantation: indications, techniques, and early results. J Thorac Cardiovasc Surg 1994; 107(4):990–1000.

18. Huddleston CB. Surgical complications of pediatric lung transplantation. Semin Thorac Cardiovasc Surg 1996; 8(3):296–304.

19. Starnes VA, Barr ML, Cohen RG. Lobar transplantation: indications, technique and outcome. J Thorac Cardiovasc Surg 1994; 108(3):403–411.

20. Mallory GB, Cohen AH. Donor considerations in living-related donor lung transplantation. Clin Chest Med 1997; 18(2):239–244.

21. Bridges ND, Mallory GB, Huddleston CB, et al. Lung transplantation in infancy and early childhood. J Heart Lung Transplant 1996; 15(9):895–902.

22. Mullins D, Livne M, Mallory GB, et al. A new technique for transbronchial biopsy in infants and small children. Pediatr Pulmonol 1995; 20(4):253–257.

23. Estenne M, Maurer JR, Boehler A, et al. Bronchiolitis obliterans syndrome 2001: an update of the diagnostic criteria. J Heart Lung Transplant 2002; 21(3):297–310.

24. Maxwell H, Rees L. Randomized controlled trial of recombinant human growth hormone in prepubertal and pubertal renal transplant recipients. Arch Dis Child 1998; 79(6):481–487.

25. Rodeck B, Kardorff R, Melter M, et al. Improvement of growth after growth hormone treatment in children who undergo liver transplantation. J Pediatr Gastroenterol Nutr 2000; 31(3):286–290.

26. Sweet SC, de la Morena MT, Schuler PM, et al. Association of growth hormone therapy with the development of bronchiolitis obliterans syndrome in pediatric lung transplant recipients. J Heart Lung Transplant 2004; 23(2S):S127.

27. Berkowitz N, Schulman LL, McGregor C, et al. Gastroparesis after lung transplantation: potential role in postoperative respiratory complications. Chest 1995; 108(6):1602–1607.

28. Minkes RK, Langer JC, Skinner MA, et al. Intestinal obstruction following lung transplantation in children with cystic fibrosis. J Pediatr Surg 1999; 34(10): 1489–1493.

29. Wong M, Mallory GB Jr, Goldstein J, et al. Neurological complications of pediatric lung transplantation. Neurol 1999; 53(7):1542–1549.

30. Jarosz JM, Howlett DC, Cox TC, et al. Cyclosporine-related reversible posterior leukoencephalopathy. MRI. Neuroradiology 1997; 39(10):711–715.

31. Cohen AH, Sweet SC, Mendeloff EN, et al. High incidence of posttransplant lymphoproliferative disease in pediatric patients with cystic fibrosis. Am J Respir Crit Care Med 2000; 161(4):1252–1255.

32. Boyle GJ, Michaels MG, Webber SA, et al. Posttransplantation lymphoproliferative disorders in pediatric thoracic organ recipients. J Pediatr 1997; 131(2): 309–313.

33. Savoldo B, Goss J, Liu Z, et al. Generation of autologous Epstein–Barr virus-specific cytotoxic T cells for adoptive immunotherapy in solid organ transplant recipients. Transplantation 2001; 72(6):1078–1086.

34. Reynaud-Gaubert M, Stoppa AM, Gaubert J, et al. Anti-CD20 monoclonal antibody therapy in Epstein-Barr Virus-associated B cell lymphoma following lung transplantation. J Heart Lung Transplant 2000; 19(5):492–495.

35. Vilozni D, Barker M, Jellouschek H, et al. An interactive computer-animated system (SpiroGame) facilitates spirometry in preschool children. Am J Resp Crit Care Med 2001; 164(12):2200–2205.

36. Cohen AH, Mallory GB, Ross K, et al. Growth of lungs after transplantation in infants and children younger than 3 years old. Am J Resp Crit Care Med 1999; 159(6):1747–1751.

37. Ro PS, Bush DM, Kramer SS, et al. Airway growth after pediatric lung transplantation. J Heart Lung Transplant 2001; 20(6):619–624.

38. Wendelin DS, Mallory GB, Mallory SB. Depilation in a 6-month-old with hypertrichosis: a case report. Pediatr Dermatol 1999; 16(4):316–318.

39. el-Shahawy MA, Gadallah MF, Massry SG. Acne: a potential side effect of cyclosporine. A therapy. Nephron 1996; 72(4):679–682.

40. Hosenpud JD, Bennett LE, Keck BM, et al. The Registry of the International Society for Heart and Lung Transplantation: eighteenth official report-2001. J Heart Lung Transplant 2001; 20(8):805–815.

41. Mendeloff EN, Huddleston CB, Mallory GB, et al. Pediatric and adult lung transplantation for cystic fibrosis. J Thorac Cardiovasc Surg 1998; 115(2):404–413.

42. Liou TG, Adler FR, Huang D. Use of lung transplantation survival models to refine patient selection in cystic fibrosis. Am J Respir Crit Care Med 2005; 171(9):1053–1059.

# 10

# Living Lobar Lung Transplantation

**Michael E. Bowdish**

*Department of Cardiothoracic Surgery, University of Southern California Keck School of Medicine, Los Angeles, California, U.S.A.*

**Mark L. Barr**

*Department of Cardiothoracic Surgery, University of Southern California and Childrens Hospital Los Angeles, Los Angeles, California, U.S.A.*

## INTRODUCTION

The number of patients awaiting lung transplantation has steadily increased over the past decade as improvements in donor management, operative technique, organ preservation, immunosuppression, and postoperative care has made lung transplantation accepted therapy for end-stage lung disease. At the end of the year 2003, there were 3836 patients on the UNOS Organ Procurement and Transplantation Network lung transplantation waiting list, representing a 147% increase from the number in 1994. Despite the increase in demand, the number of cadaveric lung transplants performed each year has increased only 51% over the same decade, despite liberalizing the standard donor criteria and considering older and sometimes more marginal donors (1–3). With this disparity in mind, our group developed living lobar lung transplantation as an alternative to cadaveric lung transplantation (4,5).

In living lobar lung transplantation, two healthy donors are selected— one to undergo removal of the right lower lobe and the other, removal of the left lower lobe. These lobes are then implanted in the recipient in place of whole right and left lungs. While the number of living lobar lung transplants performed each year remains small, as compared to kidney transplantation (where approximately 50% of transplants are now performed from living donors) and liver transplantation, living lobar lung transplantation has clearly proven itself to be beneficial to a small group of patients who would have otherwise succumbed to disease while awaiting a cadaveric donor (5,6). Since 1992, our institution has performed 141 living lobar transplants and other programs subsequently developed in North America, Europe, and Japan (7,8).

## INDICATIONS FOR LOBAR LUNG TRANSPLANTATION AND DONOR SELECTION

Living lobar lung transplant candidates should meet the standard criteria for cadaveric lung transplantation and be listed on the UNOS Organ Procurement and Transplantation Network lung transplantation waiting list (9). Potential recipients should have the expectation that they would die or become unsuitable recipients before a cadaveric organ becomes available. Overall, cystic fibrosis has been the most common indication for living lobar lung transplantation. However, other indications for living lobar lung transplantation have included primary pulmonary hypertension, pulmonary fibrosis, bronchopulmonary dysplasia and obliterative bronchiolitis, lymphangioleiomyomatosis, and idiopathic interstitial pneumonia (5,8).

The goals of donor selection are to identify donors with excellent health, adequate pulmonary reserve for lobar donation, an emotional attachment to the recipient, and a willingness to accept the risks of donation without coercion. The criteria for donation have included an age between 18 and 55, no history of thoracic procedures on the side to be donated, and excellent general health. Donors taller than the recipient are favored over donors of the same or lesser height, as they have the potential to provide larger lobes. Initially, only the mother and father of the recipient were considered as donors; however, lobes from siblings, extended family members, and unrelated individuals who can demonstrate an emotional attachment to the recipient are also presently considered. A psychosocial interview is then conducted. Potential donors are interviewed both with the recipient and the recipient's family to ascertain interpersonal dynamics. Elements of the interview include the motivation to donate, pain tolerance, feelings regarding donation should the recipient expire, and the ability of the potential donor to be separated from family and career obligations. As an element of coercion can always exist between a potential donor and the recipient and/or the recipient's family, any potential donor who discloses that they feel any pressure to donate after careful consultation and explanation of the procedure is denied for unspecified reasons, thus preventing untoward feelings between the family, recipient, and potential donor.

After the psychosocial evaluation, suitable potential donors undergo blood typing for compatibility as well as chest radiography and spirometry to assess lung size and function. This preliminary screening reduces costs as it allows the evaluation of only a limited number of potential donors. A more thorough medical workup including routine transplant seriologies (human immunodeficiency virus, venereal disease research laboratory, cytomegalovirus, Epstein–Barr virus, and hepatitis), electrocardiogram, echocardiogram, quantitative ventilation/perfusion scanning, and high-resolution chest computed tomography is completed after the preliminary screening is completed and found to be acceptable (10,11).

After identification of two suitable donors, one is chosen to undergo right lower lobectomy and the other, left lower lobectomy. The right lower lobe is usually selected from the larger donor, while, if the donors are of the same height, the donor with the more complete fissure on the left is chosen to donate that side. Occasionally, an acceptable donor will have a history of prior thoracic procedures, trauma, or infection. In this case, the contralateral side is chosen for donation. Currently, computed tomographic scanning and spirometry are used to estimate lung volume, although the optimal method of determining an appropriate size match between donor and recipient remains to be defined and further improvements in this methodology are warranted. In children, care must be exercised to ensure that the lower lobe is not oversized. While human leukocyte antigen (HLA) matching is not required for donor selection, a prospective cross-match to rule out the presence of anti-HLA antibodies is performed.

## OPERATIVE TECHNIQUE

The performance of living lobar lung transplantation involves three simultaneous operations: two donor lobectomies and the recipient bilateral pneumonectomy and lobar implantation. The operative goals of living donor lung transplantation are to avoid morbidity to the healthy volunteer lobe donor while providing adequate tissue margins for implantation in the recipient (12). The lobar vascular and bronchial anatomy of the right and left lower lobes are the most suitable for lobar transplantation.

### Donor Lobectomy, Recipient Pneumonectomy, and Allograft Implantation

The important difference in performing a lobectomy for lobar transplantation, as opposed to a lobectomy for cancer or infection, is that the lobe must be removed with adequate cuffs of bronchus, pulmonary artery, and pulmonary vein to allow successful reimplantation in the recipient, while allowing closure of these structures in the donor without compromise.

The donor lobectomy is performed through a posterolateral thoracotomy. The lobar vasculature is dissected and vascular clamps are placed just distal to the middle lobe artery and proximal to the superior segmental artery of the lower lobes. Next, the inferior pulmonary veins and right middle lobe vein (for a right lobectomy) are defined. Fissures are completed with stapling devices. The pulmonary artery and vein are then divided, followed by the lower lobe bronchi. The lobe is taken to a separate sterile table for preservation with a cold pulmonoplegic solution. The pulmonary vessels and bronchus are then repaired, chest tubes placed, and the chest closed.

The recipient operation commences in a third operating room, simultaneous with the donor operations. The operation is performed through a transverse thoracosternotomy (clamshell) incision. Dissection of the pulmonary artery and veins is performed as distally as possible to optimize cuff length for the lobar implantation. When the dissection is complete, the patient is heparinized and cardiopulmonary bypass initiated. The pulmonary vasculature is then divided, followed by the bronchus.

The lobar allografts are then implanted. The bronchus is anastomosed first with minimal peribronchial dissection. The donor pulmonary vein is then anastomosed to the superior pulmonary vein of the recipient. Last, pulmonary artery anastomosis is performed in an end-to-end fashion. After completing the bilateral implantations, the vascular clamps are removed and ventilation is begun gently. Continuous nitric oxide and intermittent aerosolized bronchodilator therapy are administered via the anesthesia circuit. The patient is weaned from cardiopulmonary bypass. Four chest tubes are then placed, the clamshell incision closed, and the patient transported directly to the intensive care unit.

### Postoperative Management

While the immunosuppression, antibiotic therapy and prophylaxis, and long-term management of the lobar recipient are very similar to standard cadaveric transplantation, the perioperative management can be quite challenging given the unique lobar physiology.

The lobar physiology of the recipient presents unique challenges compared with standard cadaveric lung transplantation as the entire cardiac output is flowing through two relatively undersized lobes. In an attempt to decrease atelectasis and optimize expansion of the lobes, the recipient is kept sedated and ventilated through a single lumen endotracheal tube with positive end-expiratory pressures of 5–10 cm water for at least 48 hours. Additionally, efforts are undertaken to decrease pulmonary artery pressures and minimize the risk of reperfusion injury and pulmonary edema. This is accomplished by maintaining the recipient in a relatively hypovolemic state, the use of nitroglycerin infusion, and the use of aerosolized nitric oxide for the first 48 to 72 hours.

Another unique aspect of managing the lobar recipient in the perioperative period is chest tube management. Depending on the degree of size mismatch between the donor lobe and the recipient pleural cavity, conventional chest tube suction in the postoperative period can result in impaired deflation mechanics. This can lead to air trapping with increasing airway pressures, a rise in pulmonary vascular resistance, and subsequently an acute rise in pulmonary arterial pressure. This problem is exaggerated as the discrepancy between the size of the lobe and the thoracic cavity increases. In an effort to avoid this problem, suction is applied at low levels (10 cm water), to each tube sequentially at one-hour intervals, in a rotational fashion for the first 24 hours postoperatively. Subsequently, each of the four chest tubes is placed on continuous suction that is gradually increased to 20 cm water over the next 48 hours. Chest tube output can be much greater than that seen after cadaveric implantation as there is an obligatory space filling of the pleural cavity with fluid, which can be exacerbated by greater topographical mismatches. The question of whether these tubes can be removed despite these higher than normal outputs is unclear. However, because of concerns of lobe compression by the pleural fluid, the chest tubes are left in place for two to three weeks, which is significantly longer than in conventional cadaveric transplantation. Any air leaks typically resolve in this time period as well.

The management of the lobar recipient with regard to immunosuppression, antibiotic therapy and prophylaxis, and long-term follow-up, is very similar to cadaveric recipients. All patients have received triple-drug immunosuppression (tacrolimus/cyclosporine, mycophenolate mofetil/ azathioprine, and prednisone) without induction therapy. Antibiotic use based on preoperative, intraoperative, and postoperative cultures is common in cystic fibrosis recipients due to the nearly universal presence of pathogenic bacterial and/or fungal species. Prophylaxis for *Pneumocystis carinii* and cytomegalovirus is given to all recipients. In all recipients, pulmonary function testing and chest roentgenography are performed with each clinic visit; however, bronchoscopy is performed only when clinically indicated by symptoms, radiography, or a decrease in spirometric results. Transbronchial biopsy is performed sparingly due to the perceived increased risk of bleeding in the lobar recipient.

## RESULTS

Although the use of live organ donors is considered ethically acceptable at most transplant centers, it creates the unique situation whereby the treatment approach affects not only the patient with end-stage organ disease, but also the live organ donor (13). The deaths of both liver and kidney donors have highlighted this issue and brought increased public attention to live organ donation (14). The need for donor safety is accentuated with living lobar lung transplantation due to the necessity of placing two donors at risk for each recipient. For these reasons, careful scrutiny of living lobar lung transplantation is needed to justify its use as a treatment for patients with end-stage lung disease.

## University of Southern California

Since our last formal report in the literature (5), we have now performed 141 living lobar lung transplants through April 2005 on 136 patients at the University of Southern California and Children's Hospital Los Angeles. Ninety recipients were adults (mean age $27 \pm 7$ years) and 46 were pediatric (mean age $14 \pm 3$ years of age). The main indication for transplantation was cystic fibrosis (86%); the remaining 14% of recipients had a variety of other diagnoses including primary pulmonary hypertension, idiopathic pulmonary fibrosis, bronchopulmonary dysplasia, and obliterative bronchiolitis. At the time of transplantation, many of the patients were critically ill with 67% hospital bound and 20% ventilator dependent—including three on jet ventilation and one patient on extracorporeal membrane oxygenation.

### Recipient Outcome

**Survival:**  Overall recipient actuarial one-, three-, and five-year survival is 73%, 58%, and 48%, respectively, and there has been no difference in actuarial survival between adult or pediatric recipients (Fig. 1). This actuarial survival compares favorably with the International Society for Heart and Lung Transplantation (ISHLT) registry data of one-, three-, and five-year survival of 74%, 58%, and 47% (2). Mean follow-up is $3.6 \pm 3.3$ years (range 0–11.8 years). Deaths occurring within 30 days of transplantation have been largely due to infection and primary graft failure. Deaths occurring between 30 days and one year after transplantation have been usually due to infectious

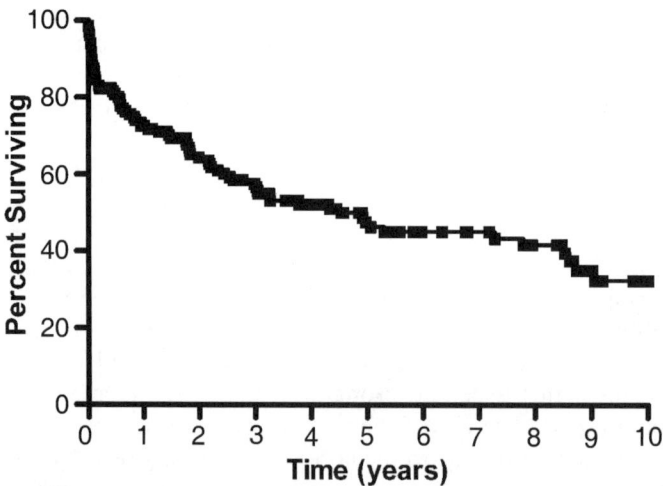

**Figure 1**   Actuarial survival curve for living lobar lung transplant recipients at the University of Southern California ($n = 136$).

etiologies. Late death (>1 year after transplantation) has been predominantly due to infection and obliterative bronchiolitis.

The predominant infections seen have presented as sepsis and/or pneumonia from *Pseudomonas* sp., *Staphylococcus* sp., and *Aspergillus* sp. As opposed to cadaveric double-lung transplantation in which rejection almost always presents in a bilateral fashion, rejection episodes in the lobar recipients have been predominantly unilateral (72%), while only 28% presented bilaterally. A total of 53% of rejection episodes were classified as grade A2 according to the ISHLT grading system, while 35% were grade A1, and 12% were grade A3. In adult recipients, overall freedom from bronchiolitis obliterans syndrome is 98%, 82%, and 76% at one, three, and five years, respectively. Age, gender, etiology, donor relationship, preoperative hospitalization status, use of preoperative steroids, and HLA-A, -B, and -DR typing did not influence survival or rejection. Patients undergoing retransplantation had an elevated risk of death (odds ratio 2.50, $P$ = n.s.). Those patients on ventilators preoperatively had significantly worse outcomes (odds ratio for death at one year 4.9, $P$ = 0.0015; overall odds ratio 3.06, $P$ = 0.03).

**Postoperative pulmonary function:** One question, which has been raised in regard to living lobar lung transplantation, is whether the relatively undersized bilateral lobar grafts would provide comparable pulmonary function to full-sized bilateral cadaveric grafts in adult recipients. In an attempt to address this question, we recently compared serial postoperative pulmonary function tests in a death-censored analysis of our initial cohort of 79 adult patients undergoing living lobar lung transplantation and 46 adult patients undergoing bilateral cadaveric lung transplantation who survived at least three months after transplantation (15). There was no significant difference in overall survival between these two groups of patients surviving at least three months after either living lobar or cadaveric lung transplantation: conditional one-, three-, and five-year actuarial survival was 83%, 81%, and 75% in cadaveric recipients and 83%, 64%, and 62% in lobar recipients, respectively ($P$ = 0.32).

Analysis of the pulmonary functions after both living-lobar and bilateral cadaveric lung transplantation showed that both groups of recipients demonstrated improvement during the first year after transplantation and that pulmonary function was equivalent between the groups by six months after transplantation. Lobar recipients demonstrated an improvement in both forced vital capacity (FVC) and forced expiratory volume in one second ($FEV_1$) by six months after transplantation, while cadaveric recipients had an improvement in FVC by 12 months after transplantation and maintained a stable $FEV_1$. These results are similar to those reported in bilateral cadaveric transplantation, which have shown improvements in $FEV_1$, FVC, and diffusing capacity for the first 6 to 12 months after transplantation, after which time, lung function tends to decline at a variable rate and is highly influenced by the presence or absence of complications (16–18). The Okayama University group has seen similar improvements in FVC and $FEV_1$ during the first year after transplantation in their series of living lobar lung transplant recipients (8).

Comparison of pulmonary functions between the living-lobar and cadaveric recipients at various time points demonstrated that FVC and $FEV_1$ were significantly lower at one and three months after transplantation in the living-lobar group as compared to the cadaveric group. However, by six months after transplantation this difference had resolved and the values then remained equivalent. These results are somewhat intriguing, but not entirely unexpected. It is generally accepted that the initial improvement seen in pulmonary function over the first year after transplantation is in large part due to improved chest wall mechanics and alveolar recruitment which occur with operative recovery (19,20). However, the process is undoubtedly multifactorial and influenced by other factors such as pulmonary compliance, episodes of infection and rejection, and other postoperative complications.

Although one might have expected the lobes in the lobar recipients to have persistently decreased flows as compared to bilateral cadaveric grafts from a strict physiologic standpoint, it seems likely that the lobes are able to provide similar flows through both careful donor and recipient selection (whereby a relatively large lobe is placed in a relatively small recipient), and through continued alveolar dilatation and recruitment in the graft, as opposed to growth (21). The explanation of the lower FVC and $FEV_1$ seen at one and three months in lobar recipients as compared to bilateral cadaveric recipients is likewise multifactorial, but is likely due to topographic and resulting mechanical issues due to the fact that the lobe is not perfectly opposed to the chest wall, as occurs with bilateral cadaveric grafts. It is possible that with time and scarring, the mechanics between the chest wall and lobe improve, resulting in an improvement in pulmonary flows as demonstrated in this study.

Exercise capacities were also comparable in the lobar and cadaveric lung transplant recipients when assessed by exercise stress testing. Although the peak oxygen consumption achieved by both groups of transplant recipients is below 80% of the normal predicted value, it is certainly adequate to permit a comfortable lifestyle and at least moderate levels of work and exercise (22). These peak exercise capacities are similar to those previously reported for recipients of double-lung and heart–lung transplants (18,23).

These results show that despite the relatively undersized grafts, lobar transplantation provides adequate pulmonary function and exercise capacity—three female recipients have even gone through full-term pregnancy without any untoward events during gestation or delivery.

Donor Outcome

There has been no perioperative or long-term mortality in the total cohort of 279 lobar donors. In a detailed study of the first 253 donors, 80.2% had no perioperative complications (24). Fifty (19.8%) of the 253 donors had one or more perioperative complications. Overall length of stay was $9.4 \pm 4.8$ days. Right-sided donors were more likely to have a perioperative complication than left sided donors (odds ratio 2.02, $P = 0.04$), likely secondary to right lower and middle lobe anatomy. Intraoperative complications occurred in nine (3.6%) donors, and were primarily related to the right middle lobe. The right middle lobe was sacrificed in four donors due to variations in either arterial or venous anatomy, while three patients required reimplantation of the right middle lobe bronchus. In addition, one donor required one packed red blood cell unit secondary to blood loss after the clamp on the left atrium was inadvertently displaced. One patient with a history of Wolf–Parkinson–White syndrome developed a persistent supraventricular tachycardia, which eventually responded to medical therapy; however, the patient subsequently required pacemaker placement.

Complications requiring reoperation occurred in eight (3.2%) donors. Three donors required reoperation for bleeding; however, none required red blood cell transfusion. The source of bleeding in these patients was most commonly an intercostal artery. One patient underwent video-assisted throacoscopy for evacuation of a loculated pleural effusion, while one required pericardiectomy for pericarditis unresponsive to medical management. The remaining three patients required reoperation for a sterile empyema, a retained sponge, and a bronchopulmonary fistula, respectively. Other perioperative complications occurred in 38 (15.0%) donors. The most common complication in this group, and overall, was the need for a thoracostomy tube for >14 days postoperatively, either for persistent drainage or airleaks, or the placement of an additional thoracostomy tube. The most significant complication in this group occurred in two patients who developed pulmonary artery thrombosis. Both patients presented with severe respiratory distress; however, neither required intubation. Both patients had positive ventilation–perfusion scans, negative lower extremity duplex scans, and contrast magnetic resonance imaging and angiography studies consistent with thrombus at the pulmonary artery suture line. Both patients were successfully managed with systemic anticoagulation and suffered no long-term sequelae. Other complications included medically treated arrhythmias and pericarditis, as well as two minor epidural related complications (hypotensive episodes resulting in syncope in two donors). One donor required bronchoscopy for right middle lobe collapse, but did not require reoperation. Four donors required readmission within 30 days of lobectomy, one for dehydration, one with shortness of breath, one with a pleural effusion managed conservatively, and one for presumed pneumonia without positive cultures.

Other Centers

Results in pediatric and adult living lobar transplantation from other centers are sparse, although programs do exist in North America, Europe, and Japan. The Washington University Group at St. Louis Children's Hospital has reported results from 31 pediatric patients in unstable condition or in a condition where survival was unlikely during the wait for a cadaveric organ (7,25). In this series, 22 (71%) patients recovered and were discharged from the hospital while nine (31%) died during the early postoperative period. The overall 1-year survival was 63.7%.

The group at Okayama University in Japan recently reported their early experience with 30 patients with end-stage lung disease who received living lobar lung transplants (8). This technique is particularly attractive in Japan due to an extreme shortage of cadaveric donors. All patients in this series were alive at the time of their report, with a mean follow-up of 22.2 months (range 1–66 months).

There have been two other reports of perioperative complications in living donor lobectomy (25,26). The Washington University group reported 62 donors utilized for 31 living lobar lung transplants in children. In this series, 10 donors (16.1%) had 12 major complications requiring subsequent intervention, three of which resulted in permanent loss of function (phrenic nerve paralysis, loss of right middle lobe, and the development of a bronchial stricture). Eleven of the 27 donors in the Okayama University group had perioperative complications; however, there has been no mortality and all donors have returned to their previous lifestyles (8).

## RECOMMENDATIONS AND FUTURE DIRECTIONS

A constant awareness of the risk to the living donors must be maintained with any live donor organ transplantation program, and comprehensive short and long-term follow-up should be strongly encouraged to maintain the viability of these potentially life-saving programs. There has been no perioperative or long-term mortality following lobectomy for living lobar lung transplantation, and the perioperative risks associated with donor lobectomy are similar to those seen with standard lung resections. However, these risks might increase if the procedure is offered on an occasional basis and not within a well-established program. An important question, which remains unanswered, is the long-term outcomes and functional effects of lobar donation. This has proven difficult to follow closely, due to the fact that many donors live far away from the medical center and are reluctant to return for routine follow-up evaluation. The death of a recipient further exacerbates this situation as there is a reluctance to insist on further routine exams for a grieving donor. Further long-term outcome data is ideally needed, similar to live donor renal and liver transplantation. Although this may not reflect the postoperative pulmonary function of the entire group of donors, initial one- and two-year postoperative pulmonary function testing, in our intermediate experience, demonstrated an average decrease of 17% in FVC, 15% in $FEV_1$, and 16% in total lung capacity from preoperative values (27). Despite these results, we still favor performing living lobar lung transplantation in the patient with a clinically deteriorating condition. We feel that prospective donors should be informed of the morbidity associated with donor lobectomy and the potential for mortality, as well of potential recipient outcomes in regard to life expectancy and quality of life after transplantation.

A major question regarding lobar lung transplantation that has been unanswered during the last decade has been defining when a potential recipient is too ill to justify placing two healthy donors at risk of donor lobectomy. Recipient age, gender, indication for primary transplant, prehospitalization status, steroid usage preoperatively, relationship of donor to recipient, and the presence or absence of rejection episodes post-operatively all do not appear to influence overall mortality (5). However, those patients on ventilators preoperatively, as well as those undergoing retransplantation after either a previous cadaveric or lobar lung transplant, have significantly elevated odds ratios for postoperative death. We would therefore recommend caution in these subgroups of patients. This experience is not that dissimilar to the cadaveric experience where intubated patients have higher one-year mortalities and retransplants have decreased three- and five-year survival (2,3). A similar experience with a smaller number of lobar transplants has been reported by the Washington University group (28).

Despite this high-risk patient group, this alternative procedure has been lifesaving in severely ill patients who would either die or become unsuitable recipients before a cadaveric organ becomes available. Although cadaveric transplantation is preferable due to the risk to the donors, living lobar lung transplantation should continue to be utilized under properly selected circumstances. While there have been no deaths in the donor cohort, a risk of death between 0.5% and 1% should be quoted pending further data. Loss of lung function should be considered an expected aspect of this procedure, and is explained as such to the potential donor during the process of obtaining informed consent. The results reported by our group as well as others are important if this procedure is to be considered as an option at more pulmonary transplant centers in view of the institutional, regional, and intra- and international differences in the philosophical and ethical acceptance of the use of live organ donors for transplantation.

## ACKNOWLEDGMENTS

Dr. Bowdish was the recipient of the 2002 American Society of Transplant Surgeons Thoracic Surgery Fellowship. Dr. Barr was funded in part by grants from the Cystic Fibrosis Foundation (CFF G965), the Heart and Lung Surgery Foundation of Los Angeles, and USC University Hospital.

## REFERENCES

1. Rosengard BR, Feng S, Alfrey EJ, et al. Report of the Crystal City meeting to maximize the use of organs recovered from the cadaver donor. Am J Transplant 2002; 2(8):701–711.
2. Trulock EP, Edwards LB, Taylor DO, et al. The registry of the international society for heart and lung transplantation: twenty-first official adult lung and heart-lung transplant report—2004. J Heart Lung Transplant 2004; 23(7): 804–815.
3. Barr ML, Bourge RC, Orens JB, et al. Thoracic organ transplantation in the United States, 1994–2003. Am J Transplant 2005; 5(4, Pt 2):934–949.
4. Starnes VA, Barr ML, Cohen RG. Lobar transplantation. Indications, technique, and outcome. J Thorac Cardiovasc Surg 1994; 108(3):403–410; discussion 410–411.
5. Starnes VA, Bowdish ME, Woo MS, et al. A decade of living lobar lung transplantation: recipient outcomes. J Thorac Cardiovasc Surg 2004; 127(1):114–122.
6. Danovitch GM, Cohen DJ, Weir MR, et al. Current status of kidney and pancreas transplantation in the United States, 1994–2003. Am J Transplant 2005; 5(4, Pt 2):904–915.
7. Mendeloff EN, Huddleston CB, Mallory GB, et al. Pediatric and adult lung transplantation for cystic fibrosis. J Thorac Cardiovasc Surg 1998; 115(2): 404–413; discussion 413–414.
8. Date H, Aoe M, Sano Y, et al. Improved survival after living-donor lobar lung transplantation. J Thorac Cardiovasc Surg 2004; 128(6):933–940.
9. Maurer JR, Frost AE, Estenne M, et al. International guidelines for the selection of lung transplant candidates. The International Society for Heart and Lung Transplantation, the American Thoracic Society, the American Society of Transplant Physicians, the European Respiratory Society. J Heart Lung Transplant 1998; 17(7):703–709.
10. Schenkel FA, Barr ML, Starnes VA. Living-donor lobar lung transplantation: donor evaluation and selection. In: Norman DJ, Turka LA, eds. Primer on Transplantation. Moorestown, NJ: American Society of Transplantation, 2001.
11. Schenkel FA, Horn MV, Woo MS, et al. Screening potential donors for living donor lobar lung transplantation. J Heart Lung Transplant 2003; 22(1S):S86.
12. Bowdish ME, Barr ML, Starnes VA. Living lobar transplantation. Chest Surg Clin N Am 2003; 13(3):505–524.
13. Abecassis M, Adams M, Adams P, et al. Consensus statement on the live organ donor. J Am Med Assoc 2000; 284(22):2919–2926.
14. Ellison MD, McBride MA, Edwards LB, et al. Living organ donation: mortality and early complications among 16,395 living donors in the U.S. Am J Transplant 2003; 3:S:Abstract 517.
15. Bowdish ME, Pessotto R, Barbers RG, et al. Long-term pulmonary function after living-donor lobar lung transplantation in adults. Ann Thorac Surg 2005; 79(2):418–425.
16. Montoya A, Mawulawde K, Houck J, et al. Survival and functional outcome after single and bilateral lung transplantation. Loyola Lung Transplant Team. Surgery 1994; 116(4):712–718.

17. Cooper JD, Patterson GA, Trulock EP. Results of single and bilateral lung transplantation in 131 consecutive recipients. Washington University Lung Transplant Group. J Thorac Cardiovasc Surg 1994; 107(2):460–470; discussion 470–471.
18. Schwaiblmair M, Reichenspurner H, Muller C, et al. Cardiopulmonary exercise testing before and after lung and heart-lung transplantation. Am J Respir Crit Care Med 1999; 159(4, Pt 1):1277–1283.
19. Arcasoy SM, Kotloff RM. Lung transplantation. N Engl J Med 1999; 340(14): 1081–1091.
20. Chaparro C, Scavuzzo M, Winton T, et al. Status of lung transplant recipients surviving beyond five years. J Heart Lung Transplant 1997; 16(5):511–516.
21. Sritippayawan S, Keens TG, Horn MV, et al. Does lung growth occur when mature lobes are transplanted into children? Pediatr Transplant 2002; 6(6): 500–504.
22. Wasserman K, Hansen J, Sue D, et al. Principles of exercise testing and interpretation. Philadelphia: Lea & Febiger, 1987.
23. Levy RD, Ernst P, Levine SM, et al. Exercise performance after lung transplantation. J Heart Lung Transplant 1993; 12(1, Pt 1):27–33.
24. Bowdish ME, Barr ML, Schenkel FA, et al. A decade of living lobar lung transplantation: perioperative complications after 253 donor lobectomies. Am J Transplant 2004; 4(8):1283–1288.
25. Battafarano RJ, Anderson RC, Meyers BF, et al. Perioperative complications after living donor lobectomy. J Thorac Cardiovasc Surg 2000; 120(5):909–915.
26. Date H, Aoe M, Nagahiro I, et al. Living-donor lobar lung transplantation for various lung diseases. J Thorac Cardiovasc Surg 2003; 126(2):476–481.
27. Starnes VA, Barr ML, Cohen RG, et al. Living-donor lobar lung transplantation experience: intermediate results. J Thorac Cardiovasc Surg 1996; 112(5):1284–1290; discussion 1290–1291.
28. Huddleston CB, Bloch JB, Sweet SC, et al. Lung transplantation in children. Ann Surg 2002; 236:270–276.

# 11

# Heart–Lung Transplantation: Is It a Viable Option in the 21st Century?

**Susan D. Moffatt-Bruce and Bruce A. Reitz**

*Department of Cardiothoracic Surgery, Stanford University Medical School, Stanford, California, U.S.A.*

## INTRODUCTION

Therapeutic lung transplantation was initiated in 1981, with the success of a heart–lung transplant procedure at Stanford University (1). This success was achieved after failed attempts in patients and after the introduction of cyclosporine immunosuppression and proof in primate studies (2–4). Heart–lung transplantation has since evolved over the last two decades to become an accepted modality of treatment for end stage lung and combined heart–lung disease.

To date more than 3000 heart–lung transplants have been reported worldwide (5). Heart–lung transplantation has evolved to have specific indications and although this form of transplantation realized a peak in numbers in 1989, a more recent decline has paralleled the increase in isolated single- and double-lung transplantations. In addition, fewer centers are continuing to perform this highly specialized transplant procedure (6,7). It is therefore a pertinent question in this day and age of outcome analysis and cost containment to ask whether or not heart–lung transplantation is a truly a viable option in the 21st century. Only after carefully reviewing indications, alternative therapies, and the ultimate results will one be able to answer this important question.

## HISTORICAL OVERVIEW

Dr. Cooley was the first to attempt heart–lung transplantation in 1968 when he transplanted a two-and-a-half-year-old girl with an atrioventricular canal defect and pulmonary hypertension; the patient unfortunately died 14 hours postoperatively (2). Dr. Lillehei and colleagues transplanted a heart and lungs into a 43-year-old man in 1969; the patient lived for eight days (3). Canine studies were ongoing during these years in an attempt to render heart–lung transplantation successful, but it was not until the late 1970s when Reitz and colleagues at Stanford achieved clinically acceptable results in primates (4). The first successful heart–lung transplant was performed in a 45-year-old woman with the diagnosis of primary pulmonary hypertension (PPH), who went on to do well for more than five years posttransplant (1). Single- and double-lung transplantation were subsequently performed successfully in 1984 and 1986, respectively (8,9).

After its inception in 1981, the number of heart–lung transplantation procedures peaked in 1989 with ~240 transplants performed (6). Since 1994, however, the number of centers that have reported heart–lung transplantation has decreased by ~40% from a maximum of 63 down to 37 in 2002. Concomitantly, the drop-off in annual activity that began in 1996 continued, and only 71 heart–lung transplantations were recorded for 2002 (6). Only four centers reported an annual volume of greater than five heart–lung transplants per year for the period between January 1, 1998, and June 30, 2003. This ongoing decline has been reported in the International Society for Heart–Lung Transplantation (ISHLT) registry but the reasons are not completely clear. The decline through the 1990s initially reflected a shift from heart–lung transplantation to lung transplantation for certain indications. An additional factor is the effect of organ allocation algorithms on the availability of combined heart–lung blocs (6,7).

## INDICATIONS FOR HEART–LUNG TRANSPLANTATION

Severe pulmonary vascular disease in the form of PPH with right heart failure and Eisenmenger's syndrome secondary to congenital heart disease have evolved to be the most common indications for heart–lung transplantation in adults (6,8,9). Despite the widespread use of bilateral lung transplantation, cystic fibrosis remained the third most common indication for heart–lung transplantation in the era between 1996 and 2003.

PPH has been associated with a rapidly declining clinical course and high mortality. Heart–lung transplantation is therefore an important treatment option. Due to donor organ shortages and the development of improved pulmonary vasodilator therapies, both single- and double-lung transplantations have been more recently used for patients with pulmonary vascular disease (10–13). In fact, a recent review of practice patterns has revealed that 83% of centers preferred double-lung transplantation to heart–lung transplantation for patients with PPH (10). Controversy over whether or not the type of transplant performed for PPH influences survival exists worldwide (12,13). Franke et al. reported that patients undergoing double-lung transplantation had a lower one-year survival rate as compared to patients after heart–lung transplantation for PPH (13). In contrast, groups in St. Louis and Stanford have revealed that, although lung and heart–lung transplantations for PPH are associated with a high early mortality, the type of transplant did not confer a significant difference in survival (11,12).

Patients with end-stage Eisenmenger's syndrome have a poor prognosis with thoracic organ transplantation being the only definitive therapy shown to extend life (14–16). Heart–lung transplantation has been particularly effective in patients with ventricular septal defects (VSDs) and multiple congenital anomalies (14). In those patients with a surgically correctable heart lesion, lung transplantation with a cardiac repair is an attractive option, thereby optimizing organ allocation (15).

Cystic fibrosis is the third most common indication for heart–lung transplantation (6). This is a challenging group of patients due to pulmonary sepsis that mandates excision of both lungs, extensive pleural adhesions, systemic comorbidities, and severe nutritional deficiencies. As the first available double-lung transplant option, heart–lung transplantation was introduced for this indication, though subsequently most patients have received double-lung transplants. The Stanford experience has revealed that both heart–lung and double-lung transplantation provide similar palliation for this suppurative condition (17,18). Due to organ shortage and allocation, double-lung transplantation will remain the preferred operation for patients with cystic fibrosis (17).

A variation on the theme of heart–lung transplantation is a combined heart–single-lung transplant (19,20). In some patients with complex congenital heart disease, the vasculature of one lung can be preserved with a surgical shunt while the second lung develops pulmonary hypertension (20).

Less common indications for heart–lung transplantation include primary cardiac sarcomas (21). The high incidence of recurrent and metastatic disease, however, limits its utility for this indication and others that include a malignancy. Combined heart–lung–liver transplantation has also been described and is appropriately considered in patients with advanced liver disease and concomitant end-stage lung disease or in those liver-failure patients with refractory portopulmonary hypertension (22,23).

Domino heart transplantation involves the explantation of the heart from a heart–lung transplant recipient with subsequent transplantation of the heart into a heart-only transplant recipient (24,25). This is a unique source of hearts from essentially live donors. Similar survival rates have been found in recipients of domino and nondomino hearts. In particular, successful domino heart transplantation into heart recipients with high pulmonary vascular resistance supports the hypothesis that heart–lung recipients may provide superior donor hearts due to right heart preconditioning. The domino heart procedure may in fact help to balance the inequity of heart–lung block allocation. It remains, however, a procedure that is poorly utilized in North America because of a lack of acceptance by most transplant centers.

### Recipient Selection Criteria

The decision to perform heart–lung transplantation is made for those patients with end-stage cardiopulmonary disease who have no other treatment possibilities, with no contraindications, and with the potential for rehabilitation. Patients are normally in New York functional class III or IV and the decision process requires a multidisciplinary team including thoracic transplant surgeons, pulmonologists, social workers, and psychologists.

The generally accepted recipient age criteria for heart–lung transplantation is <55 years and the projected life span should be <12–18 months despite optimal medical management of the underlying disease. Absolute contraindications to transplantation include irreversible dysfunction of other organs (e.g., kidney or liver), current smoking, alcohol or drug abuse, active malignancy, and HIV infection. Relative contraindications include peripheral vascular disease, severe osteoporosis, active pulmonary infection, hepatitis B or C infection, sputum with pan-resistant organisms, obesity, and chest wall deformity. These relative contraindications are considered on a case-by-case basis. Previous cardiothoracic surgery or pleurodesis were initially deemed to be absolute contraindications to transplantation due to bleeding from chest wall adhesions and difficulty preserving the vagus, recurrent laryngeal, and phrenic nerves. However, with improved surgical hemostatic devices, the use of antifibrinolytic agents, and increased experience, these patients are now eligible for transplantation.

### Management of Patients Awaiting Transplantation

Patients listed for heart–lung transplantation must continue to be seen on a routine basis to ensure that they remain in good pretransplant condition. Medications should be reviewed and signs of infection must be aggressively sought. During this time the use of oxygen and pulmonary vasodilators may improve patient comfort as well as physiologic well-being. In patients with PPH or secondary pulmonary hypertension, the use of continuous epoprostenol therapy has been extremely helpful, but requires close monitoring as patients can develop worsening disease or tachyphylaxis (10). Long-term vascular access can be an issue and signs or symptoms of infection or thrombosis must be continuously sought. Patients predisposed to pulmonary or systemic thrombosis and embolization must have their anticoagulation carefully monitored pretransplant.

## ALTERNATIVES TO HEART–LUNG TRANSPLANTATION

### Medical Alternatives to Heart–Lung Transplantation

A small proportion of patients with pulmonary hypertension, either primary or secondary, will have a dramatic hemodynamic response to acute vasodilator testing and may be candidates for calcium channel blocker therapy. The vast majority, however, will not benefit from calcium channel blockade and should be treated with one of the three U.S. Food and Drug Administration–approved prostacyclin therapies for pulmonary hypertension that include bosentan, treprostinil, and epoprostenol (26–30). The beneficial effect of prostacylin in pulmonary hypertension is linked to its powerful vasodilating capacity, and perhaps more importantly, to its inhibition of platelet aggregation, smooth muscle proliferation, and inflammatory actions (29). Investigational therapies include phophodiesterase inhibitors, prostacyclin analogs with alternative delivery routes, and selective endothelin A receptor antagonists such as sitaxsentan (31).

In the current era, heart–lung transplantation should not be considered until after the failure of medical therapy, taking into account, however, the time needed to complete a transplant evaluation and the time spent on the waiting list. In general, patients who have New York Heart Association (NYHA) class III or IV symptoms on presentation should be referred for transplant evaluation while their response to therapy is being evaluated so as to avoid delays in evaluation and listing. In the future, improvements in medical management, both in terms of delivery and lack of side effects, may preclude the need for heart–lung transplantation in selected patients with end-stage cardiopulmonary disease. That is, however, not yet the case for truly end-stage combined disease, and heart–lung transplantation remains the only option (26).

### Surgical Treatments and Interventions for Pulmonary Artery Hypertension

While it is true that considerable advances have been achieved in the medical treatment of pulmonary artery hypertension, for many patients it remains unsuccessful or unavailable. For these patients, atrial septostomy, pulmonary thromboendarterectomy, or lung or heart transplantation, in lieu of combined heart–lung transplantation, may be considered (32).

Atrial septostomy has been used as a palliative treatment in patients with advanced pulmonary artery hypertension based on its potential to decompress the failing right ventricle and increase the cardiac index and is indicated only in those refractory to medical therapy. Improvements in cardiac index immediately following the procedure range from 15% to 58% but are associated with desaturation. Unfortunately, postprocedural mortality has been reported to range from 5% to 50% (33,34). Patients with the most advanced pulmonary artery hypertension, defined by markedly elevated pulmonary vascular resistance, arterial oxygen saturation <80% at rest, and severe right heart failure appear most likely to die or worsen with atrial septostomy. The procedure should be reserved for those in whom medical therapies fail or are unavailable or who need a "bridge" to transplantation (32).

Pulmonary thromboendarterectomy may provide a potential cure for patients with pulmonary artery hypertension secondary to chronic thromboembolic disease. It is a well-accepted procedure with the goal of reducing pulmonary artery pressures, thereby leading to improved right ventricular function (35,36). There are moderate long-term data available but the 30-day mortality for this highly selective group of patients is ~14% with early mortality due to persistent pulmonary hypertension, reperfusion pulmonary edema, sepsis, and hemorrhage (32).

With limited donor resources, lung transplantation with or without cardiac repair has been examined as an alternative to heart–lung transplantation (9–13,17). When transplanting a patient with PPH, both the Washington University and the Stanford groups have reported similar outcomes for patients receiving lung versus heart–lung transplantation (11,12). One-year survival was reported as 75% with early death in both lung and heart–lung transplantations due to graft failure and infection. Although this would imply that double-lung transplantation should be attempted for all patients with PPH, care must be taken. Other groups have reported that double-lung transplant recipients actually have a lower one-year survival when compared to heart–lung transplant recipients by almost 30% (13). Regardless, recent reports have indicated that heart–lung transplant and lung transplant recipients are at similar risk of developing bronchiolitis obliterans syndrome (37). This is a very important finding in that the most common cause for late graft failure in lung transplantation is obliterative bronchiolitis and as of yet no cure has been found for this entity (6). Fortunately, both heart–lung and double-lung transplant recipients may fare slightly better than single-lung transplant recipients with broncholitis obliterans due to the increased amount of lung tissue.

Considering lung transplantation for patients with cardiac defects that have resulted in Eisenmenger's syndrome, care must be taken since this is not a homogenous group. The Toronto group has shown that patients with VSDs and multiple congenital anomalies have the best prognosis after transplantation and that heart–lung transplantation in particular provided the best survival advantage for VSD patients (14). For patients with Eisenmenger's syndrome the one-year survival for heart–lung transplant recipients was 80% as compared to 68% for patients receiving lung transplants only. These results emphasize that congenital heart defect patients need to be individualized and in particular, the reparability of the cardiac defect and the resultant level of cardiac dysfunction need to be considered carefully.

## POSTOPERATIVE COMPLICATIONS

### Rejection

Immunosuppression is started immediately upon reperfusion of the organs so to prevent rejection. Immunosuppression normally consists of induction and maintenance therapy that is cyclosporine-based. Heart–lung transplant recipients receive similar immunosuppresion to that of lung transplant recipients and therefore have similar drug monitoring regimens.

Surveillance of allograft function is the key to successful transplant outcomes. In the case of heart–lung transplants, both pulmonary and cardiac functions are followed. Bronchoscopy with endobronchial biopsies and evaluation of clinical parameters including forced expiratory volume in one second ($FEV_1$), forced expiratory flow in the middle half of an expiration ($FEF_{25-75\%}$), and arterial blood gases are performed at 2, 4, 8, and 12 weeks posttransplant and then at six months and one year. Yearly bronchoscopic surveillance occurs thereafter or when clinically indicated. Early in the experience of heart–lung transplantation, endomyocardial biopsies were done weekly but once it was recognized that cardiac rejection was uncommon in heart–lung allograft recipients, the number of cardiac biopsies was dramatically decreased (38). At our center, endomyocardial biopsies are performed roughly twice in the first six months posttransplant and then annually. Coronary angiography is performed at odd-numbered annual anniversaries posttransplant or when clinically indicated. Surveillance for heart–lung transplant recipients is therefore more involved than that for recipients of lung allografts only.

### Infectious Complications

Immunosuppression places the transplant recipient at increased risk of infectious complications. Prophylaxis against cytomegalovirus (CMV), pneumocystic carnii pneumonia (PCP), and aspergillus infections is required. Intravenous ganciclovir is used for CMV prophylaxis, whereas aerosolized Amphotericin B and oral itraconazole are used to prevent fungal infections. Trimethaprim–sulfamethoxazole is used for life to prevent PCP infection. Both lung and heart–lung transplant recipients receive similar antimicrobial prophylaxis and appear to develop infectious complications at similar rates (39). Ganciclovir prophylaxis has been shown to improve both lung and heart–lung recipient survival as well as delay the onset of bronchiolitis obliterans to similar degrees (39). The heart–lung recipient is thus more like lung recipients than heart-alone recipients.

### Posttransplant Malignancy

Allograft function depends on maintaining an immunosuppressive state that increases the incidence of developing neoplasms. Skin malignancies are very common in heart–lung transplant recipients at rates similar to that of other transplant recipients including lung-only transplant recipients (40). Common malignancies seen in the general population are not increased in heart–lung recipients but rarer tumors including posttransplant lymphoproliferative disorders (PTLD) and various sarcomas are. The Epstein–Barr Virus (EBV) has been associated with PTLD and is frequently extranodal having a predilection for brain and allograft involvement (41). Treatment includes antiviral therapy, chemotherapy, local therapy, and reduction of immunosuppression and anti-CD20 monoclonal antibodies (41). In a recent paper from Stanford, all heart and heart–lung recipients were reviewed for the incidence of PTLD. The overall incidence was 6.3% and was not statistically different between heart and heart–lung recipients. Interestingly, the incidence of PTLD has not changed despite modification of immunosuppression and viral prophylaxis over the years (42).

## ECONOMIC EVALUATION OF HEART–LUNG TRANSPLANTATION

Assessing the medical, social, and economic benefit of transplantation is problematic. However, in this day and age of cost constraints one needs to ask if it is worth the price. In a seven-center review, English economists evaluated the cost–benefit ratio of single-, double-, and heart–lung transplant recipients (43). Over a 15-year period, lung transplantation yielded mean benefits over medical therapy of 2.1, 3.3, and 3.6 quality-adjusted life-years for single-, double- and heart–lung recipients, respectively. During the same time frame, the cost of those maintained medically on the waiting list was $73,564. This can be compared to a mean cost of $176,640, $180,528, and $178,387 for single-, double- and heart–lung transplant recipients, respectively. It was therefore concluded that lung transplantation results in survival and quality-of-life gains but at substantial financial cost. It is indeed difficult to interpret these data in light of being unable to truly assess what quality of life is actually worth and which physical and financial costs are worthwhile. Interestingly, the cost of single-, double-, and heart–lung transplantation are not significantly different. This may be due to similar surveillance and immunosuppression regimens.

## RESULTS OF HEART–LUNG TRANSPLANTATION

The early mortality rate of heart–lung transplantation has been reported as being very high with a survival rate of only 70% at three months and 62% at one year as reported by the ISHLT (6). Stanford data reveal better early results with actuarial survival of 72% at one year and 67% at two years (11). This discrepancy in early survival may reflect that the ISHLT registry data include centers with low numbers and lack of experience. The survival rate of heart–lung recipients at five years is reported by the ISHLT to be 41%

and 26% at 10 years (6,11). What is clear is that over time, with improved immunosuppressive and anti-viral prophylaxis, heart–lung transplant recipients have benefited. Figure 1 demonstrates the difference in survival between those heart–lung recipients transplanted, at Stanford, between 1989 and 1992 compared to those transplanted between 1993 and 2004. The actuarial survival of heart–lung recipients of 1989–1992 at 1, 5, and 10 years was 67%, 43%, and 27%, respectively, whereas the actuarial survival of heart–lung recipients of 1993–2004 at 1, 5, and 10 years was 78%, 61%, and 38%, respectively, which was significantly better. By way of comparison, the actuarial survival rates reported for lung-only transplant recipients were 84% at three months and 74% at one year, with similar results having been reported in both North America and Europe (7). Although initially better than those of heart–lung recipients, the reported survival rates at 5 and 10 years are comparable between heart–lung and lung transplant recipients (6). Figure 2 compares heart–lung transplant outcomes to double- and single-lung transplant outcomes at Stanford between the years 1989 and 2004. Overall, the survival of double- and single-lung and heart–lung transplant recipients was similar to 10 years (Fig. 2). These results need to be interpreted in light of the fact that the time frame of 1989 to 2004 had many changes in patient management. Furthermore, comparing heart–lung and lung transplant survival rates is somewhat difficult. That is to say, transplant recipients differ in many ways, including their age, associated

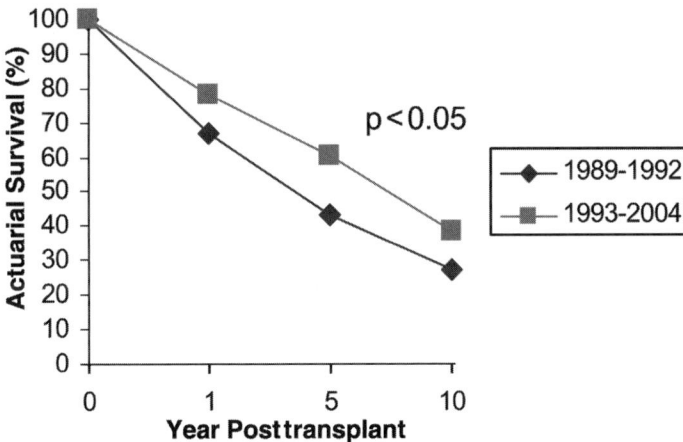

**Figure 1** Stanford University heart–lung transplant recipient survival: 1989–1992 versus 1993–2004. Between 1989 and 2004, 152 heart–lung transplants were performed at Stanford University. The survival of patients in the 1993–2004 era ($n = 93$) was significantly better than that of recipients from the 1989–1992 ($n = 59$) era ($p < 0.050$).

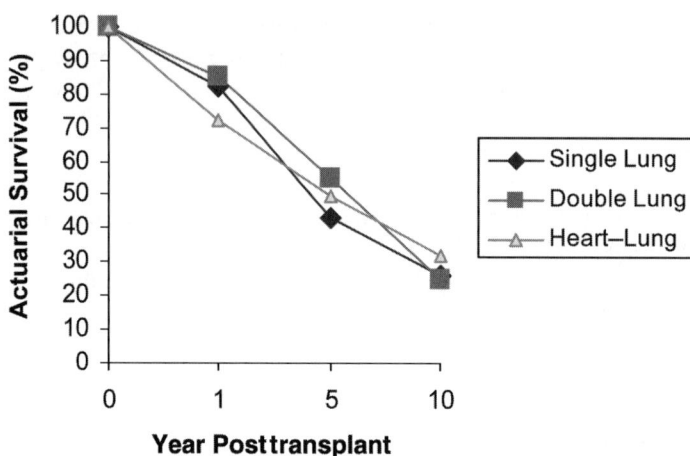

**Figure 2** Stanford University lung and heart transplant survival. The actuarial survival of single-, double-, and heart–lung transplant recipients performed since 1989 are shown. The survival of all three transplant types are similar to 10 years.

morbidities, and their indications for transplantation. Therefore, outcomes may not be simply dependent on procedure alone.

Among the pulmonary vascular disorders, the ISHLT has reported that survival over 10 years has been similar between patients with PPH and Eisenmenger's syndrome but that survival for both of these groups has been superior to other congenital anomalies (6). Patterson's group reported one- and five-year survival rates of 75% and 57% for pulmonary vascular disease recipients but found that pretransplant diagnosis did not confer a significant difference in survival. Futhermore, both Patterson's and Stanford data revealed that lung and heart–lung transplantation for pulmonary vascular disease provided similar long-term outcomes (11,12). Conversely, a large European group has found that double-lung transplantation in patients with primary and secondary pulmonary vascular disease results in lower one-year survival rates when compared to heart–lung transplantation by nearly 50%. This group has concluded that the underlying primary disease influences graft survival after lung transplantation in patients with all forms of pulmonary hypertension in addition to procedure-dependent factors (13).

Focusing on patients with congenital heart disease that survive into adulthood, the survival rate of those undergoing heart–lung transplantation and those undergoing lung transplantation with intracardiac repair was reported by the Pittsburgh group as being similar (15). Furthermore, one- and three-year survival among adults undergoing heart–lung transplantation for congenital heart disease was comparable to that obtained for all other indications.

In the first 30 days after heart–lung transplantation, technical complications, graft failure, and non-CMV infections accounted for ~80% of the deaths (6). For the remainder of the first year, graft failure and non-CMV infections were the leading causes of death. Interestingly, although acute rejection and CMV infection were common in the first year, mortality rates ascribed to these were low. After the first year, bronchiolitis obliterans syndrome was the main cause of death. Similar to heart–lung transplantation, lung transplant recipient graft failure and non-CMV infections were the principal fatal complications in the first 30 days after transplantation. Similarly, acute rejection and CMV infection, although common in the first year, did not cause many deaths. After the first year, most deaths among lung transplant recipients were caused by bronchiolitis obliterans syndrome, which is similar to heart–lung recipients.

Systemic hypertension requiring medical intervention is the most common problem among heart–lung transplant recipients at one and five years and the prevalence rates were comparable to those after lung transplantation (6). Hyperlipidemia and bronchiolitis obliterans syndrome occurred at similar rates among heart–lung and lung transplant recipients, whereas renal dysfunction and diabetes mellitus occurred at lower rates at both one and five years in heart–lung recipients compared to lung recipients. Malignancy rates were ~13% at five years among heart–lung recipients, which was similar to lung transplant recipients.

Despite the associated morbidity of transplantation, no activity limitation was reported for >85% of one-, three-, and five-year heart–lung transplant survivors. Similarly, ~80% of one-, three-, five-, and seven-year lung transplant survivors had no activity limitation reported at their follow-up (6). By way of comparison, the functional status as determined by NYHA class was significantly better among heart transplant recipients with 84% in NYHA class I at 12 and 24 months. Only 62% of lung recipients and 67% of heart–lung transplant recipients were in class I at 12 months, while 62% and 69%, respectively, were in class I at 24 months (7).

## CONCLUSIONS

Heart–lung transplantation—is it a viable option in the 21st century? To answer this question one must look at the indications for heart–lung transplantation, the alternatives to it, and ultimately the cost of and results of this form of transplantation. One must ask if this highly specialized form of transplantation, now performed in only a few centers, is worthwhile when you consider how few lives are saved by it every year. The answer is then easy.

The indications, once thought straightforward, have become blurred. As discussed, the results of lung transplantation, both single and double, are reasonable and reportedly similar to the long-term results of heart–lung transplantation. Thus, lung transplantation will continue to be preferred over heart–lung transplants because of donor availability, donor allocation, technical ability, and the experience of most teams. A suitable set of lungs for transplantation is far more likely to become available than a heart–lung bloc, since emergent heart needs are so great. Furthermore, one set of heart and lungs can be used to save as many as three people on a waiting list and therefore chances are that several recipients are more likely to receive the organs rather than one person awaiting a heart–lung bloc. As discussed, the North American literature would support the concept that with the exception of those with Eisenmenger's syndrome involving severe intracardiac defects or patients with combined end-stage heart and lung disease, lung transplantation is a suitable alternative to heart–lung transplantation (6,12). Finally, because so few heart–lung transplants are performed, those skilled in the technique must be available. A leading cause of 30-day mortality in heart–lung transplantation is technical complications. It is therefore important that this procedure be performed by those proficient in it. This would therefore imply that hopeful recipients would best be served at higher volume heart–lung centers.

Medical management of end-stage lung disease is progressing quickly. Pulmonary vasodilator therapy may provide relief for potential heart–lung recipients but as of yet it is a palliative measure rather than a curative one. Modes of administration and degrees of responsiveness have yet to be optimized and therefore heart–lung transplantation remains the gold standard for highly selected patients when all medical therapy has failed.

After all the facts are considered, the results of heart–lung transplantation have been reported as acceptable and in the long term similar to that of lung transplant recipients. There will always be patients in whom heart–lung transplantation is the only option. For this reason alone, heart–lung transplantation must continue to be considered a viable option in the 21st century.

## REFERENCES

1. Reitz BA, Wallwork JL, Hunt SA, et al. Heart–lung transplantation: successful therapy for patients with pulmonary vascular disease. N Engl J Med 1982; 306: 557–564.
2. Cooley DA, Bloodwell RD, Hallman GL, et al. Organ transplantation for advanced cardiopulmonary disease. Ann Thorac Surg 1969; 8:30–46.
3. Wildevuur CR, Benfield JR. A review of 23 human lung transplantations by 20 surgeons. Ann Thorac Surg 1970; 9:489–515.
4. Reitz BA, Burton NA, Jamieson SW, et al. Heart and lung transplantation, autotransplantation and allotransplantation in primates and extended survival. J Thorac Cardiovasc Surg 1980; 80:360–372.
5. Bennett LE, Keck BM, Daily OP, et al. Worldwide Thoracic Organ Transplantation: a report from the UNOS/ISHLT International Registry for Thoracic Organ Transplantation. Clin Transpl 2001; 1:25–40.

6. Trulock EP, Edwards LB, Taylor DO, et al. The Registry of the International Society for Heart and Lung Transplantation: twenty-first official adult lung and heart–lung transplant report- 2004. J Heart Lung Transplant 2004; 23(7):804–815.
7. Anyanwu AD, Rogers CA, Murday AJ, the Steering Group. Intrathoracic organ transplantation in the United Kingdom 1995–1999: results from the UK cardiothoracic transplant audit. Heart 2002; 87:449–454.
8. The Toronto Lung Transplant Group. Unilateral lung transplantation for pulmonary fibrosis. N Engl J Med 1986; 314:1140–1145.
9. Patterson G, Cooper J, Goldman B, et al. Techniques of successful clinical double-lung transplantation. Ann Thorac Surg 1988; 45:626–633.
10. Pielsticker EJ, Martinez FJ, Rubenfire M. Lung and heart–lung transplant practice patterns in pulmonary hypertension centers. J Heart Lung Transplant 2001; 20:1297–1304.
11. Whyte RI, Robbins RC, Altinger J, et al. Heart–lung transplantation for primary pulmonary hypertension. Ann Thorac Surg 1999; 67:937–942.
12. Mendeloff EN, Meyers BF, Sundt TM, et al. Lung transplantation for pulmonary vascular disease. Ann Thorac Surg 2002; 73:209–219.
13. Franke U, Wiebe K, Harringer W, et al. Ten years experience with lung and heart–lung transplantation in primary and secondary pulmonary hypertension. Eur J Cardiothorac Surg 2000; 18:447–452.
14. Waddell TK, Bennett L, Kennedy R, et al. Heart–lung or lung transplantation for Eisenmenger syndrome. J Heart Lung Transplant 2002; 21:731–737.
15. Pigula FA, Gandhi SK, Ristich J, et al. Cardiopulmonary transplantation for congenital heart disease in the adult. J Heart Lung Transplant 2001; 20:297–303.
16. Stoica SC, McNeil KD, Perreas K, et al. Heart–lung transplantation for Eisenmenger syndrome: early and long-term results. Ann Thorac Surg 2001; 72:1897–1891.
17. Barlow CW, Robbins RC, Moon MR, et al. Heart–lung versus double-lung transplantation for suppurative lung disease. J Thorac Cardiovasc Surg 2000; 119:466–476.
18. Vricella LA, Karamichalis JM, Ahmad S, et al. Lung and heart–lung transplantation in patients with end-stage cystic fibrosis: the Stanford experience. Ann Thorac Surg 2002; 74:13–18.
19. Conte JV, Jhaveri R, Borja MC, et al. Combined heart–single lung transplantation: a unique operation for unique indications. J Heart Lung Transplant 2002; 21:1250–1253.
20. Fann JI, Wilson MK, Theodore J, et al. Combined heart and single-lung transplantation in complex congenital heart disease. Ann Thorac Surg 1998; 65:823–825.
21. Talbot SM, Taub RN, Keohan ML, et al. Combined heart and lung transplantation for unresectable primary cardiac sarcoma. J Thorac Cardiovasc Surg 2002; 124:1145–1148.
22. Prasseedom RK, McNeil KD, Watson CJE, et al. Combined transplantation of the heart, lung and liver. Lancet 2000; 358:812–813.
23. Pirenne J, Verleden G, Nevens F, et al. Combined liver and (heart-) lung transplantation in liver transplant candidates with refractory portopulmonary hypertension. Transplantation 2002; 73:140–156.

24. Anyanwu AC, Banner NR, Radley-Smith R, et al. Long-term results of cardiac transplantation from live donors: the domino heart transplant. J Heart Lung Transplant 2002; 21:971–975.
25. Oaks TE, Aravot D, Dennis C, et al. Domino heart transplantation: the Papworth experience. J Heart Lung Transplant 1994; 13(3):433–437.
26. Huffman MD, McLaughlin VV. Pulmonary arterial hypertension: new management options. Curr Treat Options Cardiovasc Med 2004; 6(6):451–458.
27. Conte JV, Gaine SP, Orens JB, et al. The influence of continuous intravenous prostacyclin on the timing and outcome of transplantation for primary pulmonary hypertension. J Heart Lung Transplant 1998; 17:679–685.
28. Suleman N, Frost AE. Transition from epoprostenol and treprostinil to the oral endothelin receptor antagonist bosentan in patients with pulmonary hypertension. Chest 2004; 126(3):808–815.
29. Dandel M, Hetzer R. Clinical value of prostacyclin and its analogs in the management of pulmonary arterial hypertension. Curr Vasc Pharmacol 2003; 1(2): 171–181.
30. Badesch DB, McLaughlin VV, Delcroix M, et al. Prostanoid therapy for pulmonary arterial hypertension. J Am Coll Cardiol 2004; 16(12, Suppl S):56S–61S.
31. Langleben D, Hirsch AM, Shalit E, et al. Sustained symptomatic, functional and hemodynamic benefit with the selective endothelin-A receptor antagonist, Sitaxsentan, in patients with pulmonary arterial hypertension. Chest 2004; 126: 1377–1381.
32. Doyle RL, McCrory D, Channick RN, et al. Surgical treatments/interventions for pulmonary arterial hypertension. Chest 2004; 126:63S–71S.
33. Kothari SS, Yusuf A, Juneja R, et al. Graded balloon atrial septostomy in severe pulmonary hypertension. Indian Heart J 2002; 54:164–169.
34. Sandoval J, Gaspar J, Pulido T, et al. Graded balloon dilation atrial septostomy in severe primary pulmonary hypertension: a therapeutic alternative for patients nonresponsive to vasodilator treatment. J Am Coll Cardiol 1998; 32: 297–304.
35. D'Armini A, Cattadori B, Monterosso C, et al. Pulmonary thromboendarterectomy in patients with chronic thromboembolic hypertension: hemodynamic characteristics and changes. Eur J Cardiothorac Surg 2000; 18:696–702.
36. Hartz RS, Bryne J, Levitsky S, et al. Predictors of mortality in pulmonary thromboendarterectomy. Ann Thorac Surg 1996; 62:1255–1260.
37. Moffatt-Bruce SD, Karamichalis J, Robbins RC, et al. Are heart–lung transplant recipients protected from developing bronchiolitis obliterans syndrome? Ann Thorac Surg 2006; 81(1):286–291.
38. Lim TT, Botas J, Ross H, et al. Are heart–lung transplant recipients protected from developing transplant coronary artery disease? Circulation 1996; 94: 1573–1577.
39. Soghikian MV, Valentine VG, Berry GJ, et al. Impact of Ganciclovir prophylaxis on heart–lung and lung transplant recipients. J Heart Lung Transplant 1996; 15:881–887.
40. Penn I. Posttransplant malignancy. Transplant Proc 1999; 31:1260–1262.
41. Swinnen LJ. Treatment of organ transplant-related lymphoma. Hematol Oncol Clin North Am 1997; 11:963–967.

42. Gao S, Chaparro SV, Perlroth M, et al. Post-transplantation lymphoprolifera-tive disease in heart and heart–lung transplant recipients: 30-year experience at Stanford University. J Heart Lung Transplant 2003; 22:505–514.
43. Anyanwu AC, McGuire A, Rogers CA, et al. An economic evaluation of lung transplantation. J Thorac Cardiovasc Surg 2002; 123:411–420.

# 12

# Lung Allocation in the United States

**Thomas M. Egan**

*Division of Cardiothoracic Surgery, Department of Surgery, University of North Carolina at Chapel Hill, Chapel Hill, North Carolina, U.S.A.*

**Leah B. Edwards and Matthew A. Coke**

*United Network for Organ Sharing (UNOS), Richmond, Virginia, U.S.A.*

**Susan Murray and Tempie H. Shearon**

*Scientific Registry of Transplant Recipients (SRTR), University of Michigan, Ann Arbor, Michigan, U.S.A.*

**Rami Bustami**

*Scientific Registry of Transplant Recipients (SRTR), University Renal Research and Education Association (URREA), University of Michigan, Ann Arbor, Michigan, U.S.A.*

## INTRODUCTION

This chapter discusses the evolution of the new United States lung allocation system and reviews the data analyses that led to its development. Progress in lung transplantation lagged behind that of other solid organs, in part because of difficulties with bronchial anastomotic healing in the precyclosporine era and the problems with early graft failure attributed to acute rejection and the susceptibility of the newly implanted graft to infection. The introduction of cyclosporine A allowed for clinical success with heart–lung and isolated lung transplantation in the early 1980s (1,2).

## CURRENT ALGORITHM

In 1990, the responsibility for distribution of lungs for transplant was assumed by the Organ Procurement and Transplant Network (OPTN)[a], and the OPTN/UNOS Thoracic Organ Transplantation Committee decided that lungs should be distributed in a manner similar to that for hearts. In 1990, OPTN policy was amended to include policies specific to lung allocation. Prospective candidates were prioritized for lung offers based on the amount of time they had accumulated on the lung transplant waiting list. Lung offers were made first within the donation service area of the local organ procurement organization (OPO), then to candidates registered at centers within concentric 500-nautical-mile circles from the donor hospital. Within each allocation zone, offers were made first to ABO identical recipients, then ABO compatible recipients. Initially, the definition of "local" was interpreted by many programs to mean that individual programs had priority when the donor was within their own hospital. This was later clarified by OPTN policy to define "local" as within a local OPO.

In the early 1990s, there was a provision for a "UNOS/STAT" designation of thoracic organ recipients who were judged to be at imminent risk of death. The UNOS/STAT designation was not mandatory, but allowed OPOs to "jump the list" and offer an organ to a program with a patient who was desperately ill. The UNOS/STAT designation was removed from OPTN policy in 1992, and was ultimately replaced by a system that allocated hearts by urgency status codes.

The demonstration of increased mortality among patients waiting for lung transplant with a diagnosis of idiopathic pulmonary fibrosis (IPF) led the Thoracic Committee to change policy in 1995 to provide candidates listed for lung transplant with a diagnosis of IPF an automatic 90 days of additional waiting time in an attempt to direct organs to these patients because of the demonstrated higher risk of waiting-list mortality.

During the 1990s, lung transplantation became recognized as an effective therapy to palliate patients with end-stage lung disease. The number of lung transplant programs grew, but the number of suitable lung donors could not keep pace with the demand for lungs, resulting in increasing numbers of patients being listed, and increasing numbers of deaths on the lung transplant waiting list (Fig. 1). An unintended consequence of employing waiting time for allocation was the frustration experienced by OPOs trying to place lungs. The turndown rates in actual match run data appeared to be much higher for lungs than for hearts and livers, perhaps because intended lung recipients able to wait the longest could afford to wait even longer.

---

[a] The United Network for Organ Sharing (UNOS) is a private not-for-profit corporation that has operated the OPTN under contract by the Health Resource Services Administration (HRSA) since the creation of the OPTN.

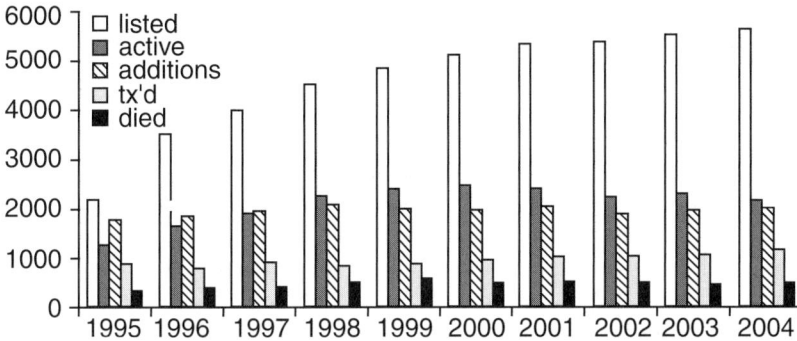

**Figure 1** Number of potential recipients listed (*open bars*), number listed in active status (*solid grey bars*), and new additions during the year (*hatched bars*) for isolated lung transplantation; number of isolated lung transplants performed by year (*dots in bars*); and number of patients dying on the lung transplant list (*black bars*) by year. *Source*: Scientific Registry of Transplant Recipients.

## IMPETUS FOR CHANGE

In 1999, the Department of Health and Human Services (DHHS) published the Final Rule (3). This required the OPTN to amend organ distribution algorithms to direct organs to those most in need, which DHHS defined as those patients most at risk of death without a transplant. The rule also required the OPTN to develop organ distribution algorithms that balanced this medical urgency with utility, i.e., the OPTN policies should prevent futile transplants in patients who were not likely to survive the procedure. Another feature of the Final Rule was that algorithms must minimize the effects of geography and waiting time on prioritization of candidates. Alternately, the OPTN could demonstrate that current organ distribution algorithms satisfied these principles.

A report was commissioned from the Institute of Medicine (IOM) to respond to publication of the Final Rule (4). Although the IOM report and subsequent press coverage and public discussion focused on liver transplantation, the Final Rule directed the OPTN to ensure that *all* organ distribution algorithms were compliant with the objectives espoused in the rule. Accordingly, the OPTN/UNOS Thoracic Committee created a Lung Allocation Subcommittee to review allocation policy and make recommendations for a system to distribute donor lungs for transplant. The Subcommittee's deliberations began in 1999. At the outset, there was consensus that waiting time was not the most appropriate criterion for distribution of potentially life-saving organs. A study of lung transplant candidates on the waiting list by Hosenpud et al. demonstrated a higher waiting-list mortality risk in the United States for patients listed with IPF or cystic fibrosis (CF) compared with patients with chronic obstructive pulmonary disease (COPD) (5).

Additionally, Hosenpud's analysis suggested that for the cohort of COPD patients transplanted, there did not appear to be a survival benefit for lung transplant, even when the analysis was carried out beyond two years (5). In another analysis of CF patients, a survival benefit of lung transplantation in the United States could not be demonstrated (6), although neither of these analyses examined the potential for a quality-of-life benefit.

Ultimately, the Subcommittee sought to develop a method of prioritizing candidates for lung transplantation based on principles of urgency and utility. The Subcommittee believed that an ideal allocation system would minimize deaths on the waiting list, while at the same time maximizing the benefit of transplant by incorporating posttransplant survival into the algorithm. The ethical issues and dilemmas discussed by members of the Subcommittee have been reviewed (7). Essentially, it was the opinion of the Subcommittee that when suitable organs became available for transplantation, they should be offered first to patients at the highest risk of mortality on the waiting list, balanced somehow with the probability of post-transplant survival. That is, if two patients had a high risk of dying on the waiting list, then the lung or lungs should be directed to the patient with the best chance of survival post transplant. The next hurdle was to establish whether there were, in fact, reliable predictors of waiting-list mortality and posttransplant survival based on clinical information among wait-listed patients.

## INITIAL ANALYSES

In order to establish if clinical variables could predict waiting-list or posttransplant survival, the initial analyses undertaken by UNOS were limited to adult ($\geq$18 years) patients on the lung transplant waiting list. A total of 3413 patients were analyzed, consisting of patients wait-listed between January 1, 1997, and December 31, 1998 (for COPD, CF, and IPF patients) and between January 1, 1995, and December 31, 1998 [for patients with primary pulmonary hypertension (PPH)], in order to obtain a cohort of sufficient size ($n = 636$ PPH patients). These four diagnoses accounted for approximately 80% of all wait-listed patients. A Cox proportional hazards regression model was fitted for each of the diagnoses using death on the waiting list as the outcome. Patients transplanted were censored at the time of transplant. Thirty variables collected at the time of listing from the candidate registration form were considered for inclusion in each model.

There was a striking effect of diagnosis on waiting-list mortality risk. Although there were equivalent *numbers* of deaths among each diagnostic group, the *percentage* of wait-listed patients dying by the time of analysis was 13.8% for COPD patients, 33% for IPF patients, 28% for CF patients, and 30% for patients with PPH. For each of these four groups, risk factors could be identified that were significant predictors of increased or decreased hazard of death on the waiting list (8).

Some surprising findings were (i) the lack of association of forced expiratory volume in one second ($FEV_1$) with increased risk of death on the waiting list for CF patients and (ii) that the severity of pulmonary hypertension was not associated with an increased risk of mortality among patients wait-listed with PPH. FEV-1 has been recognized as a major predictor of mortality among CF patients in the CF registry. And, there is a well-documented association of parameters of right heart function, including central venous pressure (CVP) and pulmonary artery (PA) pressures, with survival among patients with PPH (10). However, data on CVP and right atrial pressure were not recorded by the OPTN, and thus CVP was not available for the analysis. In addition, closer scrutiny suggested that only patients with *end-stage* CF and pulmonary hypertension were on the U.S. lung transplant waiting list, and the relatively narrow range of $FEV_1$ values in CF patients and PA pressure values in PPH patients reduced the power of these parameters to identify patients at an increased risk of death.

To determine if there were predictors of posttransplant death, 2484 patients with the same four diagnoses undergoing isolated lung transplantation between January 1, 1996, and June 30, 1999, were analyzed. These four diagnoses accounted for 83% of the transplants performed within this 3.5-year interval. A logistic regression model was fitted for each diagnosis using death within one year of lung transplant as the outcome. One-year survival was chosen for this analysis based on the premise that pretransplant factors that played a role in posttransplant survival would have a diminishing impact as time went on after transplant. Beyond one year, the cause of death and factors responsible for death were judged to be different from the immediate perioperative factors. The same clinical variables collected at the time of listing or updated at the time of transplant were considered for inclusion in the model. Once again, diagnosis was an important predictor of outcome at one year, with 80% of COPD and CF patients surviving one year, but only 66% of IPF patients and 64% of PPH patients (11) surviving.

In general, patients had a significantly increased risk of death if they were older (for both COPD and IPF), or if they were in the ICU or on a ventilator at the time of transplant. Being on a ventilator at the time of transplant for 22 CF patients was associated with a 75% survival at one year, which was not statistically significantly different from nonventilated patients. However, being on a ventilator at the time of transplant significantly reduced survival for COPD patients and even more so for patients with IPF and PPH, but the number of ventilated patients transplanted was small (10 or less in each of the other three diagnoses). Interestingly, no variable associated with poor pulmonary function or hemodynamics was associated with an increased risk of death within the first year following lung transplantation.

These initial analyses demonstrated that diagnosis and clinical data provided at the time of listing could assist in predicting both risk of death on the waiting list and posttransplant survival, and confirmed some of the findings of Hosenpud's analyses on an earlier cohort of patients. After completion of these initial analyses, the contract for the Scientific Registry of Transplant Recipients (SRTR) was awarded to the University Renal Research and Education Association at the University of Michigan, resulting in a change in staff primarily responsible for statistical analyses used in the development of the new lung allocation system.

## OTHER ISSUES TO RESOLVE

### Other Diagnoses

The Lung Allocation Subcommittee next considered how to perform analyses that would include all patients on the lung transplant waiting list, not just the 80% of patients with the four most prevalent diagnoses. One option was to attempt to identify risk factors that were independent of diagnosis, but the consensus of lung transplant clinicians on the Subcommittee was that different types of end-stage lung diseases had different natural histories and probably different risk factors for waiting-list death and posttransplant survival; this was supported by compelling data demonstrating the importance of diagnosis. Thus, the Subcommittee reviewed data for other diagnostic groups with relatively small numbers for probability of waiting-list survival and observed posttransplant survival. Based on these survival probabilities and the pathophysiology of the underlying disease (i.e., primarily obstructive, restrictive, vascular, or infectious), patients with other diagnoses listed for lung transplantation were assigned to one of the four diagnostic groups represented by the four diagnoses initially studied. Groups were designated by letter (Table 1).

This approach worked well for most diagnoses, but patients afflicted with sarcoidosis presented a particular challenge. The pathophysiology of sarcoid lung disease varies among individuals, with some having predominantly restrictive disease, and others having predominantly obstructive disease, with the frequent development of pulmonary hypertension. In fact, when patients with sarcoidosis were stratified based on their PA blood pressure, it appeared that pulmonary hypertension was associated with higher waiting-list mortality and lower posttransplant survival. Patients with sarcoidosis who had normal PA pressures had an apparently more indolent course with a waiting-list mortality and posttransplant survival similar to patients with emphysema. In contrast, patients with sarcoidosis with a mean PA pressure of >30 mmHg had waiting-list and posttransplant survival probability similar to patients with pulmonary fibrosis. Accordingly, patients with sarcoidosis with a mean PA pressure ≤30 mmHg were assigned to Group A, while those with sarcoidosis and a mean PA pressure >30 mmHg Hg were assigned to Group D.

**Table 1**  Diagnostic Groups and Their Constituent Diagnoses

---

*Group A*
Chronic obstructive pulmonary disease (COPD)
Emphysema
Alpha-one antitrypsin deficiency emphysema
Bronchiectasis, including primary ciliary dyskinesia
Lymphangioleiomyomatosis (LAM)
Sarcoidosis with mean PA pressure $\leq 30$ mmHg
*Group B*
Primary pulmonary hypertension (PPH)
Eisenmenger's syndrome
All specific pulmonary vascular diseases, including pulmonary venous obstructive
    disease, chronic pulmonary thromboembolic disease
*Group C*
Cystic fibrosis
Immune deficiency syndromes, e.g., IgG deficiency
*Group D*
Idiopathic pulmonary fibrosis
All other restrictive lung diseases, including hemosiderosis
Eosinophilic granulomatosis
Sarcoidosis with mean PA pressure $>30$ mmHg
Scleroderma/CREST
Bronchoalveolar carcinoma (BAC)
Bronchiolitis obliterans syndrome (BOS) following lung transplant
Primary graft failure following lung transplant

---

*Abbreviations*: CREST, calcinosis, Raynaud phenomenon, esophageal motility disorders, sclerodactyly, telangiectasia; PA, pulmonary artery.

Cox proportional hazards models were constructed, for both waiting-list survival and posttransplant survival, using the same cohorts, but this time using *all* patients on the U.S. lung transplant waiting list, with each patient assigned to one of four groups (Table 1). These analyses identified essentially the same clinical variables as important predictors of waiting-list mortality and posttransplant survival with similar hazard ratios. Thus, the addition of different but pathophysiologically similar diagnoses to each of the four groups did not have a dramatic impact on the models.

## Incorporation of Pediatric Patients

Based on analysis of the distribution of diagnoses, waiting-list survival probabilities, and posttransplant survival by age for patients <18 years old, it appeared that there was a "break point" at age 12. Adolescent and teenage lung transplant recipients ≥11 years old had similar diagnoses and waiting-list and posttransplant survival as young adults, while children <12 years old had different diagnoses and survival probabilities. Thus, the Subcommittee decided to group all potential recipients <12 years old together as a separate group (Group E), and include all patients ≥12 years old together in Groups A–D.

Analyses were repeated for *all* patients listed between January 1, 1997, and December 31, 1998. Because of the relatively small number of patients with pulmonary vascular disease, data were analyzed for Group B patients listed between January 1, 1995, and December 31, 1998. Group-specific Cox regression models were used to predict death on the waiting list. Patients were censored at the time of transplant. Statistically significant factors were identified for Groups A–D that were similar to the earlier analysis, and hazard ratios were calculated for these factors (12). The number of patients in Group E ($n = 131$) and the small number of waiting-list deaths ($n = 43$) made interpretation of data for this group unreliable.

Because of the difficulty with this approach for patients <12 years old, it was decided that time on the waiting list was an appropriate way to allocate lungs to this small group of patients; this decision was reached after consultation with large-volume pediatric lung transplant programs at Children's Hospital of Philadelphia and St. Louis Children's Hospital, Washington University. A separate analysis determined that recipients in this age group were most often assigned lungs from donors of a similar age. Hence, it was recommended that lungs from donors <12 years old be offered first to patients <12 years old based on waiting time, while lungs from donors ≥12 years old be offered to potential recipients based on the opportunity for enhanced survival if transplant were performed. After consultation with representatives from the OPTN/UNOS Pediatric Transplantation Committee, it was ultimately decided that lungs from donors aged 12 to17 would first be offered to candidates 12 to 17 years of age according to allocation score, and then be offered to candidates <12 years of age by waiting time before being offered to adults according to allocation score. Similarly, lungs from donors <12 years old would first be offered to candidates <12 years of age by waiting time, then to adolescents aged 12 to 17 years by allocation score, and then to adults by allocation score.

A subsequent analysis of all patients transplanted in the same time frame (January 1, 1997, to December 31, 1998, for Groups A, C, D, and E and January 1, 1995, to December 31, 1998, for Group B to increase the number of transplants) was performed to establish whether data at the time of listing or transplant could identify factors associated with increased or decreased chance of survival following transplant. Group-specific Cox models were fit with posttransplant death as the outcome to identify these factors, and hazard ratios were calculated that allowed estimation of patient-specific survival probabilities over time. Cox models were chosen in preference to logistic regression analysis because of improved handling of censored patient histories and flexibility in studying areas under patient-specific survival curves during the first year after transplantation. Again, diagnostic group was a significant predictor of survival, and within each group, factors were identified that were significant predictors of death following lung transplantation (13).

## Gameable Factors

A number of factors that were identified as statistically significant were judged by the Lung Allocation Subcommittee to be inappropriate to incorporate into an organ distribution algorithm because they were subject to manipulation by patients or their physicians. An example is a dose of prednisone $\geq 5$ mg/day for Group A patients, which was associated with an increased risk of death on the waiting list. These factors were eliminated from the models but this had little effect on the other variables that were judged appropriate for inclusion in the algorithm.

## Necessity to Provide Clinical Data

If lung allocation is based on data related to wait-listed patients' illness, then it follows that there must be some mandate to provide the data necessary to allow the algorithm to rank order patients. It also follows that candidates' relative positions on the list should change as their illnesses progress. This is accomplished by allowing centers to update wait-listed patient data at any time, but centers are *required* to update specific data elements for all wait-listed patients every six months. It is anticipated that *serial* clinical data on the same patient will be useful to identify new factors that should be incorporated into the distribution algorithm, and that serially collected patient data may affect the import of factors identified as significant in the analyses.

## Keeping the Algorithm Current

In order to keep the algorithm as current as possible, and to adapt to the population of patients being listed and transplanted with end-stage lung disease, the Lung Allocation Subcommittee recommended that analyses be undertaken to identify factors and modify their hazard ratios in the algorithm at least every six months. In order to have sufficient numbers of events to provide sufficient statistical power for significance of observations, the most recent three-year cohort of wait-listed and transplanted patients for whom one-year follow-up is available will be analyzed every six months. Parameter estimates will be modified, and new risk factors identified and incorporated into the algorithm, after approval by the Thoracic Committee and the OPTN/UNOS Board of Directors. Thus, as lung candidates are transplanted and removed from the list, and new candidates are added, and as transplant practice changes and outcomes improve, the effect of *current* risk factors for patients being listed and transplanted will be taken into account.

## THE LUNG ALLOCATION SCORE: HOW THE ALGORITHM ORDERS CANDIDATES

### The Meaning of Survival

Although it is possible to predict survival probabilities for patients on the waiting list and after transplant, two patients with identical one-year survival probabilities might have very different outcomes in the first three, six, or nine months. The Subcommittee had to decide whether to use the survival rate at a specified time point (e.g., one year) or total days of predicted survival, which would be the area under a predicted survival curve. The dilemma is depicted in Figure 2. Ultimately, the Subcommittee decided to employ area under the curve, representing total days of predicted survival within one year on the waiting list or one year posttransplant to determine an allocation score.

### Definitions

To understand how a lung allocation score is derived, a few definitions are necessary.

*Waiting-list urgency measure*: Expected number of days lived without a transplant during an additional year on the waiting list (area under the 1-year waiting-list survival curve).

*Posttransplant survival measure*: Expected number of days lived during the first year post transplant (area under the one-year posttransplant survival curve).

*Transplant benefit = posttransplant survival measure − waiting-list urgency measure*, i.e., the number of expected additional days of life over

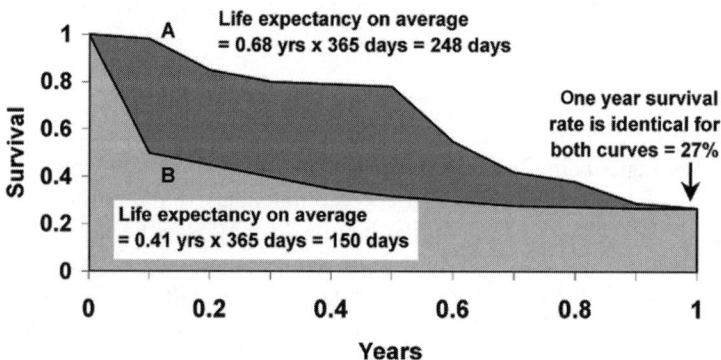

**Figure 2** Two hypothetical patient populations can have similar *interval* one-year survival, but Group A (*top line*) experiences more days of survival than Group B (*lower line*). If interval one-year survival is used, these groups are indistinguishable. If area under the curve (representing total "person-days" survived) is used, the difference between the two populations is clearer. Population A has more days of survival than population B.

the next year if a particular candidate received a transplant rather than remaining on the waiting list.

Note that the benefit might well be *negative*, i.e., patients with a high probability of survival on the waiting list or a low posttransplant survival measure might have a negative transplant benefit.

### Predicting Survival Pre- and Posttransplant

From the hazard ratios determined from Cox models, predicted waiting-list and posttransplant survival curves can be constructed for each patient based on current data in the OPTN database. An example for a hypothetical patient is presented in Figure 3. This patient clearly has a survival advantage if the patient were transplanted, because the predicted posttransplant survival exceeds the predicted waiting-list survival. This difference is defined as the "transplant benefit."

### Balancing Urgency and Benefit

The Subcommittee deliberated about how to balance urgency with posttransplant survival. The concept of somehow incorporating transplant benefit was novel, and was appealing because it might reduce the number of futile transplants performed in desperate situations when the outcome was predictably poor. The current liver allocation system (MELD) is based solely on urgency or waiting-list survival, as is the status system for heart allocation. However, there was concern that a system for lung allocation

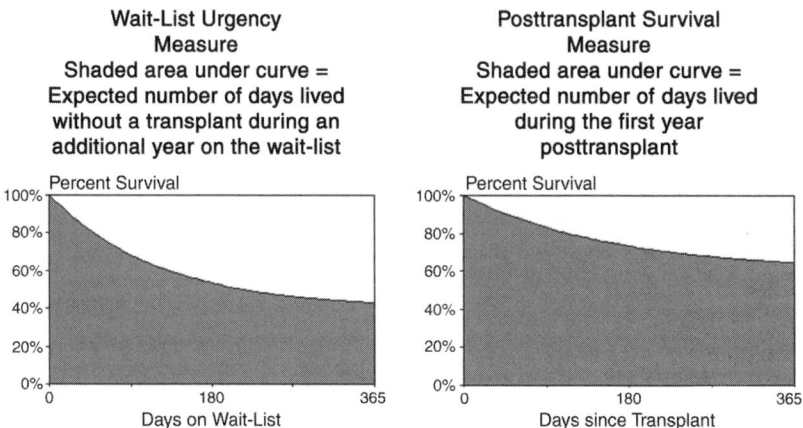

**Figure 3**  Example of a waiting-list survival curve (*left*) and posttransplant survival curve (*right*) for a hypothetical patient. Area under the waiting-list curve is a measure of transplant urgency, while area under the posttransplant survival curve is a measure of projected first-year posttransplant survival. The difference between the two is a measure of transplant benefit.

based solely on urgency would likely direct lungs to ventilated patients or critically ill candidates with a high probability of posttransplant demise.

The options for combining urgency with transplant benefit are depicted in Figure 4. Lungs could be allocated solely on the basis of benefit alone (Fig. 4A) or on the basis of urgency alone (Fig. 4B), or equal consideration

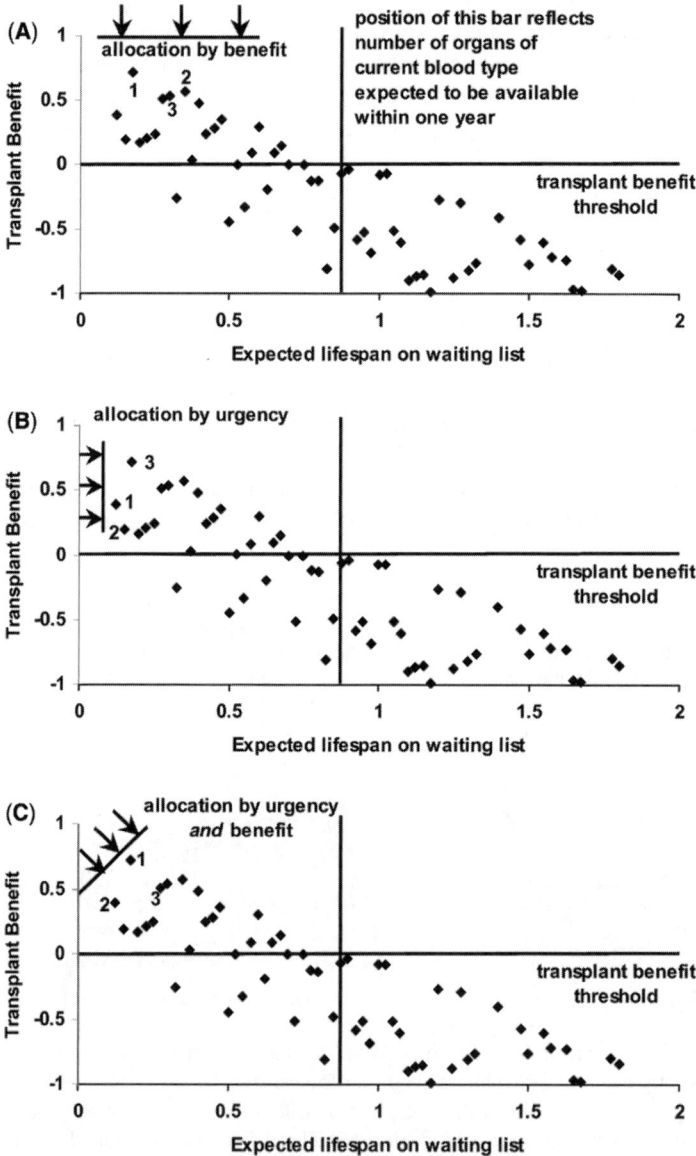

**Figure 4** (*Caption on facing page*)

could be given to urgency and benefit (Fig. 4C). Alternatively, benefit could be weighted over urgency, or urgency could be considered more than benefit. After considerable deliberation, and some mathematical modeling by the SRTR with the thoracic simulated allocation model (TSAM), the Subcommittee decided to recommend that urgency and benefit have equal weight in an allocation scheme, modeled in Figure 4C as the 45° bar descending through the points on the scatter plot representing listed patients.

## DETERMINING THE LUNG ALLOCATION SCORE

Raw allocation score = transplant benefit measure

− waiting-list urgency measure

= (Posttransplant survival measure

− waiting-list urgency measure)

− waiting-list urgency measure

= Posttransplant survival measure

− 2 × (waiting-list urgency measure)

The "2" in the equation produces the 45° angle in the graphic in Figure 4C. Other choices of weighting the importance of urgency would produce a

---

**Figure 4** (*Facing page*) Scatter plots of a hypothetical population of patients of a particular blood type of expected waiting-list survival and calculated transplant benefit (transplant benefit = expected posttransplant survival − expected waiting-list survival). Patients below the "transplant benefit threshold" have a negative transplant benefit. Only so many organs will become available within one year for this blood group, so not all listed patients can be transplanted. As time progresses, more patients can be added to the scatter plot; patients are removed if they are transplanted or if they die or are removed from the waiting list. (**A**) If organs were offered solely based on *transplant benefit*, the allocation order is depicted as a horizontal bar descending through the patient points on the scatter plot, with the allocation order as shown (1–3). (**B**) If organs were offered solely based on *urgency*, the allocation order is depicted as a vertical bar crossing through the patient points on the scatter plot, with the allocation order as shown (1–3). (**C**) If organs are offered based on a *combination* of transplant benefit and urgency, giving equal weight to both, then the allocation order is depicted as a 45° bar descending through the patient points on the scatter plot as depicted with the allocation order as shown (1–3). Different angles of this bar would give different weight to urgency or benefit. The Lung Allocation Subcommittee reviewed TSAM analyses performed by SRTR that modeled the number of total deaths (waitlist and posttransplant) for different angles: 0° (Fig. 4A), 30°, 60° and 90° (Fig. 4B). There was only a modest difference between the 0°, 30°, and 45° angles, but there were clearly more deaths predicted for 60° and 90°. The members of the Lung Allocation Subcommittee felt that balancing urgency and benefit *equally* was the most appropriate way to design the algorithm. *Abbreviations*: TSAM, thoracic simulated allocation model, resulting in adopting the 45° angle; SRTR, Scientific Registry of Transplant Recipients.

different equation. The possible range of values for the raw allocation score would be from $+365$ to $-730$ (the two extremes of 100% survival post transplant but dying today without a transplant to a 100% chance of living for a year on the waiting list but a 100% probability of dying before the first day after a transplant). Clearly, neither extreme is likely, but the Subcommittee felt that negative allocation scores would be difficult to understand. (A negative raw score simply means that the calculated posttransplant survival measure is less than twice the calculated waiting-list urgency measure.) Accordingly, it was decided to "normalize" the score and produce a range from 0 to 100 according to the following formula:

$$\text{Lung allocation score} = \frac{100 \times (\text{raw score} + 2 \times 365)}{3 \times 365}$$

This system can be used to rank order all candidates waiting for lung transplantation, and gives equal consideration to benefit and urgency. The system is "data driven," i.e., the factors important for determining the predictions of waiting-list and posttransplant survival are based on clinical criteria of individual patients that can change as their disease progresses, and as circumstances change in the treatment of patients with end-stage lung disease.

## INITIAL FEEDBACK

The proposed changes were presented to members of the pulmonary medicine and transplant communities at a Lung Allocation Consensus Conference in March 2003. Although there was agreement among the lung transplant community that waiting time was not an ideal way to allocate such a scarce resource as donor lungs, there was no consensus concerning the best way to improve the system. There was general agreement that a new system aimed at reducing deaths and incorporating posttransplant survival was a laudable goal. Participants expressed concern about the methods used to accomplish this, the use of one-year posttransplant survival instead of a longer interval, the effect of missing data and the currency of the data (because only data available at the time of listing were used to calculate waiting-list mortality). There was also considerable opposition to "grouping" diagnoses together.

The feedback obtained was incorporated into refinements of the algorithm by the Lung Allocation Subcommittee. In particular, the impact of individual diagnoses was incorporated into the algorithm by calculating parameter estimates for individual diagnoses when there were sufficient numbers of patients. A final overall Cox model combined the four diagnosis groups with parameters distinguishing diagnosis group and individual diagnoses when there were sufficient numbers for these to be estimable. Predictors that were seen to have differential effects on prognosis by diagnosis group in earlier modeling were modeled using interaction terms with diagnosis group. Otherwise, if predictors behaved similarly across diagnosis groups, a common parameter was estimated from all patients. The request for years of additional prospective data collection was felt to be impractical by the Subcommittee and members of the Division of Transplantation of HRSA, who had closely monitored all of the Subcommittee's deliberations leading to development of the algorithm.

## LUNG REVIEW BOARD

A national Lung Review Board was established to adjudicate allocation scores for exceptional cases. It was recognized that there may be circumstances when a lung transplant candidate might not be able to provide the clinical data necessary to calculate a lung allocation score (e.g., the inability to perform reliable pulmonary function tests or obtain data from a right heart catheterization). The Lung Review Board consists of adult and pediatric transplant surgeons and pulmonologists selected from lung transplant centers across the country; they oversee estimates of clinical variables that might not be obtainable from certain patients. The Lung Review Board also hears appeals from transplant programs if it is felt that the algorithm does not provide an accurate allocation score for individual patients when special circumstances justify assigning a score to individual patients separate from the predicted survival estimates provided by the algorithm.

## SUMMARY

The new system for lung allocation in the United States is in a continual state of development and improvement. There have been several debates about the proposal at national and international forums (14). The current system is committed to "self-review" every six months with updated hazard ratios and risk factors for waiting-list and posttransplant death. The OPTN is committed to reviewing the system with the lung transplant community one year after implementation. The ideal system would eliminate deaths on the waiting list but the current shortage of suitable lungs for transplant renders this an elusive goal.

## REFERENCES

1. Reitz BA, Wallwork JL, Hunt SA, et al. Heart-lung transplantation: successful therapy for patients with pulmonary vascular disease. N Engl J Med 1982; 306:557–564.
2. The Toronto Lung Transplant Group. Unilateral lung transplantation for pulmonary fibrosis. N Engl J Med 1986; 314:1140–1145.

3. Department of Health and Human Services. Organ procurement and transplantation network; final rule. In: 42 CFR—Part 121: Federal Register, October 20, 1999:56649–56661.
4. Institute of Medicine, Committee on Non-Heart-Beating Transplantation II. Non-heart-beating Organ Transplantation: Practice and Protocols. Washington, DC: National Academy Press, 2000.
5. Hosenpud JD, Bennett LE, Keck BM, Edwards EB, Novick RJ. Effect of diagnosis on survival benefit of lung transplantation for end-stage lung disease. Lancet 1998; 351:24–27.
6. Liou TG, Adler FR, Cahill BC, et al. Survival effect of lung transplantation among patients with cystic fibrosis. J Am Med Assoc 2001; 286(21):2683–2689.
7. Egan T. Ethical issues in thoracic organ distribution for transplant. Am J Transplant 2003; 3(4):366–372.
8. Egan TM, Bennett LE, Garrity ER, et al. Predictors of death on the UNOS lung transplant waiting list: results of a multivariate analysis (abstract). J Heart Lung Transplant 2001; 20(2):242.
9. Liou TG, Adler FR, Fitzsimmons SC, Cahill BC, Hibbs JR, Marshall BC. Predictive 5-year survivorship model of cystic fibrosis. Am J Epidemiol 2001; 153(4):345–352.
10. D'Alonzo GE, Barst RJ, Ayres SM, et al. Survival in patients with primary pulmonary hypertension: results from a national prospective registry. Ann Intern Med 1991; 115:343–349.
11. Egan TM, Bennett LE, Garrity ER, et al. Are there predictors of death at the time of listing for lung transplant? (abstract). J Heart Lung Transplant 2002; 21(1):154.
12. Egan T, McCullough K, Bustami R, et al. Predictors of death on the UNOS lung transplant waiting list (abstract). J Heart Lung Transplant 2003; 22:S147.
13. Egan T, McCullough K, Murray S, et al. Risk factors for death after lung transplant in the U.S. (abstract). J Heart Lung Transplant 2003; 22:S146–S147.
14. Egan TM. Pro/Con debate: the current time based lung allocation system should be replaced by one based on medical urgency and transplant survival: Pro. Chest 2005; 128(1):407–415.

# 13

# Organ Allocation and Donor Availability—The European Experience

**Hendrik Treede and Hermann Reichenspurner**
*Department of Cardiovascular Surgery, University Heart Center,*
*University of Hamburg, Hamburg, Germany*

## INTRODUCTION

In Western Europe more than 40,000 patients are currently waiting for an organ transplant. A variety of nationally or internationally based transplant organizations are responsible for organ allocation and distribution and several countries have launched national research programs to look into ways to help organ supply meet demand. Yet there is little coordination between the different national programs in Europe. One of the main barriers to joint activity is the variation in organizational structures. Some countries have a national transplantation agency, under control of the Ministry of Health, while others have implemented independent foundations.

Several countries have joined together to create a supranational organization, such as Eurotransplant (ET) and Scandia Transplant. There are also a variety of national transplantation laws setting different standards for organ donation and allocation.

This accumulation of different laws, organizational structures, and programs complicates the presentation of a pan-European experience in organ allocation and donor availability in lung and heart–lung transplantation. Therefore, there will be a focus on the leading organizations.

In 2003, a total of 945 lung transplants have been performed within the most active programs in Europe. ET as the biggest supranational transplant organization representing Germany, Netherlands, Belgium, Austria, Luxembourg, and Slovenia reported 405 transplants, followed by 145 lung transplants in Spain, 135 in the United Kingdom, 103 in Scandia Transplant member countries (Denmark, Norway, Finland, and Sweden), 92 in France, and 65 in Italy.

Within the European countries the number of organ donations per million population varies significantly. The reason for this is the existence of different donation systems.

At present, there are two systems of organ donation:

1. *Presumed consent*: This means that organ donation is automatically considered in patients' diagnosed brain dead unless they have specifically registered their wish not to donate. However, in some countries with a presumed consent law, doctors will still ask permission from relatives.
2. *Informed consent*: This is a voluntary system of organ donation whereby relatives give permission at the time of death, usually in the knowledge that the potential donor had expressed a wish to become a donor or was in possession of a donor card.

Table 1 gives an overview on legislations for organ donation in some European countries.

The important influence of organ donation regulations is becoming obvious by comparing the numbers of donors and patients on the waiting list in countries with different legislations. In the United Kingdom and Germany the rising demand for organs is confronted with falling numbers of organ donors, resulting in a serious organ shortage. Figure 1 demonstrates the development for patients in the ET region in lung and heart–lung transplantation within the last 12 years.

**Table 1**  Legal Situation for Organ Donation in European Countries

| Country | Legal situation |
| --- | --- |
| Austria | Presumed consent |
| Belgium | Presumed consent |
| United Kingdom | Informed consent |
| Germany | Informed consent |
| The Netherlands | Informed consent |
| France | Presumed consent |
| Spain | Presumed consent |
| Finland | Presumed consent |
| Norway | Presumed consent |

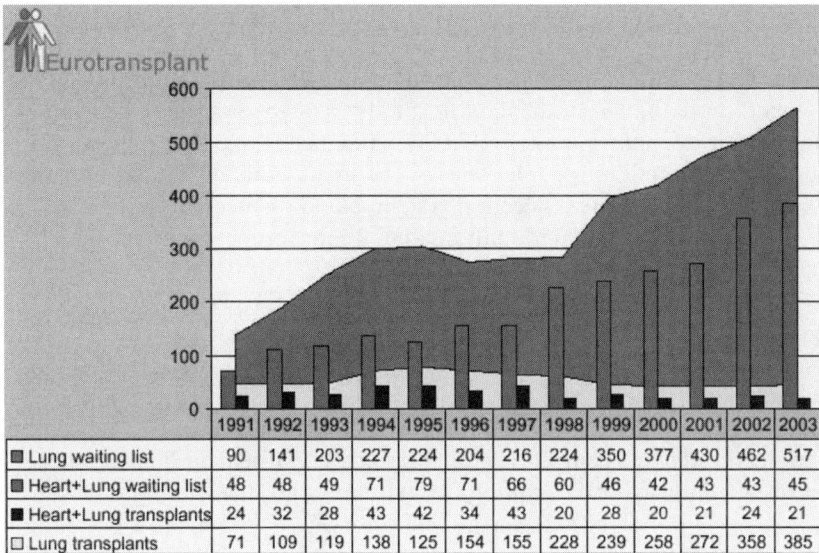

| | 1991 | 1992 | 1993 | 1994 | 1995 | 1996 | 1997 | 1998 | 1999 | 2000 | 2001 | 2002 | 2003 |
|---|---|---|---|---|---|---|---|---|---|---|---|---|---|
| Lung waiting list | 90 | 141 | 203 | 227 | 224 | 204 | 216 | 224 | 350 | 377 | 430 | 462 | 517 |
| Heart+Lung waiting list | 48 | 48 | 49 | 71 | 79 | 71 | 66 | 60 | 46 | 42 | 43 | 43 | 45 |
| Heart+Lung transplants | 24 | 32 | 28 | 43 | 42 | 34 | 43 | 20 | 28 | 20 | 21 | 24 | 21 |
| Lung transplants | 71 | 109 | 119 | 138 | 125 | 154 | 155 | 228 | 239 | 258 | 272 | 358 | 385 |

**Figure 1** Dynamics of the Eurotransplant waiting list and transplants for lung and heart–lung organs.

The situation in Spain looks remarkably different. The Organizacion Nacional de Trasplantes established in 1989 transformed Spain's transplant service from one having a shortage to one exporting surplus organs to neighbor countries. Spain rose from one of the lowest donation rates in the world to become one of the highest, rising from 14 to 25 donors per million population. The increase was the result of a nationwide implementation of a standardized donation process. Hospitals are held responsible for their performance in donation. Since 1986, a law allows obligatory donation unless a refusal is registered in the national computer database. The 46.7 kidney transplants per million population in 2003 were achieved despite the fact that Spain also reached the largest reduction in traffic accidents of the European Union (EU) during the past years. Additionally, the use of heart-beating donors is allowed and promoted by Spanish authorities. Special organ procurement programs take care about patients where resuscitations were not successful. Extracorporal membrane oxygenation is used to maintain blood and gas circulation in donors before the next of kin is asked for their consent to organ donation. Meanwhile, heart-beating donors are used in more than 30% of all lung transplantations performed at the University of Madrid.

## EUROTRANSPLANT

ET was founded in 1967 aiming for a central registration of patients on the waiting list for organ transplants in order to find a good match between tissue groups of donors and recipients. Starting with renal transplantation patients only, the organization expanded early and is now serving as an international database for every kind of clinical transplantation. At the moment, more than 75 transplant hospitals participating in ET have a joint waiting list of approximately 15,000 patients. The ET region numbers more than 118 million people. One of the main goals of ET is to secure a transparent and objective selection system, based on medical criteria, as well as the support of organ donation and donor procurement in order to increase the supply of donor organs.

As a mediator between donor and recipient, ET plays a key role in the acquisition and distribution of donor organs for transplantations. The data of all potential recipients, such as blood group, tissue characteristics (human leukocyte antigen groups), cause of the disease, clinical urgency, and the hospital where the patient is to be transplanted are passed on to ET. This information is stored in a central computer database. Subsequently, the patient is put on the (inter)national waiting list. At that point, the waiting time starts. As soon as a donor becomes available somewhere within the ET area, the regional tissue-typing laboratory determines the donor's blood group and tissue characteristics. All relevant (medical) information about the donor is then transferred on to ET's database. Subsequently, the ET staff enters the donor information into a computer program that selects the patient most suitable to receive the organ of this donor. It is crucial that the donor organ matches as much as possible with the patient. The selection criteria for the most suitable patient vary for different donor organs. For lung transplantation a combination of blood group, height and weight of the donor, clinical urgency, and waiting time are compared for donor/recipient match. The organ usually is allocated in the country where the donor has been reported. Only if no suitable recipient is found organs are offered to the other ET countries. Organs donated from children generally go to child patients to ensure the best match in size but, when there are no suitable child recipients, organs from young people are given to adults. After patient selection, ET staff immediately contacts the physicians in the patient's transplant center to send all information about the donor. These physicians are then responsible for the decision whether or not to accept the organ. If the organ is accepted, the physician immediately contacts the patient.

Patients showing a severe deterioration of their clinical status can achieve a special high urgency (HU) status on the waiting list and are preferentially considered for early transplantation. Centers applying for a HU status of a patient have to explain and substantiate the reasons for their decision. The HU status must then be agreed on by an international audit committee instituted by ET.

As soon as the donor organ has been accepted, the organ procurement and transportation is organized in cooperation with regional coordinators. If there are no suitable recipients within the ET area, ET

**Table 2**  Eurotransplant Lung Transplantation Statistics for 2003 with Total Numbers (*n*) and Lung Transplantations Per Million Population

| No. of patients | Germany | The Netherlands | Austria | Belgium |
|---|---|---|---|---|
| On waiting list (*n*) | 397 | 69 | 37 | 59 |
| Transplanted (*n*) | 192 | 34 | 89 | 68 |
| Lung Tx (pmp) | 2.3 | 2.1 | 10.9 | 6.6 |

*Abbreviations*: Tx, transplantations; pmp, per million population.

gets in touch with one of the other organizations, such as U.K. Transplant or Scandia Transplant.

The total lung transplantation numbers in the ET region in 2003 show substantial differences regarding transplant numbers and waiting list numbers between countries (Table 2). Austria and Belgium, both countries with presumed consent donor legislation, have significantly fewer patients on the waiting list due to more frequent transplantations compared to Germany and the Netherlands where informed consent legislations were implemented. The differences become even more evident when taking into account that Germany has a 10-fold higher population than Austria (83.2 million vs. 8.2 million), which is reflected by the number of lung transplantations per million population.

## LISTING AND DELISTING POLICIES

The policies for acceptance of patients as recipients of donor lungs are similar in all European countries. Patients with end-stage pulmonary diseases dependent on drugs, oxygen, and/or noninvasive mechanical ventilation fulfill the requirements for being listed as organ recipients.

The listing process requires a variety of hemodynamic data, laboratory values, patient history information, and lung function test results. Contraindications for transplants are clinically evident infections, irreversible renal or hepatic failure, history of noncurative treated cancer, systemic illnesses like amyloidosis, severe cerebral or peripheral vascular disease, ongoing nicotine, alcohol or drug abuse, and distinct noncompliance. In special cases exceptions are being made for patients who are candidates for multiorgan transplantations. Patients who are doing better can be delisted any time or set on a nontransplantable (NT) status in terms of infections or other transient problems.

Waiting times for lung transplantations vary a lot between countries and depend on patient size, blood group, and other individual characteristics. ET allows physicians to request an HU status for patients with end-stage pulmonary diseases who have an imminent need for invasive mechanical ventilation, showing a New York Health Association IV status, or suffer from recurrent severe infections in cases of cystic fibrosis. The HU request has to be explained exactly and is sent to an audit committee that decides about acceptance or refusal within 24 hours. The audit committee consists of clinical specialists in the field and is blinded to the site of the request. Decision is made by evaluation of clinical and anamnestic parameters and risk profiles that clearly underline the need for an urgent transplantation. ET coordinates the activities of the audit committees and communicates between request centers and audit staff. HU requests have to be reconfirmed every two weeks in order to keep the HU status for the patient. ET has the right to confirm the HU request data by clinical site visits. The proportion of patient's lung transplanted on a HU status in Germany in 2004 was approximately 50%.

## FUTURE EUROPEAN COOPERATION STRATEGIES

A broad variation in organizational and legislative structures between European countries and transplant organizations makes cooperation and compatibility difficult. In order to simplify structures and facilitate cooperation in the future, the EU has developed a program that aims at the identification of the best possible framework for efficient organ donation and transplantation strategies across Europe. The European Group for Coordination of Research Programs on Organ Donation and Transplantation is working on a structural basis that could help to implement the most efficient structures of every European transplant program in a working platform that exemplarily summarizes the best and most functional systems. This would allow the creation of a European network of organ donation and distribution and would thereby minimize the organ shortage and maximize the use of transplant organs.

# 14

# Allocation of Donor Organs for Lung Transplantation: The Australian Experience

**Trevor J. Williams and Gregory I. Snell**

*Department of Allergy, Immunology, and Respiratory Medicine, The Alfred Hospital, Monash University Clinical School, Melbourne, Victoria, Australia*

## INTRODUCTION

Donor organ shortage remains the major factor limiting the availability of lung transplantation to those with end-stage pulmonary and pulmonary vascular disease. Australia has a low rate of multiorgan donors (9.0 per million per year) but achieves very high rates of lung transplantation (up to 0.48 lung recipients per multiorgan donor). The preparedness to utilize marginal donors is a key factor in the high lung transplant rates. The system of organ allocation gives great discretion to the individual transplant centers and may be a key factor in the ability to seek and utilize marginal lung allografts. The organ allocation system needs to suit the overall system of delivery of medical services. Furthermore, it needs to match the overall expectations and aspirations of the population as well as complying with the relevant statutes. This chapter aims to review the Australian organ allocation system, in particular for thoracic organs, and put this into the broader perspective of the Australian health care system.

## THE AUSTRALIAN HEALTH CARE SYSTEM

Australia is a country of 20 million people with a diverse ethnic background. The original inhabitants (the Australian aborigines) have lived in Australia for 50,000 years. European settlement commenced in 1776 but continued immigration over the following 200 years has led to the diverse ethnic mix.

Geopolitically, Australian is a federation of six states and two territories. The responsibility for the provision and funding of health care is shared between the federal and state/territory governments. Provision of universal health care has been an objective of the Australian health care system for over 30 years. The state and territory governments (through direct federal grants and state taxes) are responsible for providing recurrent and infrastructure funding to maintain a system of major public (university teaching) and community hospitals. The federal government through taxes and levies is responsible for the universal health care insurance system (Medicare), which reimburses medical practitioners and other approved providers a substantial proportion of the costs of medical consultations, procedures, and investigations. Additionally, more than 40% of the population has additional private health insurance, which allows treatment by their practitioner of choice and reimbursement for private hospital costs.

The health service funding and governance, particularly for lung transplantation in Australia, is complex (Fig. 1). A combination of federal, state, and private health insurance payment cover the majority of costs. This complex governance is often inefficient, acting as an incentive to move costs from one authority to another (cost shifting), as it frequently results in disputes between the funding authorities as to who pays for what. Nevertheless, in this system, patients who on medical grounds may benefit from transplantation will be assessed, managed on the waiting list, transplanted, offered ongoing follow-up care, and provided with medications at only modest out of pocket expense. Financial capacity or insurance status is not a limiting factor in obtaining solid organ transplantation in Australia.

Presently, it is estimated that approximately 9% of the Australian gross domestic product is spent on healthcare (1). The population of 20 million is small taking into account Australia's land mass and results in a low population density. A substantial majority of Australians live in the seven state/territory capital cities, or large cities within a 200 km radius of them. Perth, the major West coast city and Western Australia's state capital is more than 3000 km from the eastern seaboard and is the most isolated of these (Fig. 2). Vast areas of Australia have an extremely low population density making access to even basic medical care difficult. Provision of highly specialized services like lung transplant programs needs to take into account these important constraints.

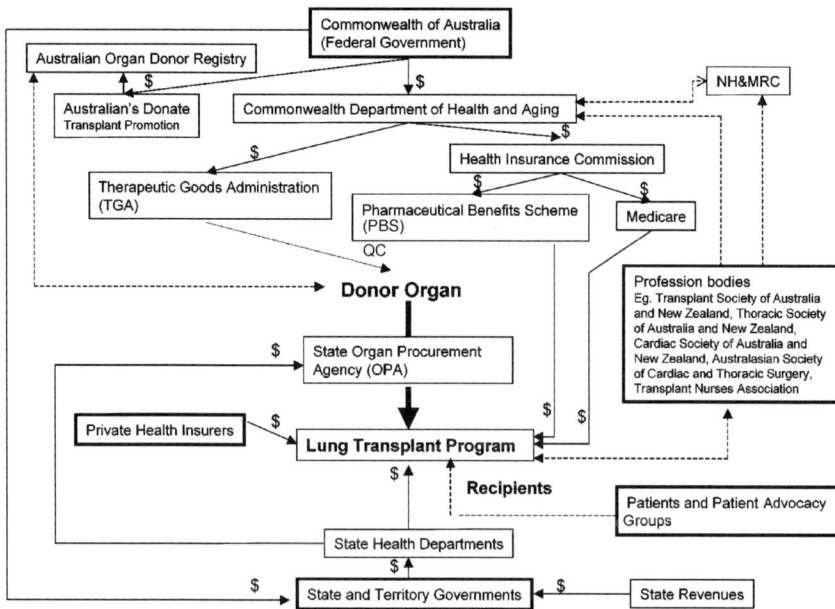

**Figure 1** A schematic diagram illustrating governance of lung transplantation within the Australian health care system. The solid lines indicate financial support and governance. Broken lines reflect consultative relationships.

## ORGAN DONATION IN AUSTRALIA

The legal basis of the use of brain death criteria in heart beating organ donation in Australia is given under the Federal Human Tissue Act 1982 (2). Two decades of renal transplantation had predated this, utilizing donors who had sustained irreversible cardiac arrest or live donors (3). From the time of the Australian Human Tissue Act 1982, which gave the legislative and legal authority for the declaration of brain death, there has been a rapid development of large renal transplant programs, liver transplant programs, cardiac transplant programs, and more recently lung transplant programs. Live donor renal transplantation (increasingly from unrelated donors) is now a common form of renal transplantation (3). Infrequent partial (lobar) liver transplantation from a live (related) donor has been performed but live donor lobar lung transplantation has yet to be performed in Australia.

Renal transplantation utilizing non–heart-beating donors has occasionally been performed in the brain death era. These have been restricted to circumstances where a patient (or next of kin) with a terminal neurological disease has specifically requested this prior to coma and death. No non–heart-beating donor lung transplantation has been performed as yet in Australia but exploration of the logistics is being actively pursued (4). Although there has

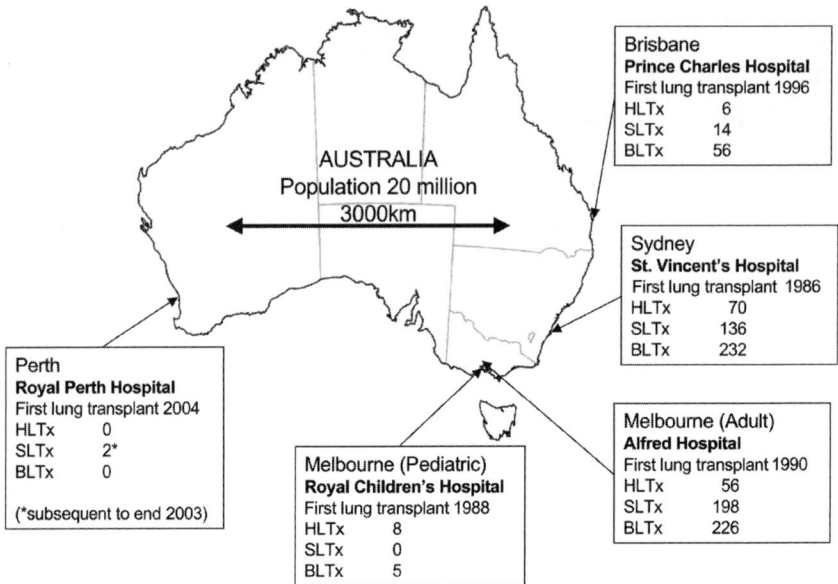

Brisbane
**Prince Charles Hospital**
First lung transplant 1996
HLTx        6
SLTx       14
BLTx       56

AUSTRALIA
Population 20 million
3000km

Sydney
**St. Vincent's Hospital**
First lung transplant 1986
HLTx       70
SLTx      136
BLTx      232

Perth
**Royal Perth Hospital**
First lung transplant 2004
HLTx        0
SLTx        2*
BLTx        0

(*subsequent to end 2003)

Melbourne (Pediatric)
**Royal Children's Hospital**
First lung transplant 1988
HLTx        8
SLTx        0
BLTx        5

Melbourne (Adult)
**Alfred Hospital**
First lung transplant 1990
HLTx       56
SLTx      198
BLTx      226

**Figure 2**   The geographic locations of lung transplant programs in Australia. The date of the first lung transplant and total transplants to the end of 2003 are shown.

been considerable discussion (5) considering opting out legislation or even compulsory organ donation, organ donation in Australia remains voluntary. Indeed, although the Human Tissue Act 1982 allows organ donation to proceed if a clear advanced directive was present despite next of kin objection, the practice still is to only proceed with the consent of the next of kin.

Responsibility for coordinating organ procurement (6,7) resides with state-based organ procurement agencies (OPAs), e.g., "Life Gift" in New South Wales and Victoria run under the auspices of the Australian Red Cross. The OPAs are responsible for obtaining (or confirming) consent from the next of kin, the relevant local authorities including the Coroner, and then liaising with the various solid organ transplant teams with the objective of obtaining the greatest number of suitable organs for transplantation as efficiently as possible. The state-based OPAs provided data regularly to the Australian and New Zealand Organ Donor Registry (ANZODR), which publishes a report annually (7,8).

Perhaps reflecting the altruistic approach to organ donation in Australia, politicians (both federal and state) and the public generally have been highly supportive of the initiative. Indeed, 83% of Australian report a willingness to be organ donor; however, only 50% of next of kin agree to donation when asked (9,10). The promotion of organ donation nationally is coordinated through one organization "Australians Donate," which in its many activities is responsible for the promotion of solid organ donation throughout Australia. As part of this initiative, a national registry of bone marrow and organ donors with a system of voluntary registration has been developed. The Australian Organ Donor register passed five million registrants by January 2005. Web-based technology allows a donor coordinator to ascertain whether an advanced directive in terms of organ donation had been made by a potential donor. Scientific support of organ transplantation in Australia is provided through the Transplant Society of Australia and New Zealand and the various special societies including the Australian Kidney Foundation, The Thoracic Society of Australia and New Zealand, The Australasian Society of Cardiac and Thoracic Surgery, and the Cardiac Society of Australia and New Zealand (6,7). Advice to government is often sought under the auspices of the Australian National Health and Medical Research Council.

Formal organ sharing arrangements exist with New Zealand, Australia's closest neighbor of approximately four million people across the Tasman Sea. Organs that cannot be used in New Zealand are offered in Australia and vice versa. Australian organs are offered preferentially to Australian nationals. Only very occasionally are lung transplants performed on non-nationals; typically they are blood group AB recipients where no suitable recipients in Australia or New Zealand are identified.

## MULTIORGAN DONORS IN AUSTRALIA

### General Description

Multiorgan donation in Australia is presently almost exclusively from heart-beating brain-dead donors according to published national protocols (11). The year 2003 provides a representative snapshot of organ donation in Australia (7,8) from the ANZODR (Fig. 3). From a population of 20 million people there were 179 cadaveric organ donors (9.0 per million). A total of 63 of the 179 were utilized as lung donors (3.2 per million). In the overall donor pool, males represented 60% with a mean age of 45.5 years. A total of 22 had undergone previous cardiopulmonary resuscitation. The initial request for donation was 54% by an intensive care consultant, 36% by a donor coordinator, and 2% by another person. In 8% of cases the family volunteered organs for donation prior to being requested. The cause of death was cerebral vascular accident (CVA) 53%, road trauma 21%, and other trauma 13%, including 3% due to gunshot wound. Other causes of death represented 13%. A total of 49% of cases required referral to the Coroner for permission to proceed to organ donation. All patients were tested serologically for cytomegalovirus (CMV) and 62% were positive. A total of 85% were tested for Epstein–Barr virus IgG and 63% were positive. All donors were tested for hepatitis B, C and HIV as per the protocol (Table 1).

## Lung Transplantation In Australia: 2003 snapshot

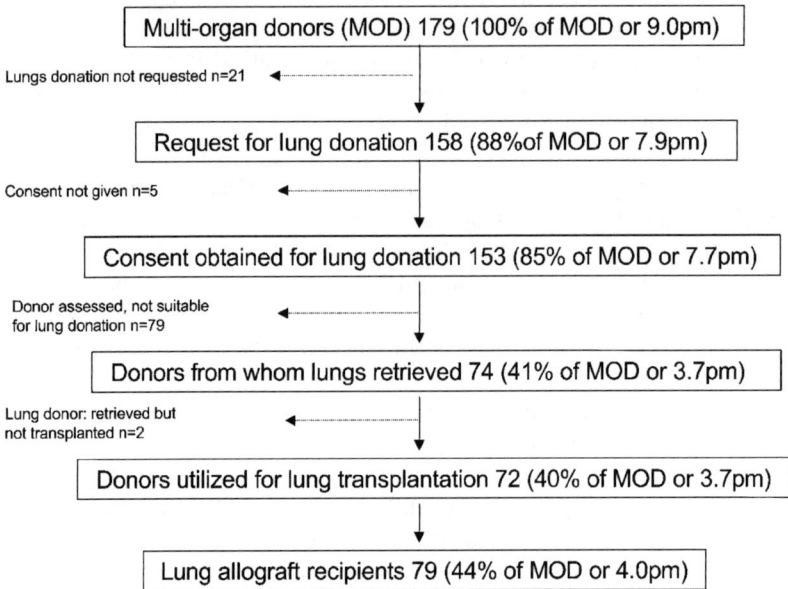

| Multi-organ donors (MOD) 179 (100% of MOD or 9.0pm) |

Lungs donation not requested n=21  ◀┄┄┄┄┄┄┄┄

| Request for lung donation 158 (88%of MOD or 7.9pm) |

Consent not given n=5  ◀┄┄┄┄┄┄┄┄

| Consent obtained for lung donation 153 (85% of MOD or 7.7pm) |

Donor assessed, not suitable
for lung donation n=79  ◀┄┄┄┄┄┄┄┄

| Donors from whom lungs retrieved 74 (41% of MOD or 3.7pm) |

Lung donor: retrieved but
not transplanted n=2  ◀┄┄┄┄┄┄┄┄

| Donors utilized for lung transplantation 72 (40% of MOD or 3.7pm) |

| Lung allograft recipients 79 (44% of MOD or 4.0pm) |

**Figure 3**  A 2003 snapshot of the utilization of multiorgan donors for lung transplantation in Australia. *Source*: From Ref. 8.

### Allocation of Thoracic Organs

Generally, thoracic donor organs are offered for transplantation in their state of origin. If the state program is unable to utilize the organs or there is no state transplant program (often the case with lung transplantation), then the organs are offered on a rotational basis to other interstate programs. For thoracic organ transplantation these offers are normally for the complete heart–lung block, allowing some continued ability to offer heart/lung transplantation where appropriate in Australia.

### LUNG TRANSPLANTATION IN AUSTRALIA

#### Programs

Lung transplantation was first performed in Australia at St Vincent's Hospital in Sydney in 1986 in the form of heart/lung transplantation (12). Early on, hearts from the heart–lung recipients were utilized as domino donors to maximize recipient numbers (13,14). The year 1990 saw the commencement of a lung transplant program in Melbourne, and for several years these were the two nationally funded programs. By late 1990, single-lung

**Table 1** Investigations for Heart–Lung or Lung Donors in Australia

| All multiorgan donors | Blood group for ABO |
|---|---|
| | HIV antibody |
| | Hepatitis B surface antigen |
| | Hepatitis B core IgG antibody (see detailed |
| | guidelines following) |
| | Hepatitis C antibody |
| | Epstein–Barr virus capsid IgG antibody |
| | Beta human chrionic gonadotrophin hormone in |
| | females of child-bearing age dying from |
| | undiagnosed intracerebral hemorrhage |
| | CMV IgG antibody |
| | HTLV I and II antibody |
| | Testing for hepatitis C and HIV using polymerase |
| | chain assays would be highly desirable for |
| | donors in high risk categories either from their |
| | medical history or laboratory tests |
| | A postmortem examination is highly desirable |
| Lung donors (in addition) | Chest X ray |
| | Arterial blood gases on 100% oxygen and 5-cm |
| | PEEP |
| Heart–lung donors (in addition) | EC |
| | Echocardiogram (if requested) |

*Abbreviations*: HTLV, human T lymphotropic virus; CMV, cytomegalovirus; PEEP, positive end-expiratory pressure.
*Source*: From Ref. 7.

transplantation was performed in Australia, and by 1992 the first double-lung transplants had been performed as bilateral sequential lung transplants (15). In 1996, a third program opened in Brisbane, and since this time approximately 100 lung transplant procedures per year have been performed throughout Australia (16). All of these programs, however, were on the eastern seaboard where the substantial majority of the population resides. Teams have regularly traveled from these lung transplant programs to assess and follow-up patients in state capital cities as far away as Perth on the west coast. In late 2004 the first single-lung transplant procedure was performed in Perth making it the fourth Australian adult lung transplant program. Occasional heart–lung and bilateral lung procedures have been performed at the Royal Children's Hospital in Melbourne. The low volume of patients and lack of a dedicated, funded program have led to a voluntary suspension of activities by that institution. At present there is no established pediatric lung transplant program in Australia, with pediatric patients cared for ad hoc by the adult programs. Neonatal lung transplantation is not performed in Australia. Some patients are referred overseas where the expertise and technology does not exist in Australia. The location and transplant activity of the Australian programs are shown in Figure 2.

All transplant programs are run out of large university teaching hospitals and are funded predominantly on a per case basis, usually through the State government. Large multidisciplinary teams have been developed at the major centers, and because of the small number of programs, the St. Vincent's and Alfred Hospital programs in particular are very experienced by international comparison. These two centers between them have performed approximately 5% of all lung transplants performed internationally (16,17).

## Selecting of Recipients

Patients are referred into the transplant center for initial discussion and evaluation. The national guidelines for recipient selection are quite simple (Table 2). The individual programs have developed selection criteria adapted from and substantially conforming to the International Society for Heart and Lung Transplantation/American Thoracic Society (ISHLT/ATS) criteria (18), although with some local variation. Equal opportunity legislation in Australia would prevent exclusion from transplantation purely on chronological age. Somewhat paradoxically, however, there is a strong prevailing view in the Australian community that younger patients should be offered transplantation by preference. The important role of the initial discussion is to outline the likelihood of the patient ever receiving a transplant within the Australian system. The risks, benefits, and the ongoing requirement of adherence to medication and careful follow-up would be also discussed at that time. Pulmonary retransplantation has been rarely performed (1–2% of all lung transplants only) but only in highly selected patients (16).

If a patient has no absolute contraindication to transplantation and chooses to seek formal evaluation this is usually done with a series of prebooked investigations, and an evaluation by the transplant team. This culminates in the presentation of the data to the multidisciplinary transplant team who would be responsible for final recommendation for listing (or not) for lung transplantation. Those listed for lung transplantation are highly

**Table 2**  Recipient Suitability Criteria in Australia

---

1. Lung disease or combined heart and lung disease, which significantly affects expected survival or quality of life of the patient and is not amenable to alternative therapy
2. Accepted onto the waiting list by a recognized heart/lung and lung transplant unit
3. The absence of contraindications including life-threatening nonpulmonary illness considered to preclude successful lung transplantation

---

*Source*: From Ref. 7.

selected from all potential recipients. In the calendar year 2003, throughout Australia 153 potential lung recipients were added to the active waiting list. The net effect of 91 transplants and 23 deaths on the waiting list (as well as several other miscellaneous causes of removal from the waiting list) was a net increase from 108 to 125 in patients actively listed for lung transplantation in Australia (16). The rate of death for lung transplant patients on the waiting list during 2003 was 19.7%.

Once listed, patients must be two to three hours from the transplant center. For practical reasons this means that they must live no more than one to two hours flight distance, which allows most patients to live in their own homes, although patients from the Western Australia and the Northern Territory have needed to relocate to one of the eastern states transplant centers to await transplantation. Patients are not listed on the waiting list of more than one lung transplant program. On the waiting list patients are reviewed regularly by members of the transplant program, which involves regular clinics held in capital cities that have no local lung transplant program.

There is sometimes concern expressed that patients waiting interstate for transplantation are disadvantaged. The ANZCOTR 2003 registry report (16) shows that in the period 1999 to 2003, patients transplanted from Victoria and New South Wales (states serviced by the two largest lung transplant programs) have more recipients relative to donors from those states. However, the greatest donor to recipient discrepancy (excess recipients) was in Western Australia, a state at that time without a program. Furthermore, our own database shows that in a state-to-state comparison, patients are transplanted in equal proportion based on referral numbers. Thus, there does not seem to be a bias in the selection of recipients; it seems more likely that having a program in a particular state increases referral of recipients.

### Donor Criteria

As with most countries around the world the criteria developed for lung transplant donors include general criteria covering all multiorgan donors and specific criteria for heart–lung and isolated lung donation (Table 3). The general criteria primarily concerned with prevention of transmission of serious infection or malignancy into the recipient (Table 1). These involve assessment for and further investigation to assess the risk for transmission of HIV, hepatitis B, hepatitis C, and Creutzfeldt–Jakob disease. Transplant coordinators attempt to glean as much information as possible about the past medical and social history of the potential donor, particularly with respect to intravenous drug use, tattooing and body piercing, sexual practice, previous blood transfusions, and use of cigarettes and alcohol. Generally, any evidence of these infections would lead to transplantation not proceeding; however, because of severe donor shortages organs, these "high-risk" organs may sometimes be used in rapidly decompensating patients who have given informed consent.

**Table 3** Organ Donor Criteria in Australia—Lung and Combined Heart/Lung

| | |
|---|---|
| Organ donor's suitability criteria | General organ donor criteria |
| | Age <60 years (lung), <50 years (heart/lung) |
| | No known lung disease |
| | Arterial blood gases on 100% oxygen and 5-cm PEEP, $PaO_2$ >300 mmHg |
| Required information for allocation | Blood group |
| | Body weight |
| | Body height |
| | Laboratory tests |

*Abbreviation*: PEEP, positive end-expiratory pressure.
*Source*: From Ref. 7.

Neoplastic disease is also specifically assessed and only organs from donors that have had no history of cancer or cancers restricted to nonmelanoma skin cancers or primary malignant brain tumors would be utilized. Specific evaluation for lung donation includes careful history about known lung disease as well as exposure to potentially toxic environmental factors including cigarette smoking. The presence or absence of secretions from suctioning the endotracheal tube, as well as blood gases performed using 100% oxygen and 5 cmH$_2$O positive end-expiratory pressure (PEEP) are also used as an important criteria. Additional information (Table 4), including blood group, body weight, body height, and laboratory investigations, particularly CMV IgG, are used to help with donor recipient matching.

Once consent has been obtained for lung donation, the transplant physician (typically a pulmonologist) will contact and where feasible visit the donor intensive care unit. Suggestions as to optimal management of the lung donor including respiratory management (including PEEP), bronchial

**Table 4** Donor/Recipient Matching (Selection) in Australia

| | |
|---|---|
| ABO compatability | Absolute requirement |
| Lymphocytotoxic cross-match | At the discretion of the heart/lung transplant unit |
| Size and weight compatibility | Usually required |
| Waiting list | The severity of the underlying lung disease is the primary selection criterion, followed by waiting time |
| HLA matching | Not required |

*Note*: Where practical, lungs from CMV IgG–negative donors will be given to CMV IgG–negative recipients.
*Abbreviations*: CMV, cytomegalovirus; HLA, human leukocyte antigen.
*Source*: From Ref. 7.

(including bronchoscopic) toilet, fluid management, and antibiotics are made, often resulting in significant improvements in gas exchange and radiographic appearance. This approach to donor management can result in 30% of donors with unacceptable gas exchange improving to acceptable levels (19).

## Donor/Recipient Matching

As outlined previously, the organ procurement network is led by state-based OPAs. A potential donor identified in the intensive care unit would lead to a telephone call to the local donor coordinator, who would travel to the donor hospital, make an initial assessment of the potential donor, and complete formalities in terms of obtaining consent from the family, the hospital, and the appropriate authorities (e.g., the coroner) after brain death has been duly certified. Once preliminaries have been completed, the heart–lung block would be offered either to the local lung transplant program or to an inter-state program on rotation if no local program was present. The heart–lung block offer would be made to the recipient coordinator, who would then liaise with the clinical staff to see if a suitable recipient (recipients) was (were) available. The recipient coordinator has 20 minutes to accept the offer or the heart–lung block would automatically be reoffered to other programs in order. It is up to the discretion of the transplant program accepting the heart–lung block to decide which combination of heart, heart–lung, and lung transplant procedures they would perform. If they were unable to use all three organs then the organ would be passed on to other programs, although the responsibility for organ procurement would rest with the initial program accepting the heart–lung block.

The organ procurement team is generally provided by the lung transplant program in that state. If there is no lung transplant program in the State or no local team available to perform the donor procedure, then a team is sent from the recipient transplant program. This sometimes results in procurements occurring at a distance of almost 4000 km from the program where the recipient procedure will occur.

As previously noted, the decision in choosing the recipient is left to the recipient program. The general guidelines are outlined in Table 4. Typically, blood group identical transplantation is performed to avoid seriously disadvantaging blood group O recipients. A negative lymphocytotoxic cross-match is usually present and appropriate size matching is required. Once these criteria are met, the sickest patient with the clearest prognostic advantage to transplantation is generally selected. Waiting time is taken into account if two equally severely ill patients are identified, although this is of secondary consideration. Where possible, CMV IgG–negative donor organs are placed in CMV IgG–negative recipients to avoid primary CMV infections.

In Australia, the approach has been to follow the selection rules and let the organs select the recipients. Cutting down larger organs to fit smaller recipients is not present practice, although it has rarely occurred where at the time of the recipient transplant procedure the donor organs appear too large.

## OUTCOMES OF LUNG TRANSPLANTATION IN AUSTRALIA

Australia has one of the lowest multiorgan donor rates of the developed world. In the five years from 1998, this ranged from 9 to 10 multiorgan donors per million population. Despite this, lung transplant servicing rates have been high, ranging over the same period between 0.41 and 0.48 lung recipients per multiorgan donor, that is 4.1 to 4.8 lung recipients per million population per year (8). This high rate of servicing has been primarily due to preparedness to use extended donors (19–23), which in a published series accounted for 57% of all lung donors in an Australian transplant center (19). Standard selection criteria for lung donors include age <55 years. Between 1999 and 2003, 12% of donors utilized in Australia would have been ≥55 years (Fig. 4). Second, although local studies suggest that smoking history >20 pack years does not affect long-term outcome (24) in practice, one Australian transplant center reports that only 8% of donors had a >20–pack year smoking history (25). The commonest departure from standard criteria, however, involved the presence of positive Gram stain of airway secretions in 38% of donors and an abnormal chest X ray in 61% of donors; this did not appear to adversely effect outcomes (19,25). Generally, donors with known or suspected chronic lung disease have not been utilized in transplantation in Australia, although following the lead from other centers (26), donors with a history of asthma are not immediately excluded. A recent report by The Alfred Lung Transplant Service has shown

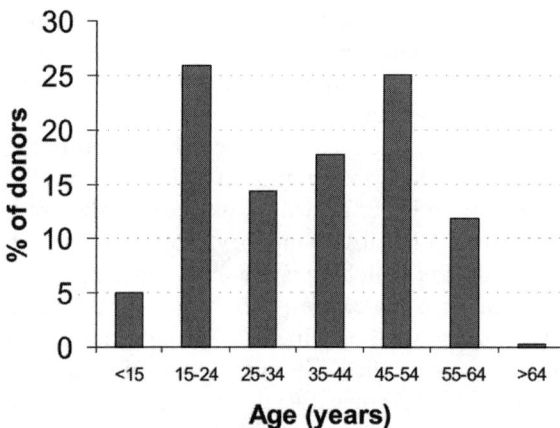

**Figure 4**  The age distribution of lung donors in Australia over the five-year-period from 1999 to 2003. *Source*: From Ref. 16.

no detectable effect on outcome utilizing asthmatic donors except where severe asthma had led to death of the donor (27). Other unusual donors who have been utilized include those who died due to carbon monoxide poisoning (28), donors with established lower-lobe pneumonia, and pulmonary donors requiring long ischemic time, sometimes exceeding nine hours of cold ischemia (29). Indeed, from 1999 to 2003 the yearly mean cold ischemic times for first lung single-lung transplant have ranged from 300 to 350 minutes, cold ischemic time for first lung engraftment in bilateral lung transplant has ranged from 340 to 380 minutes, and cold ischemic time for heart/lung transplantation has ranged from 290 to 450 minutes (16).

The second major factor has been the preparedness to use single-lung transplantation wherever possible. There has been generally a tendency to utilize donors who comply with standard criteria in single-lung transplantation, with marginal donors usually reserved for bilateral lung transplantation, although this has not been invariably practiced. Since the mid-1990s, however, the trend in Australia has been for an increase in bilateral lung transplantation with a diminution of single-lung transplantation (Fig. 5). In 2003, for example, 58 bilateral lung transplants were performed throughout Australia, but only 16 single-lung transplants (16). Despite the extensive use of marginal or extended indication lung donors, the results of lung transplantation in Australia have been good by international benchmark. Survival at one, two, and five years for heart–lung, single-lung, and bilateral lung transplants performed in Australia between 1986 and 2003 is generally in a range of 10% greater than the survival recorded in the ISHLT registry for a similar period (Table 5). Overall, five-year survival in Australia for heart–lung transplantation is 49%, for single-lung transplantation 46%,

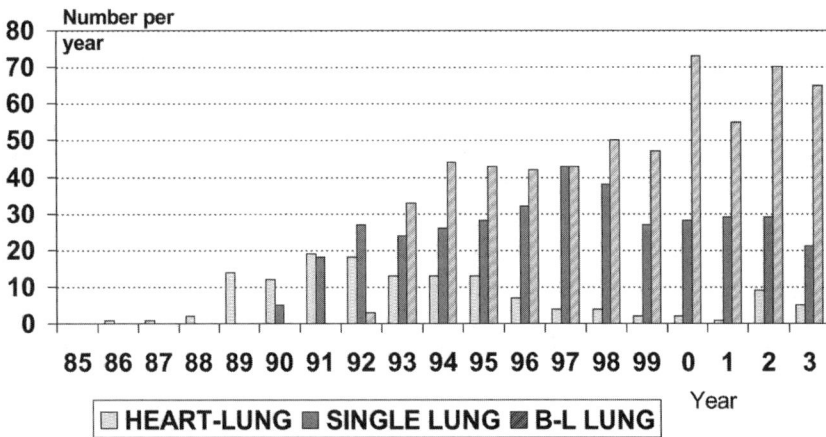

**Figure 5** Lung transplant activity in Australia from the first heart–lung transplant in 1986 to 2003. *Source*: From Ref. 16.

**Table 5**  Survival Following HLT$_X$, SLT$_X$, and BLT$_X$ Transplantation
in Australia Versus the ISHLT International Registry

| | HLT$_X$ | | SLT$_X$ | | BLT$_X$ | |
|---|---|---|---|---|---|---|
| | Australia 1986–2003 | ISHLT 1982–2002 | Australia 1990–2003 | ISHLT 1990–2002 | Australia 1992–2003 | ISHLT 1990–2002 |
| 1-year survival | 80 | 62 | 79 | 73 | 86 | 76 |
| 2-year survival | 68 | 54 | 70 | 65 | 77 | 67 |
| 5-year survival | 49 | 41 | 46 | 45 | 61 | 51 |

*Abbreviations*: HLT$_X$, SLT$_X$, and BLT$_X$: heart–lung, single-lung, and bilateral lung transplantation; ISHLT, International Society for Heart and Lung Transplantation.

and for bilateral lung transplantation 61%, covering all lung transplants
performed throughout Australia.

A third group of important factors relate to the system-wide approach
to lung transplantation in Australia (30). The major programs have the
capacity and flexibility to perform one or two lung transplants at the same
time that they are performing a heart transplant. The donor team can also
be provided if needed. Immediately upon receiving a call from the donor
coordinator, a list of suitable recipients is drawn up, awaiting further data
(e.g., CMV status, cross-match results, etc.). If there are few potential recipients in one transplant center then another center will be contacted so sufficient "backup" recipients are identified to ensure that all organs are
utilized. If no recipients are available in the first center it will be immediately
offered to the next. The 20-minute time limit on donor organ offers means
that these issues are rapidly resolved.

Although there is no priority (of lung allocation) based on clinical
urgency, programs communicate and a donor offer may be passed on if appropriate. Donor coordinators are encouraged to refer on all donors. Potential
lung recipients who are close to death will be considered for a marginal organ.
The issue of preparedness to accept a marginal donor is discussed during the
regular waiting list review so that consent to this approach can be obtained.

Australia has not seen a significant increase in waiting time for lung
transplantation (Fig. 6) or a ballooning of recipients awaiting lung transplantation (8,16). In 1993, the mean and median waiting times for lung
transplantation were 211 and 259 days, respectively. In 2003, mean waiting
time for lung transplantation was 221 days (median 217 days). As noted previously, during 2003 (the last year of published data) the number of patients
actively listed for lung transplantation in Australia increased by 16% from

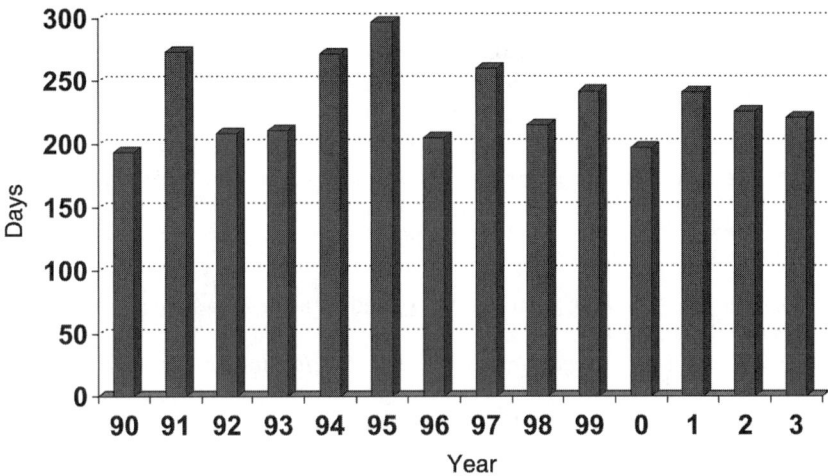

**Figure 6** Mean waiting time for lung transplantation in Australia from 1990 to 2003. *Source*: From Ref. 16.

108 to 125 throughout Australia. Australian centers have generally taken the pragmatic view that patients should only be on the waiting list if there is a high chance of transplantation with good quality of life. In the absence of a waiting list time-priority system this has led to less than half the number of patients on active lung transplant waiting list as a proportion of population in Australia compared to the United States (16,31). The relatively small Australian population is a major reason for not attempting a time-priority system for each donor as there are only a few suitable recipients. However, several other factors including a clear understanding by Australians of the limitation of donor organ availability, government funding of lung transplant programs, and a community attitude less bound by individual right than overall utility has led to an allocation system based on feasibility and clinical need. The remoteness of some lung transplant recipients from transplant centers also sometimes needs to be considered as part of an assessment of overall feasibility and quality of outcome following lung transplantation. These issues are often identified, assessed, and discussed with potential recipients prior to any detailed assessment for lung transplantation to avoid raising unrealistic expectations.

## CONCLUSION

Despite low multiorgan donor rates, high servicing rates for lung transplantation have been achieved in Australia. This has been primarily due to extensive use of marginal (or extended indication) donors, preparedness to perform single-lung transplantation where possible, and active involvement in donor management/optimization. Despite this, survival from lung transplantation significantly exceeds international benchmarks. A key to this approach, however, is a prevailing community view that is supportive of lung transplantation, recognizes that this is a therapy restricted by the extreme shortage of donor organs and thus should be reserved for patients with a reasonable prospect of success and good long-term outcome.

## REFERENCES

1.  Leeder SR. Achieving equity in the Australian healthcare system. Med J Aust 2003; 179(9):475–478.
2.  Sheil AG. Medico-legal aspects of renal transplantation. Anaesth Intensive Care 1983; 11(4):345–349.
3.  Russ GR. Renal transplantation in Australia and New Zealand 1963 to 1999. Clin Transpl:346–348.
4.  Snell GI, Levvey BJ, Williams TJ. Non-heart beating organ donation. Intern Med J 2004; 34(8):501–503.
5.  Thompson JF, Hibberd AD, Mohacsi PJ, Chapman JR, Macdonald GJ, Mahony JF. Can cadaveric organ donation rates be improved?. Anaesth Intensive Care 1995; 23(1):99–103.
6.  McBride M, Chapman JR. An overview of transplantation in Australia. Anaesth Intensive Care 1995; 23(1):60–64.
7.  The Transplant Society of Australia and New Zealand. Australian National Organ Allocation Protocols. (Accessed 2002 at www.mediserv.com.au/racp/tsanz.)
8.  Excell L, Russ GR, Wride P. ANZOD Registry Report 2004. Adelaide, South Australia: Australian and New Zealand Organ Donation Registry, 2004.
9.  Kerridge IH, Saul P, Lowe M, McPhee J, Williams D. Death, dying and donation: organ transplantation and the diagnosis of death. J Med Ethics 2002; 28(2):89–94.
10. Mathew T. The Australian experience in organ donation—2003. Ann Transplant 2004; 9(1):28–30.
11. Pearson IY. Australia and New Zealand Intensive Care Society Statement and Guidelines on Brain Death and Model Policy on Organ Donation. Anaesth Intensive Care 1995; 23(1):104–108.
12. Spratt P, Glanville AR, Macdonald P, et al. Heart/lung transplantation in Australia: early results of the St Vincent's program. Transplant Proc 1990; 22(5):2141–2142.
13. Cochrane AD, Smith JA, Esmore DS. The "domino-donor" operation in heart and lung transplantation. Med J Aust 1991; 155(9):589–593.
14. Smith JA, Roberts M, McNeil K, et al. Excellent outcome of cardiac transplantation using domino donor hearts. Eur J Cardio-Thorac Surg 1996; 10(8):628–633.
15. Esmore DS, Brown R, Buckland M, et al. Techniques and results in bilateral sequential single lung transplantation. The National Heart & Lung Replacement Service. J Card Surg 1994; 9(1):1–14.

16. Australia and New Zealand Cardiothoracic Organ Transplant Registry 2003 Report, 2003.

17. Trulock EP, Edwards LB, Taylor DO, Boucek MM, Keck BM, Hertz MI. The registry of the international society for heart and lung transplantation: twenty-first official adult lung and heart-lung transplant report–2004. J Heart Lung Transplant 2004; 23(7):804–815.

18. Maurer JR, Frost AE, Estenne M, Higenbottam T, Glanville AR. International guidelines for the selection of lung transplant candidates. The International Society for Heart and Lung Transplantation, the American Thoracic Society, the American Society of Transplant Physicians, the European Respiratory Society. J Heart Lung Transplant 1998; 17(7):703–709.

19. Gabbay E, Williams TJ, Griffiths AP, et al. Maximizing the utilization of donor organs offered for lung transplantation. Am J Respir Crit Care Med 1999; 160(1):265–271.

20. Orens JB, Boehler A, de Perrot M, et al. A review of lung transplant donor acceptability criteria. J Heart Lung Transplant 2003; 22(11):1183–1200.

21. Shumway SJ, Hertz MI, Petty MG, Bolman RM III. Liberalization of donor criteria in lung and heart-lung transplantation. Ann Thorac Surg 1994; 57(1):92–95.

22. Sundaresan S, Semenkovich J, Ochoa L, et al. Successful outcome of lung transplantation is not compromised by the use of marginal donor lungs. J Thorac Cardiovasc Surg 1995; 109(6):1075–1079.

23. Whiting D, Banerji A, Ross D, et al. Liberalization of donor criteria in lung transplantation. Am Surg 2003; 69(10):909–912.

24. Oto T, Griffiths AP, Levvey B, et al. A donor history of smoking affects early but not late outcome in lung transplantation. Transplantation 2004; 78(4):599–606.

25. de Perrot M, Snell GI, Babcock WD, et al. Strategies to optimize the use of currently available lung donors. J Heart Lung Transplant 2004; 23(10):1127–1134.

26. Corris PA, Dark JH. Aetiology of asthma: lessons from lung transplantation. Lancet 1993; 341(8857):1369–1371.

27. Oto T, Griffiths A, Levvey B, et al. Donor history of asthma is not a contraindication to lung transplantation: 12-year single-center experience. J Heart Lung Transplant 2004; 23(3):309–316.

28. Shennib H, Adoumie R, Fraser R. Successful transplantation of a lung allograft from a carbon monoxide-poisoning victim. J Heart Lung Transplant 1992; 11(1, Pt 1):68–71.

29. Snell GI, Rabinov M, Griffiths A, et al. Pulmonary allograft ischemic time: an important predictor of survival after lung transplantation. J Heart Lung Transplant 1996; 15(2):160–168.

30. Snell GI, Griffiths A, Macfarlane L, et al. Maximizing thoracic organ transplant opportunities: the importance of efficient coordination. J Heart Lung Transplant 2000; 19(4):401–407.

31. UNOS. United Network of Organ Sharing. (Accessed 2005 at http://www.unos.org/.)

# 15

# Lung Preservation Techniques

**Frank D'Ovidio and Shaf Keshavjee**

*Toronto Lung Transplant Program, University of Toronto, Toronto, Canada*

## INTRODUCTION

Organ transplantation has evolved rapidly from the initial successes to the current widespread use of donated organs for the treatment of end-stage kidney, liver, heart, and lung failure (1). The success of solid-organ transplantation has increased the need for an expanded supply of organ donors. In response to this need, the acceptable age limit for deceased donors has continued to increase, and donors over the age of 50 years are now routinely used. The use of organs from live donors (related or unrelated) and non–heart-beating donors (NHBDs; those declared dead on the basis of cardio-pulmonary criteria) has also increased. Nevertheless, there has been a progressively widening gap between the number of patients waiting for transplants and the number of transplantations performed (2).

One consequence of the increased proportion of older and "expanded" donors has been a significant increase in discarded organs after they had been procured (2). Unlike liver, kidneys, and pancreas for which temporary graft dysfunction or failure may be tolerated with supportive measures such as hemodialysis and pharmacological interventions, a reasonably well-functioning transplanted organ is crucial for successful transplantation of the heart or lung, which is required to function immediately to support life. Primary graft dysfunction accounts for approximately 30% of all deaths of heart and lung transplant recipients (3).

At a time when transplant surgeons are facing an increasing number of deaths on the waiting list, and as the size of the list continues to grow, there has never been a greater need to utilize a higher percentage of older or otherwise extended donors, with yet a relatively small incidence of primary graft dysfunction. Much of this success can be attributed to the application of improved donor management and pulmonary preservation strategies that continue to increase the number of organs available for transplant (3–13).

Primary graft dysfunction, however, remains a significant cause of early morbidity and mortality after lung transplantation and has been associated with increased risks of acute rejection and subsequent graft dysfunction in the long term (14).

The syndrome typically occurs within the first 72 hours after transplantation, and is characterized by nonspecific alveolar damage, lung edema, and hypoxemia. The clinical spectrum can range from mild hypoxemia associated with few infiltrates on chest X ray to a picture similar to full-blown acute respiratory distress syndrome (15). A recent International Society for Heart and Lung Transplantation Study Group developed a consensus document that defined and quantified grades of primary graft dysfunction as follows: Grade 0—$PaO_2/FiO_2 >300$, no infiltrates on chest X ray; Grade 1—presence of pulmonary infiltrates with a $PaO_2/FiO_2$ ratio greater than $300\,mmHg$; Grade 2—$PaO_2/FiO_2$ ratio between 300 and $200\,mmHg$; Grade 3—$PaO_2/FiO_2$ ratio lower than $200\,mmHg$ (16).

Ischemia–reperfusion injury has been identified as one of the main contributing factors to the syndrome of primary graft dysfunction. During the last 20 years knowledge about both lung preservation and the pathological changes during ischemia and reperfusion has continued to advance.

The first clinical transplantations were performed using local donors minimizing the ischemic time by transferring the donor to the transplant center if necessary at significant financial and logistical cost. Subsequently, a variety of techniques were used for lung preservation: single flush perfusion of the lungs followed by static cold storage; donor core cooling on cardiopulmonary bypass; atelectatic topical cooling of the lungs; and normothermic aurtoperfusion of the heart–lung block (17–20).

The single flush perfusion is the most commonly used technique today. It has proven to be as effective as or more effective than donor core cooling, with the advantage of being simple with minimal requirements for technical equipment (21–23).

## PRESERVATION SOLUTIONS

Organ preservation is based on a number of basic principles: prevention of intracellular and extracellular edema; prevention of intracellular acidosis; reduction of oxygen-derived free radicals; regeneration of intracellular energy metabolism; and prevention of intracellular calcium accumulation

(24,25). Colloids, hydroxyethyl starch and dextran, are used to prevent penetration of the perfusate into the interstitial space. Impermeables such as glucose, raffinose, mannitol, lactobionate, and gluconate are used to prevent intracellular edema by transgressing into the interstitial space, but not penetrating the cell membrane. Acid-neutralizing substrates such as phosphate, histidine, and bicarbonate are used to counteract the tissue acidosis following the anaerobic glycolysis during ischemia. Oxygen-derived free radicals are targeted using the scavengers such as allopurinol and glutathione. ATP precursors adenosine, ribose, and anorganic phosphate provide substrate for ATP production readily available at the time of reperfusion (6,8,26,27).

Preservation solutions that have been studied to date include primarily *intracellular*-type solutions (high-$K^+$, low-$Na^+$ solutions) such as Euro-Collins® and University of Wisconsin® solution, and *extracellular*-type solutions (low-$K^+$, high-$Na^+$ solutions) such as low-potassium dextran (LPD, Perfadex®, Vitrolife, Goteborg, Sweden) and Celsior® (Table 1).

According to a worldwide survey of 125 lung transplant centers published in 1998 by Hopkinson and colleagues, the clinical practice in pulmonary graft preservation solution was with Euro-Collins in 77% of them, University of Wisconsin solution was used in 15%, and 7% used Papworth blood-based solution (28).

**Table 1** Composition of Preservation Solutions

| Composition | Euro-Collins® | University of Wisconsin® | Celsior® | Perfadex® |
|---|---|---|---|---|
| Na (mmol/L) | 10 | 28 | 100 | 138 |
| K (mmol/L) | 115 | 125 | 15 | 6 |
| Cl (mmol/L) | 15 | 0 | 41.5 | 142 |
| Mg (mmol/L) | 0 | 0 | 13 | 0.8 |
| $SO_4$ (mmol/L) | 0 | 4 | 0 | 0.8 |
| $PO_4$ (mmol/L) | 57.5 | 25 | 0 | 0.8 |
| Ca (mmol/L) | 0 | 0 | 0.26 | 0.3 |
| $HCO_3$ (mmol/L) | 10 | 5 | 0 | 1 |
| Dextran 40 (g/L) | 0 | 0 | 0 | 50 |
| Glucose (g/L) | 3.5 | 0 | 0 | 0.9 |
| Raffinose (mmol/L) | 0 | 30 | 0 | 0 |
| Lactobionate (mmol/L) | 0 | 100 | 80 | 0 |
| Glutathione (mmol/L) | 0 | 3 | 3 | 0 |
| Adenosine (mmol/L) | 0 | 5 | 0 | 0 |
| Allopurinol (mmol/L) | 0 | 1 | 0 | 0 |
| Pentafraction (g/L) | 0 | 50 | 0 | 0 |
| Glutamate (mmol/L) | 0 | 0 | 20 | 0 |
| Histidine (mmol/L) | 0 | 0 | 30 | 0 |
| Mannitol (mmol/L) | 0 | 0 | 60 | 0 |

The experimental evidence shows that extracellular solutions are superior to intracellular solutions in lung preservation (10). The goals of intracellular solutions are to reduce the electrochemical gradient across the leaky cell membranes in an effort to prevent cellular edema by minimizing sodium influx and obligatory passive entry of water into cell in order to achieve osmotic equilibrium. Hypothermia limits the activity of the $Na^+/K^+$-ATPase pump, thus limiting the ability of cells to reestablish the normal cellular ionic gradients (7). The primary concern in the use of intracellular-type solutions is the $K^+$-induced vasoconstriction; furthermore, there are concerns that hyperkalemia may cause endothelial cell injury. The high potassium content of intracellular solutions may, therefore, lead to elevated flush perfusion pressures, capillary leakage, and uneven distribution of perfusate. Prostaglandin $E_1$ or prostacyclin is often used in combination with intracellular solutions to attempt to counteract this effect.

About a decade ago, LPD–glucose solution (Perfadex) was approved for clinical practice and the majority of lung transplant centers currently use it as their clinical lung preservation solution.

Clinical reports from six centers have compared the effect of LPD–glucose (Perfadex) with a historical control group of lungs preserved with Euro-Collins (30–35). Five of the six reports showed significantly better lung function on arrival in the intensive care unit and a trend toward lower 30-day mortality with LPD–glucose. An additional report demonstrated that, after adjustment for graft ischemic time, extracellular-type preservation solutions are associated with a decreased incidence of primary graft dysfunction after lung transplantation when compared with intracellular-type preservation solutions (36).

The beneficial effect of preservation with LPD is due to the combination of both a low-potassium concentration and the presence of dextran (37). The low-potassium concentration is less detrimental to the functional and structural integrity of endothelial cells, which may thus lead to less production of oxidants, and release of less pulmonary vasoconstrictors. Dextran improves erythrocyte deformability, prevents erythrocyte aggregation, and induces disaggregation of already aggregated cells, in addition to an antithrombotic effect induced by coating endothelial surfaces and platelets. These effects improve pulmonary microcirculation and preserve the endothelial–epithelial barrier, which may secondarily prevent the no-reflow phenomenon and reduce the degree of water and protein extravasation at the time of reperfusion. In addition, in vitro studies have demonstrated that LPD solution can exert a suppressive effect on polymorphonuclear chemotaxis, be less cytotoxic for type II pneumocytes, and maintain better activity of alveolar epithelial $Na^+/K^+$-ATPase function during the cold ischemic period when compared with Euro-Collins or University of Wisconsin solutions (38–40). These effects may result in less lipid peroxidation, and better surfactant function at the end of the ischemic time and after reperfusion (41,42).

## CONDITIONS OF ADMINISTRATION OF THE FLUSH SOLUTION

### Temperature

In the clinical setting very few programs actually measure the temperature of the flush and storage solution (43). It is generally felt that the ideal temperature is between 4°C and 10°C, a range that will sufficiently decrease cellular metabolism, but will allow the critical cellular process to continue. In particular, extracellular solutions ideally require higher preservation temperature in order to maintain an ongoing activity of ATPase to optimize the ion homeostasis and avoid diffusion of sodium and water down concentration gradients with resultant cell swelling and death (7).

In the experimental setting in small animals with a probably more rapid core cooling of the lungs, several authors have observed that lung function was significantly better after reperfusion if the lungs were initially flushed with a temperature of 15–20°C instead of 10°C or lower (44,45). Wang and colleagues showed that a temperature of 23°C for the flush solution was associated with a lower pulmonary vascular resistance during flushing and more uniform washout of the pulmonary vascular beds than a temperature of 10°C (44).

Despite some potential injuries induced by cold flushing, total injury is minimal when compared with the insult induced by warm ischemia. In fact, ultrastructural analysis of the lungs at various time points during preservation period demonstrates that the injuries induced by the flush itself appear to be minimal when compared with the insult induced by ischemia on the endothelial–epithelial barrier (46,47).

### Anterograde Flush: Volume and Pressure

The ideal volume and pressure for the administration of the solution is unknown. Although most programs agree that there is an optimal pressure at which to infuse the flush solution, most do not monitor the pressure but ensure that the flush solution bag is hung no higher than 30 cm above the donor to prevent the flush pressure from exceeding 30 cmH$_2$O.

Several studies have analyzed the effect of pressure and volume of the preservation solution during flushing. Haverich and colleagues found that lungs flushed via the pulmonary artery with anterograde high perfusate volume given at a high flow rate (60 mL/kg given in 4 minutes) resulted in significantly better cooling of the lungs and better lung function after reperfusion compared with low volume and low flow rate (20 mL/kg given in 6 minutes) or high flow rate (20 mL/kg given in 1.3 minutes) (48). Steen and colleagues have suggested the use of 150–180 mL/kg with LPD–glucose to obtain a more uniform and clean washout of the anterior part of the lungs, which is usually less uniformly flushed because of the pressure gradient in the supine position (49). The influence of the pulmonary artery pressure during the flushing period on lung preservation was systematically analyzed in an ex vivo rabbit lung reperfusion model. Flushing pressures of 10–15 mmHg were noted to achieve complete flushing of the pulmonary vascular beds and significantly better lung function after reperfusion than flushing pressures of 5, 20, and 25 mmHg (50). Furthermore, flushing pressures of 20 mmHg or higher were found to be associated with significantly less endogenous nitric oxide production, with possible detrimental effect after reperfusion (51).

Current common practice is to flush donor lungs with 50–60 mL/kg of flush solution. The flush solution bag is placed at 30 cm above the donor to achieve adequate flush pressures in the range of physiologic pulmonary artery pressure, without exceeding a maximum pressure of 30 cmH$_2$O, to avoid injury to the pulmonary vasculature.

### Retrograde Flush

Several groups have adopted a combined procedure with an anterograde flush through the pulmonary artery followed by a retrograde flush through each of the pulmonary veins in situ while the lungs are still ventilated. Experimentally, retrograde flush has been found to improve lung preservation. This effect was attributed to more effective clearance of red blood cells within the capillaries, better distribution of the flush solution along the tracheobronchial tree, and less severe impairment of surfactant function (52–54). It is hypothesized that the retrograde flush through the pulmonary veins may access and flush capillary beds in the lung that may not have been opened and flushed with the antegrade flush. The retrograde flush also likely removes embolic debris (pulmonary emboli—clot or fat emboli) from the pulmonary circulation.

The method of lung preservation that incorporates many of these concepts and is currently used in the Toronto Lung Transplant Program is summarized in Table 2.

### STORAGE OF THE LUNG

Inflation of the lungs with oxygen during the ischemic period protects the lung from injury by three mechanisms: it maintains some aerobic metabolism, preserves the integrity of pulmonary surfactant, and preserves epithelial fluid transport.

In lungs stored in an inflated state, the static pulmonary compliance, pulmonary vascular resistance, alveolar fluid clearance, total BAL protein and lactate dehydrogenase, and surfactant secretion have all been shown to be improved as compared to lungs stored in an atelectatic state (55–58).

**Table 2** Current Recommendations for Lung Preservation from the Toronto Lung Transplant Group

| | |
|---|---|
| Preservation solution | Perfadex |
| Volume of anterograde flush solution | 50–60 mL/kg |
| Volume of retrograde flush solution | 250 mL/pulmonary vein |
| PA pressure during flush delivery | 10–15 mmHg |
| Temperature of flush solution | 4–8°C |
| Lung ventilation while flushing | $V_T$: 10 mL/kg and PEEP: 5 cmH$_2$O |
| Oxygenation | ≤50% FiO$_2$ |
| Lung inflation (airway pressure) | 15–20 cmH$_2$O |
| Storage temperature | 4–8°C |

*Abbreviations*: PA, pulmonary artery; $V_T$, tidal volume; PEEP, positive end-expiratory pressure; FiO$_2$, fraction of inspired oxygen.

In our clinical practice, we perform a recruitment maneuver to fully reexpand the lungs before flushing them and we ventilate the lungs with a tidal volume of 10 mL/kg and a positive end-expiratory pressure of 5 cmH$_2$O during the flushing period. The lungs are then inflated with an oxygen fraction of 50% and a sustained peak airway pressure is brought up to 20–25 cmH$_2$O for final recruitment and then lowered to 15 cmH$_2$O for tracheal cross-clamping in an effort to obtain complete lung expansion but avoid overdistension. Overinflated lungs might be exposed to significantly more overdistension if they are transported in airplanes because of the potentially lower atmospheric pressure during the flight. Hyperinflation during storage has been shown to increase pulmonary capillary filtration coefficient. In fact, inflation during storage should be limited to 50% of the total lung capacity or to an airway pressure of 10–15 cmH$_2$O to avoid barotrauma (56,59).

Oxygen is required during storage to support aerobic metabolism. However, an inspired oxygen fraction greater than 50% may be associated with more lipid peroxidation during lung storage (60).

## Storage Temperature

Experimental lung preservation at 10°C has been shown to achieve better results than preservation at 4°C or 15°C and higher (61). However, these findings were not confirmed by other groups (17). In addition, lungs preserved at 10°C require a greater amount of metabolic substrate and the risk of lung injury can increase extremely rapidly if the temperature rises above 10°C during preservation. Hence, if a 10°C preservation temperature were used, the temperature of the organs would have to be constantly monitored because of the narrow margin of safety. For this reason, we recommend preservation of the lungs at a temperature ranging between 4°C and 8°C. Practically, this temperature is usually achieved by storing the inflated lungs floating in 2–3 L of flush solution in sterile organ storage bags. The organ bag is then stored in a standard cooler filled with ice for transportation.

## NON–HEART BEATING DONOR

NHBDs are donors who provide organs for transplantation after cardiac arrest (62). Ethical issues surrounding the use of NHBDs for transplantation are still debated (63–66).

Four types of NHBDs have been identified in the so called "Maastricht Categories" (67): categories I and II are persons who die unexpectedly—dead on arrival and following an unsuccessful resuscitation; therefore, they are so-called uncontrolled donors. Categories III and IV are referred to as "controlled donors" because the cardiac arrest is either planned in advance (category III—awaiting cardiac arrest) or occurs in a heart-beating donor (category IV—cardiac arrest in brain-dead donor).

The interest in NHBD for lung transplantation derives from the hypothesis that lungs do not necessarily rely on perfusion to deliver oxygen to the tissue for cellular respiration, since oxygen can also be derived through diffusion from air spaces (12,68).

Several groups have demonstrated that the tolerable period of warm ischemia in the lung is limited to 60 to 90 minutes in the untouched cadaver, which is too short to organize organ donation, recipient selection, and retrieval in particular in an uncontrolled donor setting (68–73). Therefore, extending this time period is a sine qua non to make NHBD lung retrieval clinically applicable. Occasional cases of successful lung transplantation with organs from controlled donors have been reported (74–76).

More interestingly, Steen and colleagues have published the first successful case of lung transplantation from an uncontrolled donor in 2001, and more recently, Varela and colleagues reported a series of five patients who underwent successful transplantation with lungs from donors all of whom had collapsed outside the hospital (77–80). Steen's initial report documents a warm ischemic time of 65 minutes until organ donation consent was obtained from the family; thereafter, chest tubes were inserted and cold Perfadex was infused into the pleural spaces to topically cool the lungs to 18°C for two hours. The lungs were then harvested and the graft function was assessed in an ex vivo reperfusion circuit at 37°C. The lungs were found to be functioning well and were then recooled in the circuit to 20°C and stored at 8°C for a further seven hours in order to prepare the recipient. Single-lung transplantation was successfully performed with a total ischemic time of approximately 13 hours.

Various novel methods have been explored in the experimental setting for cooling the lungs inside the cadaver as a way to preserve the organ in the interval between death and cold ex situ storage, such as filling the thorax with cold air, submerging the cadaver in an ice bath, and cold air ventilation

(12,81–84). Steen instead, as described, re-explored the concept of topical cooling that was the initial lung preservation method used by the Toronto group in their first successful human lung transplantations in the early 1980s (85). Similarly, other investigators have also looked at the efficacy of topical cooling using NHBD rabbits, rats, and pigs (86–88). Rega and colleagues have reported an extended duration of topical cooling up to six hours following one hour of warm ischemia showing preserved graft function, thus suggesting the potential for extension for up to seven hours of pre-harvest interval postmortem for retrieval in NHBD (89).

In Varela's report, the cadaver was transported to the operating room and connected to an extracorporeal bypass machine to provide oxygenation and deep hypothermia. Both lungs were further cooled topically with 4 L of Perfadex solution at 4°C via two chest drains on each side. Oxygenation capacity was assessed in situ after sternotomy with a single pulmonary flush of 300 mL of venous donor blood mixed with Perfadex. An additional retrograde flush was administered on the back table after lung extraction with 250 mL Perfadex in each vein (80). This experience follows the reported investigation of technique of cadaver cooling on extracorporeal bypass through cannulation of the femoral vessels for preservation of abdominal organs (90,91).

In NHBD postmortem thrombi represent a potential risk and in the experimental setting various strategies have been tested: prearrest heparinization, addition to the flush solution of urokinase or recombinant tissue-type plasminogen activator, and additional retrograde flush after antegrade flush. All have consistently shown beneficial effects implicating the potential importance of postmortem thrombi (92–97).

The assessment of a graft's function is somewhat different depending on whether it is from a controlled or uncontrolled donor. In the controlled NHBD, pulmonary graft function can be assessed after informed consent in the hours before withdrawal of life support in the same way as practiced in the brain-dead donor (chest radiograph, oxygen challenge, and bronchoscopy). In the uncontrolled NHBD, assessment of the graft is performed by ex vivo reperfusion, as reported by Steen using a special perfusate medium in a closed circuit after lung retrieval (Fig. 1), or by in situ flush as described by Varela using a donor blood-based solution before harvesting the graft (77–80,98,99).

Steen's ex vivo reperfusion of human lungs in an isolated circuit was developed as a method to assess the lung from a NHBD before transplantation. Steen developed a solution for such isolated perfusion that is now marketed under the name Steen Solution® (Vitrolife AB, Gothenburg, Sweden). A pure red blood cell concentrate at a hematocrit of approximately 15% for optimal viscosity is added to this solution to evaluate gas exchange (98). Ex vivo reperfusion has also been explored as a method to predict function after cold storage (100,101). Ex vivo perfusion provides the fascinating

**(A)**                                          **(B)**

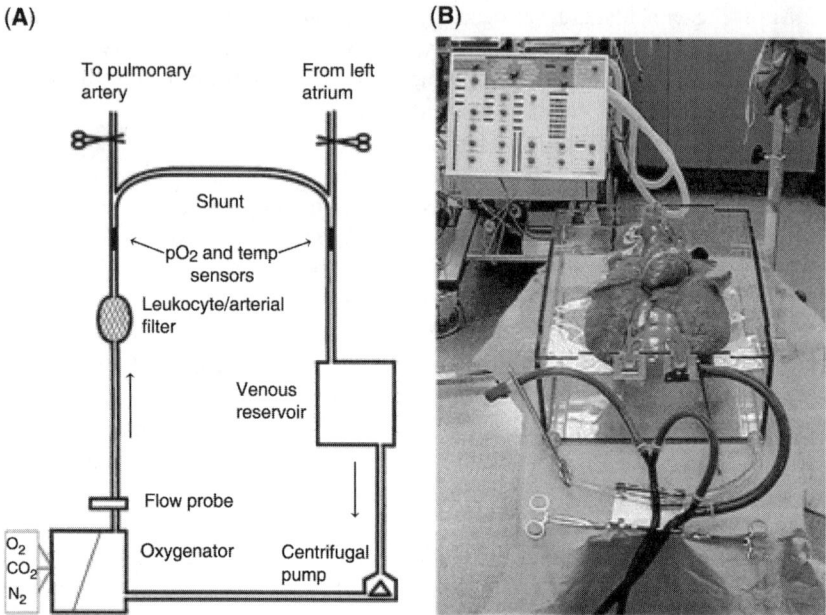

**Figure 1** Assessment of lung function ex vivo. (**A**) Schematic of the evaluation system. (**B**) The heart–lung block is placed in the evaluation box ready for cannulation. *Abbreviation*: temp, temperature. *Source*: From Ref. 98.

potential to reassess and even recondition or repair lungs from brain-dead donors who have been rejected because of poor function on initial assessment in vivo. Ex vivo reperfusion at normothermia has been shown to be possible for several hours without development of edema and gas exchange deficiencies (98). Afterward the lungs can be recooled with a red blood cell–containing oxygenated preservation medium and stored until transplantation. There is the potential for intermittent ex vivo reperfusion to preserve lungs for longer periods, thus permitting the use of lungs coming from a longer distance and hopefully to ultimately transform clinical lung transplantation into a daytime practice (102,103).

## THERAPIES UNDER INVESTIGATION

In an attempt to prevent or modulate primary graft dysfunction following lung transplantation, a variety of compounds have been tested for donor and recipient pretreatment also as additives to the preservation solution in order to improve the ischemic tolerance and limit the reperfusion injury. However, only a few have been tested in randomized double-blinded placebo-controlled trials (Table 3).

**Table 3** Clinical Series on the Prevention of Ischemia–Reperfusion Injury During Lung Transplantation

| First author | Study | Number of patients | Drug therapy | Main findings |
|---|---|---|---|---|
| Ardehali (104) | Prospective non-randomized | 28 | Inhaled NO | No prevention in the incidence of primary graft dysfunction |
| Thabut (105) | Retrospective | 23 | Inhaled NO and IV pentoxifylline | Reduction in incidence of primary graft dysfunction |
| Meade (106) | Randomized placebo controlled | 84 | Inhaled NO | No difference in oxygenation, extubation time, length of ICU stay, or 30-day mortality |
| Keshavjee (107) | Randomized placebo controlled | 59 | Complement inhibitor (TP-10) | Greater proportion of patients extubated within 24 hours after surgery |
| Wittwer (108) | Randomized placebo controlled | 24 | PAF antagonist | Trend toward better alveolo-arterial oxygen gradient during initial 32 hours of reperfusion |
| Strüber (109) | Randomized unblinded | 29 | Exogenous surfactant | No differences in clinical outcome |

*Abbreviations*: NO, nitric oxide; PAF, platelet activating factor.

## Surfactant Therapy

Surfactant dysfunction has been shown to occur during ischemia–reperfusion injury of the lung. Although some alterations in surfactant can be observed immediately after pulmonary artery flushing, most of the alterations have been shown to progressively develop during ischemic storage (110). Surfactant function was significantly improved when the lungs were preserved with extracellular preservation solution as compared to intracellular solution (41).

Experimental studies and clinical observations have shown that exogenous surfactant therapy can improve pulmonary function after lung transplantation. Exogenous surfactant has also been shown to enhance immediate recovery from transplantation injury and to be persistently beneficial for endogenous surfactant metabolism up to one week after transplantation (111). Exogenous surfactant given to the donor before retrieval has been associated with better and more reliable results than when it was administered just before or immediately after reperfusion (109). Struber and coworkers reported a randomized clinical study in 29 donors showing markedly better surfactant function in the donors who received exogenous surfactant instillation (112). However, no differences in early clinical outcome were found possibly because of the small sample size.

## Nitric Oxide

Endogenous nitric oxide has been found to be decreased after ischemia and reperfusion of the lung in human and animal studies. This finding may be associated with an increased expression of the enzyme eNOS, which may suggest that endogenously produced nitric oxide may be rapidly destroyed by oxygen-free radicals after reperfusion and/or that ischemia–reperfusion may induce the release of eNOS inhibitors in the lung (113). Multiple strategies have been developed to compensate for the fall in endogenous nitric oxide during lung transplantation. These strategies have been applied to the donor and/or to the recipient and consist of the administration of the upstream precursor molecule L-arginine, methods to increase the downstream effector molecule cyclic guanosine monophosphate, or the administration of exogenous nitric oxide. Exogenous nitric oxide has been given directly by inhalation (inhaled nitric oxide) or indirectly by infusion of a nitric oxide donor, such as FK409, nitroprusside, glyceryl trinitrate, nitroglycerin, or SIN-1. Other strategies have been directed at increasing the activity of the enzyme nitric oxide synthase by the addition of one of its cofactors (tetrahydrobiopterin, BH4) to the preservation solution, or by transfecting the donor with an adenovirus containing eNOS before lung retrieval (114,115).

These strategies have been shown to be effective experimentally and to have a prolonged effect if they are initiated before the onset of reperfusion injury. However, nitric oxide can react with superoxide anion and form peroxynitrous acid, which is a highly reactive oxidant that can induce the release of endothelin-1, damage alveolar type II cells even after a short period of ischemic time, and cause structural and functional alteration of surfactant. Hence, this reaction may explain why some authors have shown that nitric oxide administered during ischemia and/or early reperfusion may be ineffective or even harmful, in particular when it is given with a high fraction of inspired oxygen immediately after reperfusion (104).

Inhaled nitric oxide has been used clinically to treat ischemia–reperfusion injury of the lung because it can theoretically improve ventilation–perfusion mismatch and decrease pulmonary artery pressures without affecting systemic pressures. However, the role of inhaled nitric oxide in preventing ischemia–reperfusion injury during clinical lung transplantation remains controversial. In two clinical studies, one of which was a randomized double-blinded placebo-controlled trial, inhaled nitric oxide administered to recipients did not prevent primary lung graft dysfunction (106,116).

In conclusion, while inhaled nitric oxide therapy can be useful in improving gas exchange in cases of established reperfusion injury, the role of nitric oxide in the prevention of ischemia–reperfusion injury is yet to be demonstrated in clinical lung transplantation.

## Pentoxifylline

Pentoxifylline administration has been successful in ameliorating ischemia–reperfusion injury in experimental lung transplantation (105). It acts through a variety of mechanisms including inhibition of leukocyte sequestration in the lung with prevention of subsequent free radical and cytokine releases. Pentoxifylline administration may have a synergistic protective effect on lung injury during ischemia and reperfusion when it is given in association with inhaled nitric oxide (117).

Initial reports of clinical testing by Thabut and colleagues have shown that the combined administration of pentoxifylline and inhaled nitric oxide at the time of reperfusion reduced the incidence of primary graft dysfunction (118).

## Prostaglandin E$_1$

Prostaglandin E$_1$ has been shown to be beneficial when added to intracellular preservation solutions such as Euro-Collins and University of Wisconsin. The beneficial effect of prostaglandin-E$_1$ is attributed to its vasodilator properties that may lead to better distribution of the preservation solution, and to the stimulation of cyclic-3′,5′adenosine monophosphate–dependent protein kinase during the cold ischemic time, which may reduce endothelial permeability, neutrophil adhesion, and platelet aggregation on reperfusion.

The continuous intravenous administration of prostaglandin-E$_1$ to the recipient during the early phase of reperfusion has been shown to reduce ischemia–reperfusion injury of the lung in animal models of lung transplantation (119,120). Although this effect can be partially attributed to the vasodilator property of prostaglandin-E$_1$ during the initial 10 minutes of reperfusion, after a longer period of reperfusion a continuous prostaglandin-E$_1$ infusion achieved significantly better lung function than other vasodilator agents such as prostacyclin and nitroprusside (108). Hence, the continuous infusion of prostaglandin-E$_1$ clearly has a beneficial role on ischemia–reperfusion injury, some of which can be attributable to its anti-inflammatory effects. The continuous administration of prostaglandin-$E_1$ during reperfusion is associated with a shift from a proinflammatory cytokine profile including tumor necrosis factor $\alpha$ (TNF-$\alpha$), interferon-$\gamma$ (IFN-$\gamma$), and interleukin-12 (IL-12) to an anti-inflammatory cytokine profile with increased IL-10 in a rat lung transplant model (119). Other effects of prostaglandin-$E_1$, such as its antiaggregant action on platelets, may also potentially contribute to its beneficial role.

Based on experimental evidence, some centers routinely use an infusion of prostaglandin-$E_1$ during the postoperative period after lung transplantation, whereas others reserve prostaglandin-$E_1$ infusion for the treatment of severe reperfusion injury. Prospective randomized trials are required to determine whether routine prostaglandin-$E_1$ has an overall beneficial effect in the postoperative course during clinical lung transplantation. Such studies may utilize the newly developed aerosolized form of prostaglandin-$E_1$, which has been shown experimentally to reduce ischemia–reperfusion injury of the lung without having the systemic hypotensive side effect of intravenous prostaglandin-$E_1$.

## Platelet Activating Factor Antagonist

Platelet activating factor is an extraordinarily potent mediator of inflammation that can be released by a wide variety of cells including macrophages, platelets, endothelial cells, mast cells, and neutrophils. It exerts its biological effects by activating the platelet activating factor receptors, which consequently activate leukocytes, stimulate platelet aggregation, and induce the release of cytokines and the expression of cell adhesion molecules. Platelet activating factor has been difficult to analyze because it is rapidly degraded by tissue and plasma platelet activating factor acetylhydrolases. Since there are no specific inhibitors for the biosynthesis of platelet activating factor, most studies have shown the importance of platelet activating factor in ischemia–reperfusion injury by blocking its receptor.

Wittwer and colleagues have reported their clinical experience with an antagonist of platelet activating factor (BN52021, Ginkolide B) in 24 patients randomly assigned to a high dose of antagonist in the flush solution and after reperfusion ($n = 8$), a low dose of antagonist in the flush solution and after reperfusion ($n = 8$), and a control group ($n = 8$) (121). They observed a trend toward a better alveolo-arterial gradient of oxygen within the first 32 hours after reperfusion and a better chest X ray score in the two groups receiving the antagonist. In clinical kidney transplantation, a randomized, double-blinded single center trial with 29 recipients showed a significant reduction in the incidence of primary graft failure after transplantation in the group of patients receiving the antagonist of platelet activating factor (122).

## Complement Inhibitor

Studies in ischemia–reperfusion injury of the lung have shown that activation of the complement system after reperfusion may lead to cellular injury through direct and indirect mechanisms. Complement receptor-1 is a natural complement antagonist that has been shown to reduce ischemia–reperfusion injury and to improve oxygenation in a swine single-lung transplant model (107,123). A multicenter randomized, double-blinded, placebo-controlled trial that included 59 lung transplant recipients showed a significantly greater proportion of patients extubated within the first 24 hours in the group that received the complement antagonist before reperfusion (124). The effect of complement antagonist appeared to be greater in those patients who were exposed to the combined injuries of cardiopulmonary bypass and ischemia–reperfusion.

## Chemokine Receptor Antagonist

In human lung transplantation, measurable amounts of pro- and anti-inflammatory cytokines such as TNF-$\alpha$, IFN-$\gamma$, IL-8, IL-10, IL-12, and IL-18 can be measured in lung tissue during the cold ischemic time and after reperfusion (125). While most cytokine levels decreased after reperfusion, the chemokine IL-8 significantly increased after reperfusion. Donor parameters including oxygen tension, cause of brain death, smoking history, positive sputum cultures, and time on ventilator did not appear to influence the cytokine levels. However, the age of the donor was inversely correlated with the levels of IL-10 after reperfusion. Since IL-10 is an important anti-inflammatory cytokine, this may explain why lungs from older donors might be more susceptible to ischemia–reperfusion injury and are associated with higher postoperative mortality rates.

A striking relationship between IL-8 levels and graft function can also be observed after human lung transplantation (125). IL-8, a potent neutrophil chemotactic agent, rapidly increased following reperfusion. IL-8 levels in lung tissue inversely correlated with lung function and directly correlated with the early postoperative APACHE (Acute Physiology and Chronic Health Evaluation) score. In addition, high levels of IL-8 in donor lung tissue or BAL are associated with an increased risk of death from primary graft dysfunction after transplantation (125,126). The recent development of small molecules that are antagonists to the IL-8 receptor and other CXC chemokine receptors (CXCR1 and CXCR2) will be tested in clinical trials hoping to prevent primary graft dysfunction.

## REFERENCES

1. Gridelli B, Remuzzi G. Strategies for making more organs available for transplantation. N Engl J Med 2000; 343(6):404–410.

2.  UNOS. www.unos.org/resources/donorManagement.asp?index=2.
3.  Novitzky D. Donor management: state of the art. Transplant Proc 1997; 29:3773–3775.
4.  Rosendale JD, Chabalewski FL, McBride MA, et al. Increased transplanted organs from the use of a standardized donor management protocol. Am J Transplant 2002; 2:761–768.
5.  Rosendale JD, Kauffman MH, McBride M, et al. Aggressive pharmacologic donor management results in more transplanted organs. Transplantation 2003; 75:482–487.
6.  Huddleston CB, Mendeloff EN. Heart and lung preservation for transplantation. J Card Surg 2000; 15:108–121.
7.  Conte JV, Baumgartner WA. Overwiew and future practice patterns in cardiac and pulmonary preservation. J Card Surg 2000; 15:91–107.
8.  Gorler A, Haverich A. Adequate lung preservation for clinical lung transplantation: an important condition for satisfactory graft function. J Card Surg 2000; 15:141–148.
9.  de Perrot M, Liu M, Waddell TK, Keshavjee S. Ischemia–reperfusion-induced lung injury. Am J Crit Care Med 2003; 167:490–511.
10. de Perrot M, Keshavjee M. Lung preservation. Semin Thorac Cardiovasc Surg 2004; 16:300–308.
11. Van Raemdonck DEM, Rega FR, Neyrinck AP, et al. Non heart beating donors. Semin Thorac Cardiovasc Surg 2004; 16:309–321.
12. Egan TM. Non-heart-beating donors in thoracic transplantation. J Heart Lung Transplant 2004; 23:3–10.
13. de Perrot M, Weder W, Patterson GA, Keshavjee S. Strategies to increase limited donor resources. Eur Respir J 2004; 23:477–482.
14. Fiser SM, Tribble CG, Long SM. Ischemia–reperfusion injury after lung transplantation increases risk of late bronchiolitis obliterans syndrome. Ann Thorac Surg 2002; 73:1041–1047.
15. King RC, Binns OA, Rodriguez F. Reperfusion injury significantly impacts clinical outcome after pulmonary transplantation. Ann Thorac Surg 2000; 69:1681–1685.
16. International Society for Heart and Lung Transplantation Study Group. Consensus document on primary graft dysfunction. J Heart Lung Transplant. In press.
17. Kirk AJB, Colquhoun IW, Dark JH. Lung preservation: a review of current practice and future directions. Ann Thorac Surg 1993; 56:990–1000.
18. Haverich A, Scott WC, Jamieson SW. Twenty years of lung transplantation. A review. Heart Transplant 1985; 4:234–240.
19. Novick RJ, Menkis AH, McKenzie FN. New trends in lung transplantation: a collective review. J Heart Lung Transplant 1992; 11:377–392.
20. Legal YM. Lung and heart lung transplantation. Ann Thorac Surg 1990; 49:840–844.
21. Wahlers T, Haverich A, Fieguth HG, et al. Flush perfusion using Euro-Collins solution vs cooling by means of extracorporeal circulation in heart lung preservation. J Heart Transplant 1986; 5:89–98.
22. Wallwork J, Jone4s K, Cavarocchi N, et al. Distant procurement of organs for clinical heart–lung transplantation using a single flush technique. Transplantation 1987; 44:654–658.

23. Haverich A, Wahlers T, Schafers HJ, et al. Distant organ procurement in clinical lung and heart–lung transplantation. Eur J Cardiothorac Surg 1990; 4:245–249.
24. Cooper JD, Vreim CE. Biology of lung preservation for transplantation. Am Rev Respir Dis 1992; 146:803–807.
25. Belzer FO, Southard JH. Principles of solid-organ preservation by cold storage. Transplantation 1988; 45:673–676.
26. Lin PJ, Hsieh MJ, Cheng K, et al. University of Wisconsin solution extends lung preservation after prostaglandin E1 infusion. Chest 1994; 105:255–261.
27. Kayano K, Toda K, Naka Y, et al. Superior protection in orthotopic rat lung transplantation with cyclic adenosine monophosphate and nitroglycerin-containing preservation solution. J Thorac Cardiovasc Surg 1999; 118: 135–144.
28. Hopkinson DN, Bhabra MS, Hooper TL. Pulmonary graft preservation: a worldwide survey of current clinical practice. J Heart Lung Transplant 1998; 17:525–531.
29. Housen B, Beuke M, Schroeder F, et al. In vivo measurement of lung preservation solution efficacy: comparison of LPD UW, EC, and low-K-EC following short and extended ischemia. Eur J Cardiothorac Surg 1997; 12:771–780.
30. Fischer S, Matte-Martyn A, de Perrot M. Low-potassium dextran preservation solution improves lung function after human lung transplantation. J Thorac Cardiovasc Surg 2001; 121:594–596.
31. Struber M, Wilhelmi M, Harringer W. Flush perfusion with low potassium dextran solution improves early graft function in clinical lung transplantation. Eur J Cardiothorac Surg 2001; 19:190–194.
32. Muller C, Furst H, Reichenspurner H. Lung procurement by low-potassium dextran and the effect on preservation injury: Munich Lung Transplant Group. Transplantation 1999; 68:1139–1143.
33. Aziz TM, Pillay TM, Corris PA. Perfadex for clinical lung procurement: is it an advance? Ann Thorac Surg 2003; 75:990–995.
34. Rega F, Verleden G, Vanhaecke J. Switch from Euro-Collins to Perfadex for pulmonary graft preservation resulted in superior outcome in transplant recipients (abstract). J Heart Lung Transplant 2003; 22:S111.
35. Rabanal JM, Ibanez AM, Mons R. Influence of preservation solution on early lung function (Euro-Collins versus Perfadex). Transplant Proc 2003; 35:1938–1939.
36. Thabut G, Vinatier I, Brugiere O. Influence of preservation solution on early graft failure in clinical lung transplantation. Am J Respir Crit Care Med 2001; 164:1204–1208.
37. Keshavjee SH, Yamazaki F, Yokomise H. The role of dextran 40 and potassium in extended hypothermic lung preservation for transplantation. J Thorac Cardiovasc Surg 1992; 103:314–325.
38. Sakamaki F, Hoffmann H, Munzing S. Effects of lung preservation solutions on PMN activation in vitro. Transpl Int 1999; 12:113–121.
39. Maccherini M, Keshavjee SH, Slutsky AS. The effect of low-potassium-dextran versus Euro-Collins solution for preservation of isolated type II pneumocytes. Transplantation 1991; 52:621–626.
40. Suzuki S, Inoue K, Sugita M. Effects of EP4 solution and LPD solution versus Euro-Collins solution on Na(+)/K(+)-ATPase activity in rat alveolar type II

cells and human alveolar epithelial cell line A549 cells. J Heart Lung Transplant 2000; 19:887–893.

41.  Sakamaki F, Hoffmann H, Muller C. Reduced lipid peroxidation and ischemia–reperfusion injury after lung transplantation using low-potassium dextran solution for lung preservation. Am J Respir Crit Care Med 1997; 156:1073–1081.

42.  Struber M, Hohlfeld JM, Fraund S. Low-potassium dextran solution ameliorates reperfusion injury of the lung and protects surfactant function. J Thorac Cardiovasc Surg 2000; 120:566–572.

43.  Baldwin JC, First WH, Starkey TD, et al. Distant graft procurement for combined heart and lung transplantation pulmonary artery flush and simple topical hypothermia for graft preservation. Ann Thorac Surg 1987; 43:670–673.

44.  Wang LS, Nakamoto K, Hsieh CM. Influence of temperature of flushing solution on lung preservation. Ann Thorac Surg 1993; 55:711–715.

45.  Albes JM, Fischer F, Bando T. Influence of the perfusate temperature on lung preservation: is there an optimum? Eur Surg Res 1997; 29:5–11.

46.  Fehrenbach H, Riemann D, Wahlers T. Scanning and transmission electron microscopy of human donor lungs: fine structure of the pulmonary parenchyma following preservation and ischemia. Acta Anat (Basel) 1994; 151:220–231.

47.  Muller C, Hoffmann H, Bittmann I. Hypothermic storage alone in lung preservation for transplantation: a metabolic, light microscopic, and functional analysis after 18 hours of preservation. Transplantation 1997; 63:625–630.

48.  Haverich A, Aziz S, Scott WC. Improved lung preservation using Euro-Collins solution for flush-perfusion. Thorac Cardiovasc Surg 1986; 34:368–376.

49.  Steen S, Kimblad PO, Sjoberg T. Safe lung preservation for twenty-four hours with Perfadex. Ann Thorac Surg 1994; 57:450–457.

50.  Sasaki M, Muraoka R, Chiba Y. Influence of pulmonary arterial pressure during flushing on lung preservation. Transplantation 1996; 61:22–27.

51.  Tanaka H, Chiba Y, Sasaki M. Relationship between flushing pressure and nitric oxide production in preserved lungs. Transplantation 1998; 65:460–464.

52.  Struber M, Hohlfeld JM, Kofidis T. Surfactant function in lung transplantation after 24 hours of ischemia: advantage of retrograde flush perfusion for preservation. J Thorac Cardiovasc Surg 2002; 123:98–103.

53.  Sarsam MA, Yonan NA, Deiraniya Ak, et al. Retrograde pulmoplegia for lung preservation in clinical transplantation: a new technique. J Heart Lung Transplant 1993; 12:494–498.

54.  Chen CZ, Gallagher RC, Ardery P, et al. Retrograde versus anterograde flush in canine left lung preservation for six hours. J Heart Lung Transplant 1996; 15:395–403.

55.  Fukuse T, Hirata T, Nakamura T. Influence of deflated and anaerobic conditions during cold storage on rat lungs. Am J Respir Crit Care Med 1999; 160:621–627.

56.  DeCampos KN, Keshavjee S, Liu M. Optimal inflation volume for hypothermic preservation of rat lungs. J Heart Lung Transplant 1998; 17:599–607.

57.  Sakuma T, Tsukano C, Ishigaki M. Lung deflation impairs alveolar epithelial fluid transport in ischemic rabbit and rat lungs. Transplantation 2000; 69:1785–1793.

58. Baretti R, Bitu-Moreno J, Beyersdorf F, Matheis G, Francischetti I, Kreitmayr B. Distribution of lung preservation solutions in parenchyma and airways: influence of atelectasis and route of delivery. J Heart Lung Transplant 1995; 14:80–91.

59. Haniuda M, Hasegawa S, Shiraishi T. Effects of inflation volume during lung preservation on pulmonary capillary permeability. J Thorac Cardiovasc Surg 1996; 112:85–93.

60. Fukuse T, Hirata T, Ishikawa S. Optimal alveolar oxygen concentration for cold storage of the lung. Transplantation 2001; 72:300–304.

61. Date H, Lima O, Matsumura A. In a canine model, lung preservation at 10 degrees C is superior to that at 4 degrees C: a comparison of two preservation temperatures on lung function and on adenosine triphosphate level measured by phosphorus 31-nuclear magnetic resonance. J Thorac Cardiovasc Surg 1992; 103:773–780.

62. Kootstra G, Kievit J, Nederstigt A. Organ donors: heartbeating and non-heart-beating. World J Surg 2002; 26:181–184.

63. Whetstine L, Bowman K, Hawryluck L. Pro/Con ethics debate: is non-heart-beating organ donation ethically acceptable?. Crit Care 2002; 6:192–195.

64. Carlberg A. Transplanting lungs from non-heart-beating donors. Natl Cathol Bioeth Q 2002; 2:377–380.

65. Zamperetti N, Bellomo R, Ronco C. Defining death in non-heart-beating organ donors. J Med Ethics 2003; 29:127–130.

66. Van Norman GA. Another matter of life and death. Anesthesiology 2003; 98:763–773.

67. Kootstra G, Daemen JH, Oomen AP. Categories of non-heart-beating donors. Transplant Proc 1995; 27:2893–2894.

68. Egan TM, Lambert CJ, Reddick R. A strategy to increase the donor pool: use of cadaver lungs for transplantation. Ann Thorac Surg 1991; 52:1113–1121.

69. Homatas J, Bryant L, Eiseman B. Time limits of cadaver lung viability. J Thorac Cardiovasc Surg 1968; 56:132–140.

70. Loehe F, Mueller C, Annecke T. Pulmonary graft function after long-term preservation of non-heart-beating donor lungs. Ann Thorac Surg 2000; 69:1556–1562.

71. Greco R, Cordovilla G, Sanz E. Warm ischemic tolerance after ventilated non-heart-beating lung donation in piglets. Eur J Cardiothorac Surg 1998; 14:319–325.

72. Van Raemdonck DEM, Jannis NCP, De Leyn PR. Warm ischemic tolerance in collapsed pulmonary grafts is limited to 1 hour. Ann Surg 1998; 228: 788–796.

73. Rega FR, Jannis NC, Verleden GM. Should we ventilate or cool the pulmonary graft inside the non-heart-beating donor?. J Heart Lung Transplant 2003; 22:1226–1233.

74. Shennib H. Discussion on Egan TM et al. Ann Thorac Surg 1991; 52: 1120–1121.

75. Love RB, Stringham JC, Chomiak PN. Successful lung transplantation using a non-heart-beating donor (abstract). J Heart Lung Transplant 1995; 14:S88.

76. Love RB, D'Allesandro AM, Cornwell RA. Ten year experience with human lung transplantation from non-heart-beating donors (abstract). J Heart Lung Transplant 2003; 22:S87.

77. Steen S, Sjöberg T, Pierre L. Transplantation of lungs from a non-heart-beating donor. Lancet 2001; 357:825–829.

78. Varela A, Nuñez JR, Gamez AP. Are out hospital non-heart-beating donors (NHBD) better than brain death lung donors (abstract)? J Heart Lung Transplant 2004; 23:S87.

79. Nuñez JR, Varela A, del Rio F. Bipulmonary transplants with lungs obtained from two non-heart-beating donors who died out of hospital. J Thorac Cardiovasc Surg 2004; 127:297–299.

80. Gamez P, Cordoba M, Ussetti P, et al. Lung transplantation from out hospital non-heart-beating donors. One year experience and results. J Heart Lung Transplant. In press.

81. Zikria BA, Ferrer JM, Malm JR. Pulmonary hypothermia in dogs. J Appl Physiol 1968; 24:707–710.

82. Van Raemdonck DEM, Jannis NCP, Rega FRL. External cooling of warm ischemic rabbit lungs after death. Ann Thorac Surg 1996; 62:331–337.

83. Dougherty JC, Sinha S, Kibble F. Intolerance of the ischemic lung to hypothermic ventilation. J Appl Physiol 1972; 32:632–634.

84. Watanabe S, Sakasegawa K, Shimokawa S. Intrathoracic cooling of cadavers before lung transplantation with cold air: an experimental study. Transplantation 2002; 73:39–43.

85. Steen S, Sjöberg T, Ingemansson R. Efficacy of topical cooling in lung preservation: is a reappraisal due? Ann Thorac Surg 1994; 58:1657–1663.

86. Shennib H, Kuang JQ, Giaid A. Successful retrieval and function of lungs from non-heart-beating donors. Ann Thorac Surg 2001; 71:458–461.

87. Wierup P, Bolys R, Steen S. Gas exchange function one month after transplantation of lungs topically cooled for 2 hours in the non-heart-beating cadaver after failed resuscitation. J Heart Lung Transplant 1999; 18:133–138.

88. Kutschka I, Sommer SP, Hohlfeld JM. In-situ topical cooling of lung grafts: early graft function and surfactant analysis in a porcine single lung transplant model. Eur J Cardiothorac Surg 2003; 24:411–419.

89. Rega FR, Neyrinck AP, Verleden GM. How long can we preserve the pulmonary graft inside the non-heart-beating donor? Ann Thorac Surg 2004; 77:438–444.

90. Valero R, Manyalich M, Cabrer C. Organ procurement from non-heart-beating donors by total body cooling. Transplant Proc 1993; 25:3091–3092.

91. Koyama I, Shinozuka N, Miyazawa M. Total body cooling using cardiopulmonary bypass for procurement from non-heart-beating donors. Transplant Proc 2002; 34:2602–2603.

92. Boglione MM, Morandini MA, Barrenechea ME. Pre-arrest heparinization and ventilation during warm ischemia preserves lung function in non-heart-beating donors. J Pediatr Surg 1999; 34:1805–1809.

93. Umemori Y, Date H, Uno K. Improved lung function by urokinase infusion in canine lung transplantation using non-heart-beating donors. Ann Thorac Surg 1995; 59:1513–1518.

94. Akasaka S, Nishi H, Aoe M. The effects of recombinant tissue-type plasminogen activator (rt-PA) on canine cadaver lung transplantation. Surg Today 1999; 29:747–754.

95. Hayama M, Date H, Oto T. Improved lung function by means of retrograde flush in canine lung transplantation with non-heart-beating donors. J Thorac Cardiovasc Surg 2003; 125:901–906.

96. Wittwer Th, Franke UFW, Fehrenbach A. Lung retrieval from non-heart-beating donors: first experience with an innovative preservation strategy in a pig lung transplantation model. Eur Surg Res 2004; 36:1–7.

97. Wittwer T, Franke UFW, Fehrenbach A. Innovative pulmonary preservation of non-heart-beating donor grafts in experimental lung transplantation. Eur J Cardiothorac Surg 2004; 26:144–150.

98. Steen S, Liao Q, Wierup PN. Transplantation of lungs from non-heart-beating donors after functional assessment ex vivo. Ann Thorac Surg 2003; 76:244–252.

99. Aitchison JD, Orr HE, Flecknell PA. Functional assessment of non-heart-beating donor lungs: prediction of post-transplant function. Eur J Cardiothorac Surg 2001; 20:187–194.

100. Rega F, Jannis N, Verleden G. Long-term preservation with interim evaluation of lungs from a non-heart-beating donor with a warm ischemic interval of 90 minutes. Ann Surg 2003; 238:782–793.

101. Rega F, Vandezande E, Jannis N. Role of leucocyte depletion in ex vivo evaluation of pulmonary grafts from non-heart-beating donors. Perfusion 2003; 18:13–21.

102. Steen S, Kimblad PO, Sjöberg T. Safe lung preservation for twenty-four hours with Perfadex. Ann Thorac Surg 1994; 57:450–457.

103. Neyrinck A, Rega F, Jannis N. Ex vivo reperfusion of human lungs declined for transplantation: a novel approach to alleviate donor organ shortage? (abstract). J Heart Lung Transplant 2004; 23:S173.

104. Ardehali A, Laks H, Levine M. A prospective trial of inhaled nitric oxide in clinical lung transplantation. Transplantation 2001; 72:112–115.

105. Thabut G, Brugiere O, Leseche G. Preventive effect of inhaled nitric oxide and pentoxifylline on ischemia/reperfusion injury after lung transplantation. Transplantation 2001; 71:1295–1300.

106. Meade M, Granton JT, Matte-Martyn A. A randomized trial of inhaled nitric oxide to prevent ischemia–reperfusion injury after lung transplantation. Am J Respir Crit Care Med 2003; 167:1483–1489.

107. Keshavjee S, Davis RD, Zamora MR, et al. A randomized placebo controlled trial of complement inhibition in ischemia–reperfusion injury after lung transplantation in humans. J Thorac Cardiovasc Surg 2005; 129:423–428.

108. Wittwer T, Grote M, Oppelt P. Impact of PAF antagonist BN 52021 (Ginkolide B) on post-ischemic graft function in clinical lung transplantation. J Heart Lung Transplant 2001; 20:358–363.

109. Strüber M, Niedermeyer J, Warnecke G. Exogenous surfactant instillation in lung donors to reduce early graft dysfunction (abstract). J Heart Lung Transplant 2003; 22:S142.

110. Ochs M, Fehrenbach H, Nenadic I. Preservation of intraalveolar surfactant in a rat lung ischaemia/reperfusion injury model. Eur Respir J 2000; 15:526–531.

111. Erasmus ME, Hofstede GJ, Petersen AH. Effects of early surfactant treatment persisting for one week after lung transplantation in rats. Am J Respir Crit Care Med 1997; 156:567–572.

112. Novick RJ, MacDonald J, Veldhuizen RA. Evaluation of surfactant treatment strategies after prolonged graft storage in lung transplantation. Am J Respir Crit Care Med 1996; 154:98–104.

113. Liu M, Tremblay L, Cassivi SD. Alterations of nitric oxide synthase expression and activity during rat lung transplantation. Am J Physiol Lung Cell Mol Physiol 2000; 278:L1071–L1081.

114. Schmid RA, Hillinger S, Walter R. The nitric oxide synthase cofactor tetrahydrobiopterin reduces allograft ischemia–reperfusion injury after lung transplantation. J Thorac Cardiovasc Surg 1999; 118:726–732.

115. Suda T, Mora BN, D'Ovidio F. In vivo adenovirus-mediated endothelial nitric oxide synthase gene transfer ameliorates lung allograft ischemia–reperfusion injury. J Thorac Cardiovasc Surg 2000; 119:297–304.

116. Bhabra MS, Hopkinson DN, Shaw TE. Modulation of lung reperfusion injury by nitric oxide: impact of inspired oxygen fraction. Transplantation 1999; 68:1238–1243.

117. Chapelier A, Reignier J, Mazmanian M. Amelioration of reperfusion injury by pentoxifylline after lung transplantation. J Heart Lung Transplant 1995; 14:676–683.

118. Murakami S, Bacha EA, Herve P. Inhaled nitric oxide and pentoxifylline in rat lung transplantation from non-heart beating donors. J Thorac Cardiovasc Surg 1997; 113:821–829.

119. de Perrot M, Fischer S, Liu M. Prostaglandin E1 protects lung transplants from ischemia–reperfusion injury: a shift from pro- to anti-inflammatory cytokines. Transplantation 2001; 72:1505–1512.

120. Aoe M, Trachiotis GD, Okabayashi K. Administration of prostaglandin E1 after lung transplantation improves early graft function. Ann Thorac Surg 1994; 58:655–661.

121. Matsuzaki Y, Waddell TK, Puskas JD. Amelioration of post-ischemic lung reperfusion injury by prostaglandin E1. Am Rev Respir Dis 1993; 148:882–889.

122. Grino JM. BN 52021: a platelet activating factor antagonist for preventing post-transplant renal failure: a double-blind, randomized study. The BN 52021 Study Group in Renal Transplantation. Ann Intern Med 1994; 121:345–347.

123. Schmid RA, Zollinger A, Singer T. Effect of soluble complement receptor type 1 on reperfusion edema and neutrophil migration after lung allotransplantation in swine. J Thorac Cardiovasc Surg 1998; 116:90–97.

124. Pierre AF, Xavier AM, Liu M. Effect of complement inhibition with soluble complement receptor 1 on pig allotransplant lung function. Transplantation 1998; 66:723–732.

125. de Perrot M, Sekine Y, Fischer S. Interleukin-8 release during early reperfusion predicts graft function in human lung transplantation. Am J Respir Crit Care Med 2002; 165:211–215.
126. Fisher AJ, Donnelly SC, Hirani N. Elevated levels of interleukin-8 in donor lungs is associated with early graft failure after lung transplantation. Am J Respir Crit Care Med 2001; 163:259–265. Semin Thorac Cardiovasc Surg 2004; 16:300–308.

# 16

# Operative Techniques Utilized in Lung Transplantation and Strategies to Increase the Donor Pool

**Gabriel T. Schnickel and Abbas Ardehali**

*Division of Cardiothoracic Surgery, David Geffen School of Medicine at UCLA, Los Angeles, California, U.S.A.*

## INTRODUCTION

Lung transplantation has become a well-established and effective treatment option for patients with end-stage lung diseases. There has been a steady rise in the number of patients awaiting lung transplantation while the number of lung transplants performed has increased at a much slower rate. For all practical purposes the number of deceased donors has not changed significantly over the past decade, and the rate of donor procurement for lungs is less than 20% (1). These factors result in a significant number of deaths on the lung transplant waiting list, because there are not enough donor lungs for the number of patients listed for transplant. The majority of brain-dead donors are not deemed suitable to donate lungs, often due to acute lung injury associated with the cause or sequelae of brain death, such as trauma, infection, and aspiration.

Currently, the available options for increasing the number of lung donors are limited. The rigid criteria for acceptable donors are limiting factors in broadening the donor pool. By extending the criteria to include donor lungs previously considered unacceptable, the donor pool may be effectively expanded. A second alternative to increase the number of lung transplants is living lobar lung transplantation (discussed in detail by Dr. Bowdish and Barr in Chapter 10). Finally, utilizing lungs from non–heart-beating donors (NHBDs) has the potential to increase the number of donor lungs available for transplantation.

## LIVING LOBAR LUNG TRANSPLANTATION

Living lobar lung transplantation was introduced and pioneered by the University of Southern California group in 1993 to treat patients that were deemed too ill to likely survive long enough to receive cadaveric donor lungs (2). This procedure requires two donors, one to supply a left and the other to donate the right lower lobe to the recipient. These recipients must fulfill the criteria for cadaveric lung transplantation, and be listed for transplant. These patients are then selected principally on the basis of poor clinical status such that a cadaveric organ would not likely become available in time (3). An important disadvantage of this procedure is that it poses a significant risk of serious complications, or death for two healthy donors.

The University of Southern California has the largest experience with living lobar transplantation. In a review of functional outcomes in 125 (59 bilateral lobar and 43 bilateral cadaveric) adult patients transplanted between January 1993 and September 2002, surviving greater than three months, they found no significant difference in pulmonary function by six months posttransplant when comparing living lobar transplantation versus cadaveric transplantation (4). They also demonstrated no significant difference in exercise capacity and freedom from bronchiolitis obliterans syndrome (BOS) in this cohort. However, there was a significant difference in 3-month survival, which was markedly lower in the lobar group (25% mortality) versus the cadaveric group (6.5%). This may reflect the fact that most of the living lobar patients, by definition, are sicker than their cadaveric counterparts. Indeed, 73% of these patients were hospitalized, and 12% were ventilator dependent at the time of transplantation.

Although the use of living donors for liver and kidney transplantation has increased significantly, the postoperative deaths of donors emphasize the risks involved for the healthy donors (5). This is of particular and unique importance for living lobar donors, because of the need for two donors for each recipient. The largest report on postoperative outcomes in this population again comes from the University of Southern California (6). They report on the perioperative complications of 253 donor lobectomies for 128 living lobar transplants. A total of 19.8% of the donors had one or more perioperative complications, including sacrifice of the right middle lobe in 3.6% of donors in this cohort. The Washington University group found that 38 of 62 (61%) of their donors undergoing donor lobectomy had perioperative complication, including 12 major complications (7). However, neither group has reported a perioperative death in their donor populations.

Although there are limited data on the long-term pulmonary function of these lobar donors, what is available demonstrates an average decrease (among the donors) in forced vital capacity of 17%, and 16% decrease in total lung capacity from preoperative values at 12 months postoperation (6).

Considering the risk to two healthy individuals, the equivocal results compared to cadaveric transplant, and the potential application to only smaller-sized recipients, living donation is unlikely to greatly expand the number of available donors, and thereby will not have a significant effect on waiting list time.

## NON–HEART BEATING DONORS

Donors that currently provide most of the organs used for transplantation are from patients who have been declared brain-dead by neurologic criteria. These donors still have cardiac activity that continues to perfuse the remainder of their organs until the moment of cold preservation. Organs that are removed following cardiac arrest are considered NHBDs. The first lung transplant was from an NHBD in 1963, and in fact, the concept of brain death was not widely accepted until 1968 (8–10). Prior to this all organs were retrieved from NHBDs (11).

NHBDs are classified by the Maastricht Categories as either uncontrolled or controlled donors (12). NHBDs who die unexpectedly are considered uncontrolled donors, and are either dead on arrival at the hospital (category I) or undergo an unsuccessful resuscitation (category II). Controlled donors include individuals awaiting cardiac arrest (category III), or cardiac arrest in brain-dead donors (category IV).

It is estimated that one-third of all deaths in the Western world are the result of ischemic heart disease. In the United States alone 275,000 undergo sudden cardiac arrest annually (13). Considering that the lung transplant waiting list is currently 3628 patients in the United States, it would take only 1% to 2% of these patients becoming viable donors to transplant all the patients on the waiting list (1). This represents a vast potential source of donor lungs. In certain countries that do not recognize the concept of brain death, NHBDs are the only available source of solid organs for transplantation.

The concept of NHBDs in lung transplantation was reintroduced through the work of Egan et al. in 1991, which demonstrated that lung tissue remains viable after death in the absence of perfusion (14). Because of the unique properties of the lung, this may be the ideal organ for use after cardiac death. The lung parenchyma relies on diffusion from air spaces rather than perfusion of the capillary bed for the delivery of oxygen for cellular respiration. Pulmonary epithelial cells can be removed and cultured several hours following cardiac death. Subsequently, several groups demonstrated that 60 to 90 minutes is the tolerable period of warm ischemia in an untouched cadaver, with 90% of lung parenchymal cells still viable at one hour following cardiac arrest (15–18).

The use of NHBDs does impose certain restraints; 90 minutes is certainly not enough time to attain consent, retrieve the organ, and pre-op the recipient. Therefore, experimental focus shifted to extending the viable ischemic time following cardiac arrest. Work with experimental models demonstrated that viability can be extended through ventilation of the donor lungs during warm ischemia (19–21). Continuous $O_2$ supplied during ischemia confers a beneficial effect, extending tolerable warm ischemic time to four hours (16). Further experimental work found that cooling of the lungs inside the cadaver with cold air was unsuccessful. However, Steen et al., using a pig model of NHBD, demonstrated that cooling of the donor lungs with infusion of cold preservation solution into the chest cavity could extend the tolerable ischemic time to seven hours, with no difference in graft function compared to harvest at the time of cardiac death (22).

Another shortcoming of NHBDs that must be overcome is preoperative graft assessment. In the more controlled setting of HBDs, or even controlled NHBDs, the allograft may be assessed prior to procurement by a number of methods, including bronchoscopy, chest radiograph, and oxygen challenge. Postmortem functional assessment is not necessary in this setting. In the uncontrolled NHBD the donor graft must be assessed so that only lungs of proper quality will be transplanted. Two techniques have been developed to provide functional assessment in this setting: first, ex vivo reperfusion in a closed circuit after organ procurement (22) and, alternatively, in situ flush with a solution based on donor blood prior to organ retrieval (23). Both have been shown to be effective predictors of lung allograft function following reperfusion in experimental models.

There is limited clinical experience with NHBD lung transplants in humans. Love et al. reported their experience with five controlled donors transplanted between 1995 and 2002, one double-lung and four single-lung transplants (24). All recipients had good pulmonary function following transplant, with no primary graft failure. One patient died during the initial hospitalization of a bowel perforation; another died one year post-op from BOS; there were three long-term survivors at the time of the report.

Steen and colleagues reported on the first case of lung transplantation from an uncontrolled NHBD (25). The donor was a patient dying as a result of acute myocardial infarction following an unsuccessful resuscitation effort. The lungs were cooled by intrapleural infusion of cold perfadex after 65 minutes of warm ischemia. The lungs were harvested and assessed by an ex vivo reperfusion circuit, and then recooled and stored at 8°C. The recipient was a 54-year-old female with chronic obstructive pulmonary disease who had previously been listed for lung transplantation. The right lung was transplanted after a total ischemic time of 13 hours. Postoperatively, the transplanted lung showed excellent function; unfortunately, the recipient died of a cytomegalovirus infection several months posttransplant.

Following this initial work in Sweden, Varela and colleagues in Madrid, Spain, reported their one-year experience with lung transplantation from out-of-hospital NHBDs (26,27). During this period, five recipients (four double, one single) received lung transplants from NHBD donors. Following attempts at resuscitation and certification of death, the donors were taken to the operating room and placed on extracorporeal bypass with deep hypothermia. The lungs are further cooled in situ with cold low-potassium dextran (Perfadex) via intrapleural chest drain. The donor lungs are then assessed before harvest by in situ flush with donor blood mixed with Perfadex. The postoperative lung function was excellent in all recipients, though intermediate and long-term function remains to be reported at this time.

With the large number of individuals suffering from sudden cardiac arrest, employing NHBDs in lung transplantation could potentially erase the organ shortage. However, limited experience with NHBDs and the serious potential problems of prolonged warm ischemia, adequacy of in situ preservation, and functional graft assessment remain as challenges. Until more short- and long-term results are gathered, NHBDs in lung transplantation remains an investigational area with significant potential.

## NONSTANDARD DONOR LUNGS

The currently accepted criteria for an acceptable lung donor are age >55 years, clear chest radiograph, $PaO_2/FiO_2$ ratio >300 on $FiO_2$ 1.0 and positive end-expiratory pressure (PEEP) of 5, and the absence of purulent secretion on bronchoscopy. These parameters were created based on individual case reports and anecdotal evidence. While strategies in perioperative management have changed dramatically over the past decade, the criteria for acceptable donors have changed very little. An expanding waiting list and a stable number of donors suggest that to expand the donor pool, lungs previously considered marginal must be considered for transplant.

## CRITERIA FOR STANDARD DONOR LUNGS

### Age

The generally accepted age limit for donors has been 55 years. This criterion was first established at 40 years of age, but following work by Shumway et al. in 1994, the donor age limit considered acceptable was raised. Their findings suggested that short-term outcome was unrelated to advanced donor age (28). Since this initial study, multiple individual centers have found no difference when donor age was evaluated as an independent risk factor (29–32).

## Chest X Ray

A clear chest radiograph is considered standard. This criterion is somewhat subjective and may vary depending on the clinician. While a completely clear radiograph is considered the standard, some groups will accept donor lungs with a unilateral infiltrate (33). Ware et al. examined donor lungs that were rejected for transplantation based on the well-established criteria, and demonstrated that chest radiograph did not accurately predict degree of pulmonary edema or histological abnormality (34).

## $PaO_2/FiO_2$

In 1987, Harujala et al. reported on the poor outcome of a patient who received lungs from a donor with a $PaO_2/FiO_2$ ratio of $\sim$250 (35). This individual case report appears to be the basis for establishing the acceptable $PaO_2/FiO_2$ ratio for standard donor lungs at >300. Subsequently, in 1994, Shumway found no difference in the outcomes of donor lungs with $PaO_2/FiO_2$ ratio $\geq$250 (28). Examination of donor lungs rejected for transplantation based on poor oxygenation demonstrates that $PaO_2/FiO_2$ ratio can predict the ex vivo fluid balance of the donor lungs (34). However, aggressive donor management can change lungs from marginal to acceptable based on the $PaO_2/FiO_2$ ratio alone (36,37).

## Smoking

The accepted criterion for a standard donor is a smoking history of <20 pack years. The original parameter for ideal donors was no history of smoking, but early studies found no difference in outcome between patients receiving donor lungs from smokers and nonsmokers. The greatest concerns for accepting lungs from smokers are the possibility of a recipient developing cancer and loss of pulmonary reserve. Few studies have significant numbers of patients with smoking history >20 pack years. However, those that addressed this criterion have found no difference in outcome (37,38).

With regard to a donor's smoking history and a recipient's cancer risk, no evidence has demonstrated a connection, though few long-term studies have been done. The literature has scattered case reports of lung cancer in transplant recipients, but almost all of these can be attributed to recipient history of tobacco use and none in which a marginal donor was the cause (39–42). Therefore, if there is no radiological or gross evidence of malignancy, cancer should be of little concern in relation to extended criteria.

## Bronchoscopy

Bronchoscopy is an effective screening method to assess lung injury, inflammation, aspiration, and presence of infection. A clear bronchoscopy, without purulent secretion or evidence of infection, is a generally accepted criterion for ideal donors. However, only 33% of all brain-dead donors and 62% of ideal donors have what could be considered a normal bronchoscopy (43). Multiple studies have found tracheal colonization to be common in the donor population (44,45). A positive Gram stain on bronchoalveolar lavage has been considered a possible risk factor for development of a postoperative pneumonia. Bacterial pneumonia has been shown to be a common cause of early morbidity and mortality in the transplant population (46). However, recent evidence demonstrates no correlation between a positive donor Gram stain and subsequent recipient postoperative pneumonia (47).

## PROBLEMS WITH NONSTANDARD DONOR LUNGS

What is the concern about using nonstandard donor lungs for transplantation? First, there is the concern for short-term morbidity associated with primary graft dysfunction (PGD) and perioperative infections, particularly pneumonia. These potential developments are associated with high mortality and the possibility of decreased function in patients that survive. Long-term outcome, most importantly, the development of BOS, is a significant concern. BOS represents chronic lung allograft rejection and has a prevalence of 70% in patients surviving five years posttransplant (48–50).

## PRIMARY GRAFT DYSFUNCTION

Severe PGD occurs in 10% to 20% of lung transplant recipients and represents the leading cause of early death following lung transplantation, with an associated mortality of 40% (51,52). Those recipients who survive are often left with impaired residual lung function (53). Severe PGD can also be associated with an increased risk of acute rejection and late BOS (52). A major concern regarding utilization of nonstandard donor lungs is the risk of severe PGD. For this reason, addressing PGD in marginal donors is of paramount importance.

Recent advances in donor management, organ preservation, operative technique, and perioperative care have impacted the incidence of PGD in contemporary lung transplantation. Administration of steroids to the donors has been shown to improve allograft function and increase procurement rate (54). Newer lung preservation solutions, such as low-potassium dextran (Perfadex), have also been found to improve early lung allograft function. Wittwer et al. demonstrated that graft preservation with antegrade Perfadex significantly increases oxygenation capacity, decreases inspiratory pressures, and decreases lung edema compared to other preservation solutions (55). Further experimental study demonstrated that retrograde flushed preservation could further improve graft function when compared to anterograde preservation (56).

Improvements in operative management and technique have also influenced the incidence and severity of PGD. These measures include minimizing warm ischemia time, controlling reperfusion pressure, and modification of reperfusate. Bhabra et al. demonstrated, in a rat model, that poor function, reduced blood flow, elevated pulmonary artery pressure, and pulmonary edema are prevented with 10 minutes of controlled reperfusion (50% physiologic perfusion pressure) (57). Ardehali et al. found that altering the content and conditions of the initial reperfusate after surgical implantation, when compared to reperfusion with whole blood, decreases the incidence of PGD in a similar cohort of patients (58), Whiting et al. demonstrated that this technique is associated with a low incidence of PGD following transplantation of nonstandard donor lungs (59).

Improvements in ventilatory management and potential beneficial effects of induction therapy are among the advances in perioperative management of patients with lung allograft dysfunction. Collaboratively, recent findings illustrate the effectiveness of newer techniques at minimizing PGD, improving short-term outcomes, and potentially decreasing the risk for developing BOS, and therefore judicious expansion of the donor pool appears reasonable. However, caution needs to be exercised when accepting such high-risk nonstandard donors for high-risk recipients, such as those with primary pulmonary hypertension.

## INFECTIOUS COMPLICATIONS

Evidence of donor infection has always been a contraindication for acceptance. Infectious complications are the most common cause of morbidity and mortality after lung transplantation with an overall incidence of pneumonia constituting 35% to 66% of infectious episodes. The majority of these cases occur within the first posttransplant month, with bacterial pneumonia being the most frequent of these early infections (60–63). Early work in this area indicated that the vast majority of donor bronchial washings grew at least one organism (44,45). In a cohort of 29 lung transplant recipients, 43% of patients' bronchial cultures grew organisms similar to their donor, and 21% of these developed invasive pulmonary infections (45). More recent studies, in the era of standard prophylactic broad-spectrum antibiotics, have found no predictive value in type or amount of bacteria seen on donor Gram stain (47).

Fungal infections represent only 10% to 14% of postoperative infections; however, they are associated with a much higher mortality (47,60,64). Zenati et al. found that patients receiving lungs with heavy growth of *Candida* on tracheal culture were more likely to develop invasive fungal infection (45). However, routine use of prophylactic antifungal therapy has decreased the incidence of fungal infection and newer aerosolized antifungal treatments have been shown to be associated with a low rate of invasive pulmonary fungal infections with few adverse affects (67). Therefore, donor colonization, without infection, should not preclude donor lung acceptance, but care should be exercised when considering high-risk patients and donors with heavy growth of fungal species or resistant, nosocomially acquired organisms.

## LONG-TERM ALLOGRAFT FUNCTION

Long-term outcome in lung transplantation continues to remain a problem with five-year survival rates of only 42%, mainly due to BOS (67). Whether the recipients of nonstandard lungs will have similar outcomes or whether they are at an increased risk for BOS remains unclear. There are no studies, to date, that demonstrate an *increased* risk of developing BOS or a *decrease* in five-year survival among recipients of nonstandard lungs. The relative incidence of rejection episodes in nonstandard donors past the first posttransplant year remains to be demonstrated in a long-term study. Therefore, while it seems likely that nonstandard donor lungs are at no increased risk for BOS, an accurate assessment cannot be made.

## EXPERIENCE WITH NONSTANDARD LUNGS

Analysis of the lung transplants reported to the United Network for Organ Sharing over a 10-year period from 1987 to 1997 found that while donor age and ischemic time were not independent risk factors of survival, the interaction between age and prolonged ischemic time impacted one-year survival. This was more notable with a donor >55 years of age and an ischemic time greater than seven hours (30). The apparent relationship between age and ischemic time suggests that caution should be exercised in this group of donors.

Gabbay et al. reported the results of nonstandard donors at the Alfred Hospital in Melbourne, Australia, transplanted between 1995 and 1998. A total of 74 lung transplants from 64 donors in this interval did not meet the standard criteria. The most frequently breeched criteria were abnormal chest radiograph and $PaO_2/FiO_2$ ratio <300. They found that the overall survival at 30 days, one year, two years, and three years was no different between nonstandard and ideal donors transplanted over the same time period. However, multivariate analysis demonstrated that prolonged ischemic time was predictive of unfavorable outcome (37).

The Loyola University group found no difference in short-term results between ideal and marginal lungs when evaluating the incidence of operative complications, length of ICU stay, time of mechanical ventilation, and hospital survival (38). They also assessed lung function by comparing forced expiratory volume in one second ($FEV_1$) at one year. While a trend toward decreasing $FEV_1$ at one year in single-lung transplants from marginal donors was noted, it was not statistically significant and there was no difference overall between the two groups.

Washington University first reported their experience with nonstandard donor lungs in a review of 44 of 89 patients defined as nonstandard transplanted between 1991 and 1994 (68). They found no difference in short-term outcomes as defined by time on mechanical ventilation, alveolar–arterial (A–a) $O_2$ gradient, and 30-day mortality. The only difference they noted was that nonstandard donor lung transplants were more frequently performed on cardiopulmonary bypass. The authors reassessed their results after a decade of experience. Once again, now with 118 out of 450 lung transplants classified as nonstandard, they found no difference in outcome. It was found that one- and five-year survival rates of recipients of standard and nonstandard donor lungs were similar (68). This is the first large study to assess the long-term outcomes of recipients of nonstandard donor lungs.

Pierre et al. reviewed the University of Toronto experience of 128 lung transplants performed between 1997 and 2000, 63 (51%) of which were considered nonstandard. No difference in $PaO_2/FiO_2$ ratio or length of ICU stay was found. However, they did find a significant increase in 30-day mortality (6.2% vs. 17.5%) in recipients of nonstandard donor lungs. An even greater discrepancy in 30-day mortality was noted when nonstandard donor lungs were transplanted into high-risk recipients (5.3% vs. 22.2%). Although they were unable to demonstrate a statistical significance, they believe that a bilateral infiltrate and purulent secretions on bronchoscopy may be associated with higher mortality (33).

Our group at UCLA first reported our findings of 42 patients who received lungs classified as nonstandard, transplanted between 1999 and 2002 (59). We found that with the use of modified reperfusion an acceptable short-term outcome could be achieved with a low incidence of PGD. More recently, we reevaluated our experience of 100 recipients receiving nonstandard donor lungs (69). Short-term outcomes were assessed (i.e., time requiring mechanical ventilation, postoperative $PaO_2/FiO_2$ ratio, length of ICU stay, 30-day mortality, and incidence of PGD). Using these guidelines, there were no significant differences in the short-term morbidity or mortality among recipients of nonstandard versus standard lungs.

In summary, expansion of donor criteria seems warranted because of long waiting time and recent advances in organ preservation, organ resuscitation, and perioperative care. The short-term outcome associated with nonstandard donor lungs appears comparable to the standard lungs. Caution is warranted in transplanting nonstandard lungs with several risk factors to high-risk recipients (i.e., recipients with significant pulmonary hypertension). Systemic review of each risk factor and development of a scoring system for donor lungs are necessary to further elucidate the potential utility of nonstandard lungs. In addition, NHBDs hold promise as a vast source of potential donors. However, short-term and long-term studies are needed prior to widespread adoption of this approach.

## REFERENCES

1. United Network for Organ Sharing. 2003 Annual Report of the U.S. Scientific Registry for Transplant Recipients and the Organ Procurement and Transplantation Network: Transplant Data: 1993–2003. Rockville, MD: US Department of Health and Human Services/Richmond, VA: UNOS.
2. Starnes VA, Barr ML, Cohen RG. Lobar transplantation indications, technique, and outcome. J Thorac Cardiovasc Surg 1994; 108:403–411.
3. Starnes VA, Barr ML, Schenkel FA, et al. Experience with living-donor lobar transplantation for indications other than cystic fibrosis. J Thorac Cardiovasc Surg 1997; 114:917–921.
4. Bowdish ME, Pessotto R, Barbers RG, Schenkel FA, Starnes VA, Barr ML. Long-term pulmonary function after living-donor lobar lung transplantation in adults. Ann Thorac Surg 2005; 79:418–425.
5. Nathan HM, Conrad SL, Held PJ, et al. Scientific registry of transplant recipients (SRTR) report on the state of transplantation: organ donation in the United States. Am J Transplant 2003; 3(Suppl 4):2940.
6. Bowdish ME, Barr ML, Schenkel FA, et al. A decade of living lobar lung transplantation: perioperative complications after 253 donor lobectomies. Am J Transplant 2004; 4(8):1283–1288.
7. Battafarano RJ, Anderson RC, Meyers BF, et al. Perioperative complications after living donor lobectomy. J Thorac Cardiovasc Surg 2000; 120:909–915.
8. Ad hoc committee of the Harvard Medical School to examine the definition of brain death. A definition of irreversible coma. Report of the ad hoc committee of the Harvard Medical School to examine the definition of brain death. J Am Med Assoc 1968; 205:85–88.
9. Giacomini M. A change of the heart and a change of mind? Technology and the redefinition of death in 1968. Soc Sci Med 1997; 44:1465–1482.
10. Hardy JD, Webb WR, Dalton ML. Homotransplantation in man. J Am Med Assoc 1963; 186:1065–1074.
11. Pletka P, Kenyon JR, Snell M, et al. Cadaveric renal transplantation: an analysis of 65 cases. Lancet 1969; 1:1–6.
12. Kootstra G, Daemen JH, Oomen AP. Categories of non-heart-beating donors. Transplant Proc 1995; 27:2893–2894.
13. American Heart Association. Heart and Stroke Statistical Update 1998. Dallas: American Heart Association.
14. Egan TM, Lambert CJ, Reddick R. A strategy to increase the donor pool: use of cadaver lungs for transplantation. Ann Thorac Surg 1991; 52:1113–1121.
15. Homatas J, Bryant L, Eiseman B. Time limits of cadaver lung viability. J Thorac Cardiovasc Surg 1968; 56:132–140.
16. Loehe F, Mueller C, Annecke T. Pulmonary graft function after long-term preservation of non-heart-beating donor lungs. Ann Thorac Surg 2000; 69:1556–1562.
17. Greco R, Cordovilla G, Sanz E. Warm ischemic tolerance after ventilated non-heart-beating lung donation in piglets. Eur J Cardiothorac Surg 1998; 14:319–325.
18. Kuang JQ, Van Raemdonck DEM, Jannis NCP. Pulmonary cell death in warm ischemic rabbit lung is related to the alveolar oxygen reserve. J Heart Lung Transplant 1998; 17:406–414.

19. Ulicny KS Jr, Egan TM, Lambert CJ Jr. Cadaver lung donors: effect of preharvest ventilation on graft function. Ann Thorac Surg 1993; 55:1453–1459.
20. Hennington MH, D'Armini AM, Lemasters JJ. Cadaver lungs for transplantation: effect of ventilation with alveolar gas. Transplantation 1996; 61:1009–1014.
21. Steen S, Ingemansson R, Budrikis A. Successful transplantation of lungs topically cooled in the non-heart-beating donor for 6 hours. Ann Thorac Surg 1997; 63:345–351.
22. Steen S, Liao Q, Wierup PN. Transplantation of lungs from non-heart-beating donors after functional assessment ex vivo. Ann Thorac Surg 2003; 76:244–252.
23. Aitchison JD, Orr HE, Flecknell PA. Functional assessment of non-heart-beating donor lungs: prediction of post-transplant function. Eur J Cardiothorac Surg 2001; 20:187–194.
24. Love RB, D'Allesandro AM, Cornwell RA. Ten year experience with human lung transplantation from non-heart-beating donors. J Heart Lung Transplant 2003; 22:S87.
25. Steen S, Sjoberg T, Pierre L, Liao Q, Eriksson L, Algotsson L. Transplantation of lungs from a non-heart-beating donor. Lancet 2001; 357:825–829.
26. Varela A, Nuñez JR, Gamez AP. Are out hospital non-heart-beating donors (NHBD) better than brain death lung donors? (abstract). J Heart Lung Transplant 2004; 23:S87.
27. Nuñez JR, Varela A, del Rio F. Bipulmonary transplants with lungs obtained from two non-heart-beating donors who died out of hospital. J Thorac Cardiovasc Surg 2004; 127:297–299.
28. Shumway SJ, Hertz MI, Petty MG, Bolman RM. Liberalization of donor criteria in lung and heart–lung transplantation. Ann Thorac Surg 1994; 57:92–95.
29. Meyer DM, Bennett LE, Novick RJ, Hosenpud JD. Effect of donor age and ischemic time in intermediate survival and morbidity after lung transplantation. Chest 2000; 118:1255–1262.
30. Novick RJ, Bennett LE, Meyer DM, Hosenpud JD. Influence of graft ischemic time and donor age on survival after lung transplantation. J Heart Lung Transplant 1999; 18:425–431.
31. Sundaresan S, Semenkovich J, Ochoa L, et al. Successful outcome of lung transplantation is not compromised by the use of marginal donor lungs. J Thorac Cardiovasc Surg 1995; 109:1075–1079.
32. Sommers KE, Griffith BP, Hardesty RL, Keenan RJ. Early lung allograft function in twin recipients from the same donor: risk factor analysis. Ann Thorac Surg 1996; 62:784–790.
33. Pierre AF, Sekine Y, Hutcheon M, et al. Marginal lung donors: a reassessment. J Thorac Cardiovasc Surg 2002; 123:421–428.
34. Ware L, Wang Y, Rang X, et al. Assessment of lungs rejected for transplantation and implications for donor selection. Lancet 2002; 390:619–620.
35. Harjula A, Baldwin JC, Starnes VA, et al. Proper donor selection for heart–lung transplantation. The Stanford experience. J Thorac Cardiovasc Surg 1987; 94:874–880.
36. Straznicka M, Follette DM, Eisner MD, et al. Aggressive management of lung donors classified as unacceptable: excellent recipient survival one year after transplantation. J Thorac Cardiovasc Surg 2002; 124:250–258.

37. Gabbay E, Williams TJ, Griffiths, AP, et al. Maximizing the utilization of donor organs offered for lung transplantation. Am J Respir Crit Care Med 1999; 160:265–271.

38. Bhorade SM, Vigneswaran W, McCabe MA, Garrity ER. Liberalization of donor criteria may expand the donor pool without adverse consequence in lung transplantation. J Heart Lung Transplant 2000; 19:1199–1204.

39. Choi YH, Leung AN, Miro S, et al. Primary bronchogenic carcinoma after heart or lung transplantation: radiologic and clinical findings. J Thorac Imaging 2000; 15:36–40.

40. Delcambre F, Pruvot FR, Ramon P, et al. Primary bronchogenic carcinoma in transplant recipients. Transplant Proc 1996; 28:2884–2885.

41. DeSoyza AG, Dark JH, Parums DV, et al. Donor acquired small cell lung cancer following pulmonary transplantation. Chest 2001; 120:1030–1031.

42. Stagner LD, Allenspach L, Hogan K, et al. Bronchogenic carcinoma in lung transplant recipients. J Heart Lung Transplant 2001; 20:908–911.

43. Riou B, Guesde R, Jacquens Y, et al. Fiberoptic bronchoscopy in brain-dead organ donors. Am J Respir Crit Care Med 1994; 150:558–560.

44. Griffith BP, Zenati M. The pulmonary donor. Clin Chest Med 1990; 11:217–226.

45. Zenati M, Dowling RD, Dummer JS, et al. Influence of the donor lung on development of early infections in lung transplant recipients. J Heart Lung Transplant 1990; 9:502–509.

46. Low DE, Kaiser LR, Haydock DA, et al. The lung donor: infectious and pathologic factors affecting outcome in lung transplantation. J Thorac Cardiovasc Surg 1993; 106:614–621.

47. Kramer MR, Marshall SE, Starnes VA, Gamberg P, Amitai Z, Theodore J. Infectious complications in heart–lung transplantation. Analysis of 200 episodes. Arch Int Med 1993; 153:2010–2016.

48. Kelly K, Hertz MI. Obliterative bronchiolitis. Clin Chest Med 1997; 18:319–338.

49. Heng D, Sharples LD, McNeil K, et al. Bronchiolitis obliterans syndrome: incidence, natural history, prognosis, and risk factors. J Heart Lung Transplant 1998; 17:1255–1263.

50. Valentine VG, Robbins RC, Berry GJ, et al. Actuarial survival of heart–lung and bilateral sequential lung transplant recipients with obliterative bronchiolitis. J Heart Lung Transplant 1996; 15:371–383.

51. King RC, Binns OA, Rodriguez F, et al. Reperfusion injury significantly impacts clinical outcome after pulmonary transplantation. Ann Thorac Surg 2000; 69:1681–1685.

52. Christie JD, Bavaria JE, Palevsky HI, et al. Primary graft failure following lung transplantation. Chest 1998; 114:51–60.

53. Date H, Lynch JP, Sundaresan S, et al. The impact of cytolytic therapy on bronchiolitis obliterans syndrome. J Heart Lung Transplant 1998; 17:869–875.

54. Follete DM, Rudich SM, Babcock WD. Improved oxygenation and increased lung donor recovery with high-dose steroid administration after brain death. J Heart Lung Transplant 1998; 17:423–429.

55. Wittwer T, Johannes AM, Fehrenbach A, et al. Experimental lung preservation with Perfadex: effect of the NO-donor nitroglycerin on postischemic outcome. J Thorac Cardiovasc Surg 2003; 125:1208–1216.

56. Wittwer T, Franke U, Fehrenbach A, et al. Impact of retrograde graft preservation in Perfadex-based experimental lung transplantation. J Surg Res 2004; 117:239–248.
57. Bhabra MS, Hopkinson DN, Shaw TE, et al. Critical importance of the first 10 minutes of lung graft reperfusion after hypothermic storage. Ann Thorac Surg 1996; 61:1631–1635.
58. Ardehali A, Laks H, Russell H, et al. Modified reperfusion and ischemia-reperfusion injury in human lung transplantation. J Thorac Cardiovasc Surg 2003; 126:1929–1934.
59. Whiting D, Banerji A, Ross D, et al. Liberalization of lung donor criteria in lung transplantation. Am Surg 2003; 69:1–4.
60. Dauber JH, Paradis IL, Dummer JS. Infectious complications in pulmonary allograft recipients. Clin Chest Med 1990; 11:291–308.
61. Horvath J, Dummer S, Loyd J, et al. Infection in the transplanted and native lung after single lung transplantation. Chest 1993; 104:681–685.
62. Maurer JR, Tullis DE, Grossman RF, Vellend H, Winton TL, Patterson GA. Infectious complications following isolated lung transplantation. Chest 1992; 101:1056–1059.
63. Shennib H, Massard G. Airway complications in lung transplantation. Ann Thorac Surg 1994; 57:506–511.
64. Dowling RD, Zenati M, Yousem SA, et al. Donor-transmitted pneumonia in experimental lung allografts; successful prevention with donor antibiotic therapy. J Thorac Cardiovasc Surg 1992; 103:767–772.
65. Weill D, Dey GC, Young KR, et al. A positive donor gram stain does not predict the development of pneumonia, oxygenation or duration of mechanical ventilation following lung transplantation. J Heart Lung Transplant 2001; 20:255.
66. Drew RH, Ashley ED, Benjamin DK, et al. Comparative safety of amphotericin B lipid complex and amphotericin B deoxycholate as aerosolized antifungal prophylaxis in lung-transplant recipients. Transplantation 2004; 77:232–237.
67. Trulock EP. Lung transplantation. Am J Respir Crit Care Med 1997; 155:789–818.
68. Meyers BF, Lynch J, Trulock EP, et al. Lung transplantation: a decade of experience. Ann Surg 1999; 230:362–370.
69. Schnickel GT, Ross DJ, Beygui R, et al. Modified reperfusion in clinical lung transplantation: the result of 100 consecutive cases. J Thorac Cardiovasc Surg 2006; 131:218–223.

# 17

# Immunosuppressive Drugs: Cyclosporine, Tacrolimus, Sirolimus, Azathioprine, Mycophenolate Mofetil, and Corticosteroids

**Brandon S. Lu, Edward R. Garrity, Jr., and Sangeeta M. Bhorade**

*Division of Pulmonary and Critical Care Medicine, Department of Internal Medicine, Loyola University Medical Center, Maywood, Illinois, U.S.A.*

## INTRODUCTION

Lung transplantation (LTx) has become a viable option for the end-stage lung disease because of its ability to prolong survival in patients with end-stage lung diseases. In 1963, the first LTx recipient lived for 18 days post-operatively and died from renal failure (1). With improvements in surgical techniques, immunosuppression regimens, and long-term care, the current one- and five-year survival rates are 77% and 47%, respectively (2).

In this chapter, we will discuss the major immunosuppressive drugs in use today for LTx. Different immunosuppression regimens will also be discussed. It is important to realize that no drugs have been granted specific approval for use in LTx because of a lack of clinical data.

## CALCINEURIN INHIBITORS

### Cyclosporine

The clinical use of cyclosporine A (CsA) marked a major milestone in the field of LTx. Most of the 38 LTx recipients between 1963 and 1983 survived <1 month, with the exception of one patient who lived for 10 months (3–5).

In 1983, Cooper and his colleagues performed the first single LTx in the CsA era, using azathioprine (Aza) and CsA immediately postoperatively, and prednisone was added three weeks later (6). This recipient survived 6.5 years and eventually died from complications of renal failure.

Mechanism of Action

CsA is a neutral, lipophilic, cyclic undecapeptide extracted from the fungus *Tolypocladium inflatum gams* (7). Its chief mechanism of action is to block T-lymphocyte activation by inhibiting interleukin-2 (IL-2) synthesis (Fig. 1). CsA freely diffuses through cell membrane into the cytoplasm of T lymphocytes to bind with cytoplasmic proteins, called cyclophilins. The CsA–cyclophilin complex specifically and competitively binds to calcineurin, a serine–threonine phosphatase found in T lymphocytes. Calcineurin normally dephosphorylates nuclear regulatory proteins, such as nuclear factor of activated T cells (NF-AT), NF-κB, and Oct/OAP, to facilitate their passage into the nucleus where they act as transcription factors for various cytokines. By inactivating the enzymatic activity of calcineurin, the CsA–cyclophilin complex blocks the production of IL-2, IL-3, IL-4, CD40L, granulocyte–macrophage colony stimulating factor, tumor necrosis factor-α, and interferon-γ. Thus, T-lymphocyte proliferation and effector functions are suppressed (8–11).

CsA has also been shown to stimulate the production of transforming growth factor-beta (TGF-β) in LTx recipients (12). TGF-β can inhibit T-lymphocyte proliferation as well as induce a profibrotic state by upregulating fibroblast growth and proliferation. This can potentially lead to the fibrosis-promoting effect of CsA therapy (13).

Pharmacokinetics

CsA is absorbed in the upper small intestine according to a bile-dependent zero-order process, but a threefold variation can exist between individuals in the average bioavailability of the drug and the time to peak drug level. Once in the bloodstream, CsA is transported by lipoproteins and chylomicrons, with a small fraction circulating as unbound compound that has no clinical significance (7). It has a median half-life of 6.4 to 8.7 hours and is metabolized almost exclusively in the liver by the cytochrome P450 enzyme 3A4 (CYP3A4) and eliminated in the bile, with only 6% excreted in urine (7,10).

CsA was introduced as an oil-based formulation, which demonstrated unpredictable absorption, especially in the presence of biliary diversion, cholestasis, gastroparesis, and steatorrhea. Coingestion of CsA with food, normal serum low-density lipoprotein levels, and prolonged therapy promote the absorption of the drug (7). In the mid-1990s, a formulation of CsA in a microemulsion preconcentrate (CsA–ME) was introduced that spontaneously forms a homogenous emulsion in the aqueous environment of the small bowel, providing more consistent drug levels and pharmacokinetic

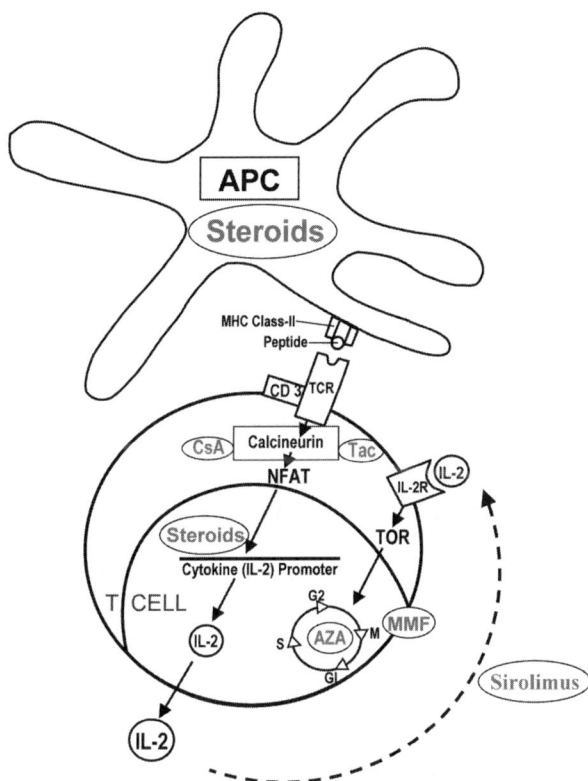

**Figure 1** T-cell activation cascade and sites of immunosuppressant action. TCR binds to a complementary MHC Class-II molecule with an associated peptide, to initiate T-cell activation. Full activation requires an additional interaction between the APC and T-cell (not shown). Intracellularly, calcineurin is activated to dephosphorylate and activate transcription factors (e.g., NF-AT) for numerous cytokines, including IL-2. IL-2 has an autocrine effect that initiates T-cell DNA synthesis and replication via the TOR. Please refer to text for exact mechanisms of action for each immunosuppressive drug. *Abbreviations:* APC, antigen presenting cell; TCR, T-cell receptor; TOR, target of rapamycin; CsA, cyclosporine A; Tac, tacrolimus; Aza, azathioprine; MMF, mycophenolate mofetil; MHC, major histocompatibility complex; IL-2R, interleukin-2 receptor. *Source:* Courtesy of B. Rosengaard, M.D.

availability than the oil-based formulation (14). In LTx recipients with CF, CsA–ME also demonstrated higher and more reliable bioavailability with less intraindividual variability than the oil-based formulation (15,16). Conversion from CsA to CSA–ME in stable LTx recipients is safe and well tolerated (17,18), and also leads to significant dose reduction (19).

The relative bioequivalence of oral to intravenous CsA is 1:3. Intravenous CsA is usually initiated immediately postoperatively at 3 mg/kg/day with the intention of converting to CsA–ME at 5 mg/kg/day to be given every 12 hours when the patient is ready for oral feeding.

### Drug Monitoring

Variability in the pharmacokinetics of CsA mandates close monitoring. Area-under-the-curve (AUC) pharmacokinetic monitoring of CsA is preferred, as it is both superior to (20) and more reproducible than (21) trough level monitoring ($C_0$). However, due to the inconvenience on the patient and the increased cost of care, AUC monitoring is rarely used. $C_0$ has been shown to correlate poorly with patient exposure to CsA, and an adequate value of $AUC_{0-4}$ has been associated with decreased allograft rejection in renal transplantation. In recent years, $C_2$ (CsA concentration at 2 hours postdose) has been studied extensively in organ transplantation. It is the best single time-point predictor of $AUC_{0-4}$, and $C_2$ monitoring has also been associated with a greater clinical benefit in stable heart transplant patients. Studies in renal and liver transplantation have confirmed the superiority of $C_2$ monitoring (22–24).

Trials examining the effectiveness of $C_2$ monitoring in LTx recipients have been sparse and inconclusive (25). In a study comparing LTx patients with cystic fibrosis to non–cystic fibrosis patients, while $C_2$ was a better predictor than $C_0$ of the $AUC_{0-6}$, only $C_0$ correlated significantly with the risk of acute rejection (26). A limited sampling strategy developed by Dumont contained $C_1$ and $C_3$ levels, but not $C_2$, and of the single-concentration strategies, $C_0$ and $C_2$ had similar coefficients of determination (0.61 and 0.60) (27). When comparing $C_0$ to $C_2$ monitoring in LTx recipients, the $C_0$ group had a greater rise in serum creatinine despite similar CsA dosage (28). Because of differences in data and opinions, there is no definitive study yet of $C_2$ use in LTx; however, the final results are likely to be similar to those of other solid organ transplants.

### Efficacy

The success of CsA is attributed to its ability to specifically and reversibly inhibit the early phase of T-lymphocyte activation and its steroid-sparing effect (29,30). Its success in improving initial and long-term survival in renal allografts (31) has been paralleled in hepatic transplantation (32), cardiac transplantation (33), heart–lung transplantation (34), and LTx (35). In 1988, the Toronto Lung Transplant Group reported their experience with 11 LTx recipients for pulmonary fibrosis using CsA, Aza, antilymphoblast globulin, and pulse doses of methylprednisolone. Eight of 11 recipients were alive at the time of reporting, with the longest survival being 44 months (35). The survival of LTx recipients had increased from days in the pre-CsA era to registry survival rates of 67% and 42% at one and five years after LTx between 1988 and 1992, and currently 77% and 47% at one and five years (2).

Aerosolized CsA, although not commercially available, has been studied extensively at Pittsburgh for use in LTx recipients. The effect of aerosolized CsA is related to the deposited aerosol dose (36) and it has been shown to be effective in reversing persistent acute allograft rejection and obliterative bronchiolitis (OB) when used in conjunction with a systemic calcineurin inhibitor (37,38).

Drug Interactions

CsA is metabolized by CYP3A4 and any drug that inhibits the enzyme will increase the level of CsA, while drugs that potentiate the system will decrease the level of CsA. A list of commonly used drugs in LTx that can potentially interact with CsA is given in Table 1.

Transplant physicians have used drug interactions to decrease the cost of CsA. Cola and itraconazole are known to enhance CsA absorption, and coadministration can reduce the daily dose and cost of CsA accordingly (39).

Toxicities

**Nephrotoxicity:** Three forms of CsA-induced renal toxicity are seen: an acute reversible form, a chronic progressive form, and the uncommon thrombotic microangiopathy that leads to thrombotic thrombocytopenic purpura and hemolytic uremic syndrome (40).

Acute renal toxicity is dose related, usually responds to dose reduction or cessation of CsA, and is reversible. The process starts early after initiation of the drug and involves vasoconstriction of the afferent preglomerular arteriole, which is likely caused by CsA stimulating the renin–angiotensin

**Table 1** Drugs that Alter Cyclosporine A/Tac Blood Levels

---

*Drugs that increase blood levels of CsA/Tac*
Antibiotics
   Erythromycin, clarithromycin, imipenem
Antifungals
   Azoles (ketoconazole, itraconazole, fluconazole)
Antiarrhythmics
   Calcium channel blockers (diltiazem, verapamil), amiodarone
Other commonly used drugs
   $H_2$ blockers, metoclopramide, colchicines
Miscellaneous
   Alcohol, grapefruit juice
*Drugs that decrease blood levels of CsA/Tac*
Phenytoin, phenobarbital, rifampin, carbamazepine, trimethoprim, sulfonamides,
   sulfinpyrazones, nafcillin, octreotide, primidone

---

*Abbreviations*: CsA, cyclosporine A; Tac, tacrolimus.

system (41). Acute tubular necrosis has also been described, but it is usually caused by CsA intoxication (42).

Chronic renal toxicity usually begins within six months after transplantation. After the initial decline in renal function, either stabilization or progression to end-stage renal failure can occur. The prevalence of LTx recipients with serum creatinine greater than 2.5 mg/dL or requiring dialysis is 10% at one year and 16.3% at five years after transplantation (2). Lesions are due to repeated episodes of renal ischemia, with a critical role for angiotensin-II (43), and structural changes of the arterioles and tubulointerstitial lesions are histologically evident (44). Potential therapies include initiating mycophenolate mofetil (MMF) or sirolimus (SRL), while reducing the dose of CsA (45,46). Table 2 lists drugs that potentiate the nephrotoxicity of CsA without increasing its blood levels (10,29).

**Cardiovascular toxicity:** CsA causes arterial hypertension by increasing systemic and renal vascular resistance, causing vasoconstriction of afferent arterioles, and also by an endothelin-related mechanism (47,48). Other mechanisms involved include nitric oxide reduction, altered cytosolic calcium translocation, and neurohormonal activation (49). The International Society for Heart & Lung Transplantation (ISHLT) reports the prevalence of hypertension to be 50.4% and 86.4% at one and five years after transplant, respectively (2). Although other factors may contribute to the development of hypertension, toxicity from immunosuppressive drugs no doubt plays a key role. Systemic hypertension is usually controlled by standard antihypertensive medications, such as angiotensin-converting enzyme inhibitors, β-blockers, and calcium channel blockers.

**Neurotoxicity:** The neurotoxicities of CsA include headache, paresthesias of the hands and feet, seizures, focal deficits, reversible posterior leukoencephalopathy, and, rarely, coma. Most side effects are related to high CsA blood levels and tend to improve when CsA treatment is discontinued. Mild tremor is seen in 35% to 55% of patients taking CsA and will often improve despite continued CsA therapy. Other uncommon neurologic symptoms include speech apraxia, sleep disturbances, anxiety, and psychosis (7,50).

**Table 2**   Drugs that Potentiate CsA Nephrotoxicity
Without Effects on Blood Concentration

| |
| --- |
| SRL |
| Aminoglycosides |
| Amphotericin B |
| Nonsteroidal anti-inflammatory drugs |
| Angiotensin converting enzyme inhibitors |

*Abbreviations*: SRL, sirolimus; CsA, cyclosporine A.

**Malignancy:** Although the risk of post-transplant malignancies (e.g., squamous cell skin cancer and benign or malignant lymphoproliferative disorders) appears to be related to the intensity of immunosuppression, CsA has been shown to independently lead to cancer progression by increasing production of TGF-β. Hojo et al. showed that CsA enhances tumor growth and this effect could be blocked by anti–TGF-β monoclonal antibodies (51).

**Dermal complications:** CsA can cause hirsutism in >20% of the patients. It can also cause gingival hyperplasia by increasing the number of gingival fibroblasts and their production of collagen (7). The risk of gingival hyperplasia appears to be related to the dose of CsA and drug withdrawal, or switching to tacrolimus (Tac), another calcineurin inhibitor, will usually lead to resolution (52). Anecdotally, metronidazole has been reported to be effective in the treatment of gingival hyperplasia (53).

**Other toxicities:** Gastrointestinal disturbances, including anorexia, nausea and vomiting, diarrhea, and abdominal discomfort, are relatively common, but usually mild. Cholestasis with hyperbilirubinemia and elevation of liver function tests are also seen (7). Glucose metabolism disorders, such as glucose intolerance and diabetes mellitus, are increased with CsA use, although less commonly than with Tac (54).

## Tacrolimus

Tac, or FK 506, is a macrolide lactone that was introduced in the 1990s and has widely gained acceptance as an alternative to CsA. Sharing similar mechanisms of action and toxicities as CsA, Tac has been shown to be at least as effective as CsA in most solid organ transplantations (55–57), including LTx (58). Because of the success seen with Tac, its use has grown exponentially in recent years, surpassing that of CsA. The ISHLT 2004 registry indicates that 60% and 55% of LTx recipients are receiving Tac by one- and five-years posttransplant, respectively, as opposed to 37% and 41% who are on CsA (2).

### Mechanism of Action

Tac is also a calcineurin inhibitor that inhibits T-lymphocyte activation. The molecular structures of Tac and CsA are vastly different, but they share very similar mechanisms of action. Both CsA and Tac enter the cell membrane freely and bind to the immunophilins: CsA to cyclophilin and Tac to FK506-binding protein (FKBP). The Tac–FKBP complex binds to calcineurin, inactivating the phosphatase. Tac has increased binding affinity for FKBP due to differences in partition coefficient, rendering Tac 50 to 100 times more potent than CsA in vitro. Tac is also 10 times more potent than CsA in vivo models of cell-mediated and humoral immunity. The inactivation of calcineurin prevents dephosphorylation of transcription factors (e.g., NF-AT, NF-κB, and Oct/OAP), thus preventing their translocation into the nucleus (54).

Pharmacokinetics

Tac has poor absorption and oral bioavailability ($\approx25\%$), which is reduced further in the presence of food, but is completely independent of the presence of bile. It is absorbed rapidly, albeit incompletely, in the small intestine and attains peak blood concentration ($C_{max}$) in approximately one to two hours. Tac is metabolized by liver and intestinal mucosal CYP3A4 and, to a lesser extent, P-glycoprotein in the intestinal mucosa, prior to elimination. Several metabolites are formed, but most have no immunosuppressive activity. Elimination half-life ranges from 12 to 19 hours and the biliary tract is the chief route of elimination; $>1\%$ of the drug is excreted as parent drug in the urine (54).

Due to the variable pharmacokinetics, narrow therapeutic index, and significant toxicity, drug level monitoring is essential to avoid over- or underimmunosuppression. Drug monitoring of Tac has routinely been performed by following trough levels, and $C_2$ levels are not superior to $C_0$ at estimating the AUC (59). Blood level monitoring is complicated by the large inter- and intraindividual variability, as well as ethnic and genetic variability (54). At Loyola University, Chicago, Tac is instituted immediately post-transplant at 0.02–0.03 mg/kg every 12 hours to achieve a $C_0$ of 10–20 ng/mL in patients with normal renal function. The target $C_0$ is lowered to 7–14 ng/mL after one year.

Efficacy

**Tac as primary therapy:**   Keenan et al. were the first to use Tac in 133 LTx recipients randomized to Tac or CsA as primary immunosuppression. After two years, OB developed in fewer patients in the Tac group, and acute rejection episodes were also fewer in the Tac group (58). Survival times were not different between the two groups, even after two additional years of follow-up (60). The authors concluded that Tac is efficacious and reduces the incidence of OB.

When Reichenspurner et al. compared a CsA/Aza/steroid regimen to two Tac-based regimens (Tac/Aza/steroid and Tac/MMF/steroid) in 78 LTx recipients, the number of acute rejections was lower in both Tac groups compared to the CsA group, and freedom from recurrent acute rejection was significantly higher in both Tac groups. While no difference in the rate of development of OB was detected, survival at three years was significantly higher in the Tac/Aza group when compared to the CsA/Aza group (61).

In a two-center, prospective, and randomized trial, 74 LTx recipients were randomized to therapy with either CsA or Tac in combination with MMF and steroid. At 12 months, neither freedom from acute rejection nor survival was different between the two groups (62). The lack of difference may be due to the small sample size or confounding variables that were not equal between the two groups (63).

The data for using Tac or CsA as primary immunosuppression are still unconvincing, and the choice of calcineurin inhibitor is mostly institution dependent.

**Tac as rescue therapy for recurrent or refractory acute rejection:** Acute rejection is a strong risk factor for the development of chronic graft failure. The risk increases when the histologic grade is severe or episodes are recurrent or persistent (64). Several studies have shown the effectiveness of conversion from CsA to Tac in cases of recurrent or refractory acute rejection (Table 3).

**Tac as rescue therapy for chronic allograft rejection:** Bronchiolitis obliterans syndrome (BOS), the clinical surrogate of chronic allograft rejection, is the single largest contributor to mortality after the first year of LTx (2). To date there are no proven therapies for patients with BOS. Augmentation of immunosuppression is usually attempted, and various studies have examined the efficacy of substituting Tac for CsA in LTx recipients who develop BOS (Table 4).

Drug Interactions

Tac, like CsA, is metabolized by CYP3A4, and thus the two drugs share similar interactions. Drugs that potentiate CYP3A4 will decrease the blood level of Tac and any drug that inhibits the system will increase the level of Tac. Table 1 lists commonly prescribed drugs that can alter Tac levels.

Caution should be exercised when administering HMG-CoA reductase inhibitors or statins with Tac as most statins are also substrates of CYP3A4.

**Table 3** Experiences in Converting CsA to Tac for Recurrent/Refractory Acute Rejection

| Author | No. of patients | Outcomes |
|---|---|---|
| Horning et al. (65) | 14 | Significantly reduced incidence of acute rejection and average histologic grade of rejection |
| Onsager et al. (66) | 15 | 11/15 (73%) experienced reversal of refractory rejection |
| Sarahrudi et al. (67) | 8 | Significantly reduced incidence of acute rejection |
| Vitulo et al. (68) | 20 | Significantly reduced incidence of acute rejection and average histologic grade of rejection |
| Sarahrudi et al. (69) | 110 | Significantly reduced histologic and clinical rejection |

*Abbreviations*: CsA, cyclosporine A; Tac, tacrolimus.

**Table 4** Experiences in Converting CsA to Tac for BOS

| Author | No. of patients | Outcomes |
|---|---|---|
| Ross et al. (70) | 10 | Significant improvement in $\Delta FEV_1$/month slopes; earlier conversion more beneficial |
| Kesten et al. (71) | 12 | Significantly reduced rate of $FEV_1$ decline; no significant change in FVC |
| Wiebe et al. (72) | 24 | Significant reduction of $FEV_1$ decline; 14/24 stabilized or increased $FEV_1$ by 10%; 10/24 dropped $FEV_1$ by >10%; all had BOS III |
| Lipson et al. (73) | 7 | 6/7 BOS stabilized or improved symptoms and $FEF_{25-75}$ |
| Mentzer et al. 1998 (74) | 9 | All nine BOS patients continued to experience impaired graft function; 4/9 patients died |
| Revell et al. (75) | 11 | Significantly reduced rate of $FEV_1$ decline; halted decline in $FEF_{25-75}$; $\Delta FEF_{25-75}$/mo from $234 \pm 194$ to $23 \pm 14.8$ ($P<0.0001$) |
| Sarahrudi et al. (67) | 11 | No significant reduction of $FEV_1$ decline; no significant change in acute rejection episodes |
| Fieguth et al. (76) | 7 | Mean $FEV_1$ rose by 31% in 12 months ($P<0.05$); 1/7 failed to improve and died |
| Verleden et al. (77) | 10 | Stabilization of $FEV_1$ by 6 months; decline in exhaled nitric oxide |
| Cairn et al. (78) | 32 | Significantly decreased decline in $FEV_1$ and $FEF_{25-75}$ for 1 year |
| Sarahrudi et al. (69) | 134 | Significantly fewer acute rejection episodes; significantly reduced rate of $FEV_1$ decline |

*Abbreviations*: CsA, cyclosporine A; Tac, tacrolimus; BOS, bronchiolitis obliterans syndrome; $FEV_1$, forced expiratory volume in one second; FEF, forced expiratory flow.

Tac will compete for the enzyme and can lead to potentially toxic levels of statins in the blood. Severe cases of rhabdomyolysis have been reported with the combination (79).

### Toxicities

Tac and CsA share many similar toxicities, including nephrotoxicity, neurotoxicity, gastrointestinal disturbances, malignancy, hypertension, and disorders in glucose metabolism, although Tac has not been as extensively studied. Malignancies, specifically post-transplant lymphoproliferative disorders, may be more common in pediatric transplant recipients who are on Tac than CsA (80). However, CsA-specific adverse reactions of hirsutism and gingival hyperplasia are only rarely seen with Tac administration.

**Cardiovascular toxicity:** Hypertension is less prevalent in patients treated with Tac than those treated with CsA, although up to 50% of patients on Tac have documented hypertension (54,62,81,82).

Tac is associated with a more favorable lipid profile than CsA, as shown by large trials in renal and liver transplant recipients (83,84). Treede et al. reported similar result in LTx recipients randomized to either a Tac- or a CsA-based immunosuppressive protocol. Nearly twice as many in the CsA group presented with cholesterol levels $\geq 300$ mg/dL, requiring statin therapy (85).

**Nephrotoxicity:** Similar to CsA, Tac is associated with acute nephrotoxicity, which is responsive to drug withdrawal, a chronic renal dysfunction that is characterized by structural lesions in the kidney, and also thrombotic microangiopathy, which leads to hemolytic uremic syndrome (86). Studies in renal transplantation, however, have shown that serum creatinine levels were typically lower in those patients receiving Tac than in those receiving CsA (54,82).

**Diabetes mellitus:** A multicenter, randomized trial demonstrated that Tac was associated with a significantly higher incidence of posttransplant diabetes mellitus when compared to CsA in renal-transplant recipients, and this was more pronounced in African Americans than in Caucasians (87). Subsequent studies, however, have found no difference in the development of diabetes mellitus in patients who received Tac compared to those who received CsA (81). In addition, several patients who developed diabetes mellitus on Tac were able to discontinue insulin therapy (83).

**Neurotoxicity:** Tac neurotoxicity has a spectrum similar to that of CsA, including visual disturbances, headache, seizures, encephalopathy, focal deficits, coma, and tremor. Neuropsychiatric symptoms, such as psychosis and speech apraxia, are rare. Symptoms may be more common with Tac than with CsA (57), and will usually subside with lowering of the dose or discontinuation of Tac (54).

## ANTIMETABOLITES

### Azathioprine

Before the advent of CsA, immunosuppression for organ transplantation was accomplished with Aza and corticosteroids (88). After Schwartz and Dameshek discovered that 6-mercaptopurine (6-MP) can suppress humoral immunity (89), Calne and Murray were able to successfully prolong renal allograft survival in canines with the use of 6-MP in 1961 (90). Since that time, Aza has become a widely used drug after solid organ transplantation.

Mechanism of Action

The structure of Aza is that of the antimetabolite 6-MP, with an additional side chain to reduce its toxicity. As a purine analog, 6-MP competes with hypoxanthine for the enzyme hypoxanthine–guanine phosphoribosyltransferase intracellularly. 6-MP is converted into a number of thio analogs that will interfere with purine synthesis (91), thus inhibiting the proliferation of B and T lymphocytes (92). Recently, Aza was unexpectedly discovered to induce T-lymphocyte apoptosis on CD28 costimulation by suppression of Rac1, a GTP-binding protein (93). This could pave the way for the development of novel immunosuppressive therapies in the future.

Pharmacokinetics

Aza is well absorbed following oral administration and reaches peak serum concentration after one to two hours. It is converted to the active drug, 6-MP, by glutathione in erythrocytes and liver, and is further competitively metabolized into several different compounds, including 6-thioguanine (6-TG), in the intestine and liver (91,94).

The oral availability of Aza is about 50%, and ≈30% of Aza and 6-MP are bound to serum proteins. The half-life of Aza is five hours, but that of 6-TG, the most abundant Aza metabolite within lymphocytes, is much longer than 24 hours (94).

Efficacy

In 1962, Murray et al. reported the first successful human renal allograft transplantation with Aza and prednisone (95). By 1967, over 230 renal transplants had been performed with Aza ± corticosteroids (96). The initial experience in LTx with Aza and corticosteroids was futile as most recipients survived <1 month after transplantation. The addition of CsA in 1983 improved survival significantly, and Aza has since been an essential part of most LTx immunosuppressive regimens. The importance of Aza in LTx was confirmed when stable lung and heart–lung recipients experienced significantly worse graft deterioration after one year of Aza withdrawal compared to the no-withdrawal group (97).

In 2000, >75% and >65% of LTx recipients were on Aza at 1 and 5 years after transplant (98), respectively. The introduction of MMF (also an antimetabolite) for LTx has decreased the use of Aza over the last five years, mainly due to the improved side effect profile of MMF. The 2004 ISHLT registry reported that a decreased number of LTx recipients (35% and 39%) were on Aza at one and five years after transplant, respectively (2).

Drug Interactions

Allopurinol may increase the levels of Aza by blocking xanthine oxidase, and thus prevent the metabolism of 6-MP to 6-thiouric acid (91). To decrease the risk of toxicity, the Aza dose should be decreased by at least two-thirds when it is coadministered with allopurinol. Even with such a dose reduction, however, Cummins (99) showed that 46% of heart and LTx recipients developed leukopenia, emphasizing the need to monitor hematologic parameters closely when the two drugs are used together. Several reports have documented an increased requirement in warfarin dose when administered with Aza (100).

### Toxicities

Bone marrow suppression and gastrointestinal toxicity are the most common and potentially lethal complications caused by Aza. Patients treated with Aza also have a higher than average risk of developing malignancy, most commonly skin cancer. Rarely, a hypersensitivity reaction can occur to Aza, which rapidly resolves after cessation of the medication. The hypersensitivity reaction can manifest as nausea, joint aches, diarrhea, fever, and rash, or polyneuritis (101,102).

**Hematologic toxicity:** Aza-induced leukopenia is common, and Pollack et al. noted leukopenia in 26% of a cohort of 160 renal-transplant recipients. Allograft and patient survival was decreased when Aza-induced leukopenia developed (103). Neutropenia will subside with dose reduction or cessation of Aza (104).

The development of Aza-related toxicity, especially leukopenia, has been attributed to a deficiency of a specific enzyme, thiopurine *S*-methyl transferase (TPMT) (105). Analysis of TPMT genotype can quickly identify patients who are at risk (106,107).

**Gastrointestinal toxicity:** Nausea, anorexia, and vomiting can occur early in the course of Aza therapy, but will abate if the drug is stopped. A more serious side effect is hepatotoxicity due to intrahepatic cholestasis or hepatic veno-occlusive disease associated with Aza use (108,109).

**Malignancy:** Aza increases the risk of malignancy in transplant recipients by 50- to 100-fold (110). Skin cancer after renal transplantation is apparently related to the duration of Aza administration (111), and a significantly increased concentration of 6-TG has been found in renal-transplant recipients with skin cancer than those without cancer (112).

## Mycophenolate Mofetil

MMF is an ester prodrug of mycophenolic acid (MPA), which was discovered over a century ago. MPA was reported to have antifungal activity over 50 years ago; today, it is used for the treatment of diseases, such as psoriasis and proliferative lupus nephritis, and for prevention of organ transplant rejection (113).

Mechanism of Action

MMF is rapidly hydrolyzed in vivo to MPA, its active compound, which selectively and reversibly inhibits inosine monophosphate dehydrogenase to prevent proliferation of both T and B lymphocytes. The inhibition of inosine monophosphate dehydrogenase, an essential enzyme in the de novo biosynthesis of guanine nucleotides, preferentially blocks proliferation of lymphocytes because they are fully dependent on both the de novo and the salvage pathways of purine biosynthesis (114).

Inhibition of guanine nucleotide synthesis not only blocks DNA synthesis, but also prevents glycosylation of adhesion molecules necessary for migration and binding of lymphocytes to endothelial cells (115). Among currently used immunosuppressants, MMF has been shown to be one of the most potent inhibitors of fibroblast proliferation after LTx. In vitro studies demonstrated the strong antiproliferative effect at concentrations achieved clinically, supporting its use in fibrotic processes, such as OB (16).

Pharmacokinetics

Esterification of MPA to MMF allows improved bioavailability of the former. After oral administration of MMF, it is hydrolyzed to MPA with 94% bioavailability and 99% protein binding. MMF is undetectable and only free MPA is active. Further metabolism is by glucuronization to MPA glucuronide with urinary (87%) and fecal excretion (6%) (113,114,117).

The plasma level of MPA demonstrates a bimodal distribution with peaks at one hour and 8 to 12 hours after ingestion (118). The half-life of MPA is 18 hours. Clinically, trough MPA plasma concentrations are followed despite large inter- and intraindividual variations and a weak correlation with MPA–$AUC_{0-12}$ (119,120).

Efficacy

Large trials have proven the superiority of MMF over Aza for the prevention of acute allograft rejection in renal transplantation (121–123). Similar results have been shown in heart-transplant recipients (124). The institution of MMF has even allowed gradual withdrawal of steroids with a significant improvement in lipid profile without increasing the incidence of acute rejection of renal allografts (125). In LTx, MMF has been used both as primary therapy and as rescue therapy for BOS.

**MMF as primary therapy:** There have been several small and nonrandomized studies that have shown a decrease in acute rejection rates in LTx with the use of MMF. These studies are summarized in Table 5. In contradistinction, Palmer et al. prospectively enrolled 81 LTx patients and randomized them to immunosuppression with Aza ($n = 38$) or MMF ($n = 43$) along with CsA and corticosteroids. The primary end point of biopsy-proven acute rejection within the first six months was not different between

**Table 5**   Early Experiences with MMF as Primary Therapy

| Author | No. of patients | Outcomes |
|---|---|---|
| Ross et al. (126) | 22 | Fewer acute rejections in MMF (11) vs. Aza (11) group ($P<0.01$); more *Aspergillus* sp. airway colonization in MMF group ($P<0.05$) |
| O'Hair et al. (127) | 44 | Patients on MMF (13) had lower acute rejection rate than patients on Aza (41) ($P = NS$) |
| Zuckermann et al. (128) | 38 | Less acute rejection in MMF (21) than Aza (17) group ($P<0.01$); significant decrease in steroids in MMF group |
| Bhorade et al. (129) | 109 | Tac-based regimen containing MMF and daclizumab had less acute rejection episodes ($P<0.05$) than Aza and no daclizumab |

*Abbreviations*: NS, not significant; MMF, mycophenolate mofetil; Aza, azathioprine; Tac, tacrolimus.

the two groups ($P = 0.82$), and neither was survival at six months ($P = 0.57$). The rate of cytomegalovirus (CMV) infection and adverse events were also not significantly different between the two groups (130). More recently, an international trial by Glanville et al. examined the development of BOS after three years of primary therapy with either MMF or Aza. In the 315 patients enrolled, there was no difference in the rate of BOS at three years and mortality ($P = NS$ for both). The difference in the rate of acute rejection was also not detected (data not shown) (131).

**MMF as rescue therapy:**   The first case report on using MMF as rescue therapy for OB was published in 1997 by Speich et al. (132). In a patient with early OB, only the addition of MMF allowed tapering of steroid dose while stabilizing lung function. Subsequently, Whyte et al. reported on stabilization of lung function in 13 LTx recipients with BOS (133).

MMF has successfully been used in patients with CsA-induced nephropathy after LTx. Zuckermann et al. described 22 LTx recipients who were switched from CsA to MMF for renal insufficiency (Cr>2.0 mg/dL) and followed for >1 year. Mean serum creatinine improved from preswitch level of $2.4 \pm 0.66$ mg/dL to $1.8 \pm 0.39$ mg/dL ($P<0.05$) at 18 months (134).

Drug Interactions

Absorption of MMF is decreased by iron, cholestyramine, and magnesium and aluminum hydroxide antacid. Acyclovir and probenecid will increase the MMF level, so Aza and MMF should not be coadministered as profound bone marrow suppression may develop. Oral contraceptives are less effective in the presence of MMF, and other forms of contraception should be sought (135). While MMF does not interact with Tac, trough levels of MMF will decrease, by up to 50%, when CsA is used as the calcineurin inhibitor (136,137). The mechanism of this interaction is not completely understood.

Toxicities

Although MMF is generally better tolerated than Aza, it is not without side effects. Dose reduction will usually lead to improvements, but is associated with an increased risk of acute rejection in renal transplantation (138).

**Gastrointestinal toxicity:**   Gastrointestinal side effects are very common with MMF administration, and they are often the reason for dose reduction or discontinuation of the drug (139). Diarrhea, abdominal pain, nausea, vomiting, and dyspepsia are more common, while intestinal perforation and gastrointestinal hemorrhage rarely occur. Oral ulcerations have also been reported in the literature (140,141). The mechanism is related to the susceptibility of enterocytes to the inhibition of the de novo pathway of purine synthesis by MMF, and the extensive enterohepatic circulation of MPA (142).

Delay in starting MMF after transplantation is associated with an increased risk of side effects, especially diarrhea. It is speculated that the higher-corticosteroid dose may confer a protective effect to the intestinal epithelium against MMF (143). Octreotide has reportedly been effective in treating MMF-associated diarrhea (144).

**Hematologic toxicity:**   Leukopenia and anemia occur commonly with MMF and will normalize with cessation or reduction of MMF dose (145). It is prudent to monitor complete blood counts regularly while patients are on MMF.

**Infection:**   MMF increases the risk of opportunistic infections, specifically the incidence and severity of CMV disease (146–148). This may be explained by the finding that MMF decreases antibody production (149), particularly the anti-CMV–IgM response in the early post-transplant period (150). Two cases of intestinal microsporidiosis have also been reported in renal-transplant recipients on MMF (151).

MMF, however, seems to exert a protective effect against *Pneumocystis carinii*. In four randomized, controlled trials of MMF in renal-transplant recipients, the rate of *P. carinii* infection was significantly lower in 1068 patients who received MMF than in the 563 patients who did not ($P = 0.00006$) (152).

Other Toxicities

Rarely reported pulmonary toxicities include pulmonary fibrosis due to recurrent respiratory failure from repeated administration of MMF (153), and interstitial pneumonitis that responded to discontinuation of MMF (154). Increased fetal loss and fetal malformation have been reported with the use of MMF (155).

## OTHER DRUGS

### Sirolimus

First discovered in the 1970s from *Streptomyces hygroscopicus*, rapamycin (now named SRL), is a macrolide antibiotic with antifungal properties (156). Further studies revealed its powerful antiproliferative and antitumor effects and its immunosuppressive properties.

#### Mechanism of Action

Structurally similar to Tac, SRL is lipophilic and enters the cytoplasm easily to bind with the same immunophilin, FKBP. However, the SRL–FKBP complex binds to the target of rapamycin (TOR) (157). The mammalian TOR (mTOR) activates protein kinase S6K1, the transcription factor CREMτ, and a translation protein 4E-BP1, all of which increase growth factor–mediated protein synthesis (158–160). mTOR is also instrumental in CD28-mediated upregulation of IL-2 transcription in T lymphocytes, and acts to decrease the synthesis of cell cycle proteins, cdc2 and cyclin A (161,162). By blocking mTOR, SRL will thus inhibit many cytokine-driven pathways, including those initiated by IL-2, and arrest cells in the G1 phase (163).

The function of SRL is not limited to its effects on T lymphocytes. Unlike CsA and Tac, which inhibit only $Ca^{2+}$-dependent signaling pathways, SRL can inhibit either $Ca^{2+}$-dependent or -independent pathways. Through a $Ca^{2+}$-independent pathway, SRL can inhibit lipopolysaccharide-induced proliferation of B lymphocytes, thereby decreasing immunoglobulin production (163). SRL can also inhibit proliferation of nonimmune cells, such as vascular smooth muscle cells and fibroblasts, induced by growth factors (164,165).

#### Pharmacokinetics

SRL has an oral bioavailability of 14% and its peak blood concentration is attained in 1.4 hours. In circulation, the drug is extensively partitioned into blood cells, with a blood/plasma ratio of 76 in healthy subjects. SRL is metabolized by CYP3A4 and P-glycoprotein into inactive metabolites with >90% excreted fecally and in urine carrying ≈2% of the metabolites. The half-life of SRL is about 60 hours and there are modest inter- and intra-individual variations in steady-state oral clearance. Therapeutic drug monitoring is regularly performed with trough drug level as it has a high correlation with drug exposure measured by AUC (166,167).

Efficacy

The effectiveness of SRL in preventing acute rejection episodes in renal-transplant recipients has been proven by large trials (168,169). The data for the treatment of rejection, either acute or chronic, in LTx, however, are minimal.

**SRL as primary therapy:**  Previous attempts at using SRL for primary therapy after LTx were terminated early due to the unacceptably high risk of airway anastomotic dehiscence (170,171). There is currently a randomized, multicenter trial examining the efficacy of SRL against Aza in a Tac-based regimen under way. Patients are switched from Aza to SRL three months after LTx, and no anastomotic dehiscence has been seen so far (172).

**SRL as rescue therapy for BOS:**  The use of SRL for the treatment of OB is supported by its antiproliferative effect on lung fibroblasts (165). Cahill et al. followed 12 LTx recipients who developed OB/BOS and were switched from either Aza or MMF to SRL, in conjunction with CsA and prednisone. As a group, the rate of change in forced expiratory volume in one second ($FEV_1$) and forced expiratory flow ($FEF_{25-75}$) did not change after institution of SRL, but individual responses varied. Serum creatinine rose in 75% of patients despite a dose reduction in CsA dose in 58% of patients, and all patients developed an anemia of chronic disease. The authors warned that SRL combination therapy should be used cautiously until optimal dosing strategies are established (173). A separate study demonstrated stabilization of $FEV_1$ in three of four patients with BOS who were started on SRL. Two of the four patients developed infectious complications, highlighting the need to monitor for excessive immunosuppression (174).

**SRL for renal impairment:**  Chronic renal impairment can be related to multiple factors in LTx, with calcineurin inhibitors being a principal cause. Snell et al. initiated SRL in 20 LTx and five heart-transplant recipients with severe renal dysfunction with concomitant decrease (52%) or cessation (48%) of calcineurin inhibitor therapy. After 30 days, four of five dialysis patients stopped dialysis and 15 of 20 patients with chronic renal failure (mean serum creatinine 3.3 mg/dL) improved their creatinine level (mean creatinine 2.38 mg/dL). Whether the improvement in renal function can be maintained will need to be followed. There were two episodes of acute rejection and one episode of chronic rejection (46). Therefore, SRL appears to be a reasonable alternative immunosuppressant in cases of renal impairment in order to decrease calcineurin inhibitor.

Drug Interactions

Similar to CsA and Tac, SRL is metabolized by CYP3A4, and therefore shares many similar drug interactions. Please refer to Table 1 for drug interactions with commonly prescribed drugs used in transplantation.

Blood concentration of SRL is elevated when it is used in combination with CsA, and the timing of drug administration influences the degree of elevation of SRL. Kaplan et al. showed that the AUC, $C_{max}$, $C_0$, and time to maximum concentration of SRL were significantly increased when the two drugs were given at the same time as compared to administering SRL four hours after CsA (175). If SRL and CsA are to be used concomitantly, a four-hour interval between dosing should be observed. The exact nature of interaction between SRL and CsA requires further investigation (168,176).

A similar study performed with SRL and Tac did not find altered pharmacokinetic profiles, in either drug, with simultaneous administration when compared to the four-hour interval dosing (177). Mean AUC for MMF has been found to be significantly higher in patients taking SRL as opposed to CsA, suggesting MMF dose reduction may be necessary when used in combination with SRL (178).

### Toxicities

SRL has toxicities primarily on the hematologic, metabolic, gastrointestinal, and pulmonary systems. Based on animal studies, SRL does not appear to have intrinsic renal toxicity. Given with CsA and prednisone, however, SRL does increase serum creatinine significantly when compared to Aza in renal-transplant recipients (168). This has been attributed to an increase in CsA concentration (179) and/or an increase in TGF-$\beta$ expression to potentiate chronic CsA nephropathy (180,181).

**Hematologic toxicity:** SRL has been reported to decrease all three cell lines resulting in anemia, leukopenia, and thrombocytopenia (168,169,182). Hemolytic uremic syndrome also occurs after kidney transplantation in patients treated with CsA, SRL, and prednisone, although at a lower rate than historic controls that did not use SRL. Most cases are reversible, and CsA and SRL may be resumed once the patient improves (183). SRL has also been reported to cause platelet-independent defect in hemostasis after renal transplantation in a patient on an SRL/MMF/prednisone regimen (184).

**Metabolic toxicity:** Dysfunction of lipid metabolism is seen with SRL use (185). Hypercholesterolemia and hyperlipemia occur in 38% to 46% of patients, but are responsive to dose reduction (168,169,182).

**Gastrointestinal toxicity:** Diarrhea and constipation are reported in 25% to 42% of patients using SRL, with nausea and vomiting being reported less commonly (168,169). Oral ulcers have also been frequently reported in renal transplantation (10–47%), and it was suggested that most are herpes simplex virus infections (169,186).

**Pulmonary toxicity:** Forty-three cases of SRL-induced pulmonary toxicity have been reported in the literature, including lymphocytic alveolitis, lymphocytic interstitial pneumonitis, bronchoalveolar obliterans organizing pneumonia, focal fibrosis, pulmonary alveolar hemorrhage, or a combination thereof (187,188).

A potential lethal pulmonary complication reported recently is airway anastomotic dehiscence. King-Biggs et al. observed an unexpectedly high incidence (4/15 patients) of anastomotic dehiscence when patients were treated with SRL, Tac, and prednisone immediately after LTx (170). Similar findings were reported by Groetzner et al. in a trial comparing the efficacy of SRL versus Tac (171). The mechanism is likely related to the inhibition of cytokine-mediated proliferation of nonimmune cells, specifically fibroblasts, by SRL (165). Therefore, it is recommended that SRL not be started until completion of bronchial wound healing or three months after LTx.

## Prednisone

Glucocorticoids (GC) were first used in transplantation when Billingham et al. established that systemically or locally applied cortisone improved the life of rabbit skin grafts by two- to fourfold (189,190). The use of GC to reverse acute renal allograft rejection was then successfully attempted in 1960 (191), and the combination of Aza and prednisone for maintenance of immunosuppression helped transform organ transplantation into an acceptable procedure (95). Despite myriad toxicities associated with the use of GC, prednisone is the single most used immunosuppressant at one and five years after LTx (97% and 96%, respectively) (2).

### Mechanism of Action

GC enter the cytoplasm easily due to their lipophilic nature and activate GC receptors, which in turn will translocate to the nucleus and bind to GC response elements in target genes. Genes responsible for the toxicity of GC are thus upregulated in this manner (192). By a distinct mechanism, the anti-inflammatory and immunosuppressive activities of GC are mediated by activated GC receptors that bind to and inhibit transcription factors, such as NF-κB and activated protein 1 (AP-1) (193). GC also increase the expression of IκBα, a protein that binds NF-κB in the cytoplasm, and prevents it from entering the nuclei (194,195). GC will therefore inhibit the production of numerous cytokines, including IL-1, IL-2, IL-6, and interferon-γ (192,196–198), in addition to suppressing lymphocyte proliferation and inducing apoptosis in lymphocytes (199,200).

### Pharmacokinetics

Of the synthetic GC, prednisone, prednisolone, and methylprednisolone are the most commonly used preparations in transplantation. Prednisone and prednisolone have four times the GC activity of cortisol, and methylprednisolone is five times more potent than cortisol. Orally administered prednisone and prednisolone are well absorbed in healthy subjects and reach peak serum concentration in two to three hours. Prednisone is converted to its active metabolite, prednisolone, in the liver, and the bioavailability of both the drugs is 92% (201). Compared to cortisol, prednisolone has approximately 60% binding affinity to cortisol-binding globulin, and prednisone has 5% (202). Like endogenous steroids, metabolism of prednisolone is mainly in the liver, with a minor contribution by the CYP3A4 enzyme. Elimination is via the urine and half-life is 200 minutes (203). Methylprednisolone is usually given intravenously for its rapid onset of action for both perioperative use and treatment of acute rejection.

Pharmacokinetic study of prednisolone in patients with cystic fibrosis revealed marked increase in prednisolone clearance, suggesting that more frequent or higher doses may be necessary (204). In solid organ transplant recipients, prednisolone metabolism was found to be slower than in healthy subjects, perhaps explaining the effectiveness of the drug at a low dose (205).

### Efficacy

GC were the first immunosuppressives used in organ transplantation, and as such, there are no randomized or controlled trials that have examined their efficacy. They are used for induction and maintenance of immunosuppression, as well as treatment of acute rejection episodes. At Loyola University, Chicago, intravenous methylprednisolone (5–10 mg/kg) is given at the time of transplant and continued postoperatively (0.2 mg/kg) until prednisone (0.5 mg/kg in divided doses) can be administered orally. Prednisone is then gradually reduced in the next several weeks to a minimal level ($\approx$0.1 mg/kg/day) and continued indefinitely. High-grade acute rejection is treated with pulse methylprednisolone (1 g/day) for three days followed by prednisone taper.

The innumerable toxicities of GC described below have compelled renal-transplant programs to move toward a steroid-free immunosuppressive regimen. While early steroid withdrawal has resulted in significantly more acute rejection episodes (206), a late withdrawal approach is still controversial (207,208). There have not been reports of steroid withdrawal in LTx.

### Drug Interactions

Although the CYP3A4 enzyme has a minor role in the metabolism of GC, drugs that augment the enzyme's activity, such as rifampin, phenobarbital, and phenytoin, will nonetheless decrease the effect of GC (209,210). Similarly, pharmacokinetic study demonstrated an increased plasma half-life of prednisolone when given with CsA, a known substrate for CYP3A4 (211). GC have also been shown to increase renal clearance of isoniazid and salicylates (212,213).

An early study showed decreased antibody response to pneumococcal vaccination in patients on GC therapy, thus limiting the protection conferred by the vaccine (214). However, that result was not reproduced in other studies involving both pneumococcal and influenza vaccines (215–217).

Toxicities

Chronic use of GC can lead to numerous well-documented toxicities including, but not limited to, osteoporosis, Cushing's syndrome, cataracts, gastrointestinal ulcers, skin cancers, impaired wound healing, myopathy, and infections (218–221). In fact, it is the toxicities that limit GC use and most LTx recipients are eventually reduced to an average daily prednisone dose of 5 mg.

**Cardiovascular toxicity:** Immunosuppression-induced hypertension frequently develops after LTx, but the calcineurin inhibitors are much more likely the cause than GC (54,82). Jackson et al. showed that taking GC at < 20 mg daily for a year, in itself, was not associated with the development of hypertension. The blood pressure before GC therapy was the only significant determinant of hypertension developing during therapy (222). GC have also not been definitively proven to cause hyperlipidemia (223–226).

**Gastrointestinal toxicity:** The risk of peptic ulcers and gastrointestinal hemorrhage is elevated in association with GC therapy, and that risk is quadrupled when nonsteroidal anti-inflammatory drugs are used in combination (227,228). Other gastrointestinal complications include perforated esophageal and intestinal ulcers and pancreatitis (229).

**Metabolic toxicity:** In a large epidemiologic study, Gurwitz et al. determined that the relative risk of developing hyperglycemia, which required treatment, was 2.23 in GC-users as compared with nonusers. They also found that the risk increased with increasing daily GC dose after adjustment for confounding variables (230). Regular monitoring of serum glucose is therefore recommended in patients on GC.

GC-induced osteoporosis is another serious toxicity of GC use. Along with inhibition of osteoblastic activity, increased osteoclastic activity leads to more bone resorption, resulting in osteoporosis (231). The severity of osteoporosis is related to the duration of GC therapy and the total cumulative GC dose (232,233). Also, alternate day prednisone therapy does not prevent the trabecular bone loss (234). The most effective treatment is using bisphosphonates (235,236).

**Other toxicities:** Psychiatric side effects occur in 6% of all patients on GC, ranging from depression (40%) to hypomania (28%), to psychosis (14%). Symptoms are reversible after termination of the drug in 90% of the cases (237).

## CONCLUSION

In conclusion, this chapter summarizes the activity, efficacy, and toxicities of currently used drugs in LTx. As more agents become available, and experience grows, attempts to tailor therapy to individual needs will be more successful. Many of the covered drugs may also have roles, as immune tolerance becomes a possibility.

## REFERENCES

1. Grover FL, Fullerton DA, Zamora MR, et al. The past, present, and future of lung transplantation. Am J Surg 1997; 173(6):523–533.
2. Trulock EP, Edwards LB, Taylor DO, et al. The registry of the International Society for Heart and Lung Transplantation: twenty-first official adult lung and heart–lung transplant report—2004. J Heart Lung Transplant 2004; 23(7):804–815.
3. Zuckermann A, Klepetko W. Use of cyclosporine in thoracic transplantation. Transplant Proc 2004; 36(2S):331S–336S.
4. Derom F, Barbier F, Ringoir S, et al. Ten-month survival after lung homo-transplantation in man. J Thorac Cardiovasc Surg 1971; 61(6):835–846.
5. Goldberg M, Lima O, Morgan E, et al. A comparison between cyclosporin A and methylprednisolone plus azathioprine on bronchial healing following canine lung autotransplantation. J Thorac Cardiovasc Surg 1983; 85(6):821–826.
6. Toronto Lung Transplant Group. Unilateral lung transplantation for pulmonary fibrosis. N Engl J Med 1986; 314(18):1140–1145.
7. Kahan BD. Cyclosporine. N Engl J Med 1989; 321(5):1725–1738.
8. Wiederrecht G, Lam E, Hung S, et al. The mechanism of action of FK-506 and cyclosporin A. Ann N Y Acad Sci 1993; 696:9–19.
9. Schreiber SL, Crabtree GR. The mechanism of action of cyclosporin A and FK506. Immunol Today 1992; 13(4):136–142.
10. Parekh K, Trulock E, Patterson GA. Use of cyclosporine in lung transplantation. Transplant Proc 2004; 36(2S):318S–322S.
11. Knoop C, Haverich A, Fischer S. Immunosuppressive therapy after human lung transplantation. Eur Respir J 2004; 23:159–171.
12. El-Gamel A, Awad M, Yonan N, et al. Does cyclosporin promote the secretion of transforming growth factor-beta 1 following pulmonary transplantation? Transplant Proc 1998; 30(4):1525–1527.
13. Ahuja SS, Shrivastav S, Danielpour D, et al. Regulation of transforming growth factor-beta 1 and its receptor by cyclosporine in human T lymphocytes. Transplantation 1995; 60(7):718–723.
14. Kahan BD, Dunn J, Fitts C, et al. Reduced inter- and intrasubject variability in cyclosporine pharmacokinetics in renal transplant recipients treated with a microemulsion formulation in conjunction with fasting, low-fat meals, or high-fat meals. Transplantation 1995; 59(4):505–511.
15. Reynaud-Gaubert M, Viard L, Girault D, et al. Improved absorption and bioavailability of cyclosporine A from a microemulsion formulation in lung transplant recipients affected with cystic fibrosis. Transplant Proc 1997; 29: 2450–2453.
16. Mikhail G, Eadon H, Leaver N, et al. An investigation of the pharmacokinetics, toxicity, and clinical efficacy of Neoral cyclosporin in cystic fibrosis patients. Transplant Proc 1997; 29(1–2):599–601.

17. Kesten S, Scavuzzo M, Laurin L, et al. Conversion from standard cyclosporine to Neoral in lung transplant recipients. Transplant Proc 1998; 30:1895–1897.
18. Aziz T, El-Gamel A, Keevil B, et al. Clinical impact of Neoral in thoracic organ transplantation. Transplant Proc 1998; 30:1900–1903.
19. Zaldonis DB, Keenan RJ, Pham SM, et al. Neoral conversion in stable thoracic transplant patients leads to dose reduction. Transplant Proc 1998; 30: 1158–1159.
20. Grevel J, Welsh MS, Kahan BD. Cyclosporine monitoring in renal transplantation: area under the curve monitoring is superior to trough-level monitoring. Ther Drug Monit 1989; 11(3):246–248.
21. Takahara S, Kokado Y, Kameoka H, et al. Clinical evaluation of trough levels and area under the curve in cyclosporine- and FK 506-treated kidney transplant recipients. Transplant Proc 1994; 26(5):2802–2806.
22. Jacksch P, Kocher A, Neuhauser P, et al. Monitoring of CyA C2 levels is predictive for AUC in lung transplant recipients. J Heart Lung Transplant 2002; 21(1):87.
23. Levy G, Thervet E, Lake J, et al. Patient management by Neoral C2 monitoring: an international consensus statement. Transplantation 2002; 73(9):S12–S18.
24. Cantarovich M, Elstein E, de Varennes B, et al. Clinical benefit of Neoral dose monitoring with cyclosporine 2-hr post-dose levels compared with trough levels in stable heart transplant patients. Transplantation 1999; 68(12):1839–1842.
25. Poirier CD. Promise of Neoral C2, basiliximab, and everolimus in lung transplantation. Transplant Proc 2004; 36(2S):509S–513S.
26. Trull A, Steel L, Sharples L, et al. Randomized, trough blood cyclosporine concentration-controlled trial to compare the pharmacodynamics of Sandimmune and Neoral in de novo lung transplant recipients. Ther Drug Monit 1999; 21(1):17–26.
27. Dumont RJ, Partovi N, Levy RD, et al. A limited sampling strategy for cyclosporine area under the curve monitoring in lung transplant recipients. J Heart Lung Transplant 2001; 20(8):897–900.
28. Morton JM, Aboyoun CL, Malouf MA, et al. Enhanced clinical utility of de novo cyclosporine C2 monitoring after lung transplantation. J Heart Lung Transplant 2004; 23(9):1035–1039.
29. Banner NR, Yacoub MH. Cyclosporine in thoracic organ transplantation. Transplant Proc 2004; 36(2S):302S–308S.
30. Lima O, Cooper JD, Peters WJ, et al. Effects of methylprednisolone and azathioprine on bronchial healing following lung autotransplantation. J Thorac Cardiovasc Surg 1981; 82(2):211–215.
31. The Canadian Multicentre Transplant Study Group. A randomized clinical trial of cyclosporine in cadaveric renal transplantation. Analysis at three years. N Engl J Med 1986; 314(19):1219–1225.
32. Starzl TE, Klintmalm GB, Porter KA, et al. Liver transplantation with use of cyclosporin a and prednisone. N Engl J Med 1981; 305(5):266–269.
33. Oyer PE, Stinson EB, Jamieson SW, et al. Cyclosporine in cardiac transplantation: a 2 1/2 year follow-up. Transplant Proc 1983; 15:2546.

34. Reitz BA, Wallwork JL, Hunt SA, et al. Heart-lung transplantation: successful therapy for patients with pulmonary vascular disease. N Engl J Med 1982; 306(10):557–564.
35. The Toronto Lung Transplant Group. Experience with single-lung transplantation for pulmonary fibrosis. J Am Med Assoc 1988; 259(12):2258–2262.
36. Corcoran TE, Smaldone GC, Dauber JH, et al. Preservation of post-transplant lung function with aerosol cyclosporin. Eur Respir J 2004; 23:378–383.
37. Iacono AT, Smaldone GC, Keenan RJ, et al. Dose-related reversal of acute lung rejection by aerosolized cyclosporine. Am J Respir Crit Care Med 1997; 155:1690–1698.
38. Iacono AT, Corcoran TE, Griffith BP, et al. Aerosol cyclosporin therapy in lung transplant recipients with bronchiolitis obliterans. Eur Respir J 2004; 23:384–390.
39. Wimberley SL, Haug MT III, Shermock KM, et al. Enhanced cyclosporine-itraconazole interaction with cola in lung transplant recipients. Clin Transplantation 2001; 15:116–122.
40. Roberts P, Follette D, Allen R, et al. Cyclosporine A-associated thrombotic thrombocytopenic purpura following lung transplantation. Transplant Proc 1998; 30:1512–1513.
41. Busauschina A, Schnuelle P, van der Woude FJ. Cyclosporine nephrotoxicity. Transplant Proc 2004; 36(2S):229S–233S.
42. Dussol B, Reynaud-Gaubert M, Saingra Y, et al. Acute tubular necrosis induced by high level of cyclosporine A in a lung transplant. Transplantation 2000; 70 (8):1234–1236.
43. Morales JM, Andres A, Rengel M, et al. Influence of cyclosporin, tacrolimus and rapamycin on renal function and arterial hypertension after renal transplantation. Nephrol Dial Transplant 2001; 16(1):121–124.
44. Myers BD, Sibley R, Newton L, et al. The long-term course of cyclosporine-associated chronic nephropathy. Kidney Int 1988; 33:590–600.
45. Zuckermann A, Ploner M, Keziban U, et al. Benefit of mycophenolate-mofetil (MMF) in patients with cyclosporine (CYA) induced nephropathy after cardiac transplantation. J Heart Lung Transplant 2001; 20(2):163.
46. Snell GI, Levvey BJ, Chin W, et al. Sirolimus allows renal recovery in lung and heart transplant recipients with chronic renal impairment. J Heart Lung Transplant 2001; 21(5):540–546.
47. Takeda Y, Miyamori I, Wu P, et al. Effects of an endothelin receptor antagonist in rats with cyclosporine-induced hypertension. Hypertension 1995; 26(6): 932–936.
48. Watschinger B, Sayegh MH. Endothelin in organ transplantation. Am J Kidney Dis 1996; 27(1):151–161.
49. Ventura HO, Malik FS, Mehra MR, et al. Mechanisms of hypertension in cardiac transplantation and the role of cyclosporine. Curr Opin Cardiol 1997; 12(4):375–381.
50. Wijdicks EFM, Wiesner RH, Krom RAF. Neurotoxicity in liver transplant recipients with cyclosporine immunosuppression. Neurology 1995; 45(11): 1962–1964.

51. Hojo M, Morimoto T, Maluccio M, et al. Cyclosporine induces cancer progression by a cell-autonomous mechanism. Nature 1999; 397:530–534.

52. Thomas DW, Newcombe RG, Osborne GR. Risk factors in the development of cyclosporine-induced gingival overgrowth. Transplantation 2000; 69(4):522–526.

53. Cecchin E, Zanello F, De Marchi S. Treatment of cyclosporine-induced gingival hypertrophy. Ann Int Med 1997; 126(5):409–410.

54. Scott LJ, McKeage K, Keam SJ, et al. Tacrolimus: a further update of its use in the management of organ transplantation. Drugs 2003; 63(12):1247–1297.

55. Taylor DO, Barr ML, Radovancevic B, et al. A randomized, multicenter comparison of tacrolimus and cyclosporine immunosuppressive regimens in cardiac transplantation: decreased hyperlipidemia and hypertension with tacrolimus. J Heart Lung Transplant 1999; 18(4):336–345.

56. Jensik SC, the FK 506 Kidney Transplant Study Group. Tacrolimus (FK 506) in kidney transplantation: three-year survival results of the US multicenter, randomized, comparative trial. Transplant Proc 1998; 30(4):1216–1218.

57. The U.S. Multicenter FK506 Liver Study Group. A comparison of tacrolimus (FK 506) and cyclosporine for immunosuppression in liver transplantation. N Engl J Med 1994; 331(17):1110–1115.

58. Keenan RJ, Konishi H, Kawai A, et al. Clinical trial of tacrolimus versus cyclosporine in lung transplantation. Ann Thorac Surg 1995; 60:580–585.

59. Jorgensen K, Povlsen J, Madsen S, et al. C2 (2-h) levels are not superior to trough levels as estimates of the area under the curve in tacrolimus-treated renal-transplant patients. Nephrol Dial Transplant 2002; 17:1487–1490.

60. Keenan RJ, Dauber JH, Iacono AT, et al. Long term followup-clinical trial of tacrolimus versus cyclosporine for lung transplantation. J Heart Lung Transplant 1998; 17(1):61A.

61. Reichenspurner H, Kur F, Treede H, et al. Optimization of the immunosuppressive protocol after lung transplantation. Transplantation 1999; 68(1):67–71.

62. Zuckermann A, Reichenspurner H, Birsan T, et al. Cyclosporine A versus tacrolimus in combination with mycophenolate mofetil and steroids as primary immunosuppression after lung transplantation: one-year results of a 2-center prospective randomized trial. J Thorac Cardiovasc Surg 2003; 125(4): 891–900.

63. Mulligan MS, Wood DE. Optimizing lung transplant immunosuppression: beyond calcineurin inhibition. J Thorac Cardiovasc Surg 2003; 125(4):784–786.

64. Estenne M, Maurer JR, Boehler A, et al. Bronchiolitis obliterans syndrome 2001: an update of the diagnostic criteria. J Heart Lung Transplant 2002; 21(3):297–310.

65. Horning NR, Lynch JP, Sundaresan SR, et al. Tacrolimus therapy for persistent or recurrent acute rejection after lung transplantation. J Heart Lung Transplant 1998; 17(8):761–767.

66. Onsager DR, Canver CC, Jahania MS, et al. Efficacy of tacrolimus in the treatment of refractory rejection in heart and lung transplant recipients. J Heart Lung Transplant 1999; 18(5):448–455.

67. Sarahrudi K, Carretta A, Wisser W, et al. The value of switching from cyclosporine to tacrolimus in the treatment of refractory acute rejection and obliterative bronchiolitis after lung transplantation. Transpl Int 2002; 15:24–28.

68. Vitulo P, Tiberio O, Cascina A, et al. Efficacy of tacrolimus rescue therapy in refractory acute rejection after lung transplantation. J Heart Lung Transplant 2002; 21(4):435.

69. Sarahrudi K, Estenne M, Corris P, et al. International experience with conversion from cyclosporine to tacrolimus for acute and chronic lung allograft rejection. J Thorac Cardiovasc Surg 2004; 127(4):1126–1132.

70. Ross DJ, Lewis MI, Kramer M, et al. FK 506 'rescue' immunosuppression for obliterative bronchiolitis after lung transplantation. Chest 1997; 112(5): 1175–1179.

71. Kesten S, Chaparro C, Scavuzzo M, et al. Tacrolimus as rescue therapy for bronchiolitis obliterans syndrome. J Heart Lung Transplant 1997; 16(9): 905–912.

72. Wiebe K, Harringer W, Franke U, et al. FK506 rescue therapy in lung transplantation. Transplant Proc 1998; 30:1508–1509.

73. Lipson DA, Palevsky HI, Kotloff RM, et al. Conversion to tacrolimus (FK506) from cyclosporine after orthotopic lung transplantation. Transplant Proc 1998; 30:1505–1507.

74. Mentzer RM Jr, Jahania MS, Lasley RD, et al. Tacrolimus as a rescue immunosuppressant after heart and lung transplantation. Transplantation 1998; 65(1):109–113.

75. Revell MP, Lewis ME, Llewellyn-Jones CG, et al. Conservation of small-airway function by tacrolimus/cyclosporine conversion in the management of bronchiolitis obliterans following lung transplantation. J Heart Lung Transplant 2000; 19(12):1219–1223.

76. Fieguth HG, Krueger S, Wiedenmann DE, et al. Tacrolimus for treatment of bronchiolitis obliterans syndrome after unilateral and bilateral lung transplantation. Transplant Proc 2002; 34:1884.

77. Verleden GM, Dupont LJ, Van Raemdonck D, et al. Effect of switching from cyclosporine to tacrolimus on exhaled nitric oxide and pulmonary function in patients with chronic rejection after lung transplantation. J Heart Lung Transplant 2003; 22(8):908–913.

78. Cairn J, Yek T, Banner NR, et al. Time-related changes in pulmonary function after conversion to tacrolimus in bronchiolitis obliterans syndrome. J Heart Lung Transplant 2003; 22(1):50–57.

79. van Gelder T. Drug interactions with tacrolimus. Drug Saf 2002; 25(10): 707–712.

80. Jain A, Nalesnik M, Reyes J, et al. Posttransplant lymphoproliferative disorders in liver transplantation. Ann Surg 2002; 236(4):429–437.

81. Margreiter R. Efficacy and safety of tacrolimus compared with ciclosporin microemulsion in renal transplantation: a randomised multicentre study. Lancet 2002; 359(9308):741–746.

82. Klein IHHT, Abrahams A, van Ede T, et al. Different effects of tacrolimus and cyclosporine on renal hemodynamics and blood pressure in healthy subjects. Transplantation 2002; 73(5):732–736.

83. Vincenti F, Jensik SC, Filo RS, et al. A long-term comparison of tacrolimus (FK506) and cyclosporine in kidney transplantation: evidence for improved allograft survival at five years. Transplantation 2002; 73(5):775–782.

84. Aguirrezabalaga J, Fernandez-Selles C, Fraguela J, et al. Lipid profiles after liver transplantation in patients receiving tacrolimus or cyclosporin. Transplant Proc 2002; 34(5):1551–1552.

85. Treede H, Klepetko W, Reichenspurner H, et al. Tacrolimus versus cyclosporine after lung transplantation: a prospective, open, randomized two-center trial comparing two different immunosuppressive protocols. J Heart Lung Transplant 2001; 20(5):511–517.

86. Shitrit D, Starobin D, Aravot D, et al. Tacrolimus-induced hemolytic uremic syndrome case presentation in a lung transplant recipient. Transplant Proc 2003; 35:627–628.

87. Neylan JF. Racial differences in renal transplantation after immunosuppression with tacrolimus versus cyclosporine. Transplantation 1998; 65(4): 515–523.

88. Shumway SJ, Frist WH. Immunosuppressants. In: Shumway SJ, Shumway NE, eds. Thoracic Transplantation. 1st ed. Cambridge, MA: Blackwell Science, 1995:55–66.

89. Schwartz R, Dameshek W. Drug-induced immunological tolerance. Nature 1959; 183(4676):183–184.

90. Calne RY, Murray JE. Inhibition of the rejection of renal homografts in dogs by Burroughs Wellcome 57–322. Surg Forum 1961; 12:118–120.

91. Elion GB. The purine path to chemotherapy. Biosci Rep 1989; 9(5):509–529.

92. Trotter JL, Rodey GE, Gebel HM. Azathioprine decreases suppressor T cells in patients with multiple sclerosis. N Engl J Med 1982; 306(6):365–366.

93. Tiede I, Fritz G, Strand S, et al. CD28-dependent Rac1 activation is the molecular target of azathioprine in primary human CD4+ T lymphocytes. J Clin Invest 2003; 111(8):1133–1145.

94. Chan GLC, Erdmann GR, Gruber SA, et al. Azathioprine metabolism: pharmacokinetics of 6-mercaptopurine, 6-thiouric acid and 6-thiogaunine nucleotides in renal transplant patients. J Clin Pharmacol 1990; 30:358–363.

95. Murray JE, Merrill JP, Harrison JH, et al. Prolonged survival of human-kidney homografts by immunosuppressive drug therapy. N Engl J Med 1963; 268(24):1315–1323.

96. Gleason RE, Murray JE. Report from kidney transplant registry: analysis of variables in the function of human kidney transplants. Transplantation 1967; 5(2):360–373.

97. Hoffmeyer F, Hoeper MM, Spiekerkotter E, et al. Azathioprine withdrawal in stable lung and heart/lung recipients receiving cyclosporine-based immunosuppression. Transplantation 2000; 70(3):522–525.

98. Hosenpud JD, Bennett LE, Keck BM, et al. The registry for the international society for heart and lung transplantation: seventeenth official report—2000. J Heart Lung Transplant 2000; 19(10):909–931.

99. Cummins D, Sekar M, Halil O, et al. Myelosuppression associated with azathioprine-allopurinol interaction after heart and lung transplantation. Transplantation 1996; 61(11):1661–1662.

100. Havrda DE, Rathbun S, Scheid D. A case report of warfarin resistance due to azathioprine and review of the literature. Pharmacotherapy 2001; 21(3):355–357.

101. King JO, Laver MC, Fairley KF. Sensitivity to azathioprine. Med J Aust 1972; 2:939–941.
102. Farthing MJ, Coxon AY, Sheaff PC. Polyneuritis associated with azathioprine sensitivity reaction. Br Med J 1980; 280(6211):367.
103. Pollack R, Nishikawa RA, Mozes MF, et al. Azathioprine-induced leukopenia—clinical significance in renal transplantation. J Surg Res 1980; 29(3): 258–264.
104. Banner NR, Lyster H. Pharmacological immunosuppression. In: Banner NR, Polak JM, Yacoub M, eds. Lung Transplantation. 1st ed. Cambridge, United Kingdom: Cambridge University Press, 2003:205–242.
105. McLeod HL, Miller DR, Evans WE. Azathioprine-induced myelosuppression in thiopurine methyltransferase deficient heart transplant recipient. Lancet 1993; 341:1151.
106. McLeod HL, Lin JS, Scott EP, et al. Thiopurine methyltransferase activity in American white subjects and black subjects. Clin Pharmacol Ther 1994; 55(1): 15–20.
107. Black AJ, McLeod HL, Capell HA, et al. Thiopurine methyltransferase genotype predicts therapy-limiting severe toxicity from azathioprine. Ann Intern Med 1998; 129(9):716–718.
108. Sparberg M, Simon N, Del Greco F. Intrahepatic cholestasis due to azathioprine. Gastroenterology 1969; 57(4):439–441.
109. Read AE, Wiesner RH, LaBrecque DR, et al. Hepatic veno-occlusive disease associated with renal transplantation and azathioprine therapy. Ann Intern Med 1986; 104(5):651–655.
110. Penn I. Cancers complicating organ transplantation. N Engl J Med 1990; 323(25):1767–1769.
111. Taylor AEM, Shuster S. Skin cancer after renal transplantation: the causal role of azathioprine. Acta Dermatol Venerol 1992; 72:115–119.
112. Lennard L, Thomas S, Harrington CI, et al. Skin cancer in renal transplant recipients is associated with increased concentrations of 6-thioguanine nucleotide in red blood cells. Br J Dermatol 1985; 113:723–729.
113. Lipsky JJ. Mycophenolate mofetil. Lancet 1996; 348(9038):1357–1359.
114. Gummert JF, Ikonen T, Morris RE. Newer immunosuppressive drugs: a review. J Am Soc Nephrol 1999; 10:1366–1380.
115. Blaheta RA, Leckel K, Wittig B, et al. Inhibition of endothelial receptor expression and of T-cell ligand activity by mycophenolate mofetil. Transpl Immunol 1998; 6(4):251–259.
116. Azzola A, Havryk A, Chhajed P, et al. Everolimus and mycophenolate mofetil are potent inhibitors of fibroblast proliferation after lung transplantation. Transplantation 2004; 77(2):275–280.
117. Lee WA, Gu L, Miksztal AR, et al. Bioavailability improvement of mycophenolic acid through amino ester derivatization. Pharm Res 1990; 7(2):161–166.
118. Bullingham R, Monroe S, Nicholls A, et al. Pharmacokinetics and bioavailability of mycophenolate mofetil in healthy subjects after single-dose oral and intravenous administration. J Clin Pharm 1996; 36(4):315–324.

119. Devyatko E, Ploner M, Zuckermann A, et al. Value of mycophenolic acid trough level monitoring after lung transplantation. Transplant Proc 2002; 34: 1881–1883.
120. Brunet M, Martorell J, Oppenheimer F, et al. Pharmacokinetics and pharmacodynamics of mycophenolic acid in stable renal transplant recipients treated with low doses of mycophenolate mofetil. Transpl Int 2000; 13(Suppl 1): S301–S305.
121. Sollinger HW. Mycophenolate mofetil for the prevention of acute rejection in primary cadaveric renal allograft recipients. Transplantation 1995; 60(3): 225–232.
122. The Tricontinental Mycophenolate Mofetil Renal Transplantation Study Group. A blinded, randomized clinical trial of mycophenolate mofetil for the prevention of acute rejection in cadaveric renal transplantation. Transplantation 1996; 61(7):1029–1037.
123. European Mycophenolate Mofetil Cooperative Study Group. Placebo-controlled study of mycophenolate mofetil combined with cyclosporin and corticosteroids for prevention of acute rejection. Lancet 1995; 345:1321–1325.
124. Kobashigawa J, Miller L, Renlund D, et al. A randomized active-controlled trial of mycophenolate mofetil in heart transplant recipients. Transplantation 1998; 66(4):507–515.
125. Squifflet J-P, Vanrenterghem Y, van Hooff JP, et al. Safe withdrawal of corticosteroids or mycophenolate mofetil: results of a large, prospective, multicenter, randomized study. Transplant Proc 2002; 34:1584–1586.
126. Ross DJ, Waters PF, Levine M, et al. Mycophenolate mofetil versus azathioprine immunosuppressive regimens after lung transplantation: preliminary experience. J Heart Lung Transplant 1998; 17(8):768–774.
127. O'Hair DP, Cantu E, McGregor C, et al. Preliminary experience with mycophenolate mofetil used after lung transplantation. J Heart Lung Transplant 1998; 17(9):864–868.
128. Zuckermann A, Klepetko W, Birsan T, et al. Comparison between mycophenolate mofetil- and azathioprine-based immunosuppressions in clinical lung transplantation. J Heart Lung Transplant 1999; 18(5):432–440.
129. Bhorade SM, Jordan A, Villanueva J, et al. Comparison of three tacrolimus-based immunosuppressive regimens in lung transplantation. Am J Transplant 2003; 3:1570–1575.
130. Palmer SM, Baz MA, Sanders L, et al. Results of a randomized, prospective, multicenter trial of mycophenolate mofetil versus azathioprine in the prevention of acute lung allograft rejection. Transplantation 2001; 71(12):1772–1776.
131. Glanville AR, Corris PA, McNeil KD, et al. Mycophenolate mofetil (MMF) vs azathioprine (AZA) in lung transplantation for the prevention of bronchiolitis obliterans syndrome (BOS): results of a 3 year international randomised trial. J Heart Lung Transplant 2003; 22(1S):S207.
132. Speich R, Boehler A, Thurnheer R, et al. Salvage therapy with mycophenolate mofetil for lung transplant bronchiolitis obliterans: importance of dosage. Transplantation 1997; 64(3):533–535.

133. Whyte RI, Rossi SJ, Mulligan MS, et al. Mycophenolate mofetil for obliterative bronchiolitis syndrome after lung transplantation. Ann Thorac Surg 1997; 64:945–948.

134. Zuckermann A, Birsan T, Thaghavi S, et al. Benefit of mycophenolate mofetil in patients with cyclosporine A-induced nephropathy after lung transplantation. Transplant Proc 1999; 31:1160–1161.

135. http://www.utdol.com/application/topic.asp?file=drug_l_z/173237&type==A&selectedTitle=2~53. (Accessed February 2005.).

136. Gerbase MW, Fathi M, Spiliopoulos A, et al. Pharmacokinetics of mycophenolic acid associated with calcineurin inhibitors: long-term monitoring in stable lung recipients with and without cystic fibrosis. J Heart Lung Transplant 2003; 22(5):587–590.

137. Vidal E, Cantarell C, Capdevila L, et al. Mycophenolate mofetil pharmacokinetics in transplant patients receiving cyclosporine or tacrolimus in combination therapy. Pharmacol Toxicol 2000 87:182–184.

138. Pelletier RP, Akin B, Henry ML, et al. The impact of mycophenolate mofetil dosing patterns on clinical outcome after renal transplantation. Clin Transplant 2003; 17:200–205.

139. Sollinger HW. Mycophenolates in transplantation. Clin Transplant 2004; 18: 485–492.

140. Garrigue V, Canet S, Dereure O, et al. Oral ulcerations in a renal transplant recipient: a mycophenolate mofetil-induced complication? Transplantation 2001; 72(5):968–969.

141. Apostolou T, Tsagalis G, Koutroubas G, et al. Mycophenolate mofetil and oral ulcerations. Transplantation 2004; 77(12):1911–1912.

142. Behrend M. Adverse gastrointestinal effects of mycophenolate mofetil: aetiology, incidence and management. Drug Saf 2001; 24(9):645–663.

143. Puig JM, Fernandez-Crespo P, Lloveras J, et al. Risk factors that influence the incidence and severity of MMF adverse events in renal transplant patients: relationship with corticosteroid dosage, renal function, sex, and patient age. Transplant Proc 1999; 31:2270–2271.

144. Mohsin N, Jha A, Kallankara S, et al. Rapid resolution of mycophenolate mofetil associated diarrhea with a small dose of octreotide: a case report. Transplant Proc 2003; 35:2754.

145. Engelen W, Verpooten GA, Van der Planken M, et al. Four cases of red blood cell aplasia in association with the use of mycophenolate mofetil in renal transplant patients. Clin Nephrol 2003; 60(2):119–124.

146. Bernabeu-Wittel M, Naranjo M, Cisneros JM, et al. Infections in renal transplant recipients receiving mycophenolate versus azathioprine-based immunosuppression. Eur J Clin Microbiol Infect Dis 2002; 21:173–180.

147. Munoz MA, Andres A, Gallego R, et al. Mycophenolate mofetil immunosuppressive therapies increase the incidence of cytomegalovirus infection in renal transplantation. Transplant Proc 2002; 34:97.

148. Sarmiento JM, Dockrell DH, Schwab TR, et al. Mycophenolate mofetil increases cytomegalovirus invasive organ disease in renal transplant patients. Clin Transplant 2000; 14:136–138.

149. Rose ML, Smith J, Dureau G, et al. Mycophenolate mofetil decreases antibody production after cardiac transplantation. J Heart Lung Transplant 2002; 21(2):282–285.

150. Zmonarski SC, Boratynska M, Madziarska K, et al. Mycophenolate mofetil severely depressed antibody response to CMV infection in early posttransplant period. Transplant Proc 2003; 35:2205–2206.

151. Guerard A, Rabodonirina M, Cotte L, et al. Intestinal microsporidiosis occurring in two renal transplant recipients treated with mycophenolate mofetil. Transplantation 1999; 68(5):699–701.

152. Husain S, Singh N. The impact of novel immunosuppressive agents on infections in organ transplant recipients and the interactions of these agents with antimicrobials. Clin Infect Dis 2002; 35(1):53–61.

153. Gross DC, Sasaki TM, Buick MK, et al. Acute respiratory failure and pulmonary fibrosis secondary to administration of mycophenolate mofetil. Transplantation 1997; 64(11):1607–1609.

154. Shrestha NK, Mossad SB, Braun W. Pneumonitis associated with the use of mycophenolate mofetil. Transplantation 2003; 75(10):1762.

155. Le Ray C, Coulomb A, Elefant E, et al. Mycophenolate mofetil in pregnancy after renal transplantation: a case of major fetal malformations. Obstet Gynecol 2004; 103(5):1091–1094.

156. Sehgal SN, Baker H, Vezina C. Rapamycin (AY-22,989), a new antifungal antibiotic. II. Fermentation, isolation, and characterization. J Antibiot 1975; 28(10):727–732.

157. Brown EJ, Albers MW, Shin TB, et al. A mammalian protein targeted by G1-arresting rapamycin-receptor complex. Nature 1994; 359(6483):756–758.

158. Feuerstein N, Firestein R, Aiyar N, et al. Late induction of CREB/ATF binding and a concomitant increase in cAMP levels in T and B lymphocytes stimulated via the antigen receptor. J Immunol 1996; 156:4582–4593.

159. Jefferies HBJ, Reinhard C, Kozma SC, et al. Rapamycin selectively represses translation of the "polypyrimidine tract" mRNA family. Proc Natl Acad Sci USA 1994; 91:4441–4445.

160. Brunn GJ, Hudson CC, Sekulic A, et al. Phosphorylation of the translational repressor PHAS-I by the mammalian target of rapamycin. Science 1997; 277(5322):99–101.

161. Lai JH, Tan TH. CD28 signaling causes a sustained down-regulation of IkBa which can be prevented by the immunosuppressant rapamycin. J Biol Chem 1994; 269(48):30077–30080.

162. Flanagan WM, Crabtree GR. Rapamycin inhibits p34cdc2 expression and arrests T lymphocyte proliferation at the G1/S transition. Ann N Y Acad Sci 1993; 696:31–37.

163. Sehgal SN. Sirolimus: its discovery, biological properties, and mechanism of action. Transplant Proc 2003; 35(Suppl 3A):7S–14S.

164. Marx S, Jayaraman T, Go LO, et al. Rapamycin-FKBP inhibits cell cycle regulators of proliferation in vascular smooth muscle cells. Circ Res 1995; 76(3): 412–417.

165. Nair RV, Huang X, Shorthourse R, et al. Antiproliferative effect of rapamycin on growth factor-stimulated human adult lung fibroblasts in vitro may explain

its superior efficacy for prevention and treatment of allograft obliterative airway disease in vivo. Transplant Proc 1997; 29:614–615.

166. Zimmerman JJ, Kahan BD. Pharmacokinetics of sirolimus in stable renal transplant patients after multiple oral dose administration. J Clin Pharmacol 1997; 37(5):405–415.

167. Kahan BD, Camardo JS. Rapamycin: clinical results and future opportunities. Transplantation 2001; 72(7):1181–1193.

168. Kahan BD. Efficacy of sirolimus compared with azathioprine for reduction of acute renal allograft rejection: a randomised multicentre study. Lancet 2000; 356:194–202.

169. MacDonald AS. A worldwide, phase III, randomized, controlled, safety and efficacy study of a sirolimus/cyclosporine regimen for prevention of acute rejection in recipients of primary mismatched renal allografts. Transplantation 2001; 71(2):271–280.

170. King-Biggs MB, Dunitz JM, Park SJ, et al. Airway anastomotic dehiscence associated with use of sirolimus immediately after lung transplantation. Transplantation 2003; 75(9):1437–1443.

171. Groetzner J, Kur F, Spelsberg F, et al. Airway anastomosis complications in de novo lung transplantation with sirolimus-based immunosuppression. J Heart Lung Transplant 2004; 23(5):632–638.

172. Bhorade SM, Ahya V, Kotloff R, et al. Comparison of sirolimus versus azathioprine in a tacrolimus based immunosuppressive regimen in lung transplantation. J Heart Lung Transplant 2004; 23(2S):S113.

173. Cahill BC, Somerville KT, Crompton JA, et al. Early experience with sirolimus in lung transplant recipients with chronic allograft rejection. J Heart Lung Transplant 2003; 22(2):169–176.

174. Ussetti P, Laporta R, de Pablo A, et al. Rapamycin in lung transplantation: preliminary results. Transplant Proc 2003; 35:1974–1977.

175. Kaplan B, Meier-Kriesche H-U, Napoli KL, et al. The effects of relative timing of sirolimus and cyclosporine microemulsion formulation coadministration on the pharmacokinetics of each agent. Clin Pharmacol Ther 1998; 63:48–53.

176. Napoli KL, Wang ME, Stepkowski SM, et al. Relative tissue distributions of cyclosporine and sirolimus after concomitant peroral administration to the rat: evidence for pharmacokinetic interactions. Ther Drug Monit 1998; 20(2):123–133.

177. McAlister VC, Mahalati K, Peltekian KM, et al. A clinical pharmacokinetic study of tacrolimus and sirolimus combination immunosuppression comparing simultaneous to separated administration. Ther Drug Monit 2002; 24(3):346–350.

178. Holt DW, Ostraat O, Grinyo JM, et al. MMF may be given at lower doses when used in association with sirolimus in renal transplant recipients. Am J Transplant 2001; 1(Suppl 1):247.

179. Podder H, Stepkowski SM, Napoli KL, et al. Pharmacokinetic interactions augment toxicities of sirolimus/cyclosporine combinations. J Am Soc Nephrol 2001; 12:1059–1071.

180. Shihab FS; Bennett WM, Yi H, et al. Sirolimus increases transforming growth factor-beta1 expression and potentiates chronic cyclosporine nephrotoxicity. Kidney Int 2004; 65(4):1262–1271.

181. Saunders RN, Bicknell GR, Nicholson ML. The impact of cyclosporine dose reduction with or without the addition of rapamycin on functional, molecular, and histological markers of chronic allograft nephropathy. Transplantation 2003; 75(6):772–780.

182. Groth CG, Brattstrom C, Claesson K, et al. New trials in transplantation: how to exploit the potential of sirolimus in clinical transplantation. Transplant Proc 1998; 30:4064–4065.

183. Langer RM, Van Buren CT, Katz SM, et al. De novo hemolytic uremic syndrome after kidney transplantation in patients treated with cyclosporine A sirolimus combination. Transplant Proc 2001; 33:3236–3237.

184. Rampino T, Marasa M, Malvezzi PM, et al. Platelet-independent defect in hemostasis associated with sirolimus use. Transplant Proc 2004; 36:700–702.

185. Morrisett JD, Abdel-Fattah G, Kahan BD. Sirolimus changes lipid concentrations and lipoprotein metabolism in kidney transplant recipients. Transplant Proc 2003; 35(Suppl 3A):143S–150S.

186. van Gelder T, ter Meulen CG, Hene R, et al. Oral ulcers in kidney transplant recipients treated with sirolimus and mycophenolate mofetil. Transplantation 2003; 75(6):788–791.

187. Pham P-TT, Pham P-CT, Danovitch GM, et al. Sirolimus-associated pulmonary toxicity. Transplantation 2004; 77(8):1215–1220.

188. McWilliams TJ, Levvey BJ, Russell PA, et al. Interstitial pneumonitis associated with sirolimus: a dilemma for lung transplantation. J Heart Lung Transplant 2003; 22(2):210–213.

189. Billingham RE, Krohn PL, Medawar PB. Effect of cortisone on survival of skin homografts in rabbits. Br Med J 1951; 1:1157–1163.

190. Billingham RE, Krohn PL, Medawar PB. Effect of locally applied cortisone acetate on survival of skin homografts in rabbits. Br Med J 1951; 2:1049–1053.

191. Goodwin WE, Kaufman JJ, Mims MM, et al. Human renal transplantation. I, Clinical experiences with six cases of renal homotransplantation. J Urol 1963; 89(1):13–24.

192. Van Laethem F, Baus E, Andris F, et al. A novel aspect of the anti-inflammatory actions of glucocorticoids: inhibition of proximal steps of signaling cascades in lymphocytes. Cell Mol Life Sci 2001; 58:1599–1606.

193. Barnes PJ, Karin M. Nuclear factor-kB—a pivotal transcription factor in chronic inflammatory diseases. N Engl J Med 1997; 336(15):1066–1071.

194. Scheinman RI, Cogswell PC, Lofquist AK, et al. Role of transcriptional activation of I kappa B alpha in mediation of immunosuppression by glucocorticoids. Science 1995; 270(5234):283–286.

195. Auphan N, DiDonato JA, Rosette C, et al. Immunosuppression by glucocorticoids: inhibition of NK-kappa B activity through induction of I kappa B synthesis. Science 1995; 270(5234):286–290.

196. Snyder DS, Unanue ER. Corticosteroids inhibit murine macrophage Ia expression and interleukin 1 production. J Immunol 1982; 129(5):1803–1805.

197. Northrop JP, Crabtree GR, Nattila PS. Negative regulation of interleukin 2 transcription by the glucocorticoid receptor. J Exp Med 1992; 175:1235–1245.

198. Zanker B, Walz G, Wieder KJ, et al. Evidence that glucocorticosteroids block expression of the human interleukin-6 gene by accessory cells. Transplantation 1990; 49(1):183–185.
199. Cupps TR, Fauci AS. Corticosteroid-mediated immunoregulation in man. Immunol Rev 1982; 65:133–155.
200. Planey SL, Litwack G. Glucocorticoid-induced apoptosis in lymphocytes. Biochem Biophys Res Commun 2000; 279:307–312.
201. Ferry JJ, Horvath AM, Bekersky I, et al. Relative and absolute bioavailability of prednisone and prednisolone after separate oral and intravenous doses. J Clin Pharmacol 1988; 28:81–87.
202. Pugeat MM, Dunn JF, Nisula BC. Transport of steroid hormones: interaction of 70 drugs with testosterone-binding globulin and corticosteroid-binding globulin in human plasma. J Clin Endocrinol Metab 1981; 53(1):69–75.
203. Ballard PL, Carter JP, Graham BS, et al. A radioreceptor assay for evaluation of the plasma glucocorticoid activity of natural and synthetic steroids in man. J Clin Endocrinol Metab 1975; 41(2):290–304.
204. Dove AM, Szefler SJ, Hill MR, et al. Altered prednisolone pharmacokinetics in patients with cystic fibrosis. J Pediatr 1992; 120(5):789–794.
205. Jeng S, Chanchairujira T, Jusko W, et al. Prednisone metabolism in recipients of kidney or liver transplants and in lung recipients receiving ketoconazole. Transplantation 2003; 75(6):792–795.
206. Hricik DE, O'Toole MA, Schulak JA, et al. Steroid-free immunosuppression in cyclosporine-treated renal transplant recipients: a meta-analysis. J Am Soc Nephrol 1993; 4(6):1300–1305.
207. Smak Gregoor PJH, de Sevaux RGL, Ligtenberg G, et al. Withdrawal of cyclosporine or prednisone six months after kidney transplantation in patients on triple drug therapy: a randomized, prospective, multicenter study. J Am Soc Nephrol 2002; 13(5):1365–1373.
208. Kasiske BL, Chakkera HA, Louis TA, et al. A meta-analysis of immunosuppression withdrawal trials in renal transplantation. J Am Soc Nephrol 2000; 11(10):1910–1917.
209. McAllister WAC, Thompson PJ, Al-Habet SM. Rifampin reduces effectiveness and bioavailability of prednisolone. Br Med J 1983; 286:923–925.
210. Bartoszek M, Brenner AM, Szefler SJ. Prednisolone and methylprednisolone kinetics in children receiving anticonvulsant therapy. Clin Pharmacol Ther 1987; 42(4):424–432.
211. Langhoff E, Madsen S, Olgaard K, et al. Clinical results and cyclosporine effect on prednisolone metabolism. Kidney Int 1984; 26:642.
212. Sarma GR, Kailasam S, Nair NGK, et al. Effect of prednisolone and rifampin on isoniazid metabolism in slow and rapid inactivators of isoniazid. Antimicrob Agents Chemother 1980; 18(5):661–666.
213. Klinenberg JR, Miller F. Effect of corticosteroids on blood salicylate concentration. J Am Med Assoc 1965; 194(6):131–134.
214. Winston DJ, Ho WG, Schiffman G, et al. Pneumococcal vaccination of recipients of bone marrow transplants. Arch Intern Med 1983; 143:1735–1737.
215. Herron A, Dettleff G, Hixon B, et al. Influenza vaccination in patients with rheumatic diseases. J Am Med Assoc 1979; 242(1):53–56.

216. Kubiet MA, Gonzalez-Rothi RJ, Cottey R, et al. Serum antibody response to influenza vaccine in pulmonary patients receiving corticosteroids. Chest 1996; 110(2):367–370.

217. Lahood N, Emerson SS, Kumar P, et al. Antibody levels and response to pneumococcal vaccine in steroid-dependent asthma. Ann Allergy 1993; 70:289–294.

218. Saag KG, Koehnke R, Caldwell JR, et al. Low dose long-term corticosteroid therapy in rheumatoid arthritis: an analysis of serious adverse events. Am J Med 1994; 96:115–123.

219. Berkowitz JS, David DS, Sakai S, et al. Ocular complications in renal transplant recipients. Am J Med 1973; 55:492–495.

220. Karagas MR, Cushing GL Jr, Greenberg ER, et al. Non-melanoma skin cancers and glucocorticoid therapy. Br J Cancer 2001; 85(5):683–686.

221. Wolfe F, Furst D, Lane N, et al. Substantial increase in important adverse events follow low dose prednisone therapy of rheumatoid arthritis (RA). Arthritis Rheum 1995; 38:S312.

222. Jackson SHD, Beevers DG, Myers K. Does long-term low-dose corticosteroid therapy cause hypertension? Clin Sci 1981; 61:381S–383S.

223. Berg AL, Nilsson-Ehle P. ACTH lowers serum lipids in steroid-treated hyperlipemic patients with kidney disease. Kidney Int 1996; 50:538–542.

224. Rigotti P. Patients with high cholesterol levels benefit most from early withdrawal of corticosteroids. Transplant Proc 2002; 34:1797–1798.

225. Svenson KLG, Lithell H, Hallgren R, et al. Serum lipoprotein in active rheumatoid arthritis and other chronic inflammatory arthritides. Arch Intern Med 1987; 147:1917–1920.

226. Lloveras J, Senti M, Puig JM, et al. Effect of time elapsed since transplantation on lipid and lipoprotein abnormalities in renal transplant patients: role of maintenance prednisone and gender influence. Transplant Proc 1997; 29: 212–215.

227. Messer J, Reitman D, Sacks HS, et al. Association of adrenocorticosteroid therapy with peptic-ulcer disease. N Engl J Med 1983; 309(1):21–24.

228. Piper JM, Ray WA, Daugherty JR, et al. Corticosteroid use and peptic ulcer disease: role of nonsteroidal anti-inflammatory drugs. Ann Intern Med 1991; 114(9):735–740.

229. Glenn F, Grafe WR Jr. Surgical complications of adrenal steroid therapy. Ann Surg 1967; 165(6):1023–1032.

230. Gurwitz JH, Bohn RL, Glynn RJ, et al. Glucocorticoids and the risk for initiation of hypoglycemic therapy. Arch Intern Med 1994; 154:97–101.

231. Adler RA, Rosen CJ. Glucocorticoids and osteoporosis. Endocrinol Metab Clin North Am 1994; 23(3):641–654.

232. Reid IR, Heap SW. Determinants of vertebral mineral density in patients receiving long-term glucocorticoid therapy. Arch Intern Med 1990; 150: 2545–2548.

233. Buckley LM, Leib ES, Cartularo KS, et al. Effects of low dose corticosteroids on the bone mineral density of patients with rheumatoid arthritis. J Rheumatol 1995; 22:1055–1059.

234. Ruegsegger P, Medici TC, Anliker M. Corticosteroid-induced bone loss. A longitudinal study of alternate day therapy in patients with bronchial asthma

using quantitative computer tomography. Eur J Clin Pharmacol 1983; 25: 615–620.

235. Reid IR, King AR, Alexander CJ, et al. Prevention of steroid-induced osteoporosis with (3-amino-1-hydroxypropylidene)-1,1-bisphosphonate (APD). Lancet 1988; 1(8578):143–146.

236. Saag KG, Emkey R, Schnitzer TJ, et al. Alendronate for the prevention and treatment of glucocorticoid-induced osteoporosis. N Engl J Med 1998; 339(5): 292–299.

237. Kershner P, Wang-Cheng R. Psychiatric side effects of steroid therapy. Psychosomatics 1989; 30:135–139.

# 18

# Lympholytic Agents (Polyclonal Antilymphocyte Antibodies, Anti-CD3 Monoclonal Antibodies, Anti-CD25 Monoclonal Antibodies)

**Brian P. Dickover, Sangeeta M. Bhorade, and Edward R. Garrity, Jr.**

*Division of Pulmonary and Critical Care Medicine, Department of Internal Medicine, Loyola University Medical Center, Maywood, Illinois, U.S.A.*

## INTRODUCTION

Successful lung transplantation (LT) is only possible with the expert use of immunosuppressive drugs that carefully navigate the path between oversuppression leading to infection and/or malignancy and undersuppression leading to rejection. These drugs are used in various combinations during the three phases of immunosuppression: induction of suppression during the initial phase of transplantation, maintenance of suppression thereafter, and reversal of established rejection (1). The agents frequently used for immunosuppression in solid organ transplantation have been corticosteroids, cyclosporine, azathioprine, tacrolimus, sirolimus, and mycophenolate mofetil. These agents are covered in detail in another chapter in this monograph. Here, we cover the so-called lympholytic immunosuppressants, namely polyclonal antilymphocyte antibodies, anti-CD3 monoclonal antibody (MAb), and anti-CD25 MAb. In particular, the use of lympholytics in the context of induction therapy in LT is emphasized with mention being made of reversal of rejection.

Lympholytic immunosuppressants are sometimes also referred to as biologic immunosuppressants. This term distinguishes them from their classic chemical counterparts by virtue of their comprising antibodies rather than inhibitory chemical pharmaceuticals. The motivation for developing biologic immunosuppressants arose from the fact that organ rejection is primarily mediated by T-cell subsets with specific surface markers (2). By targeting T-cells, investigators and clinicians hoped to increase the selectivity of the agent, thereby limiting side effects and toxicity while maintaining adequate suppression. Although biologics have been used both for induction and for treatment of rejection in kidney, liver, and heart transplantation, their role in LT is somewhat less clear (3).

Polyclonal antilymphocyte antibody in the form of antilymphocyte serum (ALS) was the first form of lympholytic therapy. Its initial use in transplantation was in the setting of rat skin homografts, where it was shown to prolong graft survival when combined with lymph drainage (4). However, the use of ALS as an anti-inflammatory has been known since the early 1900s (5). ALS was first used in renal transplantation by Thomas Starzl. The addition of ALS allowed the reduction of prednisone and azathioprine while preserving renal function (6). Its uses in LT have expanded since that initial period, as will be detailed later.

With the ability to create MAbs came an even greater level of potential immunosuppressive specificity. Polyclonal antibodies can be problematic in that they are nonspecific and are therefore directed against multiple potential lymphocytic cell-surface antigens (3). By synthesizing MAb with specificity against only one cell surface antigen, the hope prevailed that immunogenicity would be maintained with even further limiting of side effects and toxicity. In 1975, Köhler and Milstein created the first MAb, which was directed against a specific sheep red blood antigen (7). That innovation led subsequently to the development of antibodies directly targeted at the ε subunit of the human CD3 complex. Anti-CD3 MAb had its first clinical use in 1981 by Cosimi, who showed that episodes of acute renal allograft rejection could be reversed using anti-CD3 MAb while continuing to lower steroid dosages (8). It has subsequently been used in both induction therapy and antirejection therapy in renal, liver, and heart transplantation.

CD-25 refers to the α chain of the interleukin-2 receptor (IL-2R). Kirkman et al. showed in 1985 that anti-CD25 MAb produced indefinite graft survival in 50% of mice when given during the first 10 days post–heart transplant (9,10). Anti-CD25 MAb would ideally inhibit T-cell activation in a more specific way than anti-CD3 MAb. It would also be free of interaction with the entire T-cell population. As with the other lympholytic agents described, it has been proven to decrease the incidence of acute rejection in renal, liver, and heart transplantation (3). Its specific use in LT continues to develop, as will be described.

## POLYCLONAL ANTILYMPHOCYTE ANTIBODIES

The polyclonal antilymphocyte antibodies are composed specifically of ALS, antilymphocyte globulin (ALG), and antithymocyte globulin (ATG). The preparation of ALS first involves the collection of lymphocytes from the lymph nodes, thymuses, or thoracic duct lymph from the species to be immunized. Those lymphocytes are then injected intravenously, subcutaneously, or intradermally into rabbits or horses. Serum from the rabbit or horse is subsequently collected and used for therapy (11). ALG production is identical until finally the raw serum is further processed in order to obtain only the globulin component. Finally, the raw globulin is absorbed with red cells, platelets, and plasma from the recipient species in order that hemolysis, thrombocytopenia, and other toxicities, respectively, are decreased (11).

Polyclonal ALS possesses antibodies against multiple common T-cell surface antigens (Table 1). The means by which polyclonal ALS exert their effect are seemingly threefold. First, profound lymphopenia is achieved immediately after therapy through complement-mediated cell lysis of

**Table 1**  Comparison of Polyclonal Antilymphocyte Preparations

|  | Atgam® | Lympho-globuline | Thymo-globuline | ATG | MALG | RATG |
|---|---|---|---|---|---|---|
| Immunogen | Thymus | Thymus | Thymus | Jurkat cell line | Cultured lympho-blasts | Thymus |
| Species | Equine | Equine | Rabbit | Rabbit | Equine | Rabbit |
| Dosage (mg/ kg/day) | 10–30 | 10 | 1.25–2.5 | 1–5 | 15–20 | 1–5 |
| Reactivity against |  |  |  |  |  |  |
| CD2 | ++ | ++++ | + | ± | + | + |
| CD3 | ++ | + | + | 0 | + | ± |
| CD4 | +++ | + | ± | 0 | + | + |
| CD8 | ++ | +++ | ++ | 0 | + | + |
| CD11a | ++ | + | ± | 0 | + | + |
| CD18 | ++ | ++ | + | 0 | ++ | ++++ |
| CD28 | + | ++ | ± | ± | ++ | ++++ |
| CD TCR | ++ | + | + | 0 | + | N/A |

*Abbreviations*: ATG, antithymocyte globulin; MALG, Minnesota antilymphocyte globulin; RATG, rabbit antithymocyte globulin.
*Source*: From Ref. 2.

targeted T-cells. A second mechanism involves the uptake of opsonized cells by the reticuloendothelial system (RES). This mechanism is verified by the isolation of ALS-coated cells within the RES organs of treated animals (12). The third potential mechanism of action of ALS is through the modulation or suppression of expression of essential cell-surface receptors normally evident on T-cells. These cells remain in the peripheral circulation but are less able to proliferate (12).

### Induction Therapy

Initial reviews of ALS seemed to refute the efficacy of ALS when used in renal transplantation (13). However, multiple studies in the 1990s showed that antilymphocyte preparations were effective in preventing rejection in renal transplantation (14–18). Polyclonal ATG has been shown in cardiac and renal transplantation to be an effective induction agent, with differences noted between different preparations of the drug (19,20). In LT the role of ALS is at times even less clear mainly due to the increased potential for cytomegalovirus (CMV) infection and posttransplant lymphoproliferative disorder (PTLD).

Several studies have attempted to assess the efficacy of ALS as induction therapy after LT. One study showed the superiority of rabbit antithymocyte globulin (RATG) combined with cyclosporine, azathioprine, and prednisone in preventing acute rejection when compared to combination therapy without RATG (21). A single-center, randomized, prospective study in 1999 also showed a decrease in biopsy-proven acute rejection in RATG-treated patients, although 30-day, 1-year, and 2-year survival were similar in the treatment and control groups (22). A retrospective study of 212 lung and heart–lung transplant recipients showed no difference at one and five years posttransplant with respect to survival in patients who either did or did not receive ATG (23). Additionally, Wiebe et al. found no difference in the incidence of chronic rejection in patients receiving induction therapy with polyclonal antibodies versus those who did not (23). In one, monoclonal anti-CD3 antibody was shown to be superior to Minnesota ALG with respect to latency in the development of bronchiolitis obliterans syndrome (BOS) (24).

### Rejection Therapy

Hyperacute rejection is a very rare occurrence in LT, with very few case reports ever having been made (25,26). A single case report documenting successful control of hyperacute rejection using ATG in a patient who received a single-lung transplant has been published (26). Plasmapheresis with albumin and FFP along with ATG were begun along with cyclophosphamide and methylprednisolone in a patient who underwent hyperacute rejection three hours after vascular anastomosis of the graft. Mycophenolate mofetil was also stopped and cyclosporine continued, and the patient underwent a dramatic recovery over the next several days. Clearly, however, questions remain concerning the specific role of ATG in this case report given the multitude of other drugs the patient received concurrently.

ALS has been used for many years for the treatment of acute and/or steroid-resistant rejection in renal transplantation (26–30). As with induction therapy, however, the use of ALS for acute rejection in LT is less well defined. One retrospective study showed that the progression of BOS, a manifestation of chronic rejection, was not slowed down by the use of ALS (31–33). This study is in keeping with two other small studies that looked at BOS in LT patients (32,33). It is worth noting that Kriett et al. on one occasion and Calhoon et al. on another report results from LT patients who did not receive ALS at all (34,35). As such, patients who did not receive ALS fared no worse with respect to development of rejection compared to patients who did receive that treatment.

## Monitoring and Toxicity

Monitoring of levels of suppression brought on by ALS has been challenging because the same preparation can induce different levels of suppression in different individuals. Levels of cytotoxicity can be determined by adding decreasing concentrations of ALS to standardized lymphocyte preparations in order to determine the amount needed to kill 50% of cells. Several assays have been developed to determine the amount of ALS needed to inhibit rosette formation of sheep red blood cells. That inhibition results from the action of anti-CD2 antibodies that are present in the ALS (2). MAbs have also been used to monitor the number of T-cells in peripheral blood (36). T-cell subset alterations in one study were documented as long as five years after treatment with ALS (37–39). Importantly, rejection control has been shown to correlate with the maintenance of levels of mature lymphocytes at less than 10% of pretreatment values (19,38,39). Notably, elevation of levels of mature lymphocytes has been shown to be associated with unresolved rejection (2). The current recommendation includes monitoring of T-cell levels and redosing for levels greater than 100/mL (40).

Side effects of ALS are dependent on the specific preparation used (Table 2). Fever is seen in the majority of patients receiving ALS, often in association with chills and occasional diarrhea and usually during the initial infusion. Elevated levels of tumor necrosis factor (TNF), IL-1, IL-6, and interferon (IFN-$\gamma$) are associated with these side effects, not only in ALS preparations, but also in certain monoclonal cytotoxics (41,42). Up to 30% of patients have developed immune responses to foreign antibodies, and serum sickness, although rare, has also been encountered (40). Pruritic skin rashes are noted in up to 20% of patients receiving ALS, and although of concern, the rash is such that lympholytic therapy can be continued with the addition of symptomatic treatment with antihistamines (2).

**Table 2**  Clinical Toxicity of Antilymphocyte Serum Administration

| Incidence > 10% | Incidence 5–10% | Incidence ≤5% |
|---|---|---|
| *Early reactions* | | |
| Chills, fever d1 15–60%; d2 4–25% | Nausea, diarrhea 1–10% | Hypotension 2–5% |
| Thrombo- cytopenia ($< 50,000/mm^3$) 1–30% | Neutropenia ($< 2000/mm^3$) 1–10% | Dyspnea 2–5% |
| Rash/ pruritus 1–20% | Serum sickness 1–8% | Seizures 0–1% |
| Anemia 5–15% | Arthralgia 1–7% | Anaphylaxis 0–1% |
| Local phlebitis 2–15% | | |
| *Late reactions* | | |
| CMV infection | Herpes simplex infection | PTLD EBV reactivation |

*Abbreviations*: CMV, cytomegalovirus; EBV, Epstein–Barr virus; PTLD, posttransplant lymphoproliferative disorder.
*Source*: From Ref. 2.

Thrombocytopenia and anemia have occurred following the use of ALS in as many as 30% of patients. These reactions are dose related and are therefore responsive to reduction in ALS dosage (2). A poorly defined mechanism that does not involve specific antiplatelet antibodies seems to be the cause of the thrombocytopenia (43). Platelet aggregation within the pulmonary microcirculation has been noted as well.

CMV remains the most concerning infectious complication of immunosuppression with ALS. Therapy with Atgam® was shown to be associated with the majority of cases of CMV disease in liver transplant patients (44). Prophylaxis with ganciclovir is recommended, especially in cases involving CMV-positive donors and CMV-negative recipients (45). Additionally, it has been shown that reduction of concurrently administered agents such as corticosteroids decreases rates of infectious complications compared to traditional regimens (46,47).

PTLD is the most important malignancy directly related to solid organ transplantation. Its occurrence is due to primary infection in children and reactivation of latent Epstein–Barr virus (EBV) infection in adults. The administration of ALS is associated with an increased risk of PTLD, in particular when patients have received multiple courses of antirejection therapy (2,48).

The first preparations of polyclonal antibodies were manufactured and used at specific institutions and as such were not distributed outside those institutions. Continued and more widespread use of these drugs has brought about tighter regulation and limited the availability of particular agents. In some cases certain brands have been eliminated altogether. Multiple studies refer to the use of ALS in LT (49–55); however, there remain few well-designed, controlled studies upon which to base regimented therapy. Currently, the only polyclonal agents available in the United States are Atgam® and thymoglobulin. Induction therapy consists of the first dose being given intraoperatively and prior to graft implantation. Dosing regimens vary between 3 and 15 days, with or without monitoring. Use of Atgam requires skin testing prior to use due to the potential for cross-reactivity to horse serum, whereas thymoglobulin does not require such testing (40).

## ANTI-CD3 MONOCLONAL ANTIBODIES

With the advent of MAb came the ability to further narrow down antibody specificity and improve drug safety profiles while maintaining efficacy. As described earlier, the first synthesis of MAb was described by Köhler and Milstein in 1975, an accomplishment for which they were awarded the Nobel Prize (7). Anti-CD3 MAb was subsequently created and with its specificity against the ε subunit of the human CD3 complex prompted enthusiasm for its use in solid organ transplantation. The production of MAb relies on a two-step process of production that immortalizes antibody-producing cells. First, a B-lymphocyte that produces the desired antibody is isolated in cell culture. This lymphocyte has a limited lifespan and so is only capable of producing antibody for a short period of time. The second step involves combining the desired B-lymphocyte with a malignant myeloma cell. The resulting hybridoma cell line is capable of producing unlimited quantities of the desired antibody for an unspecified period of time (2,7).

OKT3 is the prototype anti-CD3 MAb and is a murine (mouse) IgG2a antibody. Similar to polyclonal antibodies, OKT3 acts by inducing opsonization and thereafter complement-mediated cytolysis and/or RES uptake of affected T-cells. Modulation of T-cells has also been noted such that following the initial profound T-cell depletion, the remaining T-cells become incapable of responding to antigenic stimulation. OKT3 brings about alterations in cell surface receptors that are responsible for this modulation (2).

### Induction Therapy

OKT3 induction therapy in renal transplantation guided the use of that drug in LT in a way similar to that seen with the use of ALS. Studies from the 1980s and early 1990s verified the role of OKT3 in preventing episodes of rejection in renal allografts (17,56–59) with one study showing that prolonged administration of OKT3 maintained prevention of rejection while decreasing the necessary total steroid dosage (56). In LT, OKT3 was shown retrospectively to induce longer periods of latency in the development of BOS when compared to patients who received Minnesota ATG (24). Wain et al. later showed that acute rejection was reduced with the use of OKT3 compared to control patients who received no induction therapy (60).

## Rejection Therapy

OKT3 was initially used in the reversal of acute renal allograft rejection (8). It was also used successfully in a group of patients with renal allograft dysfunction who were at risk for continued graft dysfunction due in part to the use of cyclosporine (36). Data in LT with respect to treatment of rejection with OKT3 are lacking. Shennib et al. described a single patient who was successfully treated for acute rejection with OKT3, which began the expansion of the use of that drug (61). That group later reported data on 28 episodes of steroid-resistant rejection that were manifest in 20 patients who were treated with OKT3 for five to seven days. An overall response of 68% was noted, with an 89% response seen in patients who were treated within six months of transplant and a 30% response in patients who were treated for more than six months after transplant (62). Obviously, it remains difficult to fashion a rejection treatment protocol using OKT3 with so few data to refer to, but it remains in the armamentarium for use potentially in the case of steroid-resistant acute rejection. Additionally, research is lacking with respect to the use of OKT3 for the treatment of BOS.

## Monitoring and Toxicity

The murine component of OKT3 renders it capable of inducing human anti-mouse antibodies (HAMA). HAMA have been shown to occur in 25% to 30% of patients after initial treatment with OKT3 (63), with the probability of a HAMA response increasing with the number of exposures encountered. The first form these antibodies can take is an anti-isotypic form that cross-reacts with all IgG2a immunoglobulins, of which OKT3 is one. The second form is anti-idiotypic, which is specific only for the antigen-binding region of OKT3 (64). Anti-isotypic HAMA possesses the potential to render patients resistant not only to OKT3 but to all IgG2a antibodies. Anti-idiotypic OKT3 HAMA limits only the use of OKT3. Production of so-called humanized OKT3 has led to the limiting of anti-isotypic HAMA. The process of humanization was first described by Boulianne et al. (65) and entails the combination of the antigen-specific murine portion of the original anti-CD3 antibody with a human IgG antibody. This humanized anti-CD3 antibody has been shown to limit antigenicity and potentially also limit first-dose side effects (66). HAMA generated following the use of humanized anti-CD3 only limit the future use of

OKT3 and not of any other potentially beneficial IgG2a immunoglobulins. On average HAMA production occurs 7 to 10 days after discontinuation of therapy and coincides with the reappearance of CD3-positive cells in the peripheral circulation. Therefore, monitoring the levels of CD3-positive cells is indicated every two to three days during periods of treatment with OKT3 (67). Varying therapeutic ranges of CD3-positive cells have been used, but a level < 10% of baseline or < 50 cells/μL are most commonly used (68,69).

The toxicity of anti-CD3 MAb therapy remains one of the major limiting factors to its use. The so-called cytokine release syndrome is the most powerful noninfectious side effect and consists of chills, headache, pyrexia, vomiting, diarrhea, and tachycardia. Pulmonary edema has also been described in a patient already volume overloaded (70). Blood levels of TNF-α and IFN-γ are elevated after the use of OKT3, in particular after the first and second doses, and the syndrome itself occurs about 45 to 60 minutes after infusion. Notably, IL-2 levels were also shown to be elevated in patients who have not received steroids (71). Alegre et al. showed that pentoxifylline significantly reduces the release of TNF-α, but the clinical relevance of that drug's use remains unclear due to seeming lack in its ability to prevent the cytokine release syndrome itself (72).

Infectious complications of OKT3 therapy classically include incidences of CMV of 20% to 60%, fungal infections 5% to 35%, herpes simplex 5% to 25%, and PTLD 0% to 8% (2). A study in LT showed specifically that OKT3 or ALG use postoperatively was associated with significantly more CMV infection than in controls who did not receive cytolytics. However, Rubin maintains that CMV is effectively prevented in at-risk populations with prophylactic ganciclovir (45). Reactivation of latent EBV is responsible for the development of PTLD and in particular is associated less with any particular agent than with the total immunosuppressive load. To that end Swinnen et al. showed retrospectively that patients were at increased risk of PTLD after two weeks of OKT3 therapy when also receiving triple therapy (73), but Debure et al. described 150 patients receiving OKT3 who did not develop lymphoma while not receiving cyclosporine (58). Regimens vary from 5 mg/day for 3 to 10 days. In the last few years, induction therapy, in general, was often used to delay the initiation of calcineurin inhibitors to avoid renal toxicity.

## ANTI-CD25 MONOCLONAL ANTIBODIES

Anti-CD25 antibodies (IL-2 inhibitors) are those antibodies directed against the α subunit of the IL-2 receptor complex. Their usefulness in transplantation immunosuppression originally stemmed from the hope that because IL-2 promotes the proliferative expansion of T-lymphocytes, blockade of its receptor might inhibit that very proliferation. IL-2 inhibitors block proliferation of T-cells that have already been activated, thereby making it a

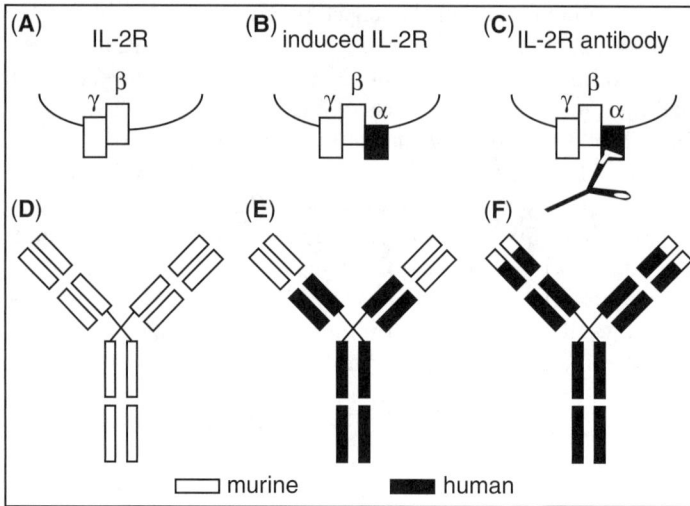

**Figure 1** Mechanism of action of therapeutic antibodies directed against CD25. The high-affinity IL-2 receptor is formed by association of the β and γ_c chains (*unshaded*, **A**) with the α chain (*shaded*, **B**) on the cell surface. Therapeutic antibodies with specificity for the α chain block binding of IL-2 to the receptor complex (**C**). The new generation of therapeutic antibodies to CD25 have been engineered from murine MAbs: parent murine MAb molecule (**D**); chimeric construct with murine variable and human constant domains (**E**); and humanized construct with murine CDR grafted to framework regions of human variable region domains (**F**). *Abbreviations*: MAb monoclonal antibody; IL, interleukin. *Source*: From Ref. 75.

late phase blocker. The two prevailing anti-CD25 antibody preparations that have any role whatsoever in LT, basiliximab and daclizumab, differ in a way that brings us back to the humanization process described in the context of anti-CD3 antibodies. Daclizumab is the humanized form of IL-2 inhibitor and is composed of about 10% murine and 90% human protein. Basiliximab, however, is composed of about 25% murine and 75% human protein (74). This difference leads to important differences in dosing that will be detailed later (Fig. 1) (75).

## Induction Therapy

The first randomized controlled trial assessing the use of an anti-CD25 antibody called 33B3.1 was published in 1990 (76). Patients were randomized to receive either 33B3.1 or RATG for two weeks after renal transplantation. 33B3.1 was shown to result in significantly fewer side effects and was comparable to RATG in preventing acute rejection. Subsequently, two randomized studies were undertaken to determine the efficacy of basiliximab. Both studies showed that basiliximab significantly reduced the number of episodes of acute rejection while maintaining equivalence or even improvement compared to placebo regarding side effects (77,78). In nonhuman primates, basiliximab was included in triple therapy and compared to cyclosporine and rapamycin and resulted in the use of lower rapamycin doses while continuing to prevent acute rejection (79). In 2002 a brief description was given of the use of basiliximab in human LT patients (80). The authors reported a delay in the onset of rejection as well as a 26% reduction in incidence of rejection at six months.

Similar to basiliximab, daclizumab was studied in renal transplantation in two large double-blind, placebo-controlled studies (81,82). When daclizumab was added to double- or triple-therapy regimens, six-month incidence of rejection was reduced to 40% and 37%, respectively, while also prolonging the time to first acute rejection (81). Similar results were achieved in the second large study (82). Results in cardiac transplantation have been comparable to those in renal transplantation (83), but there have been few studies in LT using daclizumab as an induction agent. Brock et al. compared OKT3, ATG, and daclizumab in 87 lung transplant patients between 1995 and 1999 (84). Patients underwent 59 single-lung transplants, 27 double-lung transplants, and one heart–lung transplant. The study showed no significant differences among the three groups with respect to acute rejection, and importantly, every patient who developed BOS had previously exhibited some manifestation of acute rejection. This is in keeping with previous experience that identifies acute rejection as a significant risk factor for BOS. Garrity et al. later found that triple-drug therapy with azathioprine, tacrolimus, and prednisone plus daclizumab decreased the six-month incidence of grade 2 biopsy-proven rejection from 48% to 18% when compared to historical controls who received triple-drug therapy alone (85). Grade 1 or greater biopsy-proven rejection was also significantly reduced at six months. Last, a nonsignificant prolongation of time to first rejection was noted in the daclizumab group as well.

## Rejection Therapy

The use of anti-CD25 MAb for the treatment of rejection is problematic because the $\alpha$ chain of the IL-2 receptor is not expressed on the surface of T-cells during episodes of acute rejection (74). This characteristic renders the drug incapable of suppressing episodes of rejection. One small study attempted to use the anti-CD25 antibody 33B3.1 mentioned above for the treatment of acute rejection in renal transplantation. In 10 patients with acute rejection, two responded to 33B3.1, four patients' creatinine stabilized, and four patients' creatinine continued to worsen (86). To date there are no studies of rejection treatment using anti-CD25 antibodies in LT.

## Monitoring and Toxicity

One significant advantage in the use of anti-CD25 antibodies is their seeming lack of serious side effects. Additionally, anti-CD25 antibodies do not cause a cytokine-release syndrome and have a negligible ability to elicit anti-idiotypic antibodies (78). Multiple studies have shown basiliximab and daclizumab to induce no more PTLD than traditional multidrug regimens (77,78,81,82). In a study by Brock et al. no LT patients in the daclizumab group developed PTLD compared to two patients in each of the OKT3 and ATG groups. Kidney transplant recipients have been shown to develop significantly less CMV infection with the use of basiliximab when compared to OKT3 (87). Overall rates of infection in anti-CD25 antibody-treated patients have been similar to controls in many analyses (77,78,81,82). Data from Brock et al. showed with significance that 44% of LT patients treated with daclizumab developed infections during the first postoperative year compared to 77% and 74% in the OKT3 and ATG groups, respectively (84). Bacterial infections were the most common, but daclizumab-treated patients were also shown to develop significantly fewer CMV infections. Similarly, patients in the study by Garrity et al. developed PTLD and CMV infection no more often than historical controls (85).

The main difference between basiliximab and daclizumab is in the length of their half-lives, a difference that is afforded specifically by the humanized nature of daclizumab. The chimeric agent basiliximab is generally used in a two-dose regimen, on days zero and four, and has a half-life of 13.4 days (88). It affords biological blockade of IL-2 receptors for about 36 to 49 days (89). In original work in renal transplantation the two-dose scheme appeared safer and as effective as a five-dose regimen (77,78). Humanization of daclizumab affords it less theoretical immunogenic potential than basiliximab and lengthens half-life to 20 days (90). It is regularly used in a five-dose regimen, with the first dose given intraoperatively, followed with repeat doses every two weeks. It affords nearly 90 days of successful IL-2 receptor blockade (91,92).

## FUTURE DIRECTIONS

The state of the art in transplantation is now defined by continuing incremental improvements in rejection rates, incidences of graft failure, and complications. The goal of immunotolerance via induction is not yet a reality, but progress is being made. Current experimental therapeutics includes intense lympholysis with agents such as ATG and Campath (93–95), donor bone marrow infusions (96–100), and modulators of lymphocyte trafficking such as FTY720 (101–103). It is often felt that better induction success may lead to reduced maintenance immunosuppression, and our ability to tailor both early and late treatment to the individual patient's needs. We expect continued progress in the years to come.

## CONCLUSION

Pioneering innovation was undertaken in renal transplantation with respect to immunosuppressive therapy, and that therapy has enabled the continued lowering of rejection rates while stabilizing levels of infection and malignancy that are no greater than those brought on using previous regimens. However, certain obstacles regarding immunosuppression that have been overcome in renal transplantation are sometimes still overwhelming in LT. Traditionally, postoperative infection rates have been higher in LT, and regimens that are the standard in renal transplantation have not always translated well into the setting of LT. Lympholytic therapy has emerged as an elegant addition to the growing list of immunosuppressives with our reach.

## REFERENCES

1. Halloran PF. Immunosuppressive drugs for kidney transplantation. N Engl J Med 2004; 351:2715–2729.
2. Ginns LE, Cosimi AB, Morris PJ. Transplantation. Malden, MA: Blackwell Science, 1999.
3. Bhorade SM, Villanueva J, Jordan A, et al. Modern concepts of immunosuppression for lung transplantation. In: Advanced Therapy in Thoracic Surgery. 2nd ed. BC Dekker, 2004, chap. 45.
4. Woodruff MFA, Anderson NA. Effect of lymphocyte depletion by thoracic duct fistula and administration on antilymphocytic serum on the survival of skin homografts in rats. Nature 1963; 200:702.
5. Norman DJ, Turka LA. Primer on Transplantation. 2nd ed. Ames, IA: Blackwell Publishers, 2001.
6. Starzl TE, Marchioro TL, Porter PA, et al. The use of heterologous antilymphoid agents in canine renal and liver homotransplantation and in human renal homotransplantation. Surg Gynecol Obstet 1967; 124:301–318.
7. Kohler G, Milstein C. Continuous cultures of fused cells secreting antibody of predefined specificity. Nature 1975; 256:495–497.
8. Cosimi AB, Burton RC, Colvin RB, et al. Treatment of acute renal allograft rejection with OKT3 monoclonal antibody. Transplantation 1981; 32(6):535–539.
9. Kirkman RL, Barrett LV, Gaulton GN, et al. Administration of an anti-interleukin 2 receptor monoclonal antibody prolongs cardiac allograft survival in mice. J Exp Med 1985; 162(1):358–362.
10. Kirkman RL, Barrett LV, Gaulton GN, et al. The effect of anti-interleukin-2 receptor monoclonal antibody on allograft rejection. Transplantation 1985; 40(6):719–722.
11. Starzl TE. Heterologous antilymphocyte globulin. N Engl J Med 1968; 279:700–703.
12. Thomas JM, Carver FM, Haisch CE, et al. Suppressor cells in rhesus monkeys treated with antithymocyte globulin. Transplantation 1982; 34:83–89.
13. Guttman RD. Renal transplantation (second of two parts). N Engl J Med 1979; 301:1038–1048.

14. Shield CF, Edwards EB, Davies DB, et al. Antilymphocyte induction therapy in cadaver renal transplantation: a retrospective, multicenter United Network for Organ Sharing study. Transplantation 1997; 63(9):1257–1263.

15. Steinmuller DR, Hodge E, Boshkos C, et al. Prophylaxis and treatment of post-renal transplant rejection. Cleve Clin J Med 1991; 58:125–130.

16. Frey DJ, Matas AJ, Gillingham KJ, et al. Sequential therapy—a prospective randomized trial of MALG versus OKT3 for prophylactic immunosuppression in cadaver renal allograft recipients. Transplantation 1992; 544(1):50–56.

17. Norman DJ, Kahana L, Stuart FP, et al. A randomized clinical trial of induction therapy with OKT3 in kidney transplantation. Transplantation 1993; 55(1):44–50.

18. Hanto DW, Jendrisak MD, So SKS, et al. Induction immunosuppression with antilymphocyte globulin or OKT3 in cadaver kidney transplantation. Transplantation 1994; 57(3):377–384.

19. Zuckermann AO, Grimm M, Czerny M, et al. Improved long-term results within thymoglobuline induction therapy after cardiac transplantation: a comparison of two different rabbit-antithymocyte globulines. Transplantation 2000; 69:1890–1898.

20. Brennan DC, Flavin K, Lowell JA, et al. A randomized, double-blinded comparison of thymoglobulin versus ATGAM for induction immunosuppressive therapy in adult renal transplant recipients. Transplantation 1999; 67:1011–1018.

21. Griffith BP, Hardesty RL, Armitage JM, et al. Acute rejection of lung allografts with various immunosuppressive protocols. Ann Thorac Surg 1992; 54: 846–851.

22. Palmer SM, Miralles AP, Lawrence CM, et al. Rabbit antithymocyte globulin decreases acute rejection after lung transplantation. Chest 1999; 116:127–133.

23. Wiebe K, Harringer W, Wahlers U, et al. ATG induction therapy and the incidence of bronchiolitis obliterans after lung transplantation: does it make a difference? Transplant Proc 1998; 30:1517–1518.

24. Ross DJ, Jordan SC, Nathan SD, et al. Delayed development of obliterative bronchiolits syndrome with OKT3 after unilateral lung transplantation. Chest 1996; 109:870–873.

25. Frost AE, Jammal CT, Cagle PT. Hyperacute rejection following lung transplantation. Chest 1996; 110(2):559–562.

26. Bittner HB, Dunitz J, Hertz M, et al. Hyperacute rejection in single lung transplantation—case report of successful management by means of plasmapheresis and antithymocyte globulin treatment. Transplantation 2001; 71(5):649–651.

27. Shield CF, Cosimi AB, Tolkoff-Rubin N, et al. Use of antithymocyte globulin for reversal of acute allograft rejection. Transplantation 1979; 28(6):461–464.

28. Nelson PW, Cosimi AB, Delmonico FL, et al. Antithymocyte globulin as the primary treatment for renal allograft rejection. Transplantation 1983; 36(5):587–589.

29. Richardson AJ, Higgins RM, Liddington M, et al. Antithymocyte globulin for steroid resistant rejection in renal transplant recipients immunosuppressed with triple therapy. Transplant Int 1989; 2(1):27–32.

30. Gaber AO, First MR, Tesi RJ, et al. Results of the double-blind, randomized, multicenter, phase III clinical trial of thymoglobulin versus ATGAM in the

treatment of acute graft rejection episodes after renal transplantation. Transplantation 1998; 66(1):29–37.

31. Date H, Lynch JP, Sundaresan S, et al. The impact of cytolytic therapy on bronchiolitis obliterans syndrome. J Heart Lung Transplant 1998; 17(9):869–875.

32. Kesten S, Rajagopalan N, Maurer J. Cytolytic therapy for the treatment of bronchiolitis obliterans syndrome following lung transplantation. Transplantation 1996; 61(3):427–430.

33. Snell GI, Esmore DS, William TJ. Cytolytic therapy for the bronchiolitis obliterans syndrome. Chest 1996; 109:874–878.

34. Kriett JM, Smith CM, Hayden AM, et al. Lung transplantation without the use of antilymphocyte antibody preparations. J Heart Lung Transplant 1994; 13:915–923.

35. Calhoon JH, Nichols L, Davis R, et al. Single lung transplantaion. J Thorac Cardiovasc Surg 1992; 103:21–26.

36. Delmonico FL, Auchincloss H, Rubin RH, et al. The selective use of antilymphocyte serum for cyclosporine treated patients with renal allograft dysfunction. Ann Surg 1987; 206:649–654.

37. Muller TF, Grebe SO, Neumann MC, et al. Persistent long-term changes in lymphocyte subsets induced by polyclonal antibodies. Transplantation 1997; 64(10):1432–1437.

38. Kreis H, Mansouri R, Descamps J, et al. Antithymocyted globulin in cadaver kidney transplantation: a randomized trial based on T-cell monitoring. Kidney Int 1981; 19:438–444.

39. Clark K. Monitoring antithymocyte globulin in renal transplantation. Ann R Coll Surg 1996; 78:536–540.

40. Bhorade SM, Villanueva J, Jordan A, et al. Immunosuppressive regimens in lung transplant recipients. Drugs Today 2004; 40(12):1003–1012.

41. Debets JMH, Leunissen KML, Van Hooff HJ, et al. Evidence of involvement of tumor necrosis factor in adverse reactions during treatment of kidney allograft rejection with antithymocyte globulin. Transplantation 1989; 47(3): 487–492.

42. Chatenoud L, Ferran C, Legendre C, et al. In vivo cell activation following OKT3 administration. Transplantation 1990; 49(4):697–702.

43. Henricsson A, Husberg B, Bergentz SE. The mechanism behind the effect of ALG on platelets in vivo. Clin Exp Immunol 1977; 29:515–522.

44. Stratta RJ, Shaeffer MS, Markin RS, et al. Cytomegalovirus infection and disease after liver transplantation. Dig Dis Sci 1992; 37(5):673–688.

45. Rubin RH. Preemptive therapy in immunocompromised hosts. N Engl J Med 1991; 324(15):1057–1059.

46. Cosimi AB. The clinical value of antilymphocyte antibodies. Transplant Proc 1981; 13:462–468.

47. Rubin RH, Cosimi AB, Hirsch MS, et al. Effects of antithymocyte globulin on cytomegalovirs infection in renal transplant recipients. Transplantation 1981; 31(2):143–145.

48. Malatack JJ, Gartner JC, Urbach AH, et al. Othotopic liver transplantation, Epstein–Barr virus, cyclosporine, and lymphyproliferative disease: a growing concern. J Pediatr 1991; 118:667–675.

49. Paradis IL, Duncan SR, Dauber JH, et al. Distinguishing between infection, rejection, and the adult respiratory distress syndrome after human lung transplantation. J Heart Lung Transplant 1992; 11:S232–S236.

50. De Hoyos AL, Patterson GA, Maurer JR, et al. Pulmonary transplantation: early and late results. J Thorac Cardiovasc Surg 1992; 103:295–306.

51. De Leval MR, Smyth R, Whitehead B, et al. Heart and lung transplantation for terminal cystic fibrosis. J Thorac Cardiovasc Surg 1991; 101:633–642.

52. Low DE, Trulock EP, Kaiser LR, et al. Morbidity, mortality, and early results of single versus bilateral lung transplantation for emphysema. J Thorac Cardiovasc Surg 1992; 103:1119–1126.

53. Shennib H, Noirclerc M, Ernst P, et al. Double-lung transplantation for cystic fibrosis. Ann Thorac Surg 1992; 54:27–32.

54. Novick RJ, Menkis AH, McKenzie FN, et al. Should heart-lung transplant donors and recipients be matched according to cytomegalovirus serologic status? J Heart Lung Transplant 1990; 9:699–706.

55. Egan TM, Westerman JH, Lambert CJ, et al. Isolated lung transplantation for end-stage lung disease: a viable therapy. Ann Thorac Surg 1992; 53:590–596.

56. Kreis H, Chkoff L, Chatenoud H, et al. Prolonged administration of a monoclonal anti-T3 cell antibody (Orthoclone OKT3) to kidney allograft recipients. Transplant Proc 1986; 18(4):954–956.

57. Norman DJ, Shield CF, Barry J, et al. Early use of OKT3 monoclonal antibody in renal transplantation to prevent rejection. Am J Kidney Dis 1988; 11(2):107–110.

58. Debure A, Chkoff N, Chatenoud L, et al. One-month prophylactic use of OKT3 in cadaver kidney transplant recipients. Transplantation 1988; 45(3): 546–553.

59. Kreis H, Chkoff L, Chatenoud H, et al. A randomized trial comparing the efficacy of OKT3 used to prevent or to treat rejection. Transplant Proc 1989; 21(1):1741–1744.

60. Wain JC, Wright CD, Ryan DP, et al. Induction immunosuppression for lung transplantation with OKT3. Ann Thorac Surg 1999; 67:187–193.

61. Shennib J, Mercado M, Nguyen D, et al. Successful treatment of steroid-resistant double-lung allograft rejection with Orthoclone OKT3. Am Rev Respir Dis 1991; 144:224–226.

62. Shennib H, Massard G, Reynaud M, et al. Efficacy of OKT3 therapy for acute rejection in isolated lung transplantation. J Heart Lung Transplant 1994; 13:514–519.

63. Carey G, Lisi PJ, Schroeder TJ. The incidence of antibody formation to OKT3 consequent to its use in organ transplantation. Transplantation 1995; 60(2): 151–158.

64. Chatenoud L, Jonker M, Villemain F, et al. The human immune response to the OKT3 monoclonal antibody is oligoclonal. Science 1986; 23:1406–1408.

65. Boulianne GL, Hozumi N, Shulman MJ. Production of functional chimaeric mouse/human antibody. Nature 1984; 312:643–646.

66. Alegre M, Lenschow DJ, Bluestone JA. Immunomodulation of transplant rejection using monoclonal antibodies and soluble receptors. Dig Dis Sci 1995; 40(1):58–64.

67. Cosimi AB, Colvin RB, Burton RC, et al. Use of monoclonal antibodies to T-cell subsets for immunologic monitoring and treatment in recipients of renal allografts. N Engl J Med 1981; 305(6):308–314.

68. Sheiner PA, Guarrera JV, Grunstein E, et al. Increased risk of early rejection correlates with recovery of CD3 cell count after liver transplant in patients receiving OKT3 induction. Transplantation 1997; 64(8):1214–1216.

69. Colvin RB, Preffer FI. Laboratory monitoring of therapy with OKT3 and other murine monoclonal antibodies. Clin Lab Med 1991; 11(3):693–714.

70. Group, Ortho Multicenter Transplant Study. A randomized clinical trial of OKT3 monoclonal antibody for acute rejection of cadaveric renal transplants. N Engl J Med 1985; 313(6):337–342.

71. Chatenoud L, Reuter A, Legendre C, et al. Systemic reaction to the anti-T-cell monoclonal antibody OKT3 in relation to serum levels of tumor necrosis factor and interferon-alpha. N Engl J Med 1989; 320(21):1420–1421.

72. Alegre M, Gastaldello K, Abramowicz D, et al. Evidence that pentoxifylline reduces anti-CD3 monoclonal antibody-induced cytokine release syndrome. Transplantation 1991; 52(4):674–679.

73. Swinnen L, Costanzo-Nordin MR, Fisher SG, et al. Increased incidence of lymphoproliferative disorder after immunosuppression with the monoclonal antibody OKT3 in cardiac transplantation. N Engl J Med 1990; 323(25): 1723–1728.

74. Nashan B. The interleukin-2 inhibitors and their role in low-toxicity regimens. Transplant Proc 2001; 31(suppl 8A):23S–26S.

75. Williams KA, Thiel MA, Zola H. Transplantation 1999; 68(9):1228–1229.

76. Soulillou J, Cantarovich D, Le Mauff B, et al. Randomized controlled trial of monoclonal antibody against the interleukin-2 receptor (33B3.1) as compared with rabbit antithymocyte globulin for prophylaxis against rejection of renal allografts. N Engl J Med 1990; 322(17):1175–1182.

77. Nashan B, Moore R, Amlot P, et al. Randomised trial of basiliximab versus placebo for control of acute cellular rejection in renal allograft recipients. Lancet 1997; 350:1193–1198.

78. Kahan BD, Rajagopalan PR, Hall M. Reduction of the occurence of acute cellular rejection among renal allograft recipients treated with basiliximab, a chimeric anti-interleukin-2-receptor monolconal antibody. Transplantation 1999; 67(2):276–284.

79. Hausen B, Gummert J, Berry G, et al. Prevention of acute allograft rejection in nonhuman primate lung transplant recipients: induction with chimeric anti-interleukin-2 receptor monolconal antibody improves the tolerability an potentialities the immunosuppressive activity of a regimen using low doses of both microemulsion cyclosporine and 40-*O*-(2-hydroxyethyl)-rapamycin. Transplantation 2000; 69(4):488–496.

80. Gerbase MW, De Perrot M, Spiliopoulos A, et al. Selective monoclonal versus polyclonal antibodies for induction of immunosuppression in lung recipients. Clin Pharmacol Ther 2002; 72(1):103.

81. Vincenti F, Kirkman R, Light S, et al. Interleukin-2-receptor blockade with daclizumab to prevent acute rejection in renal transplantation. N Engl J Med 1998; 338(3):161–165.

82. Nashan B, Light S, Hardie IR, et al. Reduction of acute renal allograft rejection by daclizumab. Transplantation 1999; 67(1):110–115.
83. Beniaminovitz A, Itescu S, Lietz K, et al. Prevention of rejection in cardiac transplantation by blockade of the interleukin-2 receptor with a monoclonal antibody. N Engl J Med 2000; 342(9):613–619.
84. Brock MV, Borja MC, Ferber L, et al. Induction therapy in lung transplantation: a prospective, controlled clinical trial comparing OKT3, antithymocyte globulin, and daclizumab. J Heart Lung Transplant 2001; 20:1282–1290.
85. Garrity ER, Villanueva J, Bhorade SM, et al. Low rate of acute lung allograft rejection after the use of daclizumab, an interleukin 2 receptor antibody. Transplantation 2001; 71:773–777.
86. Cantarovich D, Le Mauff B, Hourmant M, et al. Anti-interleukin 2 receptor monoclonal antibody in the treatment of ongoing acute rejection episodes of human kidney graft—a pilot study. Transplantation 1989; 47(3):454–457.
87. Kode RK, Kumar AMS, Damask AM, et al. Simulect induction significantly decreases CMV infection in kidney recipients compared to OKT3. Transplant Proc 2001; 33:1268–1269.
88. Onrust SV, Wiseman LR. Basiliximab. Drugs 1999; 57(2):207–213.
89. Chapman TM, Keating GM. Basiliximab: a review of its use as induction therapy in renal transplantation. Drugs 2003; 63(24):2803–2835.
90. Queen C, Schneider WP, Selick HE, et al. A humanized antibody that binds to the interleukin 2 receptor. Proc Nat Acad Sciences USA 1989; 86: 10,029–10,033.
91. Nashan B. The IL2 pathway in clinical immunosuppression. Transplant Proc 2001; 33(7–8):3072–3074.
92. Queen C, Schneider WP, Selick HE, et al. A humanized antibody that binds to the interleukin 2 receptor. Proc Natl Acad Sci USA 1989; 86(24):10,029–10,033.
93. Calne R, Moffatt SD, Friend PJ. Campath IH allows low-dose cyclosporine monotherapy in 31 cadaveric renal allograft recipients. Transplantation 1999; 68(10):1613–1616.
94. Knechtle SJ, Fernandez LA, Pirsch JD, et al. Campath-1H in renal transplantation: the University of Wisconsin experience. Surgery 2004; 136(4):754–760.
95. Ciancio G, Burke GW, Gaynor JJ, et al. The use of Campath-1H as induction therapy in renal transplantation: preliminary results. Transplantation 2004; 78(3):426–433.
96. Pham SM, Rao AS, Zeevi A, et al. Effects of donor bone marrow infusion in clinical lung transplantation. Ann Thorac Surg 2000; 69(2):345–350.
97. Ciancio G, Garcia-Morales R, Burke GW, et al. Donor bone marrow infusion in renal transplantation. Transplant Proc 1998; 30(4):1365–1366.
98. Rao AS, Fontes P, Iyengar A, et al. Perioperative donor bone marrow infusion in recipients of organ allografts. Transplant Proc 1997; 29(4):2192–2193.
99. Ciancio G. Donor bone marrow infusion in cadaveric renal transplantation. Transplant Proc 2003; 35(2):871–872.
100. Garcia-Morales RO, Ciancio G, Mathew J, et al. Perioperative donor bone marrow infusion in cadaver kidney transplant recipients. Transplant Proc 2001; 33(7–8):3840–3843.

101. Dragun D, FritscheL, Boehler T, et al. FTY720: early clinical experience. Transplant Proc 2004; 36(2 suppl):544S–548S.
102. Kunzendorf U, Ziegler E, Kabelitz D. FTY720—the first compound of a new promising class of immunosuppressive drugs. Nephrol Dial Transplant 2004; 19(7):1677–1681.
103. Kahan BD. FTY720: from bench to bedside. Transplant Proc 2004; 36(2 suppl):531S–543S.

# 19

# Novel and Future Approaches to Immunosuppression

**Kenneth R. McCurry**

*Division of Cardiothoracic Surgery, Department of Surgery, University of Pittsburgh School of Medicine, Pittsburgh, Pennsylvania, U.S.A.*

**Aldo Iacono**

*Division of Pulmonary Medicine, Department of Medicine, University of Maryland, Baltimore, Maryland, U.S.A.*

**Adriana Zeevi**

*Department of Pathology, University of Pittsburgh and The Starzl Transplant Institute, Pittsburgh, Pennsylvania, U.S.A.*

## INTRODUCTION

Over the last two decades, lung transplantation has progressed from initial success to a mature therapy that is the preferred option for many patients with end-stage lung disease. During the steep learning curve in the 1980s, short-term outcomes improved primarily due to advancements in surgical techniques as well as patient selection and management but then reached a relative plateau (1). In recent years, the one-year survival rate in the United States has improved slightly to approximately 80% (2) but remains well below that of most other organ transplants including kidney, liver, and heart. In addition, medium- and long-term outcomes have remained unchanged and suboptimal with U.S. and international five-year survival rates approximating the palliative levels of 45% to 50% (1,2).

Most of the morbidity and mortality following lung transplantation, indeed following transplantation of all organs, are due to deficiencies and toxicities of immunosuppressive medications and immunosuppressive strategies. The inadequacies of currently utilized immunosuppressive strategies are nowhere more apparent than in lung transplant recipients. The incidence of acute rejection following lung transplantation is greater and chronic rejection occurs with a greater incidence and at earlier time points than that following transplantation of any other organ (3–6). On the other side of the immune competence equation, complications resulting from global immune depression remain pervasive. Indeed, the two major causes of mortality following lung transplantation are infection (the most common cause of death within the first three years following transplantation) and bronchiolitis obliterans (widely believed to be the manifestation of chronic rejection and the most common cause of death more than three years from transplantation) (1). In addition to these deficiencies of immune suppression in lung transplant recipients, nonimmune, drug-specific toxicities such as renal insufficiency, osteoporosis, diabetes, hypertension, and hyperlipidemia are ubiquitous (1). Renal dysfunction occurs in up to 38% of survivors at five years from transplantation (1), frequently leading to difficulty with fluid management and graft function and with an increased risk of death in those who progress to chronic renal failure (7). In addition, of survivors at five years from transplantation, 86% have hypertension, 45% have hyperlipidemia, and 29% have diabetes (1). It is obvious from these data that alternative immunosuppressive strategies are urgently needed to improve both short- and long-term survival and to reduce morbidity.

The immunosuppressive strategies currently utilized in lung transplantation replicate the initial strategies utilized for renal and heart transplantation, and have evolved little over the last two decades. The discovery and introduction of cyclosporine facilitated the success of lung transplantation, as well as other organs, in the 1980s. In lung transplant recipients, use of cyclosporine allowed a reduction of the very high doses of steroids utilized in dual therapy with azathioprine and resulted in a reduction of bronchial anastomotic complications as well as a reduction in the incidence of acute rejection. Thus, the triple-drug immunosuppressive regimen of cyclosporine, azathioprine, and moderate to high doses of prednisone [with or without a short course of antilymphoid antibody (i.e., induction)] that was being utilized in kidney and heart transplantation was adopted for lung transplantation during this era. This conservative approach has persisted with the only significant changes being an increased use of tacrolimus and mycophenolate mofetil in lieu of cyclosporine and azathioprine, respectively, and an increased use of IL-2 receptor antagonists in lieu of antilymphoid antibody in those patients receiving induction (approximately 40% received induction worldwide in 2002) (1). The prevailing thought is that this three-drug therapy is the most effective strategy to control rejection and that the use of three drugs allows minimization of the toxicities of individual medications. In 2004, data from the International Society for Heart and Lung Transplantation (ISHLT) demonstrated that even at five years following lung transplantation >95% of patients are receiving a calcineurin inhibitor, >80% are receiving a cell-cycle inhibitor (azathioprine or mycophenolate mofetil), and >95% are receiving steroids (1). As discussed above, however, despite this heavy prophylactic immune suppression both acute and chronic rejection rates remain high. Moreover, both immune and nonimmune related toxicities are pervasive following lung transplantation. In this chapter, we will discuss two novel approaches to immunosuppression in lung transplant recipients.

## INHALATION CYCLOSPORINE

While most solid organ transplants are inaccessible to localized immune suppression, lung allografts are the exception due to ready access through the tracheobronchial tree via inhalation. Interest in the development of cyclosporine for use as an inhalational immunosuppressant began at the University of Pittsburgh with the belief that (i) the alloimmune response to lung allografts could be reduced by achieving a greater concentration of a calcineurin inhibitor in the graft and (ii) this may allow reduction of systemic immunosuppressive medications, thus reducing immune- and non–immune-related toxicities. Following conceptualization, this novel form of therapy evolved through a development stage in animal models and subsequently has been evaluated in human trials.

### Development of Inhalation Cyclosporine

Initial studies utilizing cyclosporine as an inhalant were begun in 1988 at the University of Pittsburgh. Following initial feasibility and toxicity studies in nontransplanted dogs, a subsequent study in a canine orthotopic lung transplant model demonstrated the efficacy of this approach (8). In this study, transplanted dogs received 200 mg of cyclosporine via inhalation for 8 days as the sole immunosuppressant while transplanted control dogs received no immunosuppression. Acute rejection was prevented or reduced in all treated animals while all control animals had severe acute rejection. Intragraft cyclosporine levels in inhaled cyclosporine treated animals were high while systemic levels were low without evidence of local or systemic toxicity. In addition, animals with the highest cyclosporine concentrations in the allograft had the lowest rejection grades, demonstrating a concentration-dependent effect of deposited cyclosporine on rejection risk.

A subsequent study in a rat lung transplant model utilizing inhaled cyclosporine as the sole immunosuppressive therapy reconfirmed the efficacy of this approach (9). Further studies in this model also demonstrated a dose response for inhaled cyclosporine (10,11). Animals receiving the highest inhaled dose demonstrated the lowest grades of acute rejection and also had the highest concentration of cyclosporine in the allograft.

## USE OF INHALATION CYCLOSPORINE IN HUMANS

Following the positive results obtained in the animal models described above, studies in humans were initiated. Initially, a phase 1 trial was performed at the University of Pittsburgh in patients with bronchiolitis obliterans. The rationale for initiation of a trial in this patient population was the potential efficacy of additional localized immunosuppression in improving the course of patients with established chronic rejection. Entry criteria required inexorable deterioration in lung function despite conventional immune suppression therapy. These initial human studies demonstrated a beneficial effect with regard to pulmonary function and diminution of the histological grade of rejection without systemic toxicity (12). Subsequently, between 1991 and 2001, 39 patients with bronchiolitis obliterans were treated with inhaled cyclosporine in conjunction with standard systemic maintenance immunosuppression. The outcomes in these patients were compared to 51 contemporaneous control patients with bronchiolitis obliterans who were treated with conventional immunosuppression. For further comparison, a second group of controls consisted of 100 patients with bronchiolitis obliterans selected from the Novartis Lung Transplant Registry (a multicenter registry consisting of 826 lung transplant recipients from 12 major transplant centers throughout the world). Patients treated with inhaled cyclosporine had a median survival after the onset of bronchiolitis obliterans of 4.5 years compared to 2.4 years in Pittsburgh controls and 2.3 years in multicenter controls. Factors shown to influence survival after bronchiolitis obliterans [forced expiratory volume in one second ($FEV_1$), single- vs. double-lung transplant] were included in a Cox proportional hazards model. Using this model, inhaled cyclosporine was associated with improved survival compared to both Pittsburgh controls (hazard ratio, 0.49; $P = 0.03$) and multicenter controls (hazard ratio, 0.42; $P = 0.01$). Thus, inhaled cyclosporine reduced the risk of death by approximately 50% when the model included the mentioned covariates shown to influence survival after bronchiolitis obliterans (13).

Favorable results using inhalation cyclosporine for treatment of bronchiolitis obliterans led in 1993 to its use in patients with acute rejection that failed to respond to augmented conventional immunosuppression (i.e., persistent acute rejection). An initial experience with 18 patients treated with inhaled cyclosporine was compared to 23 controls matched by histological rejection that were treated conventionally. Two patients were unable to tolerate inhaled cyclosporine. Significant improvement in histological rejection grade was seen in 14 of the remaining 16 treated patients after a mean of 37 days of inhaled cyclosporine therapy (14). Lung function [forced vital capacity (FVC) and $FEV_1$] improved significantly in treated patients, whereas that of control patients declined despite maximal therapy. In addition, the incidence of rejection ($\geq$A2) decreased from $2.49 \pm 0.98$ episodes per 100 days before initiation of inhaled cyclosporine to $0.72 \pm 0.3$ episodes per 100 days ($P < 0.05$).

Further studies in patients with refractory rejection demonstrated that longitudinal improvement in lung function was dependent on the amount of cyclosporine deposited in the allograft. The greatest improvement in $FEV_1$ was seen in patients who deposited at least 15 mg of cyclosporine in the allograft, whereas those who deposited <15 mg did not demonstrate improvement (15). These data using inhaled cyclosporine in open-label treatment for refractory rejection provided the rationale for exploring its use in a randomized trial of de novo prophylaxis in conjunction with standard triple-drug immunosuppression.

### Effect of Inhaled Cyclosporine on Graft Inflammation

Our groups as well as others have demonstrated a strong association between upregulation of proinflammatory cytokines and chemokines, such as IL-6 and IFN-$\gamma$, in lung allografts and ongoing immune activation and acute rejection (16–18). It is now recognized that these cytokines and others can activate endothelial cells and recruit effector cells, causing inflammation that may ultimately lead to tissue injury, fibrosis, and graft failure (16,19). Given our clinical results with inhaled cyclosporine, we examined the effect of inhaled cyclosporine on graft inflammation in humans treated with the drug. In an open-label study we compared cytokine mRNA expression in 12 lung transplant recipients treated with inhaled cyclosporine and 16 control lung transplant recipients who did not receive inhaled cyclosporine (all received triple-drug maintenance immunosuppression). We used semiquantitative reverse transcriptase polymerase chain reaction to measure expression of mRNA for the proinflammatory mediators Granzyme B (GB) and RANTES. GB is a serine protease produced by cytotoxic T cells (CTLs) and it is the effector molecule of the activated CTL. Upregulation of GB mRNA in bronchoalveolar lavage (BAL) is associated with severe acute cellular rejection. Chemokines, another family of cytokines, activate and attract leukocyte subsets and lead to extravasation of these cells at the site of inflammation. RANTES (a member of the C-C chemokine family) is a chemo-attractant for monocytes and lymphocytes and is believed to be important in lung allograft rejection. Our results showed that expression of GB was markedly elevated in all patients who experienced acute rejection, but recovered to baseline only in those who received inhaled cyclosporine (16).

In a subsequent randomized, controlled clinical trial (described below), we compared cytokine gene expression using the TaqMan assay in

12 lung transplant recipients who received inhaled cyclosporine and 13 control lung transplant recipients who did not. All lung transplant recipients were maintained on a triple-therapy immunosuppressive regimen consisting of tacrolimus, azathioprine, and steroids.

In this study, patients treated with inhaled cyclosporine were found to have less expression of GB or RANTES mRNA during quiescence (periods without rejection) as compared with those who did not receive inhaled cyclosporine, suggesting that patients treated with inhaled cyclosporine maintained better control over inflammation. In patients treated with inhaled cyclosporine, marked suppression of GB was also observed following a steroid bolus for treatment of acute rejection. These findings suggest that inhaled cyclosporine may exert some of its beneficial effects by reducing inflammation in lung allografts. Furthermore, these findings suggest that TaqMan-based quantitative analysis of proinflammatory cytokines in the BAL cells of lung transplant recipients is informative and may be applied for monitoring allograft rejection and the effectiveness of rejection treatment.

### Use of Inhaled Cyclosporine for De Novo Prophylaxis in a Randomized Trial and Current Status

A single-center, double-blinded, randomized, placebo-controlled trial utilizing inhaled cyclosporine in conjunction with triple-drug immunosuppression (tacrolimus, azathioprine, and steroids) was initiated in 1998 at the University of Pittsburgh. A total of 58 patients were randomized to receive either 300 mg of inhalation cyclosporine or placebo three days per week starting within six weeks of transplant and continuing for two posttransplant years (20). Analysis by intent-to-treat revealed that there was no difference in the primary end point of the rate of grade 2 or higher acute rejection. However, survival was significantly better in the inhaled cyclosporine group and there was a lower incidence of bronchiolitis obliterans and bronchiolitis obliterans syndrome (BOS) in patients who were randomized to receive inhaled cyclosporine. Furthermore, there was no difference in the rate of nephrotoxicity or infection. As of this writing, the final results of this trial have been submitted for publication. A substudy in this trial was performed to evaluate the relationship between the amount of cyclosporine deposited in the grafts and the effect (21). In this substudy, 15 patients receiving inhaled cyclosporine were evaluated with deposition tests while seven patients receiving inhaled placebo underwent mock deposition tests. In those patients receiving inhaled cyclosporine, there was a linear relationship between deposited cyclosporine dose and improvement in lung function, whereas the mock dose data from the placebo patients did not demonstrate a similar relationship. Further analysis revealed that those patients who deposited $\geq 5$ mg of cyclosporine in the periphery of their allograft experienced the greatest degree of improvement in lung function, whereas those who deposited less had longitudinal decrements in lung function comparable to those patients randomized to receive inhalation placebo. These deposition studies are consistent with similar studies in rats. Based on these data, the Food and Drug Administration (FDA) is currently considering whether inhalation cyclosporine should be approved for use in lung transplant recipients. The future availability of this therapy and the potential for its use with other novel immune suppression strategies will, undoubtedly, be determined by this decision.

## CAMPATH-1H

### Role of Induction Therapy in Lung Transplantation

Lymphocyte depletion with biological agents in the perioperative or immediate postoperative period, i.e., induction therapy, has a long experimental and clinical history. Early studies by Medawar demonstrated that lymphocyte depletion can delay rejection and in some experimental models result in tolerance (22). Induction strategies in the clinic utilizing agents such as antithymocyte globulins (ATG) or monoclonal anti-CD3 antibody (OKT3) have proceeded with the rationale of using the strongest immunosuppression at the time when the risk of acute rejection is greatest, i.e., in the first few weeks to months following transplantation (23). Concerns over increased risk of infection (especially from viral and fungal pathogens) have remained; however, in renal transplantation, prospective randomized trials have demonstrated that this strategy (induction with ATG or OKT3) significantly reduces the risk of acute rejection and also increases long-term kidney graft survival by approximately 5% compared to conventional triple-drug immunosuppression without induction (24). In immunologically high-risk patient populations (e.g., African Americans, children, and sensitized patients), the beneficial effect of this approach is even greater with as much as a 20% improvement in kidney graft survival at three to five years following transplantation. As immunologic responses to lung allografts appear to be greater in magnitude than those following most other solid organ transplants (with the exception of perhaps the small intestine), there is reason to believe that such a strategy would be beneficial in lung transplant recipients. Although induction strategies have sporadically been used in many lung transplant programs, data in lung transplant recipients are limited. There has been only one prospective, randomized study (single center) of induction therapy in lung transplant recipients (25). This study randomized 44 patients to receive triple-drug immunosuppression (cyclosporine, azathioprine, and steroids) with or without postoperative rabbit ATG induction (1.5 mg/kg/day for three days). The incidence of biopsy-proven rejection ($\geq$A2) was reduced in the induction group at one year (23% vs. 55%). There was no difference in one year survival (68% vs. 73%) while there was a nonsignificant reduction in the incidence of BOS at three years. The incidence of infection and malignancy was not different at two years of follow-up. A recent long-term follow-up of this study demonstrated that while induction with ATG delayed the onset of acute rejection, ultimately there was no difference in the cumulative incidence of rejection and no difference in the incidence of chronic rejection (26). As noted above, however, this study utilized a short course of rabbit ATG (1.5 mg/kg/day for three days) that may have resulted in variable and short-lived T cell depletion. In this regard, a retrospective study utilizing triple immunosuppression compared perioperative adminis-tration of OKT3 [10–14 days (5 mg/day)] to Minnesota antilymphocyte globulin [a polyclonal equine preparation; 5–7 days (10–15 mg/kg/day)]. This study demonstrated a longer latency period to the onset of BOS with the longer (and presumably greater T cell depletion) course of OKT3 (27).

Another potential rationale for the use of induction immuno-suppression in transplantation is to allow modification of maintenance immunosuppression to avoid global immune suppression or drug-related toxicities either through avoidance of calcineurin inhibitors or through ster-oid avoidance or minimization strategies. Once again, the renal transplant community has contributed greatly to this area in recent years with innova-tive approaches, particularly in regard to minimization or avoidance of steroids. Long-term steroid use undoubtedly contributes greatly to mor-bidity and mortality following transplantation by increasing the risk of infection as well as by increasing the frequency of complications such as dia-betes, hyperlipidemia, hypertension, osteoporosis, and cataracts. A recent economic analysis in kidney transplant recipients estimated the 10-year cost of steroid-induced complications at $5300 per transplanted patient (28). Sev-eral studies in kidney recipients (29–31) as well as a recent study in heart transplant recipients (32) have suggested that the incidence of at least some of these complications can be reduced through early steroid withdrawal. Many of the earlier studies utilizing cyclosporine-based regimens, however, documented higher rates of rejection with this approach (33). More recent studies in kidney recipients utilizing either long courses of ATG induction (10 days) or IL-2 receptor antagonists in conjunction with newer mainte-nance agents (mycophenolate mofetil, tacrolimus, and sirolimus) have demonstrated that steroid-free immunosuppression can be used in selected recipients achieving low rates of rejection although long-term results are largely unknown (34–38). There has been very limited experience with struc-tured attempts to withdraw steroids or minimize or avoid steroids in lung transplant recipients. The sole report on steroid withdrawal in lung trans-plant recipients was on a group of patients that were $70 \pm 13$ months from transplant and demonstrated some metabolic advantage (39).

Campath-1H is a lymphoid depleting agent reactive against the broadly expressed CD52 antigen. Use of this agent has garnered much attention through its ability to facilitate immunosuppressive drug minimization and avoidance strategies in transplantation and has also been suggested to facilitate recruitment of tolerance mechanisms. In the following discussion, we will describe its development and subsequent use in renal transplantation as well as early results of this novel strategy in lung transplantation.

## Development of Campath-1H

Campath-1H is a humanized monoclonal antibody reactive against CD52, which is expressed on lymphocytes and other cells of the immune system. The history of development of this antibody dates to 1980, when a team led by Herman Waldman and Geoff Hale at Cambridge University in England in search of antibodies to kill human lymphocytes through a complement-dependent process identified a set of monoclonal antibodies following immunization of rats with human lymphocytes that satisfied their criteria (40,41). This series of antibodies were found to react with a glycosyl-phosphotidylinositol (GPI)-anchored peptide known as CD52, which turned out to be one of the most prevalent proteins on the surface of human lymphocytes. These antibodies were referred to as Cambridge Pathology 1 or Campath-1 antibodies. They identified one of the IgM antibodies as being the most efficient at lysing human lymphocytes with human complement and named it Campath-1M. This antibody was evaluated in the clinic as an agent to deplete T cells from the marrow inoculum in vitro prior to marrow transplantation (the initial intent for its development) and was found to prevent graft versus host disease (42). As a result of a desire to determine the utility of Campath-1M in vivo in humans, Campath-1M and subsequently a complement fixing IgG2a anti-CD52 antibody were evaluated in patients with lymphocytic leukemia and lymphoma (43). Both were found to be ineffective and as a result an IgG2b isotype was pursued as it was felt that this isotype might provide enhanced activity through cell-mediated antibody-dependent cytotoxicity. This indeed turned out to be the case and this antibody (named Campath-1G) proved very effective in this patient population. Subsequently, Campath-1G was humanized utilizing a human IgG1 Fc framework and the resultant antibody named Campath-1H. Early studies with Campath-1H revealed very promising results in leukemia, vasculitis, multiple sclerosis, bone marrow transplantation, and in organ transplantation (43). Campath-1H was subsequently commercialized and its efficacy evaluated in the United States in patients with chronic B-cell lymphocytic leukemia. It was approved by the FDA for use in 2001 in patients with chronic B-cell lymphocytic leukemia.

## Biology of Campath-1H

CD52 is a small protein the function of which is not known. However, it is the most prevalent protein on the surface of both T and B lymphocytes and is also expressed on monocytes and NK cells. Campath-1H is uniquely different in its effects from those of other antilymphoid antibodies in that it depletes lymphocytes to a greater extent and for a longer period of time and can deplete lymphocytes from secondary lymphoid organs as well. Administration of Campath-1H to humans in the setting of transplantation results in profound depletion of peripheral blood lymphocytes, monocytes, and NK cells as well as some depletion of B cells (44,45) and, as assessed several days following its use as induction in transplantation, was demonstrated by Kirk et al. to deplete lymphocytes from lymph nodes as well (44). Knechtle et al. have reported that following the use of Campath-1H as induction in kidney transplantation, lymphocytes repopulate to 80% of baseline values at 18 to 24 months post-transplant (46). When administered to patients with rheumatoid arthritis (at up to 10 times what has been used in transplantation) CD4 counts remained <250 cells/$\mu$L for up to seven years with no increased mortality compared to age-adjusted historical controls (47).

## Campath-1H as Induction Therapy in Organ Transplantation (Non-Lung)

Both Campath-1M and Campath-1G were initially utilized in human transplantation in kidney recipients at Cambridge University in the 1980s (48,49). Both studies demonstrated efficacy but suffered from high infection rates due primarily to cytomegalovirus (CMV) disease (no antiviral treatment was available). This raised significant concerns regarding the potency of Campath-1H and its use as induction therapy in transplantation. Interest was rekindled in the 1990s when studies in nonhuman primates utilizing a different agent (CD3-immunotoxin) to produce profound T-cell depletion suggested that this approach might lead to tolerance (50,51). There were similarities between the degree of depletion achieved with CD3-immunotoxin and Campath-1H but CD3-immunotoxin was reactive only in nonhuman primates while Campath-1H was reactive only in humans. As a result, Sir Roy Calne performed the first series of transplants (kidneys) utilizing Campath-1H as induction therapy in the 1990s, utilizing a drug minimization strategy (cyclosporine monotherapy). Two doses (20 mg each) of Campath-1H were given on the day of transplant and the days after with steroid premedication. No further steroids were given and half-dose cyclosporine monotherapy (target trough level 100–150 ng/mL) was begun 48 hours following transplantation. The early results of 31 patients were reported in 1998 with excellent graft and patient survival (52,53). A subsequent follow-up report on this cohort followed for more than five years has demonstrated excellent long-term outcomes equivalent to a retrospective control cohort receiving standard (cyclosporine based) triple immunosuppression (54). There was no increase in infection or serious adverse events and long-term steroid use was avoided. The issue of true tolerance was not addressed, although this approach was termed "prope tolerance."

Based on the promising and early reports of the pilot trial of Campath-1H induction, several studies were initiated in renal transplantation in the United States. The initial two U.S. studies performed by Dr. Allan Kirk and Dr. Stuart Knechtle were designed to address whether profound lymphocyte depletion could induce tolerance. Kirk et al. utilized an approach of very aggressive preoperative lymphocyte depletion (0.3 mg/kg per dose of Campath-1H for three doses, two of which were given pretransplant) without maintenance immunosuppression (44). Although there was little evidence of lymphocyte infiltration into the grafts, all patients experienced rejection within two to three weeks. Knechtle et al. utilized an approach similar to that of Sir Roy Calne (two doses of 20 mg Campath-1H administered on the day of transplant and the day after) but substituting rapamycin monotherapy for cyclosporine monotherapy (55). Seventy percent of patients remained rejection-free, but 30% of patients experienced a significant rejection episode that was difficult to control and suggestive of humoral rejection (46,55). Knechtle et al. concluded from these studies in comparison with that of Sir Roy Calne that a calcineurin inhibitor would be preferable to rapamycin for maintenance therapy following Campath-1H induction.

Subsequently, several centers have reported their experience in renal transplantation utilizing Campath-1H induction with tacrolimus monotherapy (56) or with tacrolimus plus reduced dose mycophenolate mofetil (steroid-free) (57,58) with excellent results. These studies have demonstrated at least equivalent outcomes to approaches with standard triple immunosuppression with no increased risk of infection. One study has demonstrated a reduction in CMV disease utilizing this strategy with steroid-free immune suppression (59).

## Use of Campath-1H as Induction Therapy in Lung Transplantation

Our initial experience utilizing Campath-1H as induction therapy in lung transplant recipients began with two retransplant cases in January 2003 and February 2003. Subsequently in July 2003, we began a series of unselected, consecutive patients utilizing a drug minimization strategy (steroid minimization). We have given Campath-1H as a single infusion in the operating room prior to graft reperfusion with intravenous steroid premedication. Subsequent maintenance therapy has consisted of tacrolimus (trough target 12–15 ng/mL) and prednisone 5 mg/day. Patients receive valgancyclovir prophylaxis for six months and voriconazole as antifungal prophylaxis for four months. Our initial report consisted of 6-month outcomes in a series of 10 patients (45). Freedom from rejection ($\geq$A2), cumulative burden of rejection, and freedom from high-grade rejection ($\geq$A3) were all significantly less in the Campath-1H cohort compared to a historical control group consisting of 28 patients who received dacluzimab (an IL-2 receptor antagonist) induction with standard triple immunosuppression. There was no difference in infection rates between the two groups but with a trend toward less CMV in the Campath-1H cohort. Survival was better than in historical controls but did not reach statistical significance. Although there were no objective data to support the conclusion, our subjective impression has been that quality of life is significantly improved.

To date, we have utilized this strategy in over 140 lung transplant recipients. Based on a recent analysis of our first 56 recipients with which there is more than one-year follow-up, one-year survival is 93% significantly better than our historical results. Compared to historical cohort of 54 patients transplanted between January 1998 and January 2000, who received no induction and were treated with standard tacrolimus-based triple immunosuppression, freedom from rejection $\geq$A2 at one year was significantly greater in the Campath-1H cohort ($P = 0.0007$), as was freedom from high-grade rejection ($\geq$A3) ($P = 0.0001$). Although analysis is ongoing, our preliminary examination suggests that there is no increase in infection rates. Following further analysis and confirmation of these early, encouraging results, a prospective randomized trial of this approach in lung transplant recipients would be indicated.

## FUTURE IMMUNOSUPPRESSION AND THERAPIES

Significant improvements in outcomes following lung transplantation were made in the 1980s and early 1990s with the discovery of cyclosporine. Although slow incremental improvements continue, lung transplantation outcomes remain inferior to those of other organ transplants. Some newer immunosuppressive agents such as mycophenolate mofetil have been incorporated into lung transplant immunosuppressive strategies and have undergone evaluation in large multicenter trials utilizing traditional immunosuppressive approaches. These approaches have made little impact on survival, however. Although a greater effort and level of cooperation are certainly needed to continue the growth of multicenter, randomized trials in lung transplantation, encouragement should also be given to put forth approaches that are novel and potentially of value. In addition, continued evaluation of strategies that tailor immunosuppression to the patients' risk of rejection should also prove advantageous.

## REFERENCES

1.  Trulock EP, Edwards LB, Taylor DO, et al. The Registry of the International Society for Heart and Lung Transplantation: twenty-first official adult lung and heart–lung transplant report-2004. J Heart Lung Transplant 2004; 23(7):804–815.
2.  Barr ML, Bourge RC, Orens JB, et al. Thoracic organ transplantation in the United States, 1994–2003. Am J Transplant 2005; 5(2):934–949.

3. Brock MV, Borja MC, Ferber L, et al. Induction therapy in lung transplantation: a prospective controlled trial comparing OKT3, anti-thymocyte globulin and dacluzimab. J Heart Lung Transplant 2001; 20:1282–1290.

4. Wahlers T, Haverich A, Schafers HJ, et al. Chronic rejection following lung transplantation. Incidence, time pattern and consequences. Eur J Cardiothorac Surg 1993; 7:319–323.

5. Tamm M, Sharples L, Higenbottam T, et al. Bronchiolitis obliterans syndrome (BOS) following heart–lung transplantation. Transpl Int 1996; 9(Suppl 1): S299–S302.

6. Reichenspurner H, Girgis RE, Robbins RC, et al. Stanford experience with obliterative bronchiolitis after lung and heart–lung transplantation. Ann Thorac Surg 1996; 62:1467–1472.

7. Ojo AO, Held PJ, Port FK, et al. Chronic renal failure after transplantation of a nonrenal organ. N Engl J Med 2003; 349(10):931–940.

8. Dowling RD, Zenati M, Burckart GJ, et al. Aerosolized cyclosporine as single agent immunotherapy in canine lung allografts. Surgery 1990; 108:198–204.

9. Mitruka SN, Pham SM, Zeevi A. Aerosol cyclosporine prevents acute allograft rejection in experimental lung transplantation. J Thorac Cardiovasc Surg 1998; 115(1):28–37.

10. Keenan RJ, Duncan AJ, Yousem SA, et al. Improved immunosuppression with aerosolized cyclosporine in experimental pulmonary transplantation. Transplantation 1992; 53(1):20–25.

11. Zenati M, Duncan AJ, Burckart GJ, et al. Immunosuppression with aerosolized cyclosporine for prevention of lung rejection in a rat model. Eur J Cardiothorac Surg 1991; 5(5):266–271.

12. Iacono AT, Keenan RJ, Duncan SR, et al. Aerosolized cyclosporine in lung recipients with refractory chronic rejection. Am J Respir Crit Care Med 1996; 153:1451–1455.

13. Iacono AT, Corcoran TE, Griffith BP, et al. Aerosol cyclosporine therapy in lung transplant recipients with bronchiolitis obliterans. Eur Resp J 2004; 23:384–390.

14. Keenan RJ, Iacono AT, Dauber JH, et al. Treatment of refractory acute allograft rejection with aerosolized cyclosporine in lung transplant recipients. J Thorac Cardiovasc Surg 1997; 113(2):335–340.

15. Iacono AT, Smaldone GC, Keenan RJ, et al. Dose-related reversal of acute lung rejection by aerosol cyclosporine. Am J Respir Crit Care Med 1997; 155:1690–1698.

16. Iacono AT, Dauber J, Keenan R, et al. Interleukin-6 and interferon-gamma gene expression in lung transplant recipients with refractory acute cellular rejection: implications for monitoring and inhibition by treatment with aerosolized cyclosporine. Transplantation 1997; 64(2):263–269.

17. Keenan RJ, Zeevi A, Iacono AT, et al. Efficacy of inhaled cyclosporine in lung transplant recipients with refractory rejection: correlation of intragraft cytokine gene expression with pulmonary function and histologic characteristics. Surgery 1995; 118(2):385–391.

18. Whitehead BF, Stoehr C, Wu CJ, et al. Cytokine gene expression in human lung transplant recipients. Transplantation 1993; 56(4):956–961.

19. Jaramillo J, Smith CR, Maruyama T, et al. Anti-HLA class I antibody binding to airway epithelial cells induces production of fibrogenic growth factors and apoptotic cell death: a possible mechanism for bronchiolitis obliterans syndrome. Hum Immunol 2003; 64(5):521–529.

20. Iacono AT, Johnson BA, Corcoran TE, et al. A randomized trial of early administration of inhaled cyclosporine in lung transplant recipients. Abstracts of papers. The International Society for Heart and Lung Transplantation Twenty-Fourth Annual Meeting and Scientific Sessions, San Francisco, CA, Apr 21–24, 2004.

21. Corcoran TE, Smaldone GC, Dauber JH, et al. Preservation of post-transplant lung function with aerosol cyclosporine. Eur Respir J 2004; 23:378–383.

22. Lance EM, Medawar P. Quantitative studies on tissue transplantation immunity. IX. Induction of tolerance with antilymphocyte serum. Proc R Soc B Biol Sci 1969; 173:447–473.

23. Abramowicz D, Wissing KM, Broeders N. Induction therapy with anti-CD3 antibodies. Curr Opin Organ Transplant 1999; 4:312–317.

24. Szczech LA, Berlin JA, Aradhye S, et al. Effect of anti-lymphocyte induction therapy on renal allograft survival: a meta-analysis. J Am Soc Nephrol 1997; 8:1771–1777.

25. Palmer SM, Miralles AP, Lawrence CM, et al. Rabbit antithymocyte globulin decreases acute rejection after lung transplantation: results of a randomized, prospective study. Chest 1999; 116:127–133.

26. Hartwig MG, Snyder LG, Appel JZ, et al. Rabbit antithymocyte globulin induction therapy for lung transplantation does not effect long-term allograft function or survival. Abstracts of Papers. The International Society for Heart and Lung Transplantation Twenty-Fourth Annual Meeting and Scientific Sessions, San Francisco, CA, Apr 21–24, 2004. (J Heart Lung Transpl 2005; 24(2S):S81–S82.

27. Ross DJ, Jordan SC, Nathan SD, et al. Delayed development of obliterative bronchiolitis syndrome with OKT3 after unilateral lung transplantation. Chest 1996; 109(4):870–873.

28. Veenstra DL, Best JH, Hornberger J, et al. The incidence and long-term cost of steroid-related side effects after renal transplantation. Am J Kidney Dis 1999; 33:829–839.

29. Kasiske BL, Chakkera HA, Louis TA, et al. A meta-analysis of immunosuppression withdrawal trials in renal transplantation. J Am Soc Nephrol 2000; 11:1910–1916.

30. Hricik DE, Schulack JA. Corticosteroid withdrawal after renal transplantation in the cyclosporine era: timing, benefits and risks. Biodrugs 1997; 8:139–149.

31. Lo A, Alloway RR. Strategies to reduce toxicities and improve outcomes in renal transplant recipients. Pharmacotherapy 2002; 22(3):316–328.

32. Opelz G, Dohler B, Laux G. Long-term prospective study of steroid withdrawal in kidney and heart transplant recipients. Am J Transplant 2005; 5:720–728.

33. Hricik DE. Steroid-free immunosuppression in kidney transplantation: an editorial review. Am J Transplant 2002; 2:19–24.

34. Birkeland S. Steroid-free immunosuppression in renal transplantation: a long-term follow-up of 100 consecutive patients. Transplantation 2001; 71:1089–1090.

35. Matas AJ, Kandaswamy R, Humar A, et al. Long-term immunosuppression, without maintenance prednisone, after kidney transplantation. Ann Surg 2004; 240:510–517.
36. Vincenti F, Monaco A, Grinyo J, et al. Multicenter randomized prospective trial of steroid withdrawal in renal transplant recipients receiving basiliximab, cyclosporine emulsion and mycophenolate mofetil. Am J Transplant 2003; 3:306–311.
37. Cole E, Landsberg D, Russell D, et al. A pilot study of steroid-free immunosuppression in the prevention of acute rejection in renal allograft recipients. Transplantation 2001; 72:845–850.
38. Sarwal MM, Vidhun JR, Alexander S, et al. Continued superior outcomes with modification and lengthened follow-up of a steroid-avoidance pilot with extended dacluzimab induction in pediatric renal transplantation. Transplantation 2003; 76:1331–1339.
39. Shitrit D, Bendayan D, Sulkes J, et al. Successful steroid withdrawal in lung transplant recipients: result of a pilot study. Respir Med 2005; 99:596–601.
40. Waldmann H. A personal history of the CAMPATH-1H antibody. Med Oncol 2002; 19:S3–S9.
41. Waldmann H, Hale G. The history of alemtuzumab (Campath-1H) antibody. CLL Cutting Edge 2001; 6:2–4.
42. Waldmann H, Polliak A, Hale G, et al. Elimination of graft-versus-host disease by in-vitro depletion of alloreactive lymphocytes with a monoclonal rat anti-human lymphocyte antibody (CAMPATH-1H). Lancet 1984; 2:483–486.
43. Waldmann H, Hale G. CAMPATH: from concept to clinic. Phil Trans R Soc B. In press.
44. Kirk AD, Hale DA, Mannon RB, et al. Results from a human renal allograft tolerance trial evaluating the humanized CD52-specific monoclonal antibody alemtuzumab (Campath-1H). Transplantation 2003; 76(1):120–129.
45. McCurry KR, Iacono A, Zeevi A, et al. Early outcomes in human lung transplantation with thymoglobulin or Campath-1H for recipient pretreatment followed by posttransplant tacrolimus near-monotherapy. J Thorac Cardiovasc Surg 2005; 130(2):528–537.
46. Knechtle SJ. Present experience with Campath-1H in organ transplantation and its potential use in pediatric recipients. Pediatr Transplant 2004; 8:106–112.
47. Isaacs JD, Greer S, Sharma S, et al. Morbidity and mortality in rheumatoid arthritis patients with prolonged and profound therapy-induced lymphopenia. Arthritis Rheum 2001; 44:1998–2008.
48. Friend PJ, Hale G, Waldman H, et al. Campath-1M prophylactic use after kidney transplantation. A randomized controlled clinical trial. Transplantation 1989; 48:248–253.
49. Friend PJ, Waldman H, Hale G, et al. Reversal of allograft rejection using the monoclonal antibody, Campath-1G. Transplant Proc 1991; 23:2253–2254.
50. Knechtle SJ, Vargo D, Fechner J, et al. FN18-CRM9 immunotoxin promotes tolerance in primate renal allografts. Transplantation 1997; 63:1–6.
51. Thomas JM, Neville DM, Contreras JL, et al. Preclinical studies of allograft tolerance in rhesus monkeys: a novel anti-CD3-immunotoxin given peritransplant with donor bone marrow induces operational tolerance to kidney allografts. Transplantation 1997; 64:124–135.

52.  Calne R, Friend P, Maffat S, et al. Prope tolerance, perioperative Campath-1H, and low-dose cyclosporine monotherapy in renal allograft recipients. Lancet 1998; 351:1701–1702.
53.  Calne R, Moffat SD, Friend PJ, et al. Campath-1H allows low-dose cyclosporine monotherapy in 31 cadaveric renal allograft recipients. Transplantation 1999; 68:1613–1616.
54.  Watson CJE, Bradley JA, Friend PJ, et al. Alemtuzumab (CAMPATH-1H) induction therapy in cadaveric kidney transplantation—efficacy and safety at five years. Am J Transplant 2005; 5:1347–1353.
55.  Knechtle SJ, Pirsch JD, Fechner JH, et al. Campath-1H induction plus rapamycin monotherapy for renal transplantation: results of a pilot study. Am J Transplant 2003; 3:722–730.
56.  Shapiro R, Basu A, Tan H, et al. Kidney transplantation under minimal immunosuppression after pretransplant lymphoid depletion with thymoglobulin or Campath. J Am Coll Surg 2005; 200(4):505–515.
57.  Ciancio G, Burke GW, Gaynor JJ, et al. The use of Campath-1H as induction therapy in renal transplantation: preliminary results. Transplantation 2004; 78(3):426–433.
58.  Kaufman DB, Leventhal JR, Axelrod D, et al. Alemtuzumab induction and prednisone-free maintenance immunotherapy in kidney transplantation: comparison with basiliximab induction—long-term results. Am J Transplant 2005; 5:2539–2548.
59.  Axelrod D, Leventhal JR, Gallon LG, et al. Reduction of CMV disease with steroid-free immunosuppression in simultaneous pancreas–kidney transplant recipients. Am J Transplant 2005; 5:1423–1429.

# 20

# Primary Graft Dysfunction Following Lung Transplantation: Pathogenesis and Impact on Early and Late Outcomes

**Michael S. Mulligan**

*Division of Cardiothoracic Surgery, Department of Surgery, University of Washington, Seattle, Washington, U.S.A.*

## INTRODUCTION

Acute lung allograft dysfunction following transplantation continues to account for considerable short-term morbidity and mortality. Despite improvements in preservation and implantation techniques, primary graft dysfunction still occurs in 11% to 25% of recipients (1,2).

There are many synonymous terms that describe this phenomenon including ischemia reperfusion injury, reimplantation edema, post-transplant acute lung injury, acute respiratory distress syndrome (ARDS), and primary graft dysfunction or failure. Recently, the International Society of Heart and Lung Transplantation (ISHLT) convened a working group on primary graft dysfunction (PGD) to try and arrive at some consensus regarding definitions, risk factors, outcomes, and therapies. While "ischemia–reperfusion injury" is the term commonly used in preclinical research, PGD is currently the convention in the clinical setting.

## DEFINITION AND DIAGNOSIS

PGD typically manifests itself within several hours to 72 hours after transplantation. It is characterized by impaired oxygenation, pulmonary infiltrates on chest radiograph (Fig. 1), poor pulmonary compliance, and typically normal or low left atrial filling pressures. This is often accompanied by an increase in pulmonary vascular resistance, as well as an increase in intrapulmonary shunt. In severe cases, histologic examination of the lungs reveals diffuse alveolar damage. Although centers agree that these are the findings that characterize PGD, there continues to be a wide variation in the reported incidence of the problem. This relates to inconsistencies in thresholds for diagnosis based on injury severity. The inability to reliably define PGD has made it difficult to identify risk factors for its development and its impact on short- and long-term outcomes. Therefore, in order to improve communication between centers about PGD and facilitate its study, a consensus definition of the problem is required. In the general clinical context, the presence of bilateral diffuse pulmonary infiltrates, poor compliance, normal or low filling pressures, and a $PaO_2/FiO_2$ ratio of $<300$ has previously been defined as acute lung injury. When P/F ratio drops to $<200$, the diagnosis of ARDS is made (3).

However, reports specifically on PGD from various centers have used a variety of diagnostic criteria (1,2,4–7). Some have used a threshold P/F ratio of $<200$ while others use $<300$. If a more liberal definition is used

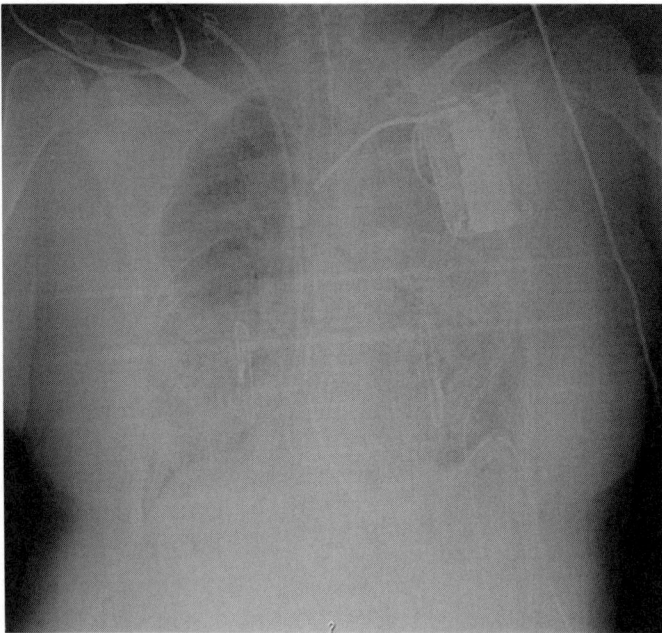

**Figure 1** CXR 24 hours post-op following bilateral lung transplantation for IPF with severe secondary pulmonary hypertension. *Abbreviations*: CXR, chest X ray, IPF, idiopathic pulmonary fibrosis.

**Table 1** Primary Graft Dysfunction Grading System

| Grade | $PaO_2/FiO_2$ | CXR: c/w pulmonary edema |
|---|---|---|
| 0 | > 300 | Absent |
| 1 | > 300 | Present |
| 2 | 200–300 | Present |
| 3 | < 200 | Present |

*Abbreviation*: CXR, chest X ray.
*Source*: From Ref. 7a.

the incidence appears higher but associations with clinical outcomes weaken. Grading of chest X ray findings has been used but these are subject to variable interpretation. Duration of ventilator dependency and even mortality has been used but these require a stringent exclusion of other causes. The variability in criteria to diagnose PGD used in these studies led to reported incidences that varied from 15% to 55%. In general, to establish the diagnosis of PGD, one must exclude confounding diagnoses such as pneumonia, congestive failure, hyperacute rejection, and venous anastomotic obstruction. Infection may be difficult to exclude and in fact frequently coexists. This is particularly true beyond 72 hours after transplantation. The most reliable assessments should therefore be made early with standardized ventilator settings. Ultimately, the consensus grading system produced by the ISHLT working group is likely to be widely adapted (Table 1) (7a).

Assessments are made within six hours of reperfusion and up to 72 hours later. Grading of PGD is not recommended beyond 72 hours. After this time, only the chest radiograph findings and the $PaO_2/FiO_2$ ratio are used. For grading purposes, the worst available P/F ratio is used. Patients on nasal cannula oxygen or less than 30% inspired oxygen are considered grade 1 or 2 depending on chest X ray findings. Patients are considered to have grade 3 PGD if they require extracorporeal membrane oxygenation (ECMO) or inhaled nitric oxide (NO) and >50% inspired oxygen beyond 48 hours.

## SCIENTIFIC PRINCIPLES

Leukocyte activation is centrally important to the development of tissue injury, and appears to occur in a biphasic pattern (8). The early phase of ischemia reperfusion injury is largely dependent on donor organ resident cell activation [in particular the alveolar macrophage (AM)], while the later phase of reperfusion injury requires recipient neutrophil and lymphocyte activation and recruitment into the allograft (8). The AM likely orchestrates the early signaling events that result in autocrine and paracrine transcriptional activation of endothelial and epithelial cells. Early endothelial activation may also promote inflammatory signaling independently. This has been demonstrated in other vascular beds, such as the heart and kidney. Subsequent upregulation of cell adhesion molecule expression and cytokine and chemokine production facilitates chemotaxis and activation of specific subpopulations of leukocytes into areas of tissue injury (8–14). Not surprisingly, clinical leukocyte depletion, especially when combined with controlled reperfusion, has only a modest protective effect on lung ischemia reperfusion injury (LIRI) after transplantation (9). It is likely that donor resident cells in the allograft are unaffected by this strategy. Furthermore, such strategies might impair the necessary immune functions of the allograft and render it more susceptible to infection.

Activation of the complement system upon allograft reperfusion contributes to tissue injury directly (via membrane attack complex–mediated cell lysis) as well as indirectly (via amplification of oxidant-induced injury). Complement depletion and inactivation are protective in animal models (15).

## Contrasting Roles of NO

NO appears to have conflicting roles in LIRI. Animal studies suggest that nitrogen centered radicals promote LIRI, and the early administration of inhaled NO (iNO) exacerbates injury possibly through the enhanced elaboration of peroxynitrite. In contrast, delayed administration of iNO was found to be protective. Additionally, exogenous NO has been found to maintain endothelial integrity and reduce neutrophil adherence, thereby limiting further amplification of postreperfusion inflammatory injury (11,15). The use of a specific peroxynitrite scavenger is also partially protective (16).

## Cytokines

Patterns of cytokine expression and functional requirements for a number of cytokines and chemokines have been demonstrated in LIRI (12). The redundancy in phlogistic cytokine activation and the complexity of cytokine networking and signaling appear to be greater in the lungs than perhaps in any other vascular bed. Our group has shown in a rodent model of warm in situ lung ischemia and reperfusion that after 90 minutes of ischemia and 15 minutes of reperfusion, tumor necrosis factor alpha (TNF-$\alpha$) and interleukin one beta (IL-1$\beta$) expression localizes exclusively to the AM (17). This occurs before intrapulmonary neutrophil accumulation is detectable and appears to be a central signaling event in the early phase of reperfusion injury. The second phase of injury is characterized by marked interstitial edema, tissue and alveolar accumulation of inflammatory cells (predominantly neutrophils), and secretion into the alveolar space of TNF-$\alpha$, IL-$\beta$, IL-6, IL-8, monocyte chemoattractant protein one (MCP-1), macrophage inflammatory protein one alpha (MIP-1$\alpha$), cytokine induced neutrophil chemoattractant (CINC), and MIP-2 (15–20). Functional requirements for the proinflammatory cytokines TNF-$\alpha$ and IL-1$\beta$, the alpha chemokines MIP-2 and CINC, and the beta chemokine MIP-1$\alpha$ have been demonstrated in animal models of LIRI (21,22). In bronchoalveolar lavage (BAL) from human lung transplant recipients, increases in TNF-$\alpha$, interferon gamma, IL-10, IL-12, and IL-18 levels were detected during ischemia, while IL-8 increased predominantly after reperfusion. High levels of IL-8 in BAL fluid or donor lung tissue were associated with an increased mortality from PGD after transplantation (15). Currently, profiles of cytokine and chemokine mRNA expression are being investigated to determine if they can be used clinically to predict acute graft dysfunction.

The Th2 cytokines IL-10, and to a lesser extent IL-4, have been shown to protect against tissue injury in multiple experimental models of LIRI. Their administration reduces both neutrophil recruitment and macrophage activation, improves oxygenation, reduces tissue edema, and shifts programmed cell death from a more inflammatory necrotic pathway to one of apoptosis (15,23). These effects can be achieved with administration of recombinant Th2 cytokines or transfection. Gene transfer via endobronchial administration of adenoviral-associated human IL-10 DNA in pigs reduces LIRI and improves graft function (24). Optimizing transfection efficiency and durability of expression could hold promise for modulating injury in human lung allografts. Airway administration and delivery in the organ perfusate are both attractive and practical options for transfection technology.

## Adhesion Molecules

Neutrophil recruitment in LIRI occurs in response to cytokines and chemokines as discussed, and is regulated by well-characterized patterns of cell-adhesion molecule expression in injured lungs. Upregulation of intercellular adhesion molecule one (ICAM-1) occurs in the later phases of lung reperfusion, and administration of anti-ICAM-1 monoclonal antibodies reduces lung injury assessed not only by neutrophil recruitment, but also by pulmonary microvascular permeability. This supports the notion that adhesion molecules are involved in reperfusion-induced endothelial injury (25). Selectins, molecules involved in the initial adhesion of activated neutrophils to endothelium, are similarly required for lung reperfusion injury to fully develop (15).

The lack of profound protection from any single intervention suggests redundancy in inflammatory activation events. To review, a partial list of these events includes complement activation, generation of reactive oxygen and nitrogen species, and elaboration of the proinflammatory cytokines and chemokines, which induce adhesion molecule expression, and promote leukocyte recruitment, which leads to tissue injury in the reperfused lung. Inhibition of a single inflammatory pathway with a well-designed intervention could confer some protection against acute lung dysfunction. However, it has become increasingly apparent that more effective strategies will likely involve administration of multiple inhibitors of synergistic, parallel inflammatory pathways, or inhibition of the inflammatory response to oxidative stress very early in the cascade before divergent redundant signaling pathways become activated.

## Role of the Alveolar Macrophage

Because of this notion of redundant inflammatory activation, the last five years of research in this field have focused more precisely on the "upstream" signaling and regulatory events that occur upon reperfusion of the allograft. Elucidating critical cellular excitation events and mapping key interactions between important lung cell populations, after oxidative stress, are required. Understanding these initial signaling events could allow targeted inhibition of the response to ischemia and reperfusion before coordinated responses begin to its ampification. The AM appears to coordinate early activation events following ischemia and reperfusion of rat lungs (26). Within 15 minutes of reperfusion, following 90 minutes of in situ warm ischemia, macrophage-derived oxidants, TNF-α, and IL-1β appear to prime pulmonary artery endothelial cells (PAEC) and type 2 pneumocytes to respond vigorously to oxidative stress (27). During the next several hours of reperfusion, the AM produces considerable additional amounts of oxidants, cytokines (TNF-α, IL-1β), and chemokines CINC, MIP-2, MIP-1 α, and MCP-1, which further promote endothelial and epithelial cell activation, upregulation of cell adhesion molecules, and recruitment of neutrophils into the interstitial and alveolar spaces (28). Macrophage depletion (with liposomes containing clodronate) or inactivation (with gadolinium) has been shown to be highly protective against the development of LIRl (16,29,30). While these findings suggest that the AM is the central coordinating cell in the inflammatory response to LIRl, the precise mechanism of activation of the AM in response to oxidative stress is still unknown.

## Cell–Cell Communication

Given the difficulty in discretely identifying activation events in individual cell populations in vivo, macrophages, endothelial cells, and epithelial cells have been cultured and examined for their response to hypoxia and reoxygenation. Primary cultures of alveolar macrophages stimulated by hypoxia and reoxygenation secrete significantly increased amounts of TNF-α, MIP-1α, MIP-2, MCP-1, and CINC by nuclear factor kappa B (NFκB) dependent-transcriptional activation (19). Primary cultures of rat PAEC respond to the same stimulus by secreting MCP-1 and CINC, as do rat alveolar epithelial cells (31). Interestingly, the amounts of cytokine and chemokine protein elaborated from the endothelial and epithelial cell are

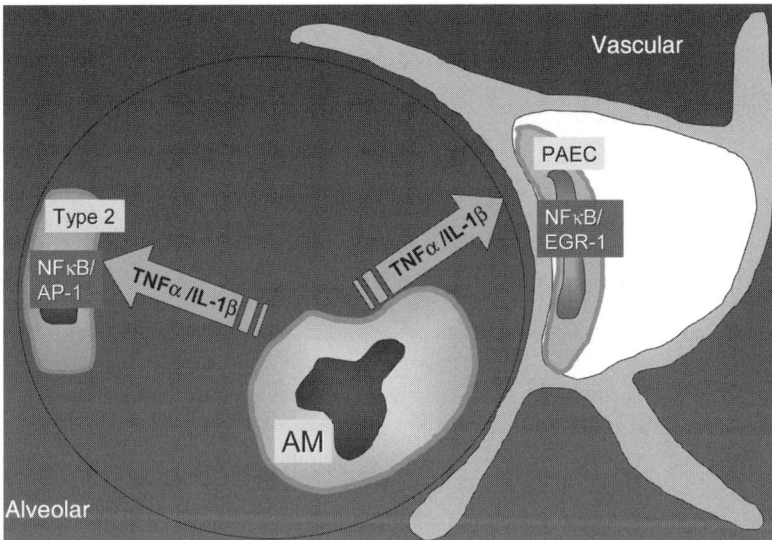

**Figure 2** Schematic of macrophage-induced endothelial and epithelial cell activation. *Abbreviations*: AM, alveolar macrophage; PAEC, pulmonary artery endothelial cells.

an order of magnitude less than that seen from the AM in response to the same oxidative stimulus. While endothelial cells depend on early transcriptional activation through NFκB and early growth response one (EGR-1), epithelial cells demonstrate early nuclear translocation of NFκB and activator protein one (AP-1) (Fig. 2) (31). All three of these transcription factors are activated in AM in response to oxidative stress. Cumulatively, they regulate the transcription of proinflammatory genes, such as cytokines, chemokines, and cell adhesion molecules. Identifying discrete associations between transcription factors and downstream activation products holds the potential for effective and specific targeting of early activation events in LIRI.

### Transcription Factor Activation

The central importance of NFκB activation has been demonstrated both in animal models of LIRI and in cultured AM subjected to oxidative stress. In a porcine lung transplant model, NFκB activation occurred early after reperfusion. An inhibitor of NFκB (pyrrolidine dithiocarbamate) administered before reperfusion improved oxygenation and reduced mean PA pressures, edema, and leukocyte infiltration (20). Indirect inhibition of AP-1 and EGR-1 also limits the inflammatory response to oxidative stress, but availability of direct specific inhibitors has limited these investigations.

## Apoptosis

Programmed cell death, in particular cellular apoptosis, is also an active area of investigation in LIRI. In biopsies from human lung allografts, up to 35% of lung cells were apoptotic two hours following graft reperfusion (32). Unfortunately, the degree of apoptosis seen on biopsy did not correlate with severity of acute allograft dysfunction. This raises a doubt as to whether anti-apoptotic agents will prove to be clinically useful in lung reperfusion injury.

## Effects of Calcineurin Inhibitors

It has been demonstrated that calcineurin inhibitors exert potent antiinflammatory effects in addition to their immunomodulatory properties. Calcineurin inhibitors confer protection from tissue injury in reperfused hearts, livers, kidneys, and lungs (33–35). When administered intratracheally, calcineurin inhibitors were markedly protective against LIRI in rodent models through inhibition of NFκB-dependent transcriptional activation (35). Likewise, cultured AM subjected to oxidative stress demonstrated diminished activation of NFκB and reduced cytokine and chemokine secretion when pretreated with a calcineurin inhibitor (20). Interestingly, these anti-inflammatory effects were seen in neutrophils and macrophages at doses of cyclosporine and tacrolimus that are an order of magnitude lower than those required to modulate immune responses in lymphocytes. The potential for off-label use of established agents, at doses that do not achieve measurable trough levels, has tremendous potential for rapid clinical translation.

## DONOR-RELATED RISK FACTORS

Donor characteristics are clearly important in the development of PGD. Unfortunately, center differences in selection criteria and a lack of consistency in diagnostic criteria for PGD have made it difficult to clearly define donor risk factors for PGD. Donor female gender and African American race appear to be associated with higher rates of PGD but how these factors exert their influence is unknown (36). Some studies have suggested that lungs from older donors (>45 years) were more frequently affected by PGD in selected studies (36,37) as were lungs from donors less than 21 years of age. The data regarding younger donors is less compelling. Age alone may ultimately not be predictive of PGD. Other studies reveal that the use of older lung donors who do not demonstrate other risk factors is quite safe (38–43). The combination of age with other risk factors, however, is definitely associated with compromised outcomes. The use of lungs from older donors who are also subjected to ischemic times greater than seven to eight hours is associated with increased recipient 30-day mortality (37). Donor smoking has been used by some to define marginal donors. Their use may impact long-term outcomes, but this does not appear to increase the incidence of PGD (44).

Brain death itself has deleterious effects on lung function and the mechanism of injury may exacerbate this problem. Specifically, lungs from donors who died from closed head injuries or intracranial hemorrhage may be associated with increased rates of PGD (45). This is a widely held conception but has been challenged by other observational studies (46).

Hemodynamic donor instability and prolonged hypotension have been suggested to increase PGD in animal models but these findings have not been systematically validated in human lung transplantation. Intuitively, excessive volume administration will cause rapid deterioration of donor lung function. As such, the donor central venous pressure should be kept below 9 mmHg. Bolus fluid administration seems to accelerate this deterioration. In general, management of hypotension in the donor should include dopamine and vasopressin. In addition to inotropic, chronotropic, and pressor support, dopamine may facilitate clearance of alveolar fluid (47). Vasopressin provides excellent afterload support, does not exacerbate pulmonary vasoconstriction, and reduces the effects of diabetes insipidus, a complication that develops in more than three-fourths of brain-dead donors.

Pneumonia in the donor would contraindicate the use of the affected lung. However, less pronounced clinical evidence of infection may also impact outcome. Cultures of upper airway secretions with tracheal aspirates do not predict the development of recipient complications. In contrast, positive cultures from donor BAL fluid are associated with impaired acute graft function after transplantation (48).

Ideally, some of the lessons learned in the preclinical laboratory would be translated into the clinical setting. Certain phlogistic and regulatory cytokines and chemokines are upregulated in lung tissue and BAL during experimental lung reperfusion injury (17). Many are known to play important functional roles (12,13). This begs the question as to whether they could be measured in donor lungs and the levels could then be used to predict the likelihood of PGD.

In human lung transplantation, levels of IL-6, IL-8, and IL–10 have been correlated with clinical outcomes. Increased levels of IL-8 in the BAL and tissue from donor lungs correlate with an increased incidence of PGD (49). The ratio of IL-6 to IL-10 levels also appears to be predictive of early mortality and PGD (50).

## Procurement and Preservation

Methods of loan, procurement, and preservation can also be optimized to limit the incidence of PGD. Bolus steroids administered to all donors increase the rate of donor lung recovery presumably by decreasing the inflammatory response and improving lung function (51,52).

The optimum temperature, volume, and pressure of the preservation solution flush as well as inflation pressure, temperature, and inspired gas content for storage have all been studied (largely in animals) and optimal conditions appear to have been defined (53–59). A lung-specific preservation solution has also been developed that has improved tolerance to prolonged cold storage. The lung preservation flush should be delivered cold and at a high flow rate with a low perfusion pressure. Ideally, the temperature should be 4°C. Although some have suggested improved preservation with a slightly warmer temperature, 4°C is more practical and reproducible. The volume of flush is optimally 50–60 cc/kg. While some centers employ pressure bags to deliver lung perfusion, it should be remembered that the flushing pressure should not be >10–15 mmHg. A high rate of flow will maintain low pressures typically by using gravity delivery with large-diameter tubing. Over distention of the lung by hyperinflation prior to cold storage is associated with alveolar stretch injury. Atelectatic storage is detrimental, so inflation is mandatory, though the composition of the inflation gas is less important. Ideally, inflation pressures for storage should not exceed 10–15 mmHg and the gas should either be room air or not >50% oxygen. Higher concentrations of inspired oxygen may be associated with an increased risk of free radical tissue injury during ischemic storage. Storage at 10°C appears to be associated with improved ultrastructural preservation in the lung when compared to 4°C. However, it is impractical to maintain a constant temperature of 10°C while it is relatively easy to achieve a constant temperature of 4°C. Specialized circulating cooling baths and significant equipment modifications would be required to consistently store lungs at 10°C. As such, centers continue to maintain preservation temperatures at 4°C.

Intracellular-type solutions were the mainstay of lung preservation since the development of lung transplantations. Euro-Collins or University of Wisconsin solution were used by virtually all centers. More recently, the development of a low-potassium dextran (LPD) solution has changed clinical lung preservation. Conceptually, these solutions were designed to provide a favorable gradient to decrease interstitial edema, decrease endothelial injury, and improve microcirculation due to the high dextran content. Prostaglandin E1 (PGE1) has been used to optimize pulmonary vasomotor relaxation as well as to decrease platelet and neutrophil adhesion in the preserved lung. PGE-1 is still a central part of clinical practice in lung procurement and preservation and LPD appears to further enhance its desired effects. The concepts were proven in preclinical animal studies. Human observational studies followed and finally a prospective randomized trial was completed demonstrating improved outcomes with LPD solutions compared to intracellular-type solutions (15). In animal studies the addition of glucose to LPD appears to support aerobic metabolism and maintain cell viability during prolonged cold storage (60). This has allowed the extension of safe ischemic periods from 12 up to 24 hours. Previously, convention warned that preservation times should not exceed four to six hours. With LPD-glucose, preservation times are now safely extended

**Table 2** Donor-Related Risk Factors for Primary
Graft Dysfunction

---

Female gender
Race
Closed head injury or intracranial hemorrhage
Hemodynamic instability
Volume overload
Culture positive BAL
Increased IL-6, IL-8 levels
Decreased IL-10 levels
Prolonged ischemia in the presence of other risk factors

---

*Abbreviations*: BAL, bronchoalveolar lavage; IL, interleukin.

to six to eight hours and many centers are accepting preservation of 12 hours or longer (15).

Data from the ISHLT registry would suggest that the combination of prolonged ischemia in the use of lungs from older donors is associated with an increased 30-day mortality. However, most of these data were collected prior to the widespread use of LPD-glucose solutions and ischemic time alone in the absence of other donor-associated risk factors is not a clear predictor of PGD. Clearly, the subject requires more study but at least in the current era it appears that we are now able to safely extend ischemic times beyond six hours.

Another fairly recent development in lung preservation is the concept of a retrograde flush. After the flush is delivered to the pulmonary artery, additional perfusate is delivered to the pulmonary veins directly or the left atrium in the setting of a heart–lung block procurement. This has been studied experimentally and examined clinically. The use of a retrograde flush removes both emboli and platelet aggregates from the pulmonary circulation, improves the distribution of a hypodermic flush, and is ultimately associated with improved graft function when compared to lungs preserved with antegrade flush alone (61,62).

As suggested, there are a number of donor-associated and procurement-related factors that can influence post-transplant graft function. Some of these associations are well supported by preclinical and clinical research. Others have been widely accepted because they seem intuitive or because they have been convention for so long. Table 2 summarizes these factors and Table 3 details recommended guidelines for procurement techniques.

## RECIPIENT-RELATED FACTORS

Although many recipient characteristics have historically been considered to affect the rate of PGD, few have been studied systematically. When

**Table 3**  Recommended Lung Preservation Techniques

Bolus systemic steroid administration (15 mg/kg)
Flush volume 50–60 cc/kg
Flush temperatures 4°C
Flush pressure not > 10–15 mmHg
LPD glucose preservation solution
Bolus PGE-1 prior to flush and mixed with perfusate
Inflation pressure for storage 10–15 mmHg
$FiO_2$ in storage gas not > 50%
Retrograde flush

*Abbreviations*: LPD, low-potassium dextran; PGE-1, prostaglandin E1.

only carefully controlled data are examined, however, certain factors consistently appear to be associated with an increased risk of PGD. Hepatic impairment in patients with pulmonary hypertension is known to affect early mortality after heart–lung transplantation. In those with a serum bilirubin >2.1 ng/dL, mortality is 58% compared to 27% for those with a serum bilirubin of between 1 and 2 ng/dL and 16% for those with a normal bilirubin level. These data suggest that hepatic dysfunction compromises early outcomes; however, data from heart–lung transplant recipients may not necessarily apply to single- or double-lung transplant recipients (63). In contrast, patients with renal dysfunction and left ventricular dysfunction do not appear to be specifically at greater risk for PGD.

Patients with panel reactive antibodies >10% have a greater risk of prolonged mechanical ventilation post lung transplantation. Whether or not this relates to PGD or immune-mediated phenomena is unclear (64). Similarly, patients undergoing retransplantation are likely immunologically sensitized. Short-term mortality is increased following retransplantation but the rate of PGD in this population does not appear to be elevated (65).

Patients with complicated pleural spaces secondary to prior thoracic surgery have long been considered to be at greater risk of PGD. However, unless dense pleural adhesions are encountered which significantly increase surgical trauma and related transfusion requirements, the rate of PGD appears to be unaffected (66).

Chronic obstructive pulmonary disease (COPD) patients appear to have the lowest risk of PGD while patients with restrictive disease have an elevated risk of PGD. This risk is increased even further among patients with primary pulmonary hypertension (PPH) (2,5,36,67). The risk of PGD in patients with CF appears to be comparable to that seen in recipients with restrictive lung diseases. Precisely why patients with the PPH have an increased risk of PGD has been the subject of much investigation and discussion. It has been postulated that since the right ventricle becomes significantly hypertrophied in response to chronically elevated pulmonary vascular resistance (PVR) and PVR abruptly decreases following transplantation, flow rates and endothelial sheer stress are increased. The resultant endothelial injury would compromise capillary membrane integrity and increase lung vascular permeability. This phenomenon appears to be more pronounced in patients with pulmonary hypertension who receive single-lung transplants as opposed to those who receive bilateral allografts. This risk is even lower among recipients who receive heart–lung transplants, presumably because the right heart is not hypertrophied and pulmonary vascular endothelial shear stress is less (68). These findings suggest that it may be appropriate to consider a bilateral lung transplantation in patients with PPH and reversible cardiac dysfunction. An attempt to decrease the inotropic response of the hypertrophied right ventricle with beta blockade may also offer a way to reduce the risk of PGD (69).

In general, secondary pulmonary hypertension does not appear to increase the risk of PGD (36). An exception to this is found among patients with COPD and advanced disease with associated secondary pulmonary hypertension. These patients do appear to have an increased risk of PGD and 30-day mortality (70). The type of transplant procedure utilized in patients with PPH may affect the incidence of PGD. However, among patients with secondary pulmonary hypertension, the impact of receiving a single-versus a double-lung transplant on the rate of PGD does not appear to be significant (71). Intuitively, patients with severe secondary pulmonary hypertension may indeed behave more like patients with PPH and one should approach those patients in a similar fashion. In that setting, maximally unloading the right heart and optimizing the size of the run-off vascular bed with bilateral lung transplantation would appear appropriate. In general terms, it is unlikely that the type of transplant performed is an important determinant of PGD (72). However, the presence of pulmonary hypertension (either primary or severe secondary) provides an exception to that.

## Cardiopulmonary Bypass

The impact of cardiopulmonary bypass (CPB) on the development of PGD is controversial. Some studies have suggested an increased rate of PGD among recipients where CPB is required for completion of their transplants (45,67,73). However, this may be confounded by the fact that many of the patients who required bypass had significant pulmonary hypertension and other complicating risk factors that confound the analyses. Excessive efforts to avoid cardiopulmonary bypass are likely harmful to those recipients who are clearly unstable from a cardiopulmonary standpoint intraoperatively. When necessary, it should be used without hesitation as it has been demonstrated to be safe, is widely accepted clinically, and is used by some centers electively for all of their transplants. Others utilize modifications of the strategy with ECMO support during and briefly after lung transplantation (74–77). Those that support the liberal utilization of CPB feel it may actually have beneficial effects on short- and long-term outcomes. CPB itself may be immunosuppressive and readily allows for controlled reperfusion of the allografts. It also facilitates leukocyte depletion with the use of in-line filters prior to reperfusion. Unfortunately, the use of CPB is frequently associated with an increased risk of bleeding and transfusion requirements.

## Blood Products

There are clear links that associate perioperative bleeding with an increased rate of PGD. The use of blood products engenders a risk of transfusion-related lung injury. This phenomenon typically occurs within hours of transfusion of a blood product. It is clinically indistinguishable from other forms of adult respiratory distress syndrome (ARDS) but thankfully resolves within several days in most patients (78). However, the combined presence of PGD and transfusion-related lung injury would have a predictably negative impact on acute recipient lung function.

## Technical Errors

Technical errors committed during the implantation procedure would certainly exacerbate PGD. Pulmonary venous anastomotic obstruction manifests almost immediately with frothy pink pulmonary edema and dense lung consolidation on chest radiograph. Patients are often hemodynamically unstable and require immediate correction. The diagnosis is easily made with transesophageal echocardiography (TEE). Surgical correction may require additional metabolic protection of the lung allograft either with systemic hypothermia and CPB or reintroduction of pneumoplegia with the lung isolated in the operative field. Some authors have suggested that thrombolytic therapy or percutaneous catheter-based therapies may play a role in selected cases of venous compromise. However, experience with these techniques is limited and, in general, surgical correction should not be delayed.

Pulmonary arterial stenosis secondary to "purse-stringing" of the suture line or excessive length of the reconstructed pulmonary artery leads to the formation of a kink. This may present as hypoxemia at rest or with exercise. This is often detectable with TEE or may be diagnosed with CT angiography with 3D reconstructions or pulmonary arteriography. Surgical correction is the mainstay of therapy. Angioplasty and possible stenting can be considered in selected cases, particularly when the diagnosis is significantly delayed.

Torsion of the allograft may affect the entire hilum or isolated lobes. This also requires prompt surgical correction. The diagnosis of lobar torsion is made by the presence of consolidation on chest X ray and bronchial luminal compromise seen at bronchoscopy.

## Mode of Graft Reperfusion

Controlled reperfusion may offer advantages in decreasing the risk of PGD as well (79,80). Two studies demonstrated benefit in terms of decreased PGD and improved graft function and overall survival. Initial reperfusion pressures are kept at <20 mmHg during the first 10 minutes. Recipient blood used to generate the perfusate is first leukocyte depleted and enriched with nitroglycerin, aspartate, glutamate, and dextrose. The use of CPB bypass facilitates this technique but it is not required. Although many centers have adopted low-pressure reperfusion during the initial 10 minutes after revascularization; modifications to the perfusate have not yet gained widespread acceptance.

## Recipient Immune Responsiveness

As outlined in the section on scientific principles of reperfusion injury, components of the innate immune system likely contribute to the development of PGD. Some recipients appear to manifest a more robust inflammatory response to the same stimulus and may develop more severe PGD. Dysfunction manifesting early after reperfusion likely relates to inherent or acquired donor lung characteristics while dysfunction that develops over the ensuing 24 hours is probably influenced primarily by recipient characteristics. The vigor of the recipient inflammatory response may be characterized by the degree of upregulation of adhesion molecule expression in pulmonary vascular beds or cytokine responses to oxidant stress. Findings from studies of ARDS patients or other solid organ transplant recipients have been extrapolated but little direct evidence exists to implicate these phenomena in PGD following lung transplantation. Assessments of BAL cytokine content predict the risk of lung dysfunction but may be a reflection of donor lung characteristics as much as recipient responses. Therefore, the influences of donor and recipient characteristics is difficult to separate. In the future, genomic analysis of recipient inflammatory responses may be predictive of a likelihood of the development of PGD.

AM resident in donor lungs appears to coordinate key signaling events in the development of lung reperfusion injury (16,17). The AM appears to be one of the earliest responders to oxidative stress in the lung. Neutrophils and lymphocytes are predominantly derived from circulating recipient populations and play a role in amplifying the later stages of lung reperfusion injury (15). Strategies to target donor AM [perhaps with inhaled medications (35)] hold promise while selected inflammatory cell targeting in the recipient would offer a complementary strategy. Leukocyte depletion by utilizing an in-line filter on cardiopulmonary bypass is favored by the Stanford group. However, this strategy has not been widely adapted and may negate some of the beneficial and required functions of these cells (i.e., resistance to infection).

**Table 4**  Recipient-Associated Risk Factors

| |
|---|
| Diagnosis of PPH |
| Marked hepatic dysfunction (bilirubin >2 mg/dL) |
| Complicated pleural space |
| Significant transfusion requirements |
| Controlled allograft reperfusion |

*Abbreviation*: PPH, primary pulmonary hypertension.

## Summary of Risk Factors

In conclusion, the most clearly established recipient factor associated with acute graft dysfunction is a diagnosis of PPH. Recipient hepatic dysfunction, the presence of dense pleural adhesions that increase the risk of postoperative bleeding, and the need for transfusion are likewise associated with a greater incidence of PGD. The type of transplant performed does not appear to have a strong influence on the risk of PGD except in the setting of PPH where double-lung transplantation and/or heart–lung transplantation appear to decrease risk compared to single-lung transplantation. Modified graft reperfusion appears to be protective. Specific modulation of the recipient inflammatory response will remain the subject of ongoing preclinical and translational investigation (Table 4).

## MANAGEMENT OF PGD

Undoubtedly, strong opinions exist regarding the optimal critical care management of the acute lung transplant recipient. However, clinical studies have not defined ideal ventilator, fluid, or pressor management.

### Fluid Management

Since patients invariably have some degree of increased lung vascular permeability, it is advisable to limit volume resuscitation. Some degree of renal embarrassment is tolerable, but adequate volume should be maintained to provide adequate visceral perfusion. Overzealous volume restriction and excessive pressor use may further compromise bronchial anastomotic blood flow and contribute to airway complications. If significant blood loss occurred intraoperatively, volume resuscitation should give first consideration to the need for red blood cells or plasma instead of crystalloid.

### Ventilation

Every attempt should be made to extubate patients as soon as possible. This is particularly true for COPD patients who received single-lung transplants and patients with septic lung disease, the former since compliance mismatch between native and allograft lungs may lead to native lung over-inflation and the latter since clearance of secretions is markedly impaired in the ventilated patient. If PGD develops, it is advisable to utilize lung protective ventilation strategies (81,82). Instead of the typical tidal volume of 10–15 cc/kg, 6–8 cc/kg is delivered, thereby avoiding exacerbation of PGD by barotrauma. Depending on the circumstances, permissive hypercapnea, inverse ratio ventilation, and prone positioning can be used (83,84). All patients should have alveolar recruitment optimized with the judicious use of positive end-expiratory pressure.

## Inhaled NO

Deficits in NO production manifest after cold ischemic storage of the lung. This appears to have detrimental effects on pulmonary vasorelaxation, capillary permeability, and adherence of neutrophils and platelets to the pulmonary endothelium (85–87). Postreperfusion pulmonary vasoconstriction and inflammatory leukocyte sequestration are common. In an effort to prevent these phenomena, the role of prophylactic inhaled NO administration has been investigated. Unfortunately, it does not appear to lower the incidence of PGD (11,88). This may relate to potentially negative effects of NO when it is present during reperfusion. In animal models, early inhaled NO administration actually exacerbated lung reperfusion injury (89). This may be due to the abrupt rise in superoxide production immediately after reperfusion. If present, NO could readily combine with superoxide to form the highly tissue toxic peroxynitrite radical. In established PGD, however, inhaled NO does appear to provide benefit. It lowers pulmonary vascular resistance without causing systemic hypotension and optimizes ventilation perfusion matching to improve oxygenation (90–92).

## Prostaglandins

Systemic prostaglandins have been used to address similar problems in PGD but their use is associated with significant hypotension and they are no longer in favor. In contrast, inhaled PGE1 has been used to treat other forms of pulmonary hypertension and may offer many of the same benefits of inhaled NO at greatly reduced cost (93).

## Other Therapies

Ischemia, preservation, and reperfusion all have detrimental effects on pulmonary surfactant composition and function (94), leading to alveolar collapse, impaired compliance, altered ventilation–perfusion matching, and ultimately hypoxemia (95). Case reports have suggested that nebulized surfactant may improve outcomes in PGD (96,97). Similar treatment of the donor prior to ischemia likewise appears to improve early graft function (98). Such treatments are seemingly easy to administer and if further clinical study validates these early findings, exogenous surfactant treatment may be adopted as an adjunctive treatment and prevention strategy for PGD.

Complement inhibition with soluble complement receptor-1 tended to decrease the duration of mechanical ventilation in clinical lung transplantation (99). This effect was not statistically significant and the specific impact on allograft function was less obvious. Currently, complement inhibition is not used clinically to prevent or treat PGD. Use of platelet activating factor antagonists administered in lung perfusates and systemically to recipients after reperfusion is associated with improved oxygenation compared to controls (100). This strategy also has yet to make its way into mainstream clinical practice.

## EXTRACORPOREAL MEMBRANE OXYGENATION

When PGD manifests in its most severe form, ECMO support may be required. If patients have adequate cardiac function and are hemodynamically stable, veno-venous ECMO will suffice. In patients with impaired cardiac function, severe PGD, and hemodynamic instability, veno-arterial ECMO will likely be required. ECMO support was more frequently required in female bilateral lung recipients transplanted for PPH at Washington University (101). Nearly 60% of their patients survived acutely. Other groups have reported short-term survival rates of up to 75% (102). Further analysis has allowed the identification of patients who are more likely to survive and therefore justify the use of this significant resource. Patients with PGD in whom ECMO support was instituted early (within one to seven days) had >70% hospital survival, whereas no survivors were reported among patients who had ECMO instituted for more than seven days after transplantation (103,104). It follows therefore that ECMO support should not be initiated for more than seven days after lung transplantation. In fact even when instituted early, ECMO support should not be prolonged in this setting since most patients cannot be weaned if they have failed to do so after seven days of support.

The morbidity associated with ECMO in this population can be considerable. Bleeding, stroke, cannulation-induced.vascular injury, and renal failure are all relatively common. Despite this, outcomes in appropriately selected patients seem better with ECMO than without. In the best circumstances appropriate patients would be identified proactively rather than waiting for marked decompensation requiring emergent institution of ECMO support. An oxygenation index has been proposed to help identify appropriate ECMO candidates (105,106). It is defined as the mean airway pressure $\times$ FiO$_2$/PaO$_2$. An index of >30 indicated the development of severe PGD and the need for very aggressive levels of support like ECMO. Such patients appear to have improved survival when ECMO is used. The extensive experience at the University of Michigan has also yielded guidelines for ECMO candidate selection among patients with ARDS. They too have had success in supporting lung transplant recipients affected by severe PGD (107). Despite the severe nature of their acute graft dysfunction, long-term outcomes among ECMO survivors are respectable. Two-year survival is approximately 50% (108–110).

## Retransplantation

Retransplantation for severe PGD can be considered in carefully selected patients with otherwise intact end-organ function. Unfortunately, short-and long-term outcomes after retransplantation remain poor. Retransplantation for bronchiolitis obliterans syndrome (BOS) >2 years after their initial operation in ambulatory patients is associated with the best outcomes. A recent multivariate analysis of 230 retransplants indicated that nonambulatory status, ventilator dependency, and retransplantation prior to 1991 were associated with poor outcomes. Retransplantation for PGD was not associated with increased morbidity and mortality (111). A comprehensive analysis of the impact of reoperation for PGD from more recent registry data from the ISHLT has not yet been done. However, most centers agree that retransplantation for PGD is associated with poor outcomes. Typically, these patients are nonambulatory, ventilated, and often have collateral organ dysfunction. When muitiorgan failure is present, mortality is prohibitive and retransplantation should not be considered.

## OUTCOMES OF PGD

As anticipated, the development of PGD is associated with increased duration of mechanical ventilation, ICU and hospital length of stay, and 30 day mortality (112,113). After a prolonged critical illness, these patients are naturally debilitated and require intensive rehabilitation to optimize their functional status. Lower long-term survival rates in PGD patients are largely explained by their increased early mortality (114).

The development of PGD is associated with a nearly threefold increase in ICU mortality (113). Scoring systems have been proposed in an attempt to predict acute outcomes (113,115). Risk factors for acute mortality have included recipient age, ischemic time, severely reduced $PaO_2/FiO_2$ ratios, hemodynamic instability, the use of CPB, pulmonary hypertension, BMI > 25 kg/m, and the use of marginal donors. Other reports and review of the ISHLT registry have suggested that it is the combination of ischemic time and advanced donor age, and not neither factor alone, that increases early mortality (36). Many reports have demonstrated equivalent outcomes with the use of marginal and ideal donors with properly selected recipients (15,116–118). Similarly, elevated BMI appears to compromise outcomes but may not influence 30-day mortality. The use of CPB and its influence on early mortality remain controversial. The remaining factors that have been proposed to increase acute mortality (severely reduced $PaO_2/FiO_2$ ratios, hemodynamic instability, and pulmonary hypertension) relate directly to PGD. As such, the primary influence on early mortality after lung transplantation may well be the development and severity of PGD.

The relationship between PGD and the development of BOS has been suggested. Lung reperfusion injury is known to increase major histocompatibility complex class II expression and would therefore render allografts more immunogenic (119). Postinflammatory pulmonary fibrosis suggests the possibility that an ARDS-like illness such as PGD could incite remodeling processes that are ultimately detrimental to lung function. Two recent single-center studies produced conflicting results regarding PGD and the subsequent development of BOS (105,114). Ultimately, differences in study methodology likely explain the disparity in conclusions. It is possible that severe PGD increases the risk of BOS. Proof of that concept will require prospective study after diagnostic criteria for PGD and severity grading have been established. Until such time, the influence of PGD on the development of BOS will remain speculative.

## REFERENCES

1.  Christie JD, Bavaria IE, Palevsky HI, et al. Primary graft failure following lung transplantation. Chest 1998; 114:51–60.
2.  King RC, Binns OA, Rodriguez F, et al. Reperfusion injury significantly impacts clinical outcome after pulmonary transplantation. Ann Thorac Surg 2000; 69:1681–1685.
3.  Bernard GR, Reines HD, Brigham KL, et al. The American European consensus conference on ARDS: definitions, mechanism, relevant outcomes and clinical trials coordination. Am J Resp Crit Care Med 1994; 149:818–824.
4.  Khan SU, Salloum J, O'Donovan PB, et al. Acute pulmonary edema after lung transplantation: the pulmonary reimplantation response. Chest 1999; 116:187–194.
5.  Thabut G, Vinatier I, Stern JB, et al. Primary graft failure following lung transplantation: predictive factors of mortality. Chest 2002; 121:1876–1882.
6.  Boujoukos AJ, Martich GD, Vega JD, et al. Reperfusion injury in single-lung transplant recipients with pulmonary hypertension and emphysema. J Heart Lung Transplant 1997; 16:439–448.
7.  Chatilla WM, Furukawa S, Gaughan JP, et al. Respiratory failure after lung transplantation. Chest 2003; 123:165–173.
7a. Christie JD, Carby M, Bag R, Corris P, Hertz M, Weill D. Report of the ISHLT working group on primary lung graft dysfunction Part II: definition. A consensus statement of the International Society for Heart and Lung Transplantation. J Heart Lung Transplant 2005; 24:1454–1459.
8.  Fiser SM, Tribble CG, Long SM, et al. Lung transplant reperfusion injury involves pulmonary macrophages and circulating leukocytes in a biphasic response. J Thorac Cardiovasc Surg 2001; 121(6):1069–1075.

9.  Clark SC, Sudarshan C, Khanna R, Roughan J, Flecknell PA, Dark JH. Controlled reperfusion and pentoxifylline modulate reperfusion injury after single lung transplantation. J Thorac Cardiovasc Surg 1998; 115(6):1335–1341.

10. Keshavjee S, Davis RD, Zamora MR, de Perrot M, Patterson GA. A randomized, placebo-controlled trial of complement inhibition in ischemia–reperfusion injury after lung transplantation in human beings. J Thorac Cardiovasc Surg 2005; 129(2):423–428.

11. Ardehali A, Laks H, Levine M, et al. A prospective trial of inhaled nitric oxide in clinical lung transplantation. Transplantation 2001; 72(1): 112–115.

12. Farivar AS, Krishnadasan B, Naidu BV, Woolley SM, Verrier ED, Mulligan MS. Alpha chemokines regulate direct lung ischemia–reperfusion injury. J Heart Lung Transplant 2004; 23(5):585–591.

13. Krishnadasan B, Farivar AS, Naidu BV, et al. Beta-chemokine function in experimental lung ischemia–reperfusion injury. Ann Thorac Surg 2004; 77(3):1056–1062.

14. Itano H, Zhang W, Ritter JH, McCarthy TJ, Mohanakumar T, Patterson GA. Adenovirus mediated gene transfer of human interleukin10 ameliorates reperfusion injury of rat lung isografts. J Thorac Cardiovasc Surg 2000; 120(5): 947–956.

15. de Perrot M, Liu M, Waddell TK, Keshavjee S. Ischemia–reperfusion-induced lung injury. Am J Respir Crit Care Med 2003; 167(4):490–511.

16. Naidu BV, Krishnadasan B, Farivar AS, et al. Early activation of the alveolar macrophage is critical to the development of lung ischemia–reperfusion injury. J Thorac Cardiovasc Surg 2003; 126(1):200–207.

17. Krishnadasan B, Naidu BV, Byrne K, Fraga C, Verrier ED, Mulligan MS. The role of proinflammatory cytokines in lung ischemia–reperfusion injury. J Thorac Cardiovasc Surg 2003; 125(2):261–272.

18. Lau CL, Patterson GA, Palmer SM. Critical care aspects of lung transplantation. J Intensive Care Med 2004; 19(2):83–104.

19. Naidu BV, Krishnadasan B, Byrne K, et al. Regulation of chemokine expression by cyclosporine A in alveolar macrophages exposed to hypoxia and reoxygenation. Ann Thorac Surg 2002; 74(3):899–905.

20. Maxey TS, Enelow RI, Gaston B, Kron IL, Laubach VE, Doctor A. Tumor necrosis factor-alpha from resident lung cells is a key initiating factor in pulmonary ischemia–reperfusion injury. J Thorac Cardiovasc Surg 2004; 127(2):541–547.

21. Farivar AS, Krishnadasan B, Naidu BV, Woolley SM, Verrier ED, Mulligan MS. Alpha chemokines regulate direct lung ischemia–reperfusion injury. J Heart Lung Transplant 2004; 23(5):585–591.

22. Krishnadasan B, Farivar AS, Naidu BV, et al. Beta-chemokine function in experimental lung ischemia–reperfusion injury. Ann Thorac Surg 2004; 77(3): 1056–1062.

23. Itano H, Zhang W, Ritter JH, McCarthy TJ, Mohanakumar T, Patterson GA. Adenovirus mediated gene transfer of human interleukin 10 ameliorates reperfusion injury of rat lung isografts. J Thorac Cardiovasc Surg 2004; 120(5): 947–956.

24. Martins S, de Perrot M, Imai Y, et al. Transbronchial administration of adenoviral-mediated interleukin-10 gene to the donor improves function in a pig lung transplant model. Gene Ther 2004; 11(24):1786–1796.

25. Chamoun F, Burne M, O'Donnell M, Rabb H. Pathophysiologic role of selectins and their ligands in ischemia–reperfusion injury. Front Biosci 2000; 5:E103–E109.

26. Naidu BV, Krishnadasan B, Farivar AS, et al. Early activation of the alveolar macrophage is critical to the development of lung ischemia–reperfusion injury. J Thorac Cardiovasc Surg 2003; 126(l):200–207.

27. Krishnadasan B, Naidu BV, Byrne K, Fraga C, Verrier ED, Mulligan MS. The role of proinflammatory cytokines in lung ischemia–reperfusion injury. J Thorac Cardiovasc Surg 2003; 125(2):261–272.

28. Naidu BV, Krishnadasan B, Byrne K, et al. Regulation of chemokine expression by cyclosporine A in alveolar macrophages exposed to hypoxia and reoxygenation. Ann Thorac Surg 2002; 74(3):899–905.

29. Maxey TS, Enelow RI, Gaston B, Kron IL, Laubach VE, Doctor A. Tumor necrosis factor-alpha from resident lung cells is a key initiating factor in pulmonary ischemia–reperfusion injury. J Thorac Cardiovasc Surg 2004; 127(2): 541–547.

30. Fiser SM, Tribble CG, Long SM, Kaza AK, Kern JA, Kron IL. Pulmonary macrophages are involved in reperfusion injury after lung transplantation. Ann Thorac Surg 2001; 71(4):1134–1138.

31. Farivar AS, Woolley SM, Fraga CH, Byrne K, Mulligan MS. Proinflammatory response of alveolar type II pneumocytes to in vitro hypoxia and reoxygenation. Am J Transplant 2004; 4(3):346–351.

32. Fischer S, Cassivi SD, Xavier AM, et al. Cell death in human lung transplantation: apoptosis induction in human lungs during ischemia and after transplantation. Ann Surg 2000; 231(3):424–431.

33. St Peter SD, Post DJ, Rodriguez-Davalos MI. Tacrolimus as a liver flush solution to ameliorate the effects of ischemia–reperfusion injury following liver transplantation. Liver Transplant 2003; 9(2):144–149.

34. Yang CW, Ahn HJ, Han HJ. Kim Preconditioning with cyclosporine A or FK506 differentially regulates mitogen-activated protein kinase expression in rat kidneys with ischemia/reperfusion injury. Transplantation 2003; 75(1):20–24.

35. Woolley SM, Farivar AS, Naidu BV, et al. Endotracheal calcineurin inhibition ameliorates injury in an experimental model of lung ischemia–reperfusion. J Thorac Cardiovasc Surg 2004; 127(2):376–384.

36. Christie JD, Kotloff RM, Pochettino A, et al. Clinical risk factors for primary graft failure following lung transplantation. Chest 2003; 124: 1232–1241.

37. Novick RJ, Bennett LE, Meyer DM, Hosenpud JD. Influence of graft ischemic time and donor age on survival after lung transplantation. J Heart Lung Transplant 1999; 18:425–431.

38. Sundaresan S, Semenkovich J, Ochoa L, et al. Successful outcome of lung transplantation is not compromised by the use of marginal donor lungs. J Thorac Cardiovasc Surg 1995; 109:1075–1079.

39. Gabbay E, Williams TJ, Griffiths AP, et al. Maximizing the utilization of donor organs offered for lung transplantation. Am J Respir Crit Care Med 1999; 160:265–271.

40. Pierre AF, Sekine Y, Hutcheon MA, Waddell TK, Keshavjee SH. Marginal donor lungs: a reassessment. J Thorac Cardiovasc Surg 2002; 123:421–428.
41. Kron IL, Tribble CG, Kern JA, et al. Successful transplantation of marginally acceptable thoracic organs. Ann Surg 1993; 217(5):518–522.
42. Meyers BF, Lynch J, Trulock EP, Guthrie TJ, Cooper JD, Patterson GA. Lung transplantation: a decade of experience. Ann Surg 1999; 230(3):362–370.
43. Bhorade SM, Vigneswaran W, McCabe MA, Garrity ER. Liberalization of donor criteria may expand the donor pool without adverse consequence in lung transplantation. J Heart Lung Transplant 2000; 19(12):1199–1204.
44. Waddell T, de Perrot M, Pierre A, Keshavjee S, Bennett-Edwards L. Impact of donor smoking on survival after lung transplantation [abstr]. J Heart Lung Transplant 2003; 22:S114–S115.
45. Sommers KE, Griffith BP, Hardesty RL, Keenan RJ. Early lung allograft function in twin recipients from the same donor: risk factor analysis. Ann Thorac Surg 1996; 62:784–790.
46. Waller DA, Thompson AM, Wrightson WN, et al. Does the mode of donor death influence the early outcome of lung transplantation? A review of lung transplantation from donors involved in major trauma. J Heart Lung Transplant 1995; 14:318–321.
47. Ware LB, Fang X, Wang Y, Sakuma T, Hall TS, Matthay MA. Selected contribution: mechanisms that may stimulate the resolution of alveolar edema in the transplanted human lung. J Appl Physiol 2002; 93:1869–1874.
48. Avlonitis VS, Krause A, Luzzi L, et al. Bacterial colonization of the donor lower airways is a predictor of poor outcome in lung transplantation. Eur J Cardiothorac Surg 2003; 24:601–607.
49. de Perrot M, Sekine Y, Fischer S, et al. Interleukin-8 release during early reperfusion predicts graft function in human lung transplantation. Am J Respir Crit Care Med 2002; 165:211–215.
50. Birks EJ, Owen VJ, Burton PB, et al. Tumor necrosis factor-alpha is expressed in donor heart and predicts right ventricular failure after human heart transplantation. Circulation 2000; 102:326–331.
51. Follette DM, Rudich SM, Babcock WD. Improved oxygenation and increased lung donor recovery with high-dose steroid administration after brain death. J Heart Lung Transplant 1998; 17:423–429.
52. Wigfield CH, Golledge HD, Shenton BK, Kirby JA, Dark JH. Ameliorated reperfusion injury in lung transplantation after reduction of brain death induced inflammatory graft damage in the donor [abstr]. J Heart Lung Transplant 2002; 21:57.
53. Hopkinson DN, Bhabra MS, Hooper TL. Pulmonary graft preservation: a worldwide survey of current clinical practice. J Heart Lung Transplant 1998; 17:525–531.
54. Wang LS, Nakamol K, Hsieh CM, Miyoshi S, Copper ID. Influence of temperature of flushing solution on lung preservation. Ann Thorac Surg 1993; 55:711–715.
55. Haverich A, Aziz S, Scott WG, Jamieson SW, Shumway NE. Improved lung preservation using Euro-Collins solution for flush-perfusion. Thorac Cardiovasc Surg 1986; 34:368–376.

56. Tanaka H, Chiba Y, Sasaki M, Matsukawa S, Muraoka R. Relationship between flushing pressure and nitric oxide production in preserved lungs. Transplantation 1998; 65:460–464.

57. DeCampos KN, Keshavjee S, Liu M, Slutsky AS. Optimal inflation volume for hypothermic preservation of rat lungs. J Heart Lung Transplant 1998; 17: 599–607.

58. Wang LS, Yoshikawa K, Miyoshi S, et al. The effect of ischemic time and temperature on lung preservation in a simple ex vivo rabbit model used for functional assessment. J Thorac Cardiovasc Surg 1989; 98:333–342.

59. Heiniuda M, Dresler CM, Mizuta T, Cooper JD, Patterson GA. Free radical-mediated vascular injury in lungs preserved at moderate hypothermia. Ann Thoracic Surg 1995; 60:1376–1381.

60. Wagner FM, Jamieson SW, Fung J, Wolf P, Reichenspurner H, Kaye MP. A new concept for successful long-term pulmonary preservation in a dog model. Transplantation 1995; 59:1530–1536.

61. Venuta F, Rendina EA, Bufi M, et al. Preimplantation retrograde pneumoplegia in clinical lung transplantation. J Thorac Cardiovasc Surg 1999; 118:107–114.

62. Nguyen DQ, Salerno CT, Bolman RM, Park SJ. Pulmonary thromboembolectomy of donor lungs prior to lung transplantation. Ann Thorac Surg 1999; 67:1787–1789.

63. Kramer MR, Marshall SE, Tiroke A, Lewiston NJ, Starnes VA, Theodore J. Clinical significance of hyperbilirubinemia in patients with pulmonary hypertension undergoing heart-lung transplantation. J Heart Lung Transplant 1991; 10:317–321.

64. Lau CL, Palmer SM, Posther KE, et al. Influence of panel-reactive antibodies on post transplant outcomes in lung transplant recipients. Ann Thorac Surg 2000; 69:1520–1524.

65. Brugiere O, Thabut G, Castier Y, et al. Lung retransplantation for bronchiolitis obliterans syndrome: long-term follow-up in a series of 15 recipients. Chest 2003; 123:1832–1837.

66. Arcasoy SM, Christie JD, Pochettino A, et al. Characteristics and outcomes of patients with sarcoidosis listed for lung transplantation. Chest 2001; 120: 873–880.

67. Cassivi SD, Meyers BF, Battafarano PJ, et al. Thirteen-year experience in lung transplantation for emphysema. Ann Thorac Surg 2002; 74:1663–1669.

68. Chapelier A, Vouhe P, Macchiarini P, et al. Comparative outcome of heart–lung and lung transplantation for pulmonary hypertension. J Thorac Cardiovasc Surg 1993; 106:299–307.

69. Franke U, Wiebe K, Harringer W, et al. Ten years experience with lung and heart–lung transplantation in primary and secondary pulmonary hypertension. Eur J Cardiothorac Surg 2000; 18:447–452.

70. Dahlberg P, Savik K, Grubbs B, et al. Preoperative pulmonary artery pressure is associated with diminished survival after single lung transplantation for chronic obstructive pulmonary diseae. J Thorac Cardiovasc Surg. In press.

71. Conte JV, Borja MJ, Patel CB, Yang SC, Jhaveri RM, Orens JB. Lung transplantation for primary and secondary pulmonary hypertension. Ann Thorac Surg 2001; 72:1673–1679.

72. Trulock EP, Edwards LB, Taylor DO, et al. The Registry of the International Society for Heart and Lung Transplantation: twentieth official adult lung and heart–lung transplant report. J Heart Lung Transplant 2003; 22:625–635.

73. Aeba R, Griffith BP, Kormos RL, et al. Effect of cardiopulmonary bypass on early graft dysfunction in clinical lung transplantation. Ann Thorac Surg 1994; 57:715–722.

74. Szeto WY, Kreisel D, Karakousis GC, et al. Cardiopulmonary bypass for bilateral sequential lung transplantation in patients with chronic obstructive pulmonary disease without adverse effect on lung function or clinical outcome. J Thorac Cardiovasc Surg 2002; 124:241–249.

75. Pereszlenyi A, Lang G, Steltzer H, et al. Bilateral lung transplantation with intra- and postoperatively prolonged ECMO support in patients with pulmonary hypertension. Eur J Cardiothorac Surg 2002; 21:858–863.

76. Ko WJ, Chen YS, Luh SP, Chu SH. Extracorporeal membrane oxygenation support for single-lung transplantation in patients with primary pulmonary hypertension. Transplant Proc 1999; 31:166–168.

77. Ko WJ, Chen YS, Lee YC. Replacing cardiopulmonary bypass with extracorporeal membrane oxygenation in lung transplantation operations. Artif Organs 2001; 25:607–612.

78. Webert KE, Blajchman MA. Transfusion-related acute lung injury. Transfus Med Rev 2003; 17:252–262.

79. Ardehali A, Laks H, Russell H, et al. Modified reperfusion and ischemia-reperfusion injury in human lung transplantation. J Thorac Cardiovasc Surg 2003; 126:1929–1934.

80. Schnickel GT, Ross DJ, Beygui R, et al. Modified reperfusion in.clinical lung transplantation: the result of 100 consecutive cases. J Thorac Cardiovasc Surg 2006; 131:218–223.

81. The Acute Respiratory Distress Syndrome Network. Ventilation with lower tidal volumes as compared with traditional tidal volumes for acute lung injury and the acute respiratory distress syndrome. N Engl J Med 2000; 342:1301–1308.

82. Kopp R, Kuhlen R, Max M, Rossaint R. Evidence-based medicine in the therapy of the acute respiratory distress syndrome. Intensive Care Med 2002; 28:244–255.

83. Pelosi P, Tubiolo D, Mascheroni D, et al. Effects of the prone position on respiratory mechanism and gas exchange during acute lung injury. Am J Respir Crit Care Med 157:387–393.

84. Gattinoni L, Tognoni G, Pesenti A, et al. Effect of prone positioning on the survival of patients with acute respiratory failure. N Engl J Med 2001; 345:568–573.

85. Bacha EA, Herve P, Murakami S, et al. Lasting beneficial effect of short-term inhaled nitric oxide on graft function after lung transplantation. Paris-Sud

University Lung Transplantation Group. J Thorac Cardiovasc Surg 1996; 112:590–598.

86. Bacha EA, Sellak H, Murakami S, et al. Inhaled nitric oxide attenuates reperfusion injury in non-heart beating-donor lung transplantation. Paris-Sud University Lung Transplantation Group. Transplantation 1997; 63:1380–1386.

87. Karamsetty MR, Klinger JR. NO: more than just a vasodilator in lung transplantation. Am J Respir Cell Mol Biol 2002; 26:1–5.

88. Meade MO, Granton JT, Matte-Martyn A, et al. The Toronto Lung Transplant Program. A randomized trial of inhaled nitric oxide to prevent ischemia–reperfusion injury after lung transplantation. Am J Respir Crit Care Med 2003; 167:1483–1489.

89. Eppinger MJ, Ward PA, Jones ML, Boiling SF, Deeb GM. Disparate effects of nitric oxide on lung ischemia–reperfusion injury. Ann Thorac Surg 1995; 60:1169–1176.

90. Date H, Triantafillou AN, Trulock EP, Pohl MS, Cooper JD, Patterson GA. Inhaled nitric oxide reduces human lung allograft dysfunction. J Thorac Cardiovasc Surg 1996; 111:913–919.

91. Adatia L, Lillehei C, Arnold JH, et al. Inhaled nitric oxide in the treatment of postoperative graft dysfunction after lung transplantation. Ann Thorac Surg 1994; 57:1311–1318.

92. MacDonald P, Mundy J, Rogers P, et al. Successful treatment of life-threatening acute reperfusion injury after lung transplantation with inhaled nitric oxide. J Thorac Cardiovasc Surg 1995; 110:861–863.

93. Fiser SM, Cope JT, Kron IL, et al. Aerosolized prostacyclin (epoprostenol) as an alternative to inhaled nitric oxide for patients with reperfusion injury after lung transplantation. J Thorac Cardiovasc Surg 2001; 121(5):981–982.

94. Hohlfeld JM, Tiryaki E, Hamm H, et al. Pulmonary surfactant activity is impaired in lung transplant recipients. Am J Respir Crit Care Med 1998; 158:706–712.

95. Veldhuizen RA, Lee J, Sandler D, et al. Alterations in pulmonary surfactant composition and activity after experimental lung transplantation. Am Rev Respir Dis 1993; 148:208–215.

96. Strueber M, Cremer J, Harringer W, et al. Nebulized synthetic surfactant in reperfusion injury after single lung transplantation. J Thorac Cardiovasc Surg 1995; 110(2):563–564.

97. Strueber M, Hirt SW, Cremer J, et al. Surfactant replacement in reperfusion injury after clinical lung transplantation. Intensive Care Med 1995; 25:862–864.

98. Strueber M, Niedermeyer J, Warnecke G, et al. Exogenous surfactant instillation in lung donors to reduce early graft dysfunction. J Heart Lung Transplant 2003; 17:S14.

99. Zamora MR, Davis RD, Keshavjee SH, et al. Complement inhibition attenuates human lung transplant reperfusion injury: a multicenter trial. Chest 1999; 116:46S.

100. Wittwer T, Grote M, Oppelt P, Franke U, Schaefers HJ, Wahlers T. Impact of PAF antagonist BN 52021 (Ginkolide B) on post-ischemic graft function in clinical lung transplantation. J Heart Lung Transplant 2001; 20:358–363.

101. Meyers BF, Sundt TM III, Henry S, et al. Selective use of extracorporeal membrane oxygenation is warranted after lung transplantation. J Thorac Cardiovasc Surg 2000; 120:20–26.
102. Zenati M, Pham SM, Keenan PJ, Griffith BP. Extracorporeal membrane oxygenation for lung transplant recipients with primary severe donor lung dysfunction. Transplant Int 1996; 9:227–230.
103. Glassman LR, Keenan RJ, Fabrizio MC, et al. Extracorporeal membrane oxygenation as an adjunct treatment for primary graft failure in adult lung transplant recipients. J Thorac Cardiovasc Surg 1995; 110:723–727.
104. Nguyen DQ, Kulick DM, Bolman RM III, Dunitz JM, Hertz MI, Park SJ. Temporary ECMO support following lung and heart–lung transplantation. J Heart Lung Transplant 2000; 19:313–316.
105. Fiser SM, Kron IL, Long SM, Kasa AK, Kern JA, Tribble CG. Early intervention after severe oxygenation index elevation improves survival following lung transplantation. J Heart Lung Transplant 2001; 20:631–636.
106. Horowitz JH, Carrico CJ, Shires T. Pulmonary response to major injury. Arch Surg 1974; 108:349–355.
107. Whyte RI, Deeb GM, McCurry KR, Anderson HL III, Bolling SF, Bartlett RH. Extracorporeal life support after heart or lung transplantation. Ann Thorac Surg 1994; 58(3):754–758; discussion 758–759.
108. Dahlberg PS, Prekker ME, Hertz MI, Herrington CS, Park SJ. Medium term results of ECMO for severe acute lung injury following lung transplantation. J Heart Lung Transplant 2003; 22(suppl 1):S159–S160 [abstr 265].
109. Jurmann MJ, Schaefers HJ, Demertzis S, Haverich A, Wahlers T, Borst HG. Emergency lung transplantation after extracorporeal membrane oxygenation. ASAIO J 1993; 39(3):M448–M452.
110. Macha M, Griffith BP, Keenan R, et al. ECMO support for adult patients with acute respiratory failure. ASAIO J 1996; 42(5):M841–M844.
111. Novick RJ, Kaye MP, Patterson GA, et al. Redo lung transplantation: a North American–European experience. J Heart Lung Transplant 1993; 12:5–16.
112. Madill J, Gutierrez C, Grossman J, et al. Nutritional assessment of the lung transplant patient: body mass index as a predictor of 90-day mortality following transplantation. J Heart Lung Transplant 2001; 20:288–296.
113. Kramer MR, Marshall SE, Tiroke A, Lewiston NJ, Starns VA, Theodore J. Clinical significance of hyperbilirubinemia in patients with pulmonary hypertension undergoing heart–lung transplantation. J Heart Lung Transplant 1991; 10:317–321.
114. Boucek MM, Edwards LB, Keck BM, et al. The Registry of the International Society for Heart and Lung Transplantation: fifth official pediatric report. J Heart Lung Transplant 2002; 21:827–840.
115. Meyers BF, Lynch JP, Battafarano RJ, et al. Lung transplantation is warranted for stable, ventilator-dependent recipients. Ann Thorac Surg 2000; 70: 1675–1678.
116. Arcasoy SM, Kotloff RM. Lung transplantation. N Engl J Med 1999; 340:1081–1091.

117. Khan SU, Salloum J, O'Donovan PB, et al. Acute pulmonary edema after lung transplantation: the pulmonary reimplantation response. Chest 1999; 116:187–119.
118. Zaas D, Palmer SM. Respiratory failure after lung transplantation: now that we know the extent of the problem, what are the solutions? Chest 2003; 123:14–16.
119. Scornik JC, Zander DS, Baz MA, Donnelly WH, Staples ED. Susceptibility of lung transplants to preformed donor-specific HLA antibodies as detected by flow cytometry. Transplantation 1999; 68:1542–1546.

# 21

# Airway Complications in Lung Transplantation

**Luis F. Angel**

*Division of Pulmonary and Critical Care and Cardiothoracic Surgery,
Departments of Medicine and Surgery, University of Texas Health Science Center at
San Antonio, San Antonio, Texas, U.S.A.*

**Irawan Susanto**

*Division of Pulmonary and Critical Care and Hospitalists, Department of Medicine,
David Geffen School of Medicine at UCLA, University of California,
Los Angeles, California, U.S.A.*

## INTRODUCTION

Airway complications in lung transplant patients may involve the large central airways as well as the small airways. Airway complications related to the proximal large central conducting airways are often related to the bronchial anastomosis, while those related to the small airways are mostly related to chronic allograft rejection. This chapter discusses complications that pertain to large central conducting airways in lung transplant recipients. We describe the surgical approaches more commonly used for bronchial anastomosis as well as the posttransplant anastomotic complications and their management.

## ANATOMIC CONSIDERATIONS AND SURGICAL TECHNIQUES

As the field of solid organ transplantation emerged, the critical importance of all anastomoses was clearly appreciated as one of the key aspects in transplant surgery. Lung transplantation has not been an exception. In the early era of lung transplantation, dehiscence and healing problems of the bronchial anastomosis were a major source of complications, occurring in most of the patients who survived for more than one week (1,2). Despite changes in the surgical techniques, this continues to be an area in which complications commonly occur, with the major impact mostly in the first few weeks or months after transplantation, when the patients are recovering from surgery and having increased levels of immunosuppression.

The key aspects of the bronchial anastomosis in lung transplantation include the length of the anastomosis, the type of surgical anastomosis, the use of omental wrap, and the impact of immunosuppression, especially high doses of steroids, on anastomotic healing.

Both vascular and bronchial anastomosis may present with problems posttransplantation; however, more commonly, the complications are associated with the bronchial anastomosis. Since the introduction of transplantation as an alternative therapy for patients with end-stage pulmonary diseases, the issue of bronchial anastomosis has been an area of significant concern due to the lack of blood supply immediately post-transplant.

The bronchial circulation originates from the bronchial arteries that are direct branches of the aorta. The bronchial artery circulation is then lost during the harvest of the donor lung. Limited bronchial artery revascularization from the recipient bronchial arteries may take three to four weeks to occur after transplantation (3). During that period of time, the viability of the donor bronchus is then dependent on the retrograde low-pressure blood flow of the poorly oxygenated blood supply from the pulmonary artery (4).

Cooper and colleagues in Toronto demonstrated in the canine model of lung transplantation that when an omental pedicle was used to wrap the bronchial anastomosis, healing of the anastomosis improved at 23 days following reimplantation (5). They also demonstrated the adverse effects of high doses of prednisone and azathioprine on the strength of the anastomosis, compared to the transplanted animals with no immunotherapy or with cyclosporin only (6). The omental wrap around the anastomosis was then considered as the preferred surgical technique. The San Antonio group later reported a low incidence of anastomotic complications in 23 patients with telescoping bronchial anastomosis without an omental wrap (7). The anastomosis was created by telescoping the donor bronchus in overlapping fashion inside the recipient bronchus. Two subsequent clinical trials confirmed the safety of the telescoping anastomosis. The first trial came from the groups in St. Louis and Toronto, in which there was no difference in anastomotic complications in the group of patients who had end-to-end anastomosis, omental wrap, and no steroids, compared to another group of patients who had telescoping anastomosis without omental wrap and received high doses of steroids (8). The second trial came from the United Kingdom, in which the incidence of bronchial anastomotic complications after single-lung transplantation was not affected by wrapping the anastomosis with either omentum or an internal mammary artery pedicle (9).

Telescoping anastomosis without an omental wrap then became a popular technique. Recent studies, however, suggest that this type of anastomosis may increase the stenotic complications (10). The technique itself tends to create a relatively narrow airway due to the forced telescoping of the donor and recipient bronchi, resulting in a propensity toward bronchial stenosis (2,11,12). Currently, most of the anastomoses are done with an end-to-end single suture in the membranous portion of the bronchus and a single or continuous suture in the cartilaginous portion of the bronchus without an omental wrap. Telescoping of the anastomosis is done only when there is a natural difference in the size of the donor and recipient bronchus, so that there is a natural, unforced telescoping overlap at the site of the anastomosis (2,13).

Regardless of the technique utilized, the bronchial anastomosis remains a very ischemic area post-transplantation (14). Despite an apparent good initial view of the bronchial anastomosis in the operating room, most of the anastomoses become very inflamed and erythematous after transplantation, and some even demonstrate some degree of necrosis. The severity of this process seems to predispose the patient to future, more serious airway complications.

Perhaps the best way to minimize the anastomotic ischemia is by direct bronchial artery revascularization, which has been reported in small series with impressive angiographic findings, and associated with low anastomotic complication rates (15). The bronchial blood flow can be measured in an experimental model and it seems to correlate with fewer complications. However, this technique has not gained widespread use, largely because it is technically demanding, which results in an increase in the ischemic time, and in turn imposes an additional challenge to the surgeon.

The length of the bronchial anastomosis is another key aspect in lung transplantation. The initial animal models of lung transplantation and the human cases reported by the Toronto group support the hypothesis that shortening the distal or donor bronchus reduces anastomotic damage, probably because of better pulmonary-to-bronchial collateral blood supply. The common surgical practice is to create a short donor bronchus and a longer recipient bronchus (16,17). The recipient main bronchus is usually divided one ring above the origin of the upper lobe bronchus, then the bronchial arteries are ligated with no electrocautery and all the dissection is done with the "minimal" or "no touch" technique (13). This has significant clinical implications later if the patients develop anastomotic complications that may require airway stenting. When the anastomosis is located close to the bifurcation to lobar bronchi, stenting of the stenotic anastomosis may be challenging. In particular, the right bronchial anastomosis is usually too close to the right upper lobe take off, such that none of the currently available airway stents can be deployed at the anastomosis without breaching the right upper lobe orifice.

## AIRWAY COMPLICATIONS

The incidence of anastomotic complications has been decreasing with improving surgical techniques and increased experience with the procedure. The reported range of anastomotic complication rate varies widely. Part of the difficulty in assessing the true anastomotic complication rate is the lack of a standardized definition or consensus of what constitutes a complication, and which method is best for assessing the severity of the complication itself, whether by direct bronchoscopic visualization, radiographic imaging, or pulmonary function studies. Some centers have reported the incidence of anastomotic complications as high as 33%, while others as low as 1.6%. Most of the recent series suggest a range between 10% and 15% with a related mortality of 2% to 3% (14,18–20). In a retrospective series, finding *Aspergillus* in the bronchial washing significantly increases the risk of anastomotic complications (21). The healing of the anastomosis is classified according to the mucosal healing and/or bronchial wall necrosis (Table 1) (21). The severity of the bronchoscopic findings of anastomotic abnormalities appears to be an independent risk factor for anastomotic complications, which supports the assumption that bronchial ischemia is the main contributor of airway complications. The anastomotic airway complications are listed on Table 2. Bronchial stenosis is the most common complication reported (Table 3), and occurs about twice as often as bronchomalacia.

### Bronchial Dehiscence

Bronchial dehiscence is a potentially disastrous complication in the post transplant period; it is difficult to treat and is associated with high mortality. Partial or complete dehiscence of the anastomosis usually occurs early after transplantation, but has been reported to occur up to four years posttransplantation (18). The cause of anastomotic dehiscence is frequently attributed to ischemic necrosis, surgical or suturing technique, postoperative hypotension, and the use of high doses of perioperative corticosteroids.

**Table 1**  Bronchial Healing Grade Classification

| | |
|---|---|
| Grade 1 | Complete primary mucosal healing, no slough or necrosis, and anastomosis healing well |
| Grade 2 | Any necrotic mucosal slough reported, but no bronchial wall necrosis |
| Grade 3 | Limited focal necrosis <2 cm from the anastomotic site |
| Grade 4 | Extensive bronchial wall necrosis >2 cm from the anastomosis |

*Source*: From Ref. 21.

**Table 2** Classification of Airway Anastomosis
Complications

| |
| --- |
| Bronchial stenosis |
| Bronchomalacia |
| Exophytic granulation tissue |
| Anastomotic dehiscence |
| Anastomotic infections |
| Segmental nonanastomotic bronchial stenosis (22) |

*Source*: From Ref. 14.

Clinically, bronchial dehiscence may cause prolonged air leak in the early posttransplant period. In some cases, the dehiscence may also lead to infection or peribronchial abscess formation. The presence of extraluminal air around the anastomosis on chest CT has been reported to have a 100% sensitivity and 94% specificity for detection of anastomotic dehiscence (24). A definitive diagnosis, however, requires direct bronchoscopic examination and confirmation (Fig. 1).

The incidence of complete anastomotic dehiscence is low. Some lung transplant centers have not reported a single case of dehiscence. The reported morbidity and mortality vary considerably according to the severity of the dehiscence and the associated necrosis or infection of the airway. The management depends on the severity of the dehiscence and the

**Table 3** Clinical Studies Evaluating Anastomotic Complications

| | Number of patients | Surgical technique | Incidence of complications (%) | Most frequent complications |
| --- | --- | --- | --- | --- |
| Herrera et al. (21) | 123 | End-to-end | 24.4 | Stenosis |
| Alvarez et al. (18) | 90 | Telescoping | 6.8 | Stenosis |
| Kshettry et al. (14) | 102 | End-to-end (25%), the rest telescoping | 15 | Stenosis and infection |
| Schmid et al. (13) | 48 | End to end | 6 | Localized dehiscence |
| Date et al. (23) | 229 | End-to-end (50%) and telescoping (50%) | 12.8 | Stenosis and dehiscence |
| Wilson et al. (20) | 100 | End-to-end | 4 | Stenosis and dehiscence |

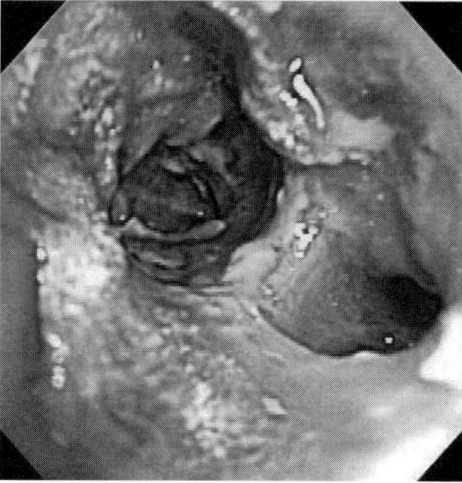

**Figure 1**  Anastomotic dehiscence.

symptoms of the patient. Patients with complete dehiscence frequently present with a persistent air leak, lung collapse, and pneumomediastinum. The management is surgical repair, with an attempt for reanastomosis of the airway or retransplant; however, the results of this urgent operation are usually poor, due to the concomitant necrosis and infection that are commonly present (18,23).

Incomplete or partial dehiscence may often respond to conservative management that includes frequent bronchoscopies to clear blood and necrotic tissue, chest or mediastinal tube drainage, and treatment of any documented infections (13,14). Aggressive antibiotic therapy in the case of documented infection may allow time for spontaneous healing of the anastomosis (13,14,18,23). In some cases, temporary stenting with a silicone or a covered metallic stent may be able to stop a persistent air leak or stabilize the anastomosis. However, bronchial stenting should not be done when there is an active infection of the anastomosis, and the use of bronchial balloon dilators should be avoided. As transplant programs mature, coupled with increasing transplant experience, meticulous surgical technique, and rigorous postoperative care, the prevalence of airway anastomosis dehiscence has consistently been decreasing.

## Rapamycin-Related Airway Complications

Rapamycin (sirolimus) has an antiproliferative mechanism of action that is different from that of the calcineurin inhibitors. The effects of rapamycin are not limited to lymphocytes; it also inhibits growth factor–induced proliferation of many cell types, including fibroblast, smooth muscle, and

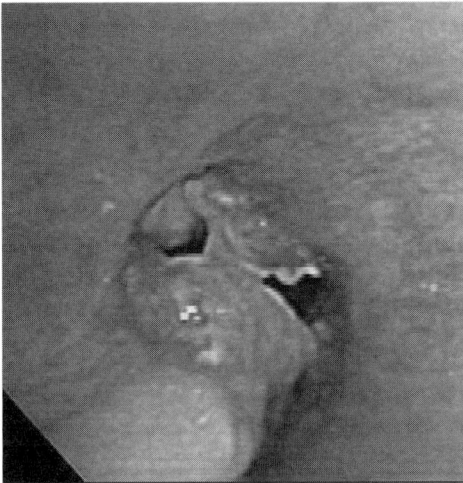

**Figure 2** Bronchial stenosis secondary to granulation tissue.

endothelial cells. These cells are essential for successful granulation tissue formation and wound healing. In clinical trials using rapamycin as one of the main immunosuppressants immediately posttransplant, airway complications were detected very early after transplantation (25). These patients suffered severe airway anastomotic complications including infection, poor healing, and dehiscence (26). As a result of these reports, the Food and Drug Administration (FDA) currently has a black box warning for the use of rapamycin for de novo therapy post lung transplant due to the risk of bronchial dehiscence.(23).

## Airway Obstruction

Airway obstruction in lung transplant recipients is the most common result of acute complications that occur at the anastomosis, such as necrosis or infection. Sometimes, airway obstruction may also be associated with a concomitant allograft rejection. Airway obstruction may manifest in the forms of bronchial stenosis, bronchomalacia, or endobronchial obstruction by granulation tissue (Table 2). Less commonly seen is bronchial web formation.

Bronchial stenosis is about twice as common as bronchomalacia as the cause or airway obstruction, and both may exist simultaneously (27). Bronchial obstruction is commonly associated with concurrent bronchial infection and/or rejection. Bronchial infection contributes to airway obstruction by eliciting excessive granulation tissue formation (Fig. 2) or by forming a stricture. Severe bronchial stenosis itself may also cause mucus

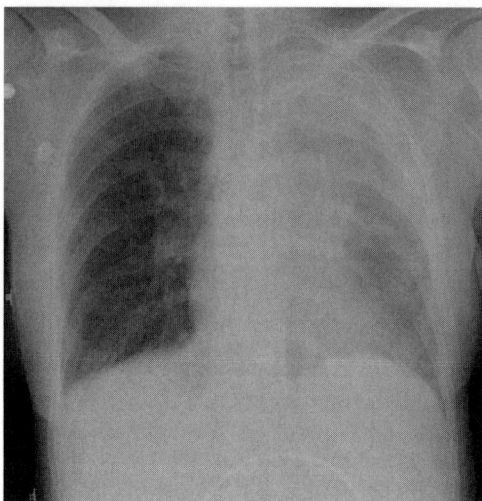

**Figure 3** Left upper lobe collapse.

and secretion retention, which may worsen the obstruction and predispose the patient to infection.

Bronchomalacia is commonly defined as >50% narrowing of the airway lumen on expiration. Therefore, for the most part, this is a bronchoscopic diagnosis, or a diagnosis suggested by the contrasting airway lumen size on dynamic inspiratory and expiratory CT scan. It is also common to find the combination of bronchial stenosis and bronchomalacia. Sometimes bronchial collapse becomes evident only after dilation of the airway stricture was successful. To adequately assess the presence of bronchomalacia, bronchoscopy should be performed under spontaneous breathing. The dynamic collapse of bronchomalacia may be missed if bronchoscopy is performed under general anesthesia with positive pressure ventilation.

The presenting symptoms and signs of obstruction include cough, dyspnea, and wheezing. While there is usually a worsening of the flow obstruction on spirometry, the flow volume loop is often nonspecific. Frequent findings on spirometry include a decrease in the $FEF_{25-75\%}$ with or without a significant decrease in the forced expiratory volume in one second ($FEV_1$). In some cases, the flow volume loop may demonstrate a decrease in the terminal flow, which normalizes upon successful dilation of the airway (28,29).

The initial management in patients with bronchial stenosis may include simple mechanical dilation, bronchoscopic airway debridement, stricture or web resection using laser or cryotherapy, and airway stenting (Figs. 3–6). Mechanical dilation of the stricture is usually the first intervention performed, but rarely provides a lasting effect. It usually provides a

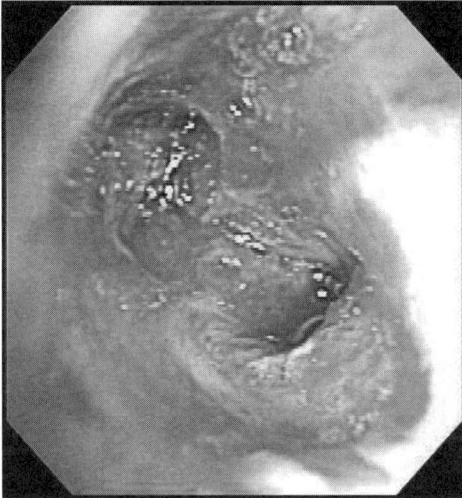

**Figure 4** Nonsegmental bronchial stenosis (left upper lobe).

temporary relief to the patients. Frequently, multiple procedures are required. Airway web formation generally can be successfully removed using endobronchial scissors, laser, or cryotherapy probes. When airway obstruction is caused primarily by granulation tissue formation, mechanical removal of the granulation using cryotherapy, and/or local injection of

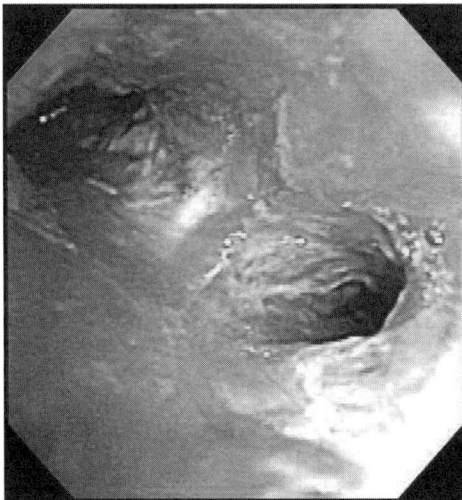

**Figure 5** Left upper lobe after balloon dilation.

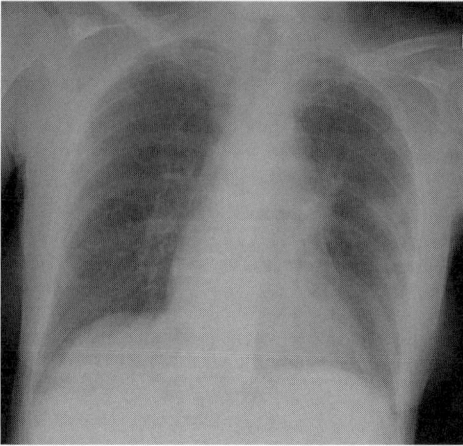

**Figure 6** Chest radiograph after dilation.

corticosteroids have generally been successful in preventing restenosis without the use of airway stents. The use of laser or electrocautery should be discouraged in patients with granulation tissue because they may potentially cause thermal burns deep beneath the mucosal tissues and induce more scarring and granulation tissue formation.

### Segmental Nonanastomotic Bronchial Stenosis

This complication is reported less frequently in lung transplant patients with an incidence around 3%. The characteristic finding is significant narrowing of the airways distal to the anastomosis. These cases are more frequently documented after three months posttransplant. It has been associated with ischemic or infectious complications in the immediate posttransplant period, although infections are not frequently seen at the time of the diagnosis. The nonanastomotic stenosis has been also reported in patients having multiple episodes of acute rejection, but it is not considered as a manifestation of chronic allograft dysfunction (22). Treatment of the underlying or associated infection and graft rejection may enhance the resolution of the stenosis (27).

Segmental nonanastomotic bronchomalacia that is symptomatic can be problematic. If there is an associated airway infection or rejection, treatment of these associated conditions may improve the bronchomalacia. Segmental bronchomalacia that persists following successful treatment of the associated or underlying infection or rejection may require long-term airway stenting. Diffuse bronchomalacia is not commonly seen, but can be a major management problem even with stenting.

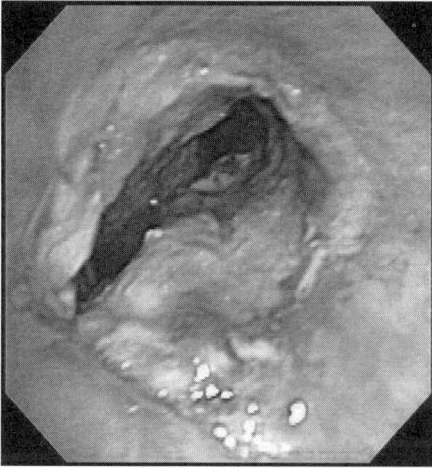

**Figure 7** Bacterial anastomotic infection with *Pseudomonas aeruginosa.*

## Infection

### Bacterial

Bacterial infections affecting the bronchial anastomosis are commonly observed in patients who have poor healing of the anastomosis. These infections are frequently polymicrobial, with gram-positive and gram-negative bacteria species, including *Staphylococcus aureus* and *Pseudomonas aeruginosa*. It is not uncommon also to have *Aspergillus* in the same setting (14). Treatment includes bronchoscopic debridement of the necrotic tissue, coupled with appropriate intravenous antimicrobial therapy, which is often required for prolonged periods of time until the cultures are negative and healing of the anastomosis is appreciated on bronchoscopy. Despite appropriate and successful treatment of the anastomotic infection, it is not uncommon to find subsequent sequelae, such as bronchial stenosis or bronchomalacia, that may require dilation or stent placement. Placement of a bronchial stent in general is not recommended during the acute phase, and is only done after the infection is under control or resolved (Fig. 7).

### Fungal

Saprophytic fungal organisms are easily airborne and thus have access to the airway lumen, and the relatively ischemic bronchial anastomosis provides an ideal environment for their proliferation. In addition to the airway ischemia, the high doses of steroids also increase the risk of infection. Patients with purulent lung disease and fungal airway colonization prior to lung transplantation, such as those with cystic fibrosis, or older patients

**Table 4** Spectrum of *Aspergillus* Disease on Lung Transplantation

|  | Definition | Frequency (%) | Therapy |
|---|---|---|---|
| Airway colonization | No clinical, endoscopic, radiologic, or pathologic evidence of invasive disease | 26 | Itraconazole or voriconazole or inhaled amphotericin B |
| Isolated tracheobronchitis | Endoscopic evidence of bronchial inflammation with no parenchymal disease | 4 | Itraconazole or voriconazole and inhaled amphotericin B |
| Invasive Aspergillosis | Radiologic evidence of nodules, cavities, infiltrates, or pleural disease with tissue invasion | 5 | Itraconazole or voriconazole systemic amphotericin B |

*Source*: From Ref. 32.

who undergo single-lung transplantation for emphysema appear to be at a higher risk of developing fungal infection (30,31). In some patients, a high inoculum of organisms may be present at the ischemic bronchial anastomosis immediately following the transplant. Table 4 summarizes the spectrum of *Aspergillus*-related diseases in lung transplant recipients.

The anastomotic and airway infections with *Aspergillus* are more common in the first few weeks up to six months post-transplantation (Fig. 8). The reported incidence varies according to different transplant programs and endemic areas, and usually ranges between 10% and 15%, but may be as high as 24% (31). The most common endoscopic findings are lesions ranging from erythema, bronchial inflammation, ulceration, and pseudomembrane formation to severe necrosis of the anastomotic area (13,30). Severe pseudomembranous tracheobronchitis may worsen a coexisting airway obstruction.

The impact of fungal infections, in particular with *Aspergillus*, is significant in lung transplant recipients. It carries a five-time relative risk for development of airway dehiscence, severe tracheobronchitis, bronchomalacia, bronchial stenosis, pneumonia, bronchopleural fistula, and even fatal hemorrhage (30,31).

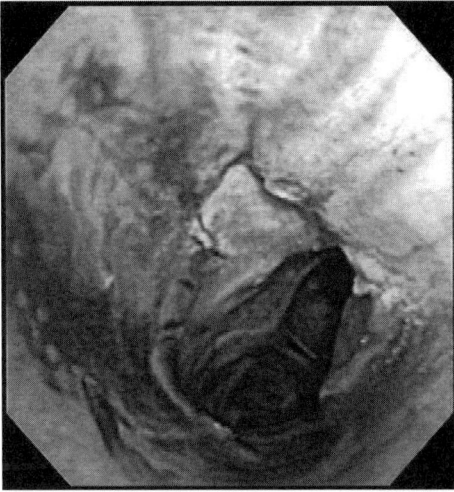

**Figure 8** Fungal anastomotic infection with *Aspergillus.*

Lung transplant centers have employed a number of strategies, including prophylaxis, mycologic surveillance, and early empiric treatment to reduce the incidence and the associated mortality of invasive aspergillosis in lung transplant recipients (33). Patients may be exposed to *Aspergillus* immediately after the transplant; therefore, environmental measures that decrease the airborne fungal spores and the use of antifungal prophylaxis are important considerations (34). The antifungal agent employed and the duration of prophylaxis remains controversial. The most commonly used agents are itraconazole and inhaled amphotericin B (33). More recently, voriconazole has been used for prophylactic and therapeutic purposes in patients at risk or with the diagnosis of *Aspergillus* infection. The vast majority of the transplant programs use one of these agents for a period of at least three months, which is the period of time when anastomotic infections with *Aspergillus* are more frequently documented.

## INTERVENTIONAL BRONCHOSCOPY FOR THE MANAGEMENT OF AIRWAY COMPLICATIONS

Bronchoscopy is an integral part of the management of patients after lung transplantation, not only as a diagnostic or surveillance method for graft infection or rejection, but also as a therapeutic tool in the management of airway complications post lung transplantation. Most of the transplant centers perform a flexible bronchoscopy immediately after the transplant to evaluate the anastomosis, and it is commonly repeated in the first 10 days to evaluate the healing of the anastomosis or for other clinical indications.

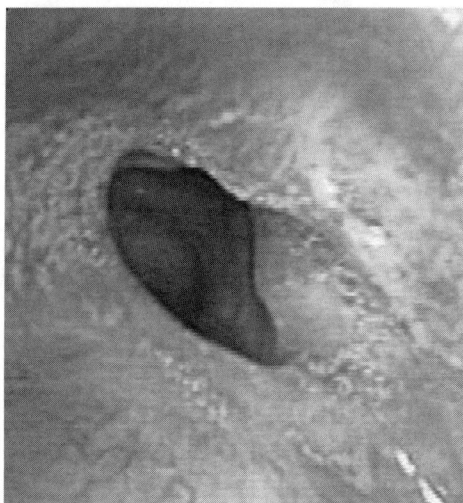

**Figure 9**  Anastomotic stenosis three months posttransplant.

Early in the post–lung transplant period, it is important not only to clear the airways from blood clots, thick secretions, and necrotic tissue, but also to define the degree of necrosis that may indicate poor anastomotic healing and obtain specimens for culture with bronchial washings and a protected specimen brush. This early diagnostic assessment helps in establishing the risk of future complications in the anastomosis and also in determining the need for continuation of empiric antimicrobial therapy or initiation of new antibiotics and antifungals for a documented infection. Early therapy in these patients is important in preventing some of the late airway complications.

Airway complications that require bronchoscopic intervention are reported to occur in around 13% of the patients, with a mean duration from transplantation to the diagnosis and interventional procedure of three months (35). The most commonly performed procedure is bronchial dilation for the treatment of bronchial stenosis. Bronchial dilations can usually be performed using a bronchial balloon dilator via a flexible bronchoscope. Rarely, the stricture is so hard that gentle radial laser cuts and rigid bronchoscopic dilation may become necessary. The dilations are usually repeated several times before a stent is placed, especially in patients with active infection, necrosis, and granulation tissue at the anastomosis. As a temporizing intervention, bronchial dilations allow more time for the acute process to heal in the setting of an acute infection, and provide the time frame for later reassessment if fibrotic stenosis would ensue. In our practice, we perform bronchial dilations first in the area of stenosis. We use cryotherapy to remove the active granulation tissue. If there is no evidence of infection, we would inject steroids locally in the stenotic area. When there

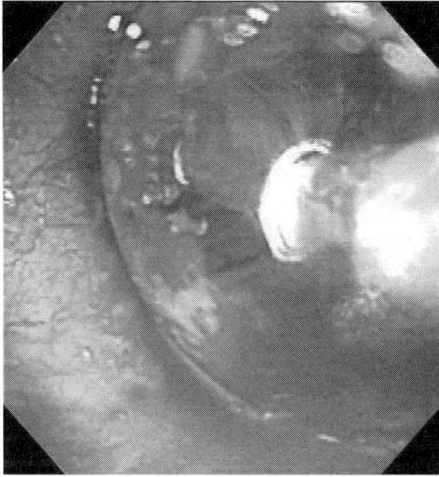

**Figure 10** Balloon dilation.

is recurrence or progression of the bronchial stenosis, the deployment of airway stents may become necessary to improve the stenosis and the pulmonary function (Figs. 9–12) (36,37). Occasionally, a circumferential hard fibrotic scar may form in the area of previous dilations. In this case, laser may be needed to cut the scar in a radial manner at two to four corners to allow the dilator to stretch the stricture, which frequently requires the use of a rigid bronchoscope or a rigid bougie, followed by a stent to keep the stricture stretched open. When laser cuts are used, it is important to do it in a radial fashion, not in a circumferential fashion, in order to preserve as much respiratory mucosa as possible to repopulate the cut area and prevent further scar formation.

There is still controversy on the ideal stent used for this particular indication. In many centers the use of stents is limited to silicone stents that require rigid bronchoscopy for placement, while in others the use of self-expandable stents has been reported with success (27,35,38). It is important to keep in mind that there is no ideal airway stent available as yet.

The advantage of a silicone stent is the ability to remove it with little damage to the respiratory mucosa, while providing a temporary prosthesis across the stenotic area for healing. The disadvantages include the need to use a rigid bronchoscope, and hence general anesthesia, for its deployment and retrieval, and the propensity for silicone stents to elicit mucus formation and mucostasis, which in turn increases the risk of airway colonization and infection by microorganisms.

The advantage of self-expandable metal stents includes the ease of placement using a flexible bronchoscope. In addition, a bare metal stent may

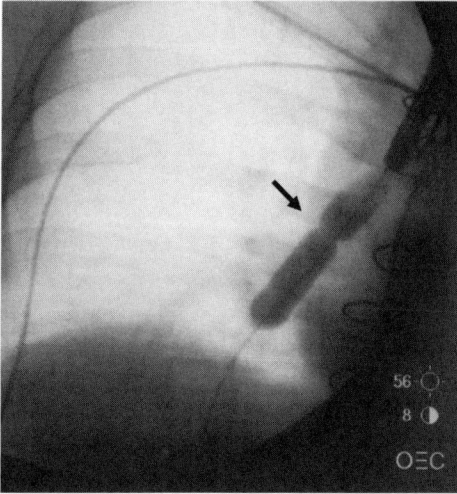

**Figure 11** Balloon dilation: area of stenosis (*arrow*).

allow partial re-epithelialization of the mucosal surface covered by the metal stent, thereby reestablishing the mucociliary transport and preventing mucostasis. However, in some cases, granulation tissue or the stenotic scar tissue can also grow past the open wire mesh and encroach into the airway lumen again (Fig. 13). These bare metal stents should be considered as permanent stents. Although bare metal stent removal is feasible and has been done, the stent is usually partially buried into the mucosal surface after a

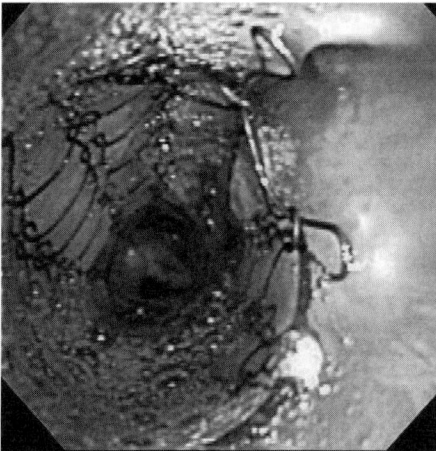

**Figure 12** Bronchial stenosis after metal stent placement.

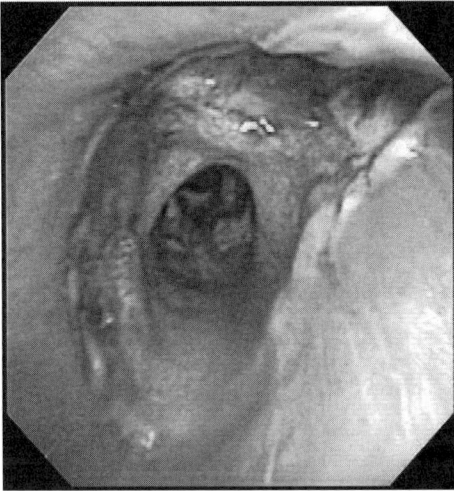

**Figure 13** Recurrent bronchial stenosis after placement of metal stent.

period of time, so that removal of the stent may be difficult and associated with significant damage to the underlying respiratory mucosa. A silicone covered metal stent has the advantage of ease of deployment using a flexible bronchoscope and the disadvantage of the risk of mucostasis.

## CONCLUSION

Ischemia, infection, and allograft rejection are common predisposing risk factors in the development of large airway complications post lung transplantation. Improved overall care and increasing experience with transplantation have decreased the incidence. Complete anastomotic dehiscence is rare, and usually requires surgical repair. Partial anastomotic dehiscence, bronchial stenosis, and bronchomalacia can usually be successfully managed conservatively using a combination of appropriate antimicrobial therapy for infection, enhanced immunosuppression for graft rejection, and interventional and therapeutic bronchoscopic techniques.

## REFERENCES

1. Cooper JD. The evolution of techniques and indications for lung transplantation. Ann Surg 1990; 212:249–255; discussion 255–246.
2. Aigner C, Jaksch P, Seebacher G, et al. Single running suture—the new standard technique for bronchial anastomoses in lung transplantation. Eur J Cardiothorac Surg 2003; 23:488–493.
3. Cooper JD, Patterson GA, Trulock EP. Results of single and bilateral lung transplantation in 131 consecutive recipients. Washington University Lung

Transplant Group. J Thorac Cardiovasc Surg 1994; 107:460–470; discussion 470–461.

4.  Barman SA, Ardell JL, Parker JC, et al. Pulmonary and systemic blood flow contributions to upper airways in canine lung. Am J Physiol 1988; 255: H1130–H1135.

5.  Morgan E, Lima O, Goldberg M, et al. Improved bronchial healing in canine left lung reimplantation using omental pedicle wrap. J Thorac Cardiovasc Surg 1983; 85:134–139.

6.  Goldberg M, Lima O, Morgan E, et al. A comparison between cyclosporin A and methylprednisolone plus azathioprine on bronchial healing following canine lung autotransplantation. J Thorac Cardiovasc Surg 1983; 85: 821–826.

7.  Calhoon JH, Grover FL, Gibbons WJ, et al. Single lung transplantation. Alternative indications and technique. J Thorac Cardiovasc Surg 1991; 101:816–824; discussion 824–815.

8.  Miller JD, DeHoyos A. An evaluation of the role of omentopexy and of early perioperative corticosteroid administration in clinical lung transplantation. The University of Toronto and Washington University lung transplant programs. J Thorac Cardiovasc Surg 1993; 105:247–252.

9.  Khaghani A, Tadjkarimi S, al-Kattan K, et al. Wrapping the anastomosis with omentum or an internal mammary artery pedicle does not improve bronchial healing after single lung transplantation: results of a randomized clinical trial. J Heart Lung Transplant 1994; 13:767–773.

10.  Garfein ES, Ginsberg ME, Gorenstein L, et al. Superiority of end-to-end versus telescoped bronchial anastomosis in single lung transplantation for pulmonary emphysema. J Thorac Cardiovasc Surg 2001; 121:149–154.

11.  Anderson MB, Kriett JM, Harrell J, et al. Techniques for bronchial anastomosis. J Heart Lung Transplant 1995; 14:1090–1094.

12.  Garfein ES, McGregor CC, Galantowicz ME, et al. Deleterious effects of telescoped bronchial anastomosis in single and bilateral lung transplantation. Ann Transplant 2000; 5:5–11.

13.  Schmid RA, Boehler A, Speich R, et al. Bronchial anastomotic complications following lung transplantation: still a major cause of morbidity? Eur Respir J 1997; 10:2872–2875.

14.  Kshettry VR, Kroshus TJ, Hertz MI, et al. Early and late airway complications after lung transplantation: incidence and management. Ann Thorac Surg 1997; 63:1576–1583.

15.  Pettersson G, Norgaard MA, Arendrup H, et al. Direct bronchial artery revascularization and en bloc double lung transplantation—surgical techniques and early outcome. J Heart Lung Transplant 1997; 16:320–333.

16.  Group TLT. Unilateral lung transplantation for pulmonary fibrosis. N Engl J Med 1986; 314:1140–1145.

17.  Pinsker KL, Koerner SK, Kamholz SL, et al. Effect of donor bronchial length on healing: a canine model to evaluate bronchial anastomotic problems in lung transplantation. J Thorac Cardiovasc Surg 1979; 77:669–673.

18.  Alvarez A, Algar J, Santos F, et al. Airway complications after lung transplantation: a review of 151 anastomoses. Eur J Cardiothorac Surg 2001; 19:381–387.

19. de Hoyos AL, Patterson GA, Maurer JR, et al. Pulmonary transplantation. Early and late results. The Toronto lung transplant group. J Thorac Cardiovasc Surg 1992; 103:295–306.

20. Wilson IC, Hasan A, Healey M, et al. Healing of the bronchus in pulmonary transplantation. Eur J Cardiothorac Surg 1996; 10:521–526; discussion 526–527.

21. Herrera JM, McNeil KD, Higgins RS, et al. Airway complications after lung transplantation: treatment and long-term outcome. Ann Thorac Surg 2001; 71: 989–993; discussion 993–984.

22. Hasegawa T, Iacono AT, Orons PD, et al. Segmental nonanastomotic bronchial stenosis after lung transplantation. Ann Thorac Surg 2000; 69:1020–1024.

23. Date H, Trulock EP, Arcidi JM, et al. Improved airway healing after lung transplantation. An analysis of 348 bronchial anastomoses. J Thorac Cardiovasc Surg 1995; 110:1424–1432; discussion 1432–1423.

24. Semenkovich JW, Glazer HS, Anderson DC, et al. Bronchial dehiscence in lung transplantation: CT evaluation. Radiology 1995; 194:205–208.

25. King-Biggs MB, Dunitz JM, Park SJ, et al. Airway anastomotic dehiscence associated with use of sirolimus immediately after lung transplantation. Transplantation 2003; 75:1437–1443.

26. Groetzner J, Kur F, Spelsberg F, et al. Airway anastomosis complications in de novo lung transplantation with sirolimus-based immunosuppression. J Heart Lung Transplant 2004; 23:632–638.

27. Susanto I, Peters JI, Levine SM, et al. Use of balloon-expandable metallic stents in the management of bronchial stenosis and bronchomalacia after lung transplantation. Chest 1998; 114:1330–1335.

28. Anzueto A, Levine SM, Tillis WP, et al. Use of the flow-volume loop in the diagnosis of bronchial stenosis after single lung transplantation. Chest 1994; 105:934–936.

29. Herlihy JP, Venegas JG, Systrom DM, et al. Expiratory flow pattern following single-lung transplantation in emphysema. Am J Respir Crit Care Med 1994; 150:1684–1689.

30. Singh N, Husain S. Aspergillus infections after lung transplantation: clinical differences in type of transplant and implications for management. J Heart Lung Transplant 2003; 22:258–266.

31. Nunley DR, Gal AA, Vega JD, et al. Saprophytic fungal infections and complications involving the bronchial anastomosis following human lung transplantation. Chest 2002; 122:1185–1191.

32. Mehrad B, Paciocco G, Martinez FJ, et al. Spectrum of Aspergillus infection in lung transplant recipients: case series and review of the literature. Chest 2001; 119:169–175.

33. Levine SM. A survey of clinical practice of lung transplantation in North America. Chest 2004; 125:1224–1238.

34. Patterson JE, Peters J, Calhoon JH, et al. Investigation and control of aspergillosis and other filamentous fungal infections in solid organ transplant recipients. Transpl Infect Dis 2000; 2:22–28.

35. Chhajed PN, Malouf MA, Tamm M, et al. Interventional bronchoscopy for the management of airway complications following lung transplantation. Chest 2001; 120:1894–1899.

36. Chhajed PN, Malouf MA, Tamm M, et al. Ultraflex stents for the management of airway complications in lung transplant recipients. Respirology 2003; 8:59–64.
37. Burch C, Angel L, Levine S. Spirometric improvement following bronchial balloon dilatation/stent placement for bronchial stenosis after lung transplantation. National Meeting of the American College of Chest Physicians, 2002.
38. Lonchyna VA, Arcidi JM Jr, Garrity ER Jr, et al. Refractory post-transplant airway strictures: successful management with wire stents. Eur J Cardiothorac Surg 1999; 15:842–849; discussion 849–850.

# 22

# Viral Infections Complicating Lung and Solid Organ Transplantation

**Martin R. Zamora**

*Division of Pulmonary Sciences and Critical Care Medicine, University of Colorado Health Sciences Center, Denver, Colorado, U.S.A.*

## INTRODUCTION

Viral infections are increasingly recognized as a serious problem in lung-transplant recipients. In addition to their direct effects of tissue injury and clinical illness, they produce indirect effects that may lead to long-term adverse sequelae in the lung allograft. The herpesviruses, which include cytomegalovirus (CMV), Epstein–Barr virus (EBV), herpes simplex virus 1 and 2 (HSV-1 and –2), varicella–zoster virus (VZV), and human herpesvirus 6, 7, and 8 (HHV-6, -7, and -8) have important immunomodulatory effects in addition to their direct infectious effects. The community-acquired respiratory viruses (CARV), such as respiratory syncytial virus (RSV), para-influenza virus (PIV), influenza A and B, adenovirus, and rhinovirus, are increasingly recognized as important pathogens in lung-transplant recipients. Newly described viruses, such as human metapneumovirus (hMPV), or emerging viruses, such as West Nile virus (WNV) or severe acute respiratory syndrome coronavirus (SARS-CoV), are being reported in increasing frequency in transplant recipients. Development of potent oral antiviral agents, molecular techniques for the detection of infection, and its response to therapy and the emergence of isolates with antiviral resistance have had significant impacts on the approach to viral infections in these patients. This chapter discusses the individual pathogens, prevention strategies in the era

of potent oral antiviral agents, the role of new diagnostic techniques, treatment regimens for established viral infection or disease, and their potential
impact on the indirect effects of these viruses on long-term allograft function, and the incidence, risk factors, and impact of antiviral resistance.
Understanding the pleiotropic effects of these viruses is important for the
development of comprehensive management strategies for viral infections
following lung transplantation.

## THE HERPESVIRUSES

The human herpesviridae (HHVs) family consists of eight members. Based
on conserved structural proteins, they can be divided into three subfamilies:
α, β, and γ. They share the ability to develop lifelong latency or persistence in
their host and to reactivate during the development of relative immunosuppression that occurs in transplant recipients. These viruses are pleiotropic.
In addition to their direct infectious effects, they exhibit a number of indirect
effects including immunomodulation, effects on angiogenesis, and tumor-
genesis. Their indirect effects may be more important than their direct effects.
The β-herpesvirinae, including CMV and HHV-6 and -7, are increasingly
recognized as major causes of morbidity and mortality in transplant recipients. CMV is associated with well-defined syndromes usually involving the
transplanted organ. HHV-6 is associated with pneumonitis, hepatitis, and
encephalitis. HHV-7 has yet to be linked to any clinical syndrome in transplant patients, but appears to facilitate the reactivation of CMV and
HHV-6. The γ-herpesvirinae, EBV, and HHV-8 are transforming viruses;
they have proven oncogenic potential. EBV causes mononucleosis and is
the etiologic agent of post-transplant lymphoproliferative disease (PTLD).
HHV-8 is the cause of Kaposi's sarcoma KS and has been termed the KS herpesvirus (KSHV). The α-herpesvirinae include HSV-1 and -2 and VZV.
HSV-1 and HSV-2 are neurotropic, causing perioral fever blisters, genital
ulcerations, and, rarely, encephalitis. Varicella-zoster causes chickenpox
(varicella) in childhood. Reactivation occurs in the immunosuppressed
patients and the elderly and typically manifests as shingles (zoster) that is
self-limited but may be complicated by postherpetic neuralgia.

### Cytomegalovirus

CMV is the most important pathogen following lung transplantation (1–3).
Anti-CMV antibodies are present in 65% to 90% of adults. Primary CMV
infection typically occurs in the first two decades of life and may present as
an asymptomatic infection or a mononucleosis-like syndrome. While cell-
mediated immunity and neutralizing antibodies develop, through mechanisms of immune system evasion, CMV establishes latency and intermittently
reactivates, producing low-level viral persistence. Host cells allowing latent
virus are hematopoietic progenitor cells, peripheral blood mononuclear cells,

leukocytes, and macrophages. CMV also infects endothelial cells, smooth muscle cells, and fibroblasts. Anti-CMV immune cells control the low-level viral persistence to keep the infection at a subclinical state but this immune stimulation may have important effects on the transplanted organ (4).

### Risk of CMV Infection and Disease in Lung-Transplant Recipients

The incidence of CMV infection and disease following lung transplantation in the postganciclovir era ranges from 30% to 86% with an associated mortality rate of 2% to 12% (1). Accepted risk factors for the development of CMV post-transplant are innate host immunity, the type of organ transplanted with its associated viral burden, viral coinfection, the net state of immunosuppression, allograft rejection, sepsis, and stress associated with critical illness. The latter three conditions are associated with cytokine production, particularly high levels of tumor necrosis factor-$\alpha$ (TNF-$\alpha$), which upregulates the CMV promoter gene leading to viral replication (2). Three potential mechanisms of CMV infection have been recognized: primary infection due to transmission by the donor organ or blood products, reactivation of latent virus, or superinfection due to the donor organ strain or new infections. Primary infection occurs in nearly all CMV-seronegative recipients of a seropositive organ. The lack of CMV-specific immunity in the seronegative patient leads to rapid viral replication. In the absence of CMV prophylaxis, CMV reactivation occurs in most seropositive transplant recipients 3 to 12 weeks posttransplant.

There is a general consensus that seronegative lung or heart–lung recipients of CMV positive organs are at the highest risk of developing severe, sometimes fatal disease (5). Presence of antibody to CMV in the recipient, whether endogenous or passively transferred, provides partial protection against the development of serious and fatal disease. Absent endogenous antibody protection, primary CMV infections, particularly CMV pneumonitis or gastrointestinal disease, may be quite severe with mortality rates of 2% to 20% (6). Lung transplantation involves the transfer of large amounts of lymphatic tissue harboring greater amounts of latent CMV than other organs, theoretically increasing the risk and severity of CMV infection (7). Therefore, many physicians and surgeons recommend that all lung-transplant recipients should be considered high-risk. Coinfection with other $\beta$-herpesviruses (HHV-6 and HHV-7) with inherent immunomodulating properties enhances CMV replication (8). Use of anti-lymphocytic antibodies for induction therapy or treatment of steroid-resistant rejection increases the rate of CMV reactivation (9).

### Clinical Syndromes

CMV infection is defined by isolation of the virus or by demonstration of its presence by immunologic or molecular techniques or by seroconversion.

Currently available techniques include the shell vial assay, pp65 antigenemia, polymerase chain reaction (PCR), or hybrid capture assays for CMV DNAemia. CMV disease is diagnosed by histologic evidence of tissue invasion or a characteristic syndrome after exclusion of other etiologies in the presence of CMV infection (10).

CMV infections in lung-transplant recipients range from asymptomatic viremia to severe, life-threatening disease. CMV infection without end organ involvement is termed CMV syndrome and manifests as fever, myalgias, arthralgias, and leukopenia or thrombocytopenia. CMV disease is due to organ invasion and characteristic syndromes including pneumonitis, gastroenteritis, colitis, hepatitis, and, rarely, encephalitis. The transplanted organ is commonly the site of infection. Therefore, CMV pneumonitis is most common in lung and heart-lung–transplant recipients. The predisposition to the transplanted organ may be related to ischemia–reperfusion injury, the viral burden in that organ, and a lack of host CMV–specific immunity to the donor strain. CMV pneumonitis manifests as fever, cough, shortness of breath or dyspnea, hypoxemia, and interstitial infiltrates on chest X ray.

In addition to its direct effects due to tissue injury and clinical illness, CMV is associated with a number of indirect effects that may lead to long-term adverse sequelae in the lung allograft. Accumulating evidence suggests that the indirect effects of CMV may be at least as important as its direct effects. CMV has been associated with, though not causally linked to, the development of acute and chronic rejection via mechanisms of enhanced allorecognition (11). Potential immunomodulatory effects of CMV may predispose patients to infection with opportunistic organisms or the development of PTLD (12,13). CMV increases the costs associated with solid organ transplants by 40% to 50% (14–16). The frequency of occurrence of these complications has prompted various strategies for the prevention, early diagnosis and treatment, and monitoring of CMV infection. While there is general consensus that seronegative recipients of seropositive organs are at the highest risk of severe disease and require prophylaxis (5) despite more than a decade of experience with lung transplantation and ganciclovir availability, management of the CMV-seropositive recipient remains controversial.

### CMV and Acute and Chronic Allograft Injury

The relationship between CMV and allograft injury is bidirectional (17). Cytokines, chemokines, and growth factors are induced in response to both CMV infection and rejection resulting in activation of the vascular endothelium and inflammatory cells. The proinflammatory cytokine, TNF, is a key signal in reactivating CMV from latency. TNF-induced activation of protein kinase C and nuclear factor-$\kappa$B (NF$\kappa$B) leads to expression of CMV immediate early proteins triggering the onset of viral replication. Since TNF is released during allograft rejection, it is not surprising that CMV reactivation occurs in response to acute rejection. Intensified immunosuppression to treat rejection can amplify viral replication; following antilymphocyte agents, the incidence of CMV disease increases from 10% to 15% to 65% (1).

CMV infection of the vascular endothelium and smooth muscle cells likely plays an important role in the pathogenesis of vascular injury seen in acute and chronic rejection. CMV upregulates endothelial adhesion molecules, such as vascular cell adhesion molecule (VCAM), intracellular adhesion molecule (ICAM), lymphocyte function antigen-1 (LFA-1), and very late antigen-4 (VLA-4), increasing the number of inflammatory cells in the graft. Injury may also occur via molecular mimicry; sequence homology and immunologic cross-reactivity between CMV immediate early antigens and the human leukocyte antigen–DR B chain have been demonstrated and CMV induces a glycoprotein homologous to major histocompatibility complex (MHC) class I antigens (18). CMV also induces antiendothelial cell antibodies that may participate directly in the development of chronic rejection. While CMV prophylaxis has been shown to decrease the incidence of acute rejection, therapy of established disease with ganciclovir alone may not prevent the long-term sequelae of CMV-induced graft injury (11). Addition of immunoglobulin preparations, which have immunomodulatory properties, may be required to limit acute inflammatory events and the progression to chronic allograft injury. Similar strategies have shown efficacy in bone marrow–transplant recipients in decreasing graft versus host disease (19).

In lung transplant recipients, CMV has been associated with chronic allograft injury or bronchiolitis obliterans syndrome (BOS), the major limiting factor to long-term survival after lung transplantation. CMV pneumonitis and positive CMV serology may be risk factors for BOS; however, these associations are still debated (11,20–23). Given that BOS is typically progressive despite augmented immunosuppressive therapy, strategies to prevent BOS are paramount in controlling this devastating complication of lung transplantation. Prevention and treatment of CMV infections may therefore be important strategies to limit the development of BOS.

### Strategies to Prevent CMV Infection

Based on the potential mechanisms of infection, four strategies to prevent CMV infection have been utilized: matching the donor–recipient pair by CMV serologic status, use of CMV negative blood products, antiviral agents to suppress viral replication, and immunoglobulin preparations to provide passive immunization. The use of CMV-negative or leukocyte-reduced blood products clearly decreases the incidence of CMV transmission and infection following lung transplantation (22). In CMV-negative bone marrow–transplant recipients, seronegative blood results in an incidence of CMV infection transmission of 1.3%, while leukocyte-reduced CMV-positive blood results in a transmission rate of 2.4% with CMV disease rates of 0% and 2.4%, respectively (24). Therefore, it seems prudent to strictly adhere to the use of

CMV-negative blood products in seronegative lung-transplant recipients. Seromatching recipients and donors may be ideal, but is impractical given the current shortage of donor organs. Furthermore, seromatching, while perhaps desirable, is most likely no longer necessary to prevent the direct effects on morbidity and mortality given the efficacy of antivirals and immunoglobulins in decreasing the incidence and severity of primary CMV infections. However, caution may still be warranted when performing CMV-mismatched transplants as the long-term sequelae of CMV infections on allograft function remains unknown. Many retrospective or case-controlled series have demonstrated the benefit of antivirals or immunoglobulin preparations alone or in combination in decreasing or delaying the onset of CMV infection following lung transplantation. However, to date, primarily due to the lack of randomized, controlled trials comparing regimens, the "ideal" strategy for the prevention, monitoring, and treatment of CMV remains controversial.

### Monitoring Techniques

Rapid and accurate diagnostic tests are critical for the appropriate management of CMV following lung transplantation. Qualitative or quantitative PCR using serum, plasma, whole-blood or circulating peripheral blood leukocytes, or the pp65 antigenemia test is efficacious in solid organ–transplant and bone marrow–transplant recipients (25–30). The hybrid capture assay, a non-PCR, molecular, quantitative, and highly sensitive assay has been shown to be effective in lung-transplant recipients (31,32). Each test has distinct advantages and disadvantages. The quantitative PCR and hybrid capture assays are fully quantitative, molecular techniques. Qualitative PCR is much less useful. PCR requires radioactive probes and most centers use "homemade primers," thereby precluding standardization. Controversy exists as to the most appropriate type of sample for PCR testing: peripheral blood cells, serum, plasma, or whole blood. Whole blood may be the preferred sample source, as Humar et al. (33) recently showed the sensitivity of quantitative plasma viral load measurements was only 38% in solid organ recipients, which was confirmed by Chemaly et al. (34) in lung-transplant recipients. The specific type of sample employed should be validated within the individual center. The pp65 antigenemia assay is only semiquantitative (read as number of positive cells), although the readings can be used in the same way by clinicians experienced in its interpretation. This assay may be more labor intensive in that the cells need to be spun and placed on slides within six hours on arrival ats the laboratory.

The value of a quantitative assay, such as viral load, is seen by its increased utilization by clinicians for assessing or predicting the severity of illness or impending illness (35). Weinberg et al. (36) evaluated serial CMV blood cultures, antigenemia, and qualitative and quantitative plasma PCR tests for their value in predicting CMV disease and for guiding preemptive therapy after lung transplantation. PCR and antigenemia tests were the most effective predictors of symptomatic CMV infections and the response to therapy. CMV PCR-measured DNA increased 5- to 10-fold immediately preceding symptoms and PCR and antigenemia levels decreased with anti-CMV therapy. A number of these monitoring tests are commercially available and regardless of which method is chosen the technique should be validated in each individual transplant center.

### Prophylaxis of CMV Infection

Prior to the development of effective antiviral agents, CMV caused illness in the majority of lung-transplant recipients and primary infection in D+/R− recipients was severe and often life-threatening (37). Following the development of ganciclovir, it soon became clear that the acute morbidity and mortality of CMV infections could be controlled with therapeutic courses of intravenous ganciclovir. Investigators then sought to determine whether prophylactic use of ganciclovir or other agents could prevent CMV infection and disease following lung transplantation. Most approaches involved universal prophylaxis in which all patients receive prophylaxis for a predetermined amount of time. This strategy aims at complete viral elimination, but is associated with increased costs, toxicities, and the possibility of the development of resistance.

While it is difficult to summarize and compare the published reports on CMV prophylaxis in lung-transplant recipients as they utilized different lengths of prophylaxis in patients receiving different immunosuppressive strategies based on the year of transplant, the published studies can be categorized as those employing ganciclovir or immunoglobulin monotherapy or combination strategies.

**Ganciclovir monotherapy:** Short courses of prophylactic ganciclovir (two to three weeks) delayed the onset of CMV infection but had limited efficacy in preventing CMV infection or disease (20,38). Extended prophylactic therapy with ganciclovir for 6 to 12 weeks suggested that prolonged ganciclovir infusion decreased the incidence of CMV infection and disease (39); however, this benefit was lost when patients were followed more than one year post-transplant (40). These reports point out the importance of long-term follow-up when comparing published reports and confirm that ganciclovir monotherapy delays rather than prevents the onset of CMV infection following lung transplantation (Table 1).

The largest prospective trial utilizing ganciclovir monotherapy was reported by Hertz et al. (41). Ganciclovir was given intravenously for three months posttransplant either daily or thrice weekly. No significant differences were seen between groups with respect to freedom from CMV infection or disease or in the incidence of BOS. CMV disease developed in 18/35 (51%) of the daily patients versus 11/37 (30%) of the thrice-weekly patients and

**Table 1**  Intravenous Ganciclovir for CMV Prophylaxis Following Lung
or Heart–Lung Transplantation (North American Centers)

| Author, institution (Ref.) | N | CMV prophylaxis | CMV onset | Outcome |
|---|---|---|---|---|
| Duncan et al., Pittsburgh (11) | 13 | GCV × 3 weeks ACY × 2 months | 72 | 5/13 Inf (38%) 2/13 Dz (15%) |
| Duncan et al., Pittsburgh (20) | 13 | GCV × 90 days | 268 | 8/13 Inf (58%) |
| Kelly et al., Seattle (40) | 21 | GCV × 6 weeks | 145 | 17/21 Inf (81%) 8/21 Dz (38%) |
| Soghikian et al., Stanford (38) | 52 L + HL | GCV × 5 weeks | 85 | 42/52 Inf (86%) 27/52 Dz (55%) |
| Hertz et al., Minneosta (41) | 35 37 | GCV qd × 90 days GCV 3 ×/week × 90 days | NR | 18/35 Dz (51%) 11/37 Dz (30%) |
| Total | 171 | | | Inf 101/171 (59.1%) Dz 66/158 (41.8%) |

*Abbreviations*: CMV, cytomegalovirus; *N*, number of patients in a series receiving intravenous ganciclovir; L + HL, lung and heart–lung transplants; GCV, ganciclovir; ACY, acyclovir; IVIG, standard intravenous immunoglobulin; NR, not reported; Inf, infection; Dz, disease.

emerged shortly after termination of prophylaxis. While prolonged thrice-weekly ganciclovir prophylaxis was as effective as daily administration at delaying the onset of CMV infections, it was still associated with patient inconvenience, catheter-related infections, and increased costs.

An alternative strategy to prolonged infusion of ganciclovir is the use of oral ganciclovir. Bhorade et al. (32) found that 12 weeks of oral ganciclovir (3 g/day) decreased the incidence of CMV to levels similar to those seen with intravenous ganciclovir. CMV disease developed in 10/34 (29%) lung transplant recipients with an average onset of four months. However, 24% of the patients developed asymptomatic, breakthrough viremia. While none of these patients developed CMV disease, this breakthrough viremia may predispose to or be a marker of the emergence of ganciclovir resistance (42).

The availability of valganciclovir (VGCV), which provides antiviral exposure similar to intravenous ganciclovir (comparable area under the curves), obviates the need for prolonged intravenous access and allows prolonged high-level antiviral exposure. VGCV was at least as effective as oral ganciclovir in preventing CMV infections and produced more complete viral suppression without the development of antiviral resistance in solid organ recipients (43).

When the published results of intravenous ganciclovir monotherapy are pooled, the incidence of CMV infection and disease following lung transplantation remains 59% and 42%, respectively (Table 1). While differing lengths of prophylaxis and types of immunosuppression were employed in these studies, taken in sum, these data suggest that while ganciclovir decreases the incidence of CMV infections compared to placebo or oral acyclovir, there is still a significant incidence of CMV infection following lung transplantation with ganciclovir monotherapy strategies.

**CMV immune globulin monotherapy:** An alternative strategy to ganciclovir monotherapy is CMV hyperimmune globulin (CMV–IVIG). Maurer reported an incidence of CMV pneumonitis of 28% in patients receiving CMV–IVIG alone (44). Similarly, Gould et al. (45) reported an incidence of CMV disease of 23%. However, a more recent study found that CMV–IVIG alone did not prevent CMV viremia or pneumonitis (46). While this suggests that a randomized, controlled trial comparing these regimens is warranted, it also begs the question as to whether combination prophylaxis with both agents may be more efficacious in the prevention of CMV following lung transplantation.

**Combination prophylaxis:** Bailey et al. (47) reported an 86% incidence of CMV pneumonitis in D+/R− recipients treated with two to three weeks of intravenous ganciclovir and standard IVIG. Maurer et al. (44) reported significant decreases in CMV pneumonitis in patients receiving CMV–IVIG and either ganciclovir or oral acyclovir (41% vs. 67%). Further, survival in the combination therapy group approached that seen when both donor and recipient were seronegative. Similarly, we have reported that CMV–IVIG in combination with ganciclovir decreased the incidence of CMV disease to 21% and of infection to 31%, decreased their severity, and delayed their onset (48). Valantine et al. (49,50) reported improved outcomes with fewer infections, decreased acute rejection and BOS at 12 and 24 months in the combined therapy group compared to a ganciclovir-only group. Similarly, Weill et al. (51) found that despite induction therapy with daclizumab, when compared to a historical, case-controlled group receiving ganciclovir alone, combination prophylaxis decreased the incidence of CMV disease from 33% to 8%.

Recently, we found that following universal prophylaxis with GCV and CMV–IVIG, VGCV was safe and effective for the prevention of CMV in lung-transplant recipients (52). Continuing VGCV for a total prophylactic period of 180 days was as effective as longer courses of prophylaxis and more efficacious than 100 days or less of prophylaxis.

Preemptive Therapy

Some centers advocate preemptive therapy based on the detection of CMV antigenemia or DNAemia in routinely collected blood samples. The advantage of this strategy is that only high-risk patients are exposed to therapy that would be expected to decrease cost and toxicity. Several small studies have suggested that this approach is indeed efficacious in lung-transplant recipients. Egan et al. (26) showed that preemptive treatment of CMV infection, as determined by antigenemia, prevented progression to CMV disease in heart- and lung-transplant recipients. Kelly et al. (53) found that preemptive therapy directed by the antigenemia assay was as effective as universal prophylaxis with six weeks of intravenous ganciclovir and concluded that it was also more cost-effective. There are several potential disadvantages of preemptive therapy: (i) in large geographic regions, it may be difficult to routinely obtain blood samples from the patients, (ii) the cost of surveillance may be high, and (iii) some patients escape detection and present with severe CMV disease. The latter was a problem in the report by Kelly et al.: 5/19 patients presented with CMV pneumonitis and the antigenemia test revealed zero positive cells (53,54). Such problems with sensitivity and specificity await clarification in larger cohorts of lung-transplant recipients. We and others have found that a high viral load was associated with a high degree of progression to symptomatic disease and that following universal prophylaxis, routine monitoring followed by preemptive therapy was effective in preventing the progression to symptomatic disease (32,35). Therefore, our center advocates universal prophylaxis followed by routine viral load monitoring at scheduled clinic visits and preemptive therapy of viremic episodes.

### Treatment

Standard therapy for CMV disease consists of two to four weeks of intravenous ganciclovir at a dosage of 5 mg/kg twice daily adjusted for renal insufficiency. Duncan et al. (11) found that treatment with intravenous ganciclovir as monotherapy did not prevent the long-term sequelae of CMV, which is of concern. Although no randomized, controlled treatment trials are available for the use of CMV–IVIG for therapy in organ transplant recipients, many centers add it to ganciclovir for the treatment of tissue invasive CMV pneumonia or colitis. Studies in bone marrow–transplant patients with CMV pneumonitis and murine models of disseminated CMV infection suggest that the combination of ganciclovir and CMV–IVIG may provide significant benefits to immunosuppressed recipients with invasive disease (1,55).

Another potential benefit for immunoglobulin therapy may be as replacement therapy in patients with occult hypogammaglobulinemia (56). In these patients, tissue-invasive CMV as well as other infectious complications were more common in the lowest IgG group. Recently, immunoglobulin replacement has been shown to decrease acute rejection and infection in heart-transplant recipients with hypogammaglobulinemia (57).

The vast majority of isolates causing first episodes of CMV infections in lung-transplant recipients are ganciclovir sensitive. Despite this, oral ganciclovir, due to its low biovailability, has no role in the treatment of symptomatic infection as it may select out resistant clones of CMV when there are high viral loads and active viral proliferation. However, oral ganciclovir may have a role in the prevention of relapsing symptomatic disease. The risk of recurrent disease ranges from 20% in seropositive recipients to 60% in those with primary disease (58). The use of oral ganciclovir for three months following a full course of intravenous therapy may decrease the risk of recurrent disease by up to 50% (59,60). Whether the use of combination therapy followed by oral ganciclovir or VGCV decreases the risk of recurrence further is presently unknown.

Antiviral Resistance

Antiviral-resistant CMV is increasing in all solid organ transplants and is particularly problematic following lung transplantation with an incidence of 3% to 16% (61). These estimates are imprecise as most of the data have been collected retrospectively and there is significant variability among centers (62), some of which is due to the fact that genotypic testing of isolates provides greater sensitivity in detecting resistance than the culture-based methods in use at most centers. Antiviral resistance has been associated not only with treatment failure, but also with poor long-term allograft function and decreased patient survival. Kruger et al. (63) found an incidence of ganciclovir resistance in their lung-transplant cohort of 5.2%, which resulted in increased positive viral blood cultures, CMV pneumonia, decreased overall survival, and the earlier onset of BOS.

The most important risk factors for antiviral resistance are D+/R− status and the intensity of immunosuppression. Suboptimal antiviral prophylaxis, which may occur with oral ganciclovir due to its poor bioavailability, is another risk factor for resistance. Finally, the intensity of the immunosuppressive regimen, particularly the use of antithymocyte globulin or OKT3 for induction therapy or treatment of rejection episodes, is associated with the development of antiviral resistance (64–66).

Resistance should be suspected in patients failing to respond to intravenous ganciclovir therapy of tissue invasive CMV infections, who have persistent viremia or recurrent viremia during or after ganciclovir prophylaxis. While neither has been validated, the lack of complete resolution of clinical symptoms or the failure of the viral load (by antigenemia or PCR) to decline after two to three weeks of therapy has been postulated to indicate the presence of a resistant isolate (62). Empiric switch therapy to foscarnet or combination therapy with ganciclovir and foscarnet should be performed while awaiting laboratory confirmation of resistance (67). Genotypic analysis is more sensitive than phenotypic or plaque-reduction assays and may provide a more rapid diagnosis of resistance.

Ganciclovir resistance occurs by two mechanisms: mutations in the *UL97* gene that codes for a phosphotransferase important in the phosphorylation of ganciclovir to its active form and mutation in the *UL54* gene that encodes the viral DNA polymerase. Foscarnet and cidofovir do not require phosphorylation for activation; thus, the *UL97* mutation does not confer cross-resistance to these agents. However, mutations of the DNA polymerase confer cross-resistance to ganciclovir and cidofovir but resistance to foscarnet is less predictable (68).

The management of antiviral-resistant CMV disease has been to switch therapy to foscarnet, which is typically effective for the treatment of ganciclovir-resistant isolates. With the emergence of cross-resistant strains, the use of cidofovir or combination antiviral therapy with or without immunoglobulin preparations may be required. One such approach has been to use intravenous ganciclovir at 50% its typical dose with once-daily foscarnet, which is gradually increased to a maximum of 125 mg/kg. This approach was effective in solid organ–transplant recipients in clearing the infection and no recurrence was seen in the 6 to 30 months of follow-up (67). The immunosuppressive agent leflunomide has been shown in vitro to have activity against resistant isolates (69) and was useful for treatment of a resistant isolate in a bone marrow–transplant recipient (70).

Two approaches have been advocated for the prevention of ganciclovir resistance. Since suboptimal prophylaxis is associated with resistance, more potent agents may be effective. VGCV, which has greater bioavailability than oral ganciclovir, may allow continual exposure to ganciclovir and may prove to be useful in the future. However, careful analysis of breakthrough viremia for resistance genotypes will be necessary. The other approach is preemptive therapy, which limits exposure to antivirals only to those at high risk as documented by active viral replication. Problems associated with this approach are the frequent monitoring that is required and patients who present with invasive CMV disease. While prolonged exposure to intravenous ganciclovir was associated with the development of resistance and it has been asserted that less antiviral for shorter time periods is beneficial, it is still debated whether prolonged exposure to potent antivirals or intermittent exposure with preemptive therapy will induce similar levels of resistance. Contrary to what is claimed by advocates of the preemptive approach, such a strategy does not always prevent the emergence of ganciclovir resistance (42). Finally, given the association of CMV pneumonia with BOS, this risk must be weighed against that of developing ganciclovir resistance with prolonged therapy.

### Future Directions in CMV Management

Most of the lung-transplant literature to date has dealt with the prevention and treatment of the direct effects of CMV. What remains to be answered is whether the prevention of CMV proliferation, or its treatment in the asymptomatic phase, will limit its indirect effects. It has been suggested that even asymptomatic viral proliferation may be associated with the development of BOS in lung-transplant recipients. Therefore, it would seem that prevention of any CMV proliferation or treatment of asymptomatic infections would be the desirable goal. Preliminary results from our institution suggest that preemptive treatment of asymptomatic CMV DNAemia is associated with a decrease in the acute and chronic effects of CMV infection following lung transplantation when compared to patients with symptomatic viremia or disease (48). The relationship between preemptive therapy and allograft response to CMV infections and augmented immunosuppression (as measured by opportunistic infections) was also investigated in this study. Preemptive therapy of CMV DNAemia decreased CMV-associated acute rejection, but not infection. This suggests that preemptive therapy of asymptomatic CMV infections attenuates the immune response in the allograft, but not the augmented immunosuppressive state induced by CMV. Clearly, further studies are necessary to investigate the role of treatment strategies on the indirect effects of CMV infection following lung transplantation.

Early clinical investigations with VGCV makes maintenance therapy more convenient; however, there appear to be potential dose-limiting properties (e.g., bone marrow suppression) (43,52). Frequent monitoring of complete blood counts and serum creatinine will be required to properly dose-adjust VGCV. Profound neutropenia may also increase the risk of fungal infection, which may counteract the benefit of preventing CMV. Future studies will be necessary to determine the role of oral VGCV in universal or preemptive prophylaxis, as a single prophylactic agent or in combination with immunoglobulin preparations and possibly for treatment of established disease.

The development of ganciclovir-resistant isolates necessitates the development of newer drugs that have high oral bioavailability, low toxicity, and mechanisms of action that will allow them to be used against ganciclovir-resistant isolates. The recognition that HHV-6 and HHV-7 are conducive to the development of CMV infection and may be additive to the indirect effects of CMV on allograft function suggests that antivirals with an expanded spectrum against these viruses would be desirable.

## Summary

Lung-transplant programs still need to refine the types of CMV prophylactic strategies that best match individual recipients of seropositive and seronegative allografts and the type of immunosuppression utilized. It seems clear that universal prophylaxis is warranted for high-risk D+/R− recipients. However, it remains unclear as to whether R+ recipients are also at higher risk than other solid organ recipients and whether they should receive universal prophylaxis or preemptive therapy. The use of antilymphocyte globulin would also appear to warrant the use of targeted, preemptive therapy with intravenous ganciclovir followed by two to three months of an oral agent. The development of high oral bioavailable drugs, such as VGCV, may provide a more convenient method of prophylaxis or treatment of CMV infections. There is a role for prophylactic hyperimmune anti-CMV immunoglobulin that may offer advantages for specific lung-transplant recipients and improve both short-term and long-term morbidity and mortality. However, better definitions for which patients likely benefit from it are needed due to the lack of pharmacoeconomic analyses of the various strategies. Combination therapy may also provide the opportunity to prevent and treat chronic and progressive allograft injury, particularly in the thoracic organs. Finally, molecular techniques should be employed for the detection of CMV infection, for determining the response to and duration of therapy, and for the determination of the emergence of ganciclovir-resistant isolates. Ongoing studies should help to answer these issues as well as generate new hypotheses in the role of CMV infection in chronic allograft failure following lung transplantation.

## Human Herpesvirus 6, 7, and 8

Emerging data suggest that these viruses are pathogenic and cause a variety of clinical syndromes on solid organ–transplant recipients (71). While a pathogenic role for HHV-8 in KS has been proven, the role of HHV-6 and HHV-7 in transplant recipients is less clear. This group may be considered to cause a "herpesvirus infection syndrome" in transplant recipients. The syndrome is characterized by reactivation of other latent viruses (CMV, HHV-6, or HHV-7), invasive fungal infections, and acceleration of the effects of other viruses, such as hepatitis C–induced fibrosis in liver-transplant recipients.

HHV-6 is a double-stranded DNA virus with 85% sequence homology to HHV-7 and 76% to CMV (72). It has two variants: variant A has been found in skin and brain tissue and variant B in brain, skin, lymph nodes, and serum. The primary target cell for HHV-6 is the CD4 T lymphocyte, but it also infects CD8 T cells, natural killer cells, macrophages, megakaryocytes, glial cells, and epithelial cells. Seroprevalence in adults is >90% with bronchial epithelial cells and salivary glands being the most likely sites of latency. The incidence in lung-transplant recipients is reported to be 57%, although another study failed to detect HHV-6 in the peripheral blood from patients who were positive for CMV DNA (73). Risk factors for HHV-6 infection include the use of OKT3 or antilymphocyte globulins and allograft rejection. Several reports have documented donor transmission of HHV-6.

Clinical manifestations of HHV-6 are directly attributable to the virus or from its immunomodulatory effects. The most frequently observed clinical features of HHV-6 are fever and skin rash and acute and chronic bone marrow suppression (72). The immunomodulatory and myelosuppressive effects of HHV-6 may be partly due to the production of cytokines, such as TNF-$\alpha$, gamma-interferon (IFN-$\gamma$), and interleukin-1$\beta$ (IL-1$\beta$). Interstitial pneumonitis, hepatitis, and encephalitis have been reported less frequently (74). HHV-6 may facilitate superinfection with opportunistic infections, such as CMV, invasive fungal disease, and late mortality in liver-transplant recipients (75). Diagnosis is made by serologic, virologic methods or in situ immunohistochemistry.

HHV-6 has similar antiviral susceptibilities to CMV (76). It is sensitive to ganciclovir and foscarnet, but less so to acyclovir. The use of intravenous ganciclovir or foscarnet reduces HHV-6 viral load and has been reported to successfully treat HHV-6–associated encephalitis (74). No data exist on superiority of either agent and the choice of therapy depends on the presence of renal insufficiency or myelosuppression.

HHV-7 may be the cause of roseola in childhood (71). It is trophic for CD4 T cells and the salivary glands are the most likely site of latency. Viremia has been detected by PCR in 39% of renal-transplant recipients. It may be a cofactor in the pathogenesis of CMV infection. Patients with CMV disease are more likely to have HHV-7 than those with asymptomatic CMV infections (75). Febrile syndromes in transplant recipients with CMV may be due to coinfection with HHV-6 or HHV-7. There is a single case report of an association of HHV-7 with bronchiolitis obliterans with organizing pneumonia in a lung-transplant recipient (77).

HHV-7 is most susceptible in vitro to cidofovir and less sensitive to ganciclovir though the data for ganciclovir are conflicting (76). Few data exist regarding the clinical efficacy of antiviral agents for HHV-7. One study in renal-transplant recipients showed that neither oral nor intravenous ganciclovir had an effect on HHV-7 viremia (78). However, a report in bone marrow–transplant recipients showed efficacy of ganciclovir and foscarnet for HHV-7 viremia (79).

As a member of the γ-herpesvirus family, HHV-8 is a transforming virus capable of causing tumors in its host (71,72). HHV-8 is a potent inducer of angiogenesis through the production of cytokines, such as IL-6, basic FGF, and IFN-G, and is the pathogenic cause of KS, hence the name KSHV. The incidence of KS in transplant recipients parallels the seroprevalence of KSHV in that region: it is low in the United States and higher in the Middle East, South Africa, and Saudi Arabia. Most KS lesions result from reactivation but donor transmission is reported. The skin is the most frequent site of involvement but visceral lesions may develop including the gastrointestinal tract, lungs, bladder, and larynx.

KS is best managed in transplant patients by a reduction in immunosuppression. Remission rates are high for visceral lesions; however, up to 50% of patients treated with cessation of immunosuppression lose their grafts. In patients who fail to respond, combination chemotherapy may be effective. Experience with antiviral agents in transplant recipients is limited, but cidofovir has been reported to be effective for the clearance of KSHV from the blood of 2/2 thoracic transplant recipients and from the skin lesions of 2/4 patients (80,81). Lymph nodes with B cells in the KSHV-related Castleman's disease stain positive for CD20; therefore, anti-CD20 therapy has been used in an HIV-positive patient with disseminated KS.

Other experimental therapies, such as inhibitors of angiogenesis and retinoids, are unproven.

## Epstein–Barr Virus

EBV is also a transforming virus: uncontrolled proliferation of EBV-infected B cells results in the spectrum of PTLD (72,82–84). PTLD results in both decreased patient and graft survival, the former due to the direct effects of the tumor and the latter a result of decreased immunosuppression to treat the disorder. The EBV genome is found in >90% of B-cell PTLD cases occurring within the first year post-transplant. An increasing number of late PTLD cases are EBV negative, so the role of the virus in these cases has been called into question. EBV-induced lymphoproliferation ranges from benign polyclonal proliferation to high-grade malignancies with monoclonal features. EBV is a double-stranded DNA virus transmitted through saliva. In low socioeconomic strata, the virus is nearly universally acquired in early childhood. In upper socioeconomic strata, it is acquired during adolescence or early adulthood resulting in the infectious mononucleosis syndrome. More than 90% of the population has immunity to EBV by age 40 years.

EBV is characterized by its ability to attain lifelong persistence in the host despite strong humoral and cellular immune responses to the virus (85). B cells are the predominant site of EBV replication in the oropharynx. Following initiation of infection of the B cells, two early genes, *EBER-1* and *EBER-2*, are expressed and allow detection of EBV in the clinical setting. The immune response to EBV infection occurs by both humoral and cell-mediated pathways. Neutralizing antibodies develop to limit the spread of cell-free virus and render the virus susceptible to antibody-dependent cell-mediated cytotoxicity. Cell-mediated responses consist of cytolysis by T cells or NK cells. Subsequently, a viral-specific CD4 or CD8 response occurs with the development of EBV-specific cytotoxic lymphocytes. Following transplantation, the cytolytic T lymphocyte (CTL) response is blunted, allowing persistent virus to proliferate.

Primary EBV infection occurs in nearly all EBV-seronegative recipients of seropositive organs. Oropharyngeal shedding occurs ≈6 weeks post-transplant and increases in EBV viral load in the peripheral blood are seen even in the presence of ganciclovir prophylaxis. Patients developing PTLD have greater viral loads than those without PTLD leading to the use of EBV viral load measurement in peripheral blood as a tool for the surveillance, diagnosis, and monitoring of therapy for EBV-related PTLD (86,87). Animal and human data suggest that early EBV-related lymphoproliferative disorders result from uncontrolled proliferation of EBV-infected B cells. This proliferation is polyclonal in nature but certain clones may develop a selective growth advantage, transforming the lesion into an oligoclonal or monoclonal lesion. Cytogenetic abnormalities may develop with ongoing proliferation resulting in a true malignancy.

### Risk Factors for the Development of PTLD

EBV infection plays a major role in the development of PTLD. However, 10–45% of lesions are EBV-negative. In any case, patients at risk of primary EBV infection have a 10- to 76-fold greater risk of developing PTLD than seropositive recipients (82,88). The incidence of PTLD is strongly correlated with the type of organ transplanted. While this may be more of a marker of the intensity of immunosuppression used for recipients of these various organs, it is possible that each organ has characteristics that may predispose them to the development of PTLD. Renal-transplant recipients have the lowest incidence of PTLD of ≈1%. Nonrenal transplant recipients have a greater risk of developing PTLD: 2.2% for liver, 3.5% for heart, 1.8% to 7.9% for lung, and up to 9.4% for heart–lung transplant recipients (89). Intestinal- or multivisceral-transplant recipients have the highest risk, with an up to 33% incidence. The use of immunosuppressive agents and the intensity of the immunosuppressive regimen are correlated with the development of PTLD. The mean time to presentation of PTLD has shifted from 48 months post-transplant to 15 months in the cyclosporine era and one-third of cases now occur in the first four months posttransplant (90). Whether this is specifically due to calcineurin inhibitors or multidrug regimens is unclear. The use of antilymphocyte globulin for induction or treatment of steroid-resistant rejection following solid organ transplantation is associated with an increased incidence of PTLD (91–93). It has been postulated that the greatest risk of PTLD does not result from any single immunosuppressive agent, but rather from the cumulative intensity of the immunosuppression (94). Data from non–renal-transplant programs show that CMV mismatching increases the risk of PTLD severalfold. In fact, patients with the combination of EBV seronegativity, CMV mismatching, and OKT3 treatment of rejection have an increased risk of >500-fold (92). Infection with HHV-8 may also increase the risk of PTLD (95,96). Hepatitis C infection has been shown to increase the risk of PTLD in liver-transplant recipients (97) but data are lacking in other solid organ transplants. Patient age has also been shown to be important in determining whether a patient develops PTLD. Younger pediatric patients appear to be at the greatest risk due their greater risk of primary EBV and CMV infections. However, older age has been shown to increase the risk in cardiac and renal transplant recipients (98).

### Clinical Presentations

PTLD occurs as a spectrum of disease ranging from self-limited lymphoproliferation to fulminant disease and localized nodular disease to widely disseminated disease. Clinical features, the response to reduced immunosuppression, therapy, and prognosis vary substantially across the spectrum of disease. In pediatric patients, the disease typically presents as a mononucleosis-like syndrome with fever and tonsillar and cervical lymph node enlargement. These patients typically respond to decreased immunosuppression or antiviral therapy. Dissemination in this patient group may be rapid and is associated with multiorgan failure and death in over 75% of cases. PTLD is most commonly limited to the allograft in early post-transplant cases. Primary presentation in the allograft occurs in 60% to 80% of cases in lung- or intestinal-transplant recipients versus 17% in renal or 8.6% in liver recipients (89,90,99). Central nervous system involvement is rare, occurring in <10% of cases. Disseminated disease may be associated with isolated leptomeningeal or cerebrospinal fluid involvement. Gastrointestinal involvement occurs in 25% to 30% of cases, may be the only site of involvement, and may be aggressive with multiple tumors. Local invasion results in bleeding, tissue necrosis, and perforation. Resection of local segments of bowel is associated with an improved prognosis and survival. Pulmonary involvement is common in cardiac, lung, and heart–lung recipients and presents as multiple pulmonary nodules. Disease occurring beyond the first year post transplant typically presents like non-Hodgkin's lymphoma (100). Patients tend to be older, have extranodal disease, mass lesions in the head and neck, and monoclonal features consistent with an immunoblastic lymphoma. These tumors may be EBV-negative and usually do not respond to decreased immunosuppression or antiviral therapy, and surgery or chemotherapy may be required.

Diagnosis

The Society for Hematopathology (101) and the World Health Organization (102) have published and updated a classification system for PTLD based on its cellular pathology. Early lesions include plasmacytic hyperplasia and an infectious mononucleosis-like syndrome. In these early forms of PTLD, lymphoid tissue architecture is intact and they tend to respond to decreased immunosuppression. Polymorphic PTLD is characterized by effacement of the tissue architecture and monoclonal B-cell lymphomas. Monomorphic PTLD is characterized by cellular atypia and is categorized by the type of lymphoma present. These are commonly B-cell lymphomas that may be immunoblastic, Burkitt-like, plasma cell myeloma, plasmacytoma-like lesions, or maltoma. T-cell malignancies include peripheral T-cell lymphoma, anaplastic large cell lymphoma, or hematosplenic $\gamma/\delta$ T-cell lymphoma. In order to develop more targeted therapy, it is important to determine the cell phenotype (B, T, or NK cell), clonality, genetic studies of antigen receptor genes, the presence of EBV by EBER stains, alteration in oncogenes or tumor suppressor genes, donor versus recipient origin, or the presence of therapy-dependent markers, such as CD20 (103).

Most PTLD lesions are monoclonal. The presence of cytogenetic abnormailities predicts lesions that may not respond to decreased immunosuppression and should be considered for chemotherapy. EBV-negative PTLD appears to be increasing (104) and tends to occur later post-transplant, has a poorer prognosis, and is resistant to decreased immunosuppression and chemotherapy. The impact of donor versus recipient origin is currently under study. The presence of EBV by EBER staining may be useful in determining whether lymphocyte proliferation in the allograft is due to PTLD or rejection.

### EBV Viral Load Determination

Determination of the EBV viral load has been reported to be useful for surveillance, diagnosis, and monitoring of therapy for PTLD (105). Low EBV viral load has a good negative predictive value; however, the specificity of high viral loads for the diagnosis of PTLD is poor with positive predictive values of 28% to 65% (106). The high viral loads do precede the development of PTLD. However, these assays suffer from lack of standardization. Optimal assay techniques, sample source (plasma vs. whole-blood vs. peripheral blood lymphocytes), and the monitoring schedule have yet to be determined. Since the natural history of an elevated EBV viral load is unknown in transplant recipients, threshold values for intervention cannot be set (107).

With identification of increasing viral loads, preemptive therapy can be implemented including a reduction in immunosuppression and use of antiviral agents with or without immunoglobulin replacement. Such an approach has been used with success in intestinal transplant and pediatric liver-transplant recipients (105,106).

### Treatment

No randomized, controlled trials of therapy for PTLD have been performed. Most treatment regimens are based on case reports or small patient series. Many patients will respond to a reduction or discontinuation of immunosuppressive therapy. The latter is not optimal in thoracic transplantation and has been associated with the development of both acute and chronic rejection, particularly in lung-transplant recipients. Remissions may occur in up to 65% of cases, but is unlikely to be effective in late cases or EBV-negative disease. Adoptive transfer of autologous EBV-specific CTLs in solid organ–transplant recipients suggests that disease may regress in response to this therapy (103,107). Acyclovir and ganciclovir are only effective during the lytic phase of EBV infections as they interfere with EBV-associated DNA polymerase (108). However, they could also be effective by treating other viral cofactors for the development of PTLD, such as CMV or HHV-8. Ganciclovir would be the preferred agent given its superior efficacy against CMV. IFN-$\alpha$ has been reported to be efficacious in anecdotal reports (109). Surgical resection or tumor debulking are necessary for the control of local complications, such as bowel perforations. Surgery and local irradiation may be useful for the management of localized disease and cranial irradiation is required for CNS involvement (110). Conventional chemotherapy is indicated for patients who fail to respond to reduced immunosuppression or antiviral agents or those with malignant, monomorphic B-cell lymphomas, or Burkitt's lymphoma occurring beyond the first posttransplant year. A recent review of chemotherapy for PTLD (109) showed that CHOP (cyclophosphamide, doxorubicin, vincristine, and prednisone) or ProMACE–Cyta-BOM (cytarabine, bleomycin, vincristine, methotrexate, and prednisone) has induced remission rates up to 69% in B-cell tumors. Cyclic administration of cyclophosphamide and corticosteroids has also been utilized to provide both antitumor and antirejection effects (111). Rituximab, a chimeric antibody directed against the CD20 antigen expressed on B cells, has been shown to induce a complete response rate of 62% when combined with reduced immunosuppression (112,113). Side effects include B-cell lymphopenia with associated hypogammaglobulinemia. Reactivation of viral infections, particularly CMV, has been reported (114).

### Prognosis

A review of factors affecting prognosis found that poorer survival was associated with poorer functional status, multiple sites of disease, primary CNS disease, T-cell origin, monoclonality, recipient organ disease, mutations in proto-oncogenes or tumor suppression genes, and EBV-negative lesions (113,115). Serial measurement of EBV viral load has been used to monitor the response to therapy. Clearance of the viral load was associated with clinical response to therapy (87).

### Preventive Strategies

Without effective therapy for PTLD, the optimal management strategy is prevention. Intensified immunosuppression should only be used for documented acute rejection. Identification of high-risk patients prior to transplant and careful monitoring posttransplant are critically important. Prophylactic antivirals for the other herpesviruses may reduce the risk of PTLD. Use of prophylactic EBV-specific antibodies is currently under study. Adoptive immunotherapy with EBV-specific CTLs has been shown to decrease EBV viral load (106) but no data on prevention are available in solid organ transplant recipients.

## HSV-1 and -2 and VZV

HSV-1 and HSV-2 and VZV are members of the α-herpesvirinae. HSV-1 is transmitted by oral secretions and causes herpes labialis (fever blisters) (116). HSV-2 is transmitted sexually and primary and secondary HSV-2 infections are characterized by painful vesicles and ulcers on the mucocutaneous surfaces of the genital or perianal areas. HSV is transmitted by direct contact with the skin or mucosal surface of a person who is actively shedding virus. Following primary infection, latency is established in the nerve cell bodies of the cutaneous nerves serving the affected areas. Reactivation allows the virus to travel along the same nerves to produce a cluster of painful vesicles. Patients may transmit the virus via autoinoculation to distant sites resulting in herpes keratitis and herpetic whitlow. Transmission of the virus via an infected donor organ has been described (117).

In patients not receiving antiviral prophylaxis, HSV disease usually occurs within two to three weeks posttransplant (118). The initial presentation of mucocutaneous disease does not differ from that seen in immunocompetent hosts; however, it is associated with longer periods of viral shedding, more invasion, slower healing, and, rarely, dissemination (119). HSV lesions may involve the lips, oral mucosa, posterior pharynx, and perioral skin. Anogenital herpes due to HSV-2 can range from self-limited lesions to deep ulcerations and may be complicated by lymphocytic meningitis. Direct extension from the oropharynx to the gastrointestinal or respiratory tracts results in esophagitis or pneumonitis. Patients with esophagitis present with dysphagia and odynophagia. Endoscopy reveals esophageal ulcerations and biopsy and culture is usually diagnostic. Patients with pneumonitis present with fever, cough, dyspnea, hypoxemia, and the chest X ray reveals diffuse infiltrates (120). Viremic dissemination to multiple organs is rare, may be difficult to diagnose, and is associated with an extremely high mortality rate. Disseminated disease has been described in liver- and kidney-transplant recipients and should be considered in patients with fever and abnormal liver function tests (121).

While experienced clinicians recognize the characteristic lesions of HSV infections, viral culture remains the gold standard for the diagnosis of HSV. Diagnosis of mucocutaneous lesions or ulcers can be made by direct immunoflourescence assay, which is more sensitive than the Tzanck smear. PCR is the method of choice for diagnosing central nervous system infections (122).

Therapy for HSV infections depends on the severity of illness (123). Intravenous acyclovir 5 mg/kg every eight hours has been shown to decrease viral shedding, the time to resolution of pain, and accelerate lesion healing. Oral acyclovir is also highly effective against HSV infection and can be used instead of the intravenous formulation for uncomplicated mucocutaneous disease. Newer agents with improved pharmacokinetic profiles have replaced oral acyclovir. Valacyclovir, a prodrug of acyclovir, and famciclovir have antiviral activity similar to acyclovir but attain higher serum concentrations and have simpler dosing schedules (124). High-dose intravenous acyclovir 10 mg/kg every eight hours is the treatment of choice for transplant recipients with visceral HSV infection (125). Antiviral therapy for mucocutaneous disease should be continued until the lesions have completely healed. Premature cessation of therapy can result in infection relapse and sets the conditions for the development of antiviral resistance. Ganciclovir, foscarnet, and cidofovir are effective against HSV and may be useful for the treatment of coinfections with CMV and HSV.

Primary VZV infection occurs in children <15 years old and is the cause of chickenpox (126). Reactivation on adults causes herpes zoster (shingles). In the transplant recipient, reactivation generally occurs >100 days posttransplant but routine use of CMV prophylaxis has altered the natural history of VZV infections. The disease manifests as typical dermatomal skin eruptions, or eruptions without a dermatomal pattern, so-called generalized zoster, or subclinical reactivation that may present as neuralgic pain typical of herpes zoster. Cutaneous dissemination may occur in up to 30% of transplant recipients and is a predictor of visceral dissemination (127).

Herpes zoster with characteristic neuralgic pain and a dermatomal rash is readily diagnosed clinically. Direct immunoflourescent antibody and PCR are very useful for the laboratory diagnosis of VZV. Intravenous acyclovir is indicated for patients with disseminated disease and prevents the progression to pneumonia (128). Once new lesion formation has ceased and fever has resolved, patients may be switched to oral therapy with acyclovir, valacyclovir, or famciclovir.

Drugs used for CMV or HSV prophylaxis are extremely effective at preventing VZV infections. Seronegative recipients with a defined exposure to VZV should receive varicella-zoster immune globulin to provide passive immunity (129). This does not prevent infection but will limit disease severity. It should be administered within 96 hours of exposure and confers up to four weeks of passive immunity. Use of a VZV vaccine has been shown to be safe and effective when given prior to solid organ transplantation (130).

## COMMUNITY-ACQUIRED RESPIRATORY VIRUSES

### Epidemiology

A growing body of evidence suggests that the CARVs are important causes of morbidity and mortality following lung transplantation. The CARVs are a diverse group of viruses belonging to several families including the *Paramyxoviridae* (RSV, PIV, hMPV), the *Orthomyxoviridae* (influenza A and B), the *Picornaviridae* (rhinovirus and enterovirus), the *Coronaviridae* (coronavirus), and the *Adenoviridae* (adenovirus). All of these viruses are single-stranded RNA viruses except for adenovirus, which is a double-stranded DNA virus. The incidence of these viruses in lung-transplant recipients has been reported to range from 2% to 15% (131–135). However, the actual incidence of the CARVs following lung transplantation is difficult to determine since most reports deal with retrospective, single-center studies with mixed populations of pediatric and adult patients, the presentation is nonspecific, often thought to be the common cold, and diagnostic methods are insensitive in adult patients. The true incidence may be much higher. In a prospective surveillance study, lung-transplant recipients with upper respiratory tract symptoms were found to have an incidence of CARVs of 27% (136). CARVs are generally transmitted directly from person to person, through fomites in respiratory secretions, or through direct contact with infected secretions. Most of these viruses can be transmitted through multiple routes, nosocomial infection is common, and hospital outbreaks have been described (137). Therefore, infection control measures are critical to contain the spread of these viruses.

Infection due to CARVs can occur within days to years post-transplant. The early onset suggests that donor organ transmission is possible (134,135,138,139). Seasonal occurrence of these viruses tends to follow the occurrence in the community. RSV typically occurs in the fall, winter, and spring and hMPV occurs in winter and spring. PIV occurs year-round, but primarily in spring, summer, and fall. Influenza occurs in late fall and winter. The other viruses occur year-round. Coinfection is common and bacterial and fungal superinfection is reported. Mortality has been reported to range from 3% to 20% with lower respiratory tract infections.

## Clinical Syndromes

In immunocompetent hosts, these viruses cause a variety of clinical syndromes including the common cold, pharyngitis, tracheobronchitis, bronchiolitis, and pneumonia. In lung-transplant recipients, infection ranges from mild upper respiratory tract infections (URTI) to life-threatening pneumonia. Symptoms include dyspnea, cough, hypoxia, and fever. Given the nonspecific nature of these symptoms, a high level of suspicion is required for diagnosis of these viruses. Chest radiograph reveals diffuse infiltrates or focal consolidation. CT scans of lung-transplant recipients infected with RSV reveal evidence of airways disease including air trapping, ground glass infiltrates, air-space consolidation, the "tree-in-bud" appearance, bronchial dilatation, and bronchial wall thickening (140). Follow-up CT scans show persistent bronchial thickening, air-trapping, and "mosaic" lung attenuation, which are manifestations of bronchiolitis obliterans or chronic rejection.

## Diagnosis

Rapid, accurate diagnosis of the CARVs is critical in the management of the lung-transplant recipient (141). It allows for the use of specific isolation procedures to prevent transmission to other immunosuppressed patients and the institution of specific antiviral therapy. A number of factors affect the ability to identify the virus in clinical specimens including the source of the specimen, the timing of collection in relation to the onset of symptoms, the rapidity and mode of transport to the laboratory, and the temperature of the transport media (142). Adult immunocompromised patients do not have high viral loads of CARVs compared to children. For instance, the viral load of RSV in adults may be three to four logs lower than in young children (143). The clinical syndrome caused by these viruses determines the preferred source of the specimen most likely to yield identification of a viral pathogen. Viruses causing respiratory tract disease (RSV, influenza) are found in respiratory secretions. Those causing systemic disease (enterovirus) may be found in throat swabs, cerebrospinal fluid (CSF), or fecal specimens. Adenovirus may be found in respiratory secretions, urine, and blood. Suspected adenoviral pneumonia warrants a bronchoscopy with bronchoalveolar lavage (BAL) and biopsy to identify adenovirus by culture or histologic localization in the lung parenchyma. Hemorrhagic cystitis should prompt urine culture or PCR.

In general, the nasal wash is the preferred method for obtaining specimens in children and adults but nasopharyngeal swabs may also be useful (144). Lower respiratory tract specimens may be obtained from tracheal aspirates and BAL fluid. Once a specimen is obtained, it should be transported to the virology laboratory as soon as possible as viral viability declines with time (145). Use of viral transport media is also recommended.

Many laboratory methods are available for the diagnosis of CARVs. They include immunoflourescence, antigen detection, radioimmunoassay, ELISA assays, in situ hybridization, PCR, direct cytology, tissue culture, and electron microscopy. All have varying sensitivity and specificity, costs, and time required for diagnosis. Cell culture remains the gold standard for the diagnosis of the respiratory viruses. Immunoflourescent assays allow rapid viral diagnosis but may be labor intensive and require a high degree of technical expertise to read the samples. Enzyme immunoassays (EIA) rely on antibodies directed against specific viral antigens. They are rapid, simple to run and to interpret. One drawback to EIA is that it cannot discern between viable and killed virus during the course of antiviral therapy (146). Sensitivity in immunocompromised adults may be as low as 15% using nasal washes, but increases to 70% to 80% with BAL samples (143). PCR is rapidly becoming the preferred test for viral diagnostics in immunosuppressed hosts. Multiplex PCR may allow for the detection of multiple viruses with a single PCR assay. Weinberg et al. (136) found that PCR had a higher sensitivity than rapid respiratory viral culture or EIA methods in the diagnosis of CARVs in lung-transplant recipients. No commercially available antigen-detection kits exist for rhinovirus, enterovirus, or coronavirus but real-time PCR assays are being developed (147,148). Isolation of these viruses by cell culture is still required.

## Treatment

Specific therapy exists for the influenza viruses. Influenza is treated with amantadine or rimantidine, but efficacy is limited due to the rapid development of antiviral resistance and the lack of efficacy against influenza B (149). The neuraminidase inhibitors, oseltamavir or zanamivir, may be more effective as they have activity against influenza B, and antiviral resistance levels are low currently (150,151). Head-to-head comparisons are not available and the appropriate length of therapy is unknown. Inhaled or intravenous ribavirin is also effective against influenza B and has been used in transplant recipients with severe influenza and respiratory failure (152).

There are no randomized control trials of treatment for the other CARVs and treatment practices vary widely among transplant centers. Aerosolized ribavirin is licensed for the treatment of RSV bronchiolitis in infants and children. The decision to treat URTI due to RSV depends on several factors including the risk of developing severe lower respiratory tract infection, unproven efficacy in transplant recipients, the potential for environmental contamination and exposure of health care workers, adverse effects of inhaled ribavirin, the high cost of these agents, and the need for hospitalization for prolonged inhaled ribavirin dosing. Conflicting reports of the efficacy of inhaled ribavirin as monotherapy exist in the transplant literature. When given early in the course of infection, with URTI symptoms, or at the early stages of pneumonia without radiographic abnormalities and prior to the onset of respiratory failure, favorable results may be obtained. Wendt et al. reported that lung-transplant recipients had good outcomes using inhaled ribavirin alone for lower respiratory tract infections (135), while Vilchez et al. reported a decrease in the incidence of post-RSV BOS to 15% with the use of inhaled ribavirin (139) compared to a reported incidence of 32% in those without therapy (131). RSV–IVIG, a human polyclonal immunoglobulin with high RSV neutralizing antibody titers, and palivizumab, a humanized monoclonal antibody directed against the fusion protein of RSV, are available. Combination therapy with inhaled ribavirin and immunoglobulin has been shown to rapidly decrease viral shedding in nontransplant patients with respiratory failure due to RSV pneumonia (153). In hematopoietic stem cell–transplant patients with pneumonia, only 4 of 13 died with combination therapy versus 100% of those who were untreated or for whom therapy was started late. Intravenous ribavirin has also been utilized, but may be associated with hemolytic anemia and liver function abnormalities (154). In preliminary studies in lung-transplant recipients, combination therapy with inhaled ribavirin, corticosteroids, and anti-RSV immunoglobulin preparations were shown to decrease the incidence of acute and chronic rejection following lower respiratory tract infections due to either RSV or PIV (155). Patients treated with this combination developed BOS in 6% of cases versus 100% in those receiving corticosteroids alone or in combination. Similar outcomes were found for the treatment of parainfluenza infections with corticosteroids, inhaled ribavirin, and either the polyclonal RSV immunoglobulin or the standard IVIG.

No definitive therapy exists for adenovirus. Supportive care with decreased immunosuppression is the cornerstone of therapy. A role for antiviral agents remains unproven. Several case reports have described the use of ribavirin, which has in vitro activity against adenovirus. Intravenous ribavirin may be associated with hepatotoxicity and hyperammonemia. We have utilized inhaled ribavirin in three patients with adenovirus pneumonia. One patient with preexisting BOS required mechanical ventilation for respiratory failure and died. Autopsy revealed necrotizing pneumonia with adenoviral inclusions and evidence of hepatic dissemination. Two patients had a lower respiratory tract infectious syndrome characterized by wheezing, mild desaturation, and cough. They improved with five days of therapy with inhaled ribavirin and IVIG. Recently, cidofovir has been described for the treatment of adenovirus in solid organ– and bone marrow–transplant recipients but conventional dosing (5 mg/kg/week × 2 weeks, then every 2 weeks) may cause nephrotoxicity (156).

## Relationship to Acute and Chronic Rejection

Concomitant acute rejection occurs in up to two-thirds of lung-transplant patients with CARV infections (133). The forced expiratory volume in one second may fall up to 25% with the acute episode, but typically recovers over weeks to months (135,139). A number of reports link these viruses to chronic allograft dysfunction or BOS in lung-transplant recipients (131–135,138). An association with BOS development at a median time of 180 to 480 days postinfection has been reported. Billings et al. (131) found that patients with CARVs had an increased relative risk of progression from early BOS to BOS grade 3 and Khalifah et al. (157) reported that lower respiratory tract infections were associated with all stages of BOS.

Recently, Chakinala and Walter reviewed the literature supporting the role of viral-mediated respiratory epithelial injury in the pathogenesis of BOS (158). Through the regulated expression of epithelial injury response genes, the respiratory epithelium coordinates immune cell function in the airways. Damage to the epithelium by acute rejection, aspiration of gastric fluid, or viruses can lead to inflammation, stimulation of profibrotic pathways, and collagen deposition in the airways—the histologic finding in BOS. Winter et al. showed that viral-induced epithelial injury following allogeneic rat lung transplantation led to excessive collagen deposition in the airways of the allogeneic animals versus syngeneic transplanted animals or uninfected allografts (159). Many epithelial injury response genes have been shown to be upregulated by viral infections including chemokines and adhesion molecules, both of which are responsible for leukocyte accumulation and inflammation in the airway. IL-8, regulated on activation, normal T-cell expressed and secreted (RANTES), and monocyte chemoattractant protein-1 (MCP-1) have been shown to be stimulated by viral infection of epithelial cells in vitro and in experimental or naturally occurring RSV infections in humans (160,161). ICAM-1 has similarly been shown to be expressed by viral infections in isolated epithelial cells and in humans (162). BAL studies in lung-transplant recipients with BOS have shown increased concentrations of IL-8, RANTES, and MCP-1 and neutrophil accumulation (163). Taken together, these observations suggest a link between CARV infections and BOS.

## PARVOVIRUS B19

PVB19 is a small, single-stranded DNA virus, typically acquired during childhood and the etiologic agent of erythema infectiosum (fifth disease) (164). Epidemiologic studies reveal that infection is global and that 30% to 60% of adults are seropositive. Infection confers lifelong immunity in immunocompetent hosts but reactivation is common in states of relative or absolute immunodeficiency.

The pathogenesis of PVB19 infection is related to its tropism and cytotoxicity for erythroid progenitor cells via the P-glycoprotein (glyboside). Therefore, infection is most commonly associated with acute and chronic hematologic disorders including anemia, pure red blood cell aplasia, thrombocytopenia, and pancytopenia. In immunocompetent individuals, PVB19 infection results in short-term viremia, the development of neutralizing antibodies, promoting the reappearance of erythroid progenitor cells, and subsequent viral clearance. Immunosuppressed patients, who may not develop specific immunity, may develop recurrent or persistent infections and chronic anemia. This has been described in both adult and pediatric lung-transplant recipients (165–167).

The clinical manifestations of PVB19 infection in children are asymptomatic, or result in a mild illness characterized by fever and flu-like symptoms. A cutaneous eruption, the so-called "slapped face" appears on the face and the extremities. The rash and arthralgias occur at the time of antiviral antibody development, suggesting that the disease manifestations may be due to immune complex deposition in the skin, joints, and visceral organs (164). Individuals with the need for rapid red blood cell turnover, such as those with sickle cell disease or thalassemia, may develop severe anemia during the acute infection. PVB19 has also been associated with a variety of medical conditions including vasculitides, chronic arthritis, and neuropathies (168). Unusual manifestations in the immunocompromised host include pneumonia, myocarditis, renal insufficiency, and decreased graft survival. Concomitant infection with CMV and HHV-6 has been described in organ-transplant recipients (164).

The infection is most commonly transmitted by direct contact with respiratory secretions from infected patients. It is also transmitted through blood transfusions, infusion of clotting factors, and contaminated donor organs. Vertical transmission from mother to fetus results in hydrops fetalis. Infection among household contacts of infected patients is very high and nosocomial infection has been described on transplant units.

Laboratory diagnosis is based on serologic methods or nucleic acid hybridization and PCR, which are more sensitive in detecting viremia. The latter is usually required in immunosuppressed patients and for the detection of persistent infections since they occur in the absence of effective antibody production (164).

Therapy consists of decreasing immunosuppression to allow recovery of antibody-mediated immunity. A growing number of reports support the use of IVIG in transplant recipients with symptomatic disease (166,167). IVIG has been shown to be effective for rapid viral clearance and shortens the time required for recovery of reticulocytosis and hemoglobin levels. The doses of IVIG range from 0.4 to 2 g/kg/day for 3 to 10 days. Monthly infusions may be required for chronic anemia due to persistent infection. Plasmapheresis has been advocated for patients failing IVIG therapy. Erythropoietin has been used for the anemia, but the response may be limited. Improved methods to detect viremia should lead to a better understanding of the pathogenesis, management, and monitoring of the response to treatment of this virus in transplant recipients.

## NEW AND EMERGING VIRUSES

### Human Metapneumovirus

hMPV is a newly recognized pathogen that is related to RSV and the other paramyxoviruses and causes upper and lower respiratory tract illness in children, the elderly, and immunocompromised patients (169–171). Although recently recognized, antibodies to hMPV were found as early as 1958 in archived serum samples from patients 8 years and older. Epidemiologic studies reveal that hMPV is ubiquitous and is the second most common pathogen detected in children with acute respiratory tract infections after RSV (169). It has a seasonal distribution, typically occurring in the winter and early spring months and overlaps the RSV season. Available data suggest that the clinical manifestations of hMPV are indistinguishable from those of RSV with potentially severe and life-threatening disease in infants, the elderly, and immunosuppressed patients (169,170). Syndromes range from mild upper respiratory tract illness to severe bronchiolitis or pneumonia. hMPV has been reported in association with fatal lower respiratory tract disease in a hematopoetic stem cell–transplant recipient (172). Anecdotal reports have described hMPV in lung-transplant recipients.

Little is known about the pathogenic mechanisms of hMPV infections in humans. The virus most likely replicates in the upper and lower respiratory tracts but the cell types affected are not known. Animal studies suggest that the epithelial cell is the most likely site of infection, but hMPV antigens are found throughout the lung tissues. Respiratory secretions of infected patients contain IL-8, but hMPV appears to induce lower levels of proinflammatory cytokines than RSV. Infection produces neutralizing antibodies that may be protective against the development of severe disease in adults. However, despite universal childhood infection, new infections can occur in adulthood due to acquisition of new genotypes or in the setting of immunosuppression. The presence of a copathogen, seen in 5% to 10% of cases, may also lead to more severe illness. The mode of transmission is through respiratory secretion and fomites. Nosocomial transmission can occur and patients should be placed in contact isolation and health care workers should employ good hand-washing practices.

hMPV grows very slowly in conventional cell culture systems. That fact and the lack of a rapid antigen detection test have led to reverse transcriptase–PCR becoming the method of choice for the diagnosis of hMPV infection. No antiviral or antibody preparation is approved for the treatment of hMPV. However, Wyde et al. (173) found that ribavirin and standard immunoglobulin had equivalent activity against hMPV and RSV, suggesting that ribavirin or combination therapy with IVIG may be effective for the treatment of severe hMPV infections. The latter approach has been reported to be more effective than ribavirin alone for the treatment of RSV infections in immunosuppressed patients (174).

## West Nile Virus

West Nile Virus (WNV) is a member of the Flavivirus family and has been identified as the cause of an outbreak of febrile illness and encephalitis in the United States in 1999 (175). The virus is transmitted from infected birds to humans by mosquitoes. Infection occurs in the summer or early fall. Most episodes present as a febrile illness, headache, and myalgias, which last three to six days. Gastrointestinal symptoms may be common in immunosuppressed patients, including nausea, vomiting, abdominal pain, and diarrhea. Neurologic involvement is the most severe complication occurring in up to 30% of transplant recipients with WNV infection. CNS manifestations include meningoencephalitis, acute flaccid paralysis, tremors, myoclonus, or parkinsonism (175). Magnetic resonance imaging is the most sensitive imaging study. The mortality rate with CNS involvement is high and many patients suffer persistent neurologic deficits.

Diagnosis relies on detection of virus-specific IgM in the serum or CSF. Humoral and cellular immune responses occur and confer protection against recurrent infection. No specific therapy exists but ribavirin, IFN-α, and IVIG may be beneficial (176,177). IVIG obtained from patients with high titers to WNV may be more effective than standard IVIG but clinical trials are under way.

WNV infection has now been reported in all types of solid organ–transplant recipients. The virus has been reported to be transmitted by donor organs and transfusion of blood products (178). Following implementation of routine screening by blood banks, post-transfusion transmission has been minimized. Immunosuppressed patients may be at risk for the development of more severe infections. DeSalvo (179) and Kumar (180) described six solid organ–transplant patients with CNS WNV infections. The diagnosis was confirmed by abnormal CSF studies and positive serum or CSF serology. Three patients had delayed antibody responses. Patients were treated with decreased immunosuppression and one received IFN-$\alpha$. Two patients died and two had persistent neurologic deficits.

The diagnosis of WNV infection may be delayed due to the nonspecific nature of the symptoms, the delayed antibody response, or the lack of availability of diagnostic tests at local centers. WNV should be considered in febrile-transplant patients with neurologic changes and gastrointestinal symptoms. Protective measures against mosquito bites including long-sleeved shirts and long pants and use of insect repellant are recommended for all transplant patients during the summer and fall months.

## SARS–Coronavirus

The SARS outbreak in the winter of 2002 involved over 8000 cases, 774 deaths, and affected 26 countries (181). The outbreak was later shown to be caused by the SARS-CoV, a previously unknown coronavirus that appears to have originated from an animal reservoir. A report in a liver-transplant recipient has been described (182). The patient presented with fever, headache, and malaise and rapidly progressed to pneumonia, respiratory failure, and death. Several family members and health care providers were infected by exposure to this patient. The virus was isolated in respiratory specimens by PCR. Screening of potential donors and SARS isolation procedures will become more important as the virus spreads worldwide.

## REFERENCES

1. Fishman JA, Rubin RH. Infection in organ-transplant recipients. N Engl J Med 1998; 338:1741–1751.
2. Paya CV, Razonable RR. Cytomegalovirus infection after solid organ transplantation. In: Bowden RA, Ljungman P, Paya CV, eds. Transplant Infections. 2nd. Philadelphia, PA: Lipincott, Williams and Wilkens, 2003.
3. Zamora MR. Cytomegalovirus and lung transplantation. Am J Transplant 2004; 4:1219–1226.
4. Dunn HS, Haney DJ, Ghanekar SA, et al. Dynamics of CD4 and CD8 T cell response to cytomegalovirus in healthy human donors. J Infect Dis 2002; 186:15–22.
5. Zamora MR, Davis RD, Leonard C, et al. Management of cytomegalovirus infection in lung transplant recipients: evidence-based recommendations Transplantation 2005; 80(2):157–163.

6. Valantine HA. Prevention and treatment of cytomegalovirus disease in thoracic organ transplant patients: evidence for a beneficial effect of hyperimmune globulin. Transplant Proc 1995; 27(Suppl 1):49–57.
7. Balthesen M, Messerle M, Reddehase MJ. Lungs are a major organ site of cytomegalovirus latency and recurrence. J Virol 1993; 67:5360–5366.
8. Mendez JC, Dockrell DH, Espy MJ, et al. Human betaherpesvirus interactions in solid organ transplant recipients. J Infect Dis 2001; 183:179–184.
9. Jamil B, Nicholls KM, Becker GJ et al. Influence of anti-rejection therapy on the timing of cytomegalovirus disease and other infections in renal transplant recipients. Clin Transplant 2000; 14:14–18.
10. van der Meer JT, Drew WL, Bowden RA, et al. Summary of the international consensus symposium on advances in the diagnosis, treatment and prophylaxis of cytomegalovirus infection. Antiviral Res 1996; 32:119–140.
11. Duncan SR, Paradis IL, Yousem SA, et al. Sequelae of cytomegalovirus pulmonary infections in lung allograft recipients. Am Rev Respir Dis 1992; 146:1419–1425.
12. Snydman DR. Infection in solid organ transplantation. Transpl Infect Dis 1999; 1:21–28.
13. Singh N, Arnow PM, Bonham A, et al. Invasive aspergillosis in liver transplant recipients in the 1990's. Transplantation 1997; 64:716–720.
14. McCarthy JM, Karim MA, Krueger H et al. The cost impact of cytomegalovirus disease in renal transplant recipients. Transplantation 1993; 55:1277–1282.
15. Falagas ME, Arbo M, Ruthhazer R, et al. Cytomegalovirus disease is associated with increased cost and hospital length of stay among orthotopic liver transplant recipients. Transplantation 1997; 63:1595–1601.
16. Kim WR, Badley AD, Weisner RH, et al. The economic impact of cytomegalovirus infection after liver transplantation. Transplantation 2000; 69:357–361.
17. Tolkhoff-Rubin NE, Fishman JA, Rubin RH. The bidirectional relationship between cytomegalovirus and allograft injury. Transplant Proc 2001; 33:1773–1775.
18. Beck S, Barrell BG. Human cytomegalovirus encodes a glycoprotein homologous to MHC class-I antigens. Nature 1988; 331:269–272.
19. Winston DJ, Antin JH, Wolff SN, et al. A multicenter, randomized, double-blind comparison of different doses of intravenous immunoglobulin for prevention of graft-versus-host disease and infection after allogeneic bone marrow transplantation. Bone Marrow Transplant 2001; 28:187–196.
20. Duncan SR, Grgurich WF, Iacono AT, et al. A comparison of ganciclovir and acyclovir to prevent cytomegalovirus after lung transplantation. Am Rev Respir Dis 1994; 150:146–152.
21. Schulman LL, Weinberg AD, McGregor CC, et al. Influence of donor and recipient HLA locus mismatching on development of obliterative bronchiolitis after lung transplantation. Am J Respir Crit Care Med 2001; 163: 437–442.
22. Ettinger NA, Bailey TC, Trulock EP, et al. Cytomegalovirus infection and pneumonitis. Am Rev Respir Dis 1993; 147:1017–1023.

23. Sharples LD, Tamm M, McNeil K, et al. Development of bronchiolitis obliterans syndrome in recipients of heart-lung transplantation—early risk factors. Transplantation 1996; 61:560–566.

24. Bowden RA, Slichter SJ, Sayers M, et al. A comparison of filtered leukocyte-reduced and cytomegalovirus (CMV) seronegative blood products for the prevention of transfusion-associated CMV infection after marrow transplant. Blood 1995; 86:3598–3603.

25. Baldanti F, Revello mg, Percivalle E, et al. Use of the human cytomegalovirus (HCMV) antigenemia assay for diagnosis and monitoring of HCMV infections and detection of antiviral drug resistance in the immunocompromised. J Clin Virol 1998; 11:51–60.

26. Egan JJ, Barber L, Lomax J, et al. Detection of human cytomegalovirus antigenemia: a rapid diagnostic technique for predicting cytomegalovirus infection/pneumonitis in lung and heart transplant recipients. Thorax 1995; 50:9–13.

27. Bewig B, Haacke TC, Tirocke A, et al. Detection of CMV pneumonitis after lung transplantation using PCR of DNA from bronchoalveolar lavage cells. Respiration 2000; 67:166–172.

28. Michaelides A, Liolios L, Glare EM, et al. Increased human cytomegalovirus (HCMV) DNA load in peripheral blood leukocytes after lung transplantation correlates with HCMV pneumonia. Transplantation 2001; 72:141–147.

29. Guiver M, Fox AJ, Mutton K, et al. Evaluation of CMV viral load using TaqMan CMV quantitative PCR and comparison with CMV antigenemia in heart and lung transplant recipients. Transplantation 2001; 71:1609–1615.

30. Masaoka T, Hiraoka A, Ohta K, et al. Evaluation of the AMPLICOR CMV, COBAS AMPLICOR CMV monitor, and antigenemia assay for cytomegalovirus disease. Jpn J Infect Dis 2001; 54:12–16.

31. Mazzulli T. Multicenter comparison of the Digene hybrid capture CMV DNA assay (version 2.0), the pp65 antigenemia assay, and cell culture for detection of cytomegalovirus viremia. J Clin Microbiol 1999; 37:958–963.

32. Bhorade SM, Sandesara C, Garrity ER, et al. Quantification of cytomegalovirus (CMV) viral load by the hybrid capture assay allows for early detection of CMV disease in lung transplant recipients. J Heart Lung Transplant 2001; 20:928–934.

33. Humar A, Paya C, Pescovitz MD, et al. Clinical utility of cytomegalovirus viral load testing for predicting CMV disease in D+/R− solid organ transplant recipients. Am J Transplant 2004; 4:644–649.

34. Chemaly RF, Yen-Lieberman B, Castilla EA, et al. Correlation between viral loads of cytomegalovirus in blood and bronchoalveolar lavage specimens from lung transplant recipients determined by histology and immunohistochemistry. J Clin Microbiol 2004; 42:2168–2172.

35. Humar A, Gregson D, Caliendo AM, et al. Clinical utility of quantitative cytomegalovirus viral load determination for predicting cytomegalovirus disease in liver transplant recipients. Transplantation 1999; 68:1305–1311.

36. Weinberg A, Hodges TN, Li S, et al. Comparison of PCR, antigenemia assay and rapid blood culture for detection and prevention of cytomegalovirus disease after lung transplantation. J Clin Microbiol 2000; 38:768–772.

37. Wreghitt T. Cytomegalovirus infections in heart and heart-lung transplant recipients. J Antimicrob Chemother 1989; 23(Suppl E):49–60.
38. Soghikian MV, Valentine VG, Berry GJ, et al. Impact of ganciclovir prophylaxis on heart-lung and lung transplant recipients. J Heart Lung Transplant 1996; 15:881–887.
39. Duncan SR, Paradis IL, Dauber JH, et al. Ganciclovir prophylaxis for cytomegalovirus infections in pulmonary allograft recipients. Am Rev Respir Dis 1992; 146:1213–1215.
40. Kelly JL, Albert RK, Wood DE et al. Efficacy of a 6-week prophylactic ganciclovir regimen and the role of serial cytomegalovirus antibody testing in lung transplant recipients. Transplantation 1995; 59:1144–1147.
41. Hertz MI, Jordan C, Savik SK, et al. Randomized trial of daily versus three-times weekly prophylactic ganciclovir after lung and heart-lung transplantation. J Heart Lung Transplant 1998; 17:913–920.
42. Limaye AP, Raghu G, Koelle DM, et al. High incidence of ganciclovir-resistant cytomegalovirus infection among lung transplant recipients receiving preemptive therapy. J Infect Dis 2002; 185:20–27.
43. Paya CV. A randomized, double-blinded, double-dummy, active comparator controlled multicenter study of the efficacy and safety of VGCV vs. oral ganciclovir for prevention of CMV in 372 high-risk (D+/R−) heart, liver and kidney recipients. (Abstract LB-4). In: Program and Abstracts of the 42nd Interscience Conference on Antimicrobial Agents and Chemotherapy, Sep 27–30, 2002. San Diego, CA: American Society for Microbiology Press, 2002.
44. Maurer JR, Snell G, deHoyos A, et al. Outcomes of lung transplantation using three different cytomegalovirus prophylactic regimens. Transplant Proc 1993; 25:1434–1435.
45. Gould FK, Freeman R, Taylor CE, et al. Prophylaxis and management of cytomegalovirus pneumonitis after lung transplantation: a review of experience in one center. J Heart Lung Transplant 1993; 12:695–699.
46. Kruger RM, Paranjothi S, Storch GA, et al. Impact of prophylaxis with cytogam alone on the incidence of CMV viremia in CMV-seropositive lung transplant recipients. J Heart Lung Transplant 2003; 22:754–763.
47. Bailey TC, Trulock EP, Ettinger NA, et al. Failure of prophylactic ganciclovir to prevent cytomegalovirus disease in recipients of lung transplants. J Infect Dis 1992; 165:548–552.
48. Zamora MR. Use of cytomegalovirus immune globulin and ganciclovir for the prevention of cytomegalovirus disease in lung transplantation. Transplant Infect Dis 2001; 3(Suppl 2):49–56.
49. Valantine HA, Luikart H, Doyle R, et al. Impact of cytomegalovirus hyperimmune globulin on outcome after cardiothoracic transplantation: a comparative study of combined prophylaxis with CMV hyperimmune globulin plus ganciclovir versus ganciclovir alone. Transplantation 2001; 72: 1647–1652.
50. Poirier CD, Doyle RL, Theodore J, et al. Comparison between CMV hyperimmune globulin and GCV for CMV prophylaxis in heart–lung and lung transplant recipients. J Heart Lung Transplant 1998: 17:96.

51. Weill D, Lock BJ, Wewers DL, et al. Combination prophylaxis with ganciclovir and cytomegalovirus (CMV) immune globulin after lung transplantation: effective CMV prevention following daclizumab induction. Am J Transplant 2003; 3:492–496.

52. Zamora MR, Nicolls MR, Hodges TN, et al. Following universal prophylaxis with intravenous ganciclovir and cytomegalovirus immune globulin, valganciclovir is safe and effective for prevention of CMV infection following lung transplantation. Am J Transplant 2004; 4:1635–1642.

53. Kelly J, Hurley D, Raghu G. Comparison of the efficacy and cost effectiveness of pre-emptive therapy as directed by CMV antigenemia and prophylaxis with ganciclovir in lung transplant recipients. J Heart Lung Transplant 2000; 19: 355–359.

54. Weill D, Zamora MR. Comparison of the efficacy and cost-effectiveness of pre-emptive therapy as directed by CMV antigenemia and prophylaxis with ganciclovir in lung transplant recipients. J Heart Lung Transplant 2000; 19:815–816.

55. Rubin RH, Lynch P, Pasternack MS, et al. Combined antibody and ganciclovir treatment of murine cytomegalovirus-infected normals and immunocompromised BALB/c mice. Antimicrob Agents Chemother 1989; 33: 1975–1979.

56. Goldfarb NS, Avery RK, Goormastic M, et al. Hypogammaglobulinemia in lung transplant recipients. Transplantation 2001; 71:242–246.

57. Yamani MH, Avery R, Mawhorter S, et al. Hypogammaglobulinemia following cardiac transplantation: a link between rejection and infection. J Heart Lung Transplant 2001; 20:425–430.

58. Rubin RH. Prevention and treatment of cytomegalovirus disease in heart transplant patients. J Heart Lung Transplant 2000; 19:731–735.

59. Turgeon N, Fishman JA, Doran M, et al. Prevention of recurrent cytomegalovirus disease in renal and liver transplant recipients: effect of oral ganciclovir. Transpl Infect Dis 2000; 2:2–10.

60. Nankivell BJ, Malouf MA, Russ GR, et al. Maintenance therapy with oral ganciclovir after treatment of cytomegalovirus infection. Clin Transplant 1998; 12:270–273.

61. Erice A. Resistance of human cytomegalovirus to antiviral drugs. Clin Microbiol Rev 1999; 12:286–297.

62. Limaye AP, Corey L, Koelle DM, et al. Emergence of ganciclovir-resistant cytomegalovirus disease among recipients of solid-organ transplants. Lancet 2000; 356:645–649.

63. Kruger RM, Shannon WD, Arens MQ, et al. The impact of ganciclovir-resistant cytomegalovirus infection after lung transplantation. Transplantation 1999; 68:1272–1279.

64. Alain S, Honderlick P, Grenet D, et al. Failure of ganciclovir treatment associated with selection of a ganciclovir-resistant cytomegalovirus strain in a lung transplant recipient. Transplantation 1997; 62:1533–1536.

65. Baldanti F, Simoncini L, Sarasini A, et al. Ganciclovir resistance as a result of oral ganciclovir in a heart transplant recipient with multiple human cytomegalovirus strains in blood. Transplantation 1998; 66:324.

66. Lurain N, Ammons H, Kapell K, et al. Molecular analysis of human cytomegalovirus strains from two lung transplant recipients with the same donor. Transplantation 1996; 62:497.

67. Mylonakis E, Kallas WM, Fishman JA. Combination antiviral therapy for ganciclovir-resistant cytomegalovirus infections in solid organ transplant recipients. Clin Infect Dis 2002; 34:1337–1341.

68. Chou S, Marousek G, Guentzel S, et al. Evolution of mutations conferring multidrug resistance during prophylaxis and therapy of cytomegalovirus disease. J Infect Dis 1998; 176:786–789.

69. Waldman WJ, Knight DA, Lurain NS, et al. Novel mechanism of inhibition of cytomegalovirus by the experimental immunosuppressive agent leflunomide. Transplantation 1999; 68:814–825.

70. Avery RK, Bolwell BJ, Yen-Lieberman B, et al. Use of leflunomide in an allogeneic bone marrow transplant recipient with refractory cytomegalovirus infection. Bone Marrow Transplant 2004; 34:1071–1075.

71. Yoshikawa T. Significance of human herpesviruses to transplant recipients. Curr Opin Inf Dis 2003; 16:601–606.

72. De Bolle L, Naesens L, De Clercq E. Update on human herpesvirus 6 biology, clinical features and therapy. Clin Microbiol Rev 2005; 18:217–245.

73. Jacobs F, Knoop C, Brancart F, et al. Human herpesvirus-6 infection after lung and heart-lung transplantation: a prospective longitudinal study. Transplantation 2003; 75:1996–2001.

74. Nash PJ, Avery RK, Wilson WH, et al. Encephalitis owing to human herpesvirus-6 after cardiac transplant. Am J Transplant 2004; 4:1200–1203.

75. Razonable RR, Rivero A, Brown RA, et al. Detection of simultaneous B-herpesvirus infections in clinical syndromes due to defined cytomegalovirus infection. Clin Transplant 2003; 17:114–120.

76. Yoshida M, Yamada M, Tsukazaki T, et al. Comparison of antiviral compounds against human herpesvirus 6 and 7. Antiviral Res 1998; 40:73–84.

77. Ross DJ, Chan RCK, Kubak B, et al. Bronchiolitis obliterans with organizing pneumonia: possible association with human herpesvirus-7 infection after lung transplantation. Transplant Proc 2001; 33:2603–2606.

78. Brennan DC, Storch GA, Singer GC, et al. The prevalence of human herpes virus-7 renal transplant recipients is unaffected by oral and intravenous ganciclovir. J Infect Dis 2000; 181:1577–1561.

79. Wang FZ, Dahl H, Linde A, et al. Lymphotrophic herpesviruses in allogeneic bone marrow transplantation. Blood 1996; 88:3615–3620.

80. Collart F, Kerbaul F, Damaj G, et al. Visceral Kaposi's sarcoma associated with human herpesvirus 8 seroconversion in a heart transplant recipient. Transplant Proc 2004; 36:3173–3174.

81. Huang PM, Chang YL, Chen JS, et al. Human herpesvirus-8 associated Kaposi's sarcoma after lung transplantation: a case report. Transplant Proc 2003; 35:447–449.

82. Preiksaitis JK, Cockfield SM. Epstein-Barr virus and lymphoproliferative disease after hematopoietic stem cell or solid organ transplantation. In: Bowden RA, Ljungman P, Paya CV, eds. Transplant Infections. 2nd. Philadelphia: Lippincott-Williams and Wilkens, 2003:326–349.

83. Gottschalk S, Rooney CM, Heslop HE. Post-transplant lymphoproliferative disorders. Annu Rev Med 2005; 56:29–44.
84. Preiksaitis JK. New developments in the diagnosis and management of post-ransplantation lymphoproliferative disorders in solid organ transplant recipients. Clin Infect Dis 2004; 39:1016–1023.
85. Moss DJ, Burrows SR, Silins, et al. The immunology of Epstein–Barr virus infection. Philos Trans R Soc Lond B Biol Sci 2001; 356:595–604.
86. Rowe DT, Webber S, Schauer EM, et al. Epstein–Barr virus load monitoring: its role in the prevention and management of post-transplant lymphoproliferative disease. Transplant Infect Dis 2001; 3:79–87.
87. Gartner BC, Fischinger J, Schafer H, et al. Epstein–Barr virus load as a tool to diagnose and monitor post-transplant lymphoproliferative disease. Recent Results Cancer Res 2002; 159:49–54.
88. Schafer H, Berger C, Aepinus C, et al. Molecular pathogenesis of Epstein–Barr virus-associated posttransplant lymphomas: new insights through latent membrane protein 1 fingerprinting. Transplantation 2001; 72:492–496.
89. Reams BD, McAdams HP, Howell DN, et al. Post-transplant lymphoproliferative disorder. Incidence, presentation and response to treatment in lung transplant recipients. Chest 2003; 124:1242–1249.
90. Penn I. The changing pattern of post-transplant malignancies. Transplant Proc 1991; 23:1101–1103.
91. Cockfield SM, Preiksaitis JK, Jewell LD, et al. Post-transplant lymphoproliferative disorder in renal allograft recipients: clinical experience and risk factor analysis in a single center. Transplantation 1993; 56:88–96.
92. Walker RC, Marshall WF, Strickler JG, et al. Pretransplant assessment of the risk of lymphoproliferative disorder. Clin Infect Dis 1995; 20:1346–1353.
93. Swinnen LJ, Costanzo-Nordin MR, Fisher SG, et al. Increased incidence of lymphoproliferative disorder after immunosuppression with the monoclonal antibody OKT3 in cardiac transplant recipients. N Engl J Med 1990; 323:1723–1728.
94. Libertiny G, Watson CJ, Gray DW, et al. Rising incidence of postransplant lymphoproliferative disease in kidney transplant recipients. Br J Surg 2001; 88:1330–1334.
95. Dotti G, Fiocchi R, Motta T. Primary effusion lymphoma after heart transplantation: a new entity associated with human herpesvirus-8. Leukemia 1999; 13:664–670.
96. Kapelushnik J, Ariad S, Benharrock D, et al. Post renal transplantation human herpesvirus-8-associated lymphoproliferative disorder and Kaposi's sarcoma. Br J Haematol 2001; 113:425–428.
97. McLaughlin K, Wajstaub S, Marotta P, et al. Increased risk for posttransplant lymphoproliferative disease in recipients of liver transplants with hepatitis C. Liver Transplant 2000; 6:570–574.
98. Opelz G, Henderson R. Incidence of non-Hodgkin's lymphoma in kidney and heart transplant recipients. Lancet 1993; 342:1514–1516.
99. Funch DP, Brady J, Ko HH, et al. Methods and objectives of a large multi-center, case-controlled study of posttransplant lymphoproliferative disorder in renal transplant recipients. Recent Results Cancer Res 2002; 159:81–88.

100. Ghobrial IM, Habermann TM, Macon WR, et al. Differences between early and late posttransplant lymphoproliferative disorders in solid organ transplant patients: are they two different diseases? Transplantation 2005; 79:244–247.
101. Harris NL, Ferry JA, Swerdlow SH. Posttransplant lymphoproliferative disorders: summary of society for hematopathology workshop. Semin Diagn Pathol 1997; 14:8–14.
102. Harris NL, Swerdlow SH, Frizerra G, et al. Posttransplant lymphoproliferative disorders. In: Jaffe ES, Harris NL, Stein H, Vardiman JW, eds. Pathology and Genetics: Tumours of Haematopoietic and Lymphoid Tumours: WHO Classification of Tumours. Lyons, France: IARC Press, 2001:264–269.
103. Gully ML, Swinnen LJ, Plaisance KT Jr, et al. Tumor origin and CD20 expression in posttransplant lymphoproliferative disorder occurring in solid organ transplant recipients: implication for immune based therapy. Transplantation 2003; 76:959–964.
104. Nelson BP, Nalesnik MA, Bahler DW, et al. Epstein–Barr virus-negative post transplant lymphoproliferative disorders. Am J Surg Pathol 2000; 24:375–385.
105. Green M, Cacciarelli T, Mazariegos GV, et al. Serial measurements of Epstein–Barr viral load in peripheral blood of pediatric liver transplant recipients during treatment for posttransplant lymphoproliferative disease. Transplantation 1998; 66:1641–1644.
106. Straathof KC, Savoldo B, Heslop H, et al. Immunotherapy for post-transplant lymphoproliferative disease. Br J Haematol 2002; 118:728–740.
107. Leung E, Shenton BK, Green K, et al. Dynamic Epstein–Barr virus gene loads in renal, hepatic and cardiothoracic transplant recipients as determined by real-time PCR light cycler. Transplant Infect Dis 2004; 6:156–164.
108. Khanna R, Bell S, Sherritt M, et al. Activation and adoptive transfer of Epstein–Barr virus-specific-cytotoxic T cells in solid organ transplant patients with posttransplant lymphoproliferative disease. Proc Natl Acad Sci USA 1999; 96:10391–10396.
109. Davis CL. Interferon and cytotoxic chemotherapy for the treatment of post transplant lymphoproliferative disorder. Transplant Infect Dis 2001; 3:108–118.
110. Paya CV, Fung JJ, Nalesnik MA, et al. Epstein–Barr virus-induced post-transplant lymphoproliferative disorders. Transplantation 1999; 68:1517–1525.
111. Gross TG. Low-dose chemotherapy for children with post-transplant lymphoproliferative disorder. Recent Results Cancer Res 2002; 159:96–103.
112. Milpied N, Vasseur B, Parquet N, et al. Humanized anti-CD20 monoclonal antibody (rituximab) in post-transplant B-lymphoproliferative disorder: a retrospective analysis in 32 patients. Ann Oncol 2000; 11:S113–S116.
113. Ghobrial IM, Habermann TM, Ristow KM, et al. Prognostic factors in patients with post-transplant lymphoproliferative disorders (PTLD) in the rituximab era. Leuk Lymphoma 2005; 46:191–196.
114. Suzan F, Ammor M, Ribrag V. Fatal reactivation of cytomegalovirus infection after use of rituximab for a post-transplantation lymphoproliferative disorder. N Engl J Med 2001; 345:1000.
115. Leblond V, Dhedin N, Mamzer Bruneel MF, et al. Identification of prognostic factors in 61 patients with post-transplantation lymphoproliferative disorders. J Clin Oncol 2001; 19:772–778.

116. Corey L, Spear PG. Infections with herpes simplex viruses, I. N Engl J Med 1986; 314:686–691.

117. Dummer JS, Armstrong J, Somers J, et al. Transmission of infection with herpes simplex virus by renal transplantation. J Infect Dis 1987; 155:202–206.

118. Holland HK, Wingard JR, Saral R, et al. Herpesvirus and enteric viral infections in bone marrow transplantation: clinical presentations, pathogenesis, and therapeutic strategies. Cancer Invest 1990; 8:509–521.

119. Singh N, Dummer JS, Kusne S, et al. Infections with cytomegalovirus and other herpesviruses in 121 liver transplant recipients: transmission by donated organ and effect of OKT3 antibodies. J Infect Dis 1988; 158:124–131.

120. Smyth RL, Higgenbottam TW, Scott JP, et al. Herpes simplex viral infection in heart-lung transplant recipients. Transplantation 1990; 49:735–739.

121. Taylor RJ, Saul SH, Dowling JN, et al. Primary disseminated herpses simplex infection with fulminant hepatitis following renal transplantation. Arch Intern Med 1981; 141:1519–1521.

122. Lakeman FD, Whitley RJ. Diagnosis of herpes simplex encephalitis: application of polymerase chain reaction to cerebrospinal fluid from brain biopsied patients and correlation with disease. National Institute of Allergy and Infectious Diseases Collaborative Antiviral Study Group. J Infect Dis 1995; 171:857–863.

123. Gnann JW Jr. Herpes simplex and varicella zoster infection after hemopoietic stem cell or solid organ transplantation. In: Bowden RA, Ljungman P, Paya CV eds. Transplant Infections. 2nd ed. Philadelphia: Lippincott-Williams and Wilkens, 2003:350–366.

124. Perry CM, Faulds D. Valacyclovir: a review of its antiviral, pharmacokinetic properties and therapeutic efficacy in herpesvirus infections. Drugs 1996; 52:754–772.

125. Gabel H, Flamholc L, Ahlfors K. Herpes simplex virus hepatitis in a renal transplant recipient: successful treatment with acyclovir. Scand J Infect Dis 1988; 20:435–438.

126. Gnann JW Jr, Whitley RJ. Clinical practice: herpes zoster. N Engl J Med 2002; 347:340–346.

127. Locksley RM, Flournoy N, Sullivan KM, et al. Infection with varicella-zoster virus after marrow transplantation. J Infect Dis 1985; 152:1172–1181.

128. Liesagang TJ. Varicella zoster viral disease. Mayo Clin Proc 1999; 74:983–998.

129. Zaia JA, Levin MJ, Preblud SR, et al. Evaluation of varicella-zoster immune globulin: protection of immunosuppressed children after household exposure to varicella. J Infect Dis 1983; 147:737–743.

130. Broyer M, Tete MJ, Guest G, et al. Varicella and zoster in children after kidney transplantation: long-term results of vaccination. Pediatrics 1997; 99:35–39.

131. Billings JL, Hertz MI, Savik K, et al. Respiratory viruses and chronic rejection in lung transplant recipients. J Heart Lung Transplant 2002; 21:559–566.

132. Holt ND, Gould FK, Taylor CE, et al. Incidence and significance of noncytomegalovirus viral respiratory infection after adult lung transplantation. J Heart Lung Transplant 1997; 16:416–419.

133. Vilchez RA, McCurry K, Dauber J, et al. The epidemiology of parainfluenza virus infection in lung transplant recipients. Clin Infect Dis 2001; 33:2004–2008.
134. Palmer SM, Henshaw NG, Howell DN, et al. Community respiratory viral infection in adult lung transplant recipients. Chest 1998; 113:944–950.
135. Wendt CH, Fox JMK, Hertz MI. Paramyxovirus infections in lung transplant recipients. J Heart Lung Transplant 1995; 14:479–485.
136. Weinberg A, Zamora MR, Li S, et al. The value of polymerase chain reaction for the diagnosis of viral respiratory tract infections in lung transplant recipients. J Clin Virol 2002; 25:171–175.
137. Raad I, Abbas J, Whimbey E. Infection control of nosocomial respiratory viral disease in the immunocompromised host. Am J Med 1997; 102:48–52.
138. Bridges ND, Spray TL, Collins MH, et al. Adenovirus infection in the lung results in graft failure after lung transplantation. J Thorac Cardiovasc Surg 1998; 116:617–623.
139. McCurdy LH, Milstone A, Dummer S. Clinical features and outcomes of paramyxoviral infections in lung transplant recipients treated with ribavirin. J Heart Lung Transplant 2003; 22:745–753.
140. Ko JP, Shepard JA, Sproule MW, et al. CT manifestations of respiratory syncytial virus infection in lung transplant recipients. J Comput Assist Tomogr 2000; 24:735–742.
141. Englund JA. Diagnosis and eopidemiology of community-acquired respiratory virus infections in the immunocompromised host. Biol Blood Marrow Transplant 2000; 7:2S–4S.
142. Barenfanger J, Drake C, Leon N, et al. Clinical and financial benefits of rapid detection of respiratory viruses: an outcomes study. J Clin Microbiol 2000; 38:2824–2828.
143. Englund JA, Piedra PA, Jewell A, et al. Rapid diagnosis of respiratory syncytial virus infection in immunocompromised adults. J Clin Microbiol 1996; 34:1649–1655.
144. Whimbey E, Englund JA, Couch RB. Community respiratory virus infections in immunocompromised patients with cancer. Am J Med 1997; 102:10–18.
145. Atmar RL, Englund JA. Laboratory methods for the diagnosis of viral diseases. In: Evans AS, Kaslow RA, eds. Viral Infections of Humans. New York: Plenum Publishing, 1997:59–88.
146. Englund JA, Whimbey EE. Community acquired respiratory viruses after hemopoietic stem cell or solid organ transplantation. In: Bowden RA, Ljungman P, Paya CV, eds. Transplant Infections. 2nd. Philadelphia: Lippincott-Williams and Wilkens, 2003:375–398.
147. Garbino J, Gerbase MW, Wunderli W, et al. Lower respiratory viral illnesses: Improved diagnosis by molecular methods and clinical impact. Am J Respir Crit Care Med 2004; 170:1197–1203.
148. Rovida F, Percivalle E, Zavattoni M, et al. Monoclonal antibodies versus reverse transcription-PCR for detection of respiratory viruses in a patient population with respiratory tract infections admitted to hospital. J Med Virol 2005; 75:336–347.

149. Englund JA. Antiviral therapy for influenza. Semin Pediatr Infect Dis 2002; 13:120–128.
150. Hayden FG, Osterhaus AD, Treanor JJ, et al. Efficacy and safety of the neuraminidase inhibitor zanamavir in the treatment of influenza virus infections. N Engl J Med 1997; 337:874–880.
151. Treanor JJ, Hayden FG, Vrooman, et al. Efficacy and safety of the oral neuraminidase inhibitor oseltamivir in treating acute influenza: a randomized controlled trial. J Am Med Assoc 2000; 283:1016–1024.
152. Knight V, Gilbert BE. Ribavirin aerosol treatment of influenza. Antiviral Chemother 1987; 1:441–457.
153. DeVincenzo JP, Hirsch RL, Fuentes RJ, et al. Respiratory syncytial virus immune globulin treatment of lower respiratory tract infection in pediatric patients undergoing bone marrow transplantation—a compassionate use experience. Bone Marrow Transplant 2000, 25:161–165.
154. Huggins JW, Hsiang CM, Cosgriff JM, et al. Prospective double-blind concurrent placebo-controlled clinical trial of intravenous ribavirin therapy of hemorrhagic fever with renal syndrome. J Infect Dis 1991; 164:1119–1127.
155. Hodges TN, Torres FP, Zamora MR. Treatment of respiratory syncytial viral and parainfluenza lower respiratory tract infections in lung transplant patients. J Heart Lung Transplant 2001; 20:170.
156. Ljungman P. Treatment of adenovirus infections in the immunocompromised host. Eur J Clin Microbiol Infect Dis 2004; 23:583–588.
157. Khalifah AP, Hachem RR, Chakinala MM, et al. Respiratory viral infections are a distinct risk factor for bronchiolitis obliterans syndrome and death. Am J Respir Crit Care Med 2004; 170:181–187.
158. Chakinala MM, Walter MJ. Community acquired respiratory virus infections following lung transplantation. Semin Thorac Cardiovasc Surg 2004; 16:342–349.
159. Winter JB, Gouw AS, Groen M, et al. Respiratory viral infections aggravate airway damage caused by chronic rejection in rat lung allografts. Transplantation 1994; 57:418–422.
160. Olszewska-Pazdrak B, Casola A, Saito T, et al. Cell-specific expression of RANTES, MCP-1 and MIP-1 alpha by lower airway epithelial cells and eosinophils infected with respiratory syncytial virus. J Virol 1998; 72:4756–4764.
161. Noah TL, Becker S. Chemokines in nasal secretions of normal adults experimentally infected with respiratory syncytial virus. Clin Immunol 2000; 97:43–49.
162. Koga T, Look DC, Taguchi M, et al. Virus-inducible expression of a host chemokine relies on replication-linked mRNA stabilization. Proc Natl Acad Sci USA 1999; 96:5680–5685.
163. Reynaud-Gaubert M, Marin V, Thirion X, et al. Upregulation of chemokines in bronchoalveolar lavage fluid as a predictive marker of post-transplant airway obliteration. J Heart Lung Transplant 2002; 21:721–730.
164. Young NS, Brown KE. Parvovirus B19. N Engl J Med 2004; 350:586–597.
165. Calvet A, Pujol MO, Bertocchi M, Bastien O, Boissonnat P, Mornex JF. Parvovirus B19 infection in thoracic organ transplant recipients. J Clin Virol 1999; 13:37–42.
166. Kariyawasam HH, Gyi KM, Hodson ME, Cohen BJ. Anaemia in lung transplant patient caused by parvovirus B19. Thorax 2000; 55:619–620.

167. Moreux N, Ranchin B, Calvet A, Bellon G, Levrey-Hadden H. Chronic parvovirus B19 infection in a pediatric lung transplanted patient. Transplantation 2002; 73:565–568.

168. Marchand S, Tchernia G, Hiesse C, et al. Human parvovirus B19 infection in organ transplant recipients. Clin Transplant 1999; 13:17–24.

169. Van den Hoogen BG, de Jong JC, Groen J, Kuiken T, de Groot R, Fouchier RA, Osterhaus AD. A newly discovered human pneumovirus isolated from young children with respiratory tract disease. Nat Med 2001; 7:719–724.

170. Crowe JE. Human Metapneumovirus as a major cause of human respiratory tract disease. Pediatr Infect Dis J 2004; 23:S215–S221.

171. Hamelin ME, Abed Y, Boivin G. Human metapneumovirus: a new player among respiratory viruses. Clin Infect Dis 2004; 38:983–990.

172. Cane PA, van den Hoogen BG, Chakrabarti S, Fegan CD, Osterhaus AD. Human metapneumovirus in a haematopoietic stem cell transplant recipient with fatal lower respiratory tract disease. Bone Marrow Transplant 2003; 31:309–310.

173. Wyde PR, Chetty SN, Jewell AM, Boivin G, Piedra PA. Comparison of the inhibition of human metapneumovirus and respiratory syncytial virus by ribavirin and immune serum globulin in vitro. Antiviral Res 2003; 60:51–59.

174. Whimbey E, Champlin RE, Englund JA, et al. Combination therapy with aerosolized ribavirin and intravenous immunoglobulin for respiratory syncytial virus disease in adult bone marrow transplant recipients. Bone Marrow Transplant 1995; 16:393–399.

175. Wadei H, Alangaden GJ, Sillix DH, et al. West Nile virus encephalitis: an emerging disease in renal transplant recipients. Clin Transplant 2004; 18:753–758.

176. Gea-Banacloche J, Johnson RT, Bagic A, et al. West Nile virus: pathogenesis and therapeutic options. Ann Intern Med 2004; 140:545.

177. Hamdan A, Green P, Mendelson E, et al. Possible benefit of intravenous immunoglobulin therapy in a lung transplant recipient with West Nile virus encephalitis. Transplant Inf Dis 2002; 4:160.

178. Iwamoto M, Jernigan DB, Guasch A, et al. Transmission of West Nile virus from an organ donor to four transplant recipients. N Engl J Med 2003; 348:2196.

179. DeSalvo D, Roy-Chaudhury P, Peddi R, et al. West Nile virus encephalitis in organ transplant recipients: another high risk group for meningoencephalitis and death. Transplantation 2004; 77:466.

180. Kumar D, Prasad GV, Zaltzman J, et al. Community-acquired West Nile virus infection in solid organ transplant recipients. Transplantation 2004; 77:399.

181. Poutenan SM, Low DE. Severe acute respiratory syndrome: an update. Curr Opin Infect Dis 2004; 17:287–294.

182. Kumar D, Tellier R, Draker R, et al. Severe acute respiratory syndrome (SARS) in a liver transplant recipient and guidelines for donor SARS screening. Am J Transplant 2003; 3:977–981.

# 23

# Coccidioidomycosis After Solid Organ Transplantation

**Bernard M. Kubak**

*Division of Infectious Diseases, Department of Medicine, David Geffen
School of Medicine at UCLA, Los Angeles, California, U.S.A.*

## INTRODUCTION

Coccidioidomycosis is geographically restricted mycosis that is responsible
for substantial morbidity and mortality in solid organ transplant recipients
(SOTRs) (1–30). While occurring less commonly than histoplasmosis in
organ transplant recipients, coccidioidomycosis is a far more serious disease
with a reported mortality in excess of 60% in some series (8,23,31). In
SOTRs, coccidioidmycosis can occur from a few weeks to several months
after transplantation and also as long as years following transplantation.
In nonimmunocompromised patients, coccidioidomycosis can result in a
clinically unapparent disease, a mild respiratory illness with a self-limited
course, or in the development of pneumonia with or without disseminated
disease depending on individual risk factors (21). Disseminated coccidioidomycosis extending beyond the pulmonary parenchyma or hilar lymph nodes
occurs in <1% of the general population (1,11,17,18,20,30). Complications
including protracted or complicated pulmonary disease or extrapulmonary disease and dissemination are infrequent, but are responsible for the substantial
public health impact of this disease. Although respiratory tract disease can affect
any individual, disseminated coccidioidomycosis is more frequent in males,
Filipinos, blacks, pregnant patients, Hispanics, and immunosuppressed patients
(15,21). African Americans more often develop disseminated osseous disease

while Filipinos manifest cutaneous or central nervous system (CNS) disease. Pregnancy, blood type, human leukocyte antigen (HLA) type, diabetes mellitus, immunocompromised states including human immunodeficiency virus infection, hematological malignancies, and organ transplantation have been reported as risk factors for disseminated disease (5,15,21,24,30–35). Notably, disease relapse is common in organ transplant recipients after apparently successful therapy and cessation of the antifungal agent (36).

Coccidioidomycosis is an emerging fungal pathogen in SOTRs most commonly reported in renal and liver transplant recipients, with a limited but increasing experience in lung and heart transplant recipients (4–10,12, 13,16–18,22–24,28,31,35,37–45). A single case report of coccidioidomycosis in a small bowel transplant recipient has been reported (46). At present, there are no reported cases of coccidioidomycosis in pancreas transplant recipients. However, it is reasonable to assume that pancreatic allograft recipients would be similarly at risk for coccidioidomycosis in endemic areas.

The endemic fungi, Histoplasma and *Coccidioides*, have the ability to remain dormant in the body for considerable periods of time (1,7,11, 13–15,21,47). Consequently, under the permissive milieu of immunosuppression that accompanies organ transplantation, reactivation can occur and organisms may proliferate leading to the clinical manifestations of disease. However, it is likely that the majority of cases are acquired as new exposure by inhalation of arthroconidida. These arthroconidia retain a hydophophic outer coating and can remain viable for long periods in the soil and the arid desert environments (14,16,19,47). Environmental disruptions of soil by natural or manmade interventions can facilitate airborne dissemination of arthroconidia by humans residing or traveling within these geographically conducive areas. Increased cases of coccidioidomycosis after earthquakes have been reported; further, increased cases have been reported in the summer seasons following winters with increased rainfall (11,19,48). Metropolitan expansion with increased residency and travel into arid desert areas by immunocompromised individuals increases the risk of exposure to *Coccidioides* spp. Further, on rare occasions in SOTRs, infection can be acquired from an unrecognized infected donor organ. The increasing clinical experience shows that coccidioidomycosis can be a serious and frequently fatal infection after solid organ transplantation, particularly in lung and heart transplant recipients.

## MYCOLOGY

Coccidioidomycosis is caused members of the genus *Coccidioides*. *Coccidioides* spp. are dimorphic fungi capable of existing as either mycelia or as spherules in tissue (20,47,49–52) (Fig. 1A). Historically, a single species *Coccidioides* was considered responsible for the clinical manifestations of this disease. Recent molecular identification techniques have identified two genetically distinct populations, *Coccidioides immitis* and *Coccidioides*

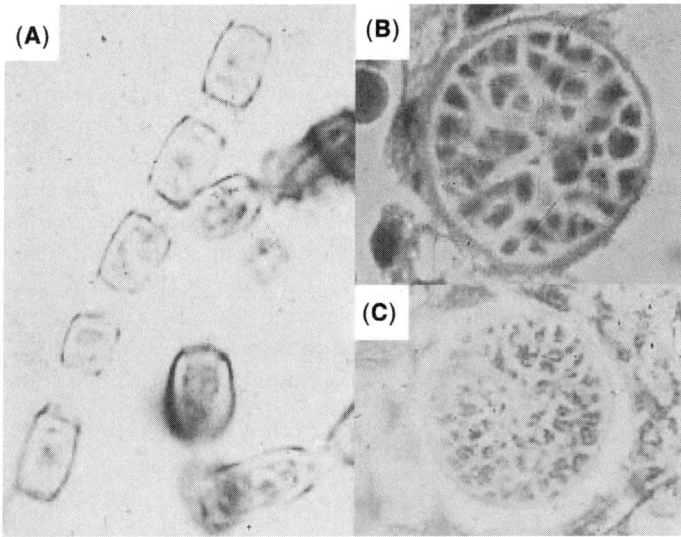

**Figure 1** (**A**) *Coccidioides immitis* culture, hyphal form: barrel-shaped arthroconidia with alternating areas of atresia. Grocott-Gomori methenamine silver (GMS) stain. (**B**) *Coccidioides immitis*, mature thick-walled spherule containing endospores. Hematoxylin & Eosin (H & E) stain. (**C**) Coccidioides in bronchoaveolar lavage from heart transplant recipient, GMS stain.

*posadasii* (21,49–54). Most of the literature and clinical laboratories have referred to *C. immitis*, as routine differentiation between the two species is currently unavailable. Reports suggest most isolates obtained from California are *C. immitis*, while *C. posadasii* has been reported in other states and from countries outside the United States. At this point in time, there does not appear to be a differences in the diseases produced by these two species (21,53). While future identification and species differentiation with evolving genomic analysis and molecular typing may yield unique differences and retrospective reevaluation between these species, current knowledge suggests the clinical manifestations of infections with either species appears similar. Literature on coccidioidomycosis in SOTRs has historically referred to *C. immitis* as the respective isolate. In vitro, *Coccidioides* spp. grow as mycelia with maturation to arthroconidia by autolysis. Patients are exposed to airborne arthroconidia with potential deposition into the lungs. A molecular remodeling in the physiological milieu of lung tissue results in spherical cells and spherule generation with internal compartments referred to as endospores (Fig. 1). Pathological analysis of infected tissues can reveal intact spherules or spherule with ruptured cell walls and released endospores. These forms are pathognomonic of coccidioidomycosis.

## EPIDEMIOLOGY AND GEOGRAPHIC OCCURRENCE

Endemic areas of coccidioidomycosis include the southwestern United States [California: in particular the Central (San Joaquin) Valley of California, areas of the San Fernando and Simi Valley, Kern County, California and the cities of Bakersfield, Porterville, and Lancaster; southern Arizona including the desert areas around Phoenix and Tucson; southern New Mexico, Nevada, areas of Utah, west Texas, the border areas along the southwestern United States and Mexico, central and western states of Mexico, Central America (Guatemala, Honduras, Nicaragua), and South America (Argentina, Paraguay, Venezuela, Colombia, and Brazil)] (20,29,30,50, 51,55). Organ transplant recipients currently and formerly residing in, and/ or visiting these areas must be evaluated for coccidioidomycosis with a compatible clinical illness.

## INCIDENCE

It has been estimated that coccidioidomycosis causes between 100,000 and 150,000 infections annually in the United States (1,15,20,21,30,55). Interestingly, even within endemic areas, it can be an unrecognized cause of community-acquired pneumonia in immunocompetent individuals. Coccidioidomycosis has been reported less frequently than histoplamosis in SOTRs. While the true incidence of coccidioidomycosis remains under ongoing review, reported ranges are from 0.3% to 10% in renal, liver, lung, and heart transplant recipients from endemic areas from different decades of reporting (5,7,8,12,22,23,38). It should be noted that the incidence of coccidioidomycosis might vary within endemic regions from year to year. This is likely due to both geographical and weather-related variations that alter the presence of *Coccidioides* in the soil and its subsequent environmental distribution and human exposures. In an earlier series of SOTRs (1970–1979) within endemic areas, a higher incidence of coccidioidomycosis was observed with a higher proportion of cases occurring in the first posttransplant year (22). In later reviews (after 1985) from a similar endemic area, a slightly lower incidence was observed (12,23). Efforts at early patient risk identification with subsequent targeted early prophylaxis may have been responsible for this reduction among other unreported variables (see section on Recommendations for Prevention). Earlier series of coccoidioidomycosis in heart transplant recipients in endemic areas describe approximately 10% incidence between 1979 and 1984 (12). Coccidioidomycosis occurred after from one to seven months after heart transplant, limited to the chest in all cases without dissemination. Mortality from coccidioidomycosis in this early series was reported at 25%, although no description of immunosuppression, rejection treatments, or comorbid illness was described.

A case of coccidioidomycosis after a heart transplant was reported in a patient previously exposed to coccidioidomycosis eight years prior (43). In this report, the patient was on immunosuppresion prior to heart transplant and presented with an unusual rash at the time of the transplant. From postoperative days 8 to 21, the rash intensified with development of cutaneous vasculitis, sepsis, renal failure, necrotic skin lesions, and pulmonary infiltrates. The patient expired three weeks after the heart transplant from disseminated coccidioidomycosis found at autopsy; sites included the myocardium, lungs, parathyroid and adrenal glands, kidneys, bone marrow, and prostate gland. Coccidioidomycosis of the myocardium is rare, and dissemination to many viscera generally represents significant underlying immunosuppression. In the case described, it is possible that this patient presented with coccidioidomycosis at the time of transplant on pretransplant corticosteroids (43).

In another series of heart transplants with coccidioidomycosis from an endemic area, 11 episodes of coccidioidomycosis were reported in nine heart tranplant recipients (23). Also, in this series of heart transplants, six patients had a history of coccidioidomycosis treated before heart transplant and were continued on ketoconazole for an undefined duration after the transplant. None of those patients developed recurrence. In the remaining patients, newly diagnosed coccidioidomycosis was seen with an incidence of 4.5%. The postransplant presentation ranged from 19 to 410 days (mean, 174 days) and was confined to the airways except for two cases of disseminated diseases. Sites of dissemination included the skin, blood, genitourinary tract, and joints, but no central nervous system disease was observed in these heart transplant recipients. All patients were treated with amphotericin B ( >1 g), then followed by chronic ketoconazole. Of note, two cases recurred in these heart transplants shortly after maintenance ketoconazole therapy was stopped for reasons of an unrelated vascular surgery and renal failure. The second patient recurred in the context of a concurrent lymphoma diagnosis from which the patient expired; disseminated coccidioidomycosis was found at autopsy.

In this group of heart transplants, one- and five-year actuarial survival was similar in the patients with and without coccidioidomycosis after transplant. In another series of heart transplant recipients with documented evidence of coccidioidomycosis 12 to 22 months before transplant, four patients had nonreactive coccidioidal tube precipitin serologies at the time of transplant (22). Three of four patients had low titers of complement fixation (CF) antibodies (1:2); three patients received posttransplant ketoconazole. None of the of aforementioned heart transplant recipients developed coccidioidomycosis. The authors suggested that these markers of past coccidioidal infection should not adversely influence a patient's eligibility for transplantation. However, despite their lower incidence of post-heart transplant coccidioidomycosis, the authors recommended that patients with a history of coccidiodomycosis infection or reactive coccidioidal serologies before transplantation may benefit from an antifungal drug after transplant. Also, periodic surveillance was suggested in these patients during periods of enhanced immunosuppression.

## IMMUNOLOGY

The primary host defense against Coccidiodes spp. is cell-mediated immunity (1,11,21). Neutrophils, mononuclear cells and natural killer cells, and humoral immunity do not appear to contribute to a measurable extent to host defenses. Speculation on the possible role of mononuclear and natural killer cells on fungal viability and the intensity of the inflammatory response and clinical presentation is still under investigation. Also, while antibodies to *Coccidioides* spp. do not seem to contribute to host defenses, these antibodies to coccidioidal antigens and infection have clinical utility in the form of several commercially available diagnostic assays. Similar to histoplasmosis, initial infection by *Coccidioides* spp. is via pulmonary inoculation by the inhalation of arthroconidia (17,18,21,30). After transformation of arthroconidia into the spherule formation within the lungs, inflammatory mechanisms ensue, producing the localized infection; further, in selected patients with altered immunological surveillance, dissemination occurs, presumably by a vascular route and/or by infected macrophages via the lymphatic system. Active organisms can be recovered from regional lymph nodes, particularly in the mediastinal, hilar, and peritrachael lymph nodes.

## PRETRANSPLANT EVALUATION

Guidelines for recipient screening prior to solid organ transplantation have been reported (5,7,56,57). It is essential to evaluate all candidates for organ transplantation for prior exposure to endemic mycoses. General pretransplant screening guidelines are listed in Table 1. The risk of coccidioidomycosis after organ transplantation has been shown to be increased by a prior history of coccidioidomycosis or positive *Coccidioides* serological findings (5).

   Also, because of the potential viability of *C. immitis* organism in healed or treated lesion within lung tissue, reactivation of disease is a genuine possibility at a time period distant from the primary exposure and infection. In SOTRs, "healed" granulomatous lesions harboring latent organisms can reactivate posttransplant either during routine immunosuppression or after multiple treatments for rejection. In a series of transplant recipients (hearts, kidneys, and liver) with coccidioidomycosis prior to solid organ transplantation, candidates identified with a positive history or reactive serological test benefited by receiving prolonged antifungal prophylaxis in the posttransplant period (22,23,38). In another group of SOTRs with prior coccidioidomycosis

**Table 1**  Pretransplant Screening

---

Prior history of coccidioidomycosis, type of disease, dissemination, and treatment
Residency and travel history within endemic areas (remote or recent, no matter how
  brief the duration)
Coccidioides IgM and IgG antibody by EIA (in patients from endemic areas)
Underlying medical conditions that may complicate the clinical presentation of
  coccidioidomycosis
  Diabetes mellitus
  Prior immunosuppression, including corticosteroids
  Spleenectomy
Chest imaging
  Evidence of prior granulomatous lesions, scarring
  Evidence of active infiltrates, nodules, effusions
  Cavities (commonly thin walled)
High-resolution chest CT (if suspicion of lesions on chest radiograph)
Bone scan (if musculoskeletal coccidioidomycosis is suspected)
CT or MRI of head with suspicion of central nervous system disease

---

*Abbreviations*: CT, computed tomography; MRI, magnetic resonance imaging; Ig, immunoglobulin; EIA, enzyme immunoassay.

who did not receive antifungal prophylactic therapy, active coccidioidomycosis developed after organ transplantation (22,23).

Untreated or unrecognized coccidioidomysosis infection in the transplant candidate can become clinically apparent in the posttransplantation
period (56,57). During pretransplant screening, the identification of prior
coccidioidomycosis in the lung, heart/lung, or heart transplant recipient
should lead to a reappraisal of transplant candidacy. If active disease is
determined in a transplant candidate during evaluation, transplantation
should be deferred. A comprehensive evaluation is required to determine
the extent of disease and dissemination. Practically, a history of prior coccidioidomycosis should include an assessment on the extent of disease, types
and duration of treatment, evaluation of pulmonary or extrapulmonary
coccidioidal lesions, and serological markers of coccidiodomycosis. The
respective treatments should be appropriate for the extent of disease after
thorough evaluation. After effective therapy, relisting the transplant candidate depends on the absence of disease and positive cultures, reductions in
serological markers, and absence of surgically correctable foci of *Coccidioides* organisms. In this event, "cured" recipients should be considered
candidates for prolonged suppressive therapy after organ transplantation
(54). The lung transplant recipient may present a unique challenge to the
transplant physician and surgeon. Specifically, residual, unrecognized, or
untreated coccidioidomycosis in the native retained lung (in single lung
transplants) or in mediastinal and hilar lymph nodes may reactivate, spread

to the new lung allograft, or disseminate. Careful scrutiny and evaluation of the recipient's native (retained) lung is required.

For the living-related donor organ transplant (i.e., segmental lung, liver lobes, kidney), a careful history of prior coccidioidomycosis and exposures and of any current signs or symptoms of infection should be obtained. Evidence of active infections should be thoroughly evaluated as indicated above. While living-related segmental lung donors represent a small percentage of lung transplant donor organs, a thorough history of pulmonary coccidioidomycosis is especially warranted in these donor organs.

## CLINICAL DISEASE

The majority of coccidioidomycosis in SOTRs occurs by reactivation of a latent infection or by a new exposure in an endemic area and primary infection (5,13,16,20,21,45,58). Typically, reactivation has been noted typically from four to six months after transplantation, although later presentations are possible. In the rare cases of donor transmission, a rapid disease presentation can occur (within 6 to 13 days). Donor transmitted coccidioidomycosis has been reported in lung, liver, and renal transplant recipients (40,59,60). Unsuspected or unrecognized disease in a donor is the main reason for donor-related transmission. A rapidly fatal fulminant presentation was observed in a bilateral lung transplant recipient (40). The donor had a history of prior travel to an endemic area two years before. The recipient developed multiorgan system failure, progressive fungal pneumonia, and brain abscesses, and expired one month after lung transplant. Widely disseminated disease with *C. immitis* isolated from multiple sites was noted on autopsy. In another case of donor-transmitted coccidioidomycosis in a double lung transplant, pneumonia developed within six days of transplant with *C. immitis* isolated from bronchoalveolar lavage fluid (59). The patient responded to high-dose fluconazole and was maintained on chronic suppressive therapy. Of note, a donor lymph node was positive for *C. immitis*. Two cases of rapidly fatal coccidioidomycosis were observed in liver and kidney transplant recipients from a single donor with a remote history of five years previously (60). The recipients developed rapidly progressive multiorgan failure within 11 to 14 days and expired within three weeks of their respective organ transplants with *C. immitis* recovered from numerous visceral abscesses. The donor's disease was treated five years prior to the current presentation. Retrospective review of the donor revealed *C. immitis* in the basilar meninges with a complement fixation titer of 1:32. These cases demonstrate the importance of a scrupulous donor history for endemic mycoses.

The diagnosis of fungal infection in general remains problematic and frequently leads to delays in clinical recognition. Factors that confound the diagnosis of coccidioidomycosis in SOTRs include: (i) an impaired host inflammatory response; (ii) failure to consider coccoidiodimycosis in the differential diagnosis especially in SOTRs from outside endemic areas with prior exposures unknown to the transplant physician; (iii) delay in clinical diagnosis due to the lack of classic clinical and radiological signs associated with infection compared to the nonimmunocompromised host; pulmonary coccidioidomycosis in lung and heart transplant patients may be difficult to differentiate from other causes of pulmonary disease including rejection, other microbial and viral pneumonias, acute respiratory distress syndrome, and heart failure; (iv) the rapid progression of coccidiodomycosis observed in some heart and lung transplant recipients; and (v) delay in laboratory diagnosis by failure to include serological assays for coccidiodomycosis in patients from nonendemic areas. Despite invasive pulmonary disease, extra-pulmonary manifestations may be the first symptoms of coccidioidomycosis in SOTRs. In a heart transplant recipient, cutaneous findings mimicking other processes were the first signs of disseminated disease (43).

In lung and heart transplant recipients, coccidioidomycosis can cause more severe disease than in nonimmunocompromised hosts (9,10,16,23, 24,40). Extrapulmonary manifestations may be the initial signs of disease. Transplant patients with coccidiodomycocis can have isolated pulmonary disease or disseminated disease in conjunction with pneumonia. The clinical sites of infections in SOTRs are listed in Table 2. Heart and lung transplant recipients with coccidioidomycosis present with fever, chills, night sweats, and anorexia (22,23,39,43). Headache is a common symptom even in patients without central nervous system involvement. Coccidioidomycosis can be subacute to chronic in its presentation. Arthralgias, myalagias, joint effusions, and bone pain (especially of the knees and ankles) are reported. Pulmonary manifestations include cough, dyspnea, pleuritic pain, and rarely hemoptysis. Rashes can be a heralding symptom in SOTRs. Skin manifestations include papules, nodules, verrucous plaques, and subcutaneous fluctuant abscesses (15,21). Progression to frank ulcers, abscesses, and fistula formation has been reported.

A necrotizing vasculitis and severe cellulitis of soft tissues has been reported in a heart transplant recipient, with pathology consisting primarily of lymphocytes and plasma cells and occasionally eosinophils (43). Histopathology of infected tissues may reveal spherules with aspects of acute and chronic inflammation. Neutrophils and eosinophils can be observed. Multinucleated giant cells, lymphocytes, and histiocytes are observed in granulomatous lesions (21). The radiological presentations of coccidioidomycosis are summarized in Table 3. Radiologic images of coccidioidomycosis in heart and lung transplants are shown in Figure 2.

Pulmonary presentations include bilateral airspace opacification, isolated or multiple nodules, cavities (single $\gg$ multiple), mass-like lesions, apical and lateral pleural thickening, bronchial plaques, and pleural effusions (15,17,18,21,28,44,45). Pleural effusions reveal elevated white counts with variable numbers of eosinophils. The fluid is exudative in nature with

**Table 2**  Reported Sites of Coccidioides Infection in Solid Organ Transplants

---

Pulmonary (pneumonia, empyema, complicated pleural effusion, pleural tissue)
Direct allograft infection (kidney, heart, liver, lung, small bowel)
Meninges (central nervous system, parenchymal vasulitis, focal intracerebral
  coccidioidal abscesses)
Liver, pancreas, spleen, peritoneum
Genitourinary (kidney, epidydimis, prostate, genital urinary fistula formation)
Cutaneous (nodules, papules, verrucous plaques, nasolabial fold, shallow ulcers
  with draining sinuses)
Musculoskeletal (axial skeletal; apendicular skeletal; cranium; skull; scapula;
  sternum; ribs; clavicle; femur; shoulder; pelvis; humerus; cervical, thoracic,
  and lumbar vertebral bodies; mandible)
Joints (synovium, spine, knee, ankle, wrist, sternoclavicular joint, acromioclavicular
  joint)
Thyroid, parathyroid
Lymph nodes (regional, hilar, mediastinal, paratracheal)
Kidney
Adrenal gland
Bone marrow
Colon
Heart, pericardium
Choroid (eye)

---

elevated total protein and lactate dehydrogenase mediastinal, hilar, and paratracheal adenopathy are observed; *C. immitis* can be recovered from these nodes. Peripheral white blood cell counts are elevated, with eosinophils noted. Limited data are available on central nervous system involvement in SOTRs. Increased cerebrospinal pressure, elevated protein, depressed or normal glucose, and a mildly elevated white blood cell count with a lymphocytic predominance, with or without eosinophils are noted. An elevated cerebrospinal fluid complement fixation titer accompanies the diagnosis.

## DIAGNOSIS

Table 3 lists the components in the clinical diagnosis of coccidioidomycosis. Definitive diagnosis of coccidioidomycosis is accomplished by growing Cocciodides spp. from respiratory specimens, tissue biopsy, joint fluid, bone, CSF, and skin lesions. The yield from blood is rare. *Coccidioides* spp. usually grows within five to seven days on standard mycologic media (14). *C. immitis* spherules can be stained with periodic acid-Schiff, hematoxylin and eosin, and calclofluor stains (Fig. 1B,C) (14,21). Biopsies of infected specimens can show intact spherules with endospores or ruptured spherules. While endospores may not be visualized fully by calclofluor staining, the cell wall of *Coccidioides*

**Table 3** Coccidioidomycosis: Laboratory and Radiological Diagnosis

| Method | Description and comments |
|---|---|
| Culture | Cultures of BAL, CSF, skin, bone, joint/synoviun, or other tissues |
| | Blood culture rarely positive |
| | Urine culture |
| Histopathology | Spherules detected by calcoflour, H and E, papanicolaos, PAS stain |
| Serology | EIA (IgG, IgM), latex agglutinin, tube precipitin (IgM—early) |
| | False-positive LA occur in specimens from CSF |
| | CF IgG in serum or in CSF (note, >1:2 CF titer in CSF may be suggestive of meningitis) |
| | Low CF titers of 1:2–1:8 may be observed in pulmonary coccidioidomycosis, with CF titers >1:16 (generally indicative of dissemination) |
| | Serum CF parallels disease severity |
| | IDCF: qualitative or semi-quantitative confirmation of CF results |
| | Coccidioidal serological assays may cross react with other fungi |
| Radiology | Chest: |
| | Airspace opacities; diffuse reticulonodular infiltrates, focal infiltrate, nodules (unifocal pulmonary disease; diffuse or multifocal intrathoracic) |
| | Single or multiple thin-walled cavity (some with air-fluid level) |
| | Hilar or mediastinal adenopathy (may be ipsilateral to parenchymal opacity) |
| | Pleura-based lesions and pleural effusions (small to moderate size) Effusions can be exudates, high lactate dehydrogensase, and total protein; white counts range 1500–18,000 cells/hpf with variable numbers of eosinophils present (5–60%) |
| | Brain: |
| | Contrast enhanced CT or MRI to assess for hydrocephalus, visualize patency of aqueduct |

*Abbreviations*: BAL, bronchioalveolar lavage; CSF, cerebrospinal fluid; H and E, hematoxylin and eosin; PAS, periodic acid-Schiff; EIA, enzyme immunoassay; IgG/IgM, immunoglobulin G/M; LA, latex agglutinin; CF, complement fixation; IDCF, immunodiffusion-complement fixation; hpf, high-power field; CT, computed tomography; MRI, magnetic resonance imaging.

spp. can be well delineated from background inflammatory cells and debris. Supplement pathological stains are usually recommended.

Serologic assays are especially useful tests for the diagnosis of cocci-dioidomycosis in nonimmunosuppressed patients (15,21,48,56). Despite the altered and reduced immune responses in SOTRs, serological assays have yielded reliable specificities with applicable clinical information (5,12,48), Of note, in patients with cycstic fibrosis, false positive coccidioidal

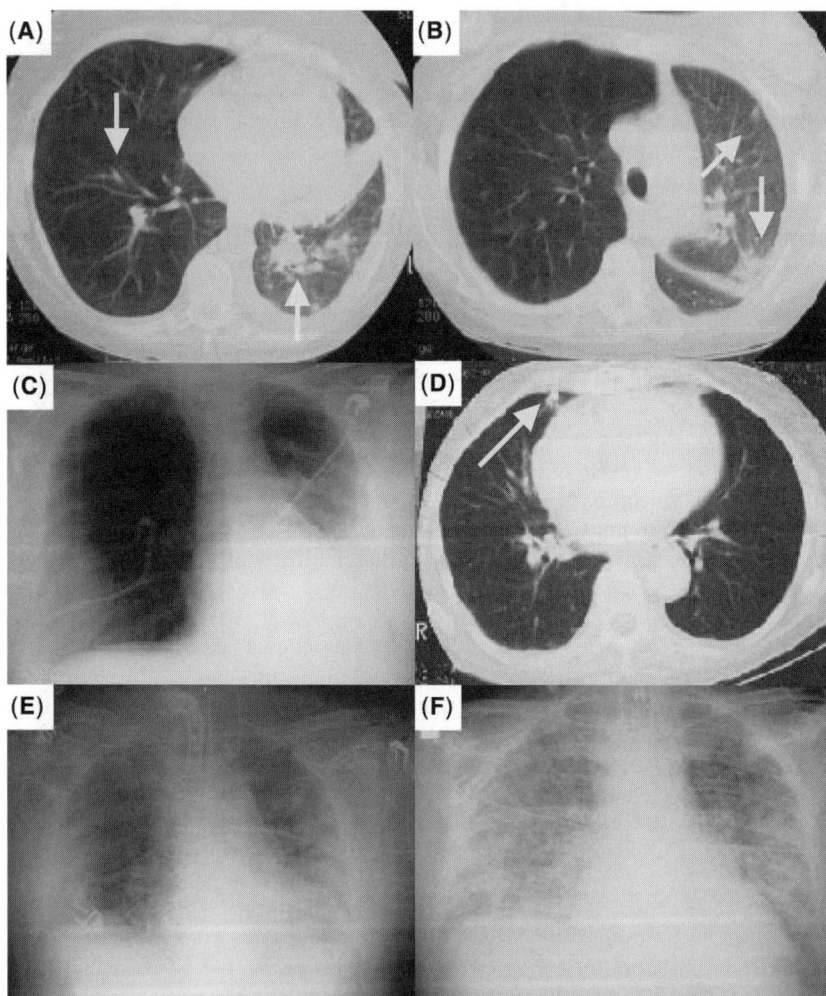

**Figure 2** (A–C) Lung transplant: ground-glass opacifications within patchy regions of the left lower and posterior left upper lobes with coalescence along the broncho-vascular bundle represent area of *Coccidoides pneumonia*. (**D**) Heart transplant: multiple scattered micronodules measuring less than 5 mm are present bilaterally with greater than 30 nodules identified; mediastinal adenopathy is seen involving the pre-vascular, paratracheal, subcarinal, periesophageal regions; the aortic pulmonic window; and the right hilum. Nodes in the anterior paratracheal region measure approximately $2 \times 3$ cm with subcarinal nodes approximately $2.5 \times 2.5$ cm. Evidence of prior granulomatous disease with 5 mm calcified nodules within the right upper lobe and right middle lobe were also noted. (**E**) Heart transplant: pneumonia is seen in the left lung. (**F**) Heart transplant: diffuse reticular nodular air space opacities throughout the lungs.

serological tests were observed (48). This is especially important in patients where cultures may be negative (e.g., cerebrospinal fluid) or where respiratory specimens are not obtainable (21). Sera from suspected patients with coccidioidomycosis can be tested for anticoccidioidal antibodies as assays have become available in most clinical reference laboratories. Serological tests for coccidioidomycosis include: enzyme-lined immunoassays for specific detection of IgM or IgG antibodies; immunodiffusion tube precipitins (IDTP); immunodiffusion; and complement fixation (CF). In the IgM immunoassay, false positive can occur and confirmation by other coccidioidal tests is usually performed. A positive result with either IgG or IgM implies the presence of antibody to *C. immitis*. An IgM is detected during an early active phase of infection while IgG may be observed in acute or chronic disease or in convalescent sera. Positive IgG and IgM strongly suggest active disease. A negative IgG and IgM resulting in a clinical scenario supportive of coccidioidomycosis does not preclude a diagnosis. Immunodifrusion assays for coccidioidomycosis are usually highly specific for and correlate with complement fixation titers.

A positive tube ID tube precipitin antibody is indicative of early infection. Complement-fixing antibodies are detected later and persist for a longer duration; CF tests are expressed as a titer. Any titer suggests past or current infection. Titer of less than 1:2 does not rule out coccidioidomycosis. Titers of 1:2–1:8 suggest recent, present, or past infection. Of note, this may also represent cross-reactive antibody to blastomyces or histoplasma. Titers of 1:16 or greater may indicate disseminated infection. Sera positive by both CF and ID are diagnostic. CF serology may be used to follow therapy. Antibody in cerebrospinal fluid is considered diagnostic for coccidioidal meningitis, although 10% of patients with coccidioidal meningitis will not have antibody in cerebrospinal fluid.

## Skin Tests

Reaction to *Coccidioides* antigens reflects delayed type dermal hypersensitivity of coccidioidal antigens (coccidioidin or spherulin). This test is highly specific for coccidoidal infection (20,21). As in other cases of dermal reactivity, in cases of severe disease, anergy may be observed. The skin testing reagents are not currently available for routine clinical use.

## TREATMENT OF COCCIDIOIDOMYCOSIS

Recommendations for the treatment of coccidioidomycosis have been established in the IDSA guidelines (2,21,25,29,36,54,61,62). Specific recommendations for the treatment of coccidioidomycosis in SOTRs are lacking; however, application of the IDSA guidelines to SOTRs with coccidiodomycosis has been generally followed. All SOTRS with coccidioidomycosis should be treated with

**Table 4**  Interactions Between Antifungal Agents Frequently Used in the Treatment of Coccidioidomycosis and Common Immunosuppressives in Solid Organ Transplant Recipients

| Antifungals | Immunosup-pressive drug[a] | Findings/implications |
|---|---|---|
| Amphotericin B deoxycholate | CsA, Tac | Increases incidence of nephrotoxicity |
| Amphotericin B lipid complex Liposomal amphotericin (ambisome) | CsA, Tac | Increases incidence of nephrotoxicity |
| Fluconazole[b], itraconazole[b], ketoconazole[b] | CsA, Tac, Sir | Increases CsA/Tac/Sir level |
| Voriconazole[c] | CsA, Tac Sir | Increases CsA/Tac/Sir level Contraindicated |
| Posaconazole | CsA, Tac, Sir | Unknown interactions, presumably similar reactions due to azole class status; specific interactions remain to be determined |
| Caspofungin[d], micafungin[d], anidulafungin[d] | CsA, Tac | Increases ALT/AST/caspofungin level and decreases Tac level |

[a]Less clinical data is available for anti-fungal interactions with Tac and Sir compared to CsA. Anti-infectives that significantly affect the metabolism of CsA by CYP3A4 have shown similar effects on Tac and Sir.

[b]Drug interaction side effects are seen mostly with high doses of fluconazole. Coadministered drugs, such as fluconazole, which are known to inhibit these enzymes, could be expected to increase plasma concentrations of tacrolimus. Patients receiving fluconazole or itraconazole concomitantly with Sir may exhibit enhanced plasma and whole blood levels of tacrolimus, resulting in tacrolimus toxicity. It is recommended that Sir not be coadministered with ketoconazole.

[c]Voriconazole is contraindicated with Sir. Sir exposure is sigificantly increased by coadministration of voriconazole. The maximum plasma concentration and area under the concentration–time curve of Sir can be increased from 7-fold and 11-fold. If utilized, readjust the dose of CsA by a half and Tac by two-thirds when taken with voriconazole. Contraindicated agents: terfenadine∗, astemizole∗, cisapride∗, pimozide∗, quinidine∗, sir, rifampin, rifabutin, carbamazepine, long-acting barbiturate, ergot alkaloids, efavirenz, ritonavir. [Voriconazole is contraindicated with these agents (starred∗) since increased plasma levels of these agents can cause serious cardiovascular events].

[d]Although limited experience exists in treating coccidioidomycosis with echinocandins, some reports suggest possible evolving usage. In this regard, caspofungin and CsA may lead to increase of AST and ALT to two to three times the upper limit of normal and increase of 35% in caspofungin have been observed. Concomitant use of caspofungin with cyclosporine is not currently recommended unless potential benefit outweighs potential risk due to reported hepatotoxicity (elevation in transaminases); further analysis with the expanding use of caspofungin and other newer echinocandins with calcineurin inhibitors may change this usage. At present, micafungin and anidulafungin have unknown reaction with calcineurin inhibitors, and their use in the treatment of coccidiodimycosis remains unknown.

*Abbreviations*: CsA, cyclosporine; Tac, tacrolimus; Sir, sirolimus; ALT, alanine aminotransferase; AST, aspartate aminotransferase.

an appropriate antifungal agent (AII) (54). However, these guidelines must be individualized in SOTRs due to the unique comorbid diseases, underlying end-organ indications for organ transplant (e.g., diabetes mellitus; pulmonary fibrosis, renal disease), concomitant nephrotoxic medications, calcineurin inhibitors, other immunosuppressive agents (e.g., sirolimus), and potential interactions with extended spectrum triazoles. Consequently, management strategies may vary in SOTRs. Antifungal agents and potential drug interactions for the treatment of coccidioidomycosis are listed in Table 4. Amphotericin B deoxycholage (AmBd) has historically been the drug of choice for the primary treatment of coccidioidomycosis, especially in severely ill patients or those with respiratory compromise (54). Doses exceeding 2.5 to 3.0 g have been required depending on the extent of dissemination and response. For patients with coccidioidomycosis, total doses up to 2.5 to 3.0 g may be required. In SOTRs with coccidioidomycosis, patients may be expected to respond less well to AmBd secondary to complications from therapy (e.g., metabolic abnormalities, nephrotoxicity, infusion-related toxicities, slow response, and relapse). In a small series of SOTRs, lipid-formulations of amphotericin B (LFAB) reported clinical cures and improvements in coccidioidomycosis (63).

More experience is required on LFAB usage for coccidioidal disease in SOTRs. However, the reduced toxicity profile and enhanced tissue penetration (i.e., lung parenchyma) offer attractive characteristics for use in SOTRs who are also receiving concomitant nephrotoxic calcineurin inhibitors. Historically, ketoconazole was the first azole to gain widespread use for coccidioidomycosis in both immunocompetent and SOTRs (21,54). The side effect profile has reduced its widespread usage and has been substituted by newer azole antifungal agents. Itraconazole (400 mg/day) and fluconazole (200–400 mg/day) have been increasingly utilized in non-SOTRs and SOTRs with an expanding and successful clinical experience (45,54,62). Both agents have been used as primary and secondary treatments for both milder forms of coccidioidomycosis and disseminated forms. Often, in SOTRs, an azole may follow primary therapy with AmBd or a LFAB for an indefinite period. Due to the risk of recurrence of coccidioidomycosis, especially after the cessation of therapy in SOTRs, lifelong prophylaxis has been considered (AIII). Voriconazole, an advanced generation triazole, has in vitro activity against *Coccidioides* spp. Its usage in the treatment of coccioidomycosis remains under investigation. Due to its enhanced penetration into CSF, its possible utility in Coccidioidal meningitis warrants investigation.

Posaconazole, an investigational oral extended-spectrum triazole, has been shown in vitro and in vivo to have potent anticoccidioides activity (37,64,65). In non-SOTRs with chronic refractory coccidioidomycosis (pulmonary, disseminated, including CNS and musculoskeletal) that had received amphotericin with or without an azole for a median duration of 306 days, 73% of patients were considered successes (partial and complete) with posaconazole at 800 mg/day (65). In another small trial of salvage

therapy for invasive fungal infections including coccidioidomycosis, posaconazole appeared well tolerated and safe for durations ≥1 year (66). In a
recent small series of six patients, none with organ transplants, with refractory coccidioidomycosis (lung, bone, skin) treated with conventional antifungal agents, a rapid response was observed in all patients, and,
moreover, within the first month after initiating treatment (64).

In a murine coccidioidomycosis model, caspofungin (cas), AmBd, and
liposomal amphotericin B prolonged survival and reduced the tissue burden
of organisms (67–69). Interestingly, combinations of LFAB and cas or
AmBd and cas enhanced the clearance of tissue organisms, with a significant
sterilization of organs for the LFAB plus cas arm. Lipid preparations were
superior to standard AmBd in other murine coccidioidomycosis models.
Caspofungin is an echinocandin class of antifungal agent. Caspofungin acts
as a noncompetitive inhibitor of beta-(1,3)-glucan synthase, blocking the
formation of the polysaccharide, beta-(1,3)-glucan, an essential cell-wall component in fungal pathogens (43,70,71). Disruption of fungal cell wall integrity
with subsequent rupture and lysis ensues. In a renal transplant recipient
with pneumonia and multiple pulmonary nodules, caspofungin was utilized
after hepatic and renal intolerance to initial fluconazole followed by a
lipid-formulation of amphotericin B. After four weeks of therapy with caspofungin, the disease was considered stabilized with improvement in the initial
hepatic and renal intolerance. There are scant in vitro data on the susceptibility of *C. immitis* to caspofungin; however, a limited role for caspofungin may
be warranted in selected patients due to intolerance to primary coccidioidal
antifungal agents (37).

Limited case reports on the use of drotrecogin alpha (activated) in
fulminant coccidioidomycosis associated with pneumonia and septic shock
have been reported (72). Both patients received a lipid formulation of
amphotericin B (liposomal amphotericin B and amphotericin B lipid complex,
respectively, followed by fluconazole). Both patients survived and remained
disease-free per the authors. In cases of prominent musculoskeletal or tissue
burden (i.e., large abscesses), or with fistula formation, surgical intervention
should be an essential adjunct to antifungal therapy. In CNS disease, shunting
may be an important part of management for decompression and in the treatment of hydrocephalus (AIII). Intrathecal amphotericin B may be required for
CNS disease and lack of response to fluconazole or itraconazole (54). Table 4
also described the potential interactions with immunosuppressive agents. Close
monitoring of drug levels is essential to prevent rejection and toxicity.

## PREVENTION

Driving through endemic desert areas, or performing activities in such areas
for brief periods have led to the development of coccidioidomycosis
(activities such as participating in model airplane exhibitions, archeological

digs, gardening activities, and hiking are have been reported as examples). Wearing masks while traveling through endemic areas may offer limited protection. Consequently, limiting activities that enhance exposures in these endemic areas is advised (21,54,56). Some transplant programs suggest the use of close surveillance and targeted prophylaxis as an alternative to universal prophylaxis for coccidiodomycosis in transplant recipients (6). Such approaches warrant further investigation and outcome analysis in other transplant recipients, especially with the newer immunosuppressive regimens and potent induction regimens.

## REFERENCES

1. Ampel NM, Wieden MA, Galgiani JN. Coccidioidomycosis: clinical update. Rev Infect Dis 1989; 11:897–911.
2. Ampel NM. Combating opportunistic infections: coccidioidomycosis. Expert Opin Pharmacother 2004; 5:255–261.
3. Arsura EL, Bellinghausen PL, Kilgore WB, Abraham JJ, Johnson RH. Septic shock in coccidioidomycosis. Crit Care Med 1998; 26:62–65.
4. Blair JE. Coccidioidal pneumonia, arthritis, and soft-tissue infection after kidney transplantation. Transplant Infect Dis 2004; 6:74–76.
5. Blair JE, Logan JL. Coccidioidomycosis in solid organ transplantation. Clin Infect Dis 2001; 33:1536–1544.
6. Blair JE, Douglas DD, Mulligan DC. Early results of targeted prophylaxis for coccidioidomycosis in patients undergoing orthotopic liver transplantation within an endemic area. Transplant Infect Dis 2003; 5:3–8.
7. Blair JE, Douglas DD. Coccidioidomycosis in liver transplant recipients relocating to an endemic area. Dig Dis Sci 2004; 49:1981–1985.
8. Blair JE, Balan V, Douglas DD, Hentz JG. Incidence and prevalence of coccidioidomycosis in patients with end-stage liver disease. Liver Transplant 2003; 9:843–850.
9. Brewer JH, Parrott CL, Rimland D. Disseminated coccidioidomycosis in a heart transplant recipient. Sabouraudia 1982; 20:261–265.
10. Britt RH, Enzmann DR, Remington JS. Intracranial infection in cardiac transplant recipients. Ann Neurol 1981; 9:107–119.
11. Bronnimann DA, Galgiani JN. Coccidioidomycosis. Eur J Clin Microbiol Infect Dis 1989; 8:466–473.
12. Calhoun DL, Galgiani JN, Sukoski C, Copeland JG. Coccidioidomycosis in recent renal or cardiac transplant recipients. In: Einstein HE, Catanzaro A, eds. Proceedings of the 4th International Conference on Coccidioidomycosis. Washington, DC: National Foundation for Infectious Diseases, 1985: 312–318.
13. Cha JM, Jung S, Bahng HS, et al. Multi-organ failure caused by reactivated coccidioidomycosis without dissemination in a patient with renal transplantation. Respirology 2000; 5:87–90.
14. Crissey JT, Lang H, Parish LC. Diseases caused by thermally dimorphic fungi. In: Manual of Medical Mycology, 1st ed. Cambride, MA: Blackwell Science, 1995:141–149.

15. Crum NF, Lederman ER, Stafford CM, Parrish JS, Wallace MR. Coccidioido-mycosis: a descriptive survey of a reemerging disease. Clinical characteristics and current controversies. Medicine (Baltimore) 2004; 83:149–175.
16. Deresinski SC, Stevens DA. Coccidioidomycosis in compromised hosts. Experience at Stanford University Hospital, Medicine (Baltimore) 1975; 54:377–395.
17. Drutz DJ, Catanzaro A. Coccidioidomycosis. Part II. Am Rev Respir Dis 1978; 117:727–771.
18. Drutz DJ, Catanzaro A. Coccidioidomycosis. Part I. Am Rev Respir Dis 1978; 117:559–585.
19. Einstein HE, Johnson RH. Coccidioidomycosis: new aspects of epidemiology and therapy. Clin Infect Dis 1993; 16:349–356.
20. Galgiani JN. Coccidioidomycosis. West J Med 1993; 153–171.
21. Galgiani JN. Coccidioides species. In: Mandell GL, Douglas RG, Bennett JE, eds. Principles and Practice of Infectious Diseases. New York: John Wiley & Sons 2005:3040–3049.
22. Hall KA, Copeland JG, Zukoski CF, Sethi GK, Galgiani JN. Markers of coccidioidomycosis before cardiac or renal transplantation and the risk of recurrent infection. Transplantation 1993; 55:1422–1424.
23. Hall KA, Sethi GK, Rosado U, Martinez JD, Huston CL, Copeland JG. Coccidioidomycosis and heart transplantation. J Heart Lung Transplant 1993; 12:525–526.
24. Hart PD, Russell E Jr, Remington JS. The compromised host and infection, II. Deep fungal infection. J Infect Dis 1969; 120:169–191.
25. Kauffman CA. Fungal infections in older adults. Clin Infect Dis 2001; 33: 550–555.
26. Kirkland TN, Fierer J. Coccidioidomycosis: a reemerging infectious disease. Emerg Infect Dis 1996; 2:192–199.
27. Kubak BM, Maree CL, Pegues DA, et al. Infections in kidney transplantation. In: Danovitch GM, ed. Handbook of Kidney Transplantation, 4th ed. Philadelphia, PA: Lippincott Williams & Wilkins, 2004:279–333.
28. Logan JL, Blair JE, Galgiani JN. Coccidioidomycosis complicating solid organ transplantation. Semin Respir Infect 2001; 16:251–256.
29. Pappagianis D. Epidemiology of coccidioidomycosis. In: Stevens DA, ed. Coccidioidomycosis: A Text New York: Plenum Medical Books, 1980:63–85.
30. Stevens DA. Coccidioidomycosis. N Engl J Med 1995; 332:1077–1082.
31. Yoshino MT, Hillman BJ, Galgiani JN. Coccidioidomycosis in renal dialysis and transplant patients: radiologic findings in 30 patients. Am J Roentgenol 1987; 149:989–992.
32. Bergstrom L, Yocum DE, Ampel NM, et al. Increased risk of coccidioidomy-cosis in patients treated with tumor necrosis factor alpha antagonists. Arthritis Rheum 2004; 50:1959–1966.
33. Blair JE, Smilack JD, Caples SM. Coccidioidomycosis in patients with hemato-logic malignancies. Arch Intern Med 2005; 165:113–117.
34. Chaim W, Burstein E. Postpartum infection treatments: a review. Expert Opin Pharmacother 2003; 4:1297–1313.
35. Cohen IM, Galgiani JN, Potter D, Ogden DA. Coccidioidomycosis in renal replacement therapy. Arch Intern Med 1982; 142:489–494.

36. Kaplan JE, Zoschke D, Kisch AL. Withdrawal of immunosuppresive agents in the treatment of disseminated coccidioidomycosis. Am J Med 1980; 68:624–628.
37. Antony S. Use of the echinocandins (caspofungin) in the treatment of disseminated coccidioidomycosis in a renal transplant recipient. Clin Infect Dis 2004; 39:879–880.
38. Holt CD, Winston DJ, Kubak B, et al. Coccidioidomycosis in liver transplant patients. Clin Infect Dis 1997; 24:216–221.
39. Magill SB, Schmahl TM, Sommer J, et al. Coccidioidomycosis-induced thyroiditis and calcitriol-mediated hypercalcemia in a heart transplantation patient. Endocrinologist 1998; 8:299–302.
40. Miller MB, Hendren R, Gilligan PH. Posttransplantation disseminated coccidioidomycosis acquired from donor lungs. J Clin Microbiol 2004; 42: 2347–2349.
41. Schroter GP, Bakshandeh K, Husberg BS, Well R III. Coccidioidomycosis and renal transplantation. Transplantation 1977; 23:485–489.
42. Serota AI. The efficacy of fluconazole in prevention of coccidioidomycosis following renal transplantation. In: Einstein HE, Catanzaro A, eds. Coccidioidomycosis: Proceedings of the 5th International Conference on Coccidioidomycosis. Bethesda, MD: National Foundation for Infectious Diseases, 1996:248–254.
43. Vartivarian SE, Coudron PE, Markowitz SM. Disseminated coccidioidomycosis. Unusual manifestations in a cardiac transplantation patient. Am J Med 1987; 83:949–952.
44. Yousem SA, Burke CM, Billingham ME. Pathologic pulmonary alterations in long-term human heart-lung transplantation. Hum Pathol 1985; 16:911–923.
45. Zeluff BJ. Fungal pneumonia in transplant recipients. Semin Respir Infect 1990; 5:80–89.
46. Kusne S, Furukawa H, Abu-Elmagd K, et al. Infectious complications after small bowel transplantation in adults: An update. Transplant Proc 1996; 28: 2761–2762.
47. Abuodeh RO, Orbach MJ, Mandel MA, Das A, Galgiani JN. Genetic transformation of *Coccidioides immitis* facilitated by *Agrobacterium tumefaciens*. J Infect Dis 2000; 181:2106–2110.
48. Dosanjh A, Theodore J, Pappagianis D. Probable false positive coccidioidal serologic results in patients with cystic fibrosis. Pediatr Transplant 1998; 2:313–317.
49. Eulalio KD, de Macedo RL, Cavalcanti MA, Martins LM, Lazera MS, Wanke B. *Coccidioides immitis* isolated from armadillos (*Dasypus novemcinctus*) in the state of Piaui, Northeast Brazil. Mycopathologia 2001; 149:57–61.
50. Fisher MC, Koenig GL, White TJ, et al. Molecular and phenotypic description of *Coccidioides posadasii* sp nov., previously recognized as the non-California population of *Coccidioides immitis*. Mycologia 2002; 94:73–84.
51. Fisher MC, Rannala B, Chaturvedi V, Taylor JW. Disease surveillance in recombining pathogens: multilocus genotypes identify sources of human Coccidioides infections. Proc Natl Acad Sci USA 2002; 99:9067–9071.
52. Huppert M, Sun SH, Harrison JL. Morphogenesis throughout saprobic and parasitic cycles of *Coccidioides immitis*. Mycopathologia 1982; 78:107–122.

53. Bialek R, Kern J, Herrmann T, et al. PCR assays for identification of *Coccidioides posadasii* based on the nucleotide sequence of the antigen 2/proline-rich antigen. J Clin Microbiol 2004; 42:778–783.
54. Galgiani JN, Ampel NM, Catanzaro A, Johnson RH, Stevens DA, Williams PL. Practice guideline for the treatment of coccidioidomycosis. Infectious Diseases Society of America. Clin Infect Dis 2000; 30:658–661.
55. Galgiani JN. Coccidioidomycosis: a regional disease of national importance. Rethinking approaches for control. Ann Intern Med 1999; 130:293–300.
56. Avery RK. Recipient screening prior to solid-organ transplantation. Clin Infect Dis 2002; 35:1513–1519.
57. Avery RK, Ljungman P. Prophylactic measures in the solid-organ recipient before transplantation. Clin Infect Dis 2001; 33(Supp 1):S15–S21.
58. Desai SA, Minai OA, Gordon SM, O'Neil B, Wiedemann HP, Arroliga AC. Coccidioidomycosis in non-endemic areas: a case series. Respir Med 2001; 95:305–309.
59. Tripathy U, Yung GL, Kriett JM, Thistlethwaite PA, Kapelanski DP, Jamieson SW. Donor transfer of pulmonary coccidioidomycosis in lung transplantation. Ann Thorac Surg 2002; 73:306–308.
60. Wright PW, Pappagianis D, Wilson M, et al. Donor-related coccidioidomycosis in organ transplant recipients. Clin Infect Dis 2003; 37:1265–1269.
61. IDSociety.org.
62. Yamada H, Kotaki H, Takahashi T. Recommendations for the treatment of fungal pneumonias. Expert Opin Pharmacother 2003; 4:1241–1258.
63. Perfect JR. Treatment of non-Aspergillus moulds in imrnunocompromised patients, with amphotericin B lipid complex. Clin Infect Dis 2005; 40(Suppl 6): S401–S408.
64. Anstead GM, Corcoran G, Lewis J, et al. Refractory coccidioidomycosis treated with posaconazole. Clin Infect Dis 2005; 40:1770–1776.
65. Stevens DA, Rendon A, Gaona V, et al. Posaconazole (POS) therapy for chronic refractory coccidioidomycosis [abstract M-663]. In Program and Abstracts of the 44th Interscience Conference on Antimicrobial Agents and Chemotherapy Washington, DC. Washington, DC: American Society for Microbiology, 2004.
66. Graybill JR, Raad I, Negroni R, et al. Posaconazole (POS) long-term safety in patients with invasive fungal infections (IFIs) [abstract M-1025]. In: Program and Abstracts of the 44th Interscience Conference on Antimicrobial Agents and Chemotherapy, Washington, DC. Washington, DC: American Society for Microbiology, 2004.
67. Gonzalez GM, Najvar LKL, Tijerina R, et al. Therapeutic efficacy of caspofungin (CAS) alone and in combination with deoxycholate amphotericin B (DAMB) or liposomal amphotericin B (LAMB) for coccidioidomycosis in a mouse model [abstract M-475]. In: Program and Abstracts of the 44th Interscience Conference on Antimicrobial Agents and Chemotherapy, Washington, DC. Washington, DC: American Society for Microbiology, 2004.
68. Gonzalez GM, Tijerina R, Najvar LK, et al. Correlation between antifungal susceptibilities of *Coccidioides immitis* in vitro and antifungal treatment with caspofungin in a mouse model. Antimicrob Agents Chemother 2001; 45: 1854–1859.

69. Gonzalez GM, Tijerina R, Najvar LK, et al. Therapeutic efficacy of amphotericin B lipid complex (AMBLC), amphotericin B colloidal dispersion (AMBCD), liposomal amphotericin B (LAMB), and conventional amphotericin B (AMB) in murine coccicioidomycosis [abstract M-194]. In: Program and Abstracts of the 44th Interscience Conference on Antimicrobial Agents and Chemotherapy, Washington, DC. Washington, DC: American Society for Microbiology, 2004.
70. Deresinski SC, Stevens DA. Caspofungin. Clin Infect Dis 2003; 36:1445–1457.
71. Walsh T, Sable C, Depauw B, et al. A randomized double blind multicenter trial of caspofungin vs. liposomal amphotericin for empirical antifungal therapy of persistently febrile neutropenic patients [abstract M-1761]. In: Program and Abstracts of the 43rd Interscience Conference on Antimicrobial Agents and Chemotherapy, Chicago IL. Washington, DC: American Society for Microbiology. 2003:477.
72. Crum NF, Groff HL, Parrish JS, Ring W. A novel use for drotrecogin alfa (activated): successful treatment of septic shock associated with coccidioidomycosis. Clin Infect Dis 2004; 39:e122–e123.

# 24

# Histoplasmosis and Blastomycosis After Solid Organ Transplantation

**Carol A. Kauffman**

*Division of Infectious Diseases, Veterans Affairs Ann Arbor Healthcare System, University of Michigan Medical School, Ann Arbor, Michigan, U.S.A.*

## INTRODUCTION

The endemic mycoses cause a relatively small number of infections in solid organ transplant recipients. This is partly because these fungi are restricted geographically; a patient must come into contact with the organism in the environment. This exposure can be immediately before the infection develops in the case of new-onset infection or decades earlier with reactivation infection. The endemic fungi, especially *Histoplasma capsulatum*, have the ability to remain dormant in the body for years; when immunosuppression occurs in the course of transplantation, the organisms begin to proliferate and cause reactivation disease. Rarely, infection can develop in a transplant recipient who has received a donor organ that contains one of the endemic fungi.

## HISTOPLASMOSIS

### Incidence of Histoplasmosis in Transplant Recipients

Histoplasmosis is the most common endemic mycosis reported in solid organ transplant recipients (1–23). However, it is still an uncommon infection in this population. The primary host defense against *H. capsulatum* is cell-mediated immunity with little contribution from humoral or neutrophil defense mechanisms; thus, transplant recipients are at increased risk of infection with this organism. Although the initial infection is pulmonary, hematogenous dissemination to the organs of the reticuloendothelial system is routine, even in healthy hosts. Only after specific cell-mediated immunity develops is the host able to contain the infection.

Histoplasmosis has been reported to occur several weeks to months after transplantation (8,14,17,22) and also as long as 14 to 20 years following transplantation (15,16,21). Most cases have been reported in kidney transplants, and only a few in liver (18–20), heart (23), or lung transplants (17). Transmission of infection from the donor organ has been documented in fewer than 10 patients (1,11,12,14,20,22).

## Clinical Disease

In solid organ transplant recipients, histoplasmosis causes more severe disease than in healthy hosts. This was verified in the two large Indianapolis outbreaks in the late 1970s and early 1980s in which patients who had received a solid organ transplant were found to be at higher risk for disseminated infection and relapse after treatment (8).

Transplant recipients with histoplasmosis can have isolated pulmonary infection (4,8,17), but most have disseminated disease. Those who have pulmonary infection present with fever, chills, cough, and shortness of breath, which can progress rapidly to marked dyspnea and hypoxemia. Chest radiographs usually show diffuse bilateral infiltrates. Mediastinal and hilar lymphadenopathy, common in healthy hosts with pulmonary histoplasmosis, are rarely seen in immunosuppressed hosts (24).

Patients with disseminated histoplasmosis present with fever, chills, fatigue, and anorexia. The illness may be acute and life-threatening or subacute to chronic in its manifestations. Hepatosplenomegaly, mouth ulcers, and skin lesions are common. The mucous membrane lesions are usually painful, nonhealing ulcers. Papules, pustules, plaques, ulcers, nodules, abscesses, and cellulitis are among the cutaneous manifestations of disseminated infection (3,6,7,14). Diffuse pulmonary infiltrates may be present or absent with disseminated histoplasmosis. Pancytopenia and elevated alkaline phosphatase are common laboratory findings; occasionally, patients are overtly jaundiced. Central nervous system involvement can either present as isolated infection or as part of disseminated disease (2,15). Meningitis is the most common central nervous system manifestation, but MRI scans reveal that many patients also have small enhancing intracranial lesions.

## Diagnosis

The definitive diagnosis of histoplasmosis is made by growing *H. capsulatum* from sputum, blood, other body fluids, or tissue biopsy (25). The yield from blood cultures is enhanced by using the lysis-centrifugation (isolator tube) system. *H. capsulatum* grows very slowly, which is a major problem when dealing with an immunosuppressed patient. Although growth in culture is extremely important, it often confirms the correct diagnosis in a patient in whom treatment has already been initiated.

In tissue, *H. capsulatum* appears as small 2–4 μm oval budding intracellular yeasts that are best seen with either periodic acid Schiff or methenamine silver stains. Biopsy of lung, mucocutaneous or cutaneous lesions, bone marrow, and liver often shows characteristic yeasts and can lead to an early diagnosis of histoplasmosis. The organisms can sometimes be seen within neutrophils or monocytes on a peripheral blood smear (6,23).

Serologic assays (complement fixation and immunodiffusion) are useful tests for the diagnosis of histoplasmosis in normal hosts, but are often not helpful in immunosuppressed patients (4,25). The detection of *H. capsulatum* capsular polysaccharide by enzyme immunoassay in urine or serum has become an extremely useful test in immunosuppressed patients with disseminated histoplasmosis (26). The assay is most sensitive when urine, rather than serum, is tested.

## Treatment

Guidelines for the treatment of histoplasmosis have been published by the Mycoses Study Group and the Infectious Diseases Society of America (27). All transplant recipients with histoplasmosis should be treated with an antifungal agent. Initial therapy should be a lipid formulation of amphotericin B (3–5 mg/kg/day) to decrease the risk of nephrotoxicity. Most patients, even those who are immunosuppressed, respond quickly to amphotericin B; therapy can then be changed to itraconazole, the preferred oral azole agent for the endemic mycoses (27). Better absorption is attained when the oral solution of itraconazole is used rather than the capsules. The oral solution is given twice daily on an empty stomach; capsules must be given with food, and medications that inhibit gastric acid secretion must be avoided. The total length of therapy is usually 6 to 12 months.

Fluconazole is a second-line agent for histoplasmosis; response to primary therapy is lower and relapse rates are higher when compared with itraconazole (28). If a patient cannot tolerate itraconazole because of side effects or poor absorption, high-dose fluconazole, 800 mg/day, can be tried (29). There is little clinical experience with voriconazole for histoplasmosis (30), so that this agent cannot be recommended. The echinocandins are not effective therapy for histoplasmosis (31).

Most solid organ transplant recipients with histoplasmosis respond well to antifungal therapy. Fatal cases are more likely to have the diagnosis established late in the course of the infection and to be seen outside the endemic area (2,10,11).

It is not clear if suppressive therapy should be used to prevent relapse of histoplasmosis. Relapses have been described among transplant recipients after amphotericin B or azoles were stopped (8,14). The agent that should be used for suppression is itraconazole, 200–400 mg daily. In individual transplant patients, the decision to use long-term suppressive azole therapy will depend on the extent of immunosuppression and the likelihood of return of cellular immune function.

## BLASTOMYCOSIS

### Incidence in Transplant Recipients

Blastomycosis is a relatively uncommon endemic mycosis; very few cases have been reported in solid organ transplant recipients (32–40). Six cases have been reported in kidney (32–35,37,38) and four in heart transplant recipients (36,37,39); only one case has been reported in a lung transplant recipient, but this case was not proved and was likely not blastomycosis (40). Neutrophils and macrophages are likely as important as T cells in the response to infection with *Blastomyces dermatitidis* (41). This dual response may help explain why blastomycosis is not as commonly seen as histoplasmosis in transplant recipients.

Almost all reported cases have occurred in those living in the endemic area. Reactivation of blastomycosis years after an initial exposure has been documented in healthy individuals (42), but this appears to occur much less often than with histoplasmosis. Cases have occurred soon after transplantation (35,39) and also several years after transplantation (33,34). There has been no documented case of blastomycosis transmitted by a donor organ.

### Clinical Disease

Blastomycosis begins as a pulmonary infection. Subsequent dissemination to skin, osteoarticular structures, and genitourinary tract is common, and skin lesions are probably the most common initial presentation of blastomycosis. The pulmonary focus may have cleared by the time skin lesions develop. Direct inoculation cutaneous blastomycosis is rare, but has been reported in a renal transplant recipient (33).

Solid organ transplant recipients are more likely than healthy hosts to develop severe pulmonary or disseminated blastomycosis. The types of pulmonary lesions in transplant recipients include lobar pneumonia, cavitary lesions, diffuse bilateral infiltrates, and adult respiratory distress syndrome. Disseminated infection presents as cutaneous lesions with or without visceral dissemination. In transplant recipients, the cutaneous lesions are more likely to be pustular or ulcerative, and evolve rather quickly when compared with the more typical verrucous lesions seen in the nonimmunocompromised host. Meningitis and intracerebral mass lesions are more common in immunosuppressed patients (41), but have not been reported specifically in transplant recipients.

## Diagnosis

Blastomycosis is definitively diagnosed by growth of the organism from tissue or body fluids (43). Sputum, bronchoalveolar lavage fluid, skin lesions, or other tissues should be cultured on fungal medium. Culture methods generally take several weeks. Histopathological examination of skin lesions, cytological examination of sputum or bronchoalveolar lavage fluid, and smears of pustular skin lesions should be performed when those organs are involved. *B. dermatitidis* is a large (5–20 µm), thick-walled yeast that retains a broad-based connection to its budding daughter cell and is readily identified with fungal stains.

Standard serological assays for blastomycosis are neither sensitive nor specific (43). A urine enzyme immunoassay for *Blastomyces* antigen has recently become available, but the usefulness of this test is not yet known (44).

## Treatment

The Mycoses Study Group, under the auspices of the Infectious Diseases Society of America, has published guidelines for the treatment of blastomycosis (45). Transplant recipients who acquire blastomycosis should be treated initially with a lipid formulation of amphotericin B. Failures have been well documented in transplant recipients who were treated with an azole (ketoconazole) (34,35). When resolution of lesions and symptoms is noted, therapy can be switched to itraconazole oral solution, 200 mg twice daily for a total of 6 to 12 months. Fluconazole and ketoconazole are not as effective as itraconazole; there is minimal experience with voriconazole (30), and this agent should not be used. The echinocandins are not effective for blastomycosis.

Long-term suppressive therapy with itraconazole is reasonable, but may not be necessary for all transplant recipients. Relapses have been well described in transplant recipients when either amphotericin B or an azole has been stopped (35,36). The need for suppressive therapy will depend on the patient's immune status.

## CONCLUSIONS

Infection with an endemic mycosis occurs as a result of new infection related to an environmental exposure, reactivation of a previously acquired infection, and least often from the donor organ. Infection can occur at any time after the transplant. Severe pulmonary infection and widespread disseminated infection are the most common manifestations of infection with histoplasmosis and blastomycosis post-transplantation. After the initial response to amphotericin B, an oral azole agent can be given for 6 to 12 months to complete the course of therapy. Itraconazole is the most active azole agent for histoplasmosis and blastomycosis. Long-term suppressive therapy may be indicated for some transplant recipients infected with *H. capsulatum* or *B. dermatitidis.*

## REFERENCES

1. Hood AB, Inglis FG, Lowenstein L, Dossetor JB, McLean LD. Histoplasmosis and thrombocytopenic purpura: transmission by renal homotransplantation. Can Med Assoc J 1965; 93:587–592.
2. Karalakulasingam R, Arora KK, Adams G, Serratoni F, Martin DG. Meningoencephalitis caused by *Histoplasma capsulatum*: occcurrence in a renal transplant recipient and review of the literature. Arch Intern Med 1976; 136:217–220.
3. Daman LA, Hashimoto K, Kaplan RJ, Trent WG. Disseminated histoplasmosis in an immunosuppressed patient. South Med J 1977; 70:355–356.
4. Kauffman CA, Israel KS, Smith JW, et al. Histoplasmosis in immunosuppressed patients. Am J Med 1978; 64:923–932.
5. Davies SF, Sarosi GA, Peterson PK. Disseminated histoplasmosis in renal transplant recipients. Am J Surg 1979; 137:686–691.
6. Farr B, Beacham BE, Atuk NO. Cutaneous histoplasmosis after renal transplantation. South Med J 1981; 74:635–637.
7. Cooper PH, Walker AW, Beacham BE. Cellulitis caused by Histoplasma organisms in a renal transplant recipient. Arch Dermatol 1982; 118:3–4.
8. Wheat LJ, Smith EJ, Sathapatayavongs B, et al. Histoplasmosis in renal allograft recipients. Two large urban outbreaks. Arch Intern Med 1983; 143: 703–707.
9. Goetz MB, Jones JM. Combined ketoconazole and amphotericin B treatment of acute disseminated histoplasmosis in a renal allograft recipient. South Med J 1985; 78:1368–1370.
10. Brett MT, Kwan JTC, Bending MR. Caecal perforation in a renal transplant patient with disseminated histoplasmosis. J Clin Pathol 1988; 41:992–995.
11. Watanabe M, Hotchi M, Nagasaki M. An autopsy case of disseminated histoplasmosis probably due to infection from the renal allograft. Acta Pathol Jpn 1988; 38:769–780.
12. Gottesdiener KM. Transplanted infections: donor-to-host transmission with the allograft. Ann Intern Med 1989; 110:1001–1016.
13. Sridhar NR, Tchervenkov KI, Weiss MA, Hijazi YM, First MR. Disseminated histoplasmosis in a renal transplant recipient: a cause of renal failure several years following transplantation. Am J Kidney Dis 1991; 17:719–721.
14. Wong SY, Allen DM. Transmission of disseminated histoplasmosis via cadaveric renal transplantation: case report. Clin Infect Dis 1992; 14:232–234.
15. Livas IC, Nechay PS, Nauseef WM. Clinical evidence of spinal and cerebral histoplasmosis twenty years after renal transplantation. Clin Infect Dis 1995; 20:692–695.

16. Peddi VR, Hariharan S, First MR. Disseminated histoplasmosis in renal allograft recipients. Clin Transplant 1996; 10:160–165.
17. Kanj SS, Welty-Wolf K, Madden J, et al. Fungal infections in lung and heart-lung transplant recipients. Report of 9 cases and review of the literature. Medicine (Baltimore) 1996; 75:142–156.
18. Shallot J, Pursell KJ, Barteloni C, et al. Disseminated histoplasmosis after orthotopic liver transplantation. Liver Transplant Surg 1997; 3:433–434.
19. Vinayek R, Balan V, Pinna A, Linden PK, Kusne S. Disseminated histoplasmosis in a patient after orthotopic liver transplantation. Clin Transplant 1998; 12:274–277.
20. Botterel F, Romand S, Saliba F, et al. A case of disseminated histoplasmosis most likely due to infection from a liver allograft. Eur J Clin Microbiol Infect Dis 1999; 18:662–664.
21. Jha V, Krishna V, Varma N, et al. Disseminated histoplasmosis 19 years after renal transplantation. Clin Nephrol 1999; 51:373–378.
22. Limaye AP, Connolly PA, Sagar M, et al. Transmission of *Histoplasma capsulatum* by organ transplantation. N Engl J Med 2000; 343:1163–1166.
23. Masri K, Mahon N, Rosario A, et al. Reactive hemophagocytic syndrome associated with disseminated histoplasmosis in a heart transplant recipient. J Heart Lung Transplant 2003; 22:487–491.
24. Wheat LJ, Conces D, Allen AD, Blue-Hnidy D, Loyd J. Pulmonary histoplasmosis syndromes: recognition, diagnosis, and management. Semin Respir Crit Care Med 2004; 25:129–144.
25. Wheat LJ. Laboratory diagnosis of histoplasmosis: a review. Semin Respir Infect 2001; 16:131–140.
26. Durkin MM, Connolly PA, Wheat LJ. Comparison of radioimmunoassay and enzyme-linked immunoassay methods for detection of *Histoplasma capsulatum* var. *capsulatum* antigen. J Clin Microbiol 1997; 35:2252–2255.
27. Wheat J, Sarosi G, McKinsey D, et al. Practice guidelines for the management of patients with histoplasmosis. Clin Infect Dis 2000; 30:688–695.
28. Wheat J, MaWhinney S, Hafner R, et al. Treatment of histoplasmosis with fluconazole in patients with acquired immunodeficiency syndrome. Am J Med 1997; 103:223–232.
29. McKinsey DS, Kauffman CA, Pappas PG, et al. Fluconazole therapy for histoplasmosis. Clin Infect Dis 1996; 23:996–1001.
30. Perfect JR, Marr KA, Walsh TJ, et al. Voriconazole treatment for less-common, emerging, or refractory fungal infections. Clin Infect Dis 2003; 36:1122–1131.
31. Kohler S, Wheat LJ, Connolly P, et al. Comparison of the echinocandin, caspofungin, with amphotericin B for treatment of histoplasmosis following pulmonary challenge in a murine model. Antimicrob Agents Chemother 2000; 44:1850–1854.
32. Pechan WB, Novick AC, Lalli A, Gephardt G. Pulmonary nodules in a renal transplant recipient. J Urol 1980; 124:111–114.
33. Butka BJ, Bennett SR, Johnson AC. Disseminated inoculation blastomycosis in a renal transplant recipient. Am Rev Respir Dis 1984; 130:1180–1183.
34. Greene NB, Baughman RP, Kim CK, Roselle GA. Failure of ketoconazole in an immunosuppressed patient with pulmonary blastomycosis. Chest 1985; 88:640–641.

35.  Hii JH, Legault L, DeVeber G, Vas SI. Successful treatment of systemic blas-
     tomycosis with high-dose ketoconazole in a renal transplant recipient. Am J
     Kidney Dis 1990; 15:595–597.
36.  Serody JS, Mill MR, Detterbeck FC, Harris DT, Cohen MS. Blastomycosis in
     transplant recipients: report of a case and review. Clin Infect Dis 1993; 16:
     54–58.
37.  Pappas PG, Threlkeld MG, Bedsole GD, Cleveland KO, Gelfand MS,
     Dismukes WE. Blastomycosis in immunocompromised patients. Medicine
     1993; 72:311–325.
38.  Winkler S, Stanek G, Hubsch P, et al. Pneumonia due to *Blastomyces dermati-
     tidis* in a European renal transplant recipient. Nephrol Dial Transplant 1996;
     11:1376–1379.
39.  Walker K, Skelton H, Smith K. Cutaneous lesions showing giant yeast forms of
     *Blastomyces dermatitidis*. J Cutan Pathol 2002; 29:616–618.
40.  Zampogna JC, Hoy MJ, Ramos-Caro FA. Primary cutaneous North American
     blastomycosis in an immunosuppressed child. Pediatr Dermatol 2003; 20:
     128–130.
41.  Pappas PG. Blastomycosis. Semin Respir Crit Care Med 2004; 25:113–122.
42.  Laskey WK, Sarosi GA. Endogenous activation in blastomycosis. Ann Intern
     Med 1978; 88:50–52.
43.  Areno JP, Campbell GD, George RB. Diagnosis of blastomycosis. Semin
     Respir Infect 1997; 12:252–262.
44.  Durkin M, Wirtt J, LeMonte A, Wheat B, Connolly P. Antigen assay with
     the potential to aid in diagnosis of blastomycosis. J Clin Microbiol 2004;
     42:4873–4875.
45.  Chapman SW, Bradsher RW, Campbell GD, Pappas PG, Kauffman CA.
     Practice guidelines for the management of patients with blastomycosis. Clin
     Infect Dis 2000; 30:679–683.

# 25

# Invasive Fungal Infections Complicating Lung and Solid Organ Transplantation: Aspergillosis, Cryptococcosis, and Molds

**Shahid Husain and Fernanda P. Silveira**

*Department of Medicine, University of Pittsburgh, Pittsburgh, Pennsylvania, U.S.A.*

## ASPERGILLUS

*Aspergillus* is a filamentous and ubiquitous fungus that can be isolated from soil, plant debris, and indoor air environment. Of the 185 species known to the *Aspergillus* genus, 20 are implicated as a cause of opportunistic infection in humans. *Aspergillus fumigatus* is the most commonly isolated species (1–4). Other common species include *Aspergillus flavus*, *Aspergillus terreus*, *Aspergillus niger*, *Aspergillus versicolor*, and *Aspergillus nidulans*. Infections with the *Aspergillus glaucus* group, *Aspergillus ustus*, *Aspergillus oryzae*, and *Aspergillus sydowi* have also been reported (5–19).

## Pathogenesis

The primary route of acquisition of an *Aspergillus* infection is via inhalation of spores. In immunocompetent mice model of pulmonary aspergillosis, inhalation of spore results in intense clearing of the conidia through alveolar macrophages and neutrophils. This is accompanied by release of cytokines (tumor necrosis factor $\alpha$ and Interleukin 6). The resultant cellular debris is then cleared by monocytes with a rapid decrease in the secretion of cytokines. In comparison, in the steroid-induced immunosuppressed mice, the initial recruitment of neutrophils, macrophages, and cytokines is delayed, causing delayed clearance of *Aspergillus* conidia. This delayed clearance results in an invasive *Aspergillus* infection with sustained release of cytokines but without the monocyte recruitment or coagulation necrosis causing respiratory failure (20).

## Incidence

The incidence of invasive aspergillosis differs among transplant recipients. In bone marrow transplant recipients the incidence varies from 2.9% to 28% (21,22). The incidence of *Aspergillus* infection in bone marrow transplant recipients (22–25) has been reported to be further increased by the introduction of antifungal prophylaxis with azoles.

Among solid organ transplant recipients, kidney/pancreas transplant recipients have the lowest rate of *Aspergillus* infection ranging from 0.4% to 5% (26,27). Small bowel transplant recipients have a reported incidence of 1% to 4% (28,29). Liver transplant recipients have a moderate risk of *Aspergillus* infection ranging from 1% to 8%, followed by heart transplant recipients at 1% to 14% (27,30,31). The lung transplant recipients have the highest incidence of *Aspergillus* infections ranging from 6% to 16% (1,32–37).

The higher incidence of invasive aspergillosis in lung transplant recipients stems from the unique characteristics of this group that render them more susceptible to pulmonary infections. These characteristics include direct exposure to the environment and impaired host defenses including decreased cough reflex and weakened mucociliary clearance (38). A further disadvantage in lung transplant recipients stems from the surgery itself. The blood supply to the allograft is compromised, relying solely on the pulmonary artery circulation until the collaterals of the bronchial artery are developed (39). This resultant relative ischemia may predispose the site of anastomosis to fungal infections particularly *Aspergillus*.

## Risk Factors

Lung transplant recipients share some common risk factors with other solid organ and heart transplant recipients while having unique risk factors of their own. These common risk factors include environmental exposure and net state of immunosuppression (Table 1).

Environmental exposure can occur in the community or in the hospital. Community exposure is typically noted in construction workers, farmers, gardeners, and residents of rural areas (42). Nosocomial exposure has two patterns: domiciliary and nondomiciliary. Domiciliary pattern of exposure typically results in case clusters while nondomiciliary exposure is difficult to detect (40,43).

**Table 1** Known Risk Factors of Invasive Aspergillosis in Thoracic Organ Transplant Recipients

| |
|---|
| *Common risk factors* |
|   Increased immunosuppression[a] |
|   Environmental exposure |
|   Technical/anatomic abnormalities |
|   Cytomegalovirus infection/disease |
| *Heart transplant* |
|   Retransplantation |
|   Posttransplant hemodialysis |
| *Lung transplant* |
|   Single-lung transplant |
|   Pre/posttransplant colonization |
|   Bronchiolitis obliterans |
|   Serum IgG levels <400 mg/dL |
|   Acute rejection |

[a]Use of high dose steroids and OKT3.
*Source*: Adapted from Refs. 1, 30, 32, 36, 40, and 41.

Net state of immunosuppression is determined by multiple factors; among these, high-dose steroid, antilymphocytic therapy, and viral infection, particularly cytomegalovirus (CMV), play an important role (44–47). CMV results in lymphocyte suppression with reversal of the helper–suppressor cell ratio and diminished function of natural killer cells (36,48,49). Lung transplant recipients may be at a higher risk of CMV infections as compared to other solid organ transplant recipients (50,51).

A unique risk factor for the development of invasive aspergillosis is the colonization of airways (42). Pre- or posttransplant colonization of airways in lung transplant recipients ranges from 29% to 48% (34,37,52–55). The highest rate of colonization was observed in cystic fibrosis patients (52). Furthermore, cystic fibrosis patients with pretransplant colonization also had the highest risk for post-transplant *Aspergillus* tracheobronchitis (52). Other unique risk factors for invasive aspergillosis include receipt of single lung transplant, development of bronchiolitis obliterans, and hypogammaglobulinemia (1,41,56). Though the positive predictive value of a positive airway culture for invasive aspergillosis ranges from 6% to 23% (95% CI 3–43%), it is to be noted that this predictive value is not a true representative of risk as most of the studies have used some sort of antifungal prophylaxis in these patients during the first six months after transplant (3). Indeed, one study in lung transplant recipients showed that patients with *Aspergillus* during the first six months were 11 times more likely to develop invasive disease than those who were not colonized (37). Additional risk factors that have been suggested to increase the susceptibility of fungal infection in general and *Aspergillus* infection in particular in lung transplant recipients include airway ischemia, positive donor bronchial cultures for molds, reperfusion injury, and placement of bronchial stents (41). Risk factors such as renal insufficiency, posttransplantation dialysis, retransplantation, prolonged intubation, and high bilirubin, which have independently been found to be associated with invasive aspergillosis in other solid organ transplant recipients have not been studied in lung transplants (44).

## Clinical Presentation

There are five distinct clinical syndromes related to *Aspergillus* and recognized in lung transplant recipients. These syndromes include *Aspergillus* colonization, *Aspergillus* tracheobronchitis, pulmonary aspergillosis, disseminated aspergillosis, and allergic bronchopulmonary aspergillosis (ABPA).

*Aspergillus* airway colonization after lung transplantation is common, being observed in as many as 46% of patients (37). In 60% of these patients, the first positive culture for *Aspergillus* is detected within three months of transplantation (1). The patients are usually asymptomatic and detection of colonization usually occurs on routine or surveillance bronchoscopy without any evidence of tissue invasion. Posttransplant colonization is considered a risk factor for subsequent invasive disease.

*Aspergillus* tracheobronchitis is observed almost exclusively in lung transplant recipients and is considered by some as an early form of invasive aspergillosis. It is characterized by local involvement of the trachea or bronchi without extension to the lungs. It is the most frequent clinical form of *Aspergillus* infection in lung recipients, corresponding to 37% of all cases (1) and tends to occur early, typically in the first three months following transplantation. Ulceration, necrosis, cartilage invasion, and formation of pseudomembrane are the pathologic features of *Aspergillus* tracheobronchitis (Fig. 1) (57). Symptoms are nonspecific and consist of dyspnea, cough, wheezing, chest pain, and hemoptysis. Fever is almost always absent. Chest radiograph and computerized tomography are often normal, but peribronchial thickening without parenchymal abnormalities may be seen (58). If not recognized and treated early, infection may extend to the lung parenchyma with dissemination. *Aspergillus* tracheobronchitis cannot be uniformly prevented by the use of nebulized amphotericin B. The performance of routine surveillance bronchoscopic examination is crucial for early detection of this condition (57).

Bronchial anastomotic infections are seen more commonly following bilateral or right lung transplantation (59). Patients with cystic fibrosis who were colonized with *Aspergillus* prior to transplantation have been shown to be at greater risk for developing bronchial anastomotic infections, particularly within the first month after transplantation (60). Lesions that involve the anastomotic site or its vicinity can result in bronchopleural fistula and eventually fatal hemorrhage. Bronchopleural fistulas have been

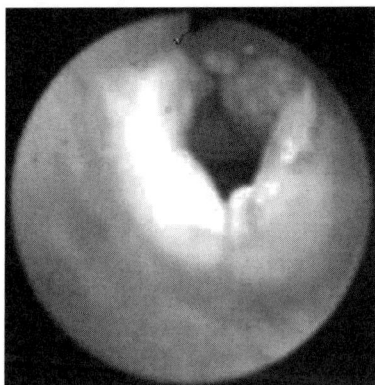

**Figure 1** *Aspergillus* tracheobronchitis in a lung transplant recipient, showing the characteristic pseudomembrane at the site of anastomosis under bronchoscopy.

documented to affect 4.4% of the lung transplant recipients with tracheo-bronchial *Aspergillus* infection (1).

Invasive pulmonary aspergillosis is the second most common invasive disease (1). This is not unexpected considering that the organisms have easy access to the respiratory tract by direct inhalation, and airway colonization is a risk factor for subsequent *Aspergillus* infection. Invasive pulmonary aspergillosis corresponds to 32% of all cases of *Aspergillus* infection among lung recipients and tends to occur later, typically seen after three months following transplantation, at a median of 5.5 months posttransplantation. Patients usually present with a dry cough and dyspnea. Hemoptysis may also occur. Fever is uncommon, being present in only 15% of the patients. This is in contrast to other patient groups at risk for pulmonary and disseminated aspergillosis, such as patients with prolonged neutropenia, in whom fever is frequently present (61). Single-lung transplant recipients are at particular risk for the development of invasive pulmonary disease. In the majority of these patients, invasive aspergillosis has occurred in the native lung, which is structurally abnormal and is a potential source of infection (35). A characteristic radiographic finding is frequently lacking.

Disseminated disease occurs in 10% of patients and also tends to occur late after transplantation, with a median time of onset of 10.6 months. *Aspergillus* may disseminate to almost any organ including the brain, eye, liver, spleen, skin, bone, heart, and pericardium. It has a predilection for the central nervous system, causing focal neurological signs, seizures, and lethargy (62).

ABPA can also develop after lung transplantation. Patients present with progressive shortness of breath and cough in association with a decline in $FEV_1$. ABPA following lung transplantation has been described only in patients with underlying cystic fibrosis (63–65). The diagnosis is difficult due to clinical and laboratorial similarities between the two entities.

## Diagnosis

The diagnosis of invasive aspergillosis in solid organ transplant recipients is challenging. A great number of patients are asymptomatic or present with nonspecific symptoms. Frequently, a combination of clinical and radiological findings, culture results, histopathologic findings, and serologic detection of antigens is necessary for diagnosis. The disease progresses rapidly, hence prompt recognition and institution of appropriate and aggressive therapy is necessary for cure.

The EORTC/MSG has standardized criteria for defining opportunistic invasive fungal infections for clinical or epidemiologic trials (66). These definitions can be applied to organ transplant recipients with limited modifications. Under the EORTC/MSG criteria, three levels of probability for defining invasive fungal infections are proposed: "proven," "probable," and "possible." The criteria for proven invasive fungal infections are valid for all host groups; those for probable fungal infections should be used only for pulmonary infections (3). The category of possible invasive fungal infection is not recommended in organ transplant recipients as it relies heavily on clinical signs and symptoms that are nonspecific for invasive fungal infections.

"Proven" aspergillosis requires demonstration of fungal invasion in histopathology as well as fungal growth in culture. Aspergillosis is called "probable" when the fungus is isolated from culture and there is radiological evidence of disease.

### Radiology

The most common radiographic findings in invasive pulmonary aspergillosis are focal areas of patchy consolidation or infiltrate. Nodular lesions with or without cavitation can be seen in 27% to 30% of patients and are highly suggestive of invasive pulmonary aspergillosis (Fig. 2A). The "halo sign," a distinct radiographic characteristic of pulmonary aspergillosis can be seen in the first week of infection, but is unusual in this transplant patient group (Fig. 2B). A chest computerized tomography is often much more helpful than a chest radiograph, since it can demonstrate the presence of small and subtle nodules, otherwise undetectable on plain radiographs. It can also reveal the presence of disease as much as five days earlier than plain films (66).

Tracheobronchitis can present with peribronchial thickening visible on chest radiographs and computerized tomography, but more commonly it is associated with normal imaging studies.

### Culture

Interpretation of a positive culture result for *Aspergillus* should take into consideration the clinical context. *Aspergillus* is ubiquitous in the air and can contaminate plates in the laboratory as well as clinical specimens. Moreover, in low-risk populations, a positive culture is almost always due to

**(A)**                              **(B)**

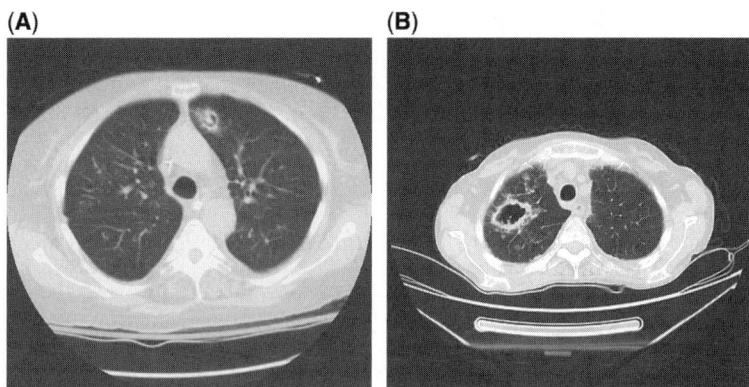

**Figure 2** Computed tomography manifestations of invasive pulmonary aspergillosis in lung transplant recipients. (**A**) shows characteristic halo sign, while (**B**) shows a large thick-walled cavitary lesion.

contamination or colonization. A more reliable diagnosis is obtained if direct examination of the clinical specimen is also positive.

In a study with liver and kidney transplant recipients, it was determined that isolation of less than two colonies of *Aspergillus* from only one site usually represented contamination. On the other hand, if two or more colonies were isolated, or if more than one site of infection was identified, particularly if the species were *A. fumigatus* or *A. flavus*, there was a greater than 70% likelihood of invasive disease. The same study also demonstrated that positive cultures from body fluids, such as pleural fluid and ascites, usually do not represent significant disease (67). However, one should be suspicious of unusual manifestations of invasive aspergillosis if clinically warranted.

The significance of a positive respiratory tract culture for *Aspergillus* has been studied in the context of solid organ transplantation. The positive predictive value of respiratory tract cultures for *Aspergillus* has ranged from 17% to 72% (45,68,69). A study that included five single-lung transplant recipients and three heart or heart–lung recipients found that a positive respiratory tract culture result predicted invasive aspergillosis in 58% of patients (70).

The use of blood cultures is limited, since fungemia is rare, even in disseminated disease. Most bloodstream isolates of *Aspergillus* are associated with pseudofungemia (68).

Histopathology

The hallmark of invasive aspergillosis is the demonstration of tissue invasion by the fungus. *Aspergillus* grows only in hyphal form in tissues. The hyphae are hyaline, frequently septate, and branch in acute angles, usually invading blood vessels and causing thrombosis. They are best visualized with silver stains and may be missed if only hematoxilin–eosin is used.

Although demonstration of tissue invasion is specific for fungal infection, this alone does not confirm the diagnosis of aspergillosis, since many other fungi, such as *Fusarium* sp., *Scedosporium apiospermum*, *Acremonium* sp., and *Paecilomyces lilacinus*, will have the same appearance as that of *Aspergillus* in tissue.

The cornerstone of diagnosis of aspergillosis is the demonstration of hyphal invasion in tissue and growth of *Aspergillus* in culture of the same tissue.

Serology

Antibody tests for *Aspergillus* lack sensitivity and specificity. A positive test does not distinguish between active and past infection or between colonization and invasive disease. Furthermore, a negative test does not rule out invasive disease, since most transplanted patients are unable to mount a significant response.

Galactomannan (GM) is a polysaccharide cell-wall component that is released by growing *Aspergillus* hyphae. A double-sandwich enzyme-linked immunosorbent assay (ELISA), known as Platelia® *Aspergillus* is now available and is capable of detecting 0.5–1 ng/mL of GM (71). Results are reported as an optical density index, and a cutoff of 0.5 is currently accepted in clinical practice.

The majority of studies with GM ELISA have been performed in patients with hematologic malignancies, allogenic stem cell transplantation, and chemotherapy-induced neutropenia. In these settings, serial monitoring of antigenemia is associated with a sensitivity of 50% to greater than 90% (71–78). Specificity ranges from 80% to 100%, with a false-positive rate of 8% to 10%. Detection of GM has preceded microbiological and radiological diagnosis in at least a week. The administration of piperacillin/tazobactam has been associated with false-positive results (79).

The data in solid organ transplantation are not as striking and only a few studies have been conducted (33,80,81). One study with 70 lung transplant recipients demonstrated a sensitivity of only 30%, with a specificity of 93% (33). Possible explanations for such a poor performance in lung transplant recipients include a high number of cases of *Aspergillus* tracheobronchitis, which is a localized form of disease without angioinvasion or frequent use of antifungal prophylaxis, and absence of neutropenia, which can be associated with a lower fungal burden. Currently, routine use of serum GM assay for the monitoring and detection of invasive aspergillosis in lung transplant recipients is not recommended.

GM can also be detected in body fluids. Galactomannuria has a lower sensitivity than antigenemia (82). The usefulness of GM detection in bronchoalveolar lavage (BAL) in solid organ transplant recipients is unknown. The assay becomes negative after a few days of antifungal therapy and airway colonization can yield false-positive results (83). The detection of cerebrospinal fluid (CSF) GM is diagnostic of cerebral aspergillosis in the appropriate clinical setting only when antigenemia is negative, since there is crossing through the blood–brain barrier (84).

Monitoring antigenemia may be useful to assess response to therapy if initially positive (85), but this has not been validated in solid organ transplant recipients. Nonetheless, a persistently high or rising titer should raise a suspicion of therapeutic failure.

$(1{\rightarrow}3)$-β-D-Glucan is a major cell wall component of yeasts and molds that can be detected in blood. It has been shown to have high sensitivity and specificity for the diagnosis of invasive fungal infections (86). The assay is not affected by the use of antifungal therapy or fungal colonization. Its use is limited by the fact that it reacts not only with *Aspergillus* but also with *Candida, Trichosporon, Fusarium, Penicillium, Saccharomyces, Acremonium,* and even *Pneumocystis jiroveci* (87).

### DNA-Based Methods

Different polymerase chain reaction assays have been developed to detect *Aspergillus* in clinical specimens. Although this technique is promising, with a sensitivity rate ranging from 55% to 100% and specificity from 65% to 100%, its clinical use cannot be yet supported. Several discrepancies exist among the studies, including the use of different DNA targets (88–95).

## Treatment

The successful management of aspergillosis depends on early and high-dose administration of effective systemic antifungal agents. Cure depends on how early in the course of the disease systemic antifungal therapy is instituted. A decrease in immunosuppression, ideally with withdrawal of steroids, plays an important role as adjunctive therapy, as well as surgical resection of focal lesions.

For years, conventional amphotericin B remained the gold standard for treatment. However, the availability of echinocandins and new azoles, which are well tolerated and efficacious antifungal agents, has given a new perspective on the management of this infection and has also stimulated research in the use of combination antifungal therapy.

Conventional amphotericin B is associated with less than 35% response rate (96). It should be administered at a dose of 1–1.5 mg/kg/ day. Infusion-related side effects, such as fever and chills, and nephrotoxicity may limit its use. The lipid preparations of amphotericin B currently available (amphotericin B liposomal, amphotericin B colloidal dispersion, and amphotericin B lipid complex) are associated with greater tolerability without well-documented improvement in efficacy. A double-blind, randomized, controlled trial of amphotericin B colloidal dispersion versus conventional amphotericin B for treatment of invasive aspergillosis in immunocompromised patients, of whom 5% were solid organ transplant recipients, showed equivalent efficacy for the two drug formulations (97). However, a nonrandomized study with liver transplant recipients who received either conventional amphotericin or amphotericin B lipid complex documented that the use of amphotericin B lipid complex was an independent predictor of survival (98). It is not well established which of the lipid formulations of amphotericin should be preferred, however, a dose of 5 mg/kg/day for all three drugs is currently recommended.

Inhaled amphotericin has been used for post-transplant prophylaxis of invasive aspergillosis and as a therapy for tracheobronchitis (99). Drug delivery to the lungs depends on the type of nebulizer used, pulmonary function test of the patient, presence or lack of bronchiolitis obliterans syndrome, and presence of the native lung. The optimal size of the aerosols generated should be 1–5 μm, since *Aspergillus* conidia that reach small airways measure 2.5–3.5 μm. Larger particles are retained in the oropharynx.

A nonhomogenous and erratic distribution is observed in the native lung and in patients with bronchiolitis obliterans syndrome (100). It has been proposed that aerosolization of lipid formulations of amphotericin B enhance drug delivery, thus achievable concentrations in the lungs would be higher (101,102). Aerosolization of amphotericin B lipid complex seems to be associated with fewer administration side effects than conventional amphotericin (l03).

Voriconazole has been the drug of choice for the treatment of invasive aspergillosis. In a randomized trial comparing it to amphotericin, voriconazole demonstrated superior efficacy and a survival benefit. However, only 14 solid organ transplant recipients were enrolled in the study and none were lung transplant recipients (104). A major advantage of voriconazole is its availability for both intravenous and oral administration, facilitating continuation of therapy once the patient is clinically stable. It also has good CSF penetration and can be used in the management of cerebral aspergillosis.

Voriconazole inhibits cytochrome P450 and significantly interacts with tacrolimus, cyclosporine, and sirolimus. Coadministration with the latter is contraindicated. Tacrolimus and cyclosporine levels should be followed closely and doses should be adjusted accordingly. Use of intravenous voriconazole is contraindicated in patients with a creatinine clearance less than 50 mL/min, due to concerns regarding accumulation of its renal excreted sulfobutyl ether β-cyclodextrin (SBECD) vehicle. Oral administration in patients with renal dysfunction is safe and the dose does not need to be adjusted.

Caspofungin, an echinocandin, blocks the synthesis of $(1 \rightarrow 3)$-β-D-glucan cell wall. It does not interact with cytochrome P450, is well tolerated, and has very low potential for toxic side effects and drug interactions. In a study evaluating the efficacy of caspofungin in patients refractory to or intolerant to conventional antifungal therapy, a favorable response to caspofungin was observed in 45% of the patients (105). Its different mode of action has also opened the perspective for use of combination antifungal therapy. Caspofungin levels are increased by coadministration with cyclosporin (106,107). Tacrolimus levels should be monitored when the two drugs are used together, since slight decreases in tacrolimus levels have been observed.

Itraconazole has been used for decades but an intravenous formulation became available only recently. Its bioavailability is unpredictable and the intravenous formulation is contraindicated in patients with significant renal dysfunction. It increases cyclosporine and tacrolimus levels by 35% to 50%. It has been substituted by the new azoles with anti-*Aspergillus* activity, such as voriconazole.

Posaconazole is a new triazole in advanced stages of clinical development, which exhibits significant in vitro fungicidal activity against *Aspergillus*. It is only available in oral formulation and requires frequent dosing. It is also active against *Zygomycetes*. Ravuconazole, also under development, has potent in vitro activity against *Aspergillus* (108).

Table 2 lists the common antifungal agents used in the management of *Aspergillus* infections and Table 3 summarizes the most common side effects and drug interactions.

Optimal duration of therapy for invasive aspergillosis is controversial owing to lack of comparative trials. It is currently accepted that therapy for invasive disease should continue for at least 12 weeks, based on the only comparative trial done to date, comparing amphotericin to voriconazole. Therapy may be longer depending on resolution of clinical and radiographic findings.

Studies in patients with localized pulmonary aspergillosis and underlying neutropenia and hematologic malignancies suggest that lung resection may be associated with a better outcome (109,110). Among lung transplant recipients, native lung pneumonectomy may be a therapeutic option if adequate response to systemic antifungals is not obtained (111). Native lung pneumonectomy not only prevents translocation of fungus to the transplanted lung but also decreases the fungal burden. For *Aspergillus* tracheobronchitis, surgical resection and stent placement may be necessary if dehiscence of the anastomosis occurs (1).

### Combination Antifungal Therapy

The use of combination antifungal therapy seems promising. Most data are derived from in vitro studies, animal models, and clinical observations. Amphotericin plus caspofungin have been shown to be sometimes synergistic in vitro (112) and successful in 35% to 60% of patients (113,114). The combination of an echinocandin and an azole is frequently synergistic in vitro (115–117), but there have been only case reports of success. Amphotericin and an azole can be antagonistic and no advantage over monotherapy has been demonstrated in smaller studies (118). At present, there is no concrete evidence to support the routine use of combination therapy.

**Table 2** Treatment of *Aspergillus* Infection in Lung Transplant Recipients

| Condition | Treatment options | Proposed duration |
|---|---|---|
| Prophylaxis | Inhaled amphotericin B 6–30 mg/day<br>or<br>Itraconazole 400 mg/day<br>or<br>Voriconazole 400 mg/day | 2 wk to lifelong |
| *Aspergillus* tracheo-bronchitis | Lipid formulations of amphotericin 2–3 mg/kg/day<br>or<br>Voriconazole 6 mg/kg q 12 hr then 3 mg/kg q 12 hr<br>or<br>Caspofungin 70 mg/day loading dose, then 50 mg/day<br>plus<br>Inhaled amphotericin 6–30 mg/day | At least 12 wk<br><br>or<br>Until normal bronchoscopy findings |
| Invasive disease | Lipid formulations of amphotericin 5 mg/kg/day<br>or<br>Voriconazole 6 mg/kg q 12 hr then 3 mg/kg q 12 hr (may switch to 200 mg Po q 12 hr)<br>or<br>Caspofungin 70 mg/day loading dose, then 50 mg/day | At least 12 wk |

## Antifungal Susceptibility Testing

The interpretation of antifungal susceptibility testing for *Aspergillus* is difficult. Much of the data have been based on nonstandardized methods. A reference method for broth dilution antifungal susceptibility testing of filamentous fungi has been proposed by the National Committee for Clinical Laboratory Standards (119). E-test methods have also been utilized (120).

Amphotericin, the newer azoles, and the echinocandins are generally active against *Aspergillus*. Fluconazole is ineffective against *Aspergillus*. *A. terreus* is usually not susceptible to amphotericin. At present, ordering antifungal susceptibility testing for *Aspergillus* is not recommended.

## Prophylaxis

Universal and preemptive prophylaxes are the two strategies employed to prevent invasive fungal infections, particularly invasive aspergillosis in lung

**Table 3** Common Side Effects and Interaction of Antifungal Agents with Immunosuppressive Agents

| Antifungal drug | Hepato- toxicity | Nephro- toxicity | Drug interactions | | Other |
|---|---|---|---|---|---|
| | | | Tacrolimus | Cyclosporine | |
| Ampho- tericin prepara- tions | − | + | − | − | Monitoring of renal function, K and Mg levels necessary |
| Voricona- zole | + | − | ↓Tacrolimus dose to 1/3 of original dose and monitor levels | ↓Cyclosporine dose to 1/2 of original dose and monitor levels | Transient and reversible visual disturbance in 1/3 of patients |
| | | | | | IV formulation contraindicated if Crcl < 50 mL/ min |
| | | | | | Dose adjustment necessary for hepatic dysfunction |
| Caspofungin | + | − | ↓AUC of tacrolimus by 20% | ↑AUC of caspofungin by 35% | Maintenance dose should be decreased in moderate-severe hepatic dysfunction |
| Itraconazole | + | − | ↑Tacrolimus levels by 35–50% | ↓Cyclosporine dose to 1/2 of original dose and monitor levels | IV formulation contra-indicated if CrCl < 30 mL/ min |

*Abbreviation*: AUC, area under the curve.

transplant recipients. The preemptive therapy is guided by the presence of positive BAL culture on surveillance bronchoscopy and has been reported to be efficacious (55).

The majority of lung transplant centers have employed the universal prophylaxis strategy (121,122). The prophylactic agent most commonly used is nebulized amphotericin. The type of nebulizers and dosage has varied between the studies, thus making it hard to determine the true efficacy of the strategy. The reported dosage of inhaled amphotericin ranges from 6 mg/day to 0.6 mg/kg/day (99,123). At our center we use 10 mg twice a day. Other agents used in lung transplant recipients include inhaled lipid complex amphotericin B, itraconazole, and voriconazole (32,103,124). Duration of therapy has varied from two weeks to lifelong.

## Avoidance of Exposure

The exposure of high-risk patients to potential sources of molds should be minimized. Hospital policies should be put into practice, focusing on periods of hospital construction or renovation. The routine use of high efficiency particulate air (HEPA) filters is not recommended for solid organ transplant recipients. Flowers and potted plants should not be permitted in patient's rooms and gardening should be discouraged.

## Prognosis

The prognosis of *Aspergillus* infection in lung transplant recipients depends on the clinical form of the disease and also on the type of transplant, i.e., single versus double lung.

Overall mortality ranges from 52% to 65%. It varies from 23.7% among patients with tracheobronchitis to as high as 86% in those with invasive pulmonary disease and 99% in patients with disseminated disease and central nervous system (CNS) involvement.

The prognosis is worse for single-lung transplant recipients, when compared to double-lung and heart–lung recipients, with mortality rates that can be as much as four times higher in the first group (35).

## *CRYPTOCOCCUS*

*Cryptococcus* is an ubiquitous encapsulated yeast. Of 37 species known to *Cryptococcus* genus only *Cryptococcus neoformans* is pathogenic. It has four serotypes (A–D) (125,126). Serotype A is named *C. neoformans* var. *grubii*, serotypes B and C are called *C. neoformans* var. *gattii*, while serotype D constitutes *C. neoformans* var. *neoformans* (127). *C. neoformans* var. *grubii* and *C. neoformans* var. *neoformans* are found all over the world in bird droppings and predominantly affect the immunocompromised host, while *C. neoformans* var. *gattii* is usually found in tropical countries and affects the immunocompetent hosts (128–142).

## Incidence and Risk Factors

The incidence of cryptococcal infection varies from 0% to 2%, although incidence as high as 6% has also been reported (143–145). In one study lung transplant recipients had the lowest incidence of cryptococcal meningitis as compared to other solid organ transplant recipients (2.3/1000 patients) (146). The risk factors for the acquisition of cryptococcal disease have not been assessed in solid organ transplant recipients. However, altered mental status, absence of headache, liver failure, and renal failure have been associated with higher mortality in patients with cryptococcal meningitis (144,146). The predictors of mortality in pulmonary cryptococcosis include acute respiratory failure requiring mechanical ventilation, pleural effusion, and bilateral pulmonary infiltrates. In multivariate regression analysis, only pleural effusion was an independent predictor of mortality (147).

## Diagnosis

The diagnosis of cryptococcal infection can be made by culture, direct microscopic examination (India ink or Gomori methenamine silver/calcofluor stains), and detection of polysaccharide antigen in body fluids and tissues. In one study, India ink was reported to be positive in 50% of cases of cryptococcal meningitis. Cryptococcal antigen was positive in 100% of CSF samples and 91% of sera collected at the time of diagnosis, while culture was positive only in 77% of cases (60). Serum cryptococcal antigen was reported to be positive in 53% to 75% of patients with pulmonary cryptococcosis (147,148). Elevated opening CSF pressure (31–60 cm/$H_2O$) was documented in 100% of patients with cryptococcal meningitis when assessed (143). Computed tomography (CT) and magnetic resonance imaging findings in cryptococcal meningitis are nonspecific and range from meningeal enhancement to space-occupying lesion. Unilateral, nodular, or cavitary infiltrate are the most common radiological presentation of pulmonary cryptococcosis. The growth of *Cryptococcus* in BAL in an asymptomatic lung transplant patient should be considered as evidence for disease unless proven otherwise (147,148). The CSF profile of patients with cryptococcal meningitis include moderate pleocytosis 0–485 white blood cells/$mm^3$, hypogylcorrhachia (40%), and increased protein in CSF (147,149).

## Clinical Presentation

In solid organ transplant recipients, CNS is the most common site of infection, involving 55% of cases, followed by skin, soft tissue, or osteoarticular infection in 13% cases and isolated pulmonary involvement in 10% of cases. Twenty-four percent of cases had multiple sites involved. Patients receiving tacrolimus are reported to have less likelihood of developing CNS infection and are more likely to develop skin and osteoarticular infection (144). The time of onset varies with the type of solid organ transplant. Median time to onset of *C. neoformans* infection in lung transplant was noted to be three months, followed by 8.8 months for liver transplant, 28 months for heart transplant, and 35 months for kidney transplant, respectively (144). Other reported cryptococcal infections in solid organ transplant recipients include prostatitis, myositis, chorioretinitis, and renal graft involvement (150,151).

Cryptococcal meningitis is a subacute meningitis with symptoms developing over a period of 1 to 12 weeks. Headache, nausea/vomiting, confusion or lethargy, and fever are the most common presenting symptoms. Meningismus, visual loss, and seizure occur in less than 10% of patients (143,146). Pulmonary cryptococcosis is mostly symptomatic, though asymptomatic cases have also been reported. The symptoms of pulmonary cryptococcosis are nonspecific and less than half of the patients present with cough, shortness of breath, and fever. A high index of suspicion in a transplant recipient with pulmonary infiltrate facilitates the early diagnosis (147,148). Anastomatic infection due to *Cryptococcus* has not been reported in lung transplant recipients.

The overall death rate due to cryptococcal infection in solid organ transplant recipients is considerably high and ranges from 42% to 50% in cases with cryptococcal meningitis.

## Treatment

The treatment of cryptococcosis has largely been extrapolated from the studies in HIV setting. Amphotericin B preferably with 5-flucytosine is the treatment of choice in patients with cryptococcal meningitis. The recommended regimens for the induction/consolidation phase include amphotericin B 0.7–1 mg/kg/day plus 5-flucytosine 100 mg/kg/day for two weeks, then fluconazole 400 mg/day for a minimum of 10 weeks or amphotericin B 0.7–1 mg/kg/day plus 5-flucytosine 100 mg/kg/day for 6 to 10 weeks (147). The amphotericin B deoxycholate can be substituted with lipid preparation of amphotericin in doses of 3–6 mg/kg/day. 5-Flucytosine is associated with leukopenia due to bone marrow suppression in 56% of patients during the first two weeks of therapy. 5-Flucytosine peak levels should be monitored especially in patients with renal insufficiency, and maintained between 30 and 80 µg/mL. Values >100 µg/mL are associated with toxicity and may warrant reduction in dosage (152). Lumbar puncture at the end of two weeks of therapy is recommended and, if negative, the patient should be treated with 400 mg/day of oral fluconazole for 8 to 10 weeks. At the completion of 10 weeks, the patient should be maintained on secondary prophylaxis with 200 mg of fluconazole. The duration of secondary prophylaxis is not known. The role of intrathecal amphotericin B therapy is not well defined in solid organ transplant recipients. It may have some value in patients with persistently raised intracranial pressure (>20 cm of water) (146). Isolated pulmonary disease in lung transplant recipients can be treated with fluconazole 400 mg/day (153). In addition to the administration of antifungal therapy, immunosuppression should be minimized. Reduction of steroid dose to the equivalent of 10 mg of prednisone may also result in improved outcome (153).

## OTHER MOLD INFECTIONS

Significant mold infections in lung transplant recipients include *Fusarium*, the dematiaceous molds, and zygomycetes.

## Fusarium

*Fusarium* is emerging as a cause of serious opportunistic infections in patients with bone marrow suppression and neutropenia (154,155). However, it has rarely been seen in solid organ transplant recipients.

Among solid organ transplant recipients, *Fusarium* infections tend to be localized, occurring at a median of nine months after transplantation, and are associated with a better outcome than that seen in bone marrow transplant recipients, with an associated 33% mortality rate (156). In lung transplant recipients, *Fusarium* infections can cause cavitary lung disease (157), pneumonia (158), and disseminated disease with endocarditis (159).

Similar to *Aspergillus*, *Fusarium* is angioinvasive and can cause tissue necrosis and pulmonary cavitation. Blood cultures can be positive in 50% to 70% of the cases. Biopsy specimens reveal fine, dichotomously branching, acutely angular, and septate hyphae. Culture is an important tool in diagnosis, since tissue morphology is undistinguishable from other hyaline molds.

*Fusarium* is relatively resistant to amphotericin. The azoles, including the newer ones, such as voriconazole, have no or very limited activity against *Fusarium*. The combination of amphotericin and surgical treatment seems to be the optimal treatment for such infection. Reduction in immunosuppression is essential to reduce morbidity and mortality.

## Dematiaceous Molds

In the past decades, these darkly pigmented fungi have been increasingly reported as pathogens, contributing to significant morbidity and mortality in immunocompromised patients (160,161). These include *Bipolaris*, *Cladophialophora*, *Ramichloridium*, *Dactylaria*, *Alternaria*, *Curvularia*, *Wangiella*, *Exophiala*, and others. Furthermore, new manifestations such as fungemia have been reported (162).

Clinical manifestations range from superficial lesions to disseminated infections. In lung transplant patients, it has been described as causing subcutaneous pheomycotic cyst, septic arthritis, pulmonary nodule, and disseminated disease (163–166).

Therapy consists of complete surgical excision of the lesion, whenever feasible, combined with systemic antifungal therapy, especially if systemic or invasive disease is present. Itraconazole is usually sufficient if only subcutaneous lesions are present; however, if the infection is systemic or involves the CNS, amphotericin B is required.

## Zygomycetes

Infection caused by the Zygomecetes occurs mostly in immunocompromised patients. The most frequent genera include *Mucor*, *Rhizopus*, *Rhizomucor*, *Absidia*, and *Cunninghamella*. These fungi are characterized by its vascular tropism with potential for invasion and dissemination and are associated with high mortality.

The most common clinical presentation of disease is rhinocerebral, which should be suspected when the patient presents with fever, maxillary swelling, and edema, accompanied by opacification of sinuses on CT. Cutaneous, pulmonary, gastrointestinal, and disseminated disease may also occur (167–169).

Zygomycetes are resistant to azoles, with the exception of posaconazole, which may have a role in the management of these infections (170,171). At present, the standard therapy constitutes of a higher than usual dose of lipid formulations of amphotericin (10 mg/kg/day) (172). Extensive debridment of necrotic tissue is recommended, even if complete resection of the infected area is not feasible.

## Scedosporium

*Scedosporium* is a filamentous fungus and contains two species, *Scedosporium apiospermum* and *Scedosporium prolificans. Psudallescheria boydii* is the sexual form of *S. apiospermum*, while no sexual form exists for *S. prolificans*. Incidence of *Scedosporium* in solid organ transplant recipients ranges from 1/1000 patients to 2.3% in lung transplant recipients (173,174). A trend for higher incidence of *Scedosporium* infection in lung transplant recipients was noted in one study (174). In solid organ transplant recipients, the majority (83%) of infections were due to *S. apiospermum,* while *S. prolificans* constituted 19% of cases (175).

Time to onset of disease varies with the species of *Scedosporium*. *S. apiospermum* infection occurs within a median of four months, while *S. prolificans* in solid organ transplant recipients can occur as early as 2.5 months (175). In lung transplant recipients the time to onset varies from two weeks to 58 months (173,174,176). Prior antifungal use, use of steroid, presence of airway stenosis, or advanced branchiolitis obliterans have been noted with higher frequency in lung transplant recipients with *Scedosporium* infection (173–175).

Forty six percent of solid organ transplant recipients have disseminated infection followed by pulmonary (43%), cutaneous (31%), and CNS involvement (29%) (175). Other manifestations include endopthalmitis, peritonitis, myocarditis, sinusitis, and mycotic aneurysm (175). The presenting symptoms are nonspecific and require a higher index of suspicion.

*Scedosporium* is diagnosed by the presence of characteristic colonies in the culture. *S. apiospermum* cannot be differentiated from *S. prolificans* in tissue sections, and *S. prolificans* has a higher mortality than *S. apiospermum* (175). Overall mortality in solid organ transplant recipients is 58%.

### Treatment

Both *Scedosporium* species are inherently resistant to amphotericin (177). Miconazole, itraconazole, voriconazole, posaconazole, ravuconazole, and caspofungin are active in vitro against *S. apiospermum* (178–180), while *S. prolificans* is resistant to ketoconazole, fluconazole, itraconazole, voriconazole, and caspofungin (177,178,181,182). The combination of terbinafine and itraconazole has been reported to be synergistic in 95% of isolates (179). Optimal treatment of the *S. prolificans* infection is still unknown. Several case reports have suggested successful outcome with the use of itraconazole and voriconazole (183–189). Concomitant surgical intervention is recommended in case of sinusitis (179). The duration of therapy remains uncertain but we usually treat for at least six months.

## REFERENCES

1. Singh N, Husain S. Aspergillus infections after lung transplantation: clinical differences in type of transplant and implications for management. J Heart Lung Transplant 2003; 22(3):258–266.
2. Singh N, Paterson DL, Gayowski T, Wagener MM, Marino IR. Preemptive prophylaxis with a lipid preparation of amphotericin B for invasive fungal infections in liver transplant recipients requiring renal replacement therapy. Transplantation 2001; 71(7):910–913.
3. Singh N. Antifungal prophylaxis in solid-organ transplant recipients: considerations for clinical trial design. Clin Infect Dis 2004; 39(suppl 4):S200–S206.
4. Baddley JW, Stroud TP, Salzman D, Pappas PG. Invasive mold infections in allogeneic bone marrow transplant recipients. Clin Infect Dis 2001; 32(9): 1319–1324.
5. Nakai K, Kanda Y, Mineishi S, et al. Primary cutaneous aspergillosis caused by *Aspergillus ustus* following reduced-intensity stem cell transplantation. Ann Hematol 2002; 81(10):593–596.
6. Gene J, Azon-Masoliver A, Guarro J, et al. Cutaneous infection caused by *Aspergillus ustus*, an emerging opportunistic fungus in immunosuppressed patients. J Clin Microbiol 2001; 39(3):1134–1136.
7. Verweij PE, van den Bergh MF, Rath PM, de Pauw BE, Voss A, Meis JF. Invasive aspergillosis caused by Aspergillus ustus: case report and review. J Clin Microbiol 1999; 37(5):1606–1609.
8. Iwen PC, Rupp ME, Bishop MR, et al. Disseminated aspergillosis caused by Aspergillus ustus in a patient following allogeneic peripheral stem cell transplantation. J Clin Microbiol 1998; 36(12):3713–3717.
9. Ricci RM, Evans JS, Meffert JJ, Kaufman L, Sadkowski LC. Primary cutaneous Aspergillus ustus infection: second reported case. J Am Acad Dermatol 1998; 38(5 Pt 2):797–798.
10. Stiller MJ, Teperman L, Rosenthal SA, et al. Primary cutaneous infection by Aspergillus ustus in a 62-year-old liver transplant recipient. J Am Acad Dermatol 1994; 31(2 Pt2):344–347.
11. Weiss LM, Thiemke WA. Disseminated Aspergillus ustus infection following cardiac surgery. Am J Clin Pathol 1983; 80(3):408–411.
12. Willinger B, Obradovic A, Selitsch B, et al. Detection and identification of fungi from fungus balls of the maxillary sinus by molecular techniques. J Clin Microbiol 2003; 41(2):581–585.

13. Sridhar H, Jayshree RS, Bapsy PP, et al. Invasive aspergillosis in cancer. Mycoses 2002; 45(9–10):358–363.
14. Yoshida K, Ando M, Ito K, et al. Hypersensitivity pneumonitis of a mushroom worker due to Aspergillus glaucus. Arch Environ Health 1990; 45(4):245–247.
15. Staib F, Seibold M, Grosse G. Aspergillus findings in AIDS patients suffering from cryptococcosis. Mycoses 1989; 32(10):516–523.
16. Sukumaran K. Ulcerative keratomycosis—case reports on three different species of fungi. Med J Malaysia 1991; 46(4):388–391.
17. Akiyama K, Takizawa H, Suzuki M, Miyachi S, Ichinohe M, Yanagihara Y. Allergic bronchopulmonary aspergillosis due to Aspergillus oryzae. Chest 1987; 91(2):285–286.
18. Byard RW, Bonin RA, Haq AU. Invasion of paranasal sinuses by *Aspergillus oryzae*. Mycopathologia 1986; 96(1):41–43.
19. Wanqing L, Hai W, Yuchong C, et al. The first case of obstructing bronchial aspergillosis caused by Aspergillus sydowi. Int J Infect Dis 2004; 8(2): 132–133.
20. Duong M, Ouellet N, Simard M, Bergeron Y, Olivier M, Bergeron MG. Kinetic study of host defense and inflammatory response to *Aspergillus fumigatus* in steroid-induced immunosuppressed mice. J Infect Dis 1998; 178(5): 1472–1482.
21. Ninin E, Milpied N, Moreau P, et al. Longitudinal study of bacterial, viral, and fungal infections in adult recipients of bone marrow transplants. Clin Infect Dis 2001; 33(1):41–47.
22. Williamson EC, Millar MR, Steward CG, et al. Infections in adults undergoing unrelated donor bone marrow transplantation. Br J Haematol 1999; 104(3):560–568.
23. Marr KA, Carter RA, Boeckh M, Martin P, Corey L. Invasive aspergillosis in allogeneic stem cell transplant recipients: changes in epidemiology and risk factors. Blood 2002; 100(13):4358–4366.
24. Jantunen E, Ruutu P, Niskanen L, et al. Incidence and risk factors for invasive fungal infections in allogeneic BMT recipients. Bone Marrow Transplant 1997; 19(8):801–808.
25. Wald A, Leisenring W, van Burik JA, Bowden RA. Epidemiology of Aspergillus infections in a large cohort of patients undergoing bone marrow transplantation. J Infect Dis 1997; 175(6):1459–1466.
26. Cornet M, Fleury L, Masio C, Bernard JF, Brucker G. Epidemiology of invasive aspergillosis in France: a six-year multicentric survey in the Greater Paris area. J Hosp Infect 2002; 51(4):288–296.
27. Singh N. Antifungal prophylaxis for solid organ transplant recipients: seeking clarity amidst controversy. Clin Infect Dis 2000; 31(2):545–553.
28. Kusne S, Furukawa H, Abu-Elmagd K, et al. Infectious complications after small bowel transplantation in adults: an update. Transplant Proc 1996; 28(5):2761–2762.
29. Reyes J, Abu-Elmagd K, Tzakis A, et al. Infectious complications after human small bowel transplantation. Transplant Proc 1992; 24(3):1249–1250.
30. Munoz P, Rodriguez C, Bouza E, et al. Risk-factors of invasive aspergillosis after heart transplantation: protective role of oral itraconazole prophylaxis. Am J Transplant 2004; 4(4):636–643.

31. Montoya JG, Chaparro SV, Celis D, et al. Invasive aspergillosis in the setting of cardiac transplantation. Clin Infect Dis 2003; 37(suppl 3):S281–S292.

32. Minari A, Husni R, Avery RK, et al. The incidence of invasive aspergillosis among solid organ transplant recipients and implications for prophylaxis in lung transplants. Transplant Infect Dis 2002; 4(4):195–200.

33. Husain S, Kwak EJ, Obman A, et al. Prospective assessment of Platelia Aspergillus galactomannan antigen for the diagnosis of invasive aspergillosis in lung transplant recipients. Am J Transplant 2004; 4(5):796–802.

34. Mehrad B, Paciocco G, Martinez FJ, Ojo TC, Iannettoni MD, Lynch JP III. Spectrum of Aspergillus infection in lung transplant recipients: case series and review of the literature. Chest 2001; 119(1):169–175.

35. Westney GE, Kesten S, De Hoyos A, Chapparro C, Winton T, Maurer JR. Aspergillus infection in single and double lung transplant recipients. Transplantation 1996; 61(6):915–919.

36. Husni RN, Gordon SM, Longworth DL, et al. Cytomegalovirus infection is a risk factor for invasive aspergillosis in lung transplant recipients. Clin Infect Dis 1998; 26(3):753–755.

37. Cahill BC, Hibbs JR, Savik K, et al. Aspergillus airway colonization and invasive disease after lung transplantation. Chest 1997; 112(5):1160–1164.

38. Chan KM, Alien SA. Infectious pulmonary complications in lung transplant recipients. Semin Respir Infect 2002; 17(4):291–302.

39. Higgins R, McNeil K, Dennis C, et al. Airway stenoses after lung transplantation: management with expanding metal stents. J Heart Lung Transplant 1994; 13(5):774–778.

40. Rubin RH. Overview: pathogenesis of fungal infections in the organ transplant recipient. Transplant Infect Dis 2002; 4(suppl 3):12–17.

41. Kubak BM. Fungal infection in lung transplantation. Transplant Infect Dis 2002; 4(suppl 3):24–31.

42. Gordon SM, Avery RK. Aspergillosis in lung transplantation: incidence, risk factors, and prophylactic strategies. Transplant Infect Dis 2001; 3(3): 161–167.

43. Hopkins CC, Weber DJ, Rubin RH. Invasive aspergillus infection: possible non-ward common source within the hospital environment. J Hosp Infect 1989; 13(1):19–25.

44. Singh N, Arnow PM, Bonham A, et al. Invasive aspergillosis in liver transplant recipients in the 1990s. Transplantation 1997; 64(5):716–720.

45. Kusne S, Torre-Cisneros J, Manez R, et al. Factors associated with invasive lung aspergillosis and the significance of positive Aspergillus culture after liver transplantation. J Infect Dis 1992; 166(6):1379–1383.

46. George MJ, Snydman DR, Werner BG, et al. The independent role of cytomegalovirus as a risk factor for invasive fungal disease in orthotopic liver transplant recipients. Am J Med 1997; 103(2):106–113.

47. Snydman DR, Falagas ME, Avery R, et al. Use of combination cytomegalovirus immune globulin plus ganciclovir for prophylaxis in CMV-seronegative liver transplant recipients of a CMV-seropositive donor organ: a muiticenter, open-label study. Transplant Proc 2001; 33(4):2571–2575.

48. Grundy JE. Virologic and pathogenetic aspects of cytomegalovirus infection. Rev Infect Dis 1990; 12(suppl 7):S711–S719.

49. Rubin RH. Impact of cytomegalovirus infection on organ transplant recipients. Rev Infect Dis 1990; 12(suppl 7):S754–S766.
50. Limaye AP. Antiviral resistance in cytomegalovirus: an emerging problem in organ transplant recipients. Semin Respir Infect 2002; 17(4):265–273.
51. Limaye AP, Raghu G, Koelle DM, Ferrenberg J, Huang ML, Boeckh M. High incidence of ganciclovir-resistant cytomegalovirus infection among lung transplant recipients receiving preemptive therapy. J Infect Dis 2002; 185(1):20–27.
52. Nunley DR, Ohori P, Grgurich WF, et al. Pulmonary aspergillosis in cystic fibrosis lung transplant recipients. Chest 1998; 114(5):1321–1329.
53. Brenier-Pinchart MP, Lebeau B, Devouassoux G, et al. Aspergillus and lung transplant recipients: a mycologic and molecular epidemiologic study. J Heart Lung Transplant 1998; 17(10):972–979.
54. Kanj SS, Tapson V, Davis RD, Madden J, Browning I. Infections in patients with cystic fibrosis following lung transplantation. Chest 1997; 112(4): 924–930.
55. Hamacher J, Spiliopoulos A, Kurt AM, Nicod LP. Pre-emptive therapy with azoles in lung transplant patients. Geneva Lung Transplantation Group. Eur Respir J 1999; 13(1):180–186.
56. Goldfarb NS, Avery RK, Goormastic M, et al. Hypogammaglobulinemia in lung transplant recipients. Transplantation 2001; 71(2):242–246.
57. Kramer MR, Denning DW, Marshall SE, et al. Ulcerative tracheobronchitis after lung transplantation. A new form of invasive aspergillosis. Am Rev Respir Dis 1991; 144(3 Pt 1):552–556.
58. Ducreux D, Chevallier P, Perrin C, et al. Pseudomembranous aspergillus bronchitis in a double-lung transplanted patient: unusual radiographic and CT features. Eur Radiol 2000; 10(10):1547–1549.
59. Hadjiiiadis D, Howell DN, Davis RD, et al. Anastomotic infections in lung transplant recipients. Ann Transplant 2000; 5(3):13–19.
60. Helmi M, Love RB, Welter D, Cornwell RD, Meyer KC. Aspergillus infection in lung transplant recipients with cystic fibrosis: risk factors and outcomes comparison to other types of transplant recipients. Chest 2003; 123(3):800–808.
61. Gerson SL, Talbot GH, Lusk E, Hurwitz S, Strom BL, Cassileth PA. Invasive pulmonary aspergillosis in adult acute leukemia: clinical clues to its diagnosis. J Clin Oncol 1985; 3(8):1109–1116.
62. Cunha BA. Central nervous system infections in the compromised host: a diagnostic approach. Infect Dis Clin North Am 2001; 15(2):567–590.
63. Casey P, Garrett J, Eaton T. Allergic bronchopulmonary aspergillosis in a lung transplant patient successfully treated with nebulized amphotericin. J Heart Lung Transplant 2002; 21(11):1237–1241.
64. Egan JJ, Yonan N, Carroll KB, Deiraniya AK, Webb AK, Woodcock AA. Allergic bronchopulmonary aspergillosis in lung allograft recipients. Eur Respir J 1996; 9(1):169–171.
65. Fitzsimons EJ, Aris R, Patterson R. Recurrence of allergic bronchopulmonary aspergillosis in the posttransplant lungs of a cystic fibrosis patient. Chest 1997; 112(1):281–282.
66. Simon DM, Levin S. Infectious complications of solid organ transplantations. Infect Dis Clin North Am 2001; 15(2):521–549.

67. Brown RS Jr, Lake JR, Katzman BA, et al. Incidence and significance of Aspergillus cultures following liver and kidney transplantation. Transplantation 1996; 61(4):666–669.
68. Perfect JR, Cox GM, Lee JY, et al. The impact of culture isolation of Aspergillus species: a hospital-based survey of aspergillosis. Clin Infect Dis 2001; 33(11):1824–1833.
69. Weiland D, Ferguson RM, Peterson PK, Snover DC, Simmons RL, Najarian JS. Aspergillosis in 25 renal transplant patients. Epidemiology, clinical presentation, diagnosis, and management. Ann Surg 1983; 198(5):622–629.
70. Horvath JA, Dummer S. The use of respiratory-tract cultures in the diagnosis of invasive pulmonary aspergillosis. Am J Med 1996; 100(2):171–178.
71. Stynen D, Goris A, Sarfati J, Latge JP. A new sensitive sandwich enzyme-linked immunosorbent assay to detect galactofuran in patients with invasive aspergillosis. J Clin Microbiol 1995; 33(2):497–500.
72. Verweij PE, Stynen D, Rijs AJ, de Pauw BE, Hoogkamp-Korstanje JA, Meis JF. Sandwich enzyme-linked immunosorbent assay compared with Pastorex latex agglutination test for diagnosing invasive aspergillosis in immunocompromised patients. J Clin Microbiol 1995; 33(7):1912–1914.
73. Pinel C, Fricker-Hidalgo H, Lebeau B, et al. Detection of circulating Aspergillus fumigatus galactomannan: value and limits of the Platelia test for diagnosing invasive aspergillosis. J Clin Microbiol 2003; 41(5):2184–2186.
74. Maertens J, Van Eldere J, Verhaegen J, Verbeken E, Verschakelen J, Boogaerts M. Use of circulating galactomannan screening for early diagnosis of invasive aspergillosis in allogeneic stem cell transplant recipients. J Infect Dis 2002; 186(9):1297–1306.
75. Sulahian A, Boutboul F, Ribaud P, Leblanc T, Lacroix C, Derouin F. Value of antigen detection using an enzyme immunoassay in the diagnosis and prediction of invasive aspergillosis in two adult and pediatric hematology units during a 4-year prospective study. Cancer 2001; 91(2):311–318.
76. Herbrecht R, Letscher-Bru V, Oprea C, et al. Aspergillus galactomannan detection in the diagnosis of invasive aspergillosis in cancer patients. J Clin Oncol 2002; 20(7):1898–1906.
77. Maertens J, Verhaegen J, Demuynck H, et al. Autopsy-controlled prospective evaluation of serial screening for circulating galactomannan by a sandwich enzyme-linked immunosorbent assay for hematological patients at risk for invasive Aspergillosis. J Clin Microbiol 1999; 37(10):3223–3228.
78. Marr KA, Balajee SA, McLaughlin L, Tabouret M, Bentsen C, Walsh TJ. Detection of galactomannan antigenemia by enzyme immunoassay for the diagnosis of invasive aspergillosis: variables that affect performance. J Infect Dis 2004; 190(3):641–649.
79. Adam O, Auperin A, Wilquin F, Bourhis JH, Gachot B, Chachaty E. Treatment with piperacillin-tazobactam and false-positive Aspergillus galactomannan antigen test results for patients with hematological malignancies. Clin Infect Dis 2004; 38(6):917–920.
80. Kwak EJ, Husain S, Obman A, et al. Efficacy of galactomannan antigen in the Platelia Aspergillus enzyme immunoassay for diagnosis of invasive aspergillosis in liver transplant recipients. J Clin Microbiol 2004; 42(1):435–438.

81. Fortun J, Martin-Davila P, Alvarez ME, et al. Aspergillus antigenemia sandwich-enzyme immunoassay test as a serodiagnostic method for invasive aspergillosis in liver transplant recipients. Transplantation 2001; 71(1):145–149.

82. Salonen J, Lehtonen OP, Terasjarvi MR, Nikoskelainen J. Aspergillus antigen in serum, urine and bronchoalveolar lavage specimens of neutropenic patients in relation to clinical outcome. Scand J Infect Dis 2000; 32(5):485–490.

83. Becker MJ, Lugtenburg EJ, Cornelissen JJ, Van Der Schee C, Hoogsteden HC, De Marie S. Galactomannan detection in computerized tomography-based bronchoalveolar lavage fluid and serum in haematological patients at risk for invasive pulmonary aspergillosis. Br J Haematol 2003; 121(3):448–457.

84. Viscoli C, Machetti M, Gazzola P, et al. Aspergillus galactomannan antigen in the cerebrospinal fluid of bone marrow transplant recipients with probable cerebral aspergillosis. J Clin Microbiol 2002; 40(4):1496–1499.

85. Boutboul F, Alberti C, Leblanc T, et al. Invasive aspergillosis in allogeneic stem cell transplant recipients: increasing antigenemia is associated with progressive disease. Clin Infect Dis 2002; 34(7):939–943.

86. Obayashi T, Yoshida M, Mori T, et al. Plasma $(1\rightarrow3)$-beta-D-glucan measurement in diagnosis of invasive deep mycosis and fungal febrile episodes. Lancet 1995; 345(8941):17–20.

87. Yoshida M, Obayashi T, Iwama A, et al. Detection of plasma $(1\rightarrow3)$-beta-D-glucan in patients with Fusarium, Trichosporon, Saccharomyces and Acremonium fungaemias. J Med Vet Mycol 1997; 35(5):371–374.

88. Buchheidt D, Baust C, Skladny H, Baldus M, Brauninger S, Hehlmann R. Clinical evaluation of a polymerase chain reaction assay to detect Aspergillus species in bronchoalveolar lavage samples of neutropenic patients. Br J Haematol 2002; 116(4):803–811.

89. Buchheidt D, Hummel M, Schleiermacher D, et al. Prospective clinical evaluation of a LightCycler-mediated polymerase chain reaction assay, a nested-PCR assay and a galactomannan enzyme-linked immunosorbent assay for detection of invasive aspergillosis in neutropenic cancer patients and haematological stem cell transplant recipients. Br J Haematol 2004; 125(2):196–202.

90. Challier S, Boyer S, Abachin E, Berche P. Development of a serum-based Taqman real-time PCR assay for diagnosis of invasive aspergillosis. J Clin Microbiol 2004; 42(2):844–846.

91. Spiess B, Buchheidt D, Baust C, et al. Development of a LightCycler PCR assay for detection and quantification of Aspergillus fumigatus DNA in clinical samples from neutropenic patients. J Clin Microbiol 2003; 41(5):1811–1818.

92. Pham AS, Tarrand JJ, May GS, Lee MS, Kontoyiannis DP, Han XY. Diagnosis of invasive mold infection by real-time quantitative PCR. Am J Clin Pathol 2003; 119(1):38–44.

93. Ferns RB, Fletcher H, Bradley S, Mackinnon S, Hunt C, Tedder RS. The prospective evaluation of a nested polymerase chain reaction assay for the early detection of Aspergillus infection in patients with leukaemia or undergoing allograft treatment. Br J Haematol 2002; 119(3):720–725.

94. Loeffler J, Kloepfer K, Hebart H, et al. Polymerase chain reaction detection of aspergillus DNA in experimental models of invasive aspergillosis. J Infect Dis 2002; 185(8):1203–1206.

95. Raad I, Hanna H, Sumoza D, Albitar M. Polymerase chain reaction on blood for the diagnosis of invasive pulmonary aspergillosis in cancer patients. Cancer 2002; 94(4):1032–1036.

96. Maschmeyer G, Ruhnke M. Update on antifungal treatment of invasive Candida and Aspergillus infections. Mycoses 2004; 47(7):263–276.

97. Bowden R, Chandrasekar P, White MH, et al. A double-blind, randomized, controlled trial of amphotericin B colloidal dispersion versus amphotericin B for treatment of invasive aspergillosis in immunocompromised patients. Clin Infect Dis 2002; 35(4):359–366.

98. Linden PK, Coley K, Fontes P, Fung JJ, Kusne S. Invasive aspergillosis in liver transplant recipients: outcome comparison of therapy with amphotericin B lipid complex and a historical cohort treated with conventional amphotericin B. Clin Infect Dis 2003; 37(1):17–25.

99. Monforte V, Roman A, Gavalda J, et al. Nebulized amphotericin B prophylaxis for Aspergillus infection in lung transplantation: study of risk factors. J Heart Lung Transplant 2001; 20(12):1274–1281.

100. Monforte V, Roman A, Gavalda J, et al. Nebulized amphotericin B concentration and distribution in the respiratory tract of lung-transplanted patients. Transplantation 2003; 75(9):1571–1574.

101. Allen SD, Sorensen KN, Nejdl MJ, Durrant C, Proffit RT. Prophylactic efficacy of aerosolized liposomal (AmBisome) and non-liposomal (Fungizone) amphotericin B in murine pulmonary aspergillosis. J Antimicrob Chemother 1994; 34(6):1001–1013.

102. Cicogna CE, White MH, Bernard EM, et al. Efficacy of prophylactic aerosol amphotericin B lipid complex in a rat model of pulmonary aspergillosis. Antimicrob Agents Chemother 1997; 41(2):259–261.

103. Drew RH, Dodds Ashley E, Benjamin DK Jr, Duane Davis R, Palmer SM, Perfect JR. Comparative safety of amphotericin B lipid complex and amphotericin B deoxycholate as aerosolized antifungal prophylaxis in lung-transplant recipients. Transplantation 2004; 77(2):232–237.

104. Herbrecht R, Denning DW, Patterson TF, et al. Voriconazole versus amphotericin B for primary therapy of invasive aspergillosis. N Engl J Med 2002; 347(6):408–415.

105. Maertens J, Raad I, Petrikkos G, et al. Efficacy and safety of caspofungin for treatment of invasive aspergillosis in patients refractory to or intolerant of conventional antifungal therapy. Clin Infect Dis 2004; 39(11):1563–1571.

106. Denning DW. Echinocandin antifungal drugs. Lancet 2003; 362(9390):1142–1151.

107. Sable CA, Nguyen BY, Chodakewitz JA, DiNubile MJ. Safety and tolerability of caspofungin acetate in the treatment of fungal infections. Transplant Infect Dis 2002; 4(1):25–30.

108. Boucher HW, Groll AH, Chiou CC, Walsh TJ. Newer systemic antifungal agents: pharmacokinetics, safety and efficacy. Drugs 2004; 64(18):1997–2020.

109. Reichenberger F, Habicht J, Kaim A, et al. Lung resection for invasive pulmonary aspergillosis in neutropenic patients with hematologic diseases. Am J Respir Crit Care Med 1998; 158(3):885–890.

110. Baron O, Guillaume B, Moreau P, et al. Aggressive surgical management in localized pulmonary mycotic and nonmycotic infections for neutropenic

patients with acute leukemia: report of eighteen cases. J Thorac Cardiovasc Surg 1998; 115(1):63–68 (discussion 68–69).

111. Sandur S, Gordon SM, Mehta AC, Maurer JR. Native lung pneumonectomy for invasive pulmonary aspergillosis following lung transplantation: a case report. J Heart Lung Transplant 1999; 18(8):810–813.

112. Arikan S, Lozano-Chiu M, Paetznick V, Rex JH. In vitro synergy of caspofungin and amphotericin B against Aspergillus and Fusarium spp. Antimicrob Agents Chemother 2002; 46(1):245–247.

113. Aliff TB, Maslak PG, Jurcic JG, et al. Refractory Aspergillus pneumonia in patients with acute leukemia: successful therapy with combination caspofungin and liposomal amphotericin. Cancer 2003; 97(4):1025–1032.

114. Kontoyiannis DP, Hachem R, Lewis RE, et al. Efficacy and toxicity of caspofungin in combination with liposomal amphotericin B as primary or salvage treatment of invasive aspergillosis in patients with hematologic malignancies. Cancer 2003; 98(2):292–299.

115. Manavathu EK, Alangaden GJ, Chandrasekar PH. In-vitro isolation and antifungal susceptibility of amphotericin B-resistant mutants of Aspergillus fumigatus. J Antimicrob Chemother 1998; 41(6):615–619.

116. Kirkpatrick WR, Perea S, Coco BJ, Patterson TF. Efficacy of caspofungin alone and in combination with voriconazole in a guinea pig model of invasive aspergillosis. Antimicrob Agents Chemother 2002; 46(8):2564–2568.

117. Marr KA, Boeckh M, Carter RA, Kim HW, Corey L. Combination antifungal therapy for invasive aspergillosis. Clin Infect Dis 2004; 39(6):797–802.

118. Lewis RE, Prince RA, Chi J, Kontoyiannis DP. Itraconazole preexposure attenuates the efficacy of subsequent amphotericin B therapy in a murine model of acute invasive pulmonary aspergillosis. Antimicrob Agents Chemother 2002; 46(10):3208–3214.

119. NCCLS. Reference method for broth dilution antifungal susceptibility testing of filamentous fungi. Approved standard M38-A. Wayne, PA: National Committee for Clinical Laboratory Standards, 2004.

120. Serrano MC, Morilla D, Valverde A, et al. Comparison of Etest with modified broth microdilution method for testing susceptibility of Aspergillus spp. to voriconazole. J Clin Microbiol 2003; 41(11):5270–5272.

121. Husain S, Kusne S, McCurry K. Differences in the antifungal prophylaxis strategies among North American and European centers in lung transplantation. Washington, DC: American Transplant Congress, May 30–Jun 4, 2003.

122. Dummer JS, Lazariashvilli N, Barnes J, Ninan M, Milstone AP. A survey of antifungal management in lung transplantation. J Heart Lung Transplant 2004; 23(12):1376–1381.

123. Calvo V, Borro JM, Morales P, et al. Antifungal prophylaxis during the early postoperative period of lung transplantation. Chest 1999; 115(5):1301–1304.

124. Husain S, Kwak EJ, Mccurry K. Role of voriconazole prophylaxis for the prevention of invasive aspergillosis (IA) at six months in lung transplant recipients. In: The International Society for Heart and Lung Transplantation 24th Annual Meeting and Scientific Sessions, San Francisco, CA, Apr 21–24, 2004.

125. Belay T, Chemiak R, O'Neill EB, Kozel TR. Serotyping of Cryptococcus neoformans by dot enzyme assay. J Clin Microbiol 1996; 34(2):466–470.

126. Belay T, Chemiak R. Determination of antigen binding specificities of Cryptococcus neoformans factor sera by enzyme-linked immunosorbent assay. Infect Immun 1995; 63(5):1810–1819.
127. Franzot SP, Salkin IF, Casadevall A. Cryptococcus neoformans var. grubii: separate varietal status for Cryptococcus neoformans serotype A isolates. J Clin Microbiol 1999; 37(3):838–840.
128. Steenbergen JN, Casadevall A. Prevalence of Cryptococcus neoformans var. neoformans (serotype D) and Cryptococcus neoformans var. grubii (serotype A) isolates in New York City. J Clin Microbiol 2000; 38(5):1974–1976.
129. Hoang LM, Maguire JA, Doyle P, Fyfe M, Roscoe DL. Cryptococcus neoformans infections at Vancouver Hospital and Health Sciences Centre (1997–2002): epidemiology, microbiology and histopathology. J Med Microbiol 2004; 53(Pt 9):935–940.
130. Igreja RP, Lazera Mdos S, Wanke B, Galhardo MC, Kidd SE, Meyer W. Molecular epidemiology of Cryptococcus neoformans isolates from AIDS patients of the Brazilian city, Rio de Janeiro. Med Mycol 2004; 42(3):229–238.
131. Correa Mdo P, Severo LC, Oliveira Fde M, Irion K, Londero AT. The spectrum of computerized tomography (CT) findings in central nervous system (CNS) infection due to Cryptococcus neoformans var. gattii in immunocompetent children. Rev Inst Med Trop Sao Paulo 2002; 44(5):283–287.
132. Lacaz Cda S, Heins-Vaccari EM, Hernandez-Arriagada GL, et al. Primary cutaneous cryptococcosis due to Cryptococcus neoformans var. gattii serotype B, in an immunocompetent patient. Rev Inst Med Trop Sao Paulo 2002; 44(4):225–228.
133. Chen SC. Cryptococcosis in Australasia and the treatment of cryptococcal and other fungal infections with liposomal amphotericin B. J Antimicrob Chemother 2002; 49(suppl 1):57–61.
134. Chen S, Sorrell T, Nimmo G, et al. Epidemiology and host- and variety-dependent characteristics of infection due to Cryptococcus neoformans in Australia and New Zealand. Clin Infect Dis 2000; 31(2):499–508.
135. Imai T, Watanabe K, Tamura M, et al. Geographic grouping of Cryptococcus neoformans var. gattii by random amplified polymorphic DNA fingerprint patterns and ITS sequence divergence. Clin Lab 2000; 46(7–8):345–354.
136. Chen SC, Currie BJ, Campbell HM, et al. Cryptococcus neoformans var gattii infection in northern Australia: existence of an environmental source other than known host eucalypts. Trans R Soc Trop Med Hyg 1997; 91(5):547–550.
137. Hamann ID, Gillespie RJ, Ferguson JK. Primary cryptococcal cellulitis caused by Cryptococcus neoformans var. gattii in an immunocompetent host. Australas J Dermatol 1997; 38(1):29–32.
138. Dromer F, Mathoulin S, Dupont B, Laporte A. Epidemiology of cryptococcosis in France: a 9-year survey (1985–1993). Clin Infect Dis 1996; 23(1):82–90.
139. Speed B, Dunt D. Clinical and host differences between infections with the two varieties of Cryptococcus neoformans. Clin Infect Dis 1995; 21(1):28–34 (discussion 35–36).
140. Mitchell DH, Sorrell TC, Allworth AM, et al. Cryptococcal disease of the CNS in immunocompetent hosts: influence of cryptococcal variety on clinical manifestations and outcome. Clin Infect Dis 1995; 20(3):611–616.

141. Rozenbaum R, Goncalves AJ. Clinical epidemiological study of 171 cases of cryptococcosis. Clin Infect Dis 1994; 18(3):369–380.
142. Fisher D, Burrow J, Lo D, Currie B. Cryptococcus neoformans in tropical northern Australia: predominantly variant gattii with good outcomes. Aust N Z J Med 1993; 23(6):678–682.
143. Singh N, Husain S. Infections of the central nervous system in transplant recipients. Transplant Infect Dis 2000; 2(3):101–111.
144. Singh N, Gayowski T, Wagener MM, Marino IR. Clinical spectrum of invasive cryptococcosis in liver transplant recipients receiving tacrolimus. Clin Transplant 1997; 11(1):66–70.
145. Jabbour N, Reyes J, Kusne S, Martin M, Fung J. Cryptococcal meningitis after liver transplantation. Transplantation 1996; 61(1):146–149.
146. Wu G, Vilchez RA, Eidelman B, Fung J, Kormos R, Kusne S. Cryptococcal meningitis: an analysis among 5,521 consecutive organ transplant recipients. Transplant Infect Dis 2002; 4(4):183–188.
147. Vilchez RA, Irish W, Lacomis J, Costello P, Fung J, Kusne S. The clinical epidemiology of pulmonary cryptococcosis in non-AIDS patients at a tertiary care medical center. Medicine (Baltimore) 2001; 80(5):308–312.
148. Mueller NJ, Fishman JA. Asymptomatic pulmonary cryptococcosis in solid organ transplantation: report of four cases and review of the literature. Transplant Infect Dis 2003; 5(3):140–143.
149. Husain S, Wagener MM, Singh N. Cryptococcus neoformans infection in organ transplant recipients: variables influencing clinical characteristics and outcome. Emerg Infect Dis 2001; 7(3):375–381.
150. Biswas J, Gopal L, Sharma T, Parikh S, Madhavan HN, Badrinath SS. Recurrent cryptococcal choroiditis in a renal transplant patient: clinicopathologic study. Retina 1998; 18(3):273–276.
151. Hill-Edgar AA, Nasr SH, Borczuk AC, D'Agati VD, Radhakrishnan J, Markowitz GS. A rare infectious cause of renal allograft dysfunction. Am J Kidney Dis 2002; 40(5):1103–1107.
152. Nguyen MH, Clancy CJ, Husain S. Cryptococcus neoformans (cryptococcosis). In: Yu VL, Weber R, Raoult D, eds. Antimicrobial Therapy and Vaccines. 2d ed. New York: Apple Tree Productions.
153. Saag MS, Graybill RJ, Larsen RA, et al. Practice guidelines for the management of cryptococcal disease. Clin Infect Dis 2000; 30(4):710–718.
154. Boutati EI, Anaissie EJ. Fusarium, a significant emerging pathogen in patients with hematologic malignancy: ten years' experience at a cancer center and implications for management. Blood 1997; 90(3):999–1008.
155. Hennequin C, Lavarde V, Poirot JL, et al. Invasive Fusarium infections: a retrospective survey of 31 cases. J Med Vet Mycol 1997; 35(2):107–114.
156. Sampathkumar P, Paya CV. Fusarium infection after solid-organ transplantation. Clin Infect Dis 2001; 32(8):1237–1240.
157. Arney KL, Tiernan R, Judson MA. Primary pulmonary involvement of Fusarium solani in a lung transplant recipient. Chest 1997; 112(4):1128–1130.
158. Herbrecht R, Kessler R, Kravanja C, Meyer MH, Waller J, Letscher-Bru V. Successful treatment of Fusarium proliferatum pneumonia with posaconazole in a lung transplant recipient. J Heart Lung Transplant 2004; 23(12):1451–1454.

159. Guinvarc'h A, Guilbert L, Marmorat-Khuong A, et al. Disseminated Fusarium solani infection with endocarditis in a lung transplant recipient. Mycoses 1998; 41(1–2):59–61.
160. Silveira F, Nucci M. Emergence of black moulds in fungal disease: epidemiology and therapy. Curr Opin Infect Dis 2001; 14(6):679–684.
161. Garcia-Diaz JB, Baumgarten K. Phaeohyphomycotic infections in solid organ transplant patients. Semin Respir Infect 2002; 17(4):303–309.
162. Nucci M, Akiti T, Barreiros G, et al. Nosocomial fungemia due to Exophiala jeanselmei var. jeanselmei and a Rhinocladiella species: newly described causes of bloodstream infection. J Clin Microbiol 2001; 39(2):514–518.
163. Chua JD, Gordon SM, Banbury J, Hall GS, Procop GW. Relapsing Exophiala jeanselmei phaeohyphomycosis in a lung transplant patient. Transplant Infect Dis 2001; 3(4):235–238.
164. Xu X, Low DW, Palevsky HI, Elenitsas R. Subcutaneous phaeohyphomycotic cysts caused by Exophiala jeanselmei in a lung transplant patient. Dermatol Surg 2001; 27(4):343–346.
165. Mazur JE, Judson MA. A case report of a dactylaria fungal infection in a lung transplant patient. Chest 2001; 119(2):651–653.
166. Burns KE, Ohori NP, Iacono AT. Dactylaria gallopava infection presenting as a pulmonary nodule in a single-lung transplant recipient. J Heart Lung Transplant 2000; 19(9):900–902.
167. Knoop C, Antoine M, Vachiery JL, et al. Gastric perforation due to mucormycosis after heart–lung and heart transplantation. Transplantation 1998; 66(7):932–935.
168. Mattner F, Weissbrodt H, Strueber M. Two case reports: fatal Absidia corymbifera pulmonary tract infection in the first postoperative phase of a lung transplant patient receiving voriconazole prophylaxis, and transient bronchial Absidia corymbifera colonization in a lung transplant patient. Scand J Infect Dis 2004; 36(4):312–314.
169. Hunstad DA, Cohen AH, St Geme JW III. Successful eradication of mucormycosis occurring in a pulmonary allograft. J Heart Lung Transplant 1999; 18(8):801–804.
170. Dannaoui E, Meis JF, Loebenberg D, Verweij PE. Activity of posaconazole in treatment of experimental disseminated zygomycosis. Antimicrob Agents Chemother 2003; 47(11):3647–3650.
171. Sun QN, Najvar LK, Bocanegra R, Loebenberg D, Graybill JR. In vivo activity of posaconazole against Mucor spp in an immunosuppressed mouse model. Antimicrob Agents Chemother 2002; 46(7):2310–2312.
172. Jimenez C, Lumbreras C, Aguado JM, et al. Successful treatment of mucor infection after liver or pancreas–kidney transplantation. Transplantation 2002; 73(3):476–480.
173. Tamm M, Malouf M, Glanville A. Pulmonary scedosporium infection following lung transplantation. Transplant Infect Dis 2001; 3(4):189–194.
174. Castiglioni B, Sutton DA, Rinaldi MG, Fung J, Kusne S. Pseudallescheria boydii (Anamorph Scedosporium apiospermum) infection in solid organ transplant recipients in a tertiary medical center and review of the literature. Medicine (Baltimore) 2002; 81(5):333–348.

175. Husain S, Munoz P, Forrest G, et al. Infections due to Scedosporium apiospermum and Scedosporium prolificans in transplant recipients: clinical characteristics and impact of antifungal agent therapy on outcome. Clin Infect Dis 2005; 40(1):89–99.

176. Raj R, Frost AE. Scedosporium apiospermum fungemia in a lung transplant recipient. Chest 2002; 121(5):1714–1716.

177. Ellis D. Amphotericin B: spectrum and resistance. J Antimicrob Chemother 2002; 49(suppl 1):7–10.

178. Meletiadis J, Mouton JW, Meis JF, Verweij PE. Combination chemotherapy for the treatment of invasive infections by Scedosporium prolificans. Clin Microbiol Infect 2000; 6(6):336–337.

179. Meletiadis J, Mouton JW, Rodriguez-Tudela JL, Meis JF, Verweij PE. In vitro interaction of terbinafine with itraconazole against clinical isolates of Scedosporium prolificans. Antimicrob Agents Chemother 2000; 44(2):470–472.

180. Pfaller MA, Marco F, Messer SA, Jones RN. In vitro activity of two echinocandin derivatives, LY303366 and MK-0991 (L-743,792), against clinical isolates of Aspergillus, Fusarium, Rhizopus, and other filamentous fungi. Diagn Microbiol Infect Dis 1998; 30(4):251–255.

181. Del Poeta M, Schell WA, Perfect JR. In vitro antifungal activity of pneumocandin L-743,872 against a variety of clinically important molds. Antimicrob Agents Chemother 1997; 41(8):1835–1836.

182. Johnson EM, Szekely A, Warnock DW. In vitro activity of Syn-2869, a novel triazole agent, against emerging and less common mold pathogens. Antimicrob Agents Chemother 1999; 43(5):1260–1263.

183. Martino R, Nomdedeu J, Altes A, et al. Successful bone marrow transplantation in patients with previous invasive fungal infections: report of four cases. Bone Marrow Transplant 1994; 13(3):265–269.

184. Lopes JO, Alves SH, Benevenga JP, Salla A, Khmohan C, Silva CB. Subcutaneous pseudallescheriasis in a renal transplant recipient. Mycopathologia 1994; 125(3):153–156.

185. Goldberg SL, Geha DJ, Marshall WF, Inwards DJ, Hoagland HC. Successful treatment of simultaneous pulmonary Pseudallescheria boydii and Aspergillus terreus infection with oral itraconazole. Clin Infect Dis 1993; 16(6):803–805.

186. Kanafani ZA, Comair Y, Kanj SS. Pseudallescheria boydii cranial osteomyelitis and subdural empyema successfully treated with voriconazole: a case report and literature review. Eur J Clin Microbiol Infect Dis 2004; 23(11):836–840.

187. Perlroth MG, Miller J. Pseudoallescheria boydii pneumonia and empyema: a rare complication of heart transplantation cured with voriconazole. J Heart Lung Transplant 2004; 23(5):647–649.

188. Nesky MA, McDougal EC, Peacock JE Jr. Pseudallescheria boydii brain abscess successfully treated with voriconazole and surgical drainage: case report and literature review of central nervous system pseudallescheriasis. Clin Infect Dis 2000; 31(3):673–677.

189. Poza G, Montoya J, Redondo C, et al. Meningitis caused by *Pseudallescheria boydii* treated with voriconazole. Clin Infect Dis 2000; 30(6):981–982.

# 26

# Bacterial Infections and Pneumocystis Infections

**Lora D. Thomas and Stephen Dummer**

*Department of Infectious Diseases, Vanderbilt University Medical Center, Nashville, Tennessee, U.S.A.*

## INTRODUCTION

It has been almost a quarter century since the first successful heart–lung transplant operation was carried out at Stanford University in 1981. In the intervening years, heart–lung and lung transplantation have become an accepted treatment for patients with end-stage lung disease. Overall clinical results in lung and heart–lung transplantation, however, still lag behind other types of transplantation. For instance, the recent three-year survival for lung transplant recipients in the United States is about 20% worse than the survival for liver or heart transplant recipients (1). There are many reasons for this reduced survival, but a significant role is undoubtedly played by the high infection rate in lung transplant recipients (2–6). It has been shown that heart–lung recipients have nearly twice the rate of infection as heart recipients managed by the same physicians (2). Most deaths after lung transplantation are associated with infection, either as a primary or as a secondary event (3). This chapter discusses bacterial infections and pneumocystis infections after lung transplantation. Bacterial pathogens are the most common infections after lung transplantation and pose the greatest infectious risk to lung recipients, particularly within the first few months after transplantation. Pneumocystis infections were common in the early days of lung transplantation but have almost totally disappeared now due to universal use of effective prophylaxis. Nonetheless, lung recipients must still be considered to be highly susceptible to pneumocystis infections and effective prophylaxis remains an important component of lung transplant management.

## BACTERIAL INFECTIONS

### Pneumonia

By far, the most common infection encountered after lung transplantation is bacterial pneumonia. In the early days of heart–lung transplantation, very high rates of postoperative pneumonia were documented. A study from Stanford University of 14 heart–lung recipients transplanted between 1981 and 1983 determined that 10 (71%) patients developed bacterial pneumonias within a median of 14 days after transplantation (4). Similar data were reported from Pittsburgh, where 23 (74%) of 31 heart–lung recipients acquired bacterial pneumonias in the early posttransplant period (7). After the introduction of single and bilateral lung transplantation in the late 1980s, substantial rates of bacterial pneumonias were still reported, with bilateral lung recipients suffering a greater burden than single-lung recipients (5). Bacterial pneumonia is responsible for substantial mortality in lung transplant centers, and >42% of all posttransplant deaths are attributable to bacterial pneumonia (6). In recent years, clinicians have become more experienced at managing these complicated patients, and the rate of postoperative pneumonias appears to have decreased. More recent data have shown a frequency of bacterial pneumonias within the first 30 days as low as 16% (8). However, even with this apparent decline in the incidence of bacterial pneumonia, pneumonias still are responsible for significant morbidity and mortality within the lung transplant population. A recent single-center study of 117 lung transplant recipients reported that 44% of postoperative deaths occurring after transplantation were related to bacterial pneumonias (9).

More than 75% of all bacterial pneumonias occur within the first six months after transplantation (5,10). Table 1 lists the findings of four lung and heart–lung transplant studies that specifically examined the pathogens associated with bacterial pneumonias after transplantation. As can be seen, the most common organisms encountered are aerobic gram-negative rods. Another study of 40 lung transplant recipients from Toronto also reported that pneumonias after transplantation were caused most frequently by gram-negative bacilli; however, this study did not indicate the specific causative organisms (5). Kanj et al. examined infections in lung transplant recipients with cystic fibrosis (CF) and similarly demonstrated that most pneumonias in this population were caused by gram-negative pathogens (predominantly *Pseudomonas aeruginosa*). This study also documented a high rate of pneumonias caused by *Staphylococcus aureus*, of which all the

**Table 1** Pneumonia Caused by Bacterial Pathogens After Lung and Heart–Lung Transplantation

| | Center (Ref.) year | | | |
|---|---|---|---|---|
| | Cleveland (10)[a] 1996 | Vanderbilt (11) 1993 | Pittsburgh (12) 1990 | Stanford (4) 1985 |
| Type of transplant | Single, double, heart–lung | Single lung | Heart–lung | Heart–lung |
| Number of patients (*n*) | 83 | 15 | 37 | 14 |
| Follow-up (mean) | Up to 5 years | 337 days | 14 days | 12 months |
| % patients with bacterial pneumonia | NA | 40 | 32 | 71 |
| Episodes of pneumonia per patient | 1.37 | 0.67 | 0.32 | 1.14 |
| Time of pneumonia after transplantation (median, range) | NA[b] | 79 days (0–315) | 8 days (1–14) | 14 days (4–720) |
| Pathogens[c] | | | | |
| Gram-negative | 50 (44%)[d] | 8 (80%) | 11 (92%) | 4 (25%) |
| *P. aeruginosa* | 31 | 5 | 5 | 1 |
| *Enterobacter* sp. | – | 1 | 3 | – |
| *Acinetobacter* sp. | – | 1 | 2 | – |
| *S. marcescens* | – | – | – | 2 |
| *P. mirabilis* | – | – | 2 | – |
| *K. pneumonia* | – | – | 1 | – |
| *H. influenzae* | – | – | 1 | 1 |
| Gram-positive | 55 (48%) | 4 (40%) | 1 (8%) | 2 (13%) |
| *S. aureus* | 24 | 4 | – | 2 |
| *S. pneumoniae* | – | – | 1 | – |
| *Other Streptococcus* | 22 | – | – | – |
| Other[e] | – | – | 1 (8%) | 3 (19%) |
| No pathogen isolated | 9 (8%) | – | – | 6 (38%) |

[a]Report only included cases where bronchoscopy with bronchoalveolar lavage, transbronchial biopsy, and protected specimen brushing were performed.
[b]Seventy-nine percent of pneumonias occurred within six months after transplant.
[c]Some infections had more than one isolate, so total percentages may exceed 100%.
[d]Nineteen episodes listed only as "other gram-negative bacilli."
[e]Includes mixed organisms (no isolate identified) and *Legionella pneumophila*.
*Abbreviation*: NA, not available.

isolates were methicillin-resistant (13). Patients who develop bronchiolitis obliterans later after transplantation may experience increased rates of pulmonary infection. These infections do not always manifest as a pneumonia on chest radiograph but may present as a syndrome of fever, cough, and dyspnea that responds to antibiotics and is probably due to underlying structural airway disease such as bronchiectasis.

Many factors contribute to the high rate of pneumonia in lung recipients. Lung donors are intubated and usually receive antibiotics, which frequently lead to airway colonization with nosocomial pathogens. It has been reported that as many as 40% of donors are colonized with *S. aureus* and nearly half are colonized with gram-negative bacilli (14). The risk of aspiration in donors is another consideration, particularly if a head injury has occurred. Silent aspiration may cause no radiographic or clinical signs in the donor lung until after transplantation. The impact of donor airway colonization on the lung recipient's outcome has been examined in multiple studies. In one study of 37 heart–lung recipients, positive donor tracheal cultures (DTC) were found in 76% of the donors, with *S. aureus* being the most common isolate. The primary factor that significantly increased a recipient's risk for developing an early postoperative intrathoracic infection was the presence of oropharyngeal flora from the DTC. Sixty-three percent of the lung recipients who experienced an early lung infection had oropharyngeal flora cultured from the DTC. Only 14% of patients without an early infection had oropharyngeal flora in their DTC ($P = 0.004$) (12). The interpretation of the authors was that oropharyngeal flora found in the donor tracheal culture might be an indicator for undetected aspiration, leading to lung injury and early infection in the recipient.

At many centers, fiber-optic bronchoscopy (FOB) with microbiological sampling is routinely performed on the donor lung. Studies that have examined the effects of organisms isolated from a donor's FOB on a recipient's outcome have had variable results. Two reports found an association between bacterial colonization of the donor lung and increased rates of pulmonary infections and reduced survival in recipients (14,15). However, another study revealed that colonization of the donor lung did not lead to more pneumonias in the postoperative period (8). Because of the potential of donors to be colonized or infected with microorganisms, routine use of broad-spectrum antibiotic coverage in the postoperative period is recommended. The initial antibiotics should cover common gram-positive and gram-negative nosocomial bacteria including methicillin-resistant *S. aureus* (MRSA) and *P. aeruginosa*. The therapy can be tailored later to the donor's and recipient's culture results. One canine study suggested that antibiotics given both intravenously and by aerosol to the organ donor before the lungs were harvested might reduce the prevalence of early bacterial pneumonias in lung recipients (16). Whether pretransplant antibiotic therapy is beneficial when administered to human donors is still undetermined.

Systemic infections, or bacteremia, in organ donors have also been evaluated as a potential source of infection in organ recipients. One study that examined the outcomes of 212 recipients of organs taken from 95 bacteremic donors found no evidence of transmission of the donor's blood pathogen to the recipients. These results are predicated on the fact that all bacteremic donors received appropriate antibiotic therapy before transplantation, as did 91% of their organ recipients posttransplantation. The study included 10 lung recipients whose donors were bacteremic. There was no difference in 30-day patient or graft survival when comparing lung recipients who had bacteremic versus nonbacteremic donors (17). Another report involving eight pediatric lung donors with systemic infections (seven with bacterial meningitis, one with bacterial epiglottitis) also showed no documented transmission of the infection to 19 organ recipients (including one heart–lung recipient) receiving standard posttransplantation antibiotic therapy (18). The results of these studies suggest that systemic bacterial infection in the donor is not a major risk to the recipient if appropriate antibiotics are given. However, some caution must be advised due to the small sample size of the studies.

Operative factors unique to heart–lung and lung transplantation may also predispose to lung infection. Injury to the recurrent laryngeal nerve during the operations may predispose to pulmonary aspiration. Vagal nerve damage may interfere with the cough reflex. It also occasionally causes gastroparesis, which may predispose to aspiration from reflux of gastric contents. Injury to the phrenic nerve may lead to poor lung expansion and atelectasis. The lymphatic drainage of the transplanted lung is interrupted by the act of transplantation. This interruption may contribute to the phenomenon of postimplantation edema (reimplantation response) in the first few days after surgery (19). Even the clearance provided by mucociliary function may be impaired in some patients (20).

Pulmonary infections in lung recipients may be difficult to diagnose, due primarily to the fact that pneumonias can present similarly to other pulmonary processes in the transplanted lung. Fever, dyspnea, cough, sputum production, as well as radiographic infiltrates can present during an infectious process, rejection, or even postimplantation edema. A retrospective study at Pittsburgh found no significant difference in type or severity of respiratory symptoms among 28 lung transplant recipients diagnosed with pulmonary infections and 60 patients diagnosed with acute rejection, although it is important to note that the symptom of fever was not included in the authors' analysis (21). Bronchoscopy with bronchoalveolar lavage (BAL) and transbronchial biopsy is often warranted to differentiate between an infectious process and rejection. Even with this aggressive approach, a pathogen is often not isolated in the setting of clinical infection, which may be due to preceding antibiotic treatment in the lung recipient. Also, the sensitivity of bronchsocopy is dependent on the technique used to sample secretions and the definition of infection. Chan et al. examined the results of 282 bronchoscopies performed on 83 lung transplant recipients who had developed new respiratory symptoms (10). Only bronchoscopies that included BAL, protected specimen brushing, and transbronchial biopsy were included in the analysis. Only 17.5% of the 114 diagnoses of bacterial infections of the lower respiratory tract were established using BAL culture, which required at least $10^5$ colony forming units (CFU)/mL of bacteria cultured from BAL fluid; the diagnostic yield was increased to over 90% with the results from protected specimen brushing, which only required a CFU of $10^3$ bacteria/mL to make the diagnosis.

### Cystic Fibrosis

The transplantation of patients with CF poses many challenges, which are primarily due to the chronic sinopulmonary infections associated with this illness. Early experience with lung transplantation in CF patients was disappointing, with a one-year survival of only 42% (22). Currently, double-lung transplantation in patients with CF has a more acceptable mortality rate, which is comparable to the mortality rate seen in lung recipients transplanted for other end-stage pulmonary diseases (23,24). However, there are still several issues in the posttransplant period that are nearly unique to patients with CF.

Essentially, all patients with CF presenting for transplantation are chronic carriers of multidrug-resistant bacteria, of which the most common is *P. aeruginosa*. One study from Duke reported that 18/21 (86%) lung recipients with CF were infected with *P. aeruginosa* pretransplant, with 15 (71%) patients possessing multidrug-resistant strains. Methicillin-resistant *S. aureus* (MRSA) was isolated from five patients (24%), and *Stenotrophomonas maltophilia* from four patients (19%) (13). A single-center Australian study documented that 52% of 54 CF patients receiving lung transplants were colonized with panresistant *P. aeruginosa*, and 19% harbored MRSA (25). Despite this high rate of pretransplant infection, it appears these infections, including multidrug-resistant *P. aeruginosa*, do not adversely affect survival or outcome after lung transplantation (13,25–27). Aris et al. investigated outcomes of lung transplant recipients with CF, in relation to the resistance patterns of isolates that colonized the patients before transplantation. During a mean follow-up of 28 months after transplantation, there was no significant difference in survival or rates of pneumonia between patients who were infected with panresistant organisms and patients with susceptible organisms. The investigators also found no significant difference in ventilator days, length of hospital stay, or postoperative antibiotic days between the two groups (26).

The strains of *P. aeruginosa* isolated from patients before and after transplantation appear to be identical (28). From this, one can infer that the sinuses or upper airways are a persistent reservoir for these pathogens after their infected lungs have been explanted. This finding has led some investigators to explore the role of sinus surgery in lung recipients with CF. A Stanford study examined the outcomes of 11 heart–lung recipients with CF (all colonized with *P. aeruginosa*) who received maxillary sinus surgery, followed by tobramycin sinus irrigations. The investigators reported that among the eight long-term survivors in the group, with more than 3200 days of follow-up, only one patient required hospitalization and intravenous antibiotics for *P. aeruginosa* pneumonia after surgery. The number of patients in this review is small, and outcomes were not compared to CF lung recipients who did not have the surgery (29). More recently, a Swiss study examined infectious outcomes of 37 CF lung transplant recipients who received sinus surgery followed by daily saline irrigations. More than half of the patients after the surgery subsequently developed negative cultures from sinus aspirates, which was associated with reduced frequency of tracheobronchitis when compared to the patients whose sinus aspirates continued to contain isolated pathogens (0.25 episodes per patient vs. 1.05 episodes per patient, $P = 0.009$). A clinical benefit was not demonstrated, because the study did not compare the outcomes of CF patients who had undergone sinus surgery with the outcomes of patients who had not undergone surgery (30).

A study from the University of North Carolina examined the types of infections among 27 lung transplant recipients with CF and 32 lung transplant recipients without CF. While both groups experienced similar rates of bronchitis and pneumonia after transplantation, bacterial sinusitis was significantly more frequent among the patients with CF. Sinusitis was encountered in 33% of patients with CF compared to 6% of patients without CF ($P = 0.02$). The investigators commented that two of the nine CF patients who experienced persistent sinus symptoms subsequently underwent surgical drainage of the sinuses (24).

A pathogen of particular concern among patients with CF is *Burkoldheria cepacia*. *B. cepacia* is a gram-negative rod that is often found in soil and water, and has become an increasingly important pulmonary pathogen in CF. A phenomenon known as "*cepacia* syndrome," which involves necrotizing pneumonia and associated bacteremia has been described in patients with CF (31). Infections from *B. cepacia* are challenging to treat because they are resistant to most antipseudomonal antibiotics. CF centers have reported carriage rates of *B. cepacia* ranging between 2% and 8% with the highest rates being described in Canada (32). Various studies have reported inferior outcomes in lung recipients with CF who are infected with *B. cepacia* before transplantation (33–35). Chaparro et al. documented reduced survival in CF patients with *B. cepacia* infection. Outcomes of 53 lung recipients with CF were analyzed, demonstrating a three-year survival rate of only 45% in 25 patients with *B. cepacia* infection compared to 86% in 28 patients without *B. cepacia* infection ($P < 0.01$).

Among the 25 patients infected with *B. cepacia*, 14 (56%) died from complications related to *B. cepacia* infection. Most patients developed progressive pulmonary infiltrates, with decline into sepsis and death, despite administration of multiple antibiotics. The majority of deaths occurred within the first three months after transplantation (33). In light of the poor outcomes encountered in these patients, many centers do not perform transplants in individuals colonized or infected with *B. cepacia*.

Multiple species of *Burkoldheria* have been isolated from patients with CF, but the most common isolate is *B. cepacia* genomovar III, also known as *Burkoldheria cenocepacia*. *B. cenocepacia* accounts for roughly half of all *B. cepacia* complex isolates recovered from CF patients (32). One particular epidemic strain of *B. cenocepacia*, known as ET-12, has been isolated from CF patients in Canada and the United Kingdom, but rarely in the United States. A U.K. study that reviewed outcomes of 11 CF lung transplant recipients who were infected with *B. cepacia* reported five deaths over a mean follow-up of 541 days. All five deaths occurred within 36 days of transplantation and four of the patients who died were infected with a *B. cenocepacia* strain, later identified as the ET-12 strain. *B. cenocepacia* was not isolated from any of the remaining six survivors, who harbored other *B. cepacia* genomovars (35,36). Similar results regarding CF patients infected with *B. cenocepacia* have been documented in the United States. Investigators of the University of North Carolina reviewed the clinical courses of 21 lung recipients with CF who had pretransplant infection with *B. cepacia*. They revealed that the risk of *B. cepacia* complex–related mortality over a mean of 1.5 years was restricted to patients with genomovar III isolates (41% mortality with genomovar III vs. 0% without genomovar III, $P = 0.035$). None of the genomovar III isolates from this American study were of the ET-12 strain (34). It still remains unclear as to whether the ET-12 strain seen predominately outside the United States adds additional risk above that conferred by the presence of genomovar III.

### Empyema

In the immediate postoperative period, accumulation of pleural fluid is an expected phenomenon in the lung recipient. Pleural infections or empyemas, however, are rarely reported. One study from Pittsburgh documented 14 (3.6%) cases of empyema in 392 lung recipients. Eleven (79%) of these empyemas were caused by bacterial pathogens. In this report, the development of empyema did not correlate with pretransplant diagnosis or the type of transplant procedure performed. While all episodes of empyema occurred within the first six months after transplantation, the mean time of occurrence was 46 days postoperatively. Organisms involved in these infections included enteric gram-negative pathogens, such as *Enterobacter* sp., *Klebsiella* sp., and *Escherichia coli*. *Staphylococcus* sp. and *Enterococcus* sp. were also described, and one case was caused by *Mycoplasma hominis*. The mortality rate associated with empyema was 28.6%; the majority of deaths were secondary to gram-negative sepsis (37). A Canadian study examining pleural complications among 138 patients after lung transplantation documented seven pleural space infections, all of which occurred in double-lung recipients. In this series, the mortality rate related to empyema (43%) was higher than in the Pittsburgh series. Three of the seven patients with empyema had CF, and all of these patients had *B. cepacia* isolated from their pleural fluid. The authors of the study did not mention if these patients were colonized with *B. cepacia* before transplantation (38).

## Mediastinitis

In the early days of heart–lung transplantation, rates of mediastinitis as high as 13.5% were reported. This was nearly double the rate seen in cardiac recipients at the same institution in the same time interval (6). Mediastinitis can result either from direct infection of a sternotomy site, or it may develop as a complication of airway dehiscence. As in the case of postoperative bacterial pneumonias, improved perioperative antibiotic prophylaxis has led to the reduced frequency of mediastinitis. More recently, a 3.8% rate of mediastinal and sternotomy infections was reported in 185 heart–lung and lung recipients (39). This rate is still about 50% higher than the rate of mediastinitis reported in two large series of isolated heart transplantation (39,40). The bacterial pathogens isolated from these infections were variable, including *Pseudomonas* sp., *B. cepacia*, *Staphylococcus epidermidis*, *E. coli*, and *Klebsiella* sp. Most cases occur within four weeks of transplantation, and the clinical findings, other than an elevated white cell count and fever, may be subtle. Early in the course of the disease, only 9% of patients with mediastinitis had sternal instability and only 24% had sternal wound drainage (39).

Anastomotic infections after heart–lung or lung transplantation are an uncommon complication, and are more often caused by fungal pathogens than by bacteria. One retrospective study from Duke reported that 5.3% of 283 lung and heart–lung recipients developed anastomotic infections after transplantation. Only one of the 15 patients who developed anastomotic infections had a bacterial source (*S. aureus*); the other infections were caused by either *Candida* or *Aspergillus* species (41).

*M. hominis* is an unusual agent that has been occasionally encountered as a causative agent in wound infections. There are a number of reports of mediastinal infections in lung recipients secondary to *M. hominis* (42–44). *M. hominis* is an important commensal in the female and, to a lesser extent, male genital tract. It is a cause of self-limited fever in women in the postpartum period and occasionally causes invasive infections. *M. hominis* should be suspected in cases of "culture-negative" wound infections. These infections can be challenging to diagnose, since gram stains of infected fluid are negative, and growth of the organism requires special media. Once diagnosed, these infections usually clear rapidly with specific therapy, but when the sternum is involved, significant damage to the bone may occur necessitating plastic surgery to provide stability to the wound.

## Bloodstream Infections

Studies of bloodstream infections in solid organ recipients have demonstrated that the source of bacteremia is commonly related to the site of transplantation. The frequency of bloodstream infections is highest among lung and liver transplant recipients, with lower rates being reported for renal and heart transplant populations (45). Not surprisingly, the source of bacteremia in lung transplant recipients is most commonly the lung. In a report on 176 lung recipients from Duke, 44 (25%) developed a bloodstream infection after transplantation. The most common sources identified were the lung (70%), intravenous lines (15%), the gastrointestinal tract (5%), the peritoneum (5%), and the urinary tract (5%). Most bloodstream infections (60%) occurred during the initial transplant hospitalization. The pathogens isolated varied according to the duration of time after transplantation. During the initial transplant hospitalization, gram-negative rods were the most common cause of bacteremia and the two most frequently encountered organisms were *P. aeruginosa* and *B. cepacia*. Bloodstream infections that occurred after discharge from the transplant hospitalization were most often caused by *S. aureus*. The primary risk factors for bacteremia after lung transplantation were CF and a history of pretransplant mechanical ventilation. Overall, the presence of a bloodstream infection was associated with reduced three-year survival (71% without vs. 44% with bloodstream infections, $P = 0.001$). There was a nonsignificant trend for improved survival for CF patients without bloodstream infections ($P = 0.09$) (46).

## Abdominal Infections

*Clostridium difficile* is a spore-forming, gram-positive pathogen that is a common cause of nosocomial and antibiotic-associated diarrhea. The spectrum of disease due to *C. difficile* ranges from asymptomatic colonization to fulminant colitis with sepsis. Immunosuppression appears to carry enhanced risk for complications associated with *C. difficile* infection, particularly in transplant settings. Researchers from the University of Pittsburgh reported on 64 fulminant cases of *C. difficile* colitis, defined as those that were fatal or required colectomy. Twenty-three percent of these cases occurred in transplant recipients, and the majority of these were in lung transplant patients. The overall incidence of *C. difficile* colitis in lung transplant recipients at Pittsburgh was 31% over a 10-year period. Thirteen percent of infected individuals (or 4% of all lung transplant recipients) developed fulminant disease.

The investigators commented that lung transplant recipients were more likely to develop fulminant symptoms compared to all other patients infected with *C. difficile* (13% vs. 1.6%, $P < 0.001$). However, the mortality rate related to *C. difficile* disease was not higher in lung recipients, in spite of more severe disease (47). *C. difficile* is primarily a nosocomial pathogen and the rates of infection vary widely between institutions. Other general reviews of infections after lung transplantation have reported lower rates of *C. difficile* infection. For instance, one study of 40 lung transplant recipients from Toronto reported only a 5% rate of *C. difficile* disease (5).

Other intra-abdominal infections occur infrequently after lung transplantation. Bacterial peritonitis related to bowel perforation has been reported, but is uncommon (5). Abdominal abscesses have also been described, with one review documenting a rate of 6% in 31 heart–lung transplant recipients with a mean follow-up of 348 days. These cases were primarily related to bowel perforation or diverticular disease (7). A retrospective study of children receiving heart, heart–lung, and lung transplants at the University of Pennsylvania found that 7% of patients developed pneumatosis intestinalis over a median of 11 months after transplantation. Causes included rotavirus (three of eight) and *C. difficile* (two of eight), but in three cases no cause could be identified (48).

Urinary tract infections are also infrequent after lung transplantation. Kramer et al. reported that only 12 (6%) of 200 infectious episodes that occurred in 73 heart–lung recipients over a mean follow-up period of 26 months were urinary tract infections (2). The specific pathogens causing the infections were not mentioned in the report.

## Miscellaneous Organisms

Infections due to *Legionella pneumophila* have been described in both immunocompetent and immunocompromised hosts. One review from Pittsburgh compared *Legionella* infections of transplant recipients and nontransplant patients. Fourteen of the 40 cases were diagnosed in solid organ recipients, one of which was a lung transplant recipient. The average yearly incidence of *Legionella* infection was estimated to be 2.07 per 1000 lung transplants. Interestingly, there was a trend for the transplant group to have a lower rate of complications and mortality related to *Legionella* infection when compared to the nontransplant group. It is possible that this observation could be explained by earlier diagnosis or a tendency to use broader spectrum antibiotics in immunocompromised patients. The risk factors associated with mortality included the presence of pleural effusion, lung abscess or cavitation, and nosocomial acquisition of *Legionella* (49).

*Rhodococcus equi* is a soil-borne, gram-positive, coccobacillus that has been emerging as an important pathogen in immunocompromised patients, particularly patients with human immunodeficiency virus (HIV) infection and acquired immunodeficiency syndrome (AIDS). This organism can often be mistaken for a contaminant or a species of *Corynebacterium*. Numerous cases have been reported in transplant recipients, including one case in a double-lung transplant recipient (50,51). This particular patient developed *Rhodococcus* infection about four years after transplantation, and presented with an indolent illness consisting of fever, dyspnea, purulent sputum, and a right lower lobe infiltrate on chest radiography. *R. equi* was isolated from the patient's blood and BAL (50). One review of *Rhodococcus* infections in transplant patients revealed that the vast majority had pulmonary infections and more than half developed cavitary disease. Extrapulmonary manifestations, such as osteomyelitis and subcutaneous abscesses, were also described in 54% of the transplant patients with pulmonary disease (51). These infections manifest late, occurring on an average over four years after organ transplantation (51,52). Transplant patients often experience relapse after treatment (30%); therefore, prolonged treatment or even lifelong maintenance therapy may be warranted (51).

*Nocardia* infections are not common after lung transplantation. This may be attributable to the almost universal use of trimethoprim–sulfamethoxazole (TMP-SMX) prophylaxis against *Pneumocystis*. However, low-dose TMP-SMX prophylaxis does not provide absolute protection against nocardiosis. Husain et al. retrospectively reviewed outcomes of 473 lung transplant patients and found a *Nocardia* infection rate of 2.1% (10 patients). These infections tended to occur late in the posttransplantation period, with a median time to onset of 34.1 months. Six of the 10 patients who developed *Nocardia* infection had concurrently been taking TMP-SMX, and all six still had isolates of *Nocardia* susceptible to TMP-SMX. The main site of infection was pulmonary, and there was a predilection for patients with single-lung transplants to have native lung involvement (three of four single-lung recipients). Radiographic characteristics of the *Nocardia* lung infections were variable (consolidation, nodules, reticulonodular pattern) but no cavitary lesions or abscesses were encountered. One patient had disseminated disease from *N. brasiliensis*, with pulmonary infiltrates, cerebellar lesions, and tibial bone involvement. The most common *Nocardia* species were *Nocardia farcinica* (30%), *Nocardia nova* (30%), and *Nocardia asteroides* (30%). Mortality related to *Nocardia* infection was 30%, and all patients infected with *N. farcinica* died in spite of therapy with multiple antibiotics (53). *Nocardia* species such as *N. farcinica* and *N. nova* may exhibit resistance to the standard antibiotics used to treat *Nocardia* infections, such as TMP-SMX, ceftriaxone, and imipenem, making them more challenging to treat (54).

Another review of *Nocardia* infections was performed at an Australian transplant center. The incidence of infection in 540 heart, lung, and heart–lung transplant recipients was 1.85%. Six of the 10 infected patients had received lung or heart–lung transplants. Six of the 10 patients were coinfected with *Aspergillus*. The most common *Nocardia* isolate was *N. nova* (60%). Seven patients died, but none of the deaths were attributed to *Nocardia* infection (55).

*Actinomyces* is a pathogen that has some similarity to *Nocardia*, but is rarely encountered as a cause of infection after lung transplantation. No formal reviews are available of actinomycosis after transplantation, but some cases in lung transplant recipients have been reported (56,57). Two cases of *Actinomyces odontolyticus* in lung transplant recipients have been described: one case involved pneumonia, the other pyogenic mediastinitis (56).

## PNEUMOCYSTIS JIROVECII

*Pneumocystis jirovecii* (previously *Pneumocystis carinii*) was first identified as a human pathogen in the 1940s when it was encountered primarily in premature infants or malnourished children. It was also encountered in the setting of impaired T-cell immunity, such as in patients with hematologic malignancies and those using high-dose corticosteroids. Increasing attention was paid to *P. jirovecii* in the 1980s when it was identified as an opportunistic infection associated with AIDS. It is believed that most humans are exposed to *P. jirovecii* by the age of four, and that both reinfection and reactivation likely play a role in disease incidence in the immunocompromised host (58). Although originally categorized as a protozoan, this organism has now been reclassified as a fungus on the basis of rRNA sequence analysis, but it is unlike most fungi in that the cell wall contains no ergosterol. The absence of ergosterol from the cell wall is likely the reason why *P. jirovecii* is resistant to most antifungal therapies.

All transplant recipients, regardless of organ type, are at increased risk of developing *Pneumocystis* pneumonia, with the greatest risk occurring two–six months after transplantation. Lung transplant recipients appear more susceptible to *P. jirovecii* infections compared to other solid organ transplant recipients. One early Pittsburgh review examined rates of *Pneumocystis* infection among different transplant recipients based on organ type, before the use of routine prophylaxis. Lung transplant recipients had a higher rate of symptomatic infection (26%) than heart (8%), liver (11%), or renal (9%) transplant recipients. Lung transplant recipients also had a higher rate of mortality associated with *Pneumocystis* infection than other transplant recipients, with 38% of infected individuals succumbing to their illness (59). A *Pneumocystis* infection rate of 88% has been documented after lung transplantation in 16 patients not taking prophylaxis (60). Many of the diagnoses in this study were made with surveillance bronchoscopy and 65% of the *Pneumocystis* infection episodes occurred in patients who were either asymptomatic or only had mild upper respiratory symptoms.

Prophylaxis with TMP-SMX dramatically reduces the incidence of *Pneumocystis* pneumonia. Kramer et al. compared the rates of *Pneumocystis* infection in lung transplant recipients based on whether the patient received TMP-SMX (160 mg/800 mg twice daily, three times per week) prophylaxis or not. Among the 48 patients who did not receive prophylaxis, 13 (27%) developed *Pneumocystis* infection, while none of the 26 patients who received prophylaxis became infected. It was also noted by the investigators that *Pneumocystis* infections did not occur >1 year after transplantation, regardless of prophylaxis status, except in those individuals who had received augmented immunosuppression for either acute or chronic rejection (61). The reduced risk of *Pneumocystis* pneumonia over time allows transplant centers to discontinue prophylaxis for *Pneumocystis* to their patients after one year. However, it is essential to reinstitute *Pneumocystis* prophylaxis whenever increased immunosuppression is given.

Since many patients are intolerant or allergic to sulfonamides, alternative prophylactic regimens have been investigated to prevent *Pneumocystis* infection. Aerosolized, inhaled pentamidine has been used in transplant patients who are intolerant to TMP-SMX. One study from UCLA reviewed the outcomes of nine lung transplant recipients who received treatments with monthly, inhaled, pentamidine (300 mg) for a mean of 10.6 months after transplantation. None of the patients experienced infections related to *Pneumocystis*. The treatments were generally well tolerated, but two patients experienced bronchospasm related to the treatments, resulting in discontinuation of therapy in one patient (62). Due to the small number of patients in this study, it is difficult to assess the true efficacy of inhaled pentamadine in preventing pneumocystosis in lung transplant recipients. A larger study involving 35 liver and kidney recipients who received monthly, aerosolized pentamadine (mean 4.28 months for liver recipients, and mean 5.71 months for kidney recipients) similarly documented an absence of *Pneumocystis* infections with this prophylactic regimen (63). However, researchers from Massachusetts General Hospital have commented informally that more than 10% of the solid organ recipients receiving aerosolized or parenteral pentamadine at their institution developed breakthrough *Pneumocystis* infection (58).

Studies in bone marrow transplant (BMT) recipients have shown significant breakthrough rates with the use of inhaled pentamidine prophylaxis. Vasconcelles et al. examined outcomes of 327 BMT recipients and showed that 9.1% of the 44 patients receiving monthly, aerosolized pentamidine developed *Pneumocystis* infections, compared to 0% of patients receiving TMP-SMX. All patients received *Pneumocystis* prophylaxis for at least one year after BMT. Although there were fewer drug toxicities associated with aerosolized pentamadine than with TMP-SMX, the investigators noted higher rates of non-*Pneumocystis* infections and mortality in the group that received only aerosolized pentamadine. At one year after BMT, 78.1% of patients taking TMP-SMX were still living, whereas only 43.2% of patients receiving aerosolized pentamadine survived ($P < 0.05$). This suggests that

TMP-SMX prophylaxis use may provide benefits that go beyond prevention of *Pneumocystis* infection (64).

Dapsone is another drug that is used for *Pneumocystis* prophylaxis in sulfonamide-allergic patients. Currently, there are no published studies that examine the efficacy of dapsone in preventing *Pneumocystis* infections in solid organ recipients. However, studies in BMT recipients and HIV patients have shown efficacy in preventing pneumocystosis. Thirty-three pediatric BMT patients at M.D. Anderson Hospital who received prophylactic oral dapsone [50 mg/m$^2$ once a week, for 6 to 12 months after BMT] had no cases of *Pneumocystis* infection (65). But a separate study of predominantly adult BMT recipients documented a substantial rate of *Pneumocystis* pneumonia with dapsone prophylaxis. In this study, 111 patients received dapsone (50 mg b.i.d. three times per week, for ≥6 months after BMT), and 535 patients received TMP-SMX (DS b.i.d. 2 days/wk, for ≥6 months after BMT). Eight patients in the dapsone group developed *Pneumocystis* pneumonia (7.2%), versus two patients (0.37%) in the TMP-SMX group ($P < 0.001$) (66).

Atovaquone is an antiprotozoal agent that also has activity against *Pneumocystis*. One report from Massachusetts General Hospital examined the records of 25 renal, 14 hepatic, and five cardiac transplant recipients intolerant to TMP-SMX who received oral atovaquone (1000 mg/day) for alternative *Pneumocystis* prophylaxis. None of the 39 patients who completed six months of therapy developed *Pneumocystis* pneumonia (58). However, in a more recent report, the investigators described two cases of breakthrough *Pneumocystis* infection in solid organ transplant recipients who were receiving atovaquone prophylaxis (67). In another prospective study, 28 liver transplant recipients who had experienced side effects related to TMP-SMX were given oral atovaquone (750 mg/day, for 12 months). No infections due to *Pneumocystis* were documented. The investigators commented that half of the patients taking atovaquone experienced adverse effects, which were primarily gastrointestinal (diarrhea, bloating, abdominal pain). However, only three of the original 28 patients discontinued atovaquone due to drug-related side effects (68). While these studies are very limited in size, they show that atovaquone has significant side effects and some breakthrough *Pneumocystis* infections can be expected when it is used for prophylaxis.

The available information on prophylaxis of *Pneumocystis* infection clearly point to TMP-SMX as the preferred agent based on its superior efficacy, low cost, and potential to provide prophylaxis for other transplant pathogens. The small size of the available studies makes it difficult to develop a rational hierarchy of the second-line agents in terms of their efficacy. Thus, the decision on which second-line agent to use in patients intolerant of sulfonamides is best made on the basis of cost, ease of use, and side-effect profile. The authors' preference is to continue the prophylaxis lifelong because of the high susceptibility of the transplanted lung to *Pneumocystis* infection. If a decision is made to discontinue *Pneumocystis* prophylaxis at ~1 year after transplantation, mechanisms should be in place to restart the prophylaxis if the patients need to have their immunosuppression augmented, particularly if this involves administration of high-dose steroids.

## REFERENCES

1.  http://www.optn.org/ (accessed January 2005)
2.  Kramer MR, Marshall SE, Starnes VA, et al. Infectious complications in heart–lung transplantation: analysis of 200 episodes. Arch Intern Med 1993; 153(17):2010–2016.
3.  Chaparro C, Maurer JR, Chamberlain D, et al. Causes of death in lung transplant recipients. J Heart Lung Transplant 1994; 13(5):758–766.
4.  Brooks RG, Hofflin JM, Jamieson SW, et al. Infectious complications in heart–lung transplant recipients. Am J Med 1985; 79(4):412–422.
5.  Maurer JR, Tullis DE, Grossman RF, et al. Infectious complications following isolated lung transplantation. Chest 1992; 101(4):1056–1059.
6.  Dauber JH, Paradis IL, Dummer JS. Infectious complications in pulmonary allograft recipients. Clin Chest Med 1990; 11(2):291–308.
7.  Thompson ME, Dummer JS, Paradis I, et al. Heart–lung transplantation. In: Yu PN, Goodwin JF, Eds. Progress in Cardiology. Philadelphia: Lea and Feibiger, 1988; 16:51–80.
8.  Weill D, Dey GC, Hicks RA, et al. A positive donor gram stain does not predict outcome following lung transplantation. J Heart Lung Transplant 2002; 21(5):555–558.
9.  Zander DS, Baz MA, Visner GA, et al. Analysis of early deaths after isolated lung transplantation. Chest 2001; 120(1):225–232.
10. Chan CC, Abi-Saleh WJ, Arroliga AC, et al. Diagnostic yield and therapeutic impact of flexible bronchoscopy in lung transplant recipients. J Heart Lung Transplant 1996; 15(2):196–205.
11. Horvath J, Dummer S, Loyd J, et al. Infection in the transplanted and native lung after single lung transplantation. Chest 1993; 104(3):681–685.
12. Zenati M, Dowling RD, Dummer JS, et al. Influence of the donor lung on development of early infections in lung transplant recipients. J Heart Transplant 1990; 9(5):502–508.
13. Kanj SS, Tapson V, Davis RD, et al. Infections in patients with cystic fibrosis following lung transplantation. Chest 1997; 112(4):924–930.
14. Avlonitis VS, Krause A, Luzzi L, et al. Bacterial colonization of the donor lower airways is a predictor of poor outcome in lung transplantation. Eur J Cardiothorac Surg 2003; 24(4):601–607.
15. Low DE, Kaiser LR, Haydock DA, et al. The donor lung: infectious and pathologic factors affecting outcome in lung transplantation. J Thorac Cardiovasc Surg 1993; 106(4):614–621.
16. Dowling RD, Zenati M, Yousem SA, et al. Donor-transmitted pneumonia in experimental lung allografts: successful prevention with donor antibiotic therapy. J Thorac Cardiovasc Surg 1992; 103(4):767–772.

17. Freeman RB, Giatras I, Falagas ME, et al. Outcome of transplantation of organs procured from bacteremic donors. Transplantation 1999; 68(8):1107–1111.

18. Little DM, Farrell JG, Cunningham PM, et al. Donor sepsis is not a contraindication to cadaveric organ donation. Q J Med 1997; 90(10):641–642.

19. Mancini MC, Borovetz HS, Griffith BP, et al. Changes in lung vascular permeability after heart–lung transplantation. J Surg Res 1985; 39(4):305–309.

20. Read RC, Shankar S, Rutman A, et al. Ciliary beat frequency and structure of recipient and donor epithelia following lung transplantation. Eur Respir J 1991; 4(7):796–801.

21. DeVito Dabbs A, Hoffman LA, Iacono AT, et al. Are symptom reports useful for differentiating between acute rejection and pulmonary infection after lung transplantation? Heart Lung 2004; 33(6):372–380.

22. Frist WH, Fox MD, Campbell PW, et al. Cystic fibrosis treated with heart–lung transplantation: North American results. Transplant Proc 1991; 23(1, Pt 2):1205–1206.

23. Egan TM, Detterbeck FC, Mill MR, et al. Improved results of lung transplantation for patients with cystic fibrosis. J Thorac Cardiovasc Surg 1995; 109(2):224–234.

24. Flume PA, Egan TM, Paradowski LJ, et al. Infectious complications of lung transplantation: impact of cystic fibrosis. Am J Respir Crit Care Med 1994; 149(6):1601–1607.

25. Dobbin C, Maley M, Harkness J, et al. The impact of pan-resistant bacterial pathogens on survival after lung transplantation in cystic fibrosis: results from a single large referral center. J Hosp Infect 2004; 56(4):277–282.

26. Aris RM, Gilligan PH, Neuringer IP, et al. The effects of panresistant bacteria in cystic fibrosis patients on lung transplant outcome. Am J Respir Crit Care Med 1997; 155(5):1699–1704.

27. De Soyza A, Archer L, Wardle J, et al. Pulmonary transplantation for cystic fibrosis: pretransplant recipient characteristics in patients dying of perioperative sepsis. J Heart Lung Transplant 2003; 22(7):764–769.

28. Walter S, Gudowius P, Bosshammer J, et al. Epidemiology of chronic *Pseudomonas aeruginosa* infections in the airways of lung transplant recipients with cystic fibrosis. Thorax 1997; 52(4):318–321.

29. Lewiston N, King V, Umetsu D, et al. Cystic fibrosis patients who have undergone heart–lung transplantation benefit from maxillary sinus antrostomy and repeated sinus lavage. Transplant Proc 1991; 23(1, Pt 2):1207–1208.

30. Holzmann D, Speich R, Kaufmann T, et al. Effects of sinus surgery in patients with cystic fibrosis after lung transplantation: a 10-year experience. Transplantation 2004; 77(1):134–136.

31. Isles A, Maclusky I, Corey M, et al. *Pseudomonas cepacia* infection in cystic fibrosis: an emerging problem. J Pediatr 1984; 104(2):206–210.

32. Husain S, Singh N. *Burkholderia cepacia* infection and lung transplantation. Semin Respir Infect 2002; 4(17):284–290.

33. Chaparro C, Maurer J, Gutierrez C, et al. Infection with *Burkholderia cepacia* in cystic fibrosis: outcome following lung transplantation. Am J Respir Crit Care Med 2001; 163(1):43–48.

34. Aris RM, Routh JC, LiPuma JJ, et al. Lung transplantation for cystic fibrosis patients with *Burkholderia cepacia* complex: survival linked to genomovar type. Am J Respir Crit Care Med 2001; 164(11):2102–2106.

35. De Soyza A, McDowell A, Archer L, et al. *Burkholderia cepacia* complex genomovars and pulmonary transplantation outcomes in patients with cystic fibrosis. Lancet 2001; 358(9295):1780–1781.
36. De Soyza A, Morris K, McDowell A, et al. Prevalence and clonality of *Burkholderia cepacia* complex genomovars in UK patients with cystic fibrosis referred for lung transplantation. Thorax 2004; 59(6):526–528.
37. Nunley DR, Grgurich WF, Keenan RJ, et al. Empyema complicating successful lung transplantation. Chest 1999; 115(5):1312–1315.
38. Herridge MS, de Hoyos AL, Chaparro C, et al. Pleural complications in lung transplant recipients. J Thorac Cardiovasc Surg 1995; 110(1):22–26.
39. Abid Q, Nkere UU, Hasan A, et al. Mediastinitis in heart and lung transplantation: 15 years experience. Ann Thorac Surg 2003; 75(5):1565–1571.
40. Montoya JG, Giraldo LF, Efron B, et al. Infectious complications among 620 consecutive heart transplant patients at Stanford University Medical Center. Clin Infect Dis 2001; 33(5):629–640.
41. Hadjiliadis D, Howell DN, Davis RD, et al. Anastomotic infections in lung transplant recipients. Ann Transplant 2000; 5(3):13–19.
42. Lyon GM, Alspaugh JA, Meredith FT, et al. *Mycoplasma hominis* pneumonia complicating bilateral lung transplantation: case report and review of the literature. Chest 1997; 112(5):1428–1432.
43. Steffenson DO, Dummer JS, Granick MS, et al. Sternotomy infections with *Mycoplasma hominis*. Ann Intern Med 1987; 106(2):204–208.
44. Hopkins PM, Winlaw DS, Chhajed PN, et al. *Mycoplasma hominis* infection in heart and lung transplantation. J Heart Lung Transplant 2002; 21(11):1225–1229.
45. Dummer JS, Ho M. Infections in solid organ transplant recipients. In: Mandell GL, Bennett JE, Dolin R, eds. Principles and Practice of Infectious Diseases. 2. 5th ed. Philadelphia: Churchill Livingstone, 2000:3148–3159.
46. Palmer SM, Alexander BD, Sanders LL, et al. Significance of blood stream infection after lung transplantation: analysis in 176 consecutive patients. Transplantation 2000; 69(11):2360–2366.
47. Dallal RM, Harbrecht BG, Boujoukas AJ, et al. Fulminant *Clostridium difficile*: an underappreciated and increasing cause of death and complications. Ann Surg 2002; 235(3):363–372.
48. Fleenor JT, Hoffman TM, Bush DM, et al. Pneumatosis intestinalis after pediatric thoracic organ transplantation. Pediatrics 2002; 109(5):E78.
49. Tkatch LS, Kusne S, Irish WD, et al. Epidemiology of *Legionella* pneumonia and factors associated with *Legionella*-related mortality at a tertiary care center. Clin Infect Dis 1998; 27(6):1479–1486.
50. Le Lay G, Martin F, Leroyer C, et al. *Rhodococcus equi* causing bacteraemia and pneumonia in a pulmonary transplant patient. J Infect 1996; 33(3):239–240.
51. Perez MG, Vassilev T, Kemmerly SA. *Rhodococcus equi* infection in transplant recipients: a case of mistaken identity and review of the literature. Transplant Infect Dis 2000; 4(1):52–56.
52. Munoz P, Burillo A, Palomo J, et al. *Rhodococcus equi* infection in transplant recipients: case report and review of the literature. Transplantation 1998; 65(3):449–453.
53. Husain S, McCurry K, Dauber J, et al. *Nocardia* infection in lung transplant recipients. J Heart Lung Transplant 2002; 21(3):354–359.

54. Nocardia infections. Guidelines for the prevention and management of infectious complications of solid organ transplantation. Am J Transplant 2004; 4(Suppl 10):47–50.
55. Roberts SA, Franklin JC, Mijch A, et al. *Nocardia* infection in heart–lung transplant recipients at Alfred Hospital, Melbourne, Australia, 1989–1998. Clin Infect Dis 2000; 31(4):968–972.
56. Bassiri AG, Girgis RE, Theodore J. *Actinomyces odontolyticus* thoracopulmonary infections: two cases in lung and heart-lung transplant recipients and a review of the literature. Chest 1996; 109(4):1109–1111.
57. Duncan SR, Paradis IL, Yousem SA, et al. Sequelae of cytomegalovirus pulmonary infections in lung allograft recipients. Am Rev Respir Dis 1992; 146(6):1419–1425.
58. Fishman JA. Prevention of infection caused by *Pneumocystis carinii* in transplant recipients. Clin Infect Dis 2001; 33(8):1397–1405.
59. Dummer JS. *Pneumocystis carinii* infections in transplant recipients. Semin Respir Infect 1990; 5(1):50–57.
60. Gryzan S, Paradis IL, Zeevi A, et al. Unexpectedly high incidence of *Pneumocystis carinii* infection after lung–heart transplantation: implications for lung defense and allograft survival. Am Rev Respir Dis 1988; 137(6):1268–1274.
61. Kramer MR, Stoehr C, Lewiston NJ, et al. Trimethoprim-sulfamethoxazole prophylaxis for *Pneumocystis carinii* infections in heart–lung and lung transplantation: how effective and for how long? Transplantation 1992; 53(3): 586–589.
62. Nathan SD, Ross DJ, Zakowski P, et al. Utility of inhaled pentamidine prophylaxis in lung transplant recipients. Chest 1994; 105(2):417–420.
63. Saukkonen K, Garland R, Koziel H. Aerosolized pentamidine as alternative primary prophylaxis against *Pneumocystis carinii* pneumonia in adult hepatic and renal transplant recipients. Chest 1996; 109(5):1250–1255.
64. Vasconcelles MJ, Bernardo MV, King C, et al. Aerosolized pentamidine as *Pneumocystis* prophylaxis after bone marrow transplantation is inferior to other regimens and is associated with decreased survival and an increased risk of other infections. Biol Blood Marrow Transplant 2000; 6(1):35–43.
65. Maltezou HC, Petropoulos D, Choroszy M, et al. Dapsone for *Pneumocystis carinii* prophylaxis in children undergoing bone marrow transplantation. Bone Marrow Transplant 1997; 20(10):879–881.
66. Souza JP, Boeckh M, Gooley TA, et al. High rates of *Pneumocystis carinii* pneumonia in allogeneic blood and marrow transplant recipients receiving dapsone prophylaxis. Clin Infect Dis 1999; 29(6):1467–1471.
67. Rodriguez M, Sifri CD, Fishman JA. Failure of low-dose atovaquone prophylaxis against *Pneumocystis jirovecii* infection in transplant recipients. Clin Infect Dis 2004; 38(8):E76–E78.
68. Meyers B, Borrego F, Papanicolaou G. *Pneumocystis carinii* pneumonia prophylaxis with atovaquone in trimethoprim-sulfamethoxazole–intolerant orthotopic liver transplant patients: a preliminary study. Liver Transplant 2001; 7(8):750–751.

# 27

# *Legionella* in Solid Organ Transplantation

## Nina M. Clark

*Section of Infectious Diseases, Department of Internal Medicine, University of Illinois at Chicago, Chicago, Illinois, U.S.A.*

## INTRODUCTION

*Legionella* species, members of the family *Legionellaceae*, are causative agents of community-acquired pneumonia (CAP) and other febrile syndromes, with *Legionella pneumophila* the etiology of approximately 90% of these infections (1,2). The first recognition of *L. pneumophila* as a causative agent of pneumonia (Legionnaires' disease) was in 1976, during an outbreak at a Philadelphia hotel where the American Legion convention was being held (3,4). Of note, none of the cases of Legionnaires' disease in this initial report occurred among transplant recipients (5).

Over the subsequent years, *Legionella* has been increasingly recognized as a CAP and nosocomial pathogen, disproportionately affecting immunocompromised persons, including those who have undergone hematopoietic stem cell or solid organ transplantation (6,7). As with other intracellular pathogens, cell-mediated immunity is the primary host defense against *Legionella*; thus, persons receiving corticosteroids and T-cell specific rejection therapies such as tacrolimus or antilymphocyte antibodies are at increased risk of Legionnaires' disease (1). As discussed later, immunocompromised persons are also at higher risk for more severe and unusual manifestations of disease (8–10).

## MICROBIOLOGY AND PATHOGENESIS

Legionellaceae are aerobic, gram-negative bacilli that appear coccobacillary in tissue and clinical specimens. The organisms do not take up Gram stain well, however, and silver stains are more effective at detecting *Legionella*. Charcoal yeast extract buffered to pH 6.9 is the optimal medium on which to grow *Legionella*, as it does not thrive on standard medium and requires specific nutrients such as L-cysteine (1). Although *L. pneumophila* produces enzymes and toxins, the clinical significance of these is unclear as they are often elaborated by strains that are not virulent in animal models (1). *L. pneumophila* can exist in variable environmental conditions, including wide ranges of temperature, pH, and concentrations of chlorine and oxygen (1,11). The presence of sediment as well as amebas and water bacteria can facilitate the growth and virulence of *Legionella* in aquatic environments (4), and this may explain the difficulty in culturing *Legionella* in vitro where facilitating organisms are absent.

It is thought that persons acquire *Legionella* by inhalation of contaminated aerosols or aspiration of contaminated water (12,13). Hematogenous spread to the lungs from another site is also possible; dissemination could occur from the gastrointestinal tract after ingesting contaminated water, for example. Upon entry into the upper respiratory tract, ciliary clearance is an important host defense against *Legionella*, an observation supported by the fact that there is an increased risk of legionellosis in cigarette smokers and persons with underlying lung diseases, including lung transplant recipients (1, 13–15). Animal studies have also shown that disruption of thoracic lymphatic vessels and bronchial arteries, as occurs in lung transplantation, increases *Legionella* concentrations in the lung following intratracheal inoculation (16).

Alveolar macrophages are critical in halting infection after organisms reach the alveoli, although *Legionella* can escape phagosome–lysosome fusion and thus can continue to replicate intracellularly (17). Polymorphonuclear leukocytes (PMNs) and monocytes also participate in phagocytosis of organisms but neutropenic patients do not seem particularly predisposed to legionellosis and *L. pneumophila* is not susceptible to killing by PMNs, thus the role of those cells in preventing disease by *Legionella* is not well defined (1). As noted above, compromised cell-mediated immunity enhances the risk of legionellosis and seems to lead to more severe disease such as is seen in transplant recipients, persons receiving corticosteroids, and persons with acquired immunodeficiency syndrome (AIDS) (1). Interleukin (IL)-1, IL-12, tumor necrosis factor, and interferon-gamma production appear to be important host responses and are triggered by the presence of *L. pneumophila* antigens (18,19).

The virulence factors for *Legionella* have not been completely defined, but it is known that all strains of *Legionella* are not similarly virulent. Multiple strains may colonize water distribution systems, but only certain strains appear to cause disease in exposed persons (20,21). In addition, certain serogroups and isolates may be more often associated with a poor outcome compared to others (10).

## EPIDEMIOLOGY

*Legionella* normally exists in natural and man-made bodies of water. In transplant recipients it can therefore cause sporadic, community-acquired disease late after transplantation, or it can cause infection in the early postoperative period from nosocomial sources. It may follow high-dose corticosteroid use for treatment of rejection (22,23). Aerosols created by air conditioners and cooling towers have been most often implicated as sources of community-acquired outbreaks of legionellosis (13,24), with whirlpool spas, shower heads, drinking water in private residences or work places, and grocery store mist machines acting as other potential sources (4,25–27). Nosocomial outbreaks of *Legionella* have occurred in hospitals (12) and the organism has been isolated from hospital water supplies, including ice machines (14,28,29), and respiratory devices such as nebulizers (30–32). Nosocomial cases have also been linked to nasogastric tube placement, which may facilitate microaspiration (30–32). While investigators have had difficulty finding evidence *of Legionella* colonizing upper airways in the absence of disease (33), there is a recent report of bronchial colonization by *Legionella* detected by polymerase chain reaction or direct fluorescent antibody in 37 of 298 samples from organ transplant recipients obtained immediately prior to organ transplantation (34).

The incidence of Legionnaires' disease depends on multiple factors, including the source and intensity of exposure and susceptibility of the exposed host (4). There are also regional differences in the incidence of *Legionella*, although on the whole, legionellosis is likely underreported (10). Between 1980 and 1998, only 6757 confirmed cases were reported to the U.S. Centers for Disease Control and Prevention (CDC), with a mean of 360 cases per year (13,35). This may be due to lack of availability and/ or implementation of accurate diagnostic methodology (36).

While *Legionella* may occur in otherwise healthy persons (37,38), it appears to have a predilection for those who use tobacco, are elderly, or have comorbidities such as chronic lung disease or immunosuppression, with corticosteroid use particularly associated (1,13,15,39). *Legionella* is generally among the top three or four causes of CAP reported in the general population and is found in 2% to 15% of all CAPs that require hospitalization (4,40). In fact, *Legionella* rarely causes pneumonia that does not require hospital admission (41). In a review of 41 European CAP studies, *Legionella* was identified as a causative organism in 1.9% of ambulatory patients with pneumonia, 4.9% of hospitalized patients, and 7.9% of those requiring intensive care unit admission (42).

Solid organ transplant recipients are reported to be at highest risk for Legionnaires' disease (6,36), although there are also wide ranges of reported incidences among this population, with some centers reporting *Legionella* as the most common cause of pneumonia among all transplant patients (43). The attack rate for nosocomial legionellosis is high in transplant recipients due to the presence of multiple risk factors including intubation, immuno-suppression, and at times, chronic lung disease and smoking history (44). Surgery with general anesthesia is also a predisposing risk factor for noso-comial *Legionella* infection; it is thought to facilitate microaspiration and transplant recipients are at the highest risk among surgical patients (23,45).

There are a number of reported series of solid organ transplant (SOT) recipients with *Legionella* pneumonia (14,22,23,43,46–59), although most are small and few specifically focus on patients with lung or heart–lung allografts. These series have most often described Legionnaires' disease in persons with cardiac or renal allografts, although lung transplant recipients have also been shown to be at increased risk for acquiring the disease (6,14,47,60). Among liver transplant recipients, splenectomy has been asso-ciated with a higher risk of *Legionella* and other pneumonia pathogens (61).

In a large International Survey of Legionellosis, *Legionella pneumophila* comprised ~92% of cases 508 sporadic community-acquired legionellosis and serogroup 1 was the most common (62). There are over 40 species of *Legionella* and 64 serogroups, with 18 species documented to cause human infection, usually pneumonia (2). The non-*pneumophila Legionella* species most frequently described in clinical specimens include *Legion-ella longbeachae*, associated with exposure to contaminated potting soil in Australia and New Zealand (30% of isolates in those countries), *Legionella dumoffii, Legionella bozemanii*, and *Legionella micdadei* (1,2). *L. pneumo-phila* and *L. micdadei* (Pittsburgh pneumonia agent) are well-described causes of pneumonia in bone marrow transplant (BMT) and SOT recipients (6,50,56,63), and patients with *L. micdadei* pneumonia are more likely to be immunocompromised than those with *L. pneumophila* infection (2). After *L. pneumophila, L. micdadei*, and *L. bozemanii* are the most common causes of legionellosis in transplant recipients (2,6). Other less frequently isolated *Legionella* spp. such as *Legionella parisiensis* (64), *Legionella cincinnatiensis* (65) and *Legionella tucsonensis* (66) have been reported to cause pneumonia in transplant recipients. *Legionella* has not infrequently been identified in concert with other pneumonia pathogens, including in transplant recipients (67–69); the diagnosis can sometimes be obscured by copathogens with fatal outcome (68).

## CLINICAL FEATURES

The incubation period for Legionnaires' disease is 2 to 10 days and the onset of illness may be accompanied by nonspecific symptoms such as fever, malaise, myalgias, and headache (1). The vast majority of infections due to *Legionella* manifest as pneumonia. *Legionella* pneumonia cannot be reliably distinguished from other types of pneumonia based on clinical, radiologic, or laboratory features (13,36,70,71), although gastrointestinal symptoms are common, especially diarrhea, seen in 25% to 50% of cases (1,4,70). Hyponatremia is said to occur more frequently in *Legionella* pneumonia than in other types of pneumonia (4,5). Patients with CAP due to *Legionella* are more likely to have severe disease as judged by vital signs, chest X ray, frequency of respiratory failure, and admission to an intensive care unit (4,72,73). Pleural effusions are common and progression of radiographic infiltrates despite appropriate antimicrobial therapy is not atypical (4). Expanding lung nodules have been described with *Legionella micdadei* (2).

Immunocompromised persons have more severe and unusual disease manifestations with *Legionella* infection, such as extrapulmonary complications, abscesses, and bacteremias (8–10,13). Soft tissue infection (74), arthritis (75), and sinusitis (76) have also been described in persons with immunocompromise. Nosocomial legionellosis has presented as wound infection related to contamination of surgical sites by *Legionella*-colonized water. The most common extrapulmonary site of infection is the heart, including postcardiotomy syndrome and prosthetic valve endocarditis, often without signs of pneumonia (4,77). Cavitary lung disease is unusual in *Legionella* infection but has been reported in patients receiving steroids, including transplant recipients (22,49,52,78). Liver allograft infection by *Legionella* (79) and *Legionella* peritonitis in a renal transplant recipient (80) have also been described.

## DIAGNOSIS

Although isolation of *Legionella* from clinical specimens such as sputum or bronchoalveolar lavage fluid is the gold standard diagnostic test, *Legionella* are fastidious and require special culture techniques, as noted earlier. Physicians must therefore alert the microbiology laboratory to handle clinical material appropriately, as routine culture methods will not recover the organism. *Legionella* grows slowly in the laboratory and the standard medium for isolation is buffered charcoal yeast extract (BCYE) agar supplemented with antimicrobials that suppress growth of competing organisms (1). Isolation of non-*pneumophila Legionella* species may be even more difficult, as BCYE has decreased sensitivity for isolation of these strains (2).

Diagnosis of Legionnaire's disease has increasingly been made by urinary antigen testing (35) given the relative ease of obtaining a sample and rapid turnaround time. In a CDC study, conducted between 1980 and 1998, the percentage of diagnoses made by urine antigen testing increased from 0% to 69% and diagnoses made by culture, direct fluorescent antibody, and serologic testing decreased significantly (35). The urine antigen test has excellent sensitivity (70–90%) and specificity (>99%) for serogroup 1 (21,81,82), which causes 70% to 80% of cases of pneumonia (10,83), though sensitivity of the antigen assay may correlate with disease severity (84). The test may remain positive for many months after infection (85), although some investigators have rarely found positive tests more than 60 days after disease onset (4). Serologic testing is often not helpful in making a timely diagnosis as it requires measurement of antibody titers in the acute and convalescent phases of illness to establish the fourfold rise in titer that indicates acute infection. Polymerase chain reaction assays for *Legionella* diagnosis are still under study (86) and not widely used as yet, but at least one assay has received U.S. Food and Drug Administration approval for detection of *L. pneumophila* serogroups 1–4 (87).

## TREATMENT AND OUTCOMES

Macrolides, fluoroquinolones, rifampin, trimethoprim–sulfamethoxazole, tetracyclines, and ketolides all have in vitro and clinical activity against *Legionella* (1,88). The traditional therapy for legionellosis, erythromycin, has been problematic in transplant recipients as it can affect cyclosporine and tacrolimus levels (89,90). Newer macrolides, particularly azithromycin, have replaced erythromycin due to fewer adverse effects, including drug interactions, and greater activity against *Legionella* (91,92).

Fluoroquinolone drugs, such as levofloxacin, have become the treatment of choice for legionellosis due to their relative lack of interactions with immunosuppressant agents and greater in vitro and clinical efficacy than the macrolides (4,91–94). Levofloxacin treatment has been associated with fewer complications, shorter hospital stays, and faster times to defervescence and clinical stability compared to macrolide use (93,94). In a recent European study, there was also a nonsignificant trend toward lower mortality with levofloxacin compared to clarithromycin or erythromycin use (93). Rifampin has been advocated as an adjunctive medication for treatment of severely ill patients (4), but rifampicin in combination with levofloxacin added no appreciable benefit and was associated with an increase in adverse effects in a recent study (94). If possible, rifampin use should be avoided in transplant recipients due to the potential for marked reductions in cyclosporine and tacrolimus levels (36).

There are anecdotal data and uncontrolled studies to support the efficacy of fluoroquinolones in transplant recipients (22,23,95,96), although comparative clinical trials are lacking. Duration of therapy is generally 10 to 14 days (5–10 days with azithromycin) although a 21-day course of therapy has been recommended for immunosuppressed patients (4,97). A recent analysis of a pharmaceutical database encompassing six CAP clinical trials noted that levofloxacin 750 mg daily for five days was efficacious at treating *Legionella* pneumonia (37), though the number of patients treated with this regimen was small and none of the patients were known to be receiving immunosuppressive medications. Data pooled from eight Multicenter International Trials have demonstrated the efficacy of 5 to 10 days of telithromycin for mild to moderate *Legionella* pneumonia (98). Failure of antimicrobials and the need for surgical treatment of lung abscess has also been described in the transplant setting (22).

It has been demonstrated that early administration of efficacious therapy plays a crucial role in the outcome of *Legionella* pneumonia (99,100). Mortality from severe Legionnaires' disease in a review of 19 published studies ranged from 0% to 25% (36); the mortality for various subgroups such as transplant recipients was not examined. In the CDC study of *Legionella* pneumonia by Marston et al. mortality was twofold higher for immunosuppressed persons (10). Interestingly, at least one study has shown a trend toward decreased mortality and less severe disease in transplant compared with nontransplant recipients (60). Multivariate analysis, however, demonstrated that intubation, nosocomial acquisition, and the presence of lung abscess or effusion were the only independent risk factors for death, leading to the conclusion that manifestations of disease rather than host immune responses may be more predictive of outcome.

Mortality from Legionnaires' disease in the United States has been decreasing. In a recent CDC surveillance study, the case fatality rate decreased from 34% to 12% between 1980 and 1998 (35). This may be related to increased awareness of the disease and recommendations for empiric treatment of atypical pneumonia pathogens including *Legionella* in patients with CAP (101).

## PREVENTION

Routine surveillance of hospital water supplies for *Legionella* has been advocated by some (4,6), particularly in hospitals with organ transplant units, but this practice is controversial as the relationship between positive water cultures and risk for legionellosis has not been established. While *Legionella* has been shown to colonize anywhere from 12% to 85% of hospital water systems (102), the organism has often been found in hospital water systems without an association with known cases *of Legionella* (103,104). In institutions where no health care–associated cases of legionellosis have been documented, it is recommended that physicians be educated to heighten their suspicion for potential cases and use appropriate methods to diagnose *Legionella*, particularly in persons at high risk of the disease, such as HSCT or SOT recipients (103). In facilities with hematopoietic stem cell transplant (HSCT) or SOT programs, the Guidelines for Preventing Health Care-Associated Pneumonia published by the CDC and the Healthcare Infection Control Practices Advisory Committee state that periodic culturing of water in transplant units can be performed but no recommendation can be made about frequency or number of sites (103). The guidelines further state that potable water should be maintained at >51°C (>124°F) or <20°C (<68°F), especially in facilities housing organ transplant recipients or other patients at high risk (103,105).

For treatment of contaminated water systems, copper–silver ionization has been effectively used to eradicate *L. pneumophila* by generating metallic ions that disrupt bacterial cell walls (106,107). Superheating water to >60°C and then flushing with hot water has also been useful (108) but scalding is a risk and it may only provide short-term control (102,109). Other techniques such as ultraviolet light treatment may be helpful as well (1), and complete eradication of *Legionella* from hospital water systems is not necessary to minimize risks of nosocomial acquisition (106). Individual electric showers have been effective at decreasing the incidence of nosocomial *Legionella* infection in hospitalized transplant recipients (23). Culturing homes of transplant recipients has been advocated to prevent community-acquired legionellosis (27), although this would not eliminate risks from other community water sources. Temporary chemoprophylaxis with ciprofloxacin has been administered during an outbreak of legionellosis on a BMT unit and was successful in ending the outbreak when combined with water decontamination (7).

## CONCLUSIONS

*Legionella* is an important cause of community-acquired and nosocomial pneumonia in immunocompromised hosts, including transplant recipients. Unfortunately, no clinical, radiographic, or laboratory features reliably distinguish Legionnaires' disease from other causes of pneumonia so that a high index of suspicion is required for making the diagnosis. Extrapulmonary features and more severe disease may be clues to *Legionella* pneumonia in immunosuppressed persons. Delayed therapy is associated with poorer outcome and fluoroquinolones have become the treatment of choice for legionellosis. When and how to implement methods to prevent nosocomial *Legionella* infection remain controversial but may be an issue most critical for settings where there are populations of immunocompromised persons, such as transplant units.

## REFERENCES

1.  Yu VL. Legionella pneumophila (Legionnaires' disease). In: Mandell GL, Bennett JE, Dolin R, eds. Principles and Practice of Infectious Diseases. Vol. 2. Philadelphia, PA: Churchill Livingstone, Inc., 2000:2424–2435.
2.  Muder RR. Other *Legionella* species. In: Mandell GL, Bennett JE, Dolin R, eds. Principles and Practice of Infectious Diseases. Vol. 2. Philadelphia, PA: Churchill Livingstone, Inc., 2000:2435–2441.

3. Fraser DW, Tsai TR, Orenstein W, et al. Legionnaires' disease: description of an epidemic of pneumonia. N Engl J Med 1977; 297:1189–1197.
4. Stout JE, Yu VL. Legionellosis. N Engl J Med 1997; 337:682–687.
5. Yu VL, Kroboth FJ, Shonnard J, Brown A, McDearman S, Magnussen M. Legionnaires' disease: new clinical perspective from a prospective pneumonia-study. Am J Med 1982; 73:357–361.
6. Chow JW, Yu VL. Legionella: a major opportunistic pathogen in transplant-recipients. Semin Respir Infect 1998; 13:132–139.
7. Oren I, Zuckerman T, Avivi I, Finkelstein R, Yigla M, Rowe JM. Nosocomial-outbreak of Legionella pneumophila serogroup 3 pneumonia in a new bone-marrow transplant unit: evaluation, treatment and control. Bone Marrow Transplant 2002; 30:175–179.
8. Babe KS Jr, Reinhardt JF. Diagnosis of legionella sepsis by examination of a peripheral blood smear. Clin Infect Dis 1994; 19:1164–1165.
9. Morley JN, Smith LC, Baltch AL, Smith RP. Recurrent infection due to *Legionella pneumophila* in a patient with AIDS. Clin Infect Dis 1994; 19: 1130–1132.
10. Marston BJ, Lipman HB, Breiman RF. Surveillance for Legionnaires' disease. Risk factors for morbidity and mortality. Arch Intern Med 1994; 154: 2417–2422.
11. Muraca P, Stout JE, Yu VL. Comparative assessment of chlorine, heat, ozone, and UV light for killing *Legionella pneumophila* within a model plumbing system. Appl Environ Microbiol 1987; 53:447–453.
12. Sabria M, Yu VL. Hospital-acquired legionellosis: solutions for a preventable infection. Lancet Infect Dis 2002; 2:368–373.
13. Roig J, Sabria M, Pedro-Botet ML. *Legionella* spp.: community acquired and nosocomial infections. Curr Opin Infect Dis 2003; 16:145–151.
14. Bangsborg JM, Uldum S, Jensen JS, Bruun BG. Nosocomial legionellosis in three heart–lung transplant patients: case reports and environmental observations. Eur J Clin Microbiol Infect Dis 1995; 14:99–104.
15. Carratala J, Gudiol F, Pallares R, et al. Risk factors for nosocomial *Legionella pneumophila* pneumonia. Am J Respir Crit Care Med 1994; 149:625–629.
16. Aeba R, Stout JE, Francalancia NA, et al. Aspects of lung transplantation that contribute to increased severity of Pneumonia. An experimental study. J Thorac Cardiovasc Surg 1993; 106:449–457.
17. Andrews HL, Vogel JP, Isberg RR. Identification of linked *Legionella pneumophila* genes essential for intracellular growth and evasion of the endocytic pathway. Infect Immun 1998; 66:950–958.
18. Brieland JK, Remick DG, LeGendre ML, Engleberg NC, Fantone JC. In vivo regulation of replicative *Legionella pneumophila* lung infection by endogenous interleukin-12. Infect Immun 1998; 66:65–69.
19. Friedman H, Yamamoto Y, Newton C, Klein T. Immunologic response and pathophysiology of *Legionella* infection. Semin Respir Infect 1998; 13:100–108.
20. Plouffe JF, Para MF, Maher WE, Hackman B, Webster L. Subtypes of *Legionella pneumophila* serogroup 1 associated with different attack rates. Lancet 1983; 2:649–650.

21. Bollin GE, Plouffe JF, Para MF, Prior RB. Difference in virulence of environmental isolates of *Legionella pneumophila*. J Clin Microbiol 1985; 21:674–677.

22. Fraser TG, Zembower TR, Lynch P, et al. Cavitary *Legionella pneumonia* in a liver transplant recipient. Transpl Infect Dis 2004; 6:77–80.

23. Prodinger WM, Bonatti H, Allerherger F, et al. *Legionella pneumonia* in transplant recipients: a cluster of cases of eight years' duration. J Hosp Infect 1994; 26:191–202.

24. Kaufmann AF, McDade JE, Patton CM, et al. Pontiac fever: isolation of the etiologic agent (*Legionella pneumophila*) and demonstration of its mode of transmission. Am J Epidemiol 1981; 114:337–347.

25. Pedro-Botet ML, Stout JE, Yu VL. Legionnaires' disease contracted from patient homes: the coming of the third plague? Eur J Clin Microbiol Infect Dis 2002; 21:699–705.

26. Den Boer JW, Yzerman EP, Schellekens J, et al. A large outbreak of Legionnaires' disease at a flower show, The Netherlands, 1999. Emerg Infect Dis 2002; 8:37–43.

27. Sax H, Dharan S, Pittet D. Legionnaires' disease in a renal transplant recipient: nosocomial or home-grown? Transplantation 2002; 74:890–892.

28. Sabria M, Garcia-Nunez M, Pedro-Botet ML, et al. Presence and chromosomal subtyping of *Legionella* species in potable water systems in 20 hospitals of Catalonia, Spain. Infect Control Hosp Epidemiol 2001; 22:673–676.

29. Best M, Yu VL, Stout J, Goetz A, Muder RR, Taylor F. Legionellaceae in the hospital water-supply. Epidemiological link with disease and evaluation of a method for control of nosocomial Legionnaires' disease and Pittsburgh pneumonia. Lancet 1983; 2:307–310.

30. Woo AH, Goetz A, Yu VL. Transmission of *Legionella* by respiratory equipment and aerosol generating devices. Chest 1992; 102:1586–1590.

31. Moiraghi A, Castellani Pastoris M, Barral C, et al. Nosocomial legionellosis associated with use of oxygen bubble humidifiers and underwater chest drains. J Hosp Infect 1987; 10:47–50.

32. Arnow PM, Chou T, Weil D, Shapiro EN, Kretzschmar C. Nosocomial Legionnaires' disease caused by aerosolized tap water from respiratory devices. J Infect Dis 1982; 146:460–467.

33. Pedro-Botet ML, Sabria M, Sopena N, Garcia Nunez M, Morera J, Reynaga E. Environmental legionellosis and oropharyngeal colonization by *Legionella* in immunosuppressed patients. Infect Control Hosp Epidemiol 2002; 23:279–281.

34. Striz I, Jaresova M, Bohmova R, Puchmajerova J, Zazula R, Korcakova L. Bronchial colonization of *Legionella* in patients before organ transplantation (abstract). Am J Respir Crit Care Med 2002; 165(Suppl):A297.

35. Benin AL, Benson RF, Besser RE. Trends in Legionnaires disease, 1980–1998: declining mortality and new patterns of diagnosis. Clin Infect Dis 2002; 35:1039–1046.

36. Vergis EN, Akbas E, Yu VL. *Legionella* as a cause of severe pneumonia. Semin Respir Crit Care Med 2000; 21:295–304.

37. Yu VL, Greenberg RN, Zadeikis N, et al. Levofloxacin efficacy in the treatment of community-acquired legionellosis. Chest 2004; 125:2135–2139.

38. Falguera M, Sacristan O, Nogues A, et al. Nonsevere community-acquired pneumonia: correlation between cause and severity or comorbidity. Arch Intern Med 2001; 161:1866–1872.

39. Matsunaga K, Klein TW, Friedman H, Yamamoto Y. In vitro therapeutic effect of epigallocatechin gallate on nicotine-induced impairment of resistance to *Legionella pneumophila* infection of established MH-S alveolar macrophages. J Infect Dis 2002; 185:229–236.

40. Muder RR, Yu VL, Fang GD. Community-acquired Legionnaires' disease. Semin Respir Infect 1989; 4:32–39.

41. Marrie TJ, Peeling RW, Fine MJ, Singer DE, Coley CM, Kapoor WN. Ambulatory patients with community-acquired pneumonia: the frequency of atypical agents and clinical course. Am J Med 1996; 101:508–515.

42. Woodhead M. Community-acquired pneumonia in Europe: causative pathogens and resistance patterns. Eur Respir J Suppl 2002; 36:20s–27s.

43. Taylor RJ, Schwentker FN, Hakala TR. Opportunistic lung infections in renal transplant patients: a comparison of Pittsburgh pneumonia agent and Legionnaires' disease. J Urol 1981; 125:289–292.

44. Singh N, Stout JE, Yu VL. Legionnaires's disease in a transplant recipient acquired from the patient's home: implications for management. Transplantation 2002; 74:755–756.

45. Korvick JA, Yu VL. Legionnaires' disease: an emerging surgical problem. Ann Thorac Surg 1987; 43:341–347.

46. Bock BV, Kirby BD, Edelstein PH, et al. Legionnaires' disease in renal-transplant recipients. Lancet 1978; 1:410–413.

47. Brooks RG, Hofflin JM, Jamieson SW, Stinson EB, Remington JS. Infectious complications in heart–lung transplant recipients. Am J Med 1985; 79:412–422.

48. Dowling JN, Pasculle AW, Frola FN, Zaphyr MK, Yee RB. Infections caused by *Legionella micdadei* and *Legionella pneumophila* among renal transplant recipients. J Infect Dis 1984; 149:703–713.

49. Ebright JR, Tarakji R, Brown WJ, Sunstrum J. Multiple bilateral lung cavities caused by *Legionella pneumophila*: case report and review. Infect Dis Clin Pract 1993; 2:195–199.

50. Ernst A, Gordon FD, Hayek J, Silvestri RC, Koziel H. Lung abscess complicating *Legionella micdadei* pneumonia in an adult liver transplant recipient: case report and review. Transplantation 1998; 65:130–134.

51. Fuller J, Levinson MM, Kline JR, Copeland J. Legionnaires' disease after heart transplantation. Ann Thorac Surg 1985; 39:308–311.

52. Gombert ME, Josephson A, Goldstein EJ, Smith PR, Butt KM. Cavitary Legionnaires' pneumonia: nosocomial infection in renal transplant recipients. Am J Surg 1984; 147:402–405.

53. Horbach I, Fehrenbach FJ. Legionellosis in heart transplant recipients. Infection 1990; 18:361–363.

54. Humphreys H, Marshall RJ, Mackay I, Caul EO. Pneumonia due to *Legionella bozemanii* and *Chlamydia psittaci*/TWAR following renal transplantation. J Infect 1992; 25:67–71.

55. Jacobs F, Liesnard C, Goldstein JP, et al. Asymptomatic *Legionella pneumophila* infections in heart transplant recipients. Transplantation 1990; 50:174–175.

56. Knirsch CA, Jakob K, Schoonmaker D, et al. An outbreak of *Legionella micdadei* pneumonia in transplant patients: evaluation, molecular epidemiology, and control. Am J Med 2000; 108:290–295.

57. Marshall W, Foster RS Jr, Winn W. Legionnaires' disease in renal transplant patients. Am J Surg 1981; 141:423–429.

58. Seu P, Winston DJ, Olthoff KM, Bruckner DA, Busuttil RW. Legionnaires' disease in liver transplant recipients. Infect Dis Clin Pract 1993; 2:109–113.

59. Wilczek H, Kallings I, Nystrom B, Hoffner S. Nosocomial Legionnaires' disease following renal transplantation. Transplantation 1987; 43:847–851.

60. Tkatch LS, Kusne S, Irish WD, Krystofiak S, Wing E. Epidemiology of *Legionella pneumonia* and factors associated with *Legionella*-related mortality at a tertiary care center. Clin Infect Dis 1998; 27:1479–1486.

61. Neumann UP, Langrehr JM, Kaisers U, Lang M, Schmitz V, Neuhaus P. Simultaneous splenectomy increases risk for opportunistic pneumonia in patients after liver transplantation. Transplant Int 2002; 15:226–232.

62. Yu VL, Plouffe JF, Pastoris MC, et al. Distribution of *Legionella* species and serogroups isolated by culture in patients with sporadic community-acquired legionellosis: an international collaborative survey. J Infect Dis 2002; 186: 127–128.

63. Schwebke JR, Hackman R, Bowden R. Pneumonia due to *Legionella micdadei* in bone marrow transplant recipients. Rev Infect Dis 1990; 12:824–828.

64. Lo Presti F, Riffard S, Vandenesch F, et al. The first clinical isolate of *Legionella parisiensis*, from a liver transplant patient with pneumonia. J Clin Microbiol 1997; 35:1706–1709.

65. Jerngan DB, Sanders LI, Waites KB, Brookings ES, Benson RF, Pappas PG. Pulmonary infection due to *Legionella cincinnatiensis* in renal transplant recipients: two cases and implications for laboratory diagnosis. Clin Infect Dis 1994; 18:385–389.

66. Thacker WL, Benson RF, Schifman RB, et al. *Legionella tucsonensis* sp. nov. isolated from a renal transplant recipient. J Clin Microbiol 1989; 27: 1831–1834.

67. Tan MJ, Tan JS, File TM Jr. Legionnaires disease with bacteremic coinfection. Clin Infect Dis 2002; 35:533–539.

68. Lerolle N, Zahar JR, Duboc V, Tissier F, Rabbat A. Pneumonia involving *Legionella pneumophila* and *Listeria monocytogenes* in an immunocompromised patient: an unusual coinfection. Respiration 2002; 69:359–361.

69. Nichols L, Strollo DC, Kusne S. Legionellosis in a lung transplant recipient obscured by cytomegalovirus infection and *Clostridium difficile* colitis. Transpl Infect Dis 2002; 4:41–45.

70. Sopena N, Sabria-Leal M, Pedro-Botet ML, et al. Comparative study of the clinical presentation of *Legionella pneumonia* and other community-acquired pneumonias. Chest 1998; 113:1195–1200.

71. Gupta SK, Imperiale TF, Sarosi GA. Evaluation of the Winthrop-University Hospital criteria to identify *Legionella pneumonia*. Chest 2001; 120:1064–1071.

72. Torres A, Serra-Batlles J, Ferrer A, et al. Severe community-acquired pneumonia. Epidemiology and prognostic factors. Am Rev Respir Dis 1991; 144: 312–318.

73. Falco V, Fernandez de Sevilla T, Alegre J, Ferrer A, Martinez Vazquez JM. *Legionella pneumophila*. A cause of severe community-acquired pneumonia. Chest 1991; 100:1007–1011.

74. Gubler JG, Schorr M, Gaia V, Zbinden R, Altwegg M. Recurrent soft tissue abscesses caused by *Legionella cincinnatiensis*. J Clin Microbiol 2001; 39: 4568–4570.

75. Bemer P, Leautez S, Ninin E, Jarraud S, Raffi F, Drugeon H. *Legionella pneumophila* arthritis: use of medium specific for Mycobacteria for isolation of *L. pneumophila* in culture of articular fluid specimens. Clin Infect Dis 2002; 35:E6–E7.

76. Schlanger G, Lutwick LI, Kurzman M, Hoch B, Chandler FW. Sinusitis caused by *Legionella pneumophila* in a patient with the acquired immune deficiency syndrome. Am J Med 1984; 77:957–960.

77. Lowry PW, Tompkins LS. Nosocomial Legionellosis: a review of pulmonary and extrapulmonary syndromes. Am J Infect Control 1993; 21:21–27.

78. Miyara T, Tokashiki K, Shimoji T, Tamaki K, Koide M, Saito A. Rapidly expanding lung abscess caused by *Legionella pneumophila* in immunocompromised patients: a report of two cases. Intern Med 2002; 41:133–137.

79. Tokunaga Y, Concepcion W, Berquist WE, et al. Graft involvement by *Legionella* in a liver transplant recipient. Arch Surg 1992; 127:475–477.

80. Avouts PJ, Ramael MR, Ysebaert DK, et al. *Legionella pneumophila* peritonitis in a kidney transplant patient. Scand J Infect Dis 1991; 23:119–122.

81. Okada C, Kura F, Wada A, Inagawa H, Lee GH, Matsushita H. Cross-reactivity and sensitivity of two *Legionella* urinary antigen kits, Biotest EIA and Binax NOW, to extracted antigens from various serogroups of *L. pneumophila* and other *Legionella* species. Microbiol Immunol 2002; 46:51–54.

82. Harrison TG, Doshi N. Evaluation of the Bartels Legionella Urinary Antigen enzyme immunoassay. Eur J Clin Microbiol Infect Dis 2001; 20:738–740.

83. Bartlett JG. Diagnostic test for etiologic agents of community-acquired pneumonia. Infect Dis Clin North Am 2004; 18:809–827.

84. Yzerman EP, den Boer JW, Lettinga KD, Schellekens J, Dankert J, Peeters M. Sensitivity of three urinary antigen tests associated with clinical severity in a large outbreak of Legionnaires' disease in The Netherlands. J Clin Microbiol 2002; 40:3232–3236.

85. Kohler RB, Winn WC Jr, Wheat LJ. Onset and duration of urinary antigen excretion in Legionnaires disease. J Clin Microbiol 1984; 20:605–607.

86. van Der Zee A, Verbakel H, de Jong C, et al. Novel PCR-probe assay for detection of and discrimination between *Legionella pneumophila* and other *Legionella* species in clinical samples. J Clin Microbiol 2002; 40:1124–1125.

87. Rapidmicrobiology.com. 2004. (Accessed May 18, 2005, at http://www.rapidmicrobiology.com/news/29h6.php.)

88. Carbon C, Moola S, Velancsics I, Leroy B, Rangaraju M, Decosta P. Telithromycin 800 mg once daily for seven to ten days is an effective and well-tolerated treatment for community-acquired pneumonia. Clin Microbiol Infect 2003; 9:691–703.

89. Jensen C, Jordan M, Shapiro R, et al. Interaction between tacrolimus and erythromycin. Lancet 1994; 344:825.

90. Jensen CW, Flechner SM, Van Buren CT, et al. Exacerbation of cyclosporine toxicity by concomitant administration of erythromycin. Transplantation 1987; 43:263–270.

91. Edelstein PH. Antimicrobial chemotherapy for legionnaires' disease: a review. Clin Infect Dis 1995; 21(Suppl 3):S265–S276.

92. Stout JE, Sens K, Mietzner S, Obman A, Yu VL. Comparative activity of quinolones, macrolides and ketolides against *Legionella* species using in vitro broth dilution and intracellular susceptibility testing. Int J Antimicrob Agents 2005; 25:302–307.

93. Mykietiuk A, Carratala J, Fernandez-Sabe N, et al. Clinical outcomes for hospitalized patients with *Legionella pneumonia* in the antigenuria era: the influence of levofloxacin therapy. Clin Infect Dis 2005; 40:794–799.

94. Blazquez Garrido RM, Espinosa Parra FJ, Alemany Frances L, et al. Antimicrobial chemotherapy for Legionnaires disease: levofloxacin versus macrolides. Clin Infect Dis 2005; 40:800–806.

95. Hooper TL, Gould FK, Swinburn CR, et al. Ciprofloxacin: a preferred treatment for *legionella* infections in patients receiving cyclosporin A. J Antimicrob Chemother 1988; 22:952–953.

96. Singh N, Muder RR, Yu VL, Gayowski T. *Legionella* infection in liver transplant recipients: implications for management. Transplantation 1993; 56: 1549–1551.

97. Plouffe JF, Breiman RF, Fields BS, et al. Azithromycin in the treatment of *Legionella pneumonia* requiring hospitalization. Clin Infect Dis 2003; 37:1475–1480.

98. Carbon C, Nusrat R. Efficacy of telithromycin in community-acquired pneumonia caused by *Legionella pneumophila*. Eur J Clin Microbiol Infect Dis 2004; 23:650–652.

99. Gacouin A, Le Tulzo Y, Lavoue S, et al. Severe pneumonia due to *Legionella pneumophila:* prognostic factors, impact of delayed appropriate antimicrobial therapy. Intensive Care Med 2002; 28:686–691.

100. Heath CH, Grove DI, Looke DF. Delay in appropriate therapy of *Legionella pneumonia* associated with increased mortality. Eur J Clin Microbiol Infect Dis 1996; 15:286–290.

101. Mandell LA, Bartlett JG, Dowell SF, File TM Jr, Musher DM, Whitney C. Update of practice guidelines for the management of community-acquired pneumonia immunocompetent adults. Clin Infect Dis 2003; 37:1405–1433.

102. Stout JE, Yu VL. Hospital-acquired Legionnaires' disease: new developments. Curr Opin Infect Dis 2003; 16:337–341.

103. Tablan OC, Anderson LJ, Besser R, Bridges C, Hajjeh R. Guidelines for preventing health-care—associated pneumonia, 2003: recommendations of CDC and the Healthcare Infection Control Practices Advisory Committee. Morb Mortal Weekly Rep 2004; 53:1–36.

104. Guidelines for prevention of nosocomial pneumonia. Centers for Disease Control and Prevention. Morb Mortal Wkly Rep Recomm Rep 1997; 46:1–79.

105. Darelid J, Lofgren S, Malmvall BE. Control of nosocomial Legionnaires' disease by keeping the circulating hot water temperature above 55 degrees C: experience from a 10-year surveillance programme in a district general hospital. J Hosp Infect 2002; 50:213–219.

106. Stout JE, Lin YS, Goetz AM, Muder RR. Controlling *Legionella* in hospital water systems: experience with the superheat-and-flush method and copper–silver ionization. Infect Control Hosp Epidemiol 1998; 19:911–914.

107. Liu Z, Stout JE, Tedesco L, et al. Controlled evaluation of copper–silver ionization in eradicating *Legionella pneumophila* from a hospital water distribution system. J Infect Dis 1994; 169:919–922.

108. Zacheus OM, Martikainen PJ. Effect of heat flushing on the concentrations of *Legionella pneumophila* and other heterotrophic microbes in hot water systems of apartment buildings. Can J Microbiol 1996; 42:811–818.

109. Perola O, Kauppinen J, Kusnetsov J, Karkkainen UM, Luck PC, Katila ML. Persistent *Legionella pneumophila* colonization of a hospital water supply: efficacy of control methods and a molecular epidemiological analysis. Acta Pathol Microbiol Immunol Scand 2005; 113:45–53.

# 28

# Mycobacterial Infections Complicating Organ Transplantation

**Rajeev Saggar**

*Division of Pulmonary and Critical Care Medicine, Department of Medicine, University of California at Irvine, Irvine, California, U.S.A.*

**Bernard M. Kubak**

*Division of Infectious Diseases, Department of Medicine, David Geffen School of Medicine at UCLA, Los Angeles, California, U.S.A.*

**David J. Ross and Joseph P. Lynch III**

*Division of Pulmonary and Critical Care Medicine and Hospitalists, Department of Internal Medicine, David Geffen School of Medicine at UCLA, Los Angeles, California, U.S.A.*

## MYCOBACTERIOSIS

Mycobacterial infections [due to both *Mycobacterium tuberculosis* and nontuberculous mycobacteria (NTM)] are rare but potentially lethal complications of hematopoietic stem cell or solid organ transplantation (1–6). Posttransplant mycobacterial infections (MBIs) may reflect acquisition of new infections (because of the intensity of immunosuppression) (7), reactivation of latent disease (particularly *M. tuberculosis*) within the recipients (1,2,8,9), or receipt of infected organs (7,10–12). Environmental sources are the reservoir for most human infections due to NTM (13–15), whereas human-to-human transmission or reactivation of latent infection are the critical factors for development of infections due to *M. tuberculosis* (1). The incidence of MBIs depend upon the intensity of immnosuppression, the prevalence of mycobacteria (both typical and NTM) in the region or country, type of transplanted organ, and risk factors and exposures to mycobacteria. In this review, we first discuss infections due to *M. tuberculosis* among organ transplant recipients (OTRs). Later, we discuss infections due to NTM.

## MYCOBACTERIUM TUBERCULOSIS

### Epidemiology and Pathogenesis

The incidence of tuberculosis in transplant recipients is 20- to 70-fold higher than in the general population (1,6,9,16,17). The onset of posttransplant tuberculosis (TB) is variable, ranging from a few weeks to greater than two years (1,6,18). Incidence rates reflect the prevalence of tuberculosis in the region. Among countries/regions with low endemic rates of tuberculosis, the incidence of *M. tuberculosis* among OTRs is low (0.2–1%), but rates are higher (2–15%) in regions with a high prevalence of TB (1,2,6,19). Incidence of TB among OTRs range from 0.35% to 1.2% in the United States (1), 0.4% to 5% in Europe (6,18), 1.5% to 3.5% in the Middle East (20,21), 1.5% to 8.2% in South Africa (22), 3.5% to 15% in Asia (2,19,23,24). The epidemiology, clinical features, and outcome of TB among OTRs were elegantly discussed in one large study (comprising 511 cases published in the English language literature from 1967 to 1997) (1), and in one recent review (6).

### Risk Factors for Tuberculosis Post–Organ Transplantation

Risk factors associating with an increased risk of developing tuberculosis following organ transplantation include: (i) residence in endemic areas with high prevalance rates of TB; (ii) intensity of immunosuppression (1,2,18); (iii) concomitant infection with cytomegalovirus (CMV) (2) or fungi (6); (iv) chronic liver disease (2); (v) diabetes mellitus (1); (vi) acute allograft rejection (1); (vii) use of OKT3 or anti-T cell antibodies (1,6); (viii) chest radiographic features consistent with old TB (25). In some studies, the use of calcineurin inhibitors (e.g., cyclosporin A or tacrolimus) (2,26), mycophenolate mofetil (26), and anti-T cell antibodies (1) were associated with the development of TB *earlier* posttransplantation.

### Incidence of Tuberculosis Among Specific Organ Allografts

#### Bone Marrow or Stem Cell Transplant Recipients

Mycobacterial infections complicate hematopoietic stem cell transplants (HSCTs) in 0.2% to 1% of patients in the United States (27–29). A retrospective review of 2241 BMT recipients at the University of Minnesota identified only two cases of *M. tuberculosis* (0.1%) (27). A survey of 29 European Bone Marrow Transplant Centers from 1994 to 1998 detected 20 cases of tuberculosis among 4525 HSCT recipients (0.5%) (30). Incidences of

*M. tuberculosis* in other series of HSCT include: France (0.4%) (31); the United Kingdom (0.3%) (32); Spain (0.6%) (33) and 0.2% (34); Turkey (1.6%) (35); Saudi Arabia (1.1%) (36); Taiwan (2.3%) (37) and 0.8% (38); and Hong Kong (5.5%) (39) and 0.4% (40). Risk factors for TB include: allogeneic HSCTs with mismatches (30), graft versus host disease (GVHD) (34,40), and total body irradiation (34,40).

### Heart Transplant Recipients

Tuberculosis is a rare complication of cardiac transplantation (41–43) with incidence rates of 0.1% to 1% in the United States (44–48) and 0.6% to 1% in Europe (18,47,49,50). Higher rates were noted in Asia (2.8–3.6%) (1,51,52).

### Hepatic Transplant Recipients

Tuberculosis is a rare complication of liver transplantation (12,16,53–59) with incidence rates according to country as follows: United States (0.9–1.2%) (16); Spain (1–1.1%) (18,25,59); South Africa (5%) (55).

### Kidney Transplant Recipients

The incidence of *M. tuberculosis* among renal transplant recipients among renal transplant recipients is low (0.15%–0.45%) (60,61). In Spain, TB incidence rates were 0.7% (18) and 1.6% (62) in two studies. Higher rates were noted in Mexico (1.8%) (63); Argentina (3.6%) (11); Saudi Arabia (3.5%) (21); Turkey (5.8%) (20); South Africa (11%) (22), India (10–12%) (23,64), and Pakistan (14.5%) (24).

### Lung Transplant Recipients

Data regarding TB following lung transplantation are limited to anecdotal case reports (7,8,10,65–69), several series (9,70–72), and one retrospective review (1). The incidence of TB among LTRs ranges from <1% to 6.5%. A retrospective review of 261 lung or heart–lung transplant recipients in Australia detected two cases of *M. tuberculosis* over a 12-year period (0.8%) (70). Analysis of 210 lung transplant recipients (LTRs) in Toronto identified two cases of *M. tuberculosis* (0.9%) (71). Schulman et al. detected two cases of TB among 94 lung and heart–lung transplant recipients (2%) (9). One case of TB was noted in a series of 59 LTRs from Chapel Hill (73). In Spain, 6 of 187 LTRs (3.2%) developed TB; an additional six cases were diagnosed from the explanted lungs at the time of transplantation (72). A prospective study in Spain detected six cases of TB among 61 LTRs (10%) over a seven-year period (74). In France, four cases of TB were detected among 61 LTRs (6.5%) (75). Lung transplantation has only recently emerged in Asia, and data from this region are limited. However, given the high rates of endemic TB in Asia (76), (including MDR-TB) (77), the development of TB following lung transplantation is a genuine threat (68). Transmission of TB from the donor lung(s) may occur. Ridgeway reported two cases of TB in single LTRs who shared a common donor (10). We documented transmission of TB from the donor to a LTR (7). Typically, TB following lung transplantation occurs within the first few months. In a review of 10 cases of TB among LTRs, the mean time to onset of TB after transplantation was 3.5 months; 9 of 10 developed TB within 12 months of transplantation (1). In order to reduce the risk of TB among LTRs, the following steps are critical: (i) the explanted lungs must be examined for granulomata or evidence for TB; (ii) bronchoalveolar lavage (BAL) fluid from the donor bronchi and receipient should be sent for mycobacterial cultures; (iii) INH prophylaxis should be routinely given to candidates for lung transplantation with any of the following criteria: positive tuberculin skin test, anergy but increased risk for TB, or evidence for old granulomatous disease on chest radiographs.

## Clinical Manifestations of *Mycobacterium tuberculosis*

Clinical manifestations of TB manifest usually within the first year following organ transplantation, but can occur greater than three years posttransplantation (1,2,6,18). In a review of 511 cases of TB post solid organ transplantation (SOT), the median time to TB onset was nine months after transplantation (range 0.5–144 months) (1). The median time to onset was longer for kidney transplant recipients (11.5 months) compared to other solid organs (range 3.5–4 months) (1). Others noted a delayed onset of TB in renal transplant patients compared to other SOT recipients (26,78); this likely reflects greater intensity of immunosuppression among other SOT recipients. Manifestations of TB among OTRs are protean, but two large series cited pulmonary involvement in 63% to 71%, extrapulmonary involvement in 12% to 16%, and disseminated disease in 33% (1,18). Factors that increase the risk of disseminated infection include nonrenal transplantation and use of OKT3 or anti-T cell antibodies (1). Extrapulmonary involvement is more common in non-endemic areas (1,21). In one large series, fever was present in 91% of patients with disseminated TB, in 66% with pulmonary TB, and 63% with extrapulmonary TB (1). Night sweats and weight loss are common presenting features (1,2,21). Pulmonary manifestations of TB among OTRs are variable (1,2,6,68). Singh et al. cited the following radiographic abnormalities among patients with pulmonary TB: focal infiltrates (40%), a miliary pattern (22%), nodules (15%), pleural effusions (13%), diffuse interstitial infiltrate (5%), cavitation (4%) (1). Gastrointestinal involvement was the most common extrapulmonary site in SOT recipients (1,6). Symptoms included fever, gastrointestinal bleeding, abdominal pain, pancreatitis, and ulcers (1,6). Liver and peritoneal involvement may also occur (1,6). Renal and genitourinary TB may present with flank pain, fever, or sterile pyuria (2). Tuberculosis in SOT recipients has been described in the skin, the muscle, the osteoarticular system, the genitourinary system, lymph nodes, pericardium, spleen, adrenals, eye, and central nervous system (CNS) (1,2,6). Importantly, TB may be asymptomatic in up to one third of patients (18,71,72). Mortality rates of 29% to 31% have been cited among SOT recipients with TB (1,6,18), but these studies included patients in whom the diagnosis was established at necropsy or untreated patients When appropriate treatment is initiated *early,* favorable outcomes are achieved in more than 90% of patients (2).

### Diagnosis

An aggressive diagnostic approach is essential to diagnose TB among OTRs. Appropriate smears and cultures should be obtained from suspected sites. Standard tests to identify acid-fast bacilli (AFB) include the Zeihl–Neelsen stain or auramine–phenol fluorochrome method (2). Cultures require special media and take three to six weeks by standard techniques (2). Polymerase chain reaction (PCR) can detect mycobacterial rRNA in clinical samples within a few hours (79) and may establish the diagnosis earlier than conventional cultures (6,78). PCR is highly specific, but sensitivities are variable (80–82). Restriction fragment length polymorphism is highly specific (83), but is limited to reference centers (2). When pulmonary infiltrates are present, bronchoscopy with BAL and/or transbronchial lung biopsies may substantiate the diagnosis. Biopsies demonstrated necrotizing granulomas and giant cells support the diagnosis of TB. Imaging modalities such as chest X-ray should be supplemented by high-resolution computed tomography (HRCT) for greater resolution in patients with high clinical suspicion (2,7,68). Increased uptake on positron emission tomography (PET) with fluorodeoxyglucose scans may be found in patients with tuberculosis, but this finding is nonspecific (84–86). Extrapulmonary organ involvement may be difficult to diagnose. Culturing bodily fluids (pleural fluid, cerebrospinal fluid, gastric fluid, urine) or percutaneous needle aspiration or biopsies of suspected sites should be performed with a low threshold.

### Treatment

In the comprehensive review of TB among SOTs by Singh and Patterson, overall mortality was 29% (146 of 499) (1). Risk factors for mortality included: disseminated TB, prior rejection, and receipt of OKT3 or anti-T cell antibodies (1). In another study of TB among SOT recipients, antilymphocyte antibodies or high doses of corticosteroids were associated with increased mortality (18). However, several studies cited high success rates ( >90–100%) with antituberculous therapy among OTRs (2,19). Early diagnosis and prompt initiation of appropriate therapy are critical for optimal outcomes.

The American Thoracic Society (ATS), Centers for Disease Control and Prevention (CDC), and Infectious Diseases Society of America (IDSA) published comprehensive guidelines for treatment of active and latent TB infections (87–89). For most patients, initial treatment (phase I) employs four drugs [i.e., isoniazid (INH), rifampin (RIF), pyrazinamide (PZA), and either ethambutol (EMB) or streptomycin (SM)] while awaiting antimicrobial susceptibility results (87). The continuation phase is given for either four months (most patients) or seven months (more complex cases) (87). For susceptible organisms, three drugs (INH, RTF, and PZA) are continued for two months; thereafter, two drugs (INH and RTF) are continued for an *additional* four (or seven) months. Different treatment schedules (daily or twice- or thrice-weekly dosing) may be used (87–89). For all patients, directed observed therapy (DOT) is recommended (90). For immunocompetent patients, a total of six months of therapy is adequate (87,88). A 9- to 12-month course is recommended for meningeal TB (87), patients exhibiting a slow response to therapy (87), or patients with imraunosuppressive disease. Additional agents or combinations may be required depending upon resistance profiles and adverse effects from the antituberculous medications. For isolates resistant to INH, six months of therapy with RTF, EMB, and PZA is recommended. Isolates displaying resistance to RIF require a longer course of therapy. Patients with *M. tuberculosis* resistant to *both* INH and RIF require at least 18 to 24 months of therapy, and should be treated by experts in the treatment of multidrug-resistant (MDR) TB (91). The ATS/CDC/IDSA guidelines (87) provided specific recommendations for "special situations" including human immunodeficiency virus (HIV) infection, extrapulmonary disease, children, pregnancy, renal insufficiency, liver disease, pregnancy, etc., but did *not specifically address* TB in SOT recipients.

Treatment of *M. tuberculosis* among SOTs recipients is controversial, owing to interactions of rifampin with calcineurin inhibitors (CNIs) and potential hepatotoxicity with INH (particularly among hepatic allograft recipients) (1,6,92). Most experts recommend that INH should be included in the treatment of all SOT recipients with TB, unless INH resistance or adverse effects preclude its use (6). Pyrazinamide is a key component of initial therapy, but may be hepatotoxic (93–95). Hepatotoxicity is more common in multidrug regimens and among hepatic transplant recipients. In one study of SOT recipients with TB, hepatotoxicity developed in 33%; the rate was higher (50%) among patients receiving four or more antituberculous drugs (18). In a review by Singh et al. hepatotoxicity associated with INH was documented in 41% of liver transplant recipients, 10% of heart transplant recipients, and 9% of renal transplant recipients (1). None of 12 lung transplant recipients developed hepatotoxicity. Careful monitoring for hepatic toxicity is warranted (particularly among hepatic transplant recipients) (6). The role of rifampin (or rifabutin) among SOT recipients is controversial, since rifamycms induce hepatic cytochrome P450 and dramatically reduce levels of CNIs or sirolimus (1,3,96,97). Rifampin is a more potent enzyme inducer than rifabutin (98). The use of rifamycins may precipitate acute allograft rejection unless dosages of CNIs are increased appropriately (often by three- to sixfold) (1,96). However, maintaining adequate CsA levels may be difficult when RIF is continued (47,99). Further, the dose of prednisolone should be doubled in patients receiving rifamycins (100). Owing to these drug interactions, some institutions avoid rifamycin altogether for OTRs with TB (6,12,18,52,101). In the review by Singh and Patterson (1), 79% of centers in Europe employed rifampin-containing regimens as compared to 92% in the United States and 91% in other regions. Mortality rates were similar with regimens containing INH *plus* RIF (21%) as compared to INH-containing regimens *without* RIF (24% mortality) (1). Similarly, in a cohort of 78 renal transplant recipients with TB, treatment success rates were similar with regimens containing rifampin (83%) or no rifampin (90%) (102). Graft survival rates were also similar between the two treatment cohorts. Fluoroquinolones have been advocated by some experts as part of multiagent initial therapy for TB among SOT recipients (6). Munoz et al. treat SOT recipients with TB as follows: three drugs (INH, EMB, and PZA) are used for stable patients *without* disseminated disease or suspected multi drug resistance (6). For more severe disease, a fluoroquinolone (usually levofloxacin) is added. For MDR-TB, streptomycin or amikacin are added (6). The ATS/CDC/IDSA guidelines (87) designated FQs as *preferrred* agents for treating MDR-tuberculosis, hut did not specifically consider FQs *as first-line* agents. Nonetheless, recent experience noted that newer FQs (moxifloxacin, levofloxacin, gatifloxacin) have early bactericidal activity (103) and are promising in clinical studies (104,105). Investigators from India cited excellent results with INH, EMB, PZA, and a FQ for two months, followed by INH and a FQ for an additional 10 months. This regimen was efficacious in 100% of >100 SOT recipients (104,106). Similarly, in Spain, all 12 lung transplant recipients with TB responded to antituberculous therapy without the use of rifamycins (72).

To date, few cases of MDR-TB have been reported among SOT recipients (6,43,68). With the rising incidence of MDR-TB in the general population (77), it is expected the number of MDR-TB cases in SOT recipients will increase in the near future. Initial treatment of MDR-TB requires five to six active agents; specific agents can then be omitted once susceptibility tests are available (6,68). Finally, pulmonary resectional surgery for MDR-TB has been tried for cases refractory to medical therapy (67,91,107).

Given the potential for allograft rejection, we agree with others that immunosuppression should be continued (6,18), provided early control of the infection can be accomplished.

Duration of therapy for TB among SOT recipients has not been studied. However, in one study, mortality rate was 33% among SOT recipients with TB who were treated for six to nine months compared to no mortality among patients treated for greater than nine months ($p = 0.03$) (18). We agree with others that treatment should be continued for at least one year (6).

## Prophylaxis

Tuberculosis may develop post organ transplantation via (i) receipt of infected donor organs, (ii) reactivation of latent disease within the recipient, or (iii) acquisition of new infection during intense immunosuppression. Preventive therapy for *high-risk* patients may reduce the incidence of TB, particularly for patients in groups (i) and (ii). Guidelines for pretransplant interventions and donor and recipient screening have been published (108–110). We believe that tuberculin skin testing (TST) with purified protein derivative (PPD) is warranted in all patients *prior to organ transplantation* to evaluate patients at risk for reactivation of tuberculosis (111). Unfortunately, TST screening underestimates the prevalence of latent tuberculous infection (LTBI), since many patients with co-morbidities or immune impairments prior to transplantation may be anergic (6,112). Unfortunately, anergy skin testing to validate negative PPD skin tests in immunocompromised individuals has been shown to be ineffective (60,113–117). We agree with Singh and Patterson (1) that prophylactic INH is warranted for OTRs in the following circumstances: positive PPD ($\geq$5 mm induration); chest radiographs consistent with old granulomatous disease; a history of inadequately treated TB; close contact with a patient with active TB; recipients of organs from donors with a history of untreated TB or positive PPD (1). This policy is not endorsed by all centers, however. Transplant candidates with a history of adequately treated TB in the past do not need new treatment courses or prolonged prophylaxis (6). Screening of *donors* for LTBI is difficult, given time constraints. Screening for LTBI among cadaveric donors is usually limited to chest X rays and inspection (and appropriate cultures) of the explanted lung (or other organs) for granulomas or "footprints" of TB. Chest CT scans are more sensitive than chest X rays, but are not used to screen donors in most centers. However, chest CT should be considered for "high-risk" donors (e.g., history of LTBI or previous TB; residence in an area with high prevalence of TB; other medical risk factors for TB) (7). For lung transplant recipients, BAL is performed to obtain cultures from donor lungs, but results (particularly cultures) are not immediately available (7). Unfortunately, a history of previous TB in organ donors may not be elicited. Recently, a whole blood gamma-interferon assay (QuantiFERON, Cellestis, Valencia, CA) was approved by the Food and Drug Administration (FDA) to detect LTBI, with sensitivity comparable to the PPD (118). However, this test has not been widely applied among OTRs.

Because of potential hepatotoxicity, the role of prophylactic therapy for SOT recipients with LTBI is controversial. Recommendations from the CDC and IDSA published in 2000 (88) endorsed one of three regimens for treating LTBI (formerly known as preventive therapy). This document was a general recommendation for patients with LTBI and did *not specifically address* OTRs. These regimens included: (i) INH for nine months, (ii) RIF for four months, or (iii) PZA plus RIF for two months. Following reports of severe (even fatal) toxicity with RIF and PZA (119,120), these recommendations were revised (87,120). Recent guidelines reserve PZA plus RIF only for patients unable to complete longer course regimens. In addition, patients receiving PZA plus RIF need to have liver function tests and symptoms monitored every two weeks throughout the course of therapy.

Because INH may be hepatotoxic, many authors do not employ preventive therapy for LTBI among hepatic transplant candidates or patients with prior hepatitis (25). Hepatotoxicity is more common among liver transplant recipients receiving INH as part of a multidrug regimen than for single-agent prophylaxis (121). For nonhepatic organ transplant candidates at high risk for LTBI, INH is usually initiated prior to transplantation (1,6). However, clinical practice patterns are variable. Randomized controlled trial assessing impact of INH prophylaxis have not been performed among OTRs. However, case series suggest that TNH prophylaxis is effective for high-risk patients, with a low incidence of adverse effects (1). Singh and Patterson reviewed data from seven publications comprising 278 OTRs who received INH prophylaxis for suspected LTBI; none developed tuberculosis (1). By contrast, TB developed in 6 of 27 *high-risk* patients who did *not* receive prophylaxis. In a retrospective study of 547 hepatic transplant recipients, 4 of 23 (17%) receiving preventive therapy with INH for LTBI developed INH-hepatotoxidty (25). Among 21 patients with radiological evidence for TB who did *not* receive INH prophylaxis, 2 (9%) developed active TB. Pretransplant TSTs were not helpful in judging risk. None of 89 patients with positive TST developed TB whereas 5 of 284 (1.8%) with negative TST developed active TB. The authors argued that INH treatment for LTBI (on the basis of positive TST only) was not justified among hepatic transplant recipients. Hepatotoxicity is much less common among nonhepatic organ transplants. Clinically significant INH hepatotoxicity developed in 3 of 119 (2.5%) renal transplant recipients receiving azathioprine-based immunosuppression (122) and in none of 83 receiving cyclosporine (123) in two studies. When INH prophylaxis is administered to OTRs, liver function studies should be monitored closely. In regions characterized by high levels of primary INH resistance (23,124), alternative regimens for prophylaxis should be considered (e.g., RIF for four months prior to transplantation).

## NONTUBERCULOSIS MYCOBACTERIOSIS

### Introduction

Infections due to nontuberculous mycobacteria (NTM) have increased dramatically over the past two decades, both in immunocompetent and immunocompromised hosts (3,5,13,14). In the 1950s, NMT were first recognized as causes of pulmonary infections in immunocompetent patients with chronic lung disorders (e.g., bronchiectasis, silicosis, healed tuberculosis) (125,126). A national surveillance study from 1979 to 1980 ( >30,000 isolates) found that approximately one-third of mycobacterial isolates were NTM; two-thirds were *M. tuberculosis* (127). In that survey, *M. avium* complex (MAC) comprised 61% of NTM, followed by *M.fortuitum* (19%) and *M. kansasii* (10%) (127). A second national survey from 1981 to 1983 noted a prevalence of NTM pulmonary disease of 1.8 case per 100,000 population (128). By the mid-1980s, a dramatic escalation of cases was noted among patients with acquired immunodeficiency syndrome (AIDS) (129,130). In this population, >95% of isolates were MAC complex (129,130). A more recent survey by the CDC from 1991 to 1992 cited a dramatic rise in the prevalence of NTM (13). In fact, *M. avium* was more common than *M. tuberculosis,* which comprised only 26% of mycobacterial isolates (13). The increased prevalence of NTM infections likely reflects several factors, including heightened awareness, development of better diagnostic techniques, the surge of infections due to HIV, and expanded pool of patients with severe immunosuppression (including OTRs).

## Epidemiology

NTMs are ubiquitous in the environment, and are frequently isolated from water and soil (13,14). Environmental sources (especially natural waters) are the reservoir for most human infections caused by NTM (13,14). Airborne transmission of NTM from environmental sources is the likely cause of respiratory disease. Gastrointestinal colonization is the likely source among children with NTM cervical lymphadenitis and patients with AIDS with disseminated NTM. Human-to-human transmission is rare (13,14). However, clusters of cases of *M. haemophilum* within hospitals suggest the possibility of person-to-person transmission (131,132).

In immunocompetent hosts, chronic pulmonary disease is the most common clinical manifestation of NTM (13,15,133). Worldwide, MAC is the most common NTM causing pulmonary disease (13). However, the prevalence of other NTMs differs according to geographical region (133). In the United States, *M. kansasii* is the second most common NTM causing pulmonary disease (13,127). By contrast, *M. xenopi* is more common in Canada and some European countries while *M. malmoense* is more prevalent in Scandanavia and northern Europe (134). The prevalence of NTM is dramatically increased among immunocompromised patients (particularly patients infected with the HIV virus) (135,136). Further, most NTM infections in HIV-infected patients typically are disseminated. *Localized* pulmonary disease in AIDS due to NTM is uncommon (<5%) (136,137). Infections have been described from myriad species of NTM in patients with HIV (138–140), but the vast majority (>95%) of NTM infections in this population are caused by *M. avium* (13,135). Infections (localized or disseminated) due to NTM may occur in immunosuppressed patients without AIDS (e.g., transplant recipients, hematological malignancies, corticosteroid use, etc). In this context, *M. avium* is most common (129,141), but *M. kansasii, M. chelonae* (17,142,143), *M. abscessus* (15), *M. haemophilum* (144,145), *M. scrofidaceum* (15) and other NTM (3,5) may cause disease in this setting.

## Nontuberculous Mycobacterial Infections Among Organ Transplant Recipients

NTM infections are uncommon, but potentially lethal, complications of HSCT or SOT recipients (2–5,146–150). A comprehensive review of the English language from 1966 to 2003 detected 276 cases of NTM infections (93 in HSCT recipients; 183 in SOT recipients) (3). More than half of NTM infections in SOT recipients involve skin, soft tissue or joints; lung occurs in 25% (3,5). The most common species of NTM in SOT recipients are: MAC, *M. fortuitum*/*M. chelonei, M. kansasii,* and *M. haemophilum* (2,3,5,147,150,151).

## Specific Organisms

### Mycobacterium avium Complex

MAC may cause pulmonary infections in immunocompetent hosts (152–154) and patients with cystic fibrosis (155) or may cause disseminated disease among immunocompromised patients (3,129,130). Lung disease due to MAC may present as apical fibrocavitary lung disease (typically in males) (154) or as bilateral nodular and interstitial disease in the right middle lobe or lingula, predominantly in females (152,153). In a comprehensive review of 276 NTM infections among transplant recipients, MAC was implicated as the cause of mycobacterial infections at the following rates: HSCT (8%); heart (21%); kidney (5%); liver [3 of 8 (38%)]; lung [7 of 22 (32%)] (3).

### Rapid-Growing NTM (*M. abscessus, M. chelonae,* or *M. fortuitum*)

Rapid-growing mycobacteria (RGM) principally cause cutaneous infections in both immunocompetent and immunocompromised hosts (143,156). Three species (*M. abscessus, M. chelonae,* or *M. fortuitum*) account for >90% of infections due to RGM (13). RGM may cause surgical wound (157–160), skin, soft tissue, or joint infections (161) in both immunocompetent (160–162) or immunosuppressed hosts (17,130,163). Pulmonary disease due to RGM is less common, but may occur in older individuals with prior lung disease or in women with no known predisposing factors (139,164). *mycobacterium abscessus* accounts for approximately 80% of respiratory infections due to RGM; *M. fortuirtum,* appoximately 15% (164), Infections due to RGM complicating kidney (17,163), kidney–pancreas (150), heart (4,5,165), or liver (3,166) transplant recipients have been described. In a review of 276 NTM infections among transplant recipients, RGM were implicated in the following percent of NTM infections: HSCT (43%); heart (9%); kidney (40%); liver [3 of 8 (38%)] lung [8 of 22 (37%)] (3).

### Mycobacterium gordonae

*Mycobacterium gordonae,* frequently isolated in tap water, whirlpools, swimming pools, and soil, is of low pathogenicity (167), but may cause disseminated or localized infections in immunocompromised hosts (168–173). Pulmonary infections due to *M. gordonae* have been reported (174–176), but most pulmonary isolates of *M. gordonae* are nonpathogenic (167). *M. gordonae* was implicated in only 3 of 276 NTM infections in transplant recipients (3).

### Mycobacterium haemophilum

*Mycobacterium haemophilum* may cause cutaneous and subcutaneous infections, arthritis, osteomyelitis, and pneumonia in immunocompromised patients (131,144,145,147,177), and lymphadenitis in immunocompetent children (178,179). Among immunocompromised patients, skin and soft tissue infections are most common (30,131,145). Erythematous or tender papules or nodules, with or without ulceration may occur (145,180). Infections due to *M. haemophilum* have been described in HSCT (30,145 181,182), cardiac (147,180,183–185), renal (144,186), and lung (3) transplant recipients. In a review of NTM infections among transplant recipients, *M. haemophilum* was implicated at the following rates: HSCT (24%), heart (15%), kidney (14%), liver (0 of 8), and lung [4 of 22 (18%)] (3). Diagnosis of *M. haemophilum* may be elusive, as the organism is fastidious and requires specialized culture techniques that are not used routinely in most mycobacteria laboratories (145,187). Identification takes up to three to four weeks (147). Identification can be confirmed by restriction fragment length polymorphisms assays (188).

### Mycobacterium kansasii

*Mycobacterium kansasii* is the second most common NTM pulmonary disease in the United States (13,127,128) and may cause pulmonary or disseminated infections in patients with AIDS (130,130) or in severely immunocompromised patients (3). *Mycobacteria kansasii* is one of the most common causes of infections due to NTM in kidney (3,62) and heart (3,5,48) transplant recipients but rarely complicates HSCT (3) or lung (70) transplantation. In a review of NTM infections among transplant recipients, *M. kansasii* was implicated at the following rates: HSCT (1%), heart (36%), kidney (22%), liver (0 of 8), and lung [1 of 22 (5%)] (3).

### Mycobacterium malmoense

*Mycobacterium malmoense* is rare in the United States (190) but is an important (and sometimes predominant) NTM in the British Isles and northern Europe (13,134,191–193). *M. malmoense* has been isolated from natural waters in Finland (13) and soils in Japan (194) and Zaire (195). Pulmonary disease due to *M. malmoense* often reveals cavities on chest radiographs, and is associated with significant morbidity and, rarely, mortality (192). Extrapulmonary and disseminated infections due to *M. malmoense* may occur (particularly in AIDS patients) (140,196,197). We were unable to find published cases of NTM due to *M. malmoense* among OTRs.

### Mycobacterium marinum

*Mycobacterium marinum,* commonly associated with water, swimming pools, and fish tanks, may cause cutaneous and soft tissue infections in both immunocompetent and immunocompromised hosts (15,198,199). Anecdotal cases of MBIs due to *M. marinum* were described among renal (149,200) and lung (201) transplant recipients. In a recent review, *M. marinum* was implicated in only 5 of 276 NTM infections in transplant recipients (3).

### Mycobacterium scrofulaceum

*Mycobacterium scrofulaceum,* a slow-growing scotochromogen, is widely distributed in tap water and soil (202), but rarely causes clinical infections. Waters, soils, and swamps in the southeastern United States are major environmental niches for *M. scrofulaceum* (203). *M. scrofulaceum* is a rare cause of cervical lymphadenitis in children (204), skin lesions in imnmnosuppressed individuals (205,206), lower respiratory tract infections in patients with cystic fibrosis (155) or chronic lung disorders (202), and disseminated NTM infections in patients with AIDS (207). *M. scrofulaceum* was implicated in a casse of pulmonary infection in a heart transplant recipient (208) and accounted for 4 of 276 NTM infections in OTRs (3).

### Mycobacterium simiae

*Mycobacterium simiae* (209,210) may be isolated from water and environmental sources within hospitals (211), but have rarely been implicated in clinical infections (13,209,212,213). *M. simiae* is most commonly isolated in the Caribbean (213), Middle East (210), and southern United States (211,214). Pulmonary infections predominate, but the vast majority (>70%) of isolates likely represent colonization (128,209). An increase in *M. simiae* isolates in a Texas military hospital was linked to contaminated water (211). Only 3 of 22 culture-positive patients met criteria for *M. simiae* pulmonary disease (211). Disseminated infections due to *M. simiae* have been noted in patients with AIDS (215–217); one case of peritonitis due to *M. simiae* was recently reported in an AIDS patient (218). Investigators from Texas identified

241 isolates of *M. simiae;* 90% of isolates were from the respiratory tract (214). Most (62%) infections due to *M. simiae* were in immunosuppressed patients, including 10 organ transplant recipients (214).

### Mycobacterium szulgai

*Mycobacterium szulgai,* a slow-growing NTM, is a rare cause of pulmonary, cutaneous, bone, or soft tissue infections (219–221). The most common site is pulmonary in patients with pre-existing lung disease (221–223). Cutaneous infections may occur in patients with impaired immune defenses (224). Keratitis due to *M. szulgai* may complicate laser-assisted in situ keratomileusis (225). Rare cases of septic arthritis (226), osteomyelitis (227), skin ulcers (227), and pneumonia (228) have been cited in AIDS patients. One case of cutaneous infection due to *M. szulgai* was described in a bone marrow transplant recipient (229).

### Mycobacterium ulcerans

*Mycobacterium ulcerans* may cause disease in certain geographic areas (e.g., tropical rain forests, Africa, Southeast Asia, Australia, South and Central America) (13,230,231). Endemic areas for *M. ulcerans* are typically low-lying swamp areas (231). Typically, *M. ulcerans* causes chronic, progressive skin ulcers (231). Most cases occur in rural west Africa where the disease is known as "Buruli" ulcer (231). We are not aware of any published cases of infections due to *M. ulcerans* among transplant recipients.

### Mycobacterium xenopi

*Mycobacterium xenopi* account for fewer than 0.3% of clinical NTM isolates (232) but have been isolated from water and environmental sources within hospitals (232–234). Three cases of infections (and 18 additional isolates) due to *M. xenopi* were ascribed to contaminated bronchoscopes; *M. xenopi* in the tap water was the source (232). Newer, more sensitive cultural techniques resulted in substantial increases in the rate of positive cultures of *M. xenopi* in clinical microbiology laboratories (235–237). However, only 3 of 422 isolates from one New York hospital from 1975 to 1998 were associated with clinical *M. xenopi* lung disease (236). Since *M. xenopi* is a common contaminant of water systems, positive cultures for this organism should be interpreted with caution (232,236). Infections due to *M. xenopi* are uncommon in the United States (13,128,232,236), but may cause slowly progressive pulmonary disease in western Europe (13,238,239). In southeast England, *M. xenopi* was the most common NTM recovered since 1977 (240). *M. xenopi* may cause disseminated infections in patients with AIDS (138,241) and in other immunocompromised populations (242,243). A nosocomial outbreak of *M. xenopi* in immunocompetent patients was described (233). Pulmonary infections may give rise to nodules, mass-like, or cavitary lesions (233). Cavitary pneumonia due to *M. xenopi* was cited in a heart transplant recipient (244). Pulmonary infections due to *M. xenopi* have also been cited among renal transplant recipients (245–247). Doucette et al. implicated *M. xenopi* in 6 of 276 NTM infections in transplant recipients (3).

## Incidence of NTM Among Organ Transplant Recipients

### Bone Marrow or Stem Cell Transplants

The incidence of NTM infection among HSCT recipients ranges from 0.4% to 4.9% (3,27,29,30,248,249). A retrospective review of 2241 BMT recipients at the University of Minnesota identified 23 cases of infections due to NTM (1%) (27). Another series reported 40 infections due to NTM among 6259 HSCTs (0.64%) (249). All 23 catheter-related infections were due to rapid growers. One series in New York City from 1993 to 2001 identified 50 NMT infections (presumed or definite) among 571 HSCTs (incidence 8.7%) but this may reflect environmental exposure (250). Of 16 "definite" MBIs, 9 were caused by *M. haemophilum* (250). A survey of 29 European Bone Marrow Transplant Centers from 1994 to 1998 detected infections due to NTMs in 11 of 4525 HSCTs (0.26%) (30). In a comprehensive review of the literature, Doucette et al. detected 93 cases of NTM infections among HSCT recipients; the most common sites of involvement were: central venous catheter-related (37%); lung (30%); cutaneous disease (18%); disseminated disease (12%) (3). The most frequently isolated organisms were: MAC ($n = 26$); *M. haemophilum* ($n = 22$); *M. fortuitum* ($n = 15$); *M. chelonae* ($n = 12$); *M. abscessus* ($n = 11$). MAC and/or *M. avium* were most often associated with pulmonary or disseminated disease whereas the rapid growers (e.g., *M. fortuitum, M. abscessus, M. chelonae*) were predominantly associated with catheter-related infections (3).

### Heart Transplant Recipients

The incidence of NTM infection among heart transplant recipients ranges from 0.24% (251) to 2.8% (48). Novick et al detected 14 cases of NTM over a 17-year period among 502 cardiac transplant recipients (2.8%); isolates included MAC ($n = 6$); *M. kansasii* ($n = 5$); other ($n = 3$) (48). Risk factors for NTM included precyclosporine immunosuppression and high rates of rejection (48). The mean time to development of NTM infections was 3.5 years. Although treatment was often complicated, only one patient died as a result of NTM. Another series of 814 heart transplant recipients identified no cases of NTM (46). A comprehensive review in 2004 identified only 34 published cases of NTM infections among heart transplant recipients (3). The most common isolates were: *M. kansasii* ($n = 12$); MAC/MAI ($n = 8$); *M. haemophilum* ($n = 5$) ; *M. chelonae* ($n = 2$); *M. scrofulaceum* ($n = 2$) (3). Most common sites of infections included: skin ($n = 10$); lung($n = 9$); disseminated ($n = 8$). Additional cases of MBIs among heart transplant recipients due to various NTMs included: *M. haemophilum* (180,183,184); *M. kansasii* (5); MAC (44); *M. xenopi* (244); *M. chelonae* (252,253); *M. scrofulaceum* (208); others (254,255)

## Hepatic Transplant Recipients

Data regarding NTM infections complicating hepatic transplantation are sparse (3–5). In their 2004 review, Doucette et al. (3) found only eight published cases of NTM infections among liver transplant recipients (165,166,256–259). Responsible organisms included: MAC (257,258); *M. chelonae* (165); *M. chelonae-abscessus* (166); *M. triplex* (259).

## Kidney Transplant Recipients

The incidence of NTM complicating renal transplantation ranges from 0.2% to 0.6% (3,17,21,22,62,260–263). In their 2004 review, Doucette et al. identified a total of 94 published cases of NTM infections among renal transplant recipients (3). Cutaneous (localized or disseminated) sites predominated; pleuropulmonary involvement was present in 10 patients (11%). The most common isolates were: *M. chelonae* ($n = 21$); *M. kansasii* ($n = 21$) ; *M. haemophilum* ($n = 13$); *M. fortuitum* ($n = 9$). Anecdotal cases of NTM among renal transplant recipients include: *M. abscessus* (163); *M. marinum* (149,200); *M. kansasii* and *M. fortuitum* (62).

## Lung Transplant Recipients

Data regarding NTM among lung or heart–lung transplant recipients are limited to one series comprising 23 cases (70), a few retrospective reviews (71,73), one comprehensive review (3), and isolated case reports (148,201 264–268). In 1989, Trulock described an infection due to *M. chelonae* in a heart–lung transplant recipient with obliterative bronchiolitis (OB) (264). Baldi et al. described a LTR with a wound infection due to *M. fortuitum* 1 month posttransplantation (265). In a retrospective review, mycobacteria were identified in 8 of 210 LTRs (3.8%) (71). Isolates included NTM in six, and *M. tuberculosis* in two. Treatment was initiated in five of six patients with NTM, but only one patient with NTM developed clinical infection (due to M. *chelonae*). Analysis of infections complications among 59 LTRs detected three isolates of mycobacteria following transplantation (73). Only one (*M. tuberculosis*) was associated with clinical infection. The others (*M. gordonae* and *M. scrofulaceum*) were identified after OB was diagnosed and were not associated with clinical symptoms; neither required treatment. In 1999, a retrospective review of 261 lung and heart–lung transplant recipients from Australia over a 12-year period detected 25 cases of MB Is (9%), which included NTM in 23 and *M. tuberculosis* in two patients (70). Sites of involvement included: lung, 19 (76%); extrapulmonary, six (24%). Isolates of NTM included: MAC ($n = 13$); *M. haemophilum* ($n = 5$); *M. abscessus*

($n = 3$); *M. kansasii* ($n = 1$); *M. asiaticum* ($n = 1$). Mean time to diagnosis from transplantation was 677 days (range 2–3086 days). Three episodes of transient colonization with *M. avium* were not treated; the remaining 22 (88%) were treated. Initial therapy for NTM included clarithromycin, rifampicin, ciprofloxacin, and/or ethambutol. All six cutaneous lesions resolved completely; 11 of 16 (69%) pulmonary infections improved with therapy. There were no deaths attributable to mycobacteriosis. In 2004, Doucette et al. reported a case of disseminated MAC in a LTR (3) and identified a total of 22 previously published cases of NTM infections among LTRs (70,71,148,201,265–268). Sites of involvement included: pleuropulmonary ($n = 12$); local cutaneous ($n = 6$); disseminated ($n = 2$); empyema or thoracotomy wound ($n = 2$) (3). The median time to onset of infection was 14.8 months (3). One of us (BMK) previously reported empyema in a LTR due to *M. abscessus* (148). Interestingly, one LTR developed subcutaneous infection due to *M. marinum* following exposure of a superficial hand burn to fish tank water (201). This was cured following surgical excision of granulomatous nodules and prolonged (12 months) antimicrobial therapy.

### Clinical Features of NTM Infections

Clinical manifestations of NTM infections are protean and include: localized or disseminated cutaneous infections (3); pulmonary involvement (244); wound infections (201); intestinal involvement (251). CT scans may be invaluable in detecting localized disease, which may be amenable to biopsy and microbiological sampling (3).

### Diagnostic Testing

The diagnosis of infections due to NTM may be difficult (13), and heightened suspicion is required. A definite diagnosis of NTM is made by isolating the causative organism from cultures *in the appropriate clinical context.* Growth of NTM in culture(s) does not necessarily indicate infection, as colonization or laboratory contamination can occur (13). However, isolation of NTM in severely immunocompromised hosts (e.g., transplant recipients) warrants an aggressive diagnostic evaluation and often, empirical institution of therapy. Biopsy and cultures of skin, subcutaneous lesions, vascular catheter sites, or surgical wounds may establish the diagnosis (3). The diagnosis of catheter-related NTM infections can often be made by routine blood cultures (3). However, mycobacterial isolator blood cultures should be used when NTM infections are considered (3). Recovery of NTM from sputum requires inoculation onto one or more solid media *and* into a liquid medium (3,13). Cultures of NTE require specialized techniques (269,270) and may take up to eight weeks for identification (13). Molecular biological techniques [e.g., polymerase chain reaction (PCR), reverse hybridization assays, DNA probes, selective growth inhibitors, etc] (271–276) may allow more rapid identification of the species. Because of differing growth requirements of different species of NTM, the laboratory should be informed as to the suspected pathogen. Mycobacterial species share common antigens (including with *M. tuberculosis*) but skin tests for NTM are not specific or commercially available (13,277).

### Treatment

Treatment of NTM needs to be individualized depending upon the species, site of infections, and degree of immunosuppression. In general, treatment of NTM disease requires the use of combinations of antimicrobial agents for prolonged periods (6 to 24 months) (3). Whenever possible, reduction of immunosuppressive therapy should be considered (3). The choice of antimicrobial agents is similar for immunocompetent and immunocompromised patients (3,13). The role of susceptibility testing for NTM is controversial, and is reviewed in detail elsewhere (13). American Thoracic Society guidelines did not recommend routine susceptibility testing for *M. avium* but advised testing for rifampin susceptibility for *M. kansasii* (13).

### Drug Interactions and Toxicities

Macrolides have significant drug interactions with CNIs or sirolimus (3). Further, rifampin (and to a lesser degree rifabutin) induces cytochrome P450 enzymes, thereby reducing levels of CNI which may precipitate allograft rejection (1). Regardless of agents utilized, careful and frequent monitoring of drug levels is essential.

### Treatment of *Mycobacterium avium*-Intracellulare Complex

Newer macrolides (e.g., clarithromycin and azithromycin) have excellent clinical and microbiological activity against MAC (278–280). The treatment regimen for MAC disease advocated by the ATS includes: daily clarithromycin (or azithromycin), rifampin (or rifabutin), and ethambutol for a minimum of 18 months (13). Intermittent streptomycin (for the first two to three months) may be added to the aforementioned above regimen for extensive disease (13).

### Treatment of *Mycobacterium kansasii*

Most isolates of *M. kansasii* are inhibited by rifampin (or ribabutin), INH, EME, ethionamide, streptomycin, clarithromycin, amikacin, and the newer fluoroquinolone (FQs) (278). Treatment advocated by the ATS for pulmonary or extrapulmonary infections due to *M. kansasii* includes INH, RTF, and ethambutol for a minimum of 18 months (13). For patients intolerant of one of those three drugs, clarithromycin can be substituted (13). Acquired resistance to RIF, EMB, and INH has been noted among treatment failures (281,282). Patients with rifampin resistance should be treated with high dose INH (900 mg/day), pyridoxine (50 mg/day), high dose ethambutol (25 mg/kg/day), and sulfamethoxazole (13). Intermittent aminoglycosides (amikacin or streptomycin) or FQs may be utilized in selected patients (13).

Treatment of *Mycobacterium haemophilum*

Antimicrobial susceptibilities of *M. haemophilum* are variable. The most active agents include rifamycins, macrolides, FQs, clofazamine, and amikacin (131,145,184,280,282,283). Isoniazid, EMB, or PZA are not active (145). Initial empirical combination therapy with rifampin (or rifabutin) *plus* clarithromycin plus ciprofloxacin is reasonable. For sicker patients, amikacin may be added (145). For immunocompromised patients, a prolonged course (≥12 months) of therapy is recommended.

Rapid-Growing Mycobacteria

Rapid-growing NTMs (e.g., *M. chetonae, M. abscessus, M. fortuitum*) are generally resistant to antituberculous agents (13), but are susceptible (especially *M. fortuitum*) to a variety of traditional antibacterial agents (e.g., amikacin, cefoxitin, ciprofloxacin, clarithomycin, doxycycline, imipenem, sulfonamides) (143,284,285). Treatment of NTM due to RGM should be based on *in vitro* susceptibility tests (13). Combination therapy with at least two active agents for 6 to 12 months is advocated (13). *M. fortuitum* is often susceptible to multiple oral antibiotics including the newer macrolides, FQs, doxycycline, and sulfonamides (13,284). By contrast, *M. abscessus* is often susceptible only to amikacin, cefoxitin, and imipenem, and the newer macrolides (13). Severe cases due to *M. fortuitum* or *M. abscessus* may require high-dose amikacin combined with cefoxitin (13). Imipenem may be active against isolates resistant to cefoxitin (13). Surgical resection may be necessary for localized disease refractory to or intolerant of drug therapy (13).

Other Mycobacteria

For other slow-growing NTM (e.g., *M. malmoense, M. xenopi, M. szulgai*), the ATS recommends susceptibility testing to five drugs (i.e., INH, RIF, EMB, clarithromycin, and ciprofloxacin) (13). The most active agents against *M. malmoense* are RIF and EMB (196). Combination therapy with four drugs (e.g., INH, RIF, EMB, and clarithromycin) for 18 to 24 months has been efficacious (13,134,191). Standard antituberculous therapy may be efficacious for *M. xenopi* (233). Combination regimens employing clarithromycin, rifampin (or rifabutin) and EMB plus or minus streptomycin) have been advocated (13). Data regarding therapy for *M. szulgai* are limited, but combination therapy with RIF, high concentrations of INH, streptomycin, and EMB may be efficacious (13). Treatment of infections due to *M. gordonae* is not clear (167), but the most active agents are RTF, EMB, macrolides, and FQs (170,173). For infections due to *M. simiae,* the newer macrolides, FQs, EMB, clofazamine, and aminoglycosides are the most active agents (209). *M. marinum* isolates are usually susceptible to RIF, EMB, clarithromycin, and sulfonamides but are resistant to INH and PZA (13). Treatment with clarithromycin, minocycline (or doxycycline) (286) Trimethoprim–sulfamethoxazole (287) (all twice daily), or RIP plus EMB (once daily) (13) may be administered, for a minimum of three months. Surgical debridement or resection is required in some cases (198).

## REFERENCES

1. Singh N, Paterson DL. *Mycobacterium tuberculosis* infection in solid-organ transplant recipients: impact and implications for management. Clin Infect Dis 1998; 27(5):1266–1277.
2. John GT, Shankar V. Mycobacterial infections in organ transplant recipients. Semin Respir Infect 2002; 17(4):274–283.
3. Doucette K, Fishman JA. Nontuberculous mycobacterial infection in hematopoietic stem cell and solid organ transplant recipients. Clin Infect Dis 2004; 38(10):1428–1439.
4. Patel R, Paya CV. Infections in solid-organ transplant recipients. Clin Microbiol Rev 1997; 10(1):86–124.
5. Patel R, Roberts GD, Keating MR, Paya CV. Infections due to nontuberculous mycobacteria in kidney, heart, and liver transplant recipients. Clin Infect Dis 1994; 19(2):263–273.
6. Munoz P, Rodriguez C, Bouza E. Mycobacterium tuberculosis infection in recipients of solid organ transplants. Clin Infect Dis 2005; 40(4):581–587.
7. Winthrop KL, Kubak BM, Pegues DA, et al. Transmission of *mycobacterium tuberculosis* via lung transplantation. Am J Transplant 2004; 4(9):1529–1533.
8. Miller RA, Lanza LA, Kline JN, Geist LJ. Mycobacterium tuberculosis in lung transplant recipients. Am J Respir Crit Care Med 1995; 152(1): 374–376.
9. Schulman LL, Scully B, McGregor CC, Austin JH. Pulmonary tuberculosis after lung transplantation. Chest 1997; 111(5):1459–1462.
10. Ridgeway AL, Warner GS, Phillips P, et al. Transmission of *Mycobacterium tuberculosis* to recipients of single lung transplants from the same donor. Am J Respir Crit Care Med 1996; 153(3):1166–1168.
11. Lattes R, Radisic M, Rial M, Argento J, Casadei D. Tuberculosis in renal transplant recipients. Transpl Infect Dis 1999; 1(2):98–104.
12. Kiuchi T, Tanaka K, Inomata Y, et al. Experience of tacrolimus-based immunosuppression in living-related liver transplantation complicated with graft tuberculosis: interaction with rifampicin and side effects. Transplant Proc 1996; 28(6):3171–3172.
13. Diagnosis and treatment of disease caused by nontuberculous mycobacteria. This official statement of the American Thoracic Society was approved by the Board of Directors, March 1997. Medical Section of the American Lung Association. Am J Respir Crit Care Med 1997; 156(2 Pt 2):S1–S25.
14. Wolinsky E. Mycobacterial diseases other than tuberculosis. Clin Infect Dis 1992; 15(1):1–10.
15. Wolinsky E. Nontuberculous mycobacteria and associated diseases. Am Rev Respir Dis 1979; 119(1):107–159.

16. Meyers BR, Halpern M, Sheiner P, Mendelson MH, Neibart E, Miller C. Tuberculosis in liver transplant patients. Transplantation 1994; 58(3):301–306.
17. Lichtenstein IH, MacGregor RR. Mycobacterial infections in renal transplant recipients: report of five cases and review of the literature. Rev Infect Dis 1983; 5(2):216–226.
18. Aguado JM, Herrero JA, Gavalda J, et al. Clinical presentation and outcome of tuberculosis in kidney, liver, and heart transplant recipients in Spain. Spanish Transplantation Infection Study Group, GESITRA. Transplantation 1997; 63(9):1278–1286.
19. John GT, Shankar V, Abraham AM, Mukundan U, Thomas PP, Jacob CK. Risk factors for posttransplant tuberculosis. Kidney Int 2001; 60(3):1148–1153.
20. Apaydin S, Altiparmak MR, Serdengecti K, Ataman R, Ozturk R, Erek E. *Mycobacterium tuberculosis* infections after renal transplantation. Scand J Infect Dis 2000; 32(5):501–505.
21. Qunibi WY, al-Sibai MB, Taher S, et al. Mycobacterial infection after renal transplantation—report of 14 cases and review of the literature. Q J Med 1990; 77(282):1039–1060.
22. Hall CM, Willcox PA, Swanepoel CR, Kahn D, Van Zyl Smit R. Mycobacterial infection in renal transplant recipients. Chest 1994; 106(2):435–439.
23. Sakhuja V, Jha V, Varma PP, Joshi K, Chugh KS. The high incidence of tuberculosis among renal transplant recipients in India. Transplantation 1996; 61(2):211–215.
24. Naqvi SA, Hussain M, Askari H, et al. Is there a place for prophylaxis against tuberculosis following renal transplantation? Transplant Proc 1992; 24(5):1912.
25. Benito N, Sued O, Moreno A, et al. Diagnosis and treatment of latent tuberculosis infection in liver transplant recipients in an endemic area. Transplantation 2002; 74(10):1381–1386.
26. Atasever A, Bacakoglu F, Toz H, et al. Tuberculosis in renal transplant recipients on various immunosuppressive regimens. Nephrol Dial Transplant 2005; 20(4):797–802.
27. Roy V, Weisdorf D. Mycobacterial infections following bone marrow transplantation: a 20 year retrospective review. Bone Marrow Transplant 1997; 19(5):467–470.
28. Ip MS, Yuen KY, Woo PC, et al. Risk factors for pulmonary tuberculosis in bone marrow transplant recipients. Am J Respir Crit Care Med 1998; 158(4):1173–1177.
29. Navari RM, Sullivan KM, Springmeyer SC, et al. Mycobacterial infections in marrow transplant patients. Transplantation 1983; 36(5):509–513.
30. Cordonnier C, Martino R, Trabasso P, et al. Mycobacterial infection: a difficult and late diagnosis in stem cell transplant recipients. Clin Infect Dis 2004; 38(9):1229–1236.
31. Rouleau M, Senik A, Leroy E, Vernant JP. Long-term persistence of transferred PPD-reactive T cells after allogeneic bone marrow transplantation. Transplantation 1993; 55(1):72–76.
32. Hoyle C, Goldman JM. Life-threatening infections occurring more than 3 months after BMT. 18 UK Bone Marrow Transplant Teams. Bone Marrow Transplant 1994; 14(2):247–252.

33. Martino R, Martinez C, Brunet S, Sureda A, Lopez R, Domingo-Albos A. Tuberculosis in bone marrow transplant recipients: report of two cases and review of the literature. Bone Marrow Transplant 1996; 18(4):809–812.

34. de la Camara R, Martino R, Granados E, et al. Tuberculosis after hematopoietic stem cell transplantation: incidence, clinical characteristics and outcome. Spanish Group on Infectious Complications in Hematopoietic Transplantation. Bone Marrow Transplant 2000; 26(3):291–298.

35. Arslan O, Gurman G, Dilek I, et al. Incidence of tuberculosis after bone marrow transplantation in a single center from Turkey. Haematologia (Budap) 1998; 29(1):59–62.

36. Aljurf M, Gyger M, Alrajhi A, et al. *Mycobacterium tuberculosis* infection in allogeneic bone marrow transplantation patients. Bone Marrow Transplant 1999; 24(5):551–554.

37. Ku SC, Tang JL, Hsueh PR, Luh KT, Yu CJ, Yang PC. Pulmonary tuberculosis in allogeneic hematopoietic stem cell transplantation. Bone Marrow Transplant 2001; 27(12):1293–1297.

38. Chen CC, Huang LM, Chang YL, King CC, Lin KH. Acute respiratory distress syndrome due to tuberculosis in a child after allogeneic bone marrow transplantation for acute lymphoblastic leukemia. J Formos Med Assoc 1999; 98(10):701–704.

39. Ip MS, Yuen KY, Chiu EK, Chan JC, Lam WK, Chan TK. Pulmonary infections in bone marrow transplantation: the Hong Kong experience. Respiration 1995; 62(2):80–83.

40. Yuen KY, Woo PC. Tuberculosis in blood and marrow transplant recipients. Hematol Oncol 2002; 20(2):51–62.

41. Ozisik K, Kaptanoglu E, Okutan O, Dural K. Pott's disease after heart transplantation: a case report. Transplant Proc 2003; 35(4):1543–1545.

42. Gavilan F, Torre-Cisneros J, Vizcaino MA, et al. Clinical microbiological case: poor radiologic evolution of pulmonary tuberculosis in a heart transplant patient. Clin Microbiol Infect 2001; 7(7):367–368, 399–401.

43. Di Perri G, Luzzati R, Forni A, et al. Fatal primary multidrug-resistant tuberculosis in a heart transplant recipient. Transpl Int 1998; 11(4):305–307.

44. Tuder RM, Renya GS, Bensch K. Mycobacterial coronary arteritis in a heart transplant recipient. Hum Pathol 1986; 17(10):1072–1074.

45. Montoya JG, Giraldo LF, Efron B, et al. Infectious complications among 620 consecutive heart transplant patients at Stanford University Medical Center. Clin Infect Dis 2001; 33(5):629–640.

46. Miller LW, Naftel DC, Bourge RC, et al. Infection after heart transplantation: a multiinstitutional study. Cardiac Transplant Research Database Group. J Heart Lung Transplant 1994; 13(3):381–392; discussion 393.

47. Korner MM, Hirata N, Tenderich G, et al. Tuberculosis in heart transplant recipients. Chest 1997; 111(2):365–369.

48. Novick RJ, Moreno-Cabral CE, Stinson EB, et al. Nontuberculous mycobacterial infections in heart transplant recipients: a seventeen-year experience. J Heart Transplant 1990; 9(4):357–363.

49. Grossi P, De Maria R, Caroli A, Zaina MS, Minoli L. Infections in heart transplant recipients: the experience of the Italian heart transplantation

program. Italian Study Group on Infections in Heart Transplantation. J Heart Lung Transplant 1992; 11(5):847–866.

50. Cisneros JM, Munoz P, Torre-Cisneros J, et al. Pneumonia after heart transplantation: a multi-institutional study. Spanish Transplantation Infection Study Group. Clin Infect Dis 1998; 27(2):324–331.

51. Hsu RB, Fang CT, Chang SC, et al. Infectious complications after heart transplantation in chinese recipients. Am J Transplant 2005; 5(8):2011–2016.

52. Chou NK, Liu LT, Ko WJ, et al. Various clinical presentations of tuberculosis in heart transplant recipients. Transplant Proc 2004; 36(8):2396–2398.

53. Nishizaki T, Yanaga K, Soejima Y, et al. Tuberculosis following liver transplantation: report of a case and review of the literature. Transpl Int 1996; 9(6):589–592.

54. Henderson C, Meyers B, Humayun Gultekin S, Liu B, Zhang DY. Intracranial tuberculoma in a liver transplant patient: first reported case and review of the literature. Am J Transplant 2003; 3(1):88–93.

55. Botha JF, Spearman CW, Millar AJ, et al. Ten years of liver transplantation at Groote Schuur Hospital. S Afr Med J 2000; 90(9):880–883.

56. Meyers BR, Papanicolaou GA, Sheiner P, Emre S, Miller C. Tuberculosis in orthotopic liver transplant patients: increased toxicity of recommended agents; cure of disseminated infection with nonconventional regimens. Transplantation 2000; 69(1):64–69.

57. Singh N, Gayowski T, Wagener M, Marino IR, Yu VL. Pulmonary infections in liver transplant recipients receiving tacrolimus. Changing pattern of microbial etiologies. Transplantation 1996; 61(3):396–401.

58. Stoblen F, Neuhaus R, Neumann K, et al. Tuberculosis in liver transplant recipients: recurrence after transplantation? Transplant Proc 1994; 26(6):3604–3605.

59. Torre-Cisneros J, de la Mata M, Rufian S, et al. Importance of surveillance mycobacterial cultures after liver transplantation. Transplantation 1995; 60(9):1054–1055.

60. Klote MM, Agodoa LY, Abbott K. Mycobacterium tuberculosis infection incidence in hospitalized renal transplant patients in the United States, 1998–2000. Am J Transplant 2004; 4(9):1523–1528.

61. Jie T, Matas AJ, Gillingham KJ, Sutherland DE, Dunn DL, Humar A. Mycobacterial infections after kidney transplant. Transplant Proc 2005; 37(2): 937–939.

62. Queipo JA, Broseta E, Santos M, Sanchez-Plumed J, Budia A, Jimenez-Cruz F. Mycobacterial infection in a series of 1261 renal transplant recipients. Clin Microbiol Infect 2003; 9(6):518–525.

63. Melchor JL, Gracida C, Ibarra A. Increased frequency of tuberculosis in Mexican renal transplant recipients: a single-center experience. Transplant Proc 2002; 34(1):78–79.

64. Malhotra KK, Dash SC, Dhawan IK, Bhuyan UN, Gupta A. Tuberculosis and renal transplantation—observations from an endemic area of tuberculosis. Postgrad Med J 1986; 62(727):359–362.

65. Carlsen SE, Bergin CJ. Reactivation of tuberculosis in a donor lung after transplantation. AJR Am J Roentgenol 1990; 154(3):495–497.

66. Paciocco G, Martinez FJ, Kazerooni EA, Bossone E, Lynch JP III. Tuberculous pneumonia complicating lung transplantation: case report and review of the literature. Monaldi Arch Chest Dis 2000; 55(2):117–121.

67. Shitrit D, Bendayan D, Saute M, Kramer MR. Multidrug resistant tuberculosis following lung transplantation: treatment with pulmonary resection. Thorax 2004; 59(1):79–80.

68. Lee J, Yew WW, Wong CF, Wong PC, Chiu CS. Multidrug-resistant tuberculosis in a lung transplant recipient. J Heart Lung Transplant 2003; 22(10):1168–1173.

69. Higenbottam T, Stewart S, Penketh A, Wallwork J. Transbronchial lung biopsy for the diagnosis of rejection in heart–lung transplant patients. Transplantation 1988; 46(4):532–539.

70. Malouf MA, Glanville AR. The spectrum of mycobacterial infection after lung transplantation. Am J Respir Crit Care Med 1999; 160(5 Pt 1):1611–1616.

71. Kesten S, Chaparro C. Mycobacterial infections in lung transplant recipients. Chest 1999; 115(3):741–745.

72. Bravo C, Roldan J, Roman A, et al. Tuberculosis in lung transplant recipients. Transplantation 2005; 79(1):59–64.

73. Flume PA, Egan TM, Paradowski LJ, Detterbeck FC, Thompson JT, Yankaskas JR. Infectious complications of lung transplantation. Impact of cystic fibrosis. Am J Respir Crit Care Med 1994; 149(6):1601–1607.

74. Roman A, Bravo C, Levy G, et al. Isoniazid prophylaxis in lung transplantation. J Heart Lung Transplant 2000; 19(9):903–906.

75. Dromer C, Nashef SA, Velly JF, Martigne C, Couraud L. Tuberculosis in transplanted lungs. J Heart Lung Transplant 1993; 12(6 Pt 1):924–9277.

76. Dye C, Scheele S, Dolin P, Pathania V, Raviglione MC. Consensus statement. Global burden of tuberculosis: estimated incidence, prevalence, and mortality by country. WHO Global Surveillance and Monitoring Project. J Am Med Arsoc 1999; 282(7):677–686.

77. Espinal MA, Laszlo A, Simonsen L, et al. Global trends in resistance to antitubercuiosis drugs. World Health Organization—International Union against Tuberculosis and Lung Disease Working Group on Anti-Tuberculosis Drug Resistance Surveillance. N Engl J Med 2001; 344(17):1294–1303.

78. Cavusoglu C, Cicek-Saydam C, Karasu Z, et al. *Mycobacterium tuberculosis* infection and laboratory diagnosis in solid-organ transplant recipients. Clin Transplant 2002; 16(4):257–261.

79. Jonas V, Longiaru M. Detection of *Mycobacterium tuberculosis* by molecular methods. Clin Lab Med 1997; 17(1):119–128.

80. Lim TK, Mukhopadhyay A, Gough A, et al. Role of clinical judgment in the application of a nucleic acid amplification test for the rapid diagnosis of pulmonary tuberculosis. Chest 2003; 124(3):902–908.

81. Middleton AM, Cullinan P, Wilson R, Kerr JR, Chadwick MV. Interpreting the results of the amplified *Mycobacterium tuberculosis* direct test for detection of *M. tuberculosis rRNA*. J Clin Microbiol 2003; 41(6):2741–2743.

82. Schluger NW. Changing approaches to the diagnosis of tuberculosis. Am J Respir Crit Care Med 2001; 164(11):2020–2024.

83. Jereb JA, Burwen DR, Dooley SW, et al. Nosocomial outbreak of tuberculosis in a renal transplant unit: application of a new technique for restriction

fragment length polymorphism analysis of *Mycobacterium tuberculosis* isolates. Infect Dis 1993; 168(5):1219–1224.

84. Bouza E, Merino P, Munoz P, Sanchez-Carrillo C, Yanez J, Cortes C. Ocular tuberculosis. A prospective study in a general hospital. Medicine (Baltimore) 1997; 76(1):53–61.

85. Kukrej N, Cook GJ, Pattison JM. Positron-emission tomography used to diagnose tuberculosis in a renal transplant patient. Am J Transplant 2002; 2(1):105–107.

86. Hara T, Kosaka N, Suzuki T, Kudo K, Niino H. Uptake rates of 18F-fluorodeoxyglucose and 11C-choline in lung cancer and pulmonary tuberculosis: a positron emission tomography study. Chest 2003; 124(3):893–901.

87. Blumberg HM, Burman WJ, Chaisson RE, et al. American Thoracic Society/Centers for Disease Control and Prevention/Infectious Diseases Society of America: treatment of tuberculosis. Am J Respir Crit Care Med 2003; 167(4):603–662.

88. Horsburgh CR Jr, Feldman S, Ridzon R. Practice guidelines for the treatment of tuberculosis. Clin Infect Dis 2000; 31(3):633–639.

89. Bass JB Jr, Farer LS, Hopewell PC, et al. Treatment of tuberculosis and tuberculosis infection in adults and children. American Thoracic Society and The Centers for Disease Control and Prevention. Am J Respir Crit Care Med 1994; 149(5):1359–1374.

90. Weis SE, Slocum PC, Blais FX, et al. The effect of directly observed therapy on the rates of drug resistance and relapse in tuberculosis. N Engl J Med 1994; 330(17):1179–1184.

91. Iseman MD. Treatment of multidrug-resistant tuberculosis. N Engl J Med 1993; 329(11):784–791.

92. Yildiz A, Sever MS, Turkmen A, et al. Tuberculosis after renal transplantation: experience of one Turkish centre. Nephrol Dial Transplant 1998; 13(7):1872–1875.

93. Kunimoto D, Warman A, Beckon A, Doering D, Melenka L. Severe hepatotoxicity associated with rifampin–pyrazinamide preventative therapy requiring transplantation in an individual at low risk for hepatotoxicity. Clin Infect Dis 2003; 36(12):e158–e161.

94. Yee D, Valiquette C, Pelletier M, Parisien I, Rocher I, Menzies D. Incidence of serious side effects from first-line antituberculosis drugs among patients treated for active tuberculosis. Am J Respir Crit Care Med 2003; 167(11): 1472–1477.

95. McNeill L, Allen M, Estrada C, Cook P. Pyrazinamide and rifampin vs isoniazid for the treatment of latent tuberculosis: improved completion rates but more hepatotoxicity. Chest 2003; 123(1):102–106.

96. Paterson DL, Singh N. Interactions between tacrolimus and antimicrobial agents. Clin Infect Dis 1997; 25(6):1430–1440.

97. Modry DL, Stinson EB, Oyer PE, Jamieson SW, Baldwin JC, Shumway NE. Acute rejection and massive cyclosporine requirements in heart transplant recipients treated with rifampin. Transplantation 1985; 39(3):313–314.

98. Li AP, Reith MK, Rasmussen A, et al. Primary human hepatocytes as a tool for the evaluation of structure–activity relationship in cytochrome P450

induction potential of xenobiotics: evaluation of rifampin, rifapentine and rifabutin. Chem Biol Interact 1997; 107(1–2):17–30.

99.  Munoz P, Palomo J, Munoz R, Rodriguez-Creixems M, Pelaez T, Bouza E. Tuberculosis in heart transplant recipients. Clin Infect Dis 1995; 21(2):398–402.

100. Chugh KS, Jha V. Tuberculosis in organ transplant recipients. Transplant Proc 2003; 35(7):2676–2677.

101. Offermann G, Keller F, Molzahn M. Low cyclosporin A blood levels and acute graft rejection in a renal transplant recipient during rifampin treatment. Am J Nephrol 1985; 5(5):385–387.

102. Park YS, Choi JY, Cho CH, et al. Clinical outcomes of tuberculosis in renal transplant recipients. Yonsei Med J 2004; 45(5):865–872.

103. Gosling RD, Uiso LO, Sam NE, et al. The bactericidal activity of moxifloxacin in patients with pulmonary tuberculosis. Am J Respir Crit Care Med 2003; 168(11):1342–1345.

104. Jha V, Sakhuja V. Rifampicin sparing treatment protocols in posttransplant tuberculosis. Int Urol Nephrol 2004; 36(2):287–288.

105. O'Brien RJ. Development of fluoroquinolones as first-line drugs for tuberculosis—at long last!. Am J Respir Crit Care Med 2003; 168(11):1266–1268.

106. Jha V, Sakhuja V, Gupta D, et al. Successful management of pulmonary tuberculosis in renal allograft recipients in a single center. Kidney Int 1999; 56(5):1944–1950.

107. Goble M, Iseman MD, Madsen LA, Waite D, Ackerson L, Horsburgh CR Jr. Treatment of 171 patients with pulmonary tuberculosis resistant to isoniazid and rifampin. N Engl J Med 1993; 328(8):527–532.

108. Delmonico FL. Cadaver donor screening for infectious agents in solid organ transplantation. Clin infect Dis 2000; 31(3):781–786.

109. Schaffner A. Pretransplant evaluation for infections in donors and recipients of solid organs. Clin Infect Dis 2001; 33(Suppl 1):S9–S14.

110. Avery RK, Ljungman P. Prophylactic measures in the solid-organ recipient before transplantation. Clin Infect Dis 2001; 33(Suppl 1):S15–S21.

111. Avery RK. Recipient screening prior to solid-organ transplantation. Clin Infect Dis 2002; 35(12):1513–1519.

112. Torre-Cisneros J, Caston JJ, Moreno J, et al. Tuberculosis in the transplant candidate: importance of early diagnosis and treatment. Transplantation 2004; 77(9):1376–1380.

113. Slovis BS, Plitman JD, Haas DW. The case against anergy testing as a routine adjunct to tuberculin skin testing. J Am Med Assoc 2000; 283(15):2003–2007.

114. Squier CL, Goetz AM, Wagener MM, Muder RR. The anergy panel: an ineffective tool to validate tuberculin skin testing. Am J Infect Control 2004; 32(4):243–245.

115. Smirnoff M, Patt C, Seckler B, Adler JJ. Tuberculin and anergy skin testing of patients receiving long-term hemodialysis. Chest 1998; 113(1):25–27.

116. Woeltje KF, Mathew A, Rothstein M, Seiler S, Fraser VJ. Tuberculosis infection and anergy in hemodialysis patients. Am J Kidney Dis 1998; 31(5):848–852.

117. Jasmer RM, Nahid P, Hopewell PC. Clinical practice. Latent tuberculosis infection. N Engl J Med 2002; 347(23):1860–1866.

118. Mazurek GH, LoBue PA, Daley CL, et al. Comparison of a whole-blood interferon gamma assay with tuberculin skin testing for detecting latent *Mycobacterium tuberculosis* infection. J Am Med Assoc 2001; 286(14): 1740–1747.

119. From the Centers for Disease Control and Prevention. Update: fatal and severe liver injuries associated with rifampin and pyrazinamide for latent tuberculosis infection, and revisions in American Thoracic Society/CDC recommendations—United States, 2001. J Am Med Assoc 2001; 286(12): 1445–1446.

120. Update: adverse event data and revised American Thoracic Society/CDC recommendations against the use of rifampin and pyrazinamide for treatment of latent tuberculosis infection—United States, 2003. MMWR Morb Mortal Wkly Rep 2003; 52(31):735–739.

121. Schluger LK, Sheiner PA, Jonas M, et al. Isoniazid hepatotoxicity after orthotopic liver transplantation. Mt Sinai J Med 1996; 63(5–6):364–369.

122. Thomas PA Jr, Mozes MF, Jonasson O. Hepatic dysfunction during isoniazid chemoprophylaxis in renal allograft recipients. Arch Surg 1979; 114(5): 597–599.

123. Antony SJ, Ynares C, Dummer JS. Isoniazid hepatotoxicity in renal transplant recipients. Clin Transplant 1997; 11(1):34–37.

124. John GT, Thomas PP, Thomas M, Jeyaseelan L, Jacob CK, Shastry JC. A double-blind randomized controlled trial of primary isoniazid prophylaxis in dialysis and transplant patients. Transplantation 1994; 57(11):1683–1684.

125. Christianson LC, Dewlett HJ. Pulmonary disease in adults associated with unclassified mycobacteria. Am J Med 1960; 29:980–991.

126. Lewis AG Jr, Lasche EM, Armstrong AL, Dunbar FP. A clinical study of the chronic lung disease due to nonphotochromogenic acid-fast bacilli. Ann Intern Med 1960; 53:273–285.

127. Good RC, Snider DE Jr. Isolation of nontuberculous mycobacteria in the United States, 1980. J Infect Dis 1982; 146(6):829–833.

128. O'Brien RJ, Geiter LJ, Snider DE Jr. The epidemiology of nontuberculous mycobacterial diseases in the United States. Results from a national survey. Am Rev Respir Dis 1987; 135(5):1007–1014.

129. Horsburgh CR Jr, Mason UG, 3rd, Farhi DC, Iseman MD. Disseminated infection with *Mycobacterium avium*-intracellulare. A report of 13 cases and a review of the literature. Medicine (Baltimore) 1985; 64(1):36–48.

130. Horsburgh CR Jr, Selik RM. The epidemiology of disseminated nontuberculous mycobacterial infection in the acquired immunodeficiency syndrome (AIDS). Am Rev Respir Dis 1989; 139(1):4–7.

131. Saubolle MA, Kiehn TE, White MH, Rudinsky MF, Armstrong D. *Mycobacterium haemophilum*: microbiology and expanding clinical and geographic spectra of disease in humans. Clin Microbiol Rev 1996; 9(4):435–447.

132. Gouby A, Branger B, Oules R, Ramuz M. Two cases of *Mycobacterium haemophilum* infection in a renal-dialysis unit. J Med Microbiol 1988; 25(4):299–300.

133. Falkinham JO, III. Epidemiology of infection by nontuberculous mycobacteria. Clin Microbiol Rev 1996; 9(2):177–215.

134. Henriques B, Hoffner SE, Petrini B, Juhlin I, Wahlen P, Kallenius G. Infection with *Mycobacterium malmoense* in Sweden: report of 221 cases. Clin Infect Dis 1994; 18(4):596–600.

135. Hoover DR, Graham NM, Bacellar H, et al. An epidemiologic analysis of *Mycobacterium avium* complex disease in homosexual men infected with human immunodeficiency virus type 1. Clin Infect Dis 1995; 20(5):1250–1258.

136. Kalayjian RC, Toossi Z, Tomashefski JF Jr, et al. Pulmonary disease due to infection by *Mycobacterium avium* complex in patients with AIDS. Clin Infect Dis 1995; 20(5):1186–1194.

137. Hoover DR, Saah AJ, Bacellar H, et al. Clinical manifestations of AIDS in the era of pneumocystis prophylaxis. Multicenter AIDS Cohort Study. N Engl J Med 1993; 329(26):1922–1926.

138. Ausina V, Barrio J, Luquin M, et al. *Mycobacterium xenopi* infections in the acquired immunodeficiency syndrome. Ann Intern Med 1988; 109(11): 927–928.

139. Rodriguez-Barradas MC, Clarridge J, Darouiche R. Disseminated *Mycobacterium fortuitum* disease in an AIDS patient. Am J Med 1992; 93(4):473–474.

140. Chocarra A, Gonzalez Lopez A, Breznes MF, Canut A, Rodriguez J, Diego JM. Disseminated infection due to *Mycobacterium malmoense* in a patient infected with human immunodeficiency virus. Clin Infect Dis 1994; 19(1):203–204.

141. Hellinger WC, Smilack JD, Greider JL Jr, et al. Localized soft-tissue infections with *Mycobacterium avium/Mycobacterium intracellulare* complex in immuno-competent patients: granulomatous tenosynovitis of the hand or wrist. Clin Infect Dis 1995; 21(1):65–69.

142. Cooper JF, Lichtenstein MJ, Graham BS, Schaffner W. *Mycobacterium chelonae*: a cause of nodular skin lesions with a proclivity for renal transplant recipients. Am J Med 1989; 86(2):173–177.

143. Wallace RJ Jr, Brown BA, Onyi GO. Skin, soft tissue, and bone infections due to *Mycobacterium chelonae chelonae*: importance of prior corticosteroid therapy, frequency of disseminated infections, and resistance to oral antimicrobials other than clarithromycin. J Infect Dis 1992; 166(2):405–412.

144. Kiehn TE, White M. *Mycobacterium haemophilum*: an emerging pathogen. Eur J Clin Microbiol Infect Dis 1994; 13(11):925–931.

145. Shah MK, Sebti A, Kiehn TE, Massarella SA, Sepkowitz KA. *Mycobacterium haemophilum* in immunocompromised patients. Clin Infect Dis 2001; 33(3):330–337.

146. Chester AC, Winn WC Jr. Unusual and newly recognized patterns of nontuberculous mycobacterial infection with emphasis on the immunocompromised host. Pathol Annu 1986; 21(Pt 1):251–270.

147. Fairhurst RM, Kubak BM, Pegues DA, et al. *Mycobacterium haemophilum* infections in heart transplant recipients: case report and review of the literature. Am J Transplant 2002; 2(5):476–479.

148. Fairhurst RM, Kubak BM, Shpiner RB, Levine MS, Pegues DA, Ardehali A. *Mycobacterium abscessus* empyema in a lung transplant recipient. J Heart Lung Transplant 2002; 21(3):391–394.

149. Farooqui MA, Berenson C, Lohr JW. *Mycobacterium marinum* infection in a renal transplant recipient. Transplantation 1999; 67(11):1495–1496.
150. Stelzmueller I, Dunst KM, Wiesmayr S, Zangerie R, Hengster P, Bonatti H. *Mycobacterium chelonae* skin infection in kidney–pancreas recipient. Emerg Infect Dis 2005; 11(2):352–354.
151. Phillips MS, von Reyn CF. Nosocomial infections due to nontuberculous mycobacteria. Clin Infect Dis 2001; 33(8):1363–1374.
152. Reich JM, Johnson RE. *Mycobacterium avium* complex pulmonary disease presenting as an isolated lingular or middle lobe pattern. The Lady Windermere syndrome. Chest 1992; 101(6):1605–1609.
153. Hartman TE, Swensen SJ, Williams DE. *Mycobacterium avium–intracellulare* complex: evaluation with CT. Radiology 1993; 187(1):23–26.
154. Primack SL, Logan PM, Hartman TE, Lee KS, Muller NL. Pulmonary tuberculosis and *Mycobacterium avium–intracellulare*: a comparison of CT findings. Radiology 1995; 194(2):413–417.
155. Oliver A, Maiz L, Canton R, Escobar H, Baquero F, Gomez-Mampaso E. Nontuberculous mycobacteria in patients with cystic fibrosis. Clin Infect Dis 2001; 32(9):1298–1303.
156. Wallace RJ Jr, Swenson JM, Silcox VA, Good RC, Tschen JA, Stone MS. Spectrum of disease due to rapidly growing mycobacteria. Rev Infect Dis 1983; 5(4):657–679.
157. Clegg HW, Foster MT, Sanders WE Jr, Baine WB. Infection due to organisms of the Mycobacterium fortuitum complex after augmentation mammaplasty: clinical and epidemiologic features. J Infect Dis 1983; 147(3):427–433.
158. Safranek TJ, Jarvis WR, Carson LA, et al. *Mycobacterium chelonae* wound infections after plastic surgery employing contaminated gentian violet skin-marking solution. N Engl J Med 1987; 317(4):197–201.
159. Lowry PW, Jarvis WR, Oberle AD, et al. *Mycobacterium chelonae* causing otitis media in an ear-nose-and-throat practice. N Engl J Med 1988; 319(15):978–982.
160. Hoffman PC, Fraser DW, Robicsek F, O'Bar PR, Mauney CU. Two outbreaks of sternal wound infection due to organisms of the *Mycobacterium fortuitum* complex. J Infect Dis 1981; 143(4):533–542.
161. Wallace RJ Jr, Musser JM, Hull SI, et al. Diversity and sources of rapidly growing mycobacteria associated with infections following cardiac surgery. J Infect Dis 1989; 159(4):708–716.
162. Bolan G, Reingold AL, Carson LA, et al. Infections with *Mycobacterium chelonei* in patients receiving dialysis and using processed hemodialyzers. J Infect Dis 1985; 152(5):1013–1019.
163. Prinz BM, Michaelis S, Kettelhack N, Mueller B, Burg G, Kempf W. Subcutaneous infection with *Mycobacterium abscessus* in a renal transplant recipient. Dermatology 2004; 208(3):259–261.
164. Griffith DE, Girard WM, Wallace RJ Jr. Clinical features of pulmonary disease caused by rapidly growing mycobacteria. An analysis of 154 patients. Am Rev Respir Dis 1993; 147(5):1271–1278.
165. Nathan DL, Singh S, Kestenbaum TM, Casparian JM. Cutaneous *Mycobacterium chelonae* in a liver transplant patient. J Am Acad Dermatol 2000; 43(2 Pt 2):333–336.

166. Chastain MA, Buckley J, Russo GG. *Mycobacterium chelonae/abscessus* complex infection in a liver transplant patient. Int J Dermatol 2001; 40(12): 769–774.

167. Eckburg PB, Buadu EO, Stark P, Sarinas PS, Chitkara RK, Kuschner WG. Clinical and chest radiographic findings among persons with sputum culture positive for *Mycobacterium gordonae*: a review of 19 cases. Chest 2000; 117(1):96–102.

168. Bonnet E, Massip P, Bauriaud R, Alric L, Auvergnat JC. Disseminated *Mycobacterium gordonae* infection in a patient infected with human immunodeficiency virus. Clin Infect Dis 1996; 23(3):644–645.

169. Bernard E, Michiels JF, Pinier Y, Bourdet JF, Dellamonica P. Disseminated infection as a result of *Mycobacterium gordonae* in an AIDS patient. Aids 1992; 6(10):1217–1218.

170. Weinberger M, Berg SL, Feuerstein IM, Pizzo PA, Witebsky FG. Disseminated infection with *Mycobacterium gordonae*: report of a case and critical review of the literature. Clin Infect Dis 1992; 14(6):1229–1239.

171. Lessnau KD, Milanese S, Talavera W. *Mycobacterium gordonae*: a treatable disease in HIV-positive patients. Chest 1993; 104(6):1779–1785.

172. Neuman HB, Andreoni KA, Johnson MW, Fair JH, Gerber DA. Terminal ileitis secondary to *Mycobacterium gordonae* in a renal transplant. Transplantation 2003; 75(4):574–575.

173. den Broeder AA, Vervoort G, van Assen S, Verduyn Lunel F, de Lange WC, de Sevaux RG. Disseminated *Mycobacterium gordonae* infection in a renal transplant recipient. Transpl Infect Dis 2003; 5(3):151–155.

174. Aguado JM, Gomez-Garces JL, Manrique A, Soriano F. Pulmonary infection by *Mycobacterium gordonae* in an immunocompromised patient. Diagn Microbiol Infect Dis 1987; 7(4):261–263.

175. Resch B, Eber E, Beitzke A, Bauer C, Zach M. Pulmonary infection due to *Mycobacterium gordonae* in an adolescent immunocompetent patient. Respiration 1997; 64(4):300–303.

176. Marchevsky A, Damsker B, Gribetz A, Tepper S, Geller SA. The spectrum of pathology of nontuberculous mycobacterial infections in open-lung biopsy specimens. Am J Clin Pathol 1982; 78(5):695–700.

177. Straus WL, Ostroff SM, Jernigan DB, et al. Clinical and epidemiologic characteristics of Mycobacterium haemophilum, an emerging pathogen in immunocompromised patients. Ann Intern Med 1994; 120(2):118–125.

178. Armstrong KL, James RW, Dawson DJ, Francis PW, Masters B. *Mycobacterium haemophilum* causing perihilar or cervical lymphadenitis in healthy children. J Pediatr 1992; 121(2):202–205.

179. Samra Z, Kaufmann L, Zeharia A, et al. Optimal detection and identification of *Mycobacterium haemophilum* in specimens from pediatric patients with cervical lymphadenopathy. J Clin Microbiol 1999; 37(3):832–834.

180. Lederman C, Spitz JL, Scully B, et al. *Mycobacterium haemophilum* cellulitis in a heart transplant recipient. J Am Acad Dermatol 1994; 30(5 Pt 1):804–806.

181. White MH, Papadopoulos EB, Small TN, Kiehn TE, Armstrong D. *Mycobacterium haemophilum* infections in bone marrow transplant recipients. Transplantation 1995; 60(9):957–960.

182. Ward MS, Lam KV, Cannell PK, Herrmann RP. Mycobacterial central venous catheter tunnel infection: a difficult problem. Bone Marrow Transplant 1999; 24(3):325–329.

183. Zappe CH, Barlow D, Zappe H, Bolton IJ, Roditi D, Steyn LM. 16S rRNA sequence analysis of an isolate of *Mycobacterium haemophilum* from a heart transplant patient. J Med Microbiol 1995; 43(3):189–191.

184. Plemmons RM, McAllister CK, Garces MC, Ward RL. Osteomyelitis due to *Mycobacterium haemophilum* in a cardiac transplant patient: case report and analysis of interactions among clarithromycin, rifampin, and cyclosporine. Clin Infect Dis 1997; 24(5):995–997.

185. Cooper DK, Lanza RP, Oliver S, et al. Infectious complications after heart transplantation. Thorax 1983; 38(11):822–828.

186. Branger B, Gouby A, Oules R, et al. *Mycobacterium haemophilum* and *Mycobacterium xenopi* associated infection in a renal transplant patient. Clin Nephrol 1985; 23(1):46–49.

187. Dawson DJ, Jennis F. Mycobacteria with a growth requirement for ferric ammonium citrate, identified as *Mycobacterium haemophilum*. J Clin Microbiol 1980; 11(2):190–192.

188. Kikuchi K, Bernard EM, Kiehn TE, Armstrong D, Riley LW. Restriction fragment length polymorphism analysis of clinical isolates of *Mycobacterium haemophilum*. J Clin Microbiol 1994; 32(7):1763–1767.

189. Sherer R, Sable R, Sonnenberg M, et al. Disseminated infection with *Mycobacterium kansasii* in the acquired immunodeficiency syndrome. Ann Intern Med 1986; 105(5):710–712.

190. Buchholz UT, McNeil MM, Keyes LE, Good RC. *Mycobacterium malmoense* infections in the United States, January 1993 through June 1995. Clin Infect Dis 1998; 27(3):551–558.

191. Banks J, Jenkins PA, Smith AP. Pulmonary infection with *Mycobacterium malmoense*—a review of treatment and response. Tubercle 1985; 66(3): 197–203.

192. Pulmonary disease caused by *M. malmoense* in HIV negative patients: 5-yr follow-up of patients receiving standardised treatment. Eur Respir J 2003; 21(3):478–482.

193. Lamden K, Watson JM, Knerer G, Ryan MJ, Jenkins PA. Opportunist myco-bacteria in England and Wales: 1982 to 1994. Commun Dis Rep CDR Rev 1996; 6(11):R147–R151.

194. Saito H, Tomioka H, Sato K, Tasaka H, Dekio S. *Mycobacterium malmoense* isolated from soil. Microbiol Immunol 1994; 38(4):313–315.

195. Portaels F, Larsson L, Jenkins PA. Isolation of *Mycobacterium malmoense* from the environment in Zaire. Tuber Lung Dis 1995; 76(2):160–162.

196. Zaugg M, Salfinger M, Opravil M, Luthy R. Extrapulmonary and dissemi-nated infections due to *Mycobacterium malmoense*: case report and review. Clin Infect Dis 1993; 16(4):540–549.

197. Claydon EJ, Coker RJ, Harris JR. *Mycobacterium malmoense* infection in HIV positive patients. J Infect 1991; 23(2):191–194.

198. Collins CH, Grange JM, Noble WC, Yates MD. *Mycobacterium marinum* infections in man. J Hyg (Lond) 1985; 94(2):135–149.

199. Ries KM, White GL Jr, Murdock RT. Atypical mycobacterial infection caused by *Mycobacterium marinum*. N Engl J Med 1990; 322(9):633.
200. Gombert ME, Goldstein EJ, Corrado ML, Stein AJ, Butt KM. Disseminated *Mycobacterium marinum* infection after renal transplantation. Ann Intern Med 1981; 94(4 pt 1):486–487.
201. Torres F, Hodges T, Zamora MR. *Mycobacterium marinum* infection in a lung transplant recipient. J Heart Lung Transplant 2001; 20(4):486–489.
202. Hautmann G, Lotti T. Diseases caused by *Mycobacterium scrofulaceum*. Clin Dermatol 1995; 13(3):277–280.
203. Kirschner RA Jr, Parker BC, Falkinham JO III. Epidemiology of infection by nontuberculous mycobacteria. *Mycobacterium avium, Mycobacterium intracellulare*, and *Mycobacterium scrofulaceum* in acid, brown-water swamps of the southeastern United States and their association with environmental variables. Am Rev Respir Dis 1992; 145(2 Pt 1):271–275.
204. Haverkamp MH, Arend SM, Lindeboom JA, Hartwig NG, van Dissel JT. Nontuberculous mycobacterial infection in children: a 2-year prospective surveillance study in the Netherlands. Clin Infect Dis 2004; 39(4): 450–456.
205. Murray-Leisure KA, Egan N, Weitekamp MR. Skin lesions caused by Myco-bacterium scrofulaceum. Arch Dermatol 1987; 123(3):369–370.
206. Sowers WF. Swimming pool granuloma due to *Mycobacterium scrofulaceum*. Arch Dermatol 1972; 105(5):760–761.
207. Sanders JW, Walsh AD, Snider RL, Sahn EE. Disseminated *Mycobacterium scrofulaceum* infection: a potentially treatable complication of AIDS. Clin Infect Dis 1995; 20(3):549.
208. LeMense GP, VanBakel AB, Crumbley AJ III, Judson MA. *Mycobacterium scrofulaceum* infection presenting as lung nodules in a heart transplant recipient. Chest 1994; 106(6):1918–1920.
209. Valero G, Peters J, Jorgensen JH, Graybill JR. Clinical isolates of *Mycobacterium simiae* in San Antonio, Texas. An 11-yr review. Am J Respir Crit Care Med 1995; 152(5 Pt 1):1555–1557.
210. Lavy A, Yoshpe-Purer Y. Isolation of *Mycobacterium simiae* from clinical spe-cimens in Israel. Tubercle 1982; 63(4):279–285.
211. Conger NG, O'Connell RJ, Laurel VL, et al. *Mycobacterium simae* outbreak associated with a hospital water supply. Infect Control Hosp Epidemiol 2004; 25(12):1050–1055.
212. Bell RC, Higuchi JH, Donovan WN, Krasnow I, Johanson WG Jr. *Mycobacterium simiae*. Clinical features and follow-up of twenty-four patients. Am Rev Respir Dis 1983; 127(1):35–38.
213. Legrand E, Devallois A, Horgen L, Rastogi N. A molecular epidemiological study of *Mycobacterium simiae* isolated from AIDS patients in Guadeloupe. J Clin Microbiol 2000; 38(8):3080–3084.
214. Al-Abdely HM, Revankar SG, Graybill JR. Disseminated *Mycobacterium simiae* infection in patients with AIDS. J Infect 2000; 41(2):143–147.
215. Huminer D, Dux S, Samra Z, et al. *Mycobacterium simiae* infection in Israeli patients with AIDS. Clin Infect Dis 1993; 17(3):508–509.

216. Torres RA, Nord J, Feldman R, LaBombardi V, Barr M. Disseminated mixed *Mycobacterium simiae–Mycobacterium avium* complex infection in acquired immunodeficiency syndrome. J Infect Dis 1991; 164(2):432–433.

217. Koeck JL, Debord T, Fabre M, Vincent V, Cavallo JD, Le Vagueresse R. Disseminated *Mycobacterium simiae* infection in a patient with AIDS: clinical features and treatment. Clin Infect Dis 1996; 23(4):832–833.

218. Keenan N, Jeyaratnam D, Sheerin NS. *Mycobacterium simiae*: a previously undescribed pathogen in peritoneal dialysis peritonitis. Am J Kidney Dis 2005; 45(5):e75–e78.

219. Marks J, Jenkins PA, Tsukamura M. *Mycobacterium szulgai*—a new pathogen. Tubercle 1972; 53(3):210–214.

220. Gur H, Porat S, Haas H, Naparstek Y, Eliakim M. Disseminated mycobacterial disease caused by *Mycobacterium szulgai*. Arch Intern Med 1984; 144(9):1861–1863.

221. Maloney JM, Gregg CR, Stephens DS, Manian FA, Rimland D. Infections caused by *Mycobacterium szulgai* in humans. Rev Infect Dis 1987; 9(6):1120–1126.

222. Benator DA, Kan V, Gordin FM. *Mycobacterium szulgai* infection of the lung: case report review of an unusual pathogen. Am J Med Sci 1997; 313(6):346–351.

223. Tortoli E, Besozzi G, Lacchini C, Penati V, Simonetti MT, Emler S. Pulmonary infection due to *Mycobacterium szulgai*, case report and review of the literature. Eur Respir J 1998; 11(4):975–977.

224. Sybert A, Tsou E, Garagusi VF. Cutaneous infection due to *Mycobacterium szulgai*. Am Rev Respir Dis 1977; 115(4):695–698.

225. Holmes GP, Bond GB, Fader RC, Fulcher SF. A Cluster of cases of *Mycobacterium szulgai* keratitis that occurred after laser-assisted in situ keratomileusis. Clin Infect Dis 2002; 34(8):1039–1046.

226. Hakawi AM, Alrajhi AA. Septic arthritis due to *Mycobacterium szulgai* in a patient with human immunodeficiency virus: case report. Scand J infect Dis 2005; 37(3):235–237.

227. Tappe D, Langmann P, Zilly M, Klinker H, Schmausser B, Frosch M. Osteomyelitis and skin ulcers caused by *Mycobacterium szulgai* in an AIDS patient. Scand J Infect Dis 2004; 36(11–12):883–885.

228. Newshan G, Torres RA. Pulmonary infection due to multidrug-resistant *Mycobacterium szulgai* in a patient with AIDS. Clin infect Dis 1994; 18(6): 1022–1023.

229. Frisk P, Boman G, Pauksen K, Petrini B, Lonnerholm G. Skin infection caused by *Mycobacterium szulgai* after allogeneic bone marrow transplantation. Bone Marrow Transplant 2003; 31(6):511–513.

230. Portaels F. Epidemiology of mycobacterial diseases. Clin Dermatol 1995; 13(3):207–222.

231. Russell FM, Starr M, Hayman J, Curtis N, Johnson PD. *Mycobacterium ulcerans* infection diagnosed by polymerase chain reaction. J Paediatr Child Health 2002; 38(3):311–313.

232. Bennett SN, Peterson DE, Johnson DR, Hall WN, Robinson-Dunn B, Dietrich S. Bronchoscopy-associated *Mycobacterium xenopi* pseudoinfections. Am J Respir Crit Care Med 1994; 150(1):245–250.

233. Costrini AM, Mahler DA, Gross WM, Hawkins JE, Yesner R, D'Esopo ND. Clinical and roentgenographic features of nosocomial pulmonary disease due to *Mycobacterium xenopi*. Am Rev Respir Dis 1981; 123(1):104–109.

234. Sniadack DH, Ostroff SM, Karlix MA, et al. A nosocomial pseudo-outbreak of *Mycobacterium xenopi* due to a contaminated potable water supply: lessons in prevention. Infect Control Hosp Epidemiol 1993; 14(11):636–641.

235. Tortoli E, Cichero P, Piersimoni C, Simonetti MT, Gesu G, Nista D. Use of BACTEC MGIT 960 for recovery of mycobacteria from clinical specimens: multicenter study. J Clin Microbiol 1999; 37(11):3578–3582.

236. Donnabella V, Salazar-Schicchi J, Bonk S, Hanna B, Rom WN. Increasing incidence of *Mycobacterium xenopi* at Bellevue hospital: an emerging pathogen or a product of improved laboratory methods? Chest 2000; 118(5):1365–1370.

237. Idigoras P, Beristain X, Iturzaeta A, Vicente D, Perez-Trallero E. Comparison of the automated nonradiometric Bactec MGIT 960 system with Lowenstein–Jensen, Coletsos, and Middlebrook 7H11 solid media for recovery of mycobacteria. Eur J Clin Microbiol Infect Dis 2000; 19(5):350–354.

238. Banks J, Hunter AM, Campbell IA, Jenkins PA, Smith AP. Pulmonary infection with *Mycobacterium xenopi*: review of treatment and response. Thorax 1984; 39(5):376–382.

239. Parrot RG, Grosset JH. Post-surgical outcome of 57 patients with *Mycobacterium xenopi* pulmonary infection. Tubercle 1988; 69(1):47–55.

240. Yates MD, Grange JM, Collins CH. The nature of mycobacterial disease in south east England, 1977–84. J Epidemiol Community Health 1986; 40(4):295–300.

241. Juffermans NP, Verbon A, Danner SA, Kuijper EJ, Speelman P. *Mycobacterium xenopi* in HIV-infected patients: an emerging pathogen. AIDS 1998; 12(13):1661–1666.

242. Jiva TM, Jacoby HM, Weymouth LA, Kaminski DA, Portmore AC. *Mycobacterium xenopi*: innocent bystander or emerging pathogen? Clin Infect Dis 1997; 24(2):226–232.

243. Miller WC, Perkins MD, Richardson WJ, Sexton DJ. Pott's disease caused by *Mycobacterium xenopi*: case report and review. Clin Infect Dis 1994; 19(6):1024–1028.

244. Bishburg E, Zucker MJ, Baran DA, Arroyo LH. *Mycobacterium xenopi* infection after heart transplantation: an unreported pathogen. Transplant Proc 2004; 36(9):2834–2836.

245. Thaunat O, Morelon E, Stern M, et al. *Mycobacterium xenopi* pulmonary infection in two renal transplant recipients under sirolimus therapy. Transpl Infect Dis 2004; 6(4):179–182.

246. Koizumi JH, Sommers HM. *Mycobacterium xenopi* and pulmonary disease. Am J Clin Pathol 1980; 73(6):826–830.

247. Weber J, Mettang T, Staerz E, Machleidt C, Kuhlmann U. Pulmonary disease due to *Mycobacterium xenopi* in a renal allograft recipient: report of a case and review. Rev Infect Dis 1989; 11(6):964–969.

248. Kurzrock R, Zander A, Vellekoop L, Kanojia M, Luna M, Dicke K. Mycobacterial pulmonary infections after allogeneic bone marrow transplantation. Am J Med 1984; 77(1):35–40.

249. Gaviria JM, Garcia PJ, Garrido SM, Corey L, Boeckh M. Nontuberculous mycobacterial infections in hematopoietic stem cell transplant recipients: characteristics of respiratory and catheter-related infections. Biol Blood Marrow Transplant 2000; 6(4):361–369.
250. Weinstock DM, Feinstein MB, Sepkowitz KA, Jakubowski A. High rates of infection and colonization by nontuberculous mycobacteria after allogeneic hematopoietic stem cell transplantation. Bone Marrow Transplant 2003; 31(11):1015–1021.
251. Munoz RM, Alonso-Pulpon L, Yebra M, Segovia J, Gallego JC, Daza RM. Intestinal involvement by nontuberculous mycobacteria after heart transplantation. Clin Infect Dis 2000; 30(3):603–605.
252. Tebas P, Sultan F, Wallace RJ Jr, Fraser V. Rapid development of resistance to clarithromycin following monotherapy for disseminated *Mycobacterium chelonae* infection in a heart transplant patient. Clin Infect Dis 1995; 20(2):443–444.
253. Wallace RJ Jr, Tanner D, Brennan PJ, Brown BA. Clinical trial of clarithromycin for cutaneous (disseminated) infection due to *Mycobacterium chelonae*. Ann Intern Med 1993; 119(6):482–486.
254. Neeley SP, Denning DW. Cutaneous Mycobacterium thermoresistibile infection in a heart transplant recipient. Rev Infect Dis 1989; 11(4):608–611.
255. Ray R, Chakravorty S, Tyagi JS, et al. Fatal atypical mycobacterial infection in a cardiac transplant recipient. Indian Heart J 2001; 53(1):100–103.
256. McDiarmid SV, Blumberg DA, Remotti H, et al. Mycobacterial infections after pediatric liver transplantation: a report of three cases and review of the literature. J Pediatr Gastroenterol Nutr 1995; 20(4):425–431.
257. Clark D, Lambert CM, Palmer K, Strachan R, Nuki G. Monoarthritis caused by *Mycobacterium avium* complex in a liver transplant recipient. Br J Rheumatol 1993; 32(12):1099–1100.
258. Neau-Cransac M, Dupon M, Carles J, Le Bail B, Saric J. Disseminated *Mycobacterium avium* infection after liver transplantation. Eur J Clin Microbiol Infect Dis 1998; 17(10):744–746.
259. Hoff E, Sholtis M, Procop G, et al. *Mycobacterium triplex* infection in a liver transplant patient. J Clin Microbiol 2001; 39(5):2033–2034.
260. Vandermarliere A, Van Audenhove A, Peetermans WE, Vanrenterghem Y, Maes B. Mycobacterial infection after renal transplantation in a Western population. Transpl Infect Dis 2003; 5(1):9–15.
261. Lloveras J, Peterson PK, Simmons RL, Najarian JS. Mycobacterial infections in renal transplant recipients. Seven cases and a review of the literature. Arch Intern Med 1982; 142(5):888–892.
262. Higgins RM, Cahn AP, Porter D, et al. Mycobacterial infections after renal transplantation. Q J Med 1991; 78(286):145–153.
263. Delaney V, Sumrani N, Hong JH, Sommer B. Mycobacterial infections in renal allograft recipients. Transplant Proc 1993; 25(3):2288–2289.
264. Trulock EP, Bolman RM, Genton R. Pulmonary disease caused by *Mycobacterium chelonae* in a heart–lung transplant recipient with obliterative bronchiolitis. Am Rev Respir Dis 1989; 140(3):802–805.
265. Baldi S, Rapellino M, Ruffini E, Cavallo A, Mancuso M. Atypical mycobacteriosis in a lung transplant recipient. Eur Respir J 1997; 10(4):952–954.

266. Sanguinetti M, Ardito F, Fiscarelli E, et al. Fatal pulmonary infection due to multid rug-resistant *Mycobacterium abscessus* in a patient with cystic fibrosis. J Clin Microbiol 2001; 39(2):816–819.

267. Swetter SM, Kindel SE, Smoller BR. Cutaneous nodules of *Mycobacterium chelonae* in an immunosuppressed patient with preexisting pulmonary colonization. J Am Acad Dermatol 1993; 28(2 Pt 2):352–355.

268. Woo MS, Downey S, Inderlied CB, Kaminsky C, Ross LA, Rowland J. Pediatric transplant grand rounds. A case presentation: skin lesions in a post-lung transplant patient. Pediatr Transplant 1997; 1(2):163–170.

269. Woods GL, Fish G, Plaunt M, Murphy T. Clinical evaluation of difco ESP culture system II for growth and detection of mycobacteria. J Clin Microbiol 1997; 35(1):121–124.

270. Wilson ML, Stone BL, Hildred MV, Reves RR. Comparison of recovery rates for mycobacteria from BACTEC 12B vials, Middlebrook 7H11-selective 7H11 biplates, and Lowenstein Jensen slants in a public health mycobacteriology laboratory. J Clin Microbiol 1995; 33(9):2516–2518.

271. Miller N, Infante S, Cleary T. Evaluation of the LiPA MYCOBACTERIA assay for identification of mycobacterial species from BACTEC 12B bottles. J Clin Microbiol 2000; 38(5):1915–1919.

272. Tortoli E, Nanetti A, Piersimoni C, et al. Performance assessment of new multiplex probe assay for identification of mycobacteria. J Clin Microbiol 2001; 39(3):1079–1084.

273. Suffys PN, da Silva Rocha A, de Oliveira M, et al. Rapid identification of Mycobacteria to the species level using INNO-LiPA Mycobacteria, a reverse hybridization assay. J Clin Microbiol 2001; 39(12):4477–4482.

274. Bottger EC. *Mycobacterium genavense*: an emerging pathogen. Eur J Clin Microbiol Infect Dis 1994; 13(11):932–936.

275. Kaminski DA, Hardy DJ. Selective utilization of DNA probes for identification of Mycobacterium species on the basis of cord formation in primary BACTEC 12B cultures. J Clin Microbiol 1995; 33(6):1548–1550.

276. Jost KC Jr, Dunbar DF, Barth SS, Headley VL, Elliott LB. Identification of *Mycobacterium tuberculosis* and *M. avium* complex directly from smear-positive sputum specimens and BACTEC 12B cultures by high-performance liquid chromatography with fluorescence detection and computer-driven pattern recognition models. J Clin Microbiol 1995; 33(5):1270–1277.

277. von Reyn CF, Green PA, McCormick D, et al. Dual skin testing with *Mycobacterium avium* sensitin and purified protein derivative: an open study of patients with *M. avium* complex infection or tuberculosis. Clin Infect Dis 1994; 19(1):15–20.

278. Heifets L. Susceptibility testing of *Mycobacterium avium* complex isolates. Antimicrob Agents Chemother 1996; 40(8):1759–1767.

279. Chaisson RE, Benson CA, Dube MP, et al. Clarithromycin therapy for bacteremic *Mycobacterium avium* complex disease. A randomized, double-blind, dose-ranging study in patients with AIDS. AIDS Clinical Trials Group Protocol 157 Study Team. Ann Intern Med 1994; 121(12):905–911.

280. Wallace RJ Jr, Brown BA, Griffith DE, et al. Initial clarithromycin monotherapy for *Mycobacterium avium-intracellulare* complex lung disease. Am J Respir Crit Care Med 1994; 149(5):1335–1341.

281. Ann CH, Wallace RJ Jr, Steele LC, Murphy DT. Sulfonamide-containing regimens for disease caused by rifampin-resistant *Mycobacterium kansasii*. Am Rev Respir Dis 1987; 135(1):10–16.

282. Wallace RJ Jr, Dunbar D, Brown BA, et al. Rifampin-resistant *Mycobacterium kansasii*. Clin Infect Dis 1994; 18(5):736–743.

283. Bernard EM, Edwards FF, Kiehn TE, Brown ST, Armstrong D. Activities of antimicrobial agents against clinical isolates of *Mycobacterium haemophilum*. Antimicrob Agents Chemother 1993; 37(11):2323–2326.

284. Swenson JM, Wallace RJ Jr, Silcox VA, Thornsberry C. Antimicrobial susceptibility of five subgroups of *Mycobacterium fortuitum* and *Mycobacterium chelonae*. Antimicrob Agents Chemother 1985; 28(6):807–811.

285. Wallace RJ Jr, Brown BA, Onyi GO. Susceptibilities of *Mycobacterium fortuitum* biovar. fortuitum and the two subgroups of *Mycobacterium chelonae* to imipenem, cefmetazole, cefoxitin, and amoxicillin–clavulanic acid. Antimicrob Agents Chemother 1991; 35(4):773–775.

286. Edelstein H. *Mycobacterium marinum* skin infections. Report of 31 cases and review of the literature. Arch Intern Med 1994; 154(12):1359–1364.

287. Black MM, Eykyn SJ. The successful treatment of tropical fish tank granuloma (*Mycobacterium marinum*) with co-trimoxazole. Br J Dermatol 1977; 97(6):689–692.

# 29

# Acute Allograft Rejection

**Jonathan B. Orens**

*Division of Pulmonary and Critical Care Medicine,
Department of Medicine, The Johns Hopkins University School of Medicine,
Baltimore, Maryland, U.S.A.*

**Sean Studer**

*University of Pittsburgh School of Medicine, Pittsburgh, Pennsylvania, U.S.A.*

**Robert D. Levy**

*University of British Columbia, Vancouver, British Columbia, Canada*

## INTRODUCTION

Acute cellular rejection (ACR) is a common complication occurring in 30% to 90% of patients during the first year following transplantation (1–12). Indeed, ACR occurs with much greater frequency in lung allografts when compared to all other solid organ transplants. Why lung allografts are more susceptible to ACR is not entirely clear, although it is speculated that lung tissue is more immunogenic. Furthermore, it is likely that nonalloimmune injury to the graft via inhalation of toxic substances or infectious agents may expose targets and or upregulate the immune system to attack. Although most cases of ACR are readily treatable with transient augmented immunosuppression, the long-term implication of ACR may be extremely important. In numerous studies, ACR has been identified as the major risk factor for bronchiolitis obliterans syndrome (BOS), the clinical hallmark of chronic allograft dysfunction and the leading cause of long-term morbidity and mortality after the first year following lung transplantation (1,13–18).

Additionally, persistent ACR may lead directly to allograft fibrosis (15). Treatment for acute rejection in the form of augmented immunosuppression increases the risk of infection and other complications.

The importance of acute humoral (antibody mediated) rejection (AHR) is established in renal and cardiac allografts, but the incidence, significance, and implications of AHR in lung transplantation are still emerging (19). This chapter will review the data regarding ACR in lung transplant recipients with respect to clinical presentation, pathobiology, diagnosis, and treatment.

## INCIDENCE OF ACR

In contrast to hyperacute rejection of the lung allograft, which is a rare complication of lung transplantation that has been reported in only three well-documented cases (20–22), ACR of the lung allograft rejection is a relatively common occurrence affecting the majority of lung transplant recipients (1,3–12). Despite improving strategies and medications for induction and maintenance immunosuppression, some degree of ACR can be demonstrated in up to 90% of lung transplant recipients (23). However, the precise incidence of ACR is difficult to ascertain due to differences in diagnostic criteria (clinical vs. histologic), varying use and intervals of surveillance lung biopsy, and differences in immunosuppression regimens. The use of transbronchial lung biopsy for diagnosis of ACR in patients with suggestive clinical or radiographic features is unchallenged. Performance of bronchoscopy only for symptomatic patients may underestimate the incidence of ACR, since clinically occult episodes may go undetected.

## DIAGNOSIS OF ACR

### Clinical Presentation

ACR may occur without signs or symptoms, particularly with minimal to mild histologic grades. When present, the signs and symptoms of ACR are nonspecific and include dyspnea, cough, fever, fatigue, wheezes, or crackles by examination, radiograph pulmonary infiltrate or deterioration in pulmonary function test (PFT) results. Chest radiographs and computed tomography (CT) scans may be normal, particularly with low grades of rejection. With higher grades of rejection, pulmonary infiltrates with either interstitial, nodular, or alveolar patterns may be present (Figs. 1–3). Chest CT scans show similar findings, all of which are nonspecific for rejection.

### Timing of Presentation

Following the immediate postoperative period, opportunistic infections and acute graft rejection are the major causes of morbidity and mortality in lung

(A) (B)

(C)

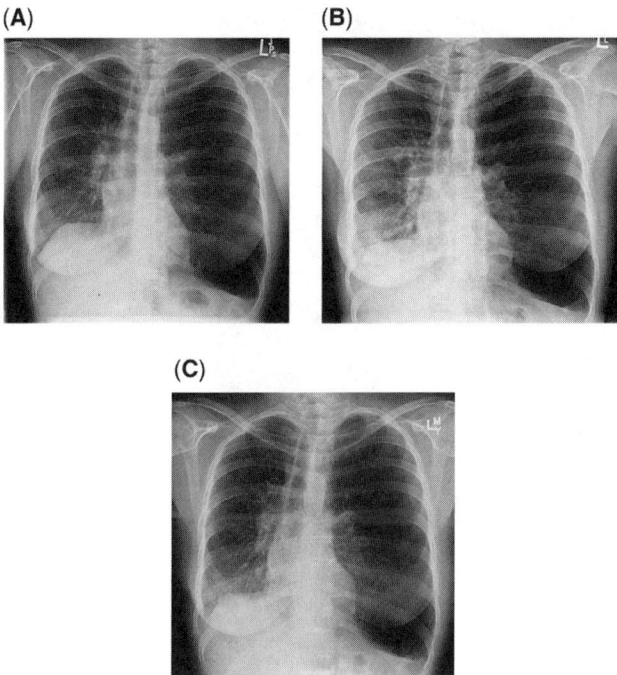

**Figure 1** Panel (**A**) is a posterio-anterior chest radiograph of a 35-year-old woman 45 days following right single-lung transplantation for emphysema related to alpha-1 antitryspin deficiency. She was seen at day 52 posttransplant with breathlessness, fever to 37.8°C, room air oxygen saturation 88%, and mild pedal edema. The chest radiograph (**B**) demonstrated hazy airspace abnormalities in the right lower lung zone, increased perihilar interstitial abnormalities, and a small right pleural effusion. Fiberoptic bronchoscopy was unremarkable on visualization. BAL was negative for infectious pathogens. Transbronchial biopsy was consistent with grade A3 acute rejection. The patient improved quickly clinically with clearing of the chest radiograph by day 55 (**C**) following treatment with intravenous methylprednisolone 500 mg daily for three days. *Abbreviation*: BAL, bronchoalveolar lavage.

and heart–lung transplant recipients (24). The latency period from the time of transplantation to the first episode of ACR may depend on individual center immunosuppressive strategies. When induction therapy is utilized perioperatively with agents such as interleukin-2 receptor antagonists or polyclonal antithymocyte globulins, the development of ACR may be delayed. Without induction therapy, ACR may be seen as early as five to seven days post-transplant. In this early period, clinical features tend to be nonspecific and can include dyspnea, low-grade fever, desaturation, weight gain, and edema. The clinical differentiation between infection and acute rejection is often problematic in view of the non-specific clinical and

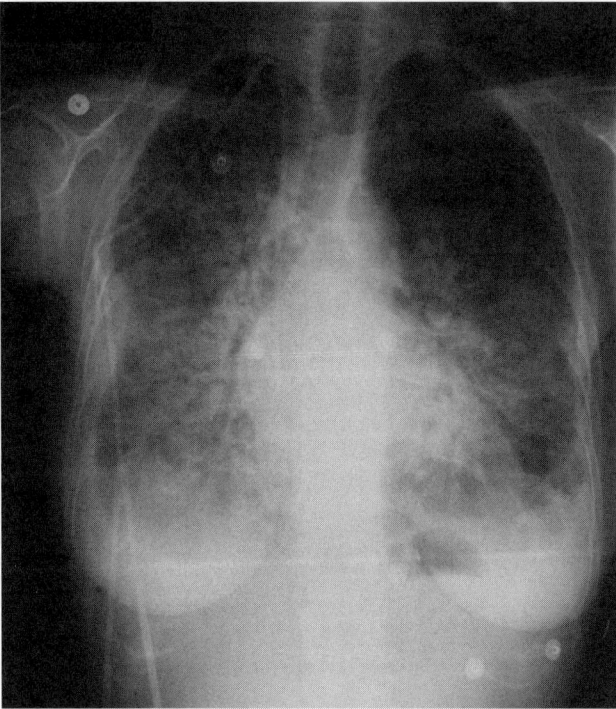

**Figure 2** Status of a 54-year-old woman post bilateral lung transplantion for sarcoidosis who presented with one week of dyspnea and lung grade fever. The patient had stopped taking her immunosuppressive medications. Note the diffuse bilateral pulmonary infiltrates. Transbronchial biopsy revealed severe acute rejection. Although the pulmonary infiltrates improved with high-dose pulse IV steroids, pulmonary function studies remained low and the patient died from chronic rejection six months after this event.

radiographic presentations (25). Most episodes of ACR occur during the first 100 days following transplantation with the incidence decreasing steadily beyond this time frame (26). It is unusual for ACR to occur more than two years after transplantation unless immunosuppressive medications are withheld.

**Pulmonary Function Testing**

In order to determine whether noninvasive clinical physiologic measures could aid in the diagnosis of acute rejection, Otulana et al., studied the lung function changes that occurred in the presence of histologically documented acute rejection (27). Acute rejection was associated with the development of

**(A)**

**(B)**

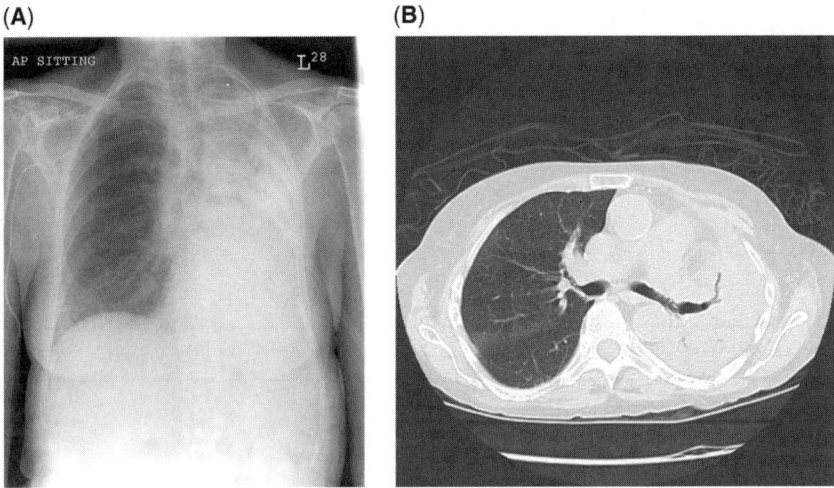

**Figure 3** Panel (**A**) is a postero-anterior chest radiograph of a 66-year-old woman five years following left single-lung transplantation who developed rapidly progressive dyspnea and nonproductive cough. Her corresponding chest computed tomography is shown in (**B**). Transbronchial biopsy was consistent with severe (grade A4) acute rejection. The patient was initially treated with solumedrol 1 mg/day for three days with no improvement. Repeat biopsy demonstrated persistent, severe acute rejection. Subsequent treatments with rabbit antilyphocyte globulin and OKT3 similarly had no effect. Radionuclide ventilation/perfusion scanning demonstrated 99% ventilation and 93% perfusion to the native lung six months later. The patient remained alive one year later.

a restrictive ventilatory abnormality, with similar reductions in forced expiratory volume in one second ($FEV_1$) and forced vital capacity (FVC), as well as less consistent decreases in total lung capacity and diffusing capacity for carbon monoxide (DLco). The pulmonary function changes in acute rejection were found to be transient, with a return to baseline after appropriate treatment of rejection (Fig. 4). Similar pulmonary function abnormalities were observed in the lung function of patients in whom the ultimate diagnosis was found to be infection. As pointed out by the authors, this pattern of change suggests a fall in lung compliance, which would be the likely outcome of both infection and acute rejection, in which the inflammatory responses are concentrated in the lung parenchyma. Similar findings were reported by Hoeper et al., who also noted that in the absence of a change in flow rates, decreased DLco was most suggestive of pulmonary viral infection (28). In summary, although pulmonary function testing cannot differentiate between acute rejection and infection, it is a highly specific noninvasive modality for detecting the occurrence of an acute lung graft

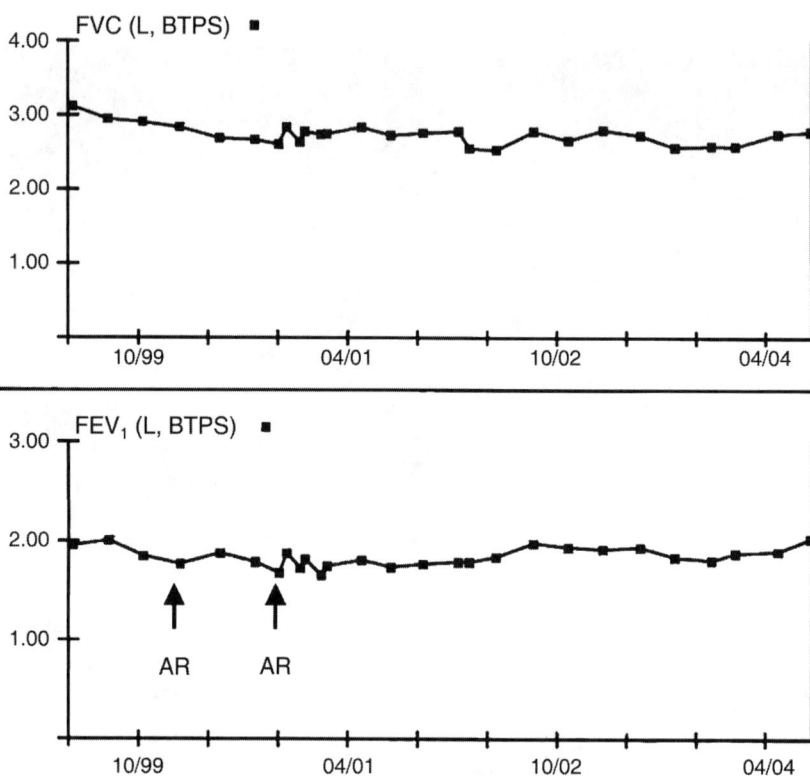

**Figure 4** Status of a 50-year-old man post single-lung transplant for alpha-1-antitrypsin deficiency–related emphysema. The patient presented on two occasions with mild dyspnea and a slight drop in $FEV_1$ and FVC (*arrows*). Transbronchial biopsy showed histologic grade A2 (mild) rejection that responded quickly to a short increased dose of oral steroids. *Abbreviations*: $FEV_1$, forced expiratory volume in one second; FVC, forced vital capacity.

complication (27). For this reason, many transplant centers have lung transplant recipients routinely measure daily $FEV_1$ and FVC with inexpensive home spirometers to aid in the early detection of graft complications (29,30).

Home daily monitoring of $FEV_1$ has become standard practice for almost all lung transplant centers. There are now several handheld "micro-spirometers" available that are portable and easy to use at home following minimal training (Fig. 5). This simple-to-perform test is sensitive to changes in graft function, particularly with the presence of rejection or infection. Regardless of symptoms, a 10% or greater decline in $FEV_1$ is an indicator to the patient to contact the transplant center for further assessment. Although home monitoring of PFTs is a standard procedure,

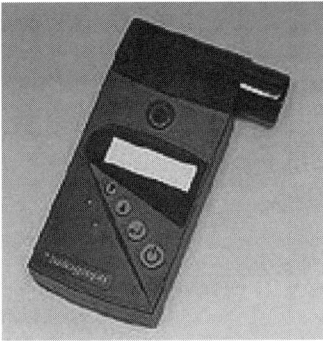

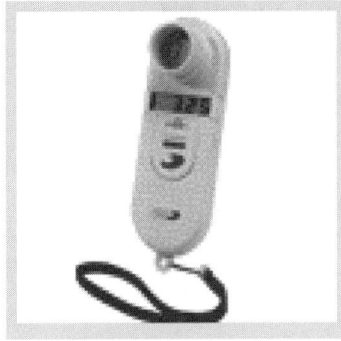

Vitalograph®                    Micro Spirometer®

**Figure 5** Examples of handheld portable spirometers currently available for home monitoring of $FEV_1$ and FVC. *Abbreviations*: $FEV_1$, forced expiratory volume in one second; FVC, forced vital capacity.

the sensitivity of spirometry to detect problems with the graft can be influenced by the underlying disease state in single-lung transplant (SLT) recipients. Becker et al. studied 30 SLT patients with varying underlying diseases (31). Although rejection was associated with a significant fall in FVC and $FEV_1$, the fall in $FEV_1$ was less in patients with underlying obstructive disease. The sensitivity and specificity of spirometry as a predictor of infection or rejection was most helpful for patients with pulmonary vascular disease, while patients with obstructive lung disease had the least clinically useful values.

## Lung Perfusion Scans

Apart from changes in lung function, acute rejection is associated with lung injury as manifested by increased pulmonary epithelial permeability and alveolocapillary leakiness (32,33). Due to hypoxic vasoconstriction associated with alveolar capillary leak, acute lung rejection may result in decreased lung perfusion, which is reversible with appropriate treatment (34). Therefore, a shift of quantitative perfusion away from the lung allograft can be useful in the detection of graft rejection in recipients of SLTs. Unfortunately, this diminished perfusion lacks sensitivity since it may not be observed despite the presence of biopsy-proven rejection.

## Clinical Monitoring

In practice, ACR is generally diagnosed by a combination of the clinical assessment and the results of transbronchial lung biopsy. While clinical monitoring in lung transplantation is a time-honored method of detecting complications, the specificity of these tools has proven to be quite limited. Dabbs et al. (35) examined symptoms in lung transplant recipients in three domains: general, respiratory, and activities of daily living. They concluded that altered symptom scores on a standardized questionnaire may signal a change in condition, but are not adequate discriminators between grades of rejection or respiratory infection. Similarly, Guilinger et al. (6) compared the clinical assessment for suspected acute rejection with the final diagnosis that included lung biopsy and observed a poor correlation with the final diagnosis.

## Transbronchial Biopsy

Given the limitations to the clinical diagnosis of ACR, bronchoscopy with transbronchial biopsy has become the accepted method and standard for diagnosing allograft rejection. The role of bronchoscopy in the management of lung transplantation cannot be understated. Bronchoscopy is simple and safe to perform and is capable of readily detecting ACR and excluding other possible complications such as infection. Transbronchial biopsies are obtained either for surveillance, to detect occult ACR, or to confirm clinically suspected rejection, or as a follow-up after treatment to ensure an adequate therapeutic response.

There are, however, drawbacks to performing transbronchial biopsies. Transbronchial biopsies are invasive, resource-intensive, carry a small risk to the patient, and cannot always be performed as frequently as desirable. Another potential shortcoming of transbronchial lung biopsies is that only a very small fraction of the total lung allograft is sampled with each biopsy, suggesting the potential for underdiagnosis due to sampling error. Typical biopsy specimens provide an area of approximately $0.5–1\,cm^2$ for histologic analysis. Given the patchy involvement of the affected lung in ACR, there is a potentially significant chance of missing early ACR. It is recommended that at least five pieces of alveolated parenchyma be obtained, each containing bronchioles and more than 100 air sacs (36). The most common complications of bronchoscopy include infection, bleeding, and pneumothorax, with the latter being of greater concern in patients undergoing transbronchial biopsies while receiving positive pressure mechanical ventilation. Burns et al. (37) studied the performance characteristics of transbronchial biopsy in 41 lung transplant recipients with respiratory failure requiring mechanical ventilation and concluded that the sensitivity of transbronchial biopsy is low in this setting. Performing surgical lung biopsy increased histopathologic diagnosis by 33% in that study.

The current clinical diagnosis of ACR is, therefore, often based on a combination of patient symptoms, physical examination findings, radiographic evaluation, spirometry, and transbronchial biopsy. The weighting of each factor in diagnosing ACR and the decision to prescribe treatment is potentially variable among individual physicians and among transplant programs. Typically, however, bronchoscopy with transbronchial biopsy is performed to confirm the clinical impression of ACR.

## NONINVASIVE MARKERS OF ACR

A number of investigators have examined the potential role for measurements of nitric oxide (NO) in expired gas samples as a marker of acute allograft rejection with contradictory results. Silkoff et al. (38) observed increased levels of expired NO during acute vascular rejection, while Fisher et al. (39) reported increased expired NO in the setting of lymphocytic bronchiolitis, but no acute vascular rejection. Studer and colleagues (40) found elevated levels of exhaled carbonyl sulfide during acute allograft rejection; however, a significant overlap with values seen in stable subjects was thought to limit the diagnostic utility of this measurement.

Bronchoalveolar lavage (BAL) fluid has been extensively studied in order to determine its usefulness for the reliable detection of acute rejection. Although BAL fluid is characterized by marked lymphocytosis in acute rejection, lymphocyte subsets are similar to those observed in stable controls (41). Hence, BAL lymphocytosis is characterized by high sensitivity but very low specificity for detection of histologic acute rejection. Rizzo et al. (42) reported that unlike BAL cellularity, increased expression of adhesion molecules and inflammatory cytokines in BAL fluid is evident during acute rejection, but further studies are needed to confirm these results as well as to evaluate the sensitivity and specificity of the findings in differentiating acute rejection from infection.

In summary, at present there are no noninvasive markers of acute allograft rejection with sufficiently high sensitivity and specificity to be useful for routine clinical purposes. Hence, the standard of care remains the maintenance of a high degree of suspicion in the correct clinical context by experienced clinicians, in conjunction with transbronchial biopsy, the gold standard for diagnosis of acute allograft rejection.

### Surveillance Bronchoscopy

In addition to bronchoscopy performed when signs or symptoms suggest allograft problems (i.e., infection or rejection), surveillance bronchoscopy is performed by many centers to look for occult problems in the allograft, particularly rejection. However, the role for surveillance transbronchial lung biopsy is not well characterized or practiced in a standardized fashion. Sixty-eight percent of programs perform routine scheduled bronchoscopies based on a 1997 survey by Kufkaka et al. (43) and Levine (44). As noted previously, low-grade ACR may develop without symptoms and there are many who believe that even low-grade asymptomatic ACR should be treated in an attempt to decrease the risk of obliterative bronchiolitis (OB)/BOS. Although much controversy exists regarding the utility of surveillance bronchoscopy, most U.S. centers perform this procedure at regularly scheduled intervals (i.e., one month posttransplant and every three months during the first year, every six months in the second year, and once a year thereafter).

Indeed, an older study by Trulock et al. (5) reported on the findings from surveillance bronchoscopy from the Washington University program and found a significant number of abnormalities even from clinically stable patients. Of the routine surveillance procedures in 90 clinically healthy patients, 39% had some degree of ACR, 14% had cytomegalovirus, 18% had nonspecific findings, 3% had "other," and only 24% were completely normal. These findings, however, must be interpreted with caution in relation to today's practice since immunosuppressive regimens and other forms of monitoring differ somewhat. Despite the common practice of surveillance bronchoscopy across United States centers, Valentine et al. (45) reported no significant difference in long-term outcomes from 91 patients when bronchoscopy was performed only when clinically indicated by symptoms or a fall in lung function or oximetry. This study was limited, however, by being retrospective and nonrandomized.

## Pathology of ACR

The Lung Rejection Study Group, sponsored by the International Society for Heart Transplantation (ISHLT), established a uniform grading system for lung transplant rejection pathology in 1990 (46). The goal was to develop a simple, easily taught, and reproducible grading system that would incorporate the favorable aspects of the multiple grading systems that existed, while providing a common platform for rejection classification. The system based solely on histopathology, excluded clinical information, and recognized both perivascular mononuclear cell infiltrates and lymphocytic bronchitis/bronchiolitis as the histopathologic characterization of acute rejection (Fig. 6). This ACR classification system was last revised in 1996 (36). The histopathologic grading system for ACR is listed in Table 1. As described in the following section regarding ACR treatment below, clinically significant (i.e., requiring treatment) rejection is often considered to be grades A2 and higher (mild to severe). However, recent evidence suggests that even grade A1 (minimal rejection) is associated with earlier onset BOS and may warrant changes in immunosuppression (47,48). Chapter 27 in this edition by Howell provides a detailed review of lung histology in lung allograft rejection including the airways grading system utilized for diagnosis of lymphocytic bronchitis and OB.

## Pathogenesis of ACR

Allograft rejection results from a reaction to donor alloantigens, expressed on the transplanted lung. The pathogenesis of this inflammatory response underlying ACR is incompletely understood but is known to involve both

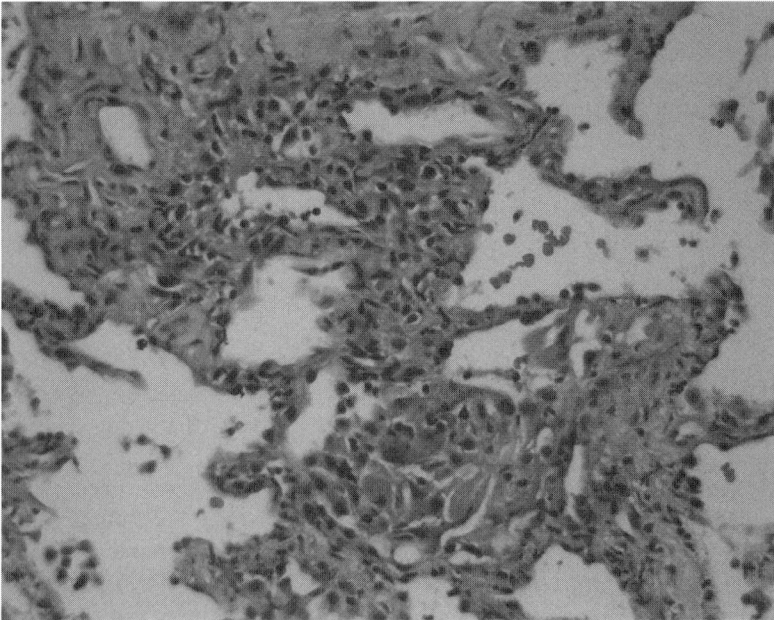

**Figure 6** Histologic specimen from a transbronchial biopsy showing moderate ACR (ISHLT grade A3). Note the mononuclear cells surrounding the vessel and extending out into the interstitium. *Abbreviations*: ACR, acute cellular rejection; ISHLT, International Society for Heart Transplantation.

**Table 1** Acute Lung Allograft Vascular Rejection Histopathologic Grading System

| AR grade | Interpretation | Histopathologic abnormality |
|---|---|---|
| Grade A0 | No rejection | No significant abnormality |
| Grade A1 | Minimal | Infrequent perivascular lymphocytic infiltrates (not evident on low microscopic power) |
| Grade A2 | Mild | Frequent perivascular infiltrates surrounding venules and arterioles (apparent on low power light microscopy) |
| Grade A3 | Moderate | Dense perivascular infiltrates extending into alveolar septae and air spaces |
| Grade A4 | Severe | Diffuse perivascular, interstitial, and air space mononuclear infiltrates with pneumocyte damage, possibly with necrosis, infarction, or vasculitis |

*Source*: From Ref. 36.

innate and adaptive immunity (49–51). The primary effector cell in ACR is the T-lymphocyte (52). T-cells react with alloantigens, most often non–self major histocompatibility complex (MHC) proteins, and become activated producing proinflammatory cytokines that result in graft infiltration with lymphocytes, macrophages, and other inflammatory effector cells (49,50,53). A more detailed discussion of the basic science of transplant immunology is the subject of Chapters 2 and 3. Recent clinical studies addressing the immunopathogenesis of ACR utilizing genomics, genetics, and cytokine expression hold the promise of advancing our understanding of ACR and leading to the development of noninvasive diagnostic tools as well as more effective therapy.

Gimino et al. (54) applied gene expression microarrays to cells in BAL of patients with ACR versus those with no evidence of rejection. As expected, gene expression patterns clearly differed between the groups. Using basic analytical tools, they identified several functional groups of genes including many previously associated with rejection; these included changes in genes associated with transforming growth factor-beta signaling, inflammatory response, G-protein–coupled receptors, apoptosis, and the Wnt family of signaling molecules. These pathways represent possible avenues for noninvasive biomarker development and provide new insights into ACR pathogenesis.

Palmer and coinvestigators (55) addressed the role of innate immunity by assessing the impact of polymorphisms in the toll-like receptor 4 on the rate of ACR in lung transplant recipients. They observed a significantly reduced rate of ACR in allograft recipients with two functional polymorphisms in TLR4 receptor compared with the wild type. This work suggests the importance of activation of innate immunity in ACR following lung transplantation and a potential novel therapeutic target for ACR prevention.

Numerous proinflammatory cytokines and chemokines have been noted to be present in BAL fluid from patients with acute rejection. The importance of each of these mediators in the pathogenesis of ACR is unclear and these are discussed in more detail in the chapter on pathogenesis of rejection. From a clinical standpoint, BAL chemokine/cytokine profiles do not distinguish acute rejection from other inflammatory processes in the graft.

## Acute Humoral Rejection

In renal and cardiac allografts the pathogenic role of anti-human leukocyte antigen (HLA) antibodies is well described. In lung transplantation, preformed HLA antibodies have been recognized for their role in hyperacute rejection (20–22), the requirement for prolonged ventilatory support postoperatively in patients with a pretransplant panel of reactive antibodies >10% (56), and their correlation with the development of BOS (56–60). AHR of the lung allograft has been reported (61), although its incidence, standards for diagnosis, and optimal treatment strategy are still evolving.

Badesch et al. (62) reported the occurrence of pulmonary capillaritis and speculated that this was a unique form of vascular rejection, although antibody staining of tissue and anti-HLA antibody screening of serum were negative. Magro and colleagues, however, observed cases of similar histopathology and demonstrated Clq, C3, and C4d in the affected tissue (63,64). Magro concluded that this represented humorally mediated acute rejection due to anti–endothelial cell antibodies. Even stronger evidence of AHR to date was a published case by Miller et al. (61) of a patient with acute allograft rejection, who failed to improve with a steroid pulse followed by treatment with rabbit antithymocyte globulin and tested positive for de novo donor-specific HLA antibodies. The patient improved after receiving plasmapheresis followed by monthly intravenous immunoglobulin and remained well. The same authors noted an elevated C4d concentration in BAL fluid of lung transplant recipients with anti-HLA antibodies, suggesting classic complement pathway activation. They proposed a possible future role for measurement of C4d in BAL to diagnose AHR. Finally, Girnita and colleagues (65) at the University of Pittsburgh observed an increased incidence of acute allograft rejection in lung transplant recipients with anti-HLA antibodies and moderate and severe rejection, raising concern that these antibodies played an important role in rejection pathogenesis. While no specific recommendations regarding diagnosis and treatment of AHR can be made at the time of this writing, screening for anti-HLA antibodies following episodes of presumptive persistent ACR may identify patients with AHR. Treatment of AHR with plasmapheresis to reduce antibody titers and intravenous (IV) immunoglobulin to maintain low titers may lead to improved outcomes.

## Prevention

### Immunosuppression

From both animal studies and from human subjects it is quite evident that the use of maintenance immunosuppression is imperative to prevent ACR. ACR will develop relatively quickly in almost all patients who stop taking their immunosuppression. Similar to treatment for ACR, maintenance therapy "cocktails," utilized to prevent rejection in lung transplant recipients is borrowed from other solid organ transplants. There have been no studies in lung transplant recipients that convincingly show the superiority of one regimen over another, particularly with regard to long-term graft survival and prevention of OB/BOS. Data from the ISHLT registry (66) show that nearly all patients are maintained on a triple immunosuppressive regimen with a combination of a calcineurin inhibitor (cyclosporine or tacrolimus), an antimetabolite (azathioprine or mycophenolate mofetil), and prednisone. Nearly 98% of patients remain on prednisone at five years posttransplant. Recently, rapamycin is being used for small minority of patients (about 8%) in place of the antimetabolite. Immunosuppressive therapy is discussed in greater detail in Chapters 17–19.

### Induction Therapy

Because of the close association between ACR and BOS/OB, there is an unproven belief that prevention of ACR will decrease the risk of BOS/OB. To this end, immunosuppressive induction therapy is used by many centers perioperatively with the hope of decreasing the risk of ACR.

According to the ISHLT registry database, induction immunosuppressive therapy is given by approximately 41% of the U.S. lung transplant centers (67). Several agents have been used for induction including the polyclonal antibodies (Atgam and Thymoglobulin), OKT-3, the interleukin-2 receptor antagonists, and most recently anti-CD 52 antibody alemtuzumab (Campath, Hex, San Antonio, Texas). OKT-3 is used less commonly today because of infectious complications and the high likelihood of treatment-limiting side effects such as fever, hypotension, and pulmonary edema associated with the cytokine release syndrome. Several centers still utilize a course of polyclonal antibodies during the first 5 to 10 days after surgery. Palmer and colleagues (68) showed that rabbit antithymocyte globulin (RATG) induction therapy decreased the rate of acute rejection after lung transplantation in a single-center, randomized, prospective study of 44 adult lung transplant recipients. RATG was administered at a dosage of 1.5 mg/kg/day for three days at the time of transplantation, along with conventional immunosuppression (cyclosporine, azathioprine, and prednisone), to one half of the patients while conventional immunosuppression alone with no induction therapy was given to the other half. The number of patients experiencing biopsy-proven grade II or greater acute rejection was significantly reduced in the group receiving RATG induction therapy (23% incidence), as compared to the patients treated with conventional immunosuppression alone (55% incidence; $P = 0.03$).

Garrity et al. (69) studied the use of daclizumab, a humanized monoclonal antibody directed against the interleukin-2 receptor. Twenty-two patients treated with daclizumab (1 mg/kg intraoperatively before reperfusion and again on days 14, 28, 42, and 56) in addition to standard immunosuppression with tacrolimus, azathioprine, and corticosteroids were compared to a control group of 21 patients who received standard immunosuppression alone. Grade 2 or greater rejection was seen in only 18% of the treated group compared to 48% in the control group ($P < 0.04$). Complications were similar between the control and treatment groups.

## Treatment

The primary goals of treatment of ACR are to resolve the ACR itself and to forestall or prevent the development of BOS. There are no studies to assess the best treatment regimen for ACR in lung transplant recipients; the current approach has been adapted from therapy for other solid organ transplants. Treatment for ACR in lung recipients does vary across programs but most centers treat initial episodes with augmentation of corticosteroids. The dose of steroids typically depends on the severity of the rejection episode, and there are no trials comparing various dosing schedules. A common treatment scheme is as follows. For minimal ACR (ISHLT grade 1), no therapy. For mild ACR (ISHLT grade 2) prednisolone 0.5–1 mg/kg/day is given orally over a two-week course with a taper. For moderate to severe rejection (ISHLT grades 3 and 4), Solumedrol 500–1000 mg IV per day for three days followed by increased oral corticosteroids over a two-week course as given for mild rejection. Although most cases of ACR respond to augmented corticosteroids, occasionally some patients fail therapy. Given the possibility of steroid failure, all documented rejection episodes are usually followed up at the completion of treatment with bronchoscopic biopsies to verify resolution. ACR that fails to respond to corticosteroids requires additional therapy. Failures may occur in two ways, persistent rejection, i.e., persistent histologic evidence of ACR, or recurrent rejection in which another episode of ACR occurs on the heels of the last episode. Persistent or recurrent rejection is typically treated aggressively with another course of IV followed by PO corticosteroids or by utilizing other agents. The polyclonal antibodies (Atgam or Thymoglobulin), OKT-3, total lymphoid irradiation (TLI), methotrexate, inhaled cyclosporine, and changing from cyclosporine-based therapy to tacrolimus have each been used as "rescue" therapy for corticosteroid resistant rejection. For all of these alternative approaches there are no large-scale data to prove efficacy. Most centers currently use the polyclonal antibodies as the next step for corticosteroid resistant rejection. Horse antithymocyte globulin (Atgam, 15 mg/kg/day) or rabbit antithymocyte globulin (Thymoglobulin, 1.5 mg/kg/day) is given for a five- to seven-day course. Major side effects include fever and thrombocytopenia. These agents may produce a profound lymphopenia and increase the risk for opportunistic infection. During the early experience in lung transplantation, OKT-3 was commonly utilized both to treat refractory rejection and as an induction agent. Shennib et al. (70) studied the utility of OKT-3 for persistent or recurrent ACR in 28 patients with 68% responding. Although OKT-3 was quite efficacious in controlling the rejection episode, the treatment was associated with infectious complications in 21%. Today, OKT-3 is used less widely because of the high likelihood of profound side effects such as fever, hypotension, and pulmonary edema associated with the cytokine release syndrome. As an alternative strategy to treat steroid resistant ACR, Cahill et al. (71) studied the utility of methotrexate. Twelve patients were treated with weekly methotrexate for a total of six weeks with 10 of the 12 showing no evidence of ACR during a mean follow-up of 12.5 months (range 1 to 42 months). Changing from cyclosporine to tacrolimus was shown to be of benefit by the Washington University group and the Wisconsin group, although each studied a small cohort of patients (14 and 15 patients, respectively) (72,73). Keenan et al. (74) reported the use of aerosolized cyclosporine to treat refractory ACR. Eighteen patients with persistent ACR who failed therapy with pulse steroids and antithymocyte globulin were treated. Aerosolized cyclosporine was administered at a dose of 300 mg/day for 10 days, then changed to dosing three days per week for maintenance. Two patients were unable to tolerate the therapy due to side effects but 14 out of 16 responded with significant improvement after a mean of 37 days. TLI was studied by Valentine et al. (75). Six patients with refractory ACR were treated with a total of 800 cGy of TLI over a five week course. Mild and transient leukopenia was the only major reported side effect. One patient died from adult respiratory distress syndrome (ARDS) four weeks after completing therapy but the remaining patients all had resolution of the ACR.

Extracorporeal photopheresis was evaluated in a retrospective study by the group from Loyola University to treat BOS in a small cohort of patients (76). In three patients with BOS and concurrent acute rejection, therapy with extracorporeal photopheresis led to the resolution of the acute rejection episode.

Finally, the group from Duke University reported the use of anti-CD 52 antibody alemtuzumab (Campath, Ilex), to successfully treat a single patient with refractory ACR (77).

## REFERENCES

1. Bando K, Paradis IL, Similo S, et al. Obliterative bronchiolitis after lung and heart–lung transplantation. An analysis of risk factors and management. J Thorac Cardiovasc Surg 1995; 110(1):4–13.
2. Glanville AR, Corris PA, McNeil K, Wahlers T. International MMF Lung Study. Group Mycophenolate mofetil (MMF) versus azithioprine for the prevention of bronchiolitis obliterans sydrome (BOS): results of a 3 year international randomised trial. J Heart Lung Transplant 2003; 22(1):S207.
3. Marshall SE, Lewiston NJ, Kramer MR, et al. Prospective analysis of serial pulmonary function studies and transbronchial biopsies in single-lung transplant recipients. Transplant Proc 1991; 23(1 Pt 2):1217–1219.
4. Sibley RK, Berry GJ, Tazelaar HD, et al. The role of transbronchial biopsies in the management of lung transplant recipients. J Heart Lung Transplant 1993; 12(2):308–324.
5. Trulock EP, Ettinger NA, Brunt EM, Pasque MK, Kaiser LR, Cooper JD. The role of transbronchial lung biopsy in the treatment of lung transplant

recipients. An analysis of 200 consecutive procedures. Chest 1992; 102(4): 1049–1054.

6. Guilinger RA, Paradis EL, Dauber JH, et al. The importance of bronchoscopy with transbronchial biopsy and bronchoalveolar lavage in the management of lung transplant recipients. Am J Respir Crit Care Med 1995; 152(6 Pt 1):2037–2043.

7. Cooper JD, Pohl MS, Patterson GA. An update on the current status of lung transplantation: report of the St. Louis International Lung Transplant Registry. Clin Transpl 1993:95–100.

8. Brock MV, Borja MC, Ferber L, et al. Induction therapy in lung transplantation: a prospective, controlled clinical trial comparing OKT3, anti-thymocyte globulin, and daclizumab. J Heart Lung Transplant 2001; 20(12): 1282–1290.

9. Hopkins PM, Aboyoun CL, Chhajed PN, et al. Prospective analysis of 1,235 transbronchial lung biopsies in lung transplant recipients. J Heart Lung Transplant 2002; 21(10):1062–1067.

10. Palmer SM, Baz MA, Sanders L, et al. Results of a randomized, prospective, multicenter trial of mycophenolate mofetil versus azathioprine in the prevention of acute lung allograft rejection. Transplantation 2001; 71(12): 1772–1776.

11. Swanson SJ, Mentzer SJ, Really JJ, et al. Surveillance transbronchial lung biopsies: implication for survival after lung transplantation. J Thorac Cardiovasc Surg 2000; 119(1):27–37.

12. Treede H, Reichenspurner H, Meiser B, et al. Influence of four different immunosuppressive protocols on acute and chronic rejection (BOS) after lung transplantation—experiences in 120 patients. J Heart Lung Transplant 2001; 20(2):176.

13. Girgis RE, Tu I, Berry GJ, et al. Risk factors for the development of obliterative bronchiolitis after lung transplantation. J Heart Lung Transplant 1996; 15(12):1200–1208.

14. Kroshus TJ, Kshettry VR, Savik K, John R, Hertz MI, Bolman RM I. Risk factors for the development of bronchiolitis obliterans syndrome after lung transplantation. J Thorac Cardiovasc Surg 1997; 114:195.

15. Estenne M, Hertz MI. Bronchiolitis obliterans after human lung transplantation. Am J Respir Crit Care Med 2002; 166(4):440–444.

16. Sharples LD, Tamm M, McNeil K, Higenbottam TW, Stewart S, Wallwork J. Development of bronchiolitis obliterans syndrome in recipients of heart–lung transplantation—early risk factors. Transplantation 1996; 61(4):560–566.

17. Sharples LD, McNeil K, Stewart S, Wallwork J. Risk factors for bronchiolitis obliterans: a systematic review of recent publications. J Heart Lung Transplant 2002; 21(2):271–281.

18. Heng D, Sharples LD, McNeil K, Stewart S, Wreghitt T, Wallwork J. Bronchiolitis obliterans syndrome: incidence, natural history, prognosis, and risk factors. J Heart Lung Transplant 1998; 17(12):1255–1263.

19. Terasaki PI. Humoral theory of transplantation. Am J Transplant 2003; 3(6): 665–673.

20. Frost AE, Jammal CT, Cagle PT. Hyperacute rejection following lung transplantation. Chest 1996; 110(2):559–562.

21. Choi JK, Keams J, Palevsky HI, et al. Hyperacute rejection of a pulmonary allograft. Immediate clinical and pathologic findings. Am J Respir Crit Care Med 1999; 160(3):1015–1018.

22. Bittner HB, Dunitz J, Hertz M, Bolman MR III, Park SJ. Hyperacute rejection in single lung transplantation—case report of successful management by means of plasmapheresis and antithymocyte globulin treatment. Transplantation 2001; 71(5):649–651.

23. Arcasoy SM. Medical complications and management of lung transplant recipients. Respir Care Clin N Am 2004; 10(4):505–529.

24. Kaye M. The Registry of the International Society for Heart and Lung Transplantation: ninth official report—1992. J Heart Lung Transplant 1992; 11(4 Pt 1):599–606.

25. Millet B, Higenbottam TW, Flower CD, Stewart S, Wallwork J. The radiographic appearances of infection and acute rejection of the lung after heart–lung transplantation. Am Rev Respir Dis 1989; 140(1):62–67.

26. Bando K, Paradis EL, Komatsu K, et al. Analysis of time-dependent risks for infection, rejection, and death after pulmonary transplantation. J Thorac Cardiovasc Surg 1995; 109(1):49–57.

27. Otulana BA, Higenbottam T, Scott J, Clelland C, Igboaka G, Wallwork J. Lung function associated with histologically diagnosed acute lung rejection and pulmonary infection in heart–lung transplant patients. Am Rev Respir Dis 1990; 142(2):329–332.

28. Hoeper MM, Hamm M, Schafers HJ, Haverich A, Wagner TO. Evaluation of lung function during pulmonary rejection and infection in heart–lung transplant patients. Hannover Lung Transplant Group. Chest 1992; 102(3):864–870.

29. Otulana BA, Higenbottam T, Ferrari L, Scott J, Igboaka G, Wallwork J. The use of home spirometry in detecting acute lung rejection and infection following heart–lung transplantation. Chest 1990; 97(2):353–357.

30. Morlion B, Knoop C, Paiva M, Estenne M. Internet-based home monitoring of pulmonary function after lung transplantation. Am J Respir Crit Care Med 2002; 165(5):694–697.

31. Becker FS, Martinez FJ, Brunsting LA, Deeb GM, Flint A, Lynch JP III. Limitations of spirometry in detecting rejection after single-lung transplantation. Am J Respir Crit Care Med 1994; 150(1):159–166.

32. Kaplan J, Trulock EP, Kaiser L, Cooper JD, Schuster D. Pulmonary vascular permeability changes during rejection and infection in heart–lung transplantation (abstract). Am Rev Respir Dis 1990; 141:A683.

33. Herve PA, Silbert D, Mensch J, et al. Increased lung clearance of 99mTcDTPA in allograft lung rejection. The Paris-Sud Lung Transplant Group. Am Rev Respir Dis 1991; 144(6):1333–1336.

34. Grossman RF, Frost A, Zamel N, et al. Results of single-lung transplantation for bilateral pulmonary fibrosis. The Toronto Lung Transplant Group. N Engl J Med 1990; 322(11):727–733.

35. Dabbs AV, Hoffman LA, Swigart V, et al. Striving for normalcy: symptoms and the threat of rejection after lung transplantation. Soc Sci Med 2004; 59(7):1473–1484.

36. Yousem SA, Berry GJ, Cagle PT, et al. Revision of the 1990 working formulation for the classification of pulmonary allograft rejection: Lung Rejection Study Group. J Heart Lung Transplant 1996; 15(1 Pt 1):1–15.
37. Burns KE, Johnson BA, Iacono AT. Diagnostic properties of transbronchial biopsy in lung transplant recipients who require mechanical ventilation. J Heart Lung Transplant 2003; 22(3):267–275.
38. Silkoff PE, Caramori M, Tremblay L, et al. Exhaled nitric oxide in human lung transplantation. A noninvasive marker of acute rejection. Am J Respir Crit Care Med 1998; 157(6 Pt 1):1822–1828.
39. Fisher AJ, Gabbay E, Small T, Doig S, Dark JH, Corns PA. Cross sectional study of exhaled nitric oxide levels following lung transplantation. Thorax 1998; 53:454.
40. Studer SM, Rosas I, Cope K, Krishnan J, Risby TH, Orens J. Patterns and significance of exhaled breath biomarkers in acute lung allograft rejection. J Heart Lung Transplant 2000; 20:1158–1166.
41. Slebos DJ, Postma DS, Koeter GH, van der BW, Boezen M, Kauffman HF. Bronchoalveolar lavage fluid characteristics in acute and chronic lung transplant rejection. J Heart Lung Transplant 2004; 23(5):532–540.
42. Rizzo M, SivaSai KS, Smith MA, et al. Increased expression of inflammatory cytokines and adhesion molecules by alveolar macrophages of human lung allograft recipients with acute rejection: decline with resolution of rejection. J Heart Lung Transplant 2000; 19:858.
43. Kukafka DS, O'Brien GM, Furukawa S, Criner GJ. Surveillance bronchoscopy in lung transplant recipients. Chest 1997; 111(2):377–381.
44. Levine SM. A survey of clinical practice of lung transplantation in North America. Chest 2004; 125(4):1224–1238.
45. Valentine VG, Taylor DE, Dhillon GS, et al. Success of lung transplantation without surveillance bronchoscopy. J Heart Lung Transplant 2002; 21(3):319–326.
46. Berry GJ, Brunt EM, Chamberlain D, et al. A working formulation for the standardization of nomenclature in the diagnosis of heart and lung rejection: Lung Rejection Study Group. The International Society for Heart Transplantation. J Heart Transplant 1990; 9(6):593–601.
47. Hadjiliadis D, Davis RD, Palmer SM. Is transplant operation important in determining posttransplant risk of bronchiolitis obliterans syndrome in lung transplant recipients? Chest 2002; 122(4);1168–1175.
48. Hopkins PM, Aboyoun CL, Chhajed PN, et al. Association of minimal rejection in lung transplant recipients with obliterative bronchiolitis. Am J Respir Crit Care Med 2004; 170(9):1022–1026.
49. Le Moine A, Goldman M, Abramowicz D. Multiple pathways to allograft rejection. Transplantation 2002; 73(9):1373–1381.
50. Parkin J, Cohen B. An overview of the immune system. Lancet 2001; 357(9270): 1777–1789.
51. Palmer SM, Burch LH, Davis RD, et al. The role of innate immunity in acute allograft rejection after lung transplantation. Am J Respir Crit Care Med 2003; 168(6):628–632.
52. Janeway CA, Travers P, Walport M, Shlomchik M. Autoimmunity and Transplantation. Immunobiology. New York: Garland Publishing, 2001.

53.  Sundaresan S, Alevy YG, Steward N, et al. Cytokine gene transcripts for tumor necrosis factor-alpha, interleukin-2, and interferon-gamma in human pulmonary allografts. J Heart Lung Transplant 1995; 14(3):512–518.
54.  Gimino VJ, Lande JD, Berryman TR, King RA, Hertz MI. Gene expression profiling of bronchoalveolar lavage cells in acute lung rejection. Am J Respir Crit Care Med 2003; 168(10):1237–1242.
55.  Palmer SM, Burch LH, Trindade AJ, et al. Innate immunity influences long-term outcomes after human lung transplant. Am J Respir Crit Care Med 2005; 171(7):780–785.
56.  Lau CL, Palmer SM, Posther KE, et al. Influence of panel-reactive antibodies on posttransplant outcomes in lung transplant recipients. Ann Thorac Surg 2000; 69(5):1520–1524.
57.  Schulman LL, Ho EK, Reed EF, et al. Immunologic monitoring in lung allograft recipients. Transplantation 1996; 61(2):252–257.
58.  Jaramillo A, Smith MA, Phelan D, et al. Development of ELISA-detected anti-HLA antibodies precedes the development of bronchiolitis obliterans syndrome and correlates with progressive decline in pulmonary function after lung transplantation. Transplantation 1999; 67(8):1155–1161.
59.  Sundaresan S, Mohanakumar T, Smith MA, et al. HLA-A locus mismatches and development of antibodies to HLA after lung transplantation correlate with the development of bronchiolitis obliterans syndrome. Transplantation 1998; 65(5):648–653.
60.  Palmer SM, Davis RD, Hadjiliadis D, et al. Development of an antibody specific to major histocompatibility antigens detectable by flow cytometry after lung transplant is associated with bronchiolitis obliterans syndrome. Transplantation 2002; 74(6):799–804.
61.  Miller GG, Destarac L, Zeevi A, et al. Acute humoral rejection of human lung allografts and elevation of C4d in bronchoalveolar lavage fluid. Am J Transplant 2004; 4(8):1323–1330.
62.  Badesch DB, Zamora M, Fullerton D, et al. Pulmonary capillaritis: a possible histologic form of acute pulmonary allograft rejection. J Heart Lung Transplant 1998; 17(4):415–422.
63.  Magro CM, Deng A, Pope-Harman A, et al. Humorally mediated posttransplantation septal capillary injury syndrome as a common form of pulmonary allograft rejection: a hypothesis. Transplantation 2002; 74(9): 1273–1280.
64.  Magro CM, Pope HA, Klinger D, et al. Use of C4d as a diagnostic adjunct in lung allograft biopsies. Am J Transplant 2003; 3(9):1143–1154.
65.  Girnita AL, McCurry KR, Iacono AT, et al. HLA-specific antibodies are associated with high-grade and persistent-recurrent lung allograft acute rejection. J Heart Lung Transplant 2004; 23(10):1135–1141.
66.  ISHLT Registry report online. (Accessed May 15, 2005, at www.ishlt.org.).
67.  Trulock EP, Edwards LB, Taylor DO, Boucek MM, Keck BM, Hertz ML. The Registry of the International Society for Heart Lung Transplantation: twenty-first official adult heart transplant. J Heart Lung Transplant 2004; 23(7):804–815.
68.  Palmer SM, Miralles AP, Lawrence CM, Gaynor JW, Davis FRD, Tapson VF. Rabbit antithymocyte globulin decreases acute rejection after lung transplantation: results of a randomized, prospective study. Chest 1999; 116(1):127–133.

69. Garrity ER Jr, Villanueva J, Bhorade SM, Husain AN, Vigneswaran WT. Low rate of acute lung allograft rejection after the use of daclizumab, an interleukin 2 receptor antibody. Transplantation 2001; 71(6):773–777.

70. Shennib H, Massard G, Reynaud M, Noirclerc M. Efficacy of OKT3 therapy for acute rejection in isolated lung transplantation. J Heart Lung Transplant 1994; 13(3):514–519.

71. Cahill BC, O'Rourke MK, Strasburg KA, et al. Methotrexate for lung transplant recipients with steroid-resistant acute rejection. J Heart Lung Transplant 1996; 15(11):1130–1137.

72. Horning NR, Lynch JP, Sundaresan SR, Patterson GA, Trulock EP. Tacrolimus therapy for persistent or recurrent acute rejection after lung transplantation. J Heart Lung Transplant 1998; 17(8):761–767.

73. Onsager DR, Canver CC, Jahania MS, et al. Efficacy of tacrolimus in the treatment of refractory rejection in heart and lung transplant recipients. J Heart Lung Transplant 1999; 18(5):448–455.

74. Keenan RJ, Iacono A, Dauber JH, et al. Treatment of refractory acute allograft rejection with aerosolized cyclosporine in lung transplant recipients. J Thorac Cardiovasc Surg 1997; 113(2):335–340.

75. Valentine VG, Robbins RC, Wehner JH, Patel HR, Berry GJ, Theodore J. Total lymphoid irradiation for refractory acute rejection in heart–lung and lung allografts. Chest 1996; 109(5):1184–1189.

76. Villanueva J, Bhorade SM, Robinson JA, Husain AN, Garrity ER Jr. Extracorporeal photopheresis for the treatment of lung allograft rejection. Ann Transplant 2000; 5(3):44–47.

77. Reams BD, Davis RD, Curl J, Palmer SM. Treatment of refractory acute rejection in a lung transplant recipient with campath 1H. Transplantation 2002; 74(6):903–904.

# 30

# Pathology of the Lung Transplant

### David N. Howell

*Department of Pathology, Duke University and Durham Veterans Affairs Medical Centers, Durham, North Carolina, U.S.A.*

### Scott M. Palmer

*Division of Pulmonary and Critical Care Medicine, Department of Medicine, Duke University Medical Center, Durham, North Carolina, U.S.A.*

## INTRODUCTION

Pathology is a cornerstone in the care of all solid organ transplant patients, but it is nowhere of more importance than in the setting of lung transplantation. The lung is unique among transplanted organs in its extensive exposure to the external environment, subjecting it to a number of infectious and physical injuries not shared by other transplants; many of these complications are best diagnosed by pathologic examination of biopsy specimens. Furthermore, flexible bronchoscopy provides a safe and convenient way to directly examine the allograft and allow for frequent and prospective pathological examination of the transplanted organ. Many forms of lung transplant pathology are at first clinically inapparent or present with nonspecific symptoms; histopathologic examination of lung transplant biopsy material thus serves a key role in the surveillance and diagnosis of lung allograft complications. Finally, since lung transplantation is a relatively young field, pathologic examination is crucial to our evolving understanding of the biology of the pulmonary allograft. It was not until the mid-1980s that Cooper and colleagues achieved the first successful long-term outcomes in a series of patients with idiopathic pulmonary fibrosis undergoing single lung transplant (1). Thus, in a relatively short time lung transplantation has evolved into an acceptable and effective therapy for many advanced lung diseases including emphysema, cystic fibrosis, and idiopathic pulmonary fibrosis, as well as more rare conditions. In this chapter, we review the broad spectrum of pathological conditions that arise in human lung transplants as well as methods for procurement and processing of samples for diagnostic analysis.

## Obtaining Tissue for Pathologic Examination

Bronchoscopic biopsy is the primary method of allograft tissue sampling employed at most centers. Bronchoscopy in lung transplant recipients requires special attention and consideration beyond that required in routine bronchoscopies of native lungs. Altered sedative requirements in cystic fibrosis patients and increased risk for bleeding in all patients represent some of the unique transplant bronchoscopic considerations. Experienced centers have found that standard guidelines for bronchoscopic practice in lung transplant recipients reduce complications (2). Routine lung transplant biopsies are performed by the transbronchial route. In general, an attempt is made to obtain at least five pieces of alveolar tissue (3). This method has both advantages and drawbacks. On the positive side, it is a safe procedure with minimal morbidity and mortality. It provides the opportunity to obtain samples from multiple areas. Furthermore, endobronchial biopsies can be performed if indicated, and transbronchial samples will also often include some airway as well as alveolar tissues, providing the opportunity to assess bronchiolar pathology. The small tissue pieces obtained bronchoscopically are amenable to rapid fixation and processing; same-day processing and interpretation are feasible. On the negative side, the total amount of tissue available for inspection in bronchoscopic biopsies is somewhat limited. Though experienced bronchoscopists usually obtain adequate samples over 95% of the time, nondiagnostic specimens are occasionally encountered. Routine sampling of endobronchial tissues in the absence of any specific endobronchial lesions appears of low yield and would not be recommended. The focus of routine surveillance or diagnostic transbronchial biopsy should be on obtaining an adequate sample of alveolar tissue.

Although most programs perform surveillance biopsies on a regular basis (e.g., biopsy every three months for at least the first posttransplant year), the utility of this approach is debated. Proponents of the surveillance approach point to the high rates of early asymptomatic rejection or infection and suggest that early diagnosis and treatment of these conditions will lead to improved patient outcomes. In contrast, one report suggested that if a patient was at least six months posttransplant with at least two consecutive biopsies negative for rejection, then the yield of subsequent biopsies was too low to justify regular surveillance (4). Furthermore, another report suggested the outcomes, including survival, were unchanged regardless of a surveillance versus clinically indicated biopsy approach (5). In contrast, more recent reports have suggested that surveillance biopsies, even when performed late posttransplant, have a surprisingly high yield for acute rejection or lymphocytic bronchiolitis. In particular, in one large series the incidence of rejection after the first 100 days posttransplant was 40% even in patients with no early rejection (6). In our opinion, there is no question that regular surveillance biopsies will uncover unsuspected pathology even in apparently stable patients relatively far out from transplant. The most appropriate therapy in patients with late asymptomatic rejection, however, remains an area of considerable controversy, and the failure of surveillance biopsies to lead to improved long-term survival likely reflects the failure of the therapies rather than the lack of yield of the biopsies.

Occasionally, open biopsies, typically obtained by video-assisted thoracoscopic surgery (VATS), will be employed to provide a much larger sample of tissue or target focal lesions. In some cases, particularly involving focal processes such as posttransplant lymphoproliferative disorder (PTLD), open biopsies have revealed abnormalities missed by prior bronchoscopic biopsies (7). Open biopsies are not without their drawbacks, however. Though thoracoscopic procedures are generally well tolerated, their morbidity exceeds that of bronchoscopic biopsy by a considerable margin. Thus the potential for uncovering an alternative diagnosis not evident on bronchoscopic examination needs to be carefully balanced with the increased risk of complications associated with surgical biopsy.

The pathologist is also called upon occasionally to examine whole lung specimens, including native pneumonectomies from patients undergoing initial transplantation, transplant pneumonectomies from patients undergoing retransplantation, and autopsy lungs. The pathologic processes in such specimens have often been presaged by biopsies or other clinical investigations, but thorough examination, including inflation of the lung with formalin via the bronchial tree and meticulous serial sectioning, frequently refines the diagnosis or yields new, unexpected findings such as focal infectious processes, tumors, or (in the case of transplanted lungs) unanticipated acute or chronic rejection. It is only possible to examine a small fraction of each lung microscopically, and guidelines for sampling are not firmly established. A reasonable strategy used at our center for transplant pneumonectomies includes preparation of tissue blocks from hilar bronchovascular structures, random samples of central and peripheral parenchyma from each lobe, and any focal lesions identified on gross examination.

Though beyond the scope of this chapter, it is also worth mentioning the vital role of histopathology in the analysis of extrapulmonary disease processes in the transplant recipient. Opportunistic infections are of particular importance to patients on long-term immunosuppressive therapy. Some opportunistic pathogens, such as cytomegalovirus (CMV), can infect the allograft as well as other organs. Others have tissue tropisms that generally exclude the transplant. For example, parvovirus B19 has been reported to infect the bone marrow and cause aplastic anemia in lung and other transplant populations (8). Toxic and allergic reactions to medications are a second major category for which tissue examination is often of central diagnostic importance, a prime example being calcineurin-inhibitor nephrotoxicity. Finally, in patients whose primary pulmonary disorders have potential for multisystemic involvement (e.g., cystic fibrosis, neoplasms), examination of biopsy tissue often plays a key role in monitoring extrapulmonary expression or extension of the disease.

## Processing and Examination of Lung Transplant Biopsies

A majority of the tissue obtained by either transbronchial or thoracoscopic biopsies is generally fixed in formalin and embedded in paraffin for routine histologic sectioning. In unusual cases, reservation of a portion of the tissue in the fresh frozen state (for immunofluorescent staining or molecular diagnostic studies) or in glutaraldehyde (for electron microscopy) may be warranted. Pathologists at most transplant centers perform a battery of histochemical and immunohistochemical stains on the paraffin-embedded portion of each biopsy prospectively. At our institution, the panel includes hematoxylin and eosin (H&E) stains on multiple sections (for examination of general tissue morphology); periodic acid-Schiff (PAS) and methenamine silver stains for fungi (the latter stain detects *Pneumocystis carinii*); and an immunoperoxidase stain for CMV. Although the role for prospective CMV immunostaining is controversial, we believe that the high rate of disease seen in this population and the high sensitivity afforded by the technique justify its routine inclusion in the analysis of lung transplant samples. Routine performance of connective tissue stains such as Masson's trichrome has also been advocated to facilitate detection of obliterative bronchiolitis (3). Though prospective performance of special stains incurs some additional expense, it has several advantages, including conservation of limited tissue (a certain amount of which is wasted in each cutting session during alignment of the block on the microtome) and rapidity. The special stains also serve as "step sections," occasionally revealing focal processes missed on the H&E stains.

Several other stains are useful for evaluation of lung transplant biopsies in selected cases. To expedite performance of these stains when they are called for, we produce and reserve three unstained slides along with the initial set of stains. Kinyoun's carbol fuchsin stain for acid-fast organisms can be used to detect mycobacteria, and is applied prospectively to transplant biopsies in some centers. In our experience, the diagnostic yield for this stain is too low to justify routine ordering. Similarly, we will not routinely perform tissue gram stains for conventional bacteria because of the low clinical utility. Immunoperoxidase stains are occasionally used to detect viruses other than CMV; immunostaining and in situ hybridization are also helpful in the diagnosis of PTLD.

In addition to the standard and elective staining procedures described previously, we routinely examine all lung transplant biopsies for foreign material by polarization microscopy. The most prevalent refractile objects identified by this procedure are small, slender silica crystals within alveolar macrophages. These are of undetermined significance, but are occasionally numerous. In a smaller percentage of cases, larger, irregular fragments of refractile material are seen within macrophages or multinucleate giant cells (Fig. 1A and B). These foreign bodies and the cells that contain them are easy to overlook on routine histologic inspection, and often signal the presence of aspiration. We have previously reported the presence of gastroesophageal reflux, which may potentiate aspiration, in over 60% of lung transplant recipients, and described its association with lung allograft dysfunction (as discussed later in this chapter). In rare cases, intravenously injected foreign material (e.g., microcrystalline cellulose contained in medications intended for oral use but administered parenterally by misguided patients) can be detected within vascular channels in allograft biopsies (9).

## ISCHEMIA–REPERFUSION LUNG INJURY

Ischemia–reperfusion lung injury (IRLI), also known as primary graft failure (PGF), represents a frequent cause of early mortality and prolonged intensive care unit stay after lung transplant. A variety of factors such as poor preservation, prolonged ischemic time, or unsuspected donor lung pathology such as contusion or aspiration play a role in its development (10). The condition is characterized by noncardiogenic pulmonary edema

**(A)**                                    **(B)**

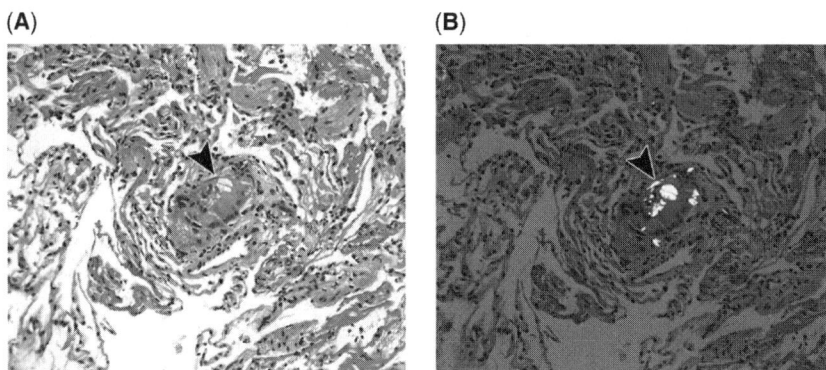

**Figure 1** Aspiration pneumonitis. (**A**) Light micrograph showing multinucleate giant cells within alveolar space (*arrowhead*). (**B**) Polarization microscopy of the same field shows refractile foreign bodies (*arrowhead*) within the giant cells (H&E stain, magnification × 180).

and progressive lung injury over the first few hours following implantation. The process can be relatively mild and self-limited or can evolve into severe diffuse alveolar damage (DAD). It appears that even long-term survivors of the condition suffer reduced pulmonary function and impaired physical conditioning, and are at an increased risk for development of bronchiolitis obliterans syndrome (11).

Though a presumptive diagnosis of IRLI is often made without biopsy, examination of tissue specimens can provide valuable information, both by identifying changes compatible with ischemia/reperfusion and by ruling out alternative (or additional) processes such as infection or rejection. The histologic findings in IRLI are similar to those in the spectrum of DAD/acute respiratory distress syndrome seen in native lungs. In the early phase, corresponding to the "exudative" phase of DAD, alveolar pneumocytes exhibit signs of injury, including swelling and nuclear reactive changes (Fig. 2A and B), often accompanied by intra-alveolar edema and patchy accumulation of neutrophils within alveolar septa. Proteins in the fibrin-rich alveolar exudate often coalesce as eosinophilic sheets, designated "hyaline membranes," lining septa (Fig. 2C). These changes, though grossly diffuse, often have significant regional variability at the microscopic level.

Over a period of days to a few weeks, the acute changes of IRLI may resolve with minimal histologic sequelae. In some patients, however, the injury progresses, in a manner similar to the "organizing" phase of DAD, with intraalveolar accumulation of plugs of immature connective tissue (Fig. 2D). The connective tissue ultimately becomes incorporated into the alveolar walls, sometimes with residual fibrous scarring. At this stage, the injury can be difficult to distinguish from the late stages of other processes, particularly infections.

In severe cases, IRLI may require maximal ventilatory support and other therapeutic measures. Inhaled nitric oxide is of benefit, as it significantly decreases pulmonary artery pressure and improves $PaO_2/FiO_2$ ratio. Recently, inhaled prostacyclin has been investigated and shown promise as an alternative to nitric oxide (12). Extracorporeal membrane oxygenation (ECMO) is a suitable treatment option if employed early (13). Initiating use of ECMO more than 24 hours after the injury has been uniformly unsuccessful in our experience.

Fortunately, severe reperfusion injury appears to be decreasing in frequency in recent years. A combination of improved preservation techniques and solutions as well as improved ventilatory strategies has likely contributed. Although the exact mechanisms for development of IRLI are unclear, the process appears to involve activation of cytokine, coagulation, and complement inflammatory cascades. Recently, elevation of IL-8 in the donor lung has been associated with an increased risk for the development of IRLI (14). If validated, these results suggest that the use of novel biomarkers might be an effective means to avoid potential donors that place recipients at high risk for IRLI.

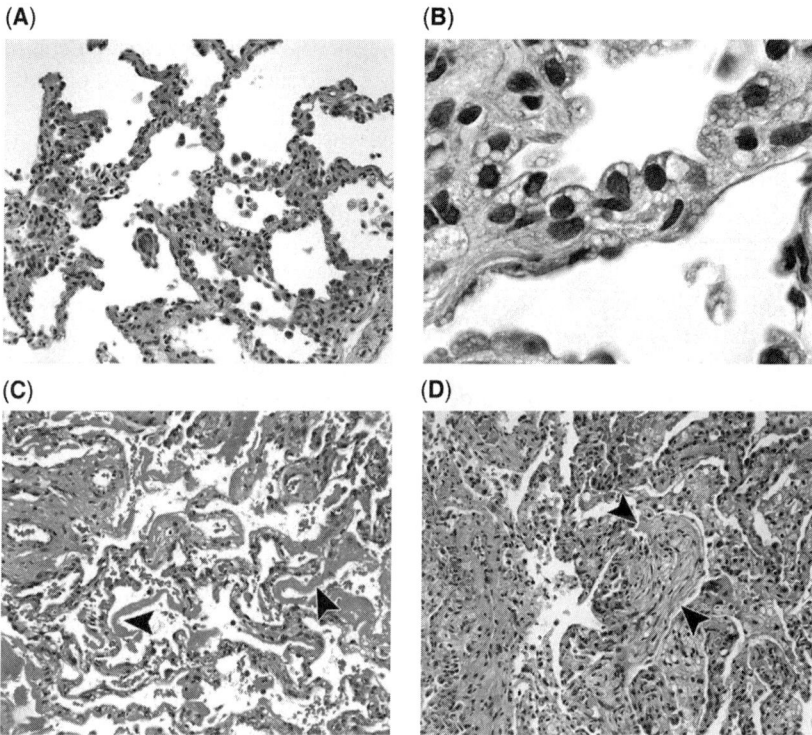

**Figure 2** Ischemia–reperfusion lung injury (IRLI). (**A**) Early IRLI, limited to swelling and vacuolization of alveolar lining cells. (**B**) High-magnification micrograph showing pneumocyte vacuolization. (**C**) More extensive early changes, with deposition of hyaline membranes (*arrowheads*) along alveolar septa. (**D**) Organizing IRLI, with intra-alveolar collections of immature fibrous tissue (*arrowheads*) (H&E stains; magnification in panels **A**, **C**, and **D** ×180; magnification in panel **B** × 900).

## INFECTION

Infection is a particularly complex topic for solid organ transplant recipients in general and lung transplant recipients in particular. The moderately intensive maintenance immunosuppressive regimens with which transplant recipients are treated render them susceptible to many of the opportunistic infections that plague individuals with more profound forms of immunocompromise, though the pattern and severity of infection may differ (to the potential confusion of the unwary pathologist). Since the ultimate goal of solid organ transplantation is to return the recipient to an active and interactive lifestyle, however, patients with successful transplants are exposed to, and often contract, the same range of community-acquired infections seen in immunocompetent individuals. In the lung transplant recipient, these susceptibilities are compounded by the extensive contact of the transplanted organ with the outside environment and deficiencies in many primary defense mechanisms (e.g., mucociliary escalator, cough reflex). In addition, patients with chronic pulmonary disorders, particularly septic lung diseases, are frequently colonized prior to transplantation with a variety of organisms that can infect the transplant. Finally, post-transplant immunoglobulin deficiency has been described after lung transplantation and is associated with an increased risk for infectious complications (15).

Transplant biopsy is a valuable approach to the diagnosis of lung transplant infections. Though it often lacks the sensitivity and specificity of alternative clinical laboratory studies (e.g., culture, molecular diagnostic testing), it has many salient advantages as a diagnostic tool. Chief among these is the ability of biopsy to detect a wide range of infectious and noninfectious processes, including multiple infections and infections superimposed on other processes such as rejection. In many cases, it may reveal an unexpected infectious process for which a more specific diagnostic test would not ordinarily have been performed. Histologic examination of biopsies can be performed rapidly; same-day processing and examination are available at most major medical centers if needed. If necessary, biopsy tissue can also be used as a substrate for more specific diagnostic tests, including immunohistochemistry and nucleic acid–based molecular methods. Furthermore, routine bacterial cultures are negative in some cases even in the presence of a clinical picture of an acute pneumonia, in which case pathological examination often provides critical confirmatory evidence for the presence of infection.

In the following sections we provide a brief survey of histologic findings in transplant infections, with illustrations of some of the more common pathologic findings. For a more complete discussion of the diagnosis and management of these infections, the reader is referred to earlier chapters in this book or to the references provided.

## Bacterial Pneumonia

Lung transplant recipients are susceptible to a variety of bacterial pneumonias, including community-acquired infections with organisms like *Staphylococcus aureus,* nosocomial infections, and, especially in patients transplanted for septic lung disease, reinfections with pretransplant pathogens such as *Pseudomonas aeruginosa* and *Burkholderia cepacia.* Biopsy can provide the first objective evidence of such infections, and frequently allows presumptive treatment while culture results are awaited. This is particularly important in patients whose differentials include both infection and rejection, since the therapeutic approaches to these processes are markedly different.

The biopsy findings in transplant pneumonia are similar to those in the native lung. Early in the course of infection, alveolar spaces are consolidated with mixtures of neutrophils, fibrin, and edema fluid (Fig. 3A), sometimes with superimposed hemorrhage. Tissue necrosis may occur in severe cases. Acute inflammation of bronchial wall, particularly the epithelium, is often present as well; neutrophils within strips of detached bronchial epithelium are occasionally a valuable diagnostic clue in biopsies with inadequate sampling of alveolar tissue. As the infection progresses, other inflammatory cell types (lymphocytes, macrophages) are recruited to the area of infection. In some cases, the inflammation may resolve with minimal residual damage. In others, the alveolar inflammatory components undergo organization, with replacement by collections of immature fibrous tissue (Fig. 3B). Foci of intra-alveolar organization ultimately become incorporated into the alveolar wall, often with development of a mature fibrous scar. The presence of organizing pneumonia has been reported in lung transplant recipients in association with bronchiolitis obliterans organizing pneumonia (BOOP), and might represent an entity histologically distinct from rejection-related bronchiolitis obliterans (see following text).

In the acute phase, bacteria (particularly gram-positive cocci) can sometimes be visualized on a tissue Gram stain or special forms of silver stain. These staining procedures have relatively low sensitivity, however, and are usually not employed. There is also concern regarding the clinical significance of visualized bacteria (i.e., colonization vs. infection) and such stains must be interpreted in light of the patient's clinical context and other histological findings. Routine histologic examination coupled with culture results is generally sufficient to achieve a diagnosis.

**(A)**                    **(B)**

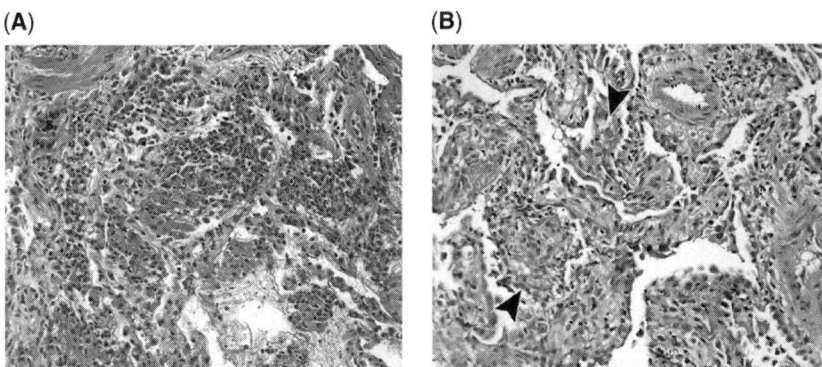

**Figure 3** Bacterial pneumonia. (**A**) Acute bacterial pneumonia, with alveolar consolidation by a mixture of neutrophils, fibrin, and cellular debris. (**B**) Organizing bacterial pneumonia, with alveolar spaces containing collections of immature fibrous tissue (*arrowheads*). Note similarity to organizing IRLI in Figure 2D (H&E stains; magnification ×180). *Abbreviation*: IRLI, ischemia–reperfusion lung injury.

## Mycobacterial Infection

Though atypical mycobacteria are detected occasionally in pulmonary cultures from lung transplant recipients, evidence of active infections in biopsy tissue is rare. In many cases, this disparity may reflect colonization rather than infection with the organisms. In other instances, focal infections may be missed by the biopsy. Even when infection is represented in the biopsy tissue, the findings are often nonspecific and the organisms difficult to identify. More research is needed to define the true frequency and clinical significance of mycobacterial disease in lung transplant recipients. *Mycobacterium avium complex* appears the most common mycobacterial isolate seen on culture after transplant and mycobacterial disease might be associated with irreversible loss of lung function (16).

The classic patterns of tissue response to mycobacterial infection, including engorgement of histiocytes with organisms (a common pattern for atypical mycobacterial infection in severely immunocompromised patients) and caseating granulomas (usually seen in *Mycobacterium tuberculosis* infection in immunocompetent individuals), are often absent in lung transplant recipients. Instead, biopsies frequently show patchy tissue necrosis or nonspecific mononuclear inflammation. Epithelioid histiocytes, a form of elongated macrophage typically found in granulomatous inflammation, may be present, but well-formed granulomas are often absent. Mycobacteria can sometimes be identified on acid-fast stains, but a diligent search is usually required.

## Other Unusual Bacteria

Bacteria with fastidious culture characteristics, unusual morphologies, and/or atypical staining properties pose a diagnostic challenge in any clinical specimen. Infections with such organisms are fortunately rare in the lung transplant population, but are easy to miss if a heightened index of suspicion is not maintained. Infections with filamentous organisms, including *Nocardia* sp. (Fig. 4A) (17) and *Actinomyces* sp. (18), have been documented in occasional transplant patients and often present with cutaneous or other extrapulmonary sites of disease. These organisms often fail to react with Gram stains, but can frequently be detected using silver or acid-fast stains. Occasional lung transplant recipients with *Legionella pneumophila* infections have also been described (19). Detection of this organism in tissues generally requires special varieties of silver stain.

## Fungal Infections

Lung transplant infections with fungi are infrequent with current prophylactic strategies but represent a potentially life-threatening complication. The most common sites of infections are at the anastomoses, where airway ischemia predisposes to the development of invasive fungal disease

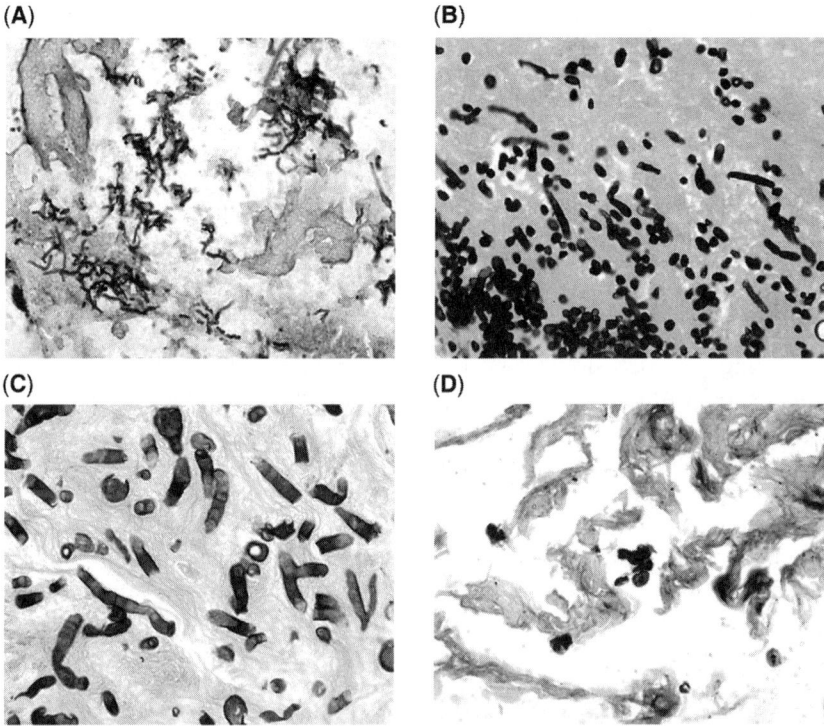

**Figure 4** Unusual bacteria and fungi. (**A**) *Nocardia* sp. masses of filamentous bacteria are seen within necrotic debris. (**B**) *Candida* sp. yeasts and occasional pseudohyphae are present in devitalized bronchial wall tissue. (**C**) *Aspergillus* sp. true hyphae with occasional branching and septa are seen in necrotic bronchial wall tissue. (**D**) *Pneumocystis carini*: a small cluster of organisms is present in an alveolar space. A central density is present in one (methenamine silver stains; magnification × 900).

(20,21). Parenchymal fungal infections also occur and are typically associated with nodular opacities or atypical lesions on radiographic studies. Although *Candida* sp. are probably the most common fungal pathogen isolated on bronchoscopic culture after lung transplant, most tissue-invasive pulmonary disease is related to more pathogenic organisms (20,21), such as *Aspergillus* sp. (21), other hyalohyphomycetes (e.g., *Scedosporium* sp.) (22), and zygomycetes such as *Cunninghamella* sp. Unfortunately, infections with *Scedosporium* sp. and *Cunninghamella* sp. are increasingly recognized in lung transplant recipients.

Anastomotic infections with fungi are often apparent to the bronchoscopist as protrusions of devitalized tissue and/or pseudomembranes, sometimes with dark discoloration. Examination of biopsy tissue typically reveals fragments of partially necrotic bronchial wall with associated fibrinopurulent debris. The organisms are often visible on H&E-stained sections, but are best visualized on PAS or methenamine silver stains. Candida forms round-to-oblong yeasts and irregular tubular structures termed pseudohyphae (Fig. 4B); *Aspergillus* forms segmented tubular hyphae with more parallel walls (Fig. 4C). Hyalohyphomycetes such as *Scedosporium* sp. often produce mixtures of true hyphae and yeasts, and have other specialized reproductive features that are sometimes identifiable in biopsies (23). Coexistence of true hyphae and yeasts may also signal the presence of a mixed infection with *Aspergillus* and *Candida*, however, so correlation of biopsy findings with culture results is essential. Zygomycetes produce thick, "ribbon-like" structures without conspicuous septation.

Fungi are occasionally encountered more distally within the transplant, either within airways or in infectious foci within alveolar tissue. In the latter situation, they are frequently associated with extensive tissue necrosis. Fungi-colonizing upper airways occasionally become attached to alveolar biopsy fragments as the bronchoscopist removes them. As such, the pathologist should attempt to document tissue invasion by the organisms before rendering a diagnosis of parenchymal infection. Ultimately, such a diagnosis requires correlation with microbiological cultures and recent clinical events.

### Pneumocystis carinii

Pneumocystosis is also an unusual complication of lung transplantation. *Pneumocystis carinii* is a fastidious organism that thrives most effectively in patients with profound immunocompromise. Routine prophylaxis of lung transplant recipients with trimethoprim/sulfamethoxazole has also played a major role in limiting pneumocystis infections (24,25). Those infections that occur are frequently in patients who discontinue or cannot tolerate prophylaxis.

Pneumocystis organisms appear as small spherical objects approximately 4–5 μm in diameter on methenamine silver stains, often with a central density (Fig. 4D). They do not react with H&E or PAS stains. *P. carinii* is approximately the same size and shape as *Histoplasma capsulatum*, with which they can easily be confused; useful distinguishing features include the PAS reactivity of *H. capsulatum* and its lack of a central density. In patients with profound immunocompromise, large clusters of pneumocystis organisms are typically present within alveolar spaces admixed with eosinophilic proteinaceous material. This pattern is generally absent in the lung transplant setting. Instead, small groups of organisms are typically seen in association with mixed inflammation, sometimes with a granulomatous pattern.

### Opportunistic Viral Infections

CMV is the leading cause of opportunistic pulmonary infection in lung transplant recipients. Infection affects over 50% of patients at risk (those with either donor or recipient positive CMV serologic status, or both) within the first year post-transplant despite ganciclovir prophylaxis (26). Pulmonary and systemic CMV disease is a significant cause of morbidity and mortality in lung transplant recipients, and may also induce immunological changes that predispose affected patients to subsequent infections or allograft rejection (26). Significant CMV pulmonary disease can be clinically and radiologically inapparent, augmenting the importance of biopsy surveillance.

As is typical of DNA viruses, CMV replicates in the nuclei of affected cells, most commonly pneumocytes and vascular endothelial cells. In patients with severe immunocompromise, intranuclear viral replication produces haloed inclusion bodies, termed "Cowdry A" or "owl's eye" inclusions; these are frequently accompanied by small cytoplasmic inclusions representing clusters of enveloped virions that have budded through the nuclear membrane. Affected cells are often markedly enlarged, the cytomegaly from which the name of the virus is derived (27). This combination of viral cytopathic effects (Fig. 5A and B), though virtually diagnostic for active CMV infection, is often absent in lung transplant recipients, particularly those with early or focal disease. Instead, cellular alterations may be limited to mild enlargement and nuclear hyperchromasia (Fig. 5C). Such infections can often be detected by immunohistochemistry for CMV immediate–early and early nuclear antigens (Fig. 5D) (28). Though CMV infections of bronchial wall are unusual, we have encountered the virus in bronchial polyps in occasional transplant recipients (29).

Infections with other viral opportunists, including herpes simplex virus and varicella zoster virus, are not uncommon in lung transplant recipients (30,31), but involvement of the allograft is fortunately infrequent in the era of modern immunosuppression. We have encountered a single fatal case of herpes simplex virus pneumonia in more than 500 transplants performed during the past decade. Both herpes simplex and varicella zoster are DNA viruses that typically induce the formation of multinucleate syncytial cells, often with milky or "ground glass" nucleoplasm (27). Tissue necrosis is common in areas of infection.

## Community-Acquired Viral Infections

Infections with a variety of community-acquired viral pathogens, including adenovirus, influenza, parainfluenza, and respiratory syncytial virus (RSV), have been reported in lung transplant recipients (32–34). With the exception of adenovirus, which is associated with considerable morbidity and mortality, these infections are usually self-limiting in the acute phase. There is some evidence, however, that community-acquired viral infection can be associated with subsequent development of acute or chronic allograft rejection (see following text).

(A)

(B)

(C)

(D)

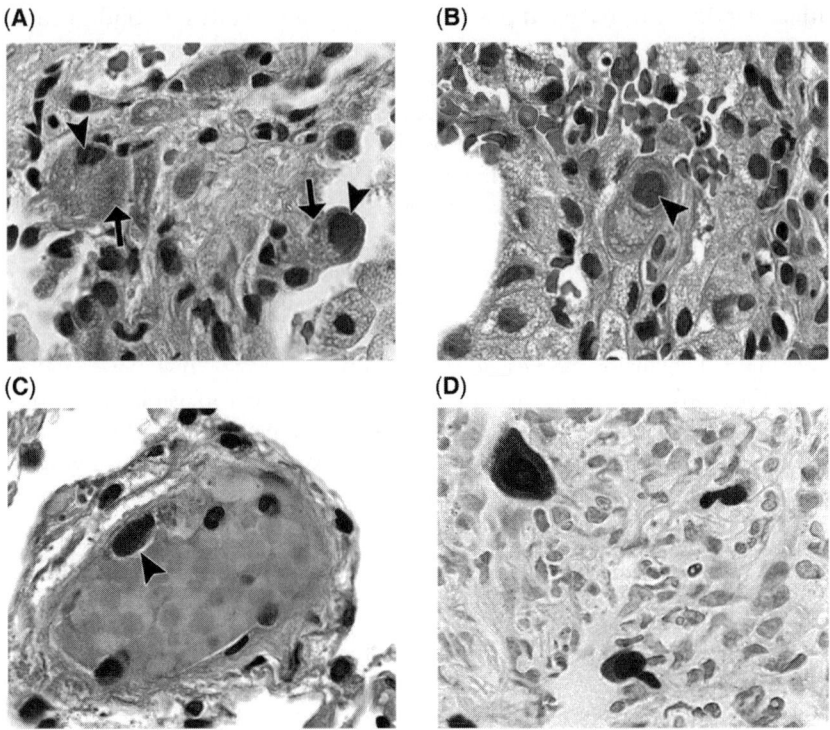

**Figure 5** Cytomegalovirus (CMV) infection. (**A** and **B**) Large (cytomegalic) cells with both intranuclear (*arrowheads*) and cytoplasmic (*arrows*) viral inclusions are present. The intranuclear inclusion in panel (**B**) has a lucent halo, a configuration often referred to as an "owl's eye" inclusion. (**C**) A CMV-infected vascular endothelial cell with subtler cytopathic effect, limited to nuclear enlargement (*arrowhead*). (**D**) The presence of CMV is confirmed by an immunoperoxidase stain (panels A–C, H&E stains; magnification×900).

Diagnosis of infections with this group of pathogens is most commonly made by culture or direct immunofluorescent staining of cytospin preparations produced from bronchoalveolar lavage (BAL) fluid. On biopsy, adenovirus often produces nuclear hyperchromasia and smudging of the chromatin pattern in infected cells (typically airway epithelium), sometimes associated with patchy necrosis. The nuclear cytopathic changes can be subtle, however, and immunoperoxidase staining with an adenovirus-specific antibody is generally necessary to establish a definitive tissue diagnosis. The histologic alterations associated with influenza, parainfluenza, and RSV in lung transplant biopsies are typically subtle and nonspecific. Though RSV derives its name from its tendency to induce formation of multinucleate syncytia in infected tissue, this characteristic finding is most commonly seen in severe infections, and is often difficult to detect in the lung transplant setting.

## REJECTION

### Humoral Allograft Rejection

The role of antibodies in the generation of allograft dysfunction, well established and reasonably well understood for renal and cardiac transplants, is currently unclear for lung transplants. For kidney and heart transplants, binding of preformed antibodies, most often directed at major histocompatibility complex (MHC) or ABO blood group antigens, to vascular endothelium, most commonly in microvasculature, triggers a sequence of events that includes activation of the complement cascade; attraction, margination, and attachment of inflammatory cells (especially neutrophils) to the endothelial surface; injury to endothelial cells and subjacent matrix with exposure of procoagulant tissue factors to the circulation and subsequent thrombosis; extravasation of erythrocytes, other blood cells, and serum components; and in severe cases, tissue necrosis. In extreme cases, termed "hyperacute rejection," these events occur within minutes of the establishment of blood flow to the graft and generally lead to irreversible graft failure. More frequently, preformed antibodies with lower concentration or avidity, or antibodies produced de novo via an anamnestic response to the graft, trigger a less fulminant form of graft dysfunction, variously termed "delayed humoral rejection," "acute humoral rejection," or "accelerated rejection," over the course of several hours to days. This form of rejection can often be treated successfully with plasmapheresis, administration of intravenous immunoglobulin, and other manipulations such as treatment with anti-CD20 antibodies (35).

Two clinicopathologic parameters have proven of great value in the diagnosis of humoral rejection in kidney and heart transplants. First, recipients with antibody-mediated graft injury frequently have circulating antibodies against one or more MHC antigens from a random donor pool (so-called "panel reactive antibodies," or PRA). (Antibodies against MHC antigens of the actual graft donor are generally undetectable in cross-matches performed at the time of transplantation by conventional microcytotoxicity methods, though they are occasionally detected retrospectively by more sensitive techniques such as flow cytometry.) Second, transplant biopsies from affected individuals usually show vascular deposition of C4d and C3d, complement cleavage products that bind covalently to vessel walls and are particularly amenable to immunologic detection (35,36). (Deposits of other complement components and immunoglobulins are surprisingly difficult to detect, and are of questionable significance when they are seen.)

In contrast to kidney and heart transplants, humoral rejection has been reported infrequently in lung transplant recipients. This could conceivably reflect true rarity of the phenomenon, under-recognition, or a combination of the two. Possible rationales for a low frequency of humoral rejection in lung allografts include infrequent humoral sensitization of the recipient population (37), dilution of preformed antibodies in the vast pulmonary vascular bed, and paucity of relevant target antigens in the pulmonary vasculature.

Hyperacute rejection of lung transplants has been reported in only a handful of cases (37–41), though these have shared interesting commonalities, including production of copious blood-tinged bronchial secretions and/or development of diffuse pulmonary infiltrates within a few hours of transplantation and positive PRA and retrospective crossmatch studies. All five patients received single lung transplants for chronic obstructive pulmonary disorder (COPD), with uneventful implantation of the contralateral donor lungs into other recipients in several cases. In four patients, histologic examination of biopsy or autopsy tissue showed microvascular thrombosis and neutrophil accumulation, often accompanied by stigmata of diffuse alveolar damage and focal intra-alveolar neutrophil infiltrates in patients surviving for a day or more. In some cases, deposition of immunoglobulin and complement components was identified by immunostaining, though the specificity and significance of the staining were unclear; all of the cases were reported prior to the general availability of immunostains for C4d. Possible examples of antibody-mediated rejection with a less fulminant course have also been described in a small number of patients (37,42,43).

Magro and coworkers recently described a group of patients with a different form of alveolar septal capillary injury that they attributed to anti-endothelial antibodies directed against non-MHC antigens (44). Biopsies in this series of patients, none of whom had positive PRA determinations, reportedly showed alveolar septal necrosis in the absence of significant inflammation, but with deposition of a variety of immunoreactants including C4d as assessed by immunofluorescent staining. The histologic and immunohistologic signs of injury correlated with clinical signs and symptoms of allograft dysfunction, and were reported to improve in several patients treated with plasmapheresis. These findings have yet to be confirmed by other investigators.

## Acute Cellular Allograft Rejection

Acute cellular rejection is mediated by T lymphocytes, which respond to alloantigenic stimulation by donor antigen-presenting cells ("direct" antigen presentation) or recipient antigen-presenting cells that have ingested alloantigens ("indirect" antigen presentation) by producing proinflammatory cytokines (primarily CD4-positive T lymphocytes) or mediating cytotoxicity (primarily CD8-positive lymphocytes). Post-transplant development of anti-MHC antibodies has also been reported recently to be associated with development of high-grade or recurrent acute cellular rejection (45), but may represent an epiphenomenon rather than an etiologic factor. While adaptive immunity to alloantigens is clearly central to the pathogenesis of acute cellular rejection, recent evidence suggests that patients with blunted potential for innate, or nonantigen-specific immunity as a result of mutations in TLR4, a lipopolysaccharide receptor, have a decreased incidence of acute rejection compared to individuals with wild-type TLR4 (46). As such, effector mechanisms in acute cellular rejection may involve a complex interplay of adaptive and innate immunity.

The histologic approach to diagnosis and grading of acute cellular rejection used by most pathologists was developed by a study group sponsored by the International Society for Heart and Lung Transplantation (ISHLT) in 1990 (47) and revised in 1995 (3). In these grading schemas, the hallmark lesion of acute cellular rejection is perivascular cuffing of mononuclear inflammatory cells (lymphocytes and monocytes/macrophages) within alveolar tissue; this parameter is designated with the prefix "A" in the revised version of the system, and assigned a grade of 0–4 (Table 1, Fig. 6A–D). A grade of A0 indicates the absence of perivascular inflammation. A grade of Al (minimal acute rejection) designates the presence of small perivascular collars of inflammatory cells two to three cells thick, inconspicuous at scanning magnification and generally centered on venules. At least one focus of microscopically conspicuous perivascular inflammation merits a grade of A2 (mild acute rejection); if the inflammation extends into adjacent alveolar septa, a grade of A3 (moderate acute rejection) is assigned. In severe (grade A4) rejection, extensive perivascular and interstitial inflammation are accompanied by signs of more advanced tissue injury, including alveolar pneumocyte damage; intraalveolar accumulation of mixed inflammatory cells, necrotic cell debris, fibrin, and hemorrhage; and in some cases, frank tissue necrosis or infarction.

**Table 1**  Acute Cellular Rejection (Perivascular/Interstitial Inflammation)

| Grade | Mononuclear inflammation | | Other findings |
| | Perivascular | Alveolar septa | |
| --- | --- | --- | --- |
| A0 | None | None | |
| Al | Inconspicuous | None | |
| A2 | Conspicuous | None | |
| A3 | Conspicuous | Present | |
| A4 | Conspicuous | Present | Intra-alveolar inflammation, pneumocyte injury, necrosis, infarction |

**(A)**

**(B)**

**(C)**

**(D)**

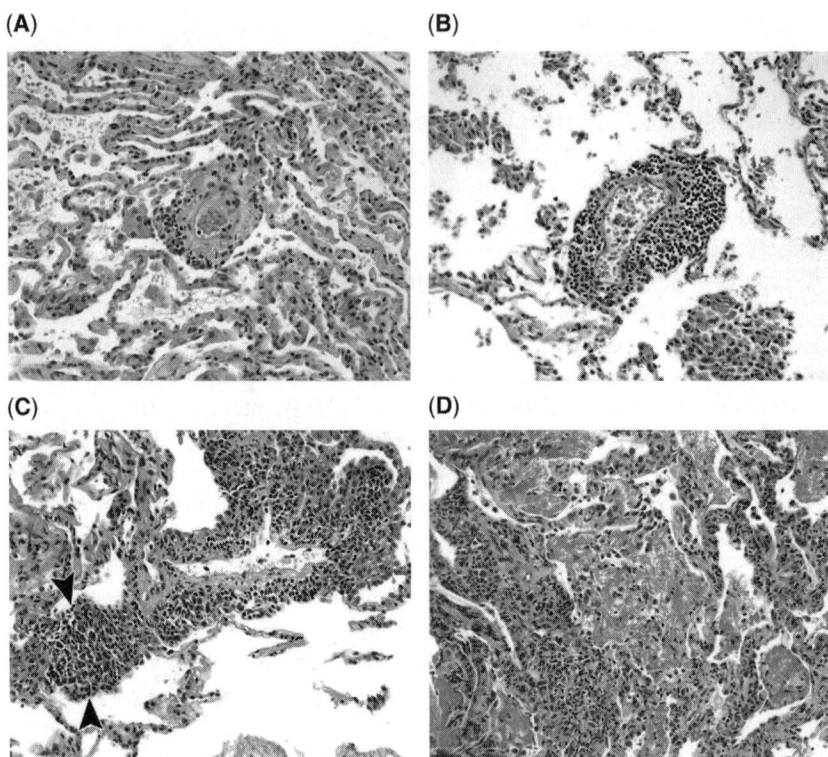

**Figure 6** Acute cellular allograft rejection. (**A**) Grade A1. An inconspicuous cluster of mononuclear inflammatory cells partially surrounds a small vessel. (**B**) Grade A2. A conspicuous collar of mononuclear inflammatory cells, in some places more than three cells thick, surrounds a vessel. (**C**) Grade A3. Intense perivascular inflammation extends into alveolar septa (*arrowheads*). (**D**) Grade A4. Extensive perivascular and alveolar septal inflammation is accompanied by fibrinous exudates and mixed inflammation within alveolar spaces (H&E stains; magnification×180).

In addition to the definitions noted in the preceding text, several ancillary criteria are useful in corroborating the grade of rejection. The infiltrates in grade A1 rejection are frequently sparse, while progressively higher grades tend to involve a greater percentage of vessels. In addition to venules, rejection of higher grades often involves arterioles and small arteries and veins. Inflammation and injury of vascular endothelium (endothelialitis) is also more common in higher grades of rejection. Small lymphocytes generally predominate in the infiltrates of grade A1 rejection; with progressively higher grades, one often sees greater admixtures of activated lymphocytes, eosinophils, and (particularly in grade A4) neutrophils. Though these accessory findings are not central to the grading scheme, a marked disparity between any of them and the amount of perivascular/interstitial inflammation present should trigger a consideration of diagnoses other than rejection; some special examples are noted in the following paragraphs.

Though perivascular inflammation is the principle diagnostic hallmark for acute cellular rejection, its specificity for rejection is imperfect. Several studies have indicated that perivascular inflammatory infiltrates can accompany infection with organisms such as CMV and *P. carinii,* and often resolve with appropriate antibiotic treatment in the absence of antirejection therapy (48,49). Whether this inflammation represents superimposed rejection potentiated by the infectious process (and subsequently abrogated by clearance of the infection) or a phenomenon unrelated to rejection is a matter of speculation. It is clear, however, that the finding of perivascular inflammation does not obviate the necessity of a thorough clinicopathologic search for infection.

Acute cellular rejection is frequently associated with mononuclear inflammation of airways, referred to as lymphocytic bronchitis/bronchiolitis; some investigators have proposed that this lesion is a precursor to, or at least a predictor for, subsequent development of bronchiolitis obliterans (50). The revised ISHLT working formulation encourages reporting of lymphocytic bronchitis/bronchiolitis in the context of rejection, and proposes a grading scheme with a "B" prefix, with grades on a 0–4 scale (Table 2, Fig. 7A–D); a grade of BX is assigned if bronchial/bronchiolar changes are upgradable.

In occasional biopsies, mononuclear airway inflammation is encountered in the absence of significant perivascular inflammation. Though this finding does not allow a formal diagnosis of rejection by ISHLT criteria, it presumably reflects the presence of rejection in many cases. Since perivascular inflammation is often quite focal, it may be present but not sampled in biopsy tissue that nonetheless shows evidence of bronchial inflammation. In unusual cases, "pure" forms of acute cellular bronchial rejection without associated perivascular inflammation may exist (50,51). That notwithstanding,

**Table 2**   Airway Inflammation

| Grade | Mononuclear inflammation | | Other |
| | Submucosa | Epithelium | |
| --- | --- | --- | --- |
| B0 | None | None | |
| Bl | Rare, scattered cells | None | |
| B2 | Band of cells | None | |
| B3 | Dense band of cells | Extensive | Epithelial cell apoptosis |
| B4 | Dense band of cells | Extensive | Epithelial necrosis, ulceration, sloughing |
| BX | Ungradable | | |

**(A)**                                              **(B)**

**(C)**                                              **(D)**

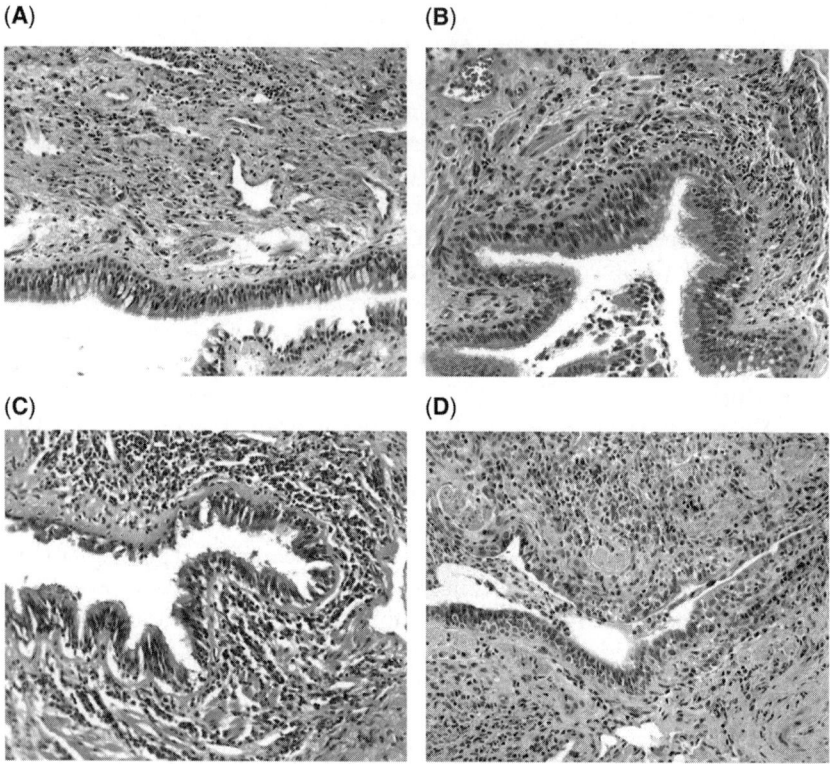

**Figure 7** Lymphocytic bronchitis/bronchiolitis. (**A**) Grade B1. Scattered mononuclear inflammatory cells are present within the airway wall. (**B**) Grade B2. A denser, band-like mononuclear infiltrate is present in the airway wall. (**C**) Grade B3. An intense inflammatory infiltrate fills the lamina propria and extends focally into the epithelium, which is nonetheless intact. (**D**) Grade B4. Intense inflammation of the airway wall is accompanied by epithelial inflammation, injury, and focal detachment, with necrotic debris and inflammatory cells in the airway lumen (H&E stains; magnification×180).

a wide variety of other conditions, including infections (particularly with viruses) and chronic aspiration, can cause lymphocyte-rich airway inflammation, and must be included in the differential diagnosis when such inflammation is encountered. Since the initiating agent in these conditions gains access via the airway lumen, they often cause a disproportionate amount of injury to the epithelium, frequently with associated neutrophil infiltrates. This feature is useful in distinguishing them from all but the highest grades of acute airway rejection.

A special form of airway lymphoid aggregate with potential for confusion with rejection-associated lymphocytic bronchitis is bronchus-associated lymphoid tissue (BALT) (52). This lesion does not appear to be associated with acute rejection or development of bronchiolitis obliterans, and has even been speculated to signal the development of immunologic tolerance to the allograft (52). It consists of a dense, often large lymphoid aggregate within the lamina propria, typically nestled immediately beneath the epithelium, with minimal signs of associated tissue injury. The immunophenotypes of its constituent cells recapitulate those of a normal lymphoid follicle, with a core of B lymphocytes surrounded by T lymphocytes; as such, immunostaining for T- and B-cell markers is occasionally useful in distinguishing BALT from infiltrates of rejection and other processes such as PTLD.

Aggregates of mononuclear inflammatory cells are occasionally seen around vessels coursing in the zone between alveolar tissue and the periphery of the smooth-muscle walls of airways. In our experience, symptomatic patients with such lesions frequently respond to steroid therapy, suggesting that they are part of the histologic spectrum of rejection. There is some ambiguity as to whether the involved vessels belong to the alveolar compartment (thus meriting an "A" designation in the ISHLT schema) or the airway (in which case a "B" designation would be more appropriate). Our practice has been to use the "A" designation (and issue a diagnosis of acute rejection) if any portion of the infiltrate touches on the alveolar compartment. However, we have also frequently seen such lesions in association with active bronchiolitis obliterans in pneumonectomies from patients undergoing retransplantation. As such, they could conceivably represent a transitional lesion in the progression from acute to chronic rejection, as has been proposed for lymphocytic bronchitis/bronchiolitis (50,51).

Though cells other than lymphocytes and monocytes/macrophages are often seen in patients with acute cellular rejection, they merit special consideration if they are unusually prevalent. Eosinophils, as noted earlier, are frequently encountered in biopsies from patients with acute rejection, particularly those with higher rejection grades (53,54). In rare patients, they may be the predominant inflammatory cell type present (53). However, since tissue eosinophilia can be associated with a wide variety of conditions, including infections, allergic and drug reactions, and connective tissue disorders, the presence of large numbers of eosinophils in a transplant biopsy should trigger a careful search for etiologies other than rejection. In one series of nine transplant recipients whose biopsies contained inflammatory infiltrates with a majority population of eosinophils, five were shown to have steroid-responsive rejection, while the other four had fungal, bacterial, or viral infections (53). Occasional patients with intense bronchial wall infiltrates of eosinophils have also been described in case reports (55) and encountered in our own anecdotal experience. Though steroid therapy sometimes elicits clinical and histologic improvement in such patients, it is unclear whether this lesion represents an unusual pattern of rejection or some other steroid-responsive process.

Neutrophils are also frequently present in patients with high-grade acute cellular rejection, where they generally accompany intense mononuclear cell infiltrates. They can be seen in a wide range of other conditions, however. Acute bronchitis/bronchiolitis has been reported in association with procurement/preservation injury, infection, and bronchiolitis obliterans (56) and gastroesophageal reflux disease/aspiration (57) in addition to acute cellular rejection. Such etiologies should be considered in cases where airway neutrophils outnumber mononuclear inflammatory cells. Likewise, significant numbers of intraalveolar neutrophils generally favor a diagnosis of infection unless unusually severe rejection is present.

A final cellular component frequently seen in modest numbers in the infiltrates of patients with rejection is the plasma cell. Plasma cells are particularly common in the airway wall, and may be more prevalent in patients with ongoing, recurrent, or late episodes of rejection. There is no clear evidence that these cells play a specific role in allograft injury (e.g., by producing alloantibodies). An early report, however, suggested that large numbers of B lymphocytes in early acute rejection predict nonresponsiveness to interventional immunosuppressive therapy (58). Interestingly, a much more recent report in renal transplantation described the molecular heterogeneity of acute allograft rejection using microarray analysis and concluded the presence of clusters of B cells in a biopsy sample was strongly associated with severe graft rejection (59). These studies raise the possibility that additional immunohistochemical analysis of the lymphocytic infiltrate in acute rejection might provide clinically important diagnostic and therapeutic information, although more research is needed. Finally, if large numbers of B-lymphocytes or plasma cells are present, and particularly if they are associated with infiltrates in an irregular distribution and exhibit cytologic atypia, an alternative diagnosis of PTLD should be entertained.

## Chronic Allograft Rejection

Chronic rejection of pulmonary allografts takes two forms: a progressive, fibrosing injury of small airways termed constrictive bronchiolitis obliterans or obliterative bronchiolitis (OB), and an intimal vasculopathy affecting large arteries and veins. As opposed to humoral and acute cellular rejection, the pathogenesis of which has been substantially if incompletely elucidated, the mechanisms underlying chronic rejection are currently poorly understood. This lack of mechanistic understanding has been one of the major impediments to the design of successful therapeutic interventions for chronic rejection. As noted in the following text, however, correlations have been documented between chronic rejection and several antecedent or coexisting conditions, some of which may ultimately shed light on the pathogenesis of the chronic rejection process. It is likely that in many cases chronic rejection reflects the cumulative effect of multiple injuries (60); some investigators have also suggested that forms with acute and chronic onset represent different disease entities with similar histologic patterns (61).

Constrictive bronchiolitis obliterans occurs as part of a clinicopathologic syndrome termed bronchiolitis obliterans syndrome (BOS), manifested by progressive signs of small airways obstruction in the absence of documented infection, acute rejection, or other known causes of allograft dysfunction (62). The hallmark of constrictive bronchiolitis obliterans is fibrosis and distortion of the walls of bronchioles. The damage may be eccentric or concentric, and is often associated with epithelial atrophy and loss of the subjacent smooth muscle layer. In advanced lesions, total obliteration of the bronchiolar lumen may occur; a distinction between "total" and "subtotal" lesions was made in the original ISHLT working formulation (47), but was omitted in the revised version (3). In the latter version, bronchiolitis obliterans is notated with the letter "C," and is subclassified by the presence or absence of associated inflammation, conditions designated as "active" (Ca) (Fig. 8A) or "inactive" (Cb) (Fig. 8B) bronchiolitis obliterans, respectively (3). The lesions of bronchiolitis obliterans are typically patchy, and are often not represented in transbronchial biopsies. Even so, biopsy can play a valuable role in arriving at a clinicopathologic diagnosis of BOS by ruling out alternative causes of allograft dysfunction.

Constrictive bronchiolitis obliterans should be distinguished clinically and histologically from BOOP. Though both lesions center on bronchioles, the typical lesion of BOOP is a fibromyxoid plugging of small airways that extends into alveolar ducts and alveoli. Bronchiolitis obliterans obstructive pneumonia and BOOP-like lesions have been reported to occur in lung transplant recipients in a variety of settings, including acute cellular rejection,

**(A)**                    **(B)**

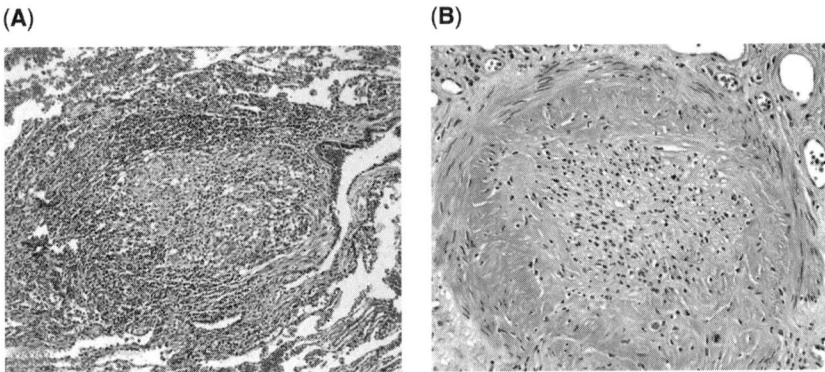

**Figure 8** Chronic rejection—obliterative bronchiolitis. (**A**) Active lesion. The lumen of a bronchiole is obliterated, with intense inflammation of the bronchiolar wall. (**B**) Inactive lesion. The lumen of this bronchiole is likewise obliterated, but inflammation is minimal (H&E stains; magnification × 180).

lymphocytic bronchitis, aspiration, and various infections (63–66), so it clearly does not have an obligate relationship with chronic rejection. In one study, however, several transplant recipients with biopsy-documented BOOP were found to have constrictive bronchiolitis obliterans on previous or subsequent biopsies (66). As such, BOOP may be a predisposing factor for or complication of BOS in selected patients.

Chronic vascular rejection, designated with a "D" in the revised ISHLT working formulation, is a fibrosing process that focuses primarily in the intimal layers of larger arteries and veins. Such vessels are not generally represented in transplant biopsies, as a result of which the diagnosis of chronic vascular rejection is most commonly made on transplant pneumonectomies or autopsy specimens. The intima of affected vessels is expanded by fibrous tissue, often admixed with foamy macrophages (Fig. 9). Other inflammatory cells are frequently absent or inconspicuous, though active mononuclear inflammation is occasionally present. In advanced cases, subtotal or total obliteration of vascular lumens may occur (3).

One of the most salient predictors of the development of chronic pulmonary allograft rejection is antecedent acute cellular rejection and/or lymphocytic bronchitis/bronchiolitis (50,51,67–71). The link between acute cellular rejection of higher grade (A2 and above) and bronchiolitis obliterans has been established in numerous studies (67–69). More recently, patients with recurrent bouts of minimal (grade A1) acute cellular rejection have been reported to develop bronchiolitis obliterans earlier and with greater frequency than controls with no history of acute cellular rejection (70).

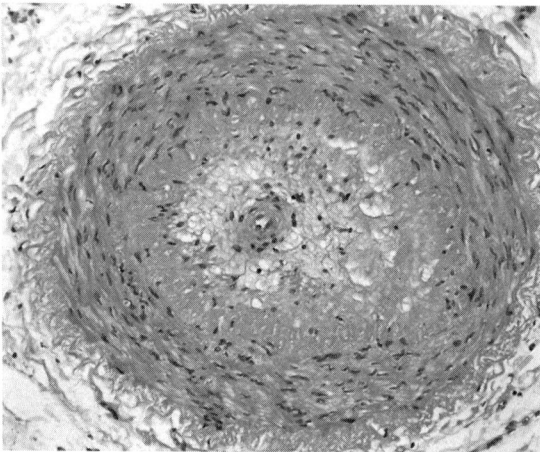

**Figure 9** Chronic rejection—vascular form. The lumen of a small artery is virtually obliterated by intimal expansion. In this example, there is minimal inflammation, but considerable intimal arteritis is occasionally seen (H&E stain; magnification × 180).

It is not clear whether acute rejection and lymphocytic bronchitis/ bronchiolitis are directly involved in the pathogenesis of bronchiolitis obliterans, markers of recipient alloreactivity with disparate acute and chronic mechanisms, or some combination of the two. For lymphocytic bronchiolitis, it is reasonably easy to posit a mechanism by which the acute inflammatory process could lead to chronic injury, possibly via elaboration of profibrotic cytokines within the airway wall (71). A direct pathogenetic link between perivascular inflammation and bronchiolitis obliterans is more difficult to envision, though inflammatory damage to small vessels providing the vascular supply to bronchioles could conceivably engender ischemic injury to the small airways. Indeed, one recent study has documented a decrease in the number of small vessels supplying bronchioles affected by bronchiolitis obliterans in autopsy lungs (72).

A link between humoral immunity and chronic rejection of lung transplants has also been suggested by the development of bronchiolitis obliterans in transplant recipients who produce new antibodies to donor class I (73,74) or class II (75) MHC antigens. A few studies have also suggested a role for antibodies against non-MHC antigens expressed by airway epithelium or vascular endothelium (76,77). As with antecedent acute cellular rejection, it has not been established whether antidonor antibodies are directly involved in the pathogenesis of bronchiolitis obliterans or simply serve as a marker for the development of chronic rejection.

Given the ubiquitous distribution of class I antigens, mechanisms by which antibodies against them could elicit chronic allograft damage after binding to the epithelium of bronchioles or the endothelium of vessels providing their blood supply are not difficult to envision. Indeed, exposure of cultured airway epithelial cells to anti–class I antibodies in tissue culture has been reported variously to induce cellular proliferation (78), apoptosis, and production of fibrogenic growth factors (79). Constitutive expression of class II antigens in the lung is generally limited to hematopoietic cells, including antigen-presenting cells and B lymphocytes, which are unlikely to serve as primary targets for antibody-mediated damage. Inducible expression of class II antigens occurs on a variety of cells, however, including human bronchial epithelial cells (80) and vascular endothelial cells, in response to stimuli such as interferon-gamma. Induction of class II antigen expression by cytokines produced during previous inflammatory processes (for example, acute cellular rejection or infection) could conceivably expose target antigens for circulating anti–class II antibodies.

Processes not directly related to alloimmunity, particularly infections, have also been posited to play a role in the development of bronchiolitis obliterans. Since BOS may in turn facilitate the development of infections as airflow obstruction and bronchiectasis develop, self-perpetuating cycles of airway injury are a distinct possibility. Patients with CMV infection have been reported to have an increased risk of developing BOS in numerous studies (81,82), and recent data suggest that treatment of CMV pneumonia abrogates the risk of development of BOS (83). Infections with community-acquired viruses, including influenza virus, parainfluenza virus, adenovirus, and RSV, have also been reported to predispose lung transplant recipients to development of BOS with increased frequency or severity (34,82,84–86). Association of bacterial infections with BOS, as either a potentiating or an exacerbating factor, may also occur (82). It was reported recently that prophylactic maintenance treatment of a small group of patients with early BOS with azithromycin significantly improved their pulmonary function (87). Fungal infections have also been associated with development of BOS (22).

Infections could conceivably lead to bronchiolitis obliterans by a number of mechanisms. Direct injury of small airways as a result of infection could ultimately cause chronic damage, particularly if repeated or smoldering infections were involved. CMV has a tropism for vascular endothelium, and could potentially damage small vessels in a manner that engendered ischemic injury to bronchioles. In addition to these nonimmunologic mechanisms, infections may facilitate immune-mediated damage to the allograft via indirect routes. Nonantigen-specific effector mechanisms (e.g., activated macrophages) generated in the immune response to a pathogen may on occasion cause collateral damage to allograft tissues. As mentioned earlier, cytokines elaborated during the immune response to infectious agents have the potential to cause upregulation of graft alloantigens, particularly class II MHC antigens that could serve subsequently as targets for rejection. Infection of cultured fibroblasts with CMV can also cause upregulation of class I MHC antigens (88). Antibodies or effector T lymphocytes generated against antigenic epitopes on pathogens may on occasion cross-react with structurally similar epitopes on host tissues, leading to autoimmune injury. Activation of innate immune pathways by microbes, particularly bacteria, could also facilitate airway injury (46). Respiratory syncytial virus has been shown to bind directly to TLR4 and result in production of inflammatory cytokines, perhaps providing a link between viral infection, activation of innate immunity, and upregulation of subsequent adaptive responses (89).

Mechanical or ischemic injuries to bronchioles have also been proposed as possible initiating factors for BOS. In particular, aspiration is a likely source of chronic, repetitive injury to bronchioles. Aspiration might be of particular concern in the setting of the denervated posttransplant recipient, where normal cough and mucociliary clearance are impaired. We have demonstrated that the severity of gastroesophageal reflux, when measured objectively using a 24-hour esophageal pH probe, increased significantly after lung transplantation, presumably as a result of the surgery, medications or both (90). Furthermore, we have retrospectively demonstrated an association between the presence and severity of posttransplant gastroesophageal reflux disease (GERD) and posttransplant allograft dysfunction, including an association with GERD and BOS (91). Finally, we have demonstrated that patients with GERD and BOS can experience an improvement in lung function after surgical treatment of GERD with fundoplication (57,92,93). Mechanisms by which GERD and aspiration could potentiate BOS are conceptually similar to those described previously for infections, and might include direct bronchiolar injury or secondary activation of immune and inflammatory responses directed to the airways. Transplant ischemia–reperfusion injury has also been reported to increase the risk of subsequent development of BOS (94). Finally, we have anecdotally observed episodes of rejection that appear precipitated by inhalational toxin or smoke exposures. The role for nonalloimmune injury in the development of chronic graft dysfunction thus warrants additional study in lung transplantation, and might in part explain the much higher rates of rejection observed in lung transplant as compared to other solid organs.

## TUMORS AND TUMOR-LIKE CONDITIONS

### Posttransplant Lymphoproliferative Disorder

PTLD is an unusual complication of lung transplantation, but can be associated with significant morbidity and mortality. Incidence rates for PTLD ranging from 1.6% to 5.0% have been reported in recent series (7,95–99), though it may occur more frequently in pediatric transplant recipients, particularly those with negative Epstein–Barr virus (EBV) serology who receive EBV positive allografts, where an incidence of 23% has been reported by one group (100). In the vast majority of cases, PTLD represents a disregulated proliferation of B lymphocytes driven by transformation with EBV in the setting of post-transplant immunosuppression (7,101); antiviral prophylaxis has been reported to decrease the incidence of the disorder (98), and certain types of immunosuppression (e.g., antithymocyte globulin) have been reported to increase the risk. In a small group of cases where the source of the proliferating cells has been examined, origin from recipient lymphocytes has been seen most frequently (101,102), though a few examples of donor-derived PTLD have been documented (101,103). Rare cases of T-cell PTLD have been described in the setting of pulmonary transplantation, generally without evidence of EBV involvement (7). PTLD can involve the transplanted lung, native lung (in the case of a single transplant recipient), systemic lymphoid tissues, and other organs in various combinations.

EBV-driven PTLD includes a spectrum of clinical and pathological subtypes ranging from benign, polyclonal processes to frank lymphomas. One durable classification scheme divides PTLD into a polyclonal, polymorphous group, where the proliferating cells (mixed B lymphocytes and plasma cells) have minimal cytologic abnormality; a monoclonal, polymorphous group, where the proliferating cells are clonal but nonetheless have cytologic variability and usually lack features of frank malignancy; and a monoclonal, monomorphous group, histologically similar to immunoblastic lymphoma or plasmacytoma (104). The first two categories sometimes regress with diminution of immunosuppressive therapy; the latter, as well as most cases of T-cell PTLD, generally behave clinically as aggressive lymphomas.

Pulmonary PTLD often presents as multiple nodules first noted on chest X-ray, though endobronchial lesions detected by bronchoscopy have been described as an alternative presentation (105,106). Since the lesions are often focal, they can be missed in transbronchial biopsies; diagnosis may require thoracoscopic wedge biopsy (7). On histologic examination, PTLD is generally manifested as sheets of lymphoid cells with varying degrees of polymorphism and atypia, depending on the subtype (Fig. 10A and B). Necrosis is common; in some cases, entire nodules may undergo

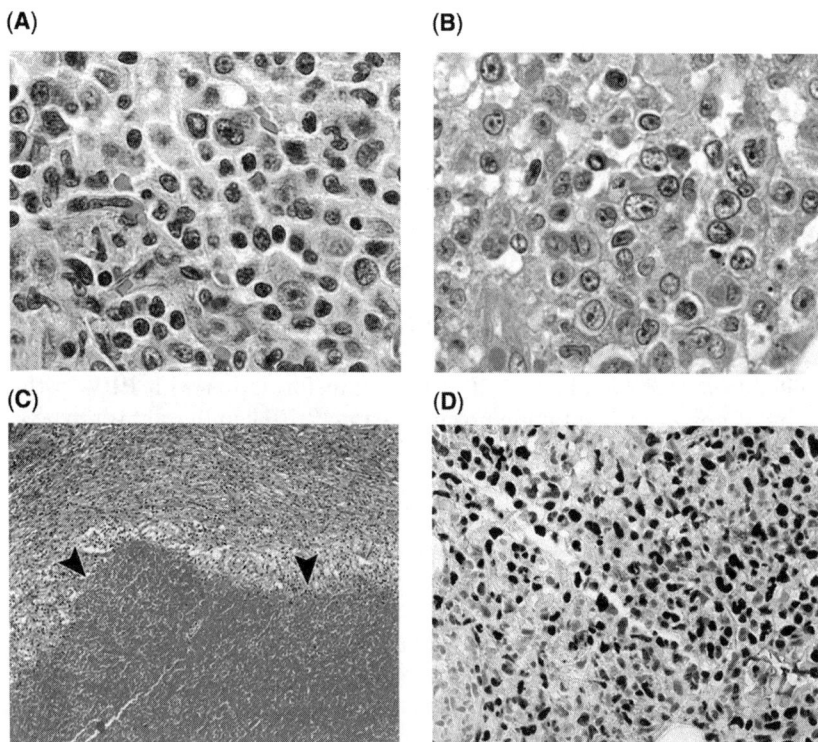

**Figure 10** Posttransplant lymphoproliferative disorder (PTLD). (**A**) Polymorphous form, with mixture of cell types. (**B**) Monomorphous form, with monotonous population of cells with more atypical features. (**C**) Involuted PTLD nodule with almost complete necrosis (*arrowheads*). (**D**) Immunoperoxidase stain for EBV nuclear antigen-2 (EBNA-2); same case as panel (**B**), (panels **A–C**, H&E stains; magnification in panels **A** and **B** × 900; magnification in panel **C** × 90; magnification in panel **D** × 360). *Abbreviation*: EBV, Epstein–Barr virus.

spontaneous or therapy-induced involution (Fig. 10C). The nodules of PTLD are frequently fairly well circumscribed, though perivascular infiltrates of mixed lymphocytes resembling those seen in acute cellular rejection are occasionally seen at the periphery (107); biopsies that miss the PTLD nodules but sample adjacent inflammatory responses may yield a false diagnosis of rejection.

As mentioned earlier, ancillary techniques are of great value in the diagnosis of PTLD. The lineage of the proliferating cells can be assessed by immunohistochemical staining for markers such as CD20 (for B cells) and CD3 (for T cells). Immunoperoxidase stains for EBV antigens, including latent membrane protein-1 (LMP-1) and Epstein–Barr nuclear antigen-2 (EBNA-2) (Fig. 10D) are positive in a majority of cases (7), though in situ hybridization for EBV RNA is generally considered more sensitive (101). Polymerase chain reaction–based assays for clonal immunoglobulin gene rearrangements are often useful for distinguishing polyclonal from mono-clonal forms of PTLD; immunoperoxidase staining for immunoglobulin kappa and lambda light chains can also be used to assess clonality, but gen-erally requires fresh-frozen tissue. A variety of techniques, including HLA typing (103) and genomic analysis of polymorphic loci (102,108), can be used to determine the origin of PTLD from recipient or donor.

Although there is no single treatment that has proven effective for all types of PTLD, therapy usually involves a combination of reduced immunosup-pression and chemotherapy. We have recently reported moderate success with the use of reduced immunosuppression and anti-CD20 antibody (Rituximab) in the treatment of several cases of advanced PTLD (7). Older reports suggest that treatment with more traditional chemotherapy regimens is associated with relatively high rates of death due to infectious complications, probably as a result of the added immunosuppressive effects of the chemotherapy.

## Carcinoma

Primary and metastatic carcinomas are rare in the transplant lung, owing in part no doubt to the careful pretransplant clinical and radiographic screen-ing of recipients and donors and also to the fact that most recipients and donors are younger than the peak incidence ages for a majority of solid tumors. Occasional patients with bronchioloalveolar carcinoma (BAC) (109–112) and other bronchogenic carcinomas (112–114), diagnosed pre-transplant or discovered ex post facto in pneumonectomy specimens, have received lung allografts. For BAC, a high recurrence rate has been docu-mented, presumably as a result of aerogenous seeding of tumor from a reser-voir in the recipient tracheobronchial stump, though long-term survival has been achieved for several patients. Good long-term survival has also been reported for patients found to have incidental stage I bronchogenic carcino-mas on pneumonectomy, though the prognosis for patients with carcinomas of higher stage is poor (112).

Primary tumors arising in extrapulmonary sites have metastasized to the transplant on rare occasions (115). We have encountered one squamous cell carcinoma in a female transplant recipient that apparently arose as a metastasis from a cervical primary. Patients receiving single lung transplants, particularly for centrilobular emphysema, occasionally develop primary carcinomas in the residual native lung (115,116).

In a handful of cases, clinically inapparent carcinomas and other malignant tumors in donor lungs have spread and metastasized in the recipients posttransplant (117,118). Occurrence of carcinomas in other recipients of transplants from the same donor is a clue to this pathogenetic sequence. Donor or recipient origin of the tumor can be assessed by molecular diagnostic methods (117).

## Benign Tumors

Small, benign proliferations of epithelioid cells, including pulmonary tumorlets (carcinoid tumorlets) (119) and minute pulmonary meningothelial-like nodules (also known as minute pulmonary chemodectomas) (120), are encountered from time to time in pulmonary allograft biopsies. These are frequently multiple, and may be present in sequential biopsies, but are of no known clinical significance. Both consist of small nests of cytologically bland cells. Those of carcinoid tumorlets have a nested pattern, often described as "organoid," that has some similarity to normal endocrine tissues, while those of meningothelial-like inclusions have a spindled pattern reminiscent of a benign meningioma. The two can be distinguished by the staining of carcinoid tumorlets, but not meningothelial-like inclusions, for neuroendocrine granule proteins such as synaptophysin and chromogranin.

## RECURRENT PRIMARY DISEASE

Recurrence of primary pulmonary pathology in lung transplants is fortunately limited to a relatively small group of diseases, most of which are not common indications for transplantation (Table 3). The recurrence of bronchioloalveolar cell carcinoma has already been mentioned. Sarcoidosis

**Table 3** Diseases Reported to Recur in Lung Transplants

Bronchioloalveolar cell carcinoma
Sarcoidosis
Lymphangioleiomyomatosis
Diffuse panbronchiolitis
Giant cell interstitial pneumonitis
Pulmonary alveolar proteinosis
Alpha-1-antitrypsin deficiency

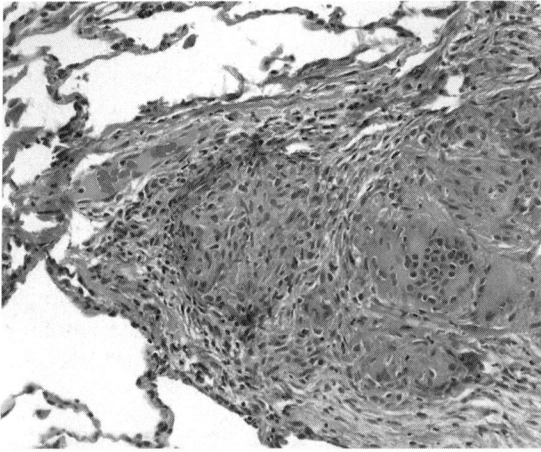

**Figure 11** Recurrent sarcoidosis in lung transplant. A large, noncaseating granuloma is present in alveolar tissue. Special stains and cultures for microorganisms were negative (H&E stain; magnification × 180).

(Fig. 11) (121–125), lymphangioleiomyomatosis (126–128), diffuse panbronchiolitis (129), giant cell interstitial pneumonitis (130), and pulmonary alveolar proteinosis (131,132) have also been reported to recur in transplanted lungs. In most cases, the histopathology of the recurrent disease is similar to that seen in the native lung, though the biopsy findings in transplant sarcoidosis may be modulated somewhat by maintenance immunosuppression. Recently, a case of recurrent emphysema has been reported in a patient with alpha-1-antitrypsin deficiency who began smoking again posttransplant (133), and radiographic recurrence of this disorder has been reported in nonsmoking lung transplant recipients (134). Alpha-1-antitrypsin replacement therapy could conceivably offer a long-term advantage in this select patient population.

For disorders involving infiltration of the lung by proliferating cells, including BAC (109) and lymphangioleiomyomatosis (127), the abnormal cells have been determined to be of recipient origin in all cases studied to date. Residual disease in the recipient tracheobronchial tree is a potential source for disease recurrence and other complications. Recurrence of BAC due to seeding of transplants from an upper airway source is noted above. Failure of lung allografts in a patient with Williams–Campbell syndrome, a rare form of bronchial cartilage deficiency, has been reported and attributed in part to proximal bronchomalacia engendered by the primary disease (135). Though cystic fibrosis is not known to recur in lung transplants, residual pathogenic microbes in the upper airways are a well-documented source of transplant infections.

In patients receiving transplants for emphysema associated with cigarette smoking, resumption of smoking occurs occasionally after transplantation. Though recurrence of emphysema is unlikely, vigilant monitoring for resumption of cigarette abuse is warranted by the wide range of other pathologic processes with known or hypothetical links to smoking. A histologic clue is often provided by the presence in biopsy tissue of alveolar macrophages containing fine brown pigment, distinct in appearance from hemosiderin, which is coarser, more refractile, and golden-brown in hue. Recognition of these "smoker's macrophages" by the pathologist should trigger clinical testing for nicotine metabolites. It should be noted, however, that pigmented macrophages present in the lungs of a smoking donor can persist for several years post-transplant (136). As such, their presence is not absolute proof of smoking by the recipient.

## SUMMARY

Pathologic examination of the transplanted lung provides a unique window into allograft function. Successful histopathologic assessment requires extensive familiarity with a wide range of pulmonary disorders. Differential diagnosis includes consideration of infection (both typical and unusual opportunistic pathogens), rejection (both cellular and humoral), recurrent native disease, and malignancy. Pathological correlation with a patient's post-transplant clinical status and physiological function is often necessary to fully appreciate the significance of any specific pathological findings. Ultimately, successful outcomes after lung transplant are critically dependent upon effective and accurate clinical–pathological diagnosis.

## REFERENCES

1. Grossman RF, Frost A, Zamel N, et al. Results of single-lung transplantation for bilateral pulmonary fibrosis. The Toronto Lung Transplant Group. N Engl J Med 1990; 322(11):727–733.
2. Dransfield MT, Garver RI, Weill D. Standardized guidelines for surveillance bronchoscopy reduce complications in lung transplant recipients. J Heart Lung Transplant 2004; 23(1):110–114.
3. Yousem SA, Berry GJ, Cagle PT, et al. Revision of the 1990 working formulation for the classification of pulmonary allograft rejection: Lung Rejection Study Group. J Heart Lung Transplant 1996;15(1 Pt 1):1–15.
4. Baz MA, Layish DT, Govert JA, et al. Diagnostic yield of bronchoscopies after isolated lung transplantation. Chest 1996; 110(1):84–88.
5. Valentine VG, Taylor DE, Dhillon GS, et al. Success of lung transplantation without surveillance bronchoscopy. J Heart Lung Transplant 2002; 21(3):319–326.
6. Chakinala MM, Ritter J, Gage BF, et al. Yield of surveillance bronchoscopy for acute rejection and lymphocytic bronchitis/bronchiolitis after lung transplantation. J Heart Lung Transplant 2004; 23(12):1396–1404.

7. Reams BD, McAdams HP, Howell DN, et al. Posttransplant lymphoproliferative disorder: incidence, presentation, and response to treatment in lung transplant recipients. Chest 2003; 124(4):1242–1249.

8. Kariyawasam HH, Gyi KM, Hodson ME, et al. Anaemia in lung transplant patient caused by parvovirus B19. Thorax 2000; 55(7):619–620.

9. Fields TA, McCall SJ, Reams BD, et al. Pulmonary embolization of microcrystalline cellulose in a lung transplant recipient. J Heart Lung Transplant 2005; 24(5):624–627.

10. de Perrot M, Liu M, Waddell TK, et al. Ischemia–reperfusion-induced lung injury. Am J Respir Crit Care Med 2003; 167(4):490–511.

11. Christie JD, Sager JS, Kimmel SE, et al. Impact of primary graft failure on outcomes following lung transplantation. Chest 2005; 127(1):161–165.

12. Fiser SM, Cope JT, Kron IL, et al. Aerosolized prostacyclin (epoprostenol) as an alternative to inhaled nitric oxide for patients with reperfusion injury after lung transplantation. J Thorac Cardiovasc Surg 2001; 121(5):981–982.

13. Meyers BF, Sundt TM III, Henry S, et al. Selective use of extracorporeal membrane oxygenation is warranted after lung transplantation. J Thorac Cardiovasc Surg 2000; 120(1):20–26.

14. Fisher AJ, Donnelly SC, Hirani N, et al. Elevated levels of interleukin-8 in donor lungs is associated with early graft failure after lung transplantation. Am J Respir Crit Care Med 2001; 163(1):259–265.

15. Goldfarb NS, Avery RK, Goormastic M, et al. Hypogammaglobulinemia in lung transplant recipients. Transplantation 2001; 71(2):242–246.

16. Malouf MA, Glanville AR. The spectrum of mycobacterial infection after lung transplantation. Am J Respir Crit Care Med 1999; 160(5 Pt 1):1611–1616.

17. Husain S, McCurry K, Dauber J, et al. Nocardia infection in lung transplant recipients. J Heart Lung Transplant 2002; 21(3):354–359.

18. Galaria, II, Marcos A, Orloff M, et al. Pulmonary actinomycosis in solid organ transplantation. Transplantation 2003; 75(11):1914–1915.

19. Nichols L, Strollo DC, Kusne S. Legionellosis in a lung transplant recipient obscured by cytomegalovirus infection and Clostridium difficile colitis. Transplant Infect Dis 2002; 4(1):41–45.

20. Palmer SM, Perfect JR, Howell DN, et al. Candidal anastomotic infection in lung transplant recipients: successful treatment with a combination of systemic and inhaled antifungal agents. J Heart Lung Transplant 1998; 17(10):1029–1033.

21. Hadjiliadis D, Howell DN, Davis RD, et al. Anastomotic infections in lung transplant recipients. Ann Transplant 2000; 5(3):13–19.

22. Tamm M, Malouf M, Glanville A. Pulmonary scedosporium infection following lung transplantation. Transplant Infect Dis 2001; 3(4):189–194.

23. Liu K, Howell DN, Perfect JR, et al. Morphologic criteria for the preliminary identification of Fusarium, Paecilomyces, and Acremonium species by histopathology. Am J Clin Pathol 1998; 109(1):45–54.

24. Fishman JA. Prevention of infection caused by Pneumocystis carinii in transplant recipients. Clin Infect Dis 2001; 33(8):1397–1405.

25. Faul JL, Akindipe OA, Berry GJ, et al. Recurrent Pneumocystis carinii colonization in a heart–lung transplant recipient on long-term trimethoprim–sulfamethoxazole prophylaxis. J Heart Lung Transplant 1999; 18(4):384–387.

26. Zamora MR. Cytomegalovirus and lung transplantation. Am J Transplant 2004; 4(8):1219–1226.
27. Caruso JL, Howell DN. Surgical pathology and diagnostic cytopathology of viral infections. In: Lennette EH, Smith TF, eds. Laboratory Diagnosis of Viral Infections. 3rd ed. New York: Marcel Dekker, 1998:21–43.
28. Solans EP, Garrity ER Jr, McCabe M, et al. Early diagnosis of cytomegalovirus pneumonitis in lung transplant patients. Arch Pathol Lab Med 1995; 119(1):33–35.
29. Naber JM, Palmer SM, Howell DN. Cytomegalovirus infection presenting as bronchial polyps in lung transplant recipients. J Heart Lung Transplant 2005; 24(12):2109–2113.
30. Gourishankar S, McDermid JC, Jhangri GS, et al. Herpes zoster infection following solid organ transplantation: incidence, risk factors and outcomes in the current immunosuppressive era. Am J Transplant 2004; 4(1):108–115.
31. Shreeniwas R, Schulman LL, Berkmen YM, et al. Opportunistic bronchopulmonary infections after lung transplantation: clinical and radiographic findings. Radiology 1996; 200(2):349–356.
32. Palmer SM Jr, Henshaw NG, Howell DN, et al. Community respiratory viral infection in adult lung transplant recipients. Chest 1998; 113(4):944–950.
33. Matar LD, McAdams HP, Palmer SM, et al. Respiratory viral infections in lung transplant recipients: radiologic findings with clinical correlation. Radiology 1999; 213(3):735–742.
34. Garantziotis S, Howell DN, McAdams HP, et al. Influenza pneumonia in lung transplant recipients: clinical features and association with bronchiolitis obliterans syndrome. Chest 2001; 119(4):1277–1280.
35. Michaels PJ, Fishbein MC, Colvin RB. Humoral rejection of human organ transplants. Springer Semin Immunopathol 2003; 25(2):119–140.
36. Baldwin WM III, Kasper EK, Zachary AA, et al. Beyond C4d: other complement-related diagnostic approaches to antibody-mediated rejection. Am J Transplant 2004; 4(3):311–318.
37. Scornik JC, Zander DS, Baz MA, et al. Susceptibility of lung transplants to preformed donor-specific HLA antibodies as detected by flow cytometry. Transplantation 1999; 68(10):1542–1546.
38. Frost AE, Jammal CT, Cagle PT. Hyperacute rejection following lung transplantation. Chest 1996; 110(2):559–562.
39. Choi JK, Kearns J, Palevsky HI, et al. Hyperacute rejection of a pulmonary allograft. Immediate clinical and pathologic findings. Am J Respir Crit Care Med 1999; 160(3):1015–1018.
40. Bittner HB, Dunitz J, Hertz M, et al. Hyperacute rejection in single lung transplantation—case report of successful management by means of plasmapheresis and antithymocyte globulin treatment. Transplantation 2001; 71(5):649–651.
41. Christie JD, Bavaria JE, Palevsky HI, et al. Primary graft failure following lung transplantation. Chest 1998; 114(1):51–60.
42. Badesch DB, Zamora M, Fullerton D, et al. Pulmonary capillaritis: a possible histologic form of acute pulmonary allograft rejection. J Heart Lung Transplant 1998; 17(4):415–422.

43. Lau CL, Palmer SM, Posther KE, et al. Influence of panel-reactive antibodies on posttransplant outcomes in lung transplant recipients. Ann Thorac Surg 2000; 69(5):1520–1524.

44. Magro CM, Deng A, Pope-Harman A, et al. Humorally mediated post-transplantation septal capillary injury syndrome as a common form of pulmonary allograft rejection: a hypothesis. Transplantation 2002; 74(9): 1273–1280.

45. Girnita AL, McCurry KR, Iacono AT, et al. HLA-specific antibodies are associated with high-grade and persistent-recurrent lung allograft acute rejection. J Heart Lung Transplant 2004; 23(10):1135–1141.

46. Palmer SM, Burch LH, Davis RD, et al. The role of innate immunity in acute allograft rejection after lung transplantation. Am J Respir Crit Care Med 2003; 168(6):628–632.

47. Berry GJ, Brunt EM, Chamberlain D, et al. A working formulation for the standardization of nomenclature in the diagnosis of heart and lung rejection: Lung Rejection Study Group. The International Society for Heart Transplantation. J Heart Transplant 1990; 9(6):593–601.

48. Tazelaar HD. Perivascular inflammation in pulmonary infections: implications for the diagnosis of lung rejection. J Heart Lung Transplant 1991; 10(3):437–441.

49. Sibley RK, Berry GJ, Tazelaar HD, et al. The role of transbronchial biopsies in the management of lung transplant recipients. J Heart Lung Transplant 1993; 12(2):308–324.

50. Yousem SA. Lymphocytic bronchitis/bronchiolitis in lung allograft recipients. Am J Surg Pathol 1993; 17(5):491–496.

51. Ross DJ, Marchevsky A, Kramer M, et al. "Refractoriness" of airflow obstruction associated with isolated lymphocytic bronchiolitis/bronchitis in pulmonary allografrs. J Heart Lung Transplant 1997; 16(8):832–838.

52. Hasegawa T, Iacono A, Yousem SA. The significance of bronchus-associated lymphoid tissue in human lung transplantation: is there an association with acute and chronic rejection? Transplantation 1999; 67(3):381–385.

53. Yousem SA. Graft eosinophilia in lung transplantation. Hum Pathol 1992; 23(10):1172–1177.

54. Dosanjh AK, Robinson TE, Strauss J, et al. Eosinophil activation in cardiac and pulmonary acute allograft rejection. J Heart Lung Transplant 1998; 17(10):1038.

55. Mogayzel PJ Jr, Yang SC, Wise BV, et al. Eosinophilic infiltrates in a pulmonary allograft: a case and review of the literature. J Heart Lung Transplant 2001; 20(6):692–695.

56. Ohori NP, Iacono AT, Grgurich WF, et al. Significance of acute bronchitis/bronchiolitis in the lung transplant recipient. Am J Surg Pathol 1994; 18(12): 1192–1204.

57. Lau CL, Palmer SM, Howell DN, et al. Laparoscopic antireflux surgery in the lung transplant population. Surg Endosc 2002; 16(12):1674–1678.

58. Yousem SA, Martin T, Paradis IL, et al. Can immunohistological analysis of transbronchial biopsy specimens predict responder status in early acute rejection of lung allografts? Hum Pathol 1994; 25(5):525–529.

59. Sarwal M, Chua MS, Kambham N, et al. Molecular heterogeneity in acute renal allograft rejection identified by DNA microarray profiling. N Engl J Med 2003; 349(2):125–138.

60. Egan JJ. Obliterative bronchiolitis after lung transplantation: a repetitive multiple injury airway disease. Am J Respir Crit Care Med 2004; 170(9): 931–932.

61. Jackson CH, Sharples LD, McNeil K, et al. Acute and chronic onset of bronchiolitis obliterans syndrome (BOS): are they different entities? J Heart Lung Transplant 2002; 21(6):658–666.

62. Estenne M, Maurer JR, Boehler A, et al. Bronchiolitis obliterans syndrome 2001: an update of the diagnostic criteria. J Heart Lung Transplant 2002; 21(3):297–310.

63. Abernathy EC, Hruban RH, Baumgartner WA, et al. The two forms of bronchiolitis obliterans in heart-lung transplant recipients. Hum Pathol 1991; 22(11):1102–1110.

64. Yousem SA, Duncan SR, Griffith BP. Interstitial and airspace granulation tissue reactions in lung transplant recipients. Am J Surg Pathol 1992; 16(9): 877–884.

65. Siddiqui MT, Garrity ER, Husain AN. Bronchiolitis obliterans organizing pneumonia-like reactions: a nonspecific response or an atypical form of rejection or infection in lung allograft recipients? Hum Pathol 1996; 27(7): 714–719.

66. Chaparro C, Chamberlain D, Maurer J, et al. Bronchiolitis obliterans organizing pneumonia (BOOP) in lung transplant recipients. Chest 1996; 110(5): 1150–1154.

67. Girgis RE, Tu I, Berry GJ, et al. Risk factors for the development of obliterative bronchiolitis after lung transplantation. J Heart Lung Transplant 1996; 15(12):1200–1208.

68. Heng D, Sharpies LD, McNeil K, et al. Bronchiolitis obliterans syndrome: incidence, natural history, prognosis, and risk factors. J Heart Lung Transplant 1998; 17(12):1255–1263.

69. Sharples LD, McNeil K, Stewart S, et al. Risk factors for bronchiolitis obliterans: a systematic review of recent publications. J Heart Lung Transplant 2002; 21(2):271–281.

70. Hopkins PM, Aboyoun CL, Chhajed PN, et al. Association of minimal rejection in lung transplant recipients with obliterative bronchiolitis. Am J Respir Crit Care Med 2004; 170(9):1022–1026.

71. El-Gamel A, Sim E, Hasleton P, et al. Transforming growth factor beta (TGF-beta) and obliterative bronchiolitis following pulmonary transplantation. J Heart Lung Transplant 1999; 18(9):828–837.

72. Luckraz H, Goddard M, McNeil K, et al. Microvascular changes in small airways predispose to obliterative bronchiolitis after lung transplantation. J Heart Lung Transplant 2004; 23(5):527–531.

73. Jaramillo A, Smith MA, Phelan D, et al. Development of ELISA-detected anti-HLA antibodies precedes the development of bronchiolitis obliterans syndrome and correlates with progressive decline in pulmonary function after lung transplantation. Transplantation 1999; 67(8):1155–1161.

74. Smith MA, Sundaresan S, Mohanakumar T, et al. Effect of development of antibodies to HLA and cytomegalovirus mismatch on lung transplantation survival and development of bronchiolitis obliterans syndrome. J Thorac Cardiovasc Surg 1998; 116(5):812–820.

75. Palmer SM, Davis RD, Hadjiliadis D, et al. Development of an antibody specific to major histocompatibility antigens detectable by flow cytometry after lung transplant is associated with bronchiolitis obliterans syndrome. Transplantation 2002; 74(6):799–804.

76. Jaramillo A, Naziruddin B, Zhang L, et al. Activation of human airway epithelial cells by non-HLA antibodies developed after lung transplantation: a potential etiological factor for bronchiolitis obliterans syndrome. Transplantation 2001; 71(7):966–976.

77. Magro CM, Ross P Jr, Kelsey M, et al. Association of humoral immunity and bronchiolitis obliterans syndrome. Am J Transplant 2003; 3(9):1155–1166.

78. Reznik SI, Jaramillo A, Zhang L, et al. Anti-HLA antibody binding to hla class I molecules induces proliferation of airway epithelial cells: a potential mechanism for bronchiolitis obliterans syndrome. J Thorac Cardiovasc Surg 2000; 119(1):39–45.

79. Jaramillo A, Smith CR, Maruyama T, et al. Anti-HLA class I antibody binding to airway epithelial cells induces production of fibrogenic growth factors and apoptotic cell death: a possible mechanism for bronchiolitis obliterans syndrome. Hum Immunol 2003; 64(5):521–529.

80. Saunders NA, Smith RJ, Jetten AM. Differential responsiveness of human bronchial epithelial cells, lung carcinoma cells, and bronchial fibroblasts to interferon-gamma in vitro. Am J Respir Cell Mol Biol 1994; 11(2):147–152.

81. Duncan SR, Paradis IL, Yousem SA, et al. Sequelae of cytomegalovirus pulmonary infections in lung allograft recipients. Am Rev Respir Dis 1992; 146(6):1419–1425.

82. Husain S, Singh N. Bronchiolitis obliterans and lung transplantation: evidence for an infectious etiology. Semin Respir Infect 2002; 17(4):310–314.

83. Tamm M, Aboyoun CL, Chhajed PN, et al. Treated cytomegalovirus pneumonia is not associated with bronchiolitis obliterans syndrome. Am J Respir Crit Care Med 2004; 170(10):1120–1123.

84. Khalifah AP, Hachem RR, Chakinala MM, et al. Respiratory viral infections are a distinct risk for bronchiolitis obliterans syndrome and death. Am J Respir Crit Care Med 2004; 170(2):181–187.

85. Vilchez RA, Dauber J, Kusne S. Infectious etiology of bronchiolitis obliterans: the respiratory viruses connection—myth or reality? Am J Transplant 2003; 3(3):245–249.

86. Billings JL, Hertz MI, Savik K, et al. Respiratory viruses and chronic rejection in lung transplant recipients. J Heart Lung Transplant 2002; 21(5):559–566.

87. Gerhardt SG, McDyer JF, Girgis RE, et al. Maintenance azithromycin therapy for bronchiolitis obliterans syndrome: results of a pilot study. Am J Respir Crit Care Med 2003; 168(1):121–125.

88. Grundy JE, Ayles HM, McKeating JA, et al. Enhancement of class I HLA antigen expression by cytomegalovirus: role in amplification of virus infection. J Med Virol 1988; 25(4):483–495.

89. Kurt-Jones EA, Popova L, Kwinn L, et al. Pattern recognition receptors TLR4 and CD14 mediate response to respiratory syncytial virus. Nat Immunol 2000; 1(5):398–401.

90. Young LR, Hadjiliadis D, Davis RD, et al. Lung transplantation exacerbates gastroesophageal reflux disease. Chest 2003; 124(5):1689–1693.

91. Hadjiliadis D, Duane Davis R, Steele MP, et al. Gastroesophageal reflux disease in lung transplant recipients. Clin Transplant 2003; 17(4):363–368.

92. Palmer SM, Miralles AP, Howell DN, et al. Gastroesophageal reflux as a reversible cause of allograft dysfunction after long transplantation. Chest 2000; 118(4):1214–1217.

93. Cantu E III, Appel JZ III, Hartwig MG, et al. Early fundoplication prevents chronic allograft dysfunction in patients with gastroesophageal reflux disease. Ann Thorac Surg 2004; 78(4):1142–1151; discussion 1142–1151.

94. Fiser SM, Tribble CG, Long SM, et al. Ischemia-reperfusion injury after lung transplantation increases risk of late bronchiolitis obliterans syndrome. Ann Thorac Surg 2002; 73(4):1041–1047; discussion 1047–1048.

95. Levine SM, Angel L, Anzueto A, et al. A low incidence of posttransplant lymphoproliferative disorder in 109 lung transplant recipients. Chest 1999; 116(5):1273–1277.

96. Angel LF, Cai TH, Sako EY, et al. Posttransplant lymphoproliferative disorders in lung transplant recipients: clinical experience at a single center. Ann Transplant 2000; 5(3):26–30.

97. Wigle DA, Chaparro C, Humar A, et al. Epstein–Barr virus serology and posttransplant lymphoproliferative disease in lung transplantation. Transplantation 2001; 72(11):1783–1786.

98. Malouf MA, Chhajed PN, Hopkins P, et al. Anti-viral prophylaxis reduces the incidence of lymphoproliferative disease in lung transplant recipients. J Heart Lung Transplant 2002; 21(5):547–554.

99. Ramalingam P, Rybicki L, Smith MD, et al. Posttransplant lymphoproliferative disorders in lung transplant patients: the Cleveland Clinic experience. Mod Pathol 2002; 15(6):647–656.

100. Cohen AH, Sweet SC, Mendeloff E, et al. High incidence of posttransplant lymphoproliferative disease in pediatric patients with cystic fibrosis. Am J Respir Crit Care Med 2000; 161(4 Pt 1):1252–1255.

101. Gulley ML, Swinnen LJ, Plaisance KT Jr, et al. Tumor origin and CD20 expression in posttransplant lymphoproliferative disorder occurring in solid organ transplant recipients: implications for immune-based therapy. Transplantation 2003; 76(6):959–964.

102. Wood BL, Sabath D, Broudy VC, et al. The recipient origin of posttransplant lymphoproliferative disorders in pulmonary transplant patients. A report of three cases. Cancer 1996; 78(10):2223–2228.

103. Mentzer SJ, Longtine J, Fingeroth J, et al. Immunoblastic lymphoma of donor origin in the allograft after lung transplantation. Transplantation 1996; 61(12):1720–1725.

104. Knowles DM, Cesarman E, Chadburn A, et al. Correlative morphologic and molecular genetic analysis demonstrates three distinct categories of posttransplantation lymphoproliferative disorders. Blood 1995; 85:552–565.

105. Egan JJ, Hazleton PS, Yonan N, et al. Necrotic, ulcerative bronchitis, the presenting feature of lymphoproliferative disease following heart–lung transplantation. Thorax 1995; 50(2):205–207.

106. Legere BM, Saad CP, Mehta AC. Endobronchial post-transplant lymphoproliferative disorder and its management with photodynamic therapy: a case report. J Heart Lung Transplant 2003; 22(4):474–477.

107. Rosendale E, Yousem SA. Discrimination of Epstein–Barr virus-related post-transplant lymphoproliferations from acute rejection in lung allograft recipients. Arch Pathol Lab Med 1995; 119(5):418–423.

108. Nuckols JD, Baron PW, Stenzel TT, et al. The pathology of liver-localized post-transplant lymphoproliferative disease: a report of three cases and a review of the literature. Am J Surg Pathol 2000; 24:733–741.

109. Garver RI Jr, Zorn GL, Wu X, et al. Recurrence of bronchioloalveolar carcinoma in transplanted lungs. N Engl J Med 1999; 340(14):1071–1074.

110. Paloyan EB, Swinnen LJ, Montoya A, et al. Lung transplantation for advanced bronchioloalveolar carcinoma confined to the lungs. Transplantation 2000; 69(11):2446–2448.

111. Zorn GL Jr, McGiffin DC, Young KR Jr, et al. Pulmonary transplantation for advanced bronchioloalveolar carcinoma. J Thorac Cardiovasc Surg 2003; 125(1):45–48.

112. de Perrot M, Chernenko S, Waddell TK, et al. Role of lung transplantation in the treatment of bronchogenic carcinomas for patients with end-stage pulmonary disease. J Clin Oncol 2004; 22(21):4351–4356.

113. de Perrot M, Fischer S, Waddell TK, et al. Management of lung transplant recipients with bronchogenic carcinoma in the native lung. J Heart Lung Transplant 2003; 22(1):87–89.

114. Abrahams NA, Meziane M, Ramalingam P, et al. Incidence of primary neoplasms in explanted lungs: long-term follow-up from 214 lung transplant patients. Transplant Proc 2004; 36(9):2808–2811.

115. Lee P, Minai OA, Mehta AC, et al. Pulmonary nodules in lung transplant recipients: etiology and outcome. Chest 2004; 125(1):165–172.

116. Arcasoy SM, Hersh C, Christie JD, et al. Bronchogenic carcinoma complicating lung transplantation. J Heart Lung Transplant 2001; 20(10):1044–1053.

117. De Soyza AG, Dark JH, Parums DV, et al. Donor-acquired small cell lung cancer following pulmonary transplantation. Chest 2001; 120(3):1030–1031.

118. Knoop C, Jacobovitz D, Antoine M, et al. Donor-transmitted tumors in lung allograft recipients: report on two cases. Transplantation 1994; 57(11):1679–1680.

119. Finkelstein SD, Hasegawa T, Colby T, et al. 11q13 allelic imbalance discriminates pulmonary carcinoids from tumorlets. A microdissection-based genotyping approach useful in clinical practice. Am J Pathol 1999; 155(2):633–640.

120. Ionescu DN, Sasatomi E, Aldeeb D, et al. Pulmonary meningothelial-like nodules: a genotypic comparison with meningiomas. Am J Surg Pathol 2004; 28(2):207–214.

121. Johnson BA, Duncan SR, Ohori NP, et al. Recurrence of sarcoidosis in pulmonary allograft recipients. Am Rev Respir Dis 1993; 148(5):1373–1377.

122. Walker S, Mikhail G, Banner N, et al. Medium term results of lung transplantation for end stage pulmonary sarcoidosis. Thorax 1998; 53(4):281–284.

123. Nunley DR, Hattler B, Keenan RJ, et al. Lung transplantation for end-stage pulmonary sarcoidosis. Sarcoidosis Vasc Diffuse Lung Dis 1999; 16(1):93–100.
124. Burke M, Stewart S, Ashcroft T, et al. Biopsy diagnosis of disease recurrence after transplantation (TX) for pulmonary sarcoidosis: a multicentre study. J Heart Lung Transplant 2001; 20(2):154–155.
125. Slebos DJ, Verschuuren EA, Koeter GH, et al. Bronchoalveolar lavage in a patient with recurrence of sarcoidosis after lung transplantation. J Heart Lung Transplant 2004; 23(8):1010–1013.
126. Nine JS, Yousem SA, Paradis IL, et al. Lymphangioleiomyomatosis: recurrence after lung transplantation. J Heart Lung Transplant 1994; 13(4):714–719.
127. Bittmann I, Rolf B, Amann G, et al. Recurrence of lymphangioleiomyomatosis after single lung transplantation: new insights into pathogenesis. Hum Pathol 2003; 34(1):95–98.
128. Pechet TT, Meyers BF, Guthrie TJ, et al. Lung transplantation for lymphangioleiomyomatosis. J Heart Lung Transplant 2004; 23(3):301–308.
129. Baz MA, Kussin PS, Van Trigt P, et al. Recurrence of diffuse panbronchiolitis after lung transplantation. Am J Respir Crit Care Med 1995; 151(3 Pt 1): 895–898.
130. Frost AE, Keller CA, Brown RW, et al. Giant cell interstitial pneumonitis. Disease recurrence in the transplanted lung. Am Rev Respir Dis 1993; 148(5):1401–1404.
131. Parker LA, Novotny DB. Recurrent alveolar proteinosis following double lung transplantation. Chest 1997; 111(5):1457–1458.
132. Santamaria F, Brancaccio G, Parenti G, et al. Recurrent fatal pulmonary alveolar proteinosis after heart-lung transplantation in a child with lysinuric protein intolerance. J Pediatr 2004; 145(2):268–272.
133. Mal H, Guignabert C, Thabut G, et al. Recurrence of pulmonary emphysema in an alpha-1 proteinase inhibitor-deficient lung transplant recipient. Am J Respir Crit Care Med 2004; 170(7):811–814.
134. Sathyapala SA, Gupta NK, Westwood JP, et al. Recurrence of alpha 1-antitrypsin deficiency emphysema on computed tomography (CT) after lung transplantation. J Heart Lung Transplant 2005; 24:S103.
135. Palmer SM Jr, Layish DT, Kussin PS, et al. Lung transplantation for Williams–Campbell syndrome. Chest 1998; 113(2):534–537.
136. Marques LJ, Teschler H, Guzman J, et al. Smoker's lung transplanted to a nonsmoker. Long-term detection of smoker's macrophages. Am J Respir Crit Care Med 1997; 156(5):1700–1702.

# 31

# Obliterative Bronchiolitis

**Geert M. Verleden and Lieven J. Dupont**

*Department of Respiratory Medicine and Lung Transplantation Unit,
University Hospital Gasthuisberg, Leuven, Belgium*

## INTRODUCTION

Lung and heart–lung transplantation (LTx and HLTx) are now accepted operative therapeutic interventions for well-selected patients with end-stage heart–lung or lung disease. Although the procedure remains a palliation therapy, most of the patients are doing well with, nowadays, a mean actuarial five-year survival of 40% to 50% (1), even increasing to over 60% to 70% for selected indications such as cystic fibrosis and emphysema in some high volume centers (2,3). Although the surgical techniques and the immunosuppressive drug regimen have improved and new techniques for early detection of chronic rejection have emerged, long-term survival is hampered by the development of chronic rejection. Indeed, obliterative bronchiolitis (OB) or bronchiolitis obliterans syndrome (BOS), the clinical correlate of OB, is now regarded as a manifestation of chronic rejection (4), leading to obliteration and scarring of the terminal bronchioles, and remains the leading cause of morbidity and of late mortality after HLTx or LTx (1).

In this chapter, we give an overview of the incidence, risk factors, symptomatology, diagnosis, and treatment of OB.

## INCIDENCE AND PREVALENCE OF OB/BOS

In the Stanford University experience, the overall prevalence of OB in patients surviving more than three months after transplantation was 64%

after HLTx and 68% after LTx (5). In St. Louis, the actuarial one-, three-, and five-year freedom from OB was 82%, 42%, and 25%, respectively, in adults (6). Whitehead et al. reported data in children with as much as 76% after one year and 37% after three years being free of OB (7). In the recent International Society for Heart and Lung Transplantation (ISHLT) registry report, the one-, three-, and five-year freedom from OB in adult patients followed up between April 1994 and June 2003 was 89.8%, 69.2%, and 55.3%, respectively (1). These figures illustrate a clear improvement with more patients being free of OB in recent years, compared to the original St. Louis data. The overall incidence of OB is estimated at 12% at one year and over 50% at five years (8).

Chronic rejection after LTx is the single most important factor responsible for late mortality with as much as 40% to 50% of deaths >3 to 5 years after transplantation being due to chronic rejection (1).

## CLINICAL PRESENTATION

Clinically, OB was first described in 1984 in a patient who developed a progressive decline in forced expiratory volume in one second ($FEV_1$) after an HLTx (9). Chronic allograft rejection is indeed consistently characterized by a reduction in pulmonary function parameters, most specifically in $FEV_1$, attributed to airways obstruction. There is no significant reversibility after inhalation of short-acting $\beta_2$-agonists. The onset of symptoms is mostly insidious, with progressive exertional dyspnoe, often accompanied by cough. Sometimes a respiratory tract infection seems to have triggered the onset of OB, with acute dyspnoe, wheezing, and the development of airways obstruction. In the later course of the disease, superinfections are frequently seen and colonization of the airways with *Pseudomonas aeruginosa* and *Aspergillus fumigatus* is common. At that time, high-resolution computed axial tomography (CAT) scan of the thorax often reveals bronchiectasis and other signs of chronic infection (10). Auscultation of the lungs is often normal, however, occasional rhales and in later stages squeaks may be heard. Once established, OB may develop progressively and lead to severe airways obstruction with respiratory insufficiency and death, resulting from an infectious exacerbation (Fig. 1A). In other patients, the progression may be arrested, either spontaneously or in response to treatment (Fig. 1B) (11,12). Patients may also develop what is called a "late acute chronic rejection," mostly preceded by an acute rejection episode (13). After antirejection treatment there is some recuperation of the $FEV_1$ but after a short time period (sometimes only a couple of weeks) there is a fast and progressive decline in $FEV_1$, which may plateau at low volumes (Fig. 1C). This clinical presentation of OB often has a poor prognosis leading to death of the patient in a couple of months, without any medical treatment being helpful. Only retransplantation may be of benefit in this situation. Sometimes, episodes of progressive loss of lung function may disperse with stable intervals.

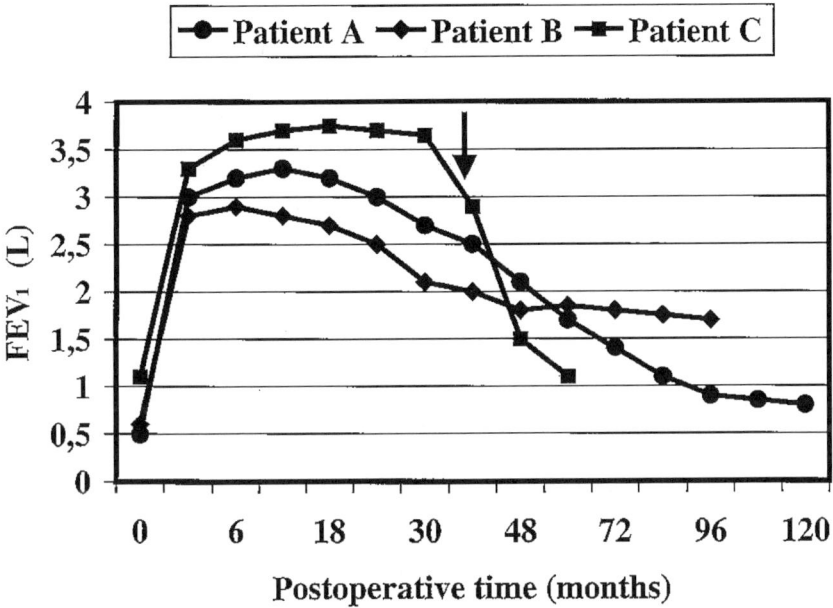

**Figure 1** (-•-) Natural evolution of FEV$_1$ in a patient with slowly progressing BOS and biopsy-proven OB. During the last months of evolution, there appears to be a spontaneous arrest in the FEV$_1$ decline. (-◆-) Another patient with BOS, who has a spontaneous arrest of the FEV$_1$ decline, with a plateau, reached after several months. (-■-) Typical FEV$_1$ evolution in a patient with late acute BOS. After a very stable period of several years, there is a documented acute rejection episode (*arrow*), quickly followed by a very rapid decline in the FEV$_1$, indicative of BOS. *Abbreviations*: FEV$_1$, forced expiratory volume in one second; BOS, bronchiolitis obliterans syndrome; OB, obliterative bronchiolitis.

OB/BOS not only represents the most important cause of late mortality, but also causes a significant morbidity, loss of health-related quality of life (HRQOL), and constitutes a tremendous cost. In two recent studies from the same group (14,15), the relationship between HRQOL and BOS was specifically assessed. HRQOL was measured both cross-sectionally and longitudinally by standardized patient self-administered questionnaires, including the Nottingham Health Profile (NHP), the State-trait Anxiety Inventory (STAI), the Zung Self-Rating Depression Scale, and the Index of Well-Being (IWB). Data were collected at one, four, and seven months, and every six months afterwards for as long as 49 months post-LTx (14) or 18 months after the onset of BOS (15).

The number of patients who completed the questionnaires varied from 72 at 4 months, to 27 at 49 months after LTx (14) or 29 patients with 18 months follow-up after BOS onset (15). Cross-sectionally, the patients with

BOS reported persistently and significantly more restrictions on the dimensions energy and physical mobility of the NHP compared with patients without BOS. Other domains, i.e., pain, sleep, social interaction, and emotional reactions, were not affected. Additionally, patients with BOS reported significantly more depressive symptoms and anxiety one and two years after LTx. Results from the longitudinal analysis support these findings, although no change in depressive symptoms could be found after onset of BOS.

In a parallel follow-up study, costs were prospectively investigated in relation to the development of BOS. The difference in costs between patients who remained stable and those who developed BOS was largely accounted for by an increase in used health care resources, in particular hospitalization and medication (16).

Such studies clearly demonstrate that BOS is not only associated with a significant loss of HRQOL but also with substantial extra costs, which further emphasizes the need to focus efforts on prevention of BOS to enhance the cost-effectiveness of LTx.

## HISTOLOGY OF CHRONIC REJECTION

Bronchiolitis obliterans syndrome is a term used to describe the graft deterioration secondary to persistent airflow obstruction in LTx recipients (4). The current consensus is that chronic rejection causes or at least significantly contributes to this functional deterioration and that the associated pathological lesion is that of OB (17). It is, however, evident that BOS not always is a manifestation of chronic rejection as newer treatment modalities such as azithromycine or fundoplication may greatly improve the pulmonary function of some patients with BOS (see further in this chapter) (18). BOS is defined clinically and functionally and does not necessarily require histological confirmation (19). Indeed, the patchy nature of OB particularly in its early stages means that transbronchial biopsy often has a poor yield, which, however, increases significantly by the use of serial sections and connective tissue stains together with the experience of the reading histopathologist in identifying subtle early changes and some helpful surrogate markers. Transbronchial biopsies and less frequently thoracoscopic or open lung biopsies can also be useful in the clinical setting of BOS in confirming or excluding alternative or concomitant diagnoses, particularly where these are amenable to treatment (20).

Obliterative bronchiolitis is essentially a scarring process affecting the small noncartilage containing airways of the lung graft (17). The 2001 BOS recommendations are that the pathological term "obliterative bronchiolitis" (bronchiolitis obliterans) should be used only when histology demonstrated dense fibrous scar tissue affecting the small airways (21). The presence of a lymphocytic submucosal infiltrate or intraluminal granulation tissue is insufficient for a diagnosis of OB. Furthermore, the obliterative lesion can be defined as active when it is associated with the mononuclear cell infiltrate and inactive when inflammatory cells are absent (17). Histologically, the small airway fibrosis involves both membranous and respiratory bronchioles and can be eccentric or concentric in distribution, thereby reducing the bronchiolar lumen (22). The initial pathological process appears to be lymphocytic infiltration of the submucosa of the airways and epithelium which is known as lymphocytic bronchiolitis (17,23). Refractory airflow obstruction has been described in association with isolated lymphocytic bronchiolitis/bronchitis in lung allografts and it is likely that it can represent the progenitor lesion (24). Epithelial damage is common in both lymphocytic bronchiolitis and OB with epithelial cell necrosis leading to denudation and frank ulceration of the mucosa. The resulting inflammatory reaction involving fibroblasts and myofibroblast migration into the lumen leads to the formation of intraluminal granulation tissue, often polypoid, which can result in subtotal or total obliteration of the small airway. It is assumed that the active inflammatory and fibroblastic phase of OB precedes the acellular hyaline plaques of inactive disease, although for instance late acute BOS may represent an immediate scarring of the airways without significant inflammation (25). The airway scarring can extend into the interstitium but is easily distinguished from intra-alveolar granulation tissue of organizing pneumonia which is also frequently observed as a consequence of associated infections or aspiration. Organizing pneumonia with or without OB can also be seen in cases of aspiration, which is a recognized cause of both these pathologies (26).

## RISK FACTORS FOR CHRONIC REJECTION

Obliterative brochiolitis affects all lung transplant recipients irrespective of age, gender, race, type of lung transplantation procedure, and underlying diagnosis. Several risk factors for the development of OB/BOS have been identified, of which late or recurrent/refractory acute rejection and lymphocytic bronchitis/bronchiolitis were the most convincing (27). Together with noncompliance, human leukocyte antigen (HLA) mismatches at the A locus, and total HLA mismatches, these factors constitute the immunological risk factors. Several nonimmunological risk factors have been proposed: cytomegalovirus (CMV) pneumonitis (28) and ischemia–reperfusion (29) (commonly associated factors although evidence for these factors was inconsistent). Other possible nonimmunological factors included early nonspecific bronchial hyper-responsiveness (30), donor and recipient age, graft ischemic time, transplantation for primary pulmonary hypertension (31), gastroesophageal reflux (26), and bacterial/fungal/non-CMV viral infection (32).

### Immunological Risk Factors

*Acute Rejection and Lymphocytic Bronchitis/Bronchiolitis*

The single most important clinical risk factor for OB is acute rejection, defined as a perivascular infiltration of activated lymphocytes into the graft.

Of the most recent reports from 14 transplant centers that investigated this relationship, 12 reported a significant association with acute rejection. In two of these studies, the effect was only evident for later acute rejection episodes (28,29). In a recent study, it was demonstrated that patients with multiple A1 acute rejection episodes also developed an earlier onset of OB, challenging the fact that such rejections should not be treated in asymptomatic patients (33,34). Further evidence of the role of acute rejection was provided by an association between OB/BOS and decreased immunosuppression (35). Nonetheless, there are some patients who develop OB/BOS without having experienced any (documented or treated) acute rejection episode, which may indicate that it may not be the only factor involved. On the other hand, severe or unresponsive acute rejection may directly lead to chronic rejection with a short time interval between them.

Nonfibrosing lymphocytic inflammation of the airways (lymphocytic bronchitis/bronchiolitis) is frequently seen in bronchial biopsies of lung transplant recipients and is now thought to be a manifestation of acute rejection (23,36), although it may also represent a manifestation or a progenitor of chronic rejection (24).

### Human Leukocyte Antigen Mismatches

The association between mismatches at specific loci of the major histocompatibility complex (MHC) is not clear. In the largest published series to date, comprising 3549 lung transplants, no significant association could be found between HLA mismatches and the development of OB. There was, however, an association between mismatch at the HLA-A locus and acute rejection episodes (37). Pittsburgh, on the other hand, reported an association between OB and fewer mismatches, which was marginally significant (28); other centers found an association between BOS onset and mismatches at the A locus (28,38), or with two DR mismatches (39), or with total mismatches at the A-, B-, and DR-loci (28,36,40). In general, single center studies have limited power due both to the small absolute effect of mismatching and to the lack of prospective tissue matching, resulting in few beneficial transplants. As a consequence, there remains some doubt whether HLA mismatch is really important in the development of OB.

### Nonimmunological Risk Factors

#### Cytomegalovirus Infection and Other Infections

Infections are increasingly recognized as a potential risk factor for the development of OB/BOS. CMV infection, pneumonitis, and serology mismatching have all been implicated in earlier onset BOS and some studies have shown the introduction of ganciclovir prophylaxis to be protective. In a recent study from Australia, freedom from BOS for patients with or without CMV pneumonia was similar after one, three, and five years, and it was therefore concluded that CMV pneumonia treated with ganciclovir was a risk factor neither for BOS nor patient survival (41), again questioning the exact role of CMV.

In addition, a small number of centers have implicated community respiratory virus infections, especially influenza virus, parainfluenza virus, respiratory syncytial virus, and adenovirus as risk factors for BOS (42–44).

Bacterial and fungal infections may all play a role in the development of OB, although there is certainly no direct causal association (32). On the other hand, patients with OB experience more bacterial and fungal infections, which may then cause further deterioration of the $FEV_1$.

More recently, it was demonstrated that treatment with azithromycin may improve the pulmonary function of some patients with BOS (45,46). A comparable improvement of $FEV_1$ has been demonstrated in patients with bronchiolitis obliterans complicating bone marrow transplantation (47). Whether this is due to an antibacterial or rather an anti-inflammatory effect of these drugs remains unanswered at this time (18).

### Airway Ischemia

In earlier reports it was suggested that bronchial arterial revascularization might reduce the incidence (48,49) or postpone the development of OB (50). However, this has up to now not been substantiated in humans, although it was shown that bronchial arterial revascularization protects pulmonary endothelium and type II pneumocytes in the early phase after lung transplantation in dogs, which may have consequences in the long term (51).

### Gastroesophageal Reflux

Gastroesophageal reflux (GER) is nowadays regarded as a hypothetical risk factor for the development of BOS and has been demonstrated to be a reversible cause of allograft dysfunction or BOS after lung transplantation (52). Moreover, lung transplantation on its own significantly increased the incidence of GER, as measured objectively by 24-hour pH studies, despite a lack of symptoms in most patients. In fact, before lung transplantation, 35% of the patients had an abnormal acid contact time, whereas after transplantation, this increased to 65% to 69.8% (53). This was, however, not confirmed in a longer retrospective study, in which the preoperative incidence of reflux was 63%, while 76% of patients had an abnormal pH study postoperatively (54). After fundoplication, there was a significant survival difference, together with an improvement of the pulmonary function (55). Of the 43 patients who underwent fundoplication in the series by Davis et al., 26 met the criteria for BOS at the time of the operation (13 patients in stage 1, seven in stage 2, and six in stage 3). After the fundoplication, 16 patients had improved their BOS stage: 10/13 BOS 1 patients and 3/7 BOS 2 patients no longer met the criteria for BOS, whereas another two from the BOS 2 group improved to BOS 1. Of the six patients in BOS 3, only one improved (55). These studies are, however, limited by their retrospective design and nonrandom patient selection, which might induce a selection bias. Additional prospective studies are needed to corroborate these results.

A larger, but still retrospective study by Cantu et al. from the same center showed that patients who had a fundoplication within three months after LTx had a significantly greater freedom from BOS and increased survival, compared to patients with reflux and no surgery, patients without reflux, and patients who underwent fundoplication at a later stage after LTx (54).

The mechanism by which LTx increases the incidence of GER is probably multifactorial, including vagus nerve dysfunction and effects of immunosuppressive medication on the gastric emptying and the lower esophageal sphincter function. In fact, it has previously been demonstrated that immunosuppressive agents may indeed influence gastric emptying. For instance, cyclosporine A causes a slower solid emptying pattern, whereas tacrolimus produces a significantly faster solid emptying (56). That is why conversion from cyclosporine to tacrolimus may improve gastric discomfort in transplant patients (57).

How GER might induce chronic allograft dysfunction is not quite clear, although lung denervation with impaired cough reflex and abnormal mucociliairy clearance may have a role to play. These factors might increase the acid contact time and so prolong the injury time to the airways, leading to sustained inflammation. Recently, it has also been demonstrated that GER is associated with an increased number of acute rejection episodes and that the presence of GER increased the rapidity and severity of the initial acute rejection. Furthermore, early fundoplication decreased the number of late rejections (58). In the retrospective study by Cantu et al., there was no association between GER and the occurrence of acute rejection episodes (54).

### Other Risk Factors

Younger age at transplantation (59), transplantation for primary pulmonary hypertension (31), and single lung transplantation (40) have been associated with BOS or OB.

Donor age, ischemic time, and their interaction were significantly related to OB/BOS in an ISHLT registry report of over 5000 transplants (60). One study of 500 lung transplant recipients showed increased incidence of BOS in patients with organs from donors with traumatic brain injury death (61) but this needs confirmation. However, despite extensive study, recipient and donor characteristics such as age, sex, blood group matching, procurement time, and ischemic time were not associated with OB/BOS in any study. It has also been suggested that reperfusion injury may predispose to allograft dysfunction (62), other studies could not corroborate these results (63).

## DIAGNOSIS

Obliterative bronchiolitis is the histological manifestation of chronic graft failure following lung transplantation, however, it is difficult to diagnose with transbronchial biopsies (TBB). In fact, it was demonstrated that the sensitivity of TBB for OB was only 28%, whereas the specificity was 75% (64). In another study only 15% of TBB showed signs of OB, whereas all investigated patients had clinical OB (65). That is exactly why in 1993 a committee sponsored by the International Society for Heart and Lung Transplantation proposed a clinical definition, called bronchiolitis obliterans syndrome (BOS) (4). The aim of the clinical classification was to standardize nomenclature, to facilitate the description of the natural history of graft failure, to enhance accurate recording of outcome following transplantation, and to measure the impact of therapeutic interventions. Based on pulmonary function criteria, rather than histology, BOS has initially been divided in four stages (Table 1). Within each BOS category, there is a subtype a and b, based on no pathologic evidence of OB or no pathologic material for evaluation (a) or pathologic evidence of OB (b). Importantly, it emphasized specifically for the first time that a histological diagnosis was not required to make a diagnosis of graft failure.

Although BOS has been proposed as a clinical description of OB, it is obvious that not all patients in whom airflow obstruction develops have BOS and hence OB. In fact, several confounding factors have to be excluded before a patient may be diagnosed as having BOS. These factors may originate from the graft itself or from the native lung and include infection, acute rejection, anastomotic problems, disease recurrence, aging, native lung hyperinflation, disease progression, and factors that induce a restrictive defect such as pleural disease, steroid myopathy, pain, etc. (4).

In a recent revision of these BOS criteria (21), besides $FEV_1$ the $FEF_{25-75}$ has also been included in the staging parameters, because it

**Table 1** BOS Stages, Based on Percentage of the Best Postoperative $FEV_1$[a]

| BOS stage | $FEV_1$ (%) |
|---|---|
| 0 | 80 or more |
| 1 | 66–79 |
| 2 | 51–65 |
| 3 | <50 |

[a]Best postoperative $FEV_1$ is defined as the average of two postoperative best $FEV_1$ measurements, three to six weeks apart.
*Abbreviations*: BOS, bronchiolitis obliterans syndrome; $FEV_1$, forced expiratory volume in one second.
*Source*: From Ref. 4.

**Table 2**  The New BOS Classification

| BOS stage | FEV$_1$/FEF$_{25-75}$ (% of baseline)[a] |
|-----------|------------------------------------------|
| 0 | FEV$_1$ >90 and FEF$_{25-75}$ >75 |
| Potential BOS | FEV$_1$ 81–90 and/or FEF$_{25-75}$ <76 |
| 1 | FEV$_1$ 66–80 |
| 2 | FEV$_1$ 51–65 |
| 3 | FEV$_1$ <50 |

[a]Same definition as in Table 1.
*Abbreviations*: BOS, bronchiolitis obliterans syndrome; FEV$_1$, forced expiratory volume in one second; FEF$_{25-27}$, forced midexpiration flow rate.
*Source*: From Ref. 21.

became clear that the latter parameter declined earlier than the FEV$_1$ (66–68). On the other hand, it has been intensively debated whether a 20% drop in FEV$_1$ is not too late to establish a diagnosis of BOS. Therefore, in the revised criteria, the key change was the introduction of a new subcategory referred to as "potential" BOS stage (BOS 0-p) (Table 2). The aim of this new classification was firstly to increase the sensitivity of physiological change for the diagnosis of BOS. It remains to be seen whether BOS 0-p achieves sufficiently high positive and negative predictive values for the diagnosis of BOS 1, and in fact in a recent study it was demonstrated that the FEV$_1$ criteria for BOS 0-p is a reasonable predictor of BOS stage 1 (57% of the patients who developed BOS 0-p by the FEV$_1$ stage, progressed to stage 1). However, the FEF$_{25-75}$ criterion for BOS stage 0-p is not predictive of BOS stage 1, since only 37% of those who developed BOS stage 0-p by the FEF$_{25-75}$ criterion, progressed to stage 1 (69). Therefore, reaching BOS stage 0-p should certainly alert the physician (and the patient), but does not allow to make a definitive prediction as to the further evolution of the pulmonary function parameters.

The second aim of the new classification was to highlight emerging surrogate markers for the diagnosis of OB including high-resolution CT scan (HRCT), indices of ventilation, and exhaled nitric oxide (FE$_{NO}$).

## High-Resolution CT Scan

High-resolution CT may demonstrate early signs of chronic rejection such as diminution of peripheral vascular markings, thickening of septal lines, and volume reduction. Hyperlucency, air trapping, and mosaic phenomenon appeared during more advanced BOS (70). The findings of two substantial studies by Worthy et al. (71) and Leung et al. (72) suggested that air trapping on expiratory CT scans is an accurate indicator of the bronchiolar obliterations that underlie BOS. This was only based on small numbers of patients, without a control group. Bankier et al. reviewed 111 CT examinations performed in 38 lung transplant patients over a period of seven years. They also determined air trapping scores in eight healthy volunteers. Functional impairment was assessed with the BOS classification. They found that the extent of air trapping increased with BOS severity ($P = 0.001$). A threshold of 32% of air trapping was optimal for distinguishing between patients with and those without BOS and provided a sensitivity of 83%, a specificity of 89%, and an accuracy of 88%. Moreover, patients without BOS who had air trapping exceeding 32% of the parenchyma were at significantly increased risk of developing BOS ($P = 0.004$) (73). Using spirometrically gated CT, it was shown in another study that the accuracy for diagnosing OB/BOS was 84% (74). Others, however, demonstrated that none of the typical HRCT characteristics of OB/BOS (mosaic perfusion, air trapping, bronchiectasis, and tree in bud) could accurately predict the development of OB/BOS (75,76).

## Indexes of Ventilation

Unlike the conventional single-breath test, single-breath washouts using mixtures containing two inert gases with different diffusivities, such as $SF_6$ and He, may provide information about the sites where ventilation inhomogeneities arise. Indeed, whereas the slope of a single gas is determined by both interregional and intra-acinar inequalities, the slope difference ($S_{SF_6} - S_{He}$) primarily reflects diffusion-dependent peripheral inhomogeneity. In addition, because theoretical models suggest that the diffusion front for He is located more proximally in the acinus than the diffusion front for $SF_6$, $S_{He}$ is expected to be more sensitive (i.e., to increase more) than $S_{SF_6}$ when inhomogeneities arise at the level of terminal and respiratory bronchioles; as a result, $S_{SF_6} - S_{He}$ is expected to decrease in disease processes affecting these bronchioles. This is the concept that has been used in the studies looking at the role of ventilation distribution in the diagnosis of OB/BOS.

In a prospective study by Estenne et al. (77), a total of 1929 single-breath tests (median, 30 tests per patient) were performed in 57 heart–lung and bilateral-lung transplant recipients who were followed for a median of 1215 (range = 164–2829) days. Eighteen of these patients were in stage BOS $\geq 1$ at the end of the study period. In stable patients, the distribution of ventilation was normal. On the other hand, in most patients who developed BOS, $S_{N_2}$ and $S_{He}$ increased above the confidence interval before the $FEV_1$ criterion for the diagnosis of BOS 1 was reached. The median time interval between the change in the slope of the alveolar plateau and the 20% drop in $FEV_1$ was 356 days for He and 178 days for $N_2$. Reynaud-Gaubert et al. (78) have also conducted a prospective trial aimed at assessing the role of $N_2$ single-breath tests for the detection of BOS. They studied 45 patients who underwent 47 bilateral-lung or heart–lung procedures, 22 of whom developed BOS; 765 pulmonary function tests were analyzed. On average, $S_{N_2}$ increased significantly 151 days before the spirometric criteria for BOS 1 was reached. In a study of 15 bilateral-lung transplant recipients, Arens and colleagues (79) reported that 9 of 11 stable patients without BOS and four patients with BOS had a significant increase in $S_{N_2}$. In the study of Estenne et al. (77), only 7 of 39 patients without BOS (at the end of the study period) demonstrated a significant alteration in ventilation distribution; the corresponding value found by Reynaud-Gaubert and colleagues (78) was 8 of 25 patients. It is possible, though speculative at this stage, that alterations in ventilation distribution seen in patients without BOS reflect early lesions which will later produce a gradual decline in $FEV_1$. Data on ventilation distribution reported so far seem to be very promising in that they indicate that the $N_2$ or He single-breath test detects post-transplant BO much earlier than conventional pulmonary function tests, in particular the $FEV_1$. However, so far these tests are restricted to patients who underwent heart–lung or bilateral-lung transplantation. Future studies will have to examine the relative performance of the single-breath test in the early detection of BOS and also its potential use in recipients of single-lung grafts.

### Fractional Concentration of Exhaled Nitric Oxide (FE$_{NO}$)

It is already known for some years that patients with BOS have an increased $FE_{NO}$ compared to stable lung transplant recipients and also compared to healthy volunteers (80–82). Furthermore, neither the transplantation procedure itself (single, sequential-single, or heart–lung procedure) nor the diseased native lung in single lung transplant recipients seems to influence the $FE_{NO}$, which makes it a useful test in all lung transplant recipients (83). Moreover, in a prospective study, Verleden et al. demonstrated that an increase of $FE_{NO}$ above a cutoff level of 15 ppb at two consecutive measure moments with three to six weeks in between occurs at a mean of 263 ($\pm$169) days before BOS 1 is diagnosed (based on an irreversible decline in $FEV_1$ of 20% or more), with an accuracy of 0.88 for the diagnosis of OB/BOS (84). Decreasing levels of eNO may also accompany the stabilization of the $FEV_1$ after switching the immunosuppressive therapy from cyclosporine A to tacrolimus in an attempt to treat chronic rejection, indicating that there is a reduction in airways inflammation in the patients who responded to the treatment shift (85). As a consequence, $FE_{NO}$ measurements seem to be a reliable tool in the early detection of BOS, especially since it is a noninvasive and highly reproducible test that can be used in all lung transplant recipients. Further studies are definitely needed to establish its exact role in the detection and management of BOS.

### TREATMENT OF OB/BOS

There are, as yet, no double-blind, randomized studies available that have looked at the effect of a certain intervention (mostly addition of a new immunosuppressive drug or replacement of an immunosuppressive drug) on the further evolution of OB/BOS. Therefore, it remains very difficult to define whether any intervention really constitutes a true effect on the $FEV_1$ evolution or rather is a reflection of the natural history of OB/BOS. Keeping this in mind, it remains difficult to interpret all the literature data that are available concerning the medical treatment of OB/BOS, because all available studies have looked at an apparent arrest in decline in $FEV_1$, which is, however, difficult to interpret because of the lack of a control group.

"The best treatment for a disease is to prevent its occurrence," remains a statement that can also be used in lung transplantation. Therefore, it is of interest to give an overview of different treatment regimes that may have a more preventive effect on the development of OB/BOS on the one hand, and an overview of what is already published in the literature regarding the treatment of established OB/BOS, on the other.

### Prevention of Known Risk Factors

Since the acceptable cold ischemic time of a lung remains rather short (varying between four and eight hours) and because of the increasing donor organ shortage (especially lungs and heart–lungs) worldwide, it is not possible today to routinely perform a prospective HLA cross-match, to overcome the problem of severe HLA mismatch after LTx. Moreover, as already mentioned in this chapter, there is no clear relationship between gross HLA mismatch and a higher incidence of chronic allograft dysfunction. Therefore, this will not be discussed further.

Since acute rejection during the first months after transplantation and especially the occurrence of refractory and recurrent acute rejection (RAR) is one of the major risk factors to develop OB/BOS, several studies have looked at the effect of newer immunosuppressive drugs to better treat RAR, hoping to reduce the prevalence of OB/BOS.

Nowadays more and more transplant centers are using mofetil mycophenolate (MMF) in de novo therapy or intend to switch to MMF in cases of RAR. Several authors have demonstrated that initial treatment with MMF in combination with either cyclosporine or tacrolimus may reduce the incidence of acute rejection episodes (86–88), although this could not be corroborated in other studies (89–91). Based on these data, results with MMF seem controversial and at best, a trend towards a reduced acute rejection rate and/or survival rate has been reported for MMF in comparison to azathioprine, either in combination with cyclosporine or with tacrolimus.

Tacrolimus as a comparator to cyclosporine is used for basic immunosuppression in lung transplanted patients since 1990. Several studies have addressed the possibility of tacrolimus as initial therapy to reduce the number of acute rejection episodes compared to initial cyclosporine therapy. Horning et al. looked at the effect of tacrolimus crossover therapy (instead of cyclosporine) for persistent or recurrent acute rejections and found that the number of acute rejection episodes significantly decreased from $4.4 \pm 2.1$ to $0.4 \pm 0.5$, while the average histologic grade of rejection as well as the incidence of acute rejection also significantly declined (92). Since then, numerous authors have reported a reduction in acute rejection and the refractory acute rejection rate; after switching from cyclosporine A to tacrolimus (93–96). In other studies, there was no clear effect of tacrolimus on the acute rejection rate; however, there was a significant reduction of the development of OB/BOS (97,98). Yet, other authors demonstrated a reduction in the acute rejection grade using tacrolimus instead of cyclosporine (99). As a consequence, tacrolimus-based initial immunosuppressive therapy may have some beneficial effects over cyclosporine-based initial therapy, as well on the acute rejection rate as on the occurrence of OB/BOS. What is accepted now is that a shift from cyclosporine to tacrolimus is certainly beneficial in case of RAR.

Cytolytic induction therapy has also been the subject of numerous studies. In fact, several authors have compared rabbit antithymocyte globulin (rATG) with OKT3 as induction therapy and found no clear benefit of either of the two agents with regard to acute rejection or BOS development, although the latency to develop BOS was longer in the OKT3 group (100). On the other hand, Reichenspurner et al. demonstrated in their study that the linearized rate of acute rejection per 100 patient-days was significantly higher in the OKT3-group versus the rATG-group (1.16 vs. 0.49, $P < 0.0002$). At the same time, the incidence of infections was also lower in the rATG-group (101). Comparing rATG induction therapy with no induction therapy, several authors could not demonstrate a clear difference in the development of OB/BOS (102,103), although rATG reduced the acute rejection rate in one study (103).

Daclizumab, an interleukin-2 receptor blocker, produced a reduced incidence of grade 2 or higher acute rejection during the first six months after transplantation (18% in the daclizumab group and 48% in the control group, $P < 0.04$) compared with historical controls (104), which was also found in a pediatric lung transplant population (105). Only one study has compared the three different induction therapies, rATG, OKT3, and daclizumab, and concluded that in all three drug regimens there was no significant difference in the freedom from acute rejection or OB/BOS (106). The conclusion of these studies seems to be that the number of acute rejection episodes following transplantation may be reduced by cytolytic therapy, whereas it is still debated whether there is an effect on the prevalence of chronic allograft dysfunction.

An alternative immunomodulating strategy that has been applied for the management of RAR and BOS is total lymphoid irradiation (TLI). Valentine et al. reported the use of TLI in the management of RAR in HLT and LTx recipients. Six patients with persistent rejection unresponsive to high-dose steroid therapy were treated with 800 cGy of TLI during a five-week period. TLI was started at a mean of 142 (37–707) days post-transplant. Three patients died between 28 and 457 days after the TLI due to severe rejection or BOS. Two patients have been free from acute rejection with a reversal of the morphological changes for more than four years; another patient had stable OB four years later. TLI was not associated with a reduction in the subsequent development of BOS (107).

Takao et al. investigated the effects of nebulized budesonide on acute and chronic lung function in HLTx patients with three or more episodes of acute rejection within any three-month period or who had steroid-resistant acute rejection using a prospective, open, randomized, parallel-group study design in which seven patients received 2 mg inhaled budesonide twice a day for one year in addition to their current immunosuppressive therapy. The other seven patients received no additional medication and comprised the control group. The number of acute rejection episodes in de budesonide group was lower than in the control group, although this did not reach significance. In the budesonide group, neither OB nor lung function deterioration has been found, whereas three patients from the control group developed OB (108). De Soyza et al. demonstrated that inhaled budesonide is able to reverse the decrease in $FEV_1$ and the increase in $FE_{NO}$, accompanying lymphocytic bronchiolitis (109), which is regarded as a manifestation of acute rejection (23,36).

The possible role of extracorporeal photochemotherapy (ECP) in acute lung rejection has only been documented in one case report. The patient presented with a simultaneous infection and acute rejection and institution of anti-infectious therapy together with ECP resulted in resolution of the acute rejection (110).

Methotrexate also significantly reduced the incidence of RAR during a follow-up of 12.5 months (111). Ganciclovir prophylaxis has been demonstrated to delay the onset of OB. In this study, the development of OB was significantly delayed in the group of HLTx patient who received ganciclovir prophylaxis ($1072 \pm 280$ days in the prophylaxis group vs. $432 \pm 189$ days in the nonprophylaxis group, $P < 0.01$) (112). This has also been confirmed in a rat trachea allograft model, in which ganciclovir prophylaxis-inhibited cytomegalovirus induced tracheal obliteration probably via an inhibitory effect on IL-2 and TNF-$\alpha$ release (113).

## Treatment of Established OB/BOS

### Changes in Immunosuppressive Regimens

Most of the current studies have looked at a change of the maintenance immunosuppressive regimen. In fact, already in 1987 it has been described that after the institution of azathioprine, the rate of decline in $FEF_{25-75}$ improved considerably in HLTx patients with OB (9). Since then, different drugs and experimental therapies have been investigated with regard to their effect on the decline in $FEV_1$ in OB/BOS patients.

Several papers deal with the effect of switching from cyclosporine to tacrolimus in (H)LTx patients with progressive OB/BOS (85,98,114–120). All studies are open, nonrandomized without a control group and often retrospective. They all conclude that after the switch, there seems to be an arrest in decline of the $FEV_1$ in about 50% to 90% of the patients and the results seem to be better when the switch is performed earlier in the progression of OB/BOS.

Other authors have looked at the conversion from azathioprine to MMF. In a first paper, 13 patients with OB were treated with MMF (1.5 g twice a day) for one week to 24 months. After the initiation of MMF, the $FEV_1$ decline arrested in 10 patients, whereas two patients died of progressive disease. Seven patients experienced gastrointestinal side effects and one patient developed a fungal infection (121). Speich et al. had a similar experience, although they specifically pointed out that the MMF dose seems very important: reduction of MMF from 3 to 2 g/day resulted in deterioration of the lung function, whereas increasing again to 3 g/day improved the pulmonary function data (122). In the study by Roman et al., switching from cyclosporine and azathioprine to tacrolimus and MMF arrested the decline in or improved $FEV_1$ in 3/12 and 6/12 patients, respectively. Only two patients had a progressive decline in $FEV_1$ after the switch (123). Dupont et al. switched 16 LTx patients with established OB/BOS from azathioprine to MMF at a mean of $1348 \pm 888$ days following lung transplantation and demonstrated a significant reduction of the mean rate of decline of the $FEV_1$ per month after this conversion (from $-1.3 \pm 1.4\%$ of baseline $FEV_1$/month to $+0.4 \pm 1.6\%$, $P < 0.05$) (124).

There seems to be no role today for inhaled steroids in the treatment of OB/BOS, since two randomized double-blind placebo controlled trials of three months duration, using either 750 μg fluticasone propionate twice daily in 30 clinically stable lung transplant recipients or inhaled CFC driven beclomethasone dipropionate 400 μg twice daily, (CFC-BDP) in comparison with a device designed to promote small airway deposition of ICS (HFA driven beclomethasone 200 μg twice daily, HFA-BDP), had no beneficial effects either on airway inflammation, airflow limitation, or incidence of BOS (125,126), or on small airway reticular basement membrane thickening (127).

Attempts using methotrexate or cyclophosphamide have only been successful in very few patients, carrying the risk for neoplastic disorders and/or severe infectious complications. Dusmet et al. treated 10 patients with persistent or progressive OB/BOS with methotrexate after the failure of conventional therapy (pulse steroids, antilymphocyte products, or both) to improve the $FEV_1$. Two patients had no further decline in $FEV_1$, in five there was only a reduction of 10% or less, only one patient had no benefit at all (128). In the study by Verleden et al., seven patients with OB/BOS were treated with cyclophosphamide, which was used instead of azathioprine. During a mean follow-up of $21 \pm 8$ months, the $FEV_1$ increased in five patients, whereas there was an arrest in the decline of the $FEV_1$ in another two. Only one patient died of progressive OB/BOS 18 months after the introduction of cyclophosphamide (129).

Three studies have evaluated the effect of cytolytic therapy in the treatment of progressive OB/BOS. Using rATG, antilymphocyte globulin, or OKT3, there was an arrest in the decline of the $FEV_1$ in 40% to 90% of the patients, although the stage of BOS nevertheless progressed over time in most patients (130–132).

In 1996 a first clinical study in lung transplant patients with chronic rejection using aerosolized cyclosporine was published, demonstrating the usefulness of this delivery mode of cyclosporine. From the nine patients with OB/BOS in whom it was used, there were seven responders, who experienced a stabilization in their pulmonary function compared with nine historical control patients who further deteriorated, suggesting that this therapy might be effective for refractory chronic rejection (133). In a recent study from the same group, it was shown that aerosolized cyclosporine compared to placebo in addition to systemic immunosuppressive therapy resulted in a better survival; however, no data on the prevalence of chronic rejection in both groups were mentioned (134).

Rapamycin is a new antiproliferative drug that has successfully been used after liver and kidney transplantation; however, little data is available in lung transplantation. In a recently published study by Cahill et al., rapamycin was added to the existing therapy in 12 patients with OB/BOS without having an effect on the decline in pulmonary function. Nonetheless, among individuals with rapidly declining pulmonary mechanics, sirolimus resulted in stabilization or improvement in pulmonary function (135). In a second small study, addition of rapamycin resulted in an arrest in the decline of $FEV_1$ and even an improvement of the $FEV_1$ in three out of four patients with OB/BOS (136,137). Larger studies and more experience with the use of rapamycin after lung transplantation will reveal the potential effect on obliterative bronchiolitis in the future.

Recently, azithromycin (azi) has been shown to produce an amelioration of the $FEV_1$ in lung transplant patients in different stages of BOS. Gerhardt et al. treated six lung transplant patients with BOS with azi and showed a significant improvement of the $FEV_1$ (+17.1%, or an absolute increase of 0.5 L) after a mean follow-up of 13.7 weeks (45). This study was further corroborated by Verleden et al., who also treated eight lung transplant patients with progressive chronic allograft dysfunction (four patients were in BOS stage 1, two in stage 2, and two in stage 3) with azi and who demonstrated a comparable improvement of the $FEV_1$ after 12 weeks (+18.3%). The $FEV_1$ started to increase after two to four weeks of treatment (46). In both studies, there were patients who no longer met the criteria for BOS, or who at least improved their BOS stage. The study of Gerhardt et al. (45) was in fact the first to show a significant improvement of the $FEV_1$ in BOS patients using medical treatment. Not only an improvement in pulmonary function, but also a major amelioration of bronchiectasis on CT scan has been demonstrated by using azi (138). The possible mechanisms of action of azithromycin in lung transplant patients with BOS remain unclear at the present time, although several explanations have been hypothesized such as inhibition of the transcription of quorum sensing genes, which may prevent production of tissue-damaging proteins and which have indeed been detected in clinically stable lung transplant recipients without any signs of infection (139), a positive effect on GER, since macrolide antibiotics are known as motilin agonists, an inhibitory effect on neutrophils and IL-8, which are characteristically found in increased amounts in the bronchoalveolar lavage fluid of patients with BOS. To date, there are no clear arguments favoring one or the other mechanism, although recently it was demonstrated in stable chronic obstructive pulmonary disease (COPD) patients that clarithromycin significantly inhibits the IL-8 production in induced sputum after a 14-day treatment period (140). Furthermore, azi also reduced airway neutrophilia in patients with OB/BOS (141).

### Other Treatment Options: TLI and ECP

Chacon et al. have previously reported the benefits of TLI treatment in 12 subjects with BOS (142). Although the individual response to TLI was variable, the administration of TLI resulted in a significant slowing in the rate of decline in lung function. An uncontrolled retrospective study by Melville et al. compared TLI with a switch from cyclosporine to tacrolimus in the management of BOS. In this series, 11 patients were converted from cyclosporine to tacrolimus as treatment of BOS, leading to a significant reduction in the decline in $FEV_1$. This was in agreement with a cohort of 20 patients who received treatment with TLI for BOS resulting in a significant and comparable median reduction in the fall in $FEV_1$ (143).

In the study by Fisher et al., TLI was well tolerated, with a low incidence of serious side effects, and resulted in a significant reduction in the decline in $FEV_1$ (144). No immediate life-threatening complications have been described in connection with TLI treatment. The immunosuppressive effects of low dose TLI have been associated with leukopenia, necessitating adjustments in the maintenance dose of azathioprine.

Compared to cardiac transplantation, experience with ECP in lung transplantation is still scarce. Slovis et al. described three lung transplant recipients with OB/BOS who had stabilization of airflow obstruction after the use of ECP (145). Salerno et al. reported stabilization of $FEV_1$ in 5/8 patients with OB/BOS of whom seven were in BOS grade 3 before start of ECP therapy (146). Villanueva et al. published their experience in 14 patients with OB/BOS. They demonstrated that seven of the eight patients with lower BOS stages (0 and 1) remained alive (one died from lung cancer), whereas two have progressed to BOS stage 2. On the other hand, from the six patients with BOS stages 2 or 3, four died of BOS (147). O'Hagan et al. reported on five pediatric patients with refractory BO of whom four temporarily stabilized their lung function with ECP (148).

### Retransplantation

Despite all possible treatments, patients with OB/BOS may further progress and some of them may qualify for retransplantation, immediately raising an ethical dilemma: since the gap between patients on the waiting list and the availability of suitable lungs is increasing, it may be debated whether retransplantation is a real therapeutic option in patients with unremitting chronic rejection after lung transplantation (149), or in other words, can we justify a policy of retransplantation that affords a patient a second chance, while depriving another of a first (150)?

In the recent ISHLT registry, only 1.8% of all lung transplantations are retransplants and 0.8% of these were performed because of OB/BOS, whereas 1% was done for other reasons (1).

In the largest cohort so far reported (151), 230 retransplantations from 47 lung transplant programs have been included. Indications for retransplantation were: chronic rejection in 146 patients, acute graft failure in 52, intractable airway complications in 14, histologically confirmed severe rejection in nine, and miscellaneous conditions in nine. The overall actuarial survival of retransplantation was 47% at one year, which is far beyond the one-year survival after a first transplantation, although patients undergoing retransplantation for OB/BOS had a significantly better survival when a center-adjusted analysis was performed. It became also clear from this data that a longer interval between the first transplantation and the redo operation (especially longer than two years) was associated with a better survival. In another single center study, the one-, two-, and five-year actuarial survival was 60%, 53%, and 45% respectively (152). In this study, a lot of patients died later on because of infection from the graft that was left in place. As a consequence, the authors concluded that they now favor replacement of the primary graft (or perform a sequential single lung transplantation if indicated) (152).

The prevalence of chronic rejection after retransplantation for OB/BOS was comparable to the one after a first transplantation, although a higher prevalence of OB/BOS has been demonstrated after retransplantation in the Hannover experience (153). Also in children, although the experience is rather limited, one center mentioned development of chronic allograft dysfunction in two of eight children who were retransplanted because of OB/BOS (154).

In general, it may be concluded that the best intermediate-term functional results occurred in more experienced centers, in nonventilated patients, and in patients undergoing retransplantation more than two years after the first transplantation (155).

## REFERENCES

1.  Trulock EP, Edwards LB, Taylor DO, et al. The registry of the international society for heart and lung transplantation: twenty-first official adult heart–lung report—2004. J Heart Lung Transplant 2004; 23:804–815.
2.  Vricella LA, Karamichalis JM, Ahmad S, et al. Lung and heart–lung transplantation in patients with end-stage cystic fibrosis: the Stanford experience. Ann Thorac Surg 2002; 74:13–18.
3.  Cassivi SD, Meyers BF, Battafarano RJ, et al. Thirteen-year experience in lung transplantation for emphysema. Ann Thorac Surg 2002; 74:1663–1670.
4.  Cooper JD, Billingham M, Egan T, et al. A working formulation for the standardization of nomenclature for clinical staging of chronic dysfunction in lung allografts. J Heart Lung Transplant 1993; 12:713–716.
5.  Reichenspurner H, Girgis RE, Robbins BC, et al. Stanford experience with obliterative bronchiolitis after lung and heart–lung transplantation. Ann Thorac Surg 1996; 62:1547–1573.
6.  Meyers BF, Lynch J, Trulock EP, et al. Lung transplantation: a decade of experience. Ann Surg 1999; 230:362–370.
7.  Whitehead B, Rees P, Sorensen K, et al. Incidence of obliterative bronchiolitis after heart–lung transplantation in children. J Heart Lung Transplant 1993; 12:903–908.
8.  Tamm M, Sharples L, Higenbottam T, et al. Bronchiolitis obliterans syndrome (BOS) following heart–lung transplantation. Transpl Int 1996; 9(Suppl 1): S299–S302.
9.  Glanville AR, Baldwin JC, Burke CM, et al. Obliterative bronchiolitis after heart–lung transplantation: apparent arrest by augmented immunosuppression. Ann Int Med 1987; 107:300–304.
10. Loubeyre P, Reven D, Delignette A, et al. Bronchiectasis detected with thin section CT as a predictor of chronic lung allograft rejection. Radiology 1995; 194:213–216.
11. Verleden GM. Bronchiolitis obliterans syndrome after lung transplantation: medical treatment. Monaldi Arch Chest Dis 2000; 55:140–145.
12. Verleden GM, Bankier A, Boehler A, et al. Bronchiolitis obliterans syndrome after lung transplantation: diagnosis and treatment. Eur Respir Monogr 2005; 29:19–43.
13. Jackson CH, Sharples LD, McNeil K, et al. Acute and chronic onset of bronchiolitis obliterans syndrome (BOS): are they different entities? J Heart Lung Transplant 2002; 21:658–666.
14. Van den Berg JW, Geertsma A, van der Bij W, et al. Bronchiolitis obliterans syndrome after lung transplantation and health-related quality of life. Am J Respir Crit Care Med 2000; 161:1937–1941.
15. Vermeulen KM, Groen H, van der Bij W, et al. The effect of bronchiolitis obliterans syndrome on health related quality of life. Clin Transplant 2004; 18:377–383.

16. Van den Berg JW, van Enckevort PJ, TenVergert EM, et al. Bronchiolitis obliterans syndrome and additional costs of lung transplantation. Chest 2000; 118:1648–1652.
17. Yousem SA, Berry GH, Cagle PT, et al. Revision of the 1990 working formulation for the classification of pulmonary allograft rejection: Lung Rejection Study Group. J Heart Lung Transplant 1996; 15:1–15.
18. Verleden GM, Dupont J, Van Raemdonck D. Is it bronchiolitis obliterans syndrome or is it chronic rejection: a reappraisal? Eur Respir J 2005; 25:221–224.
19. Yousem SA, Paradis I, Griffith BP. Can transbronchial biopsy aid in the diagnosis of bronchiolitis obliterans in lung transplant recipients? Transplantation 1994; 57:151–152.
20. Sibley RK, Berry GJ, Tazelaar HD, et al. The role of transbronchial biopsies in the management of lung transplant recipients. J Heart Lung Transplant 1993; 12:308–324.
21. Estenne M, Maurer J, Boehler A, et al. Bronchiolitis obliterans syndrome 2001: an update of the diagnostic criteria. J Heart Lung Transplant 2002; 21:297–310.
22. Stewart S. The pathology of lung transplantation. Semin Diagn Pathol 1992; 9:210–219.
23. Yousem SA. Lymphocytic bronchitis/bronchiolitis in lung allograft recipients. Am J Surg Pathol 1993; 17:491–496.
24. Ross DJ, Marchevsky A, Kramer M, et al. "Refractoriness" of airflow obstruction associated with isolated lymphocytic bronchiolitis/bronchitis in pulmonary allografts. J Heart Lung Transplant 1997; 16:832–838.
25. Verbeken EK, Stewart S. Bronchiolitis obliterans syndrome and bronchiolitis obliterans in lung transplantation: will a pathologist and a physician ever meet? Eur Respir Monogr 2004; 29:55–65.
26. Palmer SM, Miralles AP, Howell DN, et al. Gastroesophageal reflux as a reversible cause of allograft dysfunction after lung transplantation. Chest 2000; 118:1214–1217.
27. Sharples LD, Mc Neil K, Stewart S, et al. Risk factors for bronchiolitis obliterans: a systematic review of recent publications. J Heart Lung Transplant 2002; 21:271–281.
28. Kroshus TJ, Kshettry VR, Savik K, et al. Risk factors for the development of bronchiolitis obliterans syndrome after lung transplantation. J Thorac Cardiovasc Surg 1997; 114:195–202.
29. Bando K, Paradis IL, Similo S, et al. Obliterative bronchiolitis after lung and heart–lung transplantation. An analysis of risk factors and management. J Thorac Cardiovasc Surg 1995; 110:4–13.
30. Stanbrook MB, Kesten S. Bronchial hyperreactivity after lung transplantation predicts early bronchiolitis obliterans. Am J Respir Crit Care Med 1999; 160:2034–2039.
31. Kshettry VR, Kroshus TJ, Savik K, et al. Primary pulmonary hypertension as a risk factor for the development of obliterative bronchiolitis in lung allograft recipients. Chest 1996; 110:704–709.
32. Ward CW, De Soyza T, Keating DT, et al. Infection and bronchiolitis obliterans syndrome in lung transplant recipients. Eur Respir Monogr 2004; 29:44–54.

33. Hopkins PM, Aboyoun CL, Chhajed PN, et al. Association of minimal rejection in lung transplant recipients with obliterative bronchiolitis. Am J Respir Crit Care Med 2004; 170:1022–1026.

34. Egan JJ. Obliterative bronchiolitis after lung transplantation. A repetitive multiple injury airway disease. Am J Respir Crit Care Med 2004; 170: 931–932.

35. Husain AN, Siddique MT, Holmes EW, et al. Analysis of risk factors for the development of bronchiolitis obliterans syndrome. Am J Respir Crit Care Med 1999; 159:829–633.

36. Heng D, Sharples L, McNeil K, et al. Bronchiolitis obliterans syndrome: incidence, natural history, prognosis, and risk factors. J Heart Lung Transplant 1998; 17:1255–1263.

37. Quantz MA, Bennett LE, Meyer DM, et al. Does human leukocyte antigen matching influence the outcome of lung transplantation? An analysis of 3,549 lung transplantations. J Heart Lung Transplant 2000; 19:473–479.

38. Schulman LL, Weinberg AD, McGregor C, et al. Mismatches at the HLA-DR and HLA-B loci are risk factors for acute rejection after lung transplantation. Am J Respir Crit Care Med 1998; 157:1833–1837.

39. van den Berg JW, Hepkema BG, Geertsma A, et al. Long-term outcome of lung transplantation is predicted by the number of HLA-DR mismatches. Transplantation 2001; 71:368–373.

40. Hadjiliadis D, Davis RD, Palmer SM. Is transplant operation important in determining posttransplant risk of bronchiolitis obliterans syndrome in lung transplant recipients? Chest 2002; 122:1168–1175.

41. Tamm M, Aboyoun CL, Chajet PN, et al. Treated Cytomegalovirus pneumonia is not associated with bronchiolitis obliterans syndrome. Am J Respir Crit Care Med 2004; 170:1120–1123.

42. Billings JL, Hertz MI, Savik K. Respiratory viruses and chronic rejection in lung transplant recipients. J Heart Lung Transplant 2002; 21:559–566.

43. Garbino J, Gerbase MW, Wunderli W, et al. Respiratory viruses and severe lower respiratory tract complications in hospitalized patients. Chest 2004; 125:1033–1039.

44. Khalifah AP, Hachem RR, Chakinala MM, et al. Respiratory viral infections are a distinct risk factor for bronchiolitis obliterans syndrome and death. Am J Respir Crit Care Med 2004; 170:181–187.

45. Gerhardt S, McDyer JF, Girgis RE, et al. Maintenance azithromycin therapy for bronchiolitis obliterans syndrome. Am J Respir Crit Care Med 2003; 168:121–125.

46. Verleden GM, Dupont LJ. Azithromycin therapy for patients with bronchiolitis obliterans syndrome after lung transplantation. Transplantation 2004; 77:1465–1467.

47. Khalid M, Al Saghir A, Saleemi S, et al. Azithromycin in bronchiolitis obliterans complicating bone marrow transplantation: a preliminary study. Eur Respir J 2005; 25:490–493.

48. Baudet EM, Dromer C, Dubrez J, et al. Intermediate term results after en-bloc double-lung transplantation with bronchial arterial revascularization. J Thorac Cardiovasc Surg 1996; 112:1292–1299.

49. Yacoub M, Al-Kttan KM, Tadjkarimi S, et al. Medium term results of direct bronchial revascularization using IMA for single lung transplantation (SLT) with direct revascularization. Eur J Cardiothor Surg 1997; 11:1030–1036.

50. Norgaard M, Andersen C, Pettersson G. Does bronchial artery revascularization influence results concerning bronchiolitis obliterans syndrome and/or obliterative bronchiolitis after lung transplantation? Eur J Cardiothorac Surg 1998; 14:311–317.

51. Nowak K, Kamler M, Bock M, et al. Bronchial artery revasculariazation affects graft recovery after lung transplantation. Am J Respir Crit Care Med 2002; 165:216–220.

52. Palmer SM, Miralles AP, Howell DN, et al. Gastroesophageal reflux as a reversible cause of allograft dysfunction after lung transplantation. Chest 2000; 118:1214–1217.

53. Young LR, Hadjiliadis D, Davis D, et al. Lung transplantation exacerbates gastroesophageal reflux disease. Chest 2003; 124:1689–1693.

54. Cantu E III, Appel JZ III, Hartwig MG, et al. Early fundoplication prevents chronic allograft dysfunction in patients with gastroesophageal reflux disease. Ann Thorac Surg 2004; 78:1142–1151.

55. Davis D, Lau CL, Eubanks SS, et al. Improved lung allograft function after fundoplication in patients with gastroesophageal reflux disease undergoing lung transplantation. J Thorac Cardiovasc Surg 2003; 125:533–542.

56. Maes BD, Vanwalleghem J, Kuypers D, et al. Differences in gastric motor activity in renal transplant patients treated with FK-506 versus ciclosporine. Transplantation 1999; 68:1482–1485.

57. Verleden GM, Besse T, Maes B. Successful conversion from cyclosporine to tacrolimus for gastric motor dysfunction in a lung transplant recipient. Transplantation 2002; 73:1974–1976.

58. Hartwig MG, Cantu E, Appel JZ, et al. Non-alloimmune injury mediated by gastroesophageal reflux precipitates alloimmune injury in lung transplant patients. J Heart Lung Transplant 2004; 23:S43.

59. Girgis RE, Tu I, Berry GJ, et al. Risk factors for the development of obliterative bronchiolitis after lung transplantation. J Heart Lung Transplant 1996; 15:1200–1208.

60. Hosenpud JD, Bennett LE, Keck BM, et al. The registry of the International Society of Heart and Lung Transplantation: Seventeenth Official Report—2000. J Heart Lung Transplant 2000; 19:909–931.

61. Ciccone AM, Stewart KC, Meyers BF, et al. Does donor cause of death affect the outcome of lung transplantation? J Thorac Cardiovasc Surg 2002; 123:429–434.

62. Fiser SM, Tribble CG, Long SM, et al. Ischemia-reperfusion injury after lung transplantation increases risk of late bronchiolitis obliterans syndrome. Ann Thorac Surg 2002; 73:1041–1047.

63. Fisher AJ, Wardle J, Dark JH, et al. Non-immune acute graft injury after lung transplantation and the risk of subsequent bronchiolitis obliterans syndrome (BOS). J Heart Lung Transplant 2002; 21:1206–1212.

64. Pomerance A, Madden B, Burke MM, et al. Transbronchial biopsy in heart and lung transplantation: clinicopathologic correlations. J Heart Lung Transplant 1995; 14:761–763.

65.  Kramer MR, Stoehr C, Wang JL, et al. The diagnosis of obliterative bronchiolitis after heart–lung and lung transplantation: low yield of transbronchial biopsies. J Heart Lung Transplant 1993; 12:675–681.

66.  Patterson GM, Wilson S, Whang JL, et al. Physiologic definitions of obliterative bronchiolitis in heart–lung and double lung transplantation: a comparison of the forced expiratory flow between 25% and 75% of the forced vital capacity and forced expiratory volume in one second. J Heart Lung Transplant 1996; 15:175–181.

67.  Reynaud-Gaubert M, Thomas P, Badier M, et al. Early detection of airway involvement in obliterative bronchiolitis after lung transplantation. Functional and bronchoalveolar lavage findings. Am J Respir Crit Care Med 2000; 161(6):1924–1929.

68.  Ouwens JP, van der Mark TW, Koëter GH, et al. Bronchiolar airflow impairment after lung transplantation: an early and common manifestation. J Heart Lung Transplant 2002; 21:1056–1061.

69.  Hachem RR, Chakinala MM, Yusen RD, et al. The predictive value of bronchiolitis obliterans syndrome stage 0-p. Am J Respir Crit Care Med 2004; 169:468–472.

70.  Ikonen T, Kivisaari L, Taskinen E, et al. High-resolution CT in long-term follow-up after lung transplantation. Chest 1997; 111:370–376.

71.  Worthy SA, Park CS, Kim JS, et al. Bronchiolitis obliterans after lung transplantation: high-resolution CT findings in 15 patients. AJR Am J Roentgenol 1997; 169:673–677.

72.  Leung AN, Fisher K, Valentine V, et al. Bronchiolitis obliterans after lung transplantation: detection using expiratory HRCT. Chest 1998; 113:365–370.

73.  Bankier AA, Van Muylem A, Knoop C, et al. Bronchiolitis obliterans syndrome in heart–lung transplant recipients: diagnosis with expiratory CT. Radiology 2001; 218:533–539.

74.  Knollmann FD, Ewert R, Wundrich T, et al. Bronchiolitis obliterans syndrome in lung transplant recipients: use of spirometrically gated CT. Radiology 2002; 225:655–662.

75.  Lee E-S, Gotway MB, Reddy GP, et al. Early bronchiolitis obliterans following lung transplantation. Radiology 2000; 216:472–477.

76.  Millet WT Jr, Kotlof RM, Blumenthal NP, et al. Utility of high resolution computed tomography in predicting bronchiolitis obliterans syndrome following lung transplantation: preliminary findings. J Thorac Imaging 2001; 16:76–80.

77.  Estenne M, Van Muylem A, Knoop C, et al. Detection of obliterative bronchiolitis after lung transplantation by indexes of ventilation distribution. Am J Respir Crit Care Med 2000; 162:1047–1051.

78.  Reynaud-Gaubert M, Thomas P, Badier M, et al. Early detection of airway involvement in obliterative bronchioltiis after lung transplantation. Functional and bronchoalveolar lavage cell findings. Am J Respir Crit Care Med 2000; 161:1924–1929.

79.  Arens R, McDonough M, Zhao H, et al. Altered lung mechanics after double-lung transplantation. Am J Respir Crit Care Med 1998; 158:1403–1409.

80.  Fisher AJ, Gabbay E, Small T, et al. Cross sectional study of exhaled nitric oxide levels following lung transplantation. Thorax 1998; 53:454–458.

81. Verleden GM, Dupont LJ, Lamont J, et al. Is there a role for measuring exhaled nitric oxide in lung transplant recipients with chronic rejection? J Heart Lung Transplant 1998; 17:231–232.

82. Gabbay E, Walters EH, Orsida B, et al. Post-lung transplant bronchiolitis obliterans syndrome is characterized by increased exhaled nitric oxide levels and epithelial inducible nitric oxide synthase. Am J Respir Crit Care Med 2000; 162:2182–2187.

83. Verleden GM, Dupont LJ, Delcroix M, et al. Exhaled nitric oxide after lung transplantation: impact of the native lung. Eur Respir J 2003; 21:429–432.

84. Verleden GM, Dupont L, Van Raemdonck D, et al. Accuracy of exhaled nitric oxide measurements for the diagnosis bronchiolitis obliterans syndrome after lung transplantation. Transplantation 2004; 78:730–733.

85. Verleden GM, Dupont J, Van Raemdonck D, et al. The effect of switching cyclosporine A to tacrolimus on exhaled nitric oxide and pulmonary function in patients with chronic rejection after lung transplantation. J Heart Lung Transplant 2003; 22:908–913.

86. Reichenspurner H, Kur F, Treede H, et al. Optimization of an immunosuppressive protocol after lung transplantation. Transplantation 1999; 68:67–71.

87. Ross DJ, Waters PF, Levine M, et al. Mycophenolate mofetil versus azathioprine immunosuppressive regimens after lung transplantation: preliminary experience. J Heart Lung Transplant 1998; 17:768–774.

88. Gerbase MW, Spiliopoulos A, Fathi M, et al. Low doses of mycophenolate mofetil with low doses of tacrolimus prevent acute rejection and long-term function loss after lung transplantation. Transplant Proc 2001; 33: 2146–2147.

89. O'Hair DP, Cantu E, McGregor C, et al. Preliminary experience with mycophenolate mofetil used after lung transplantation. J Heart Lung Transplant 1998; 17:864–868.

90. Palmer SM, Baz MA, Sanders L, et al. Results of a randomised, prospective, multicenter trial of mycophenolate mofetil and azathioprine in the prevention of acute rejection. Transplantation 2001; 71:1772–1776.

91. Corris P, Glanville A, McNeil K, et al. One year analysis of an ungoing international randomized study of mycophenolate mofetil (MMF) vs azathioprine (AZA) in lung transplantion. J Heart Lung Transplant 2001; 20(Suppl): 149–150.

92. Horning N, Lynch J, Sundaresan S, et al. Tacrolimus therapy for persistent or recurrent acute rejection after lung transplantation. J Heart Lung Transplant 1998; 17:761–767.

93. Onsager DR, Canver CC, Jahania MS, et al. Efficacy of tacrolimus in the treatment of refractory rejection in heart and lung transplant recipients. J Heart Lung Transplant 1999; 18:448–455.

94. Vitulo P, Oggionni T, Cascina A, et al. Efficacy of tacrolimus rescue therapy in refractory acute rejection after lung transplantation. J Heart Lung Transplant 2002; 21:435–439.

95. Sarahrudi K, Carretta A, Wisser W, et al. The value of switching from cyclosporine to tacrolimus in the treatment of refractory acute rejection and obliterative bronchiolitis after lung transplantation. Transpl Int 2002; 15:24–28.

96. Sarahrudi K, Estenne M, Corris P, et al. International experience with conversion from cyclosporine to tacrolimus for acute and chronic allograft rejection. J Thorac Cardiovasc Surg 2004; 127:1126–1132.

97. Zuckermann A, Reichenspurner H, Jaksch P, et al. Long term follow up of a prospective randomised trial comparing tacrolimus versus cyclosporine in combination with MMF after lung transplantation. J Heart Lung Transplant 2003; 22(Suppl):S76–S77.

98. Keenan RJ, Konishi H, Kawai A, et al. Clinical trial of tacrolimus versus cyclosporine in lung transplantation. Ann Thorac Surg 1995; 60:580–585.

99. Kur F, Reichenspurner H, Meiser BM, et al. Tacrolimus (FK506) as primary immunosuppressant after lung transplantation. J Thorac Cardiovasc Surg 1999; 47:174–178.

100. Ross DJ, Jordan SC, Nathan SD, et al. Delayed development of obliterative bronchiolitis syndrome with OKT3 after unilateral lung transplantation. A plea for multicenter immunosuppressive trials. Chest 1996; 109:870–873.

101. Reichenspurner H, Robbins R, Miller J, et al. RATG-induction therapy significantly reduces incidence of acute pulmonary rejection compared to OKT3 treatment. J Heart Lung Transplant 1996; 15:S103.

102. Wiebe K, Harringer W, Wahlers T, et al. ATG induction therapy and the incidence of bronchiolitis obliterans after lung transplantation: does it make a difference? Transplant Proc 1998; 30:1517–1518.

103. Palmer SM, Miralles AP, Lawrence CM, et al. Rabbit antithymocyte globulin decreases acute rejection after lung transplantation. Chest 1999; 116:127–133.

104. Garrity ER, Villanueva J, Bhorade SM, et al. Low rate of acute lung allograft rejection after the use of daclizumab, an interleukin 2 receptor antibody. Transplantation 2001; 71:773–777.

105. Sweet SC, De La Morena MT, Shapiro SD, et al. Interleukin-2-receptor blockade with daclizumab decreases the incidence of acute rejection in pediatric lung transplant recipients. J Heart Lung Transplant 2001; 20:221–222.

106. Brock MV, Borja MC, Ferber L, et al. Induction therapy in lung transplantation: a prospective, controlled clinical trial comparing OKT3, anti-thymocyte globulin and daclizumab. J Heart Lung Transplant 2001; 20:1282–1290.

107. Valantine VG, Robbins RC, Wehner JH, et al. Total lymphoid irradiation for refractory acute rejection in heart–lung and lung allografts. Chest 1996; 109: 1184–1189.

108. Takao M, Higenbottam TW, Audley T, et al. Effects of inhaled nebulized steroids (budesonide) on acute and chronic lung function in heart–lung transplant recipients. Transplant Proc 1995; 27:1284–1285.

109. De Soyza A, Fisher AJ, Small T, et al. Inhaled corticosteroids and the treatment of lymphocytic bronchiolitis following lung transplantation. Am J Respir Crit Care Med 2001; 164:1209–1212.

110. Andreu G, Achkar A, Couetil JP, et al. Extracorporeal photochemotherapy treatment for acute lung rejection episode. J Heart Lung Transplant 1995; 14:793–796.

111. Cahill BC, O'Rourke MK, Strasburg KA, et al. Methotrexate for lung transplant recipients with steroid-resistant acute rejection. J Heart Lung Transplant 1996; 15:1130–1137.

112. Soghikian MV, Valentine VG, Berry GJ, et al. Impact of ganciclovir prophylaxis on heart–lung and lung transplant recipients. J Heart Lung Transplant 1996; 15:881–887.

113. Tikkanen JM, Kallio EA, Bruggeman CA, et al. Prevention of cytomegalovirus infection-enhanced experimental obliterative bronchiolitis by antiviral prophylaxis or immunosuppression in rat tracheal allografts. Am J Respir Crit Care Med 2001; 15:672–679.

114. Ross DJ, Lewis MI, Kramer M, et al. FK 506 rescue immunosuppression for obliterative bronchiolitis after lung transplantation. Chest 1997; 112: 1175–1179.

115. Kesten S, Chaparro C, Scavuzzo M, et al. Tacrolimus as rescue therapy for bronchiolitis obliterans syndrome. J Heart Lung Transplant 1997; 16: 905–912.

116. Reichenspurner H, Meiser BM, Kur F, et al. First experience with FK 506 for treatment of chronic pulmonary rejection. Transplant Proc 1995; 27:2009.

117. Knoop C, Antoine M, Vachiery JL, et al. FK 506 rescue therapy for irreversible airway rejection in heart–lung transplant recipients: report on five cases. Transplant Proc 1994; 26:3240–3241.

118. Wiebe K, Harringer W, Franke U, et al. FK506 rescue therapy in lung transplantation. Transplant Proc 1998; 30:1508–1509.

119. Lipson DA, Palevsky HI, Kotloff RM, et al. Conversion to tacrolimus (FK506) from cyclosporine after orthotopic lung transplantation. Transplant Proc 1998; 30:1505–1507.

120. Revell MP, Lewis ME, Llewellyn-Jones CG, et al. Conservation of small-airway function by tacrolimus/cycosporine conversion in the management of bronchiolitis obliterans following lung transplantation. J Heart Lung Transplant 2000; 19:1219–1223.

121. Whyte RI, Rossi SJ, Mulligan MS, et al. Mycophenolate mofetil for obliterative bronchiolitis syndrome after lung transplantation. Ann Thorac Surg 1997; 64:945–948.

122. Speich R, Boehler A, Thurnheer R, et al. Salvage therapy with mycophenolate mofetil for lung transplant bronchiolitis obliterans: importance of dosage. Transplantation 1997; 15:533–535.

123. Roman A, Bravo C, Monforte V, et al. Preliminary results of rescue therapy with tacrolimus and mycophenolate mofetil in lung transplanted patients with bronchiolitis obliterans. Transplant Proc 2002; 34:146–147.

124. Dupont LJ, Delcroix M, Vanhaecke J, et al. Azathioprine/mycophenolate conversion in the management of bronchiolitis obliterans syndrome (BOS) following (heart)–lung transplantation. J Heart Lung Transplant 2003; 22(Suppl):S123.

125. Whitford H, Walters EH, Levvey B, et al. Addition of inhaled corticosteroids to systemic immunosuppression after lung transplantation: a double-blind, placebo-controlled trial. Transplantation 2002; 73:1793–1797.

126. Whitford H, Orsida B, Kotsimbos T, et al. Bronchoalveolar lavage cellular profiles in lung transplantation: the effect of inhaled corticosteroids. Ann Transplant 2000; 5:31–37.

127. Ward C, De Soyza A, Fisher A, et al. Reticular basement membrane thickening in airways of lung transplant recipients is not affected by inhaled corticosteroids. Clin Exp Allergy 2004; 34:1905–1909.

128. Dusmet M, Maurer J, Winton T, et al. Methotrexate can halt the progression of bronchiolitis obliterans syndrome in lung transplant recipients. J Heart Lung Transplant 1996; 15:948–954.

129. Verleden GM, Buyse B, Delcroix M, et al. Cyclophosphamide rescue therapy for chronic rejection after lung transplantation. J Heart Lung Transplant 1999; 18:1139–1142.

130. Snell GI, Esmore DS, Williams JW. Cytolytic therapy for the bronchiolitis obliterans syndrome complicating lung transplantation. Chest 1996; 109: 874–878.

131. Kesten S, Rajagopalan N, Maurer J. Cytolytic therapy for the treatment of bronchiolitis obliterans syndrome following lung transplantation. Transplantation 1996; 61:427–430.

132. Date H, Lynch JP, Sundaresan S, et al. The impact of cytolytic therapy on bronchiolitis obliterans syndrome. J Heart Lung Transplant 1998; 17:869–875.

133. Iacono AT, Keenan RJ, Duncan SR, et al. Aerosolized cyclosporine in lung recipients with refractory chronic rejection. Am J Respir Crit Care Med 1996; 153:1451–1455.

134. Iacono AT, Capra WB, Shrewsbury B, et al. Long-term follow up of a double-blind, randomized, placebo-controlled trial of cyclosporine inhalation solution (CyIS) in lung transplant recipients. J Heart Lung Transplant 2005; 24(Suppl 2S):S82–S83.

135. Cahill BC, Somerville T, Karwande SW, et al. Early experience with sirolimus in lung transplant recipients with chronic allograft rejection. J Heart Lung Transplant 2003; 22:169–176.

136. Ussetti R, Laporta A, de Pablo A, et al. Rapamycin in lung transplantation: preliminary results. Transplant Proc 2003; 35:1974–1977.

137. Ussetti R, Carreno, MC, de Pablo A, et al. Rapamycin and chronic lung rejection. J Heart Lung Transplant 2004; 23:917–918.

138. Verleden GM, Dupont LJ, Vanhaecke J, et al. Effect of azithromycin on bronchiectasis and pulmonary function in a heart lung transplant patient with severe chronic allograft dysfunction. J Heart Lung Transplant 2005; 24(8):1155–1158.

139. Ward C, Camara M, Forrest I, et al. Preliminary findings of quorum signal molecules in clinically stable lung allograft recipients. Thorax 2003; 58: 444–446.

140. Basyigit I, Yildiz F, Yildirim E, et al. The effect of clarithromycin on inflammatory markers in chronic obstructive pulmonary disease: preliminary data. Ann Pharmacother 2004; 38:1400–1405.

141. Verleden GM, Dupont LJ, Vanaudenaerde BM, et al. Azithromycin reduces airway neutrophilia in patients with bronchiolitis obliterans syndrome. J Heart Lung Transplant 2005; 24(Suppl 2S):S59.

142. Chacon RA, Corris PA, Dark JH, et al. Tests of airway function in detecting and monitoring treatment of obliterative bronchiolitis after lung transplantation. J Heart Lung Transplant 2000; 19:263–269.

143. Melville A, Wardle J, Parry G, et al. Comparison of total lymphoid irradiation (TLI) versus tacrolimus for the treatment of obliterative bronchiolitis (OB) in lung transplants. J Heart Lung Transplant 2001; 20(Suppl):S208.

144. Fisher AJ, Rutherford RM, Bozzino J, et al. The safety and efficacy of total lymphoid irradiation in progressive bronchiolitis obliterans syndrome after lung transplantation. Am J Transplant 2005; 5:537–543.

145. Slovis BS, Loyd JE, King LE Jr. Photophoresis for chronic rejection of lung allografts. N Engl J Med 1995; 332:962.

146. Salerno CT, Park SJ, Kreykes NS, et al. Adjuvant treatment of refractory lung transplant rejection with extracorporeal photopheresis. J Thorac Cardiovasc Surg 1999; 117:1063–1069.

147. Villanueva J, Bhorade SM, Robinson JA, et al. Extracorporeal photopheresis for the treatment of lung allograft rejection. Ann Transplant 2000; 5:44–47.

148. O'Hagan AR, Stillwell PC, Arroliga A, et al. Photopheresis in the treatment of refractory bronchiolitis obliterans complicating lung transplantation. Chest 1999; 115:1459–1462.

149. Shennib H, Novick R, Mulder D, et al. Is lung retransplantation indicated? Report on four cases. Eur Respir J 1993; 6:354–357.

150. Kotloff RM. Lung retransplantation. All for one or one for all? Chest 2003; 123:1781–1782.

151. Novick R, Stitt LW, Al-Kattan K, et al. Pulmonary retransplantation: predictors of graft function and survival in 230 patients. Ann Thorac Surg 1998; 65:227–234.

152. Brugière O, Thabut G, Castier Y, et al. Lung retransplantation for bronchiolitis obliterans syndrome. Chest 2003; 123:1832–1837.

153. Schäfers HJ, Hausen B, Walters T, et al. Retranspantation of the lung. A single center experience. Eur J Cardiothorac Surg 1995; 9:291–295.

154. Huddleston CB, Mendeloff EN, Cohen AH, et al. Lung retransplantation in children. Ann Thorac Surg 1998; 66:199–204.

155. Novick RJ, Stitt L. Pulmonary retransplantation. Semin Thorac Cardiovasc Surg 1998; 10:227–236.

# 32

# The Role for Alloimmune and Nonalloimmune Injury and Cytokine Responses in the Pathogenesis of Bronchiolitis Obliterans Syndrome

**Robert Aris**

*Division of Pulmonary and Critical Care Medicine and Cystic Fibrosis/Pulmonary Research and Treatment Center, University of North Carolina at Chapel Hill, Chapel Hill, North Carolina, U.S.A.*

**John A. Belperio**

*Division of Pulmonary and Critical Care Medicine, Department of Medicine, David Geffen School of Medicine at UCLA, Los Angeles, California, U.S.A.*

**Scott M. Palmer**

*Division of Pulmonary and Critical Care Medicine, Department of Medicine, Duke University Medical Center, Durham, North Carolina, U.S.A.*

## INTRODUCTION

Lung transplantation is now an effective therapeutic option for patients with many different end-stage pulmonary disorders (1,2). Although short-term survival has improved significantly since the first successful lung transplant operations, long-term outcomes remain disappointing, with five-year survival rates of only 42%, as compared to >70% for other solid organ transplantations at five years (1,2). Most late deaths are due directly or indirectly to the development of bronchiolitis obliterans syndrome (BOS), generally thought to be a manifestation of chronic lung allograft rejection (1–6). Lung transplantation is characterized by unusually high rates of allograft rejection, likely in part due to the intense recipient alloimmune and nonalloimmune responses generated to the transplanted donor lung tissue. In this chapter we focus on the two critical factors driving alloimmune [donor human leukocyte antigen (HLA)] and nonalloimmune (recipient gastroesophageal reflux) responses and highlight mechanisms by which these factors drive the production of cytokines that ultimately lead to the development of BOS.

Rejection is a recipient (host) response to a foreign antigen (i.e., the newly transplanted donor lung allograft). Allograft major histocompatibility complex (MHC)/HLA is a surface antigen that is recognized by the recipient's immune system as foreign, allowing for T cell activation by costimulatory molecules, which stimulates an intense cytokine (cytokines, growth factors, and chemokines) mediated inflammatory/immune response. This is further escalated early on by a reverse response, in which the allograft immune system reacts against the recipient, intensifying this inflammatory/immune cascade. Moreover, nonimmune lung injury such as gastroesophageal reflux disease (GERD) can perpetuate this inflammatory cascade and contribute to the fibro-obliteration of the allograft airway known as obliterative bronchiolitis (OB), the histopathological correlate of BOS (1–6). Histopathologic features of OB begin with a peribronchiolar leukocyte infiltration that invades/disrupts the basement membrane, submucosa, and lumenal epithelium (3,4). This is followed by fibroproliferation with increased numbers of mesenchymal cells, extracellular matrix deposition (ECM), and granulation tissue formation within/around the lumen of the allograft airway (3,4). Ultimately, smooth muscle cells, myofibroblasts, and mature collagen obliterate the airway (3,4). HLA mismatching leads to allospecific recognition, allowing for leukocyte activation and cytokine expression while nonimmune injury (i.e., GERD) can perpetuate the production of cytokines, all of which are thought to have specific roles during the pathogenesis of BOS.

## THE ROLE OF HLA MISMATCHES IN THE PATHOGENESIS OF BOS

Systematic HLA antigen matching of donors and recipients unequivocally improves outcomes after hematopoeitic cell, kidney, and heart transplantation. Several smaller studies and a more recent, larger study have noted an association between HLA mismatching and lung graft (7,8) and patient survival (9,10). In addition, several studies have found associations between the number of HLA mismatches and acute (11–13) and chronic rejection (or BOS) (11,14,15). However, the association between HLA mismatches and BOS has been controversial, because more studies have found no association than those that have found one (9,16,17). As a result, the most recent consensus from the International Society of Heart and Lung Transplantation (ISHLT) does not recognize HLA-mismatching as an established risk factor for BOS and the lung allocation algorithm does not endeavor to match HLA proteins (18).

The conflicting results on the role of HLA mismatches in the development of BOS are predominantly due to the small sample sizes and methodologic differences among studies. First, the influence of HLA molecules and/or HLA peptides on inducing an alloimmune response is likely not uniform across different HLA antigens or among different organ grafts. That is to say, every mismatch may not be immunologically equal, making it harder to determine the influence of mismatching in small data sets. Second, many previous analyses have used a bivariate analysis (i.e., present or absent) of the BOS outcome measure. Thus, the patients with BOS were viewed as being homogenous irrespective of the time of onset, severity (or stage), or progression of BOS. For example, a patient may be BOS stage 0 at four months posttransplant and yet the same patient may be at BOS stage 3 at two years posttransplant. Thus, the length of follow-up in such a case would affect the analysis of any predictor of BOS. Last, other studies failed to account for effects of other known predictors of BOS, including, but not limited to, acute rejection and cytomegalovirus (CMV) infection.

In a recent study, Chalermskulrat el al. hypothesized that immune responses are involved in the development of BOS and that mismatched donor HLA alloantigens provide the immunologic stimulus that increases the likelihood and, more importantly, the severity of BOS (19). They studied the associations between other pre- and posttransplant risk factors (recipient age, donor age, CMV mismatch, cold ischemic time, use of cardiopulmonary bypass, ventilatory days, episodes of acute rejection and CMV pneumonitis, mean trough cyclosporine A level, episodes of subtherapeutic cyclosporine A levels, and histopathology of OB and diffuse alveolar damage) and the severity of BOS at a single time point (namely four years posttransplant). In addition, they excluded recipients whose graft function deteriorated or who died due to causes other than BOS before four years to minimize the influence of the "no outcome" patients. The independent risk factors for the severity of BOS as determined in univariate analyses were then integrated into two proportional odds models, one that included pre- and posttransplant variables and another that included only pretransplant variables.

In univariate analyses, the number of combined HLA-A and B mismatches was strongly associated with the BOS stage at four years ($P = 0.002$). This association remained significant after inclusion of other potential risk factors for BOS in multiple linear regression models. Pretransplant and posttransplant proportional odds models confirmed that the increasing number of combined HLA-A and B mismatches increased the overall severity of BOS [adjusted odds ratio (AOR) = 1.84, $P = 0.035$ and

AOR = 1.69, $P = 0.067$, respectively]. A trend toward significance was seen with HLA-DR mismatching as well. The results of this study demonstrate that the degree of HLA class I loci mismatching independently predicted the severity of BOS at four years (or three years, confirmed by separate analyses) after lung transplantation after controlling for other pre- and/or posttransplant variables that were either known or believed to predict BOS. Although other studies have reported that HLA-A mismatches predicted the occurrence of BOS using a posttransplant model, this analysis showed, for the first time, that prior to the time of transplant, one can objectively, albeit imperfectly, predict the severity of posttransplant BOS on the basis of donor–recipient HLA incompatibility. As a simple example, one HLA-A or B mismatch between recipient and donor will create a 1.84 times higher chance of the recipient experiencing a higher stage of BOS after lung transplant than recipients with no mismatches. This finding, if authenticated, may yield an important strategy (i.e., donor–recipient HLA matching) to mitigate the influence of BOS on the premature demise of lung transplant recipients.

This study, like many before it reviewed by Estenne et al. (18), found that acute rejection was an important clinical risk factor for BOS. As acute rejection has been shown to be associated with HLA mismatches in multiple studies (9,13), HLA mismatches and acute rejection are probably not truly independent predictors. Yet, in the posttransplant multivariate analysis discussed above, adjusting for the occurrence of acute rejection did not fundamentally negate the relationship between HLA mismatches and BOS stage.

After acute rejection, few other clinical variables have stood the test of time in predicting BOS. In some studies, CMV pneumonitis, low cyclosporine levels, ischemia–reperfusion injury, including ventilator days, histologic evidence of diffuse alveolar damage, and the use of cardiopulmonary bypass have predicted BOS, but most of these predictor variables could not be confirmed in subsequent studies. While it is quite likely that the innate and adaptive immune systems interface in the pathogenesis of BOS, it has been difficult to confirm that any of the innate events that occur clinically, as mentioned earlier, are directly linked to BOS. It seems plausible that the magnitude of the effect of innate events and the variability with which the innate effects influence the adaptive responses confound the analysis of these interactions in clinical research in the area of BOS causality.

The association between HLA mismatches and BOS is supported by a number of observations in clinical, animal model, and in vitro studies. First, several previous studies have shown that mismatches at the HLA class I loci were associated with BOS (13,14). In other clinical studies, associations have been described between BOS and serum anti-HLA alloantibodies directed against donor-mismatched class I or class II peptides, with the former being more common (11,14,20–22). In fact, the presence of anti-HLA antibodies, detected by any of a variety of different methods, can be found in the serum months before measures of airflow decrease and the patient is diagnosed with BOS. Nonetheless, not all patients who develop antibodies against HLA epitopes develop BOS in the studies reported to date, suggesting that factors in addition to humoral responses are involved in the pathogenesis of BOS. Other clinical studies using in vitro techniques have demonstrated that indirect allorecognition of HLA class I or class II peptides were associated with BOS (20,23). While alloantibodies can be demonstrated in vivo in patients with BOS, their precise function is not clear and is under investigation. In addition, the cell or tissue target of these alloantibodies is not known and it is not clear if they engage airway antigens, fix complement, or induce antibody-dependent cellular toxicity.

In vitro studies of human airway epithelial cells have also indicated that antibodies directed against either HLA class I or non-HLA epitopes leads to the activation of signal transduction (inducing intracellular $Ca^{2+}$ influx as well as tyrosine phosphorylation of several proteins), proliferation, and transcription and secretion of profibrotic factors [transforming growth factor beta (TGF-$\beta$), platelet-derived growth factor (PDGF), heparin binding epidermal growth factor, fibroblast growth factor, and insulin-like growth factor 1 (IGF-1)] (24–26). In some airway epithelial cells, alloantibodies ultimately caused apoptosis, but in other cases the cellular activation caused the proliferation of lung fibroblasts in vitro (24–26). These findings indicate that anti-HLA antibodies may play an important role in the pathogenesis of BOS including their ability to both activate and injure airway epithelial cells. These studies add credence to the correlation of HLA mismatching and BOS in the clinical studies described earlier.

Animal models have given us an enormous amount of information about the pathogenesis of BOS and have confirmed and extended the findings of the clinical studies on the differential role of HLA antigens in BOS. Kelly and colleagues demonstrated that mice mismatched at a single MHC class I locus were more likely to reject tracheal allografts than mice mismatched at a single MHC class II locus (27). Smith and colleagues reported that a single HLA (A2) protein when introduced into mice by transgenics would lead to efficient rejection of tracheal allografts and that anti-HLA-A2 antibodies could be detected weeks before the development of OB in this model (28), reproducing the findings of the clinical studies cited earlier.

Chalermskulrat et al. demonstrated that MHC class I proteins were more important alloantigens than class II using genetically deficient donor mice and the heterotopic tracheal transplant model (29). The class I deficient donors survived approximately one to two weeks longer than wild-type and class II deficient grafts. Nonetheless, the MHC I deficient and doubly deficient (MHCI/II) grafts were rejected at later time points, indicating the hierarchical importance of these foreign proteins and the potential importance of minor antigens. Richards et al. also confirmed that MHC class I proteins were important regulators of allograft rejection using the novel model of adoptively transferring l(d)-specific TCR-Tg 2C CD8(+) T cells into C57BL6 mice engrafted with BALB/C tracheas (30). This notion of a hierarchical order for alloantigens received further support from the work of Richards et al. (31) and Higuchi et al. (32) who demonstrated that a minor antigen mismatched tracheal allograft would be rejected but with much slower kinetics than MHC mismatched grafts (10,31,32).

The current standard of practice is for donor lungs and heart–lung blocks to be allocated to recipients without consideration of HLA mismatching. Because of its high polymorphicity, the likelihood that HLA loci will be well matched between donor and recipient by chance alone is extremely small, as only 4.6% of the recipients in the ISHLT registry had two or fewer HLA mismatches (9). It is likely, however, that better HLA matches will be achieved by chance alone in countries and areas that have less ethnic (genetic) diversity. The United States, possibly the most ethnically diverse country in the world, contributes the largest number of cases to the ISHLT registry and is probably largely responsible for the low number of matches in the lung database. In light of the acceptance of increasingly longer cold ischemic times for most lung grafts (with the possible exception of marginal donors) (16), the ability to perform HLA matching may become a viable approach and have a considerable impact on lung transplant outcomes once the HLA typing technology is more advanced. Nonetheless, it must be remembered that morbidity and mortality due to causes other than lung rejection are likely to "dilute" the final impact of HLA matching on patient and graft survival.

## THE ROLE OF GASTROESOPHAGEAL REFLUX IN THE PATHOGENESIS OF BOS

Although alloantigenic processes have been clearly implicated in the development of acute rejection and BOS (as outlined in the previous section), intensification or alternation of immunosuppressive regimens has had little impact on the progression of BO/BOS (33,34). Furthermore, several nonalloimmune stimuli have been linked with the development of BOS, including respiratory viral infection, prolonged donor graft ischemia, early post-transplant primary graft failure, type of transplant operation (with an earlier onset of BOS in single-lung transplant recipients), and gastroesophageal reflux (35). Nonalloimmune injury could directly damage the allograft, leading to chronic scarring and dysfunction, or could activate or augment adaptive responses, thus leading to more traditional rejection responses in OB. In either case, BOS might best be viewed as a heterogenous condition of chronic graft dysfunction with certain final common cytokines (as described in the next section).

Among the nonalloimmune stimuli implicated in the development of BOS, perhaps the notion that GERD contributes to chronic graft dysfunction is most intriguing. Increasing evidence has suggested that gastroesophageal reflux may contribute to bronchoconstriction in asthma (36). Further, increased prevalence of reflux is observed in several lung diseases such as cystic fibrosis and idiopathic pulmonary fibrosis (37,38). GERD has been associated with the development of chronic bronchial disease in patients with neurological impairments leading to recurrent aspiration (39). Furthermore, the impaired cough and mucociliary clearance observed after lung transplant might render recipients particularly vulnerable to the adverse effects of acid aspiration and reflux (40).

Gastrointestinal complications have been recognized for some time to occur after lung transplantation. Lubetkin and colleagues reported a 51% prevalence of gastrointestinal complications, including reflux, colitis, and ulceration, in a cohort of lung transplant patients they followed for three years (41). Other investigators have demonstrated that delayed gastric emptying is also common. Reid and colleagues were the first to suggest an association between OB and chronic aspiration (42). In a series of 11 heart–lung transplant patients, antireflux therapy, the specifics of which were not defined, resulted in improvement in pulmonary function. Similarly, an early report suggested that two forms of BOS exist after lung or heart–lung transplant (43). In a small autopsy series of heart–lung transplant recipients, four of seven patients had early onset BOS of a more focal and cellular nature. Interestingly, those patients all had evidence of aspiration with foreign material upon examination of the lungs at autopsy. Unfortunately, the potential significance of these early findings was not appreciated and few further investigations were pursued into the potential relationship between GERD and BOS until our recent work.

We have pursued the hypothesis that gastroesophageal reflux contributes to the development of posttransplant lung injury and BOS. Our work has developed along the following lines. First, we have demonstrated that lung transplantation exacerbates gastroesophageal reflux. In a prospective study of patients undergoing objective 24-hour pH studies, Young found that acid contact time significantly increased after transplantation (44). Second, we have found abnormal acid contact times in over 70% of post-transplant recipients in studies involving over 200 lung transplant patients (44–46). Third, we noted an association between the presence and severity of post-transplant gastroesophageal reflux and the development of BOS and severity of lung allograft dysfunction (45). Fourth, we have recently demonstrated that fundoplication is safe and well tolerated in a large series of lung transplant recipients (47). Fifth, we have shown that on average, lung allograft function improves in patients after fundoplication. In 43 stable lung transplant patients who underwent fundoplication, the average pre-antireflux surgery forced expiratory volume in one second ($FEV_1$) was 1.87 L and when re-evaluated at least six months after antireflux surgery, the $FEV_1$ had increased to 2.19 L, representing an increase of 24.1% (46). Of the patients undergoing fundoplication, 26 patients (60%) had met the criteria for BOS at the time of their antireflux operation. Of these, 13 patients met the criteria for BOS 1 (50%), seven for BOS 2 (27%), and six for BOS 3 (23%). Ten of the 13 patients (77%) with BOS 1 improved their $FEV_1$ enough so that they no longer met the criteria for BOS after fundoplication, 43% of patients with BOS 2 improved their $FEV_1$ enough so that they no longer met the criteria for BOS, while another 28% improved to BOS 1. Only 17% of BOS 3 patients at the time of fundoplication showed improvement in their BOS score. Although retrospective and subject to a number of potential biases, these data imply that early BOS could be related to GERD and that lung function is improved by fundoplication in patients with GERD. Finally, we have demonstrated that early fundoplication prior to the onset of BOS appears to delay the development of this condition as compared to matched controls (48).

Given the dismal outcomes and lack of effective therapies for lung transplant recipients with BOS, further studies of the mechanisms by which GERD might contribute to BOS are sorely needed. We believe that aspiration of gastric material is common among all posttransplant lung recipients and drives the development of lung inflammation. Surgical fundoplication provides a mechanical barrier that prevents aspiration from occurring and reduces inflammatory stimuli in the lung. In support of this hypothesis, the Toronto transplant group has recently developed an assay to measure bile acids in the bronchoalveolar lavages and demonstrated a striking correlation between the detection of bile acids in the lung, airway neutrophilia, and the early onset of posttransplant BOS in a series of 85 lung recipients (Dr. S. Keshavjee, personal communication). The presence of bile acids in the lung presumably occurs as a result of gastroesophageal reflux and provides a potential mechanistic link between the elevated acid contact times and the development of BOS observed in our transplant population. While results in this area are intriguing, much more clinical and basic research is needed to definitively link GERD to the development of BOS.

## THE ROLE OF CYTOKINES DURING THE PATHOGENESIS OF BOS

Critical to airway wound repair is a delicate balance between pro- and anti-inflammatory cytokines. Changes in this balance can influence airway tissue remodeling. The specific mechanisms that lead to the eventual fibro-obliteration of allograft airways may involve the interactions between type 1 and 2 cells/cytokines. Naive cells (i.e., CD4+ T cells and mononuclear phagocytes) can differentiate into at least two distinct cell subsets (type 1 or 2 cells), which have distinct cytokine profiles/functions. Type 1 cells/cytokines are mainly involved in cell mediated immunity, whereas type 2 cells/cytokines are associated with humoral immunity. The nature of the antigen and the pattern of cytokines released into the microenvironment are the most important factors dictating whether the inflammatory response is directed toward a type 1 [i.e., IL-1, tumor necrosis factor alpha (TNF-α), IL-12, IL-23, and interferon gamma (IFN-γ)] or type 2 (IL-10, TGF-β, IL-4, IL-5, and IL-6) response. In addition, type 1 and 2 cells can cross regulate each other through their respective cytokines (Fig. 1) (49,50). While type 1 cytokines are considered the predominate regulators of rejection by promoting cytotoxic T cell responses and delayed type hypersensitivity, simply driving an allogeneic response toward a type 2 cytokine cascade may not be as beneficial as initially thought. In fact, induction of long-term tolerance to an allograft may depend on the inhibition of both type 1 and type 2 inflammatory responses (51).

## THE ROLE OF THE IL-1 CYTOKINE FAMILY DURING THE PATHOGENESIS OF BOS

The IL-1 family consists of two agonists (IL-1α and IL-1β), two receptors (biologically active IL-1RI and inert IL-1RII), and a specific naturally occurring receptor antagonist (IL-1Ra) with a proven ability to attenuate IL-1 activity (52). IL-1Ra and IL-1 are known to have near-equal affinity for the IL-1 receptor (IL-1RI) (53,54). Excess IL-1Ra can enhance a local profibrotic environment through the inhibition of the normal "fibrolytic activity" mediated by IL-1. For instance, the inhibition of IL-1 by IL-1Ra has been shown to cause a reduction in the production of $PGE_2$, nitric oxide, and metalloproteinase (MMP), resulting in the promotion of excess deposition of ECM (55,56). With regard to lung transplantation, elevated levels of IL-1Ra in human bronchoalveolar lavage fluid (BALF) were found to be associated with BOS (57). Similar results were found in human BALF just prior to the development of BOS (i.e., future-BOS) (57). Importantly, the elevated levels of IL-1Ra were not accompanied by significant elevations in IL-1β. Thus, the elevated ratio of IL-1Ra to IL-1β in both lung transplantation recipients with BOS and those with future-BOS is consistent with a persistent alteration in IL-1 activity in the allograft airways producing a persistent profibrotic environment. Moreover, in cardiac transplantation recipients, an intronic variable number of tandem repeats (VNTR) polymorphism (IL1RN) of the gene encoding IL-1Ra, which is suspected to be associated with increased expression of IL-1Ra with or without decreased IL-1 levels, has been shown to be an important risk factor for the development of chronic cardiac rejection (58,59). These findings support a contention that inhibition of IL-1 biology may impair the ability of the allograft airway to repair/remodel, leading to the development of BOS.

## THE ROLE OF TNF-α DURING THE PATHOGENESIS OF BOS

TNF-α is a proximal proinflammatory cytokine with numerous effects on multiple inflammatory and immunologic responses, including enhanced

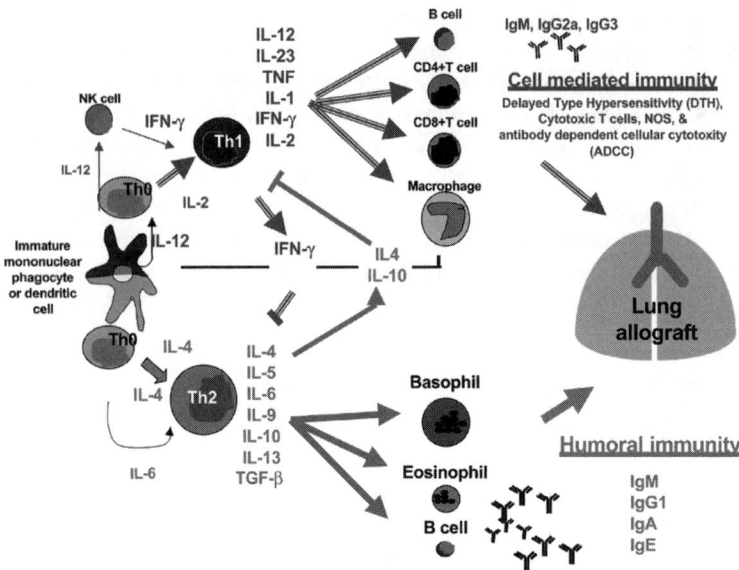

**Figure 1** Development of a type 1 and a type 2 immune response. Immature mononuclear phagocytes and dendritic cells present alloantigen to the T helper cells (Th0 cells) allowing for polarization (type 1 vs. 2) of T cells and mononuclear phagocytes depending on the cytokine microenvironment produced by the alloantigen and donor/recipient genetic factors. Type 1 differentiation is developed by an IL-12–rich microenvironment predominantly produced by mononuclear phagocytes and dendritic cells. The type 1 cells produce IL-2, IL-23, IFN-γ, lymphotoxin, IL-1, and TNF-α, promoting the development of cytotoxic T cells, delayed-type hypersensitivity reaction, and facilitating antibody-dependent cellular cytotoxicity (i.e., the effector mechanisms against the lung allograft). Type 2 differentiation is produced by an IL-4–rich microenvironment polarizing T cells and mononuclear phagocytes toward a type 2 cell that produces IL-3, IL-4, IL-5, IL-6, IL-9, IL-10, and IL-13, affecting immunoglobulin isotypes and stimulating IgE and IgG1 production by B cells and eosinophils and ultimately creating a profibrotic allograft airway microenvironment. Type 1 cells secreting IFN-γ can inhibit differentiation of type 2 cells, and type 2 cells secreting IL-4 and IL-10 can inhibit differentiation of type 1 cells. Both the type 1 and type 2 responses are likely to be involved in the pathogenesis of BOS. *Abbreviations*: IL, interleukin; IFN, interferon; TNF, tumor necrosis factor; BOS, bronchiolitis obliterans syndrome.

cytolytic activity of natural killer (NK) cells, upregulation of MHC Class II antigen and IL-2 receptors, and induction of T-cell proliferation (60,61). In addition, TNF-α has been shown to play a key role in the fibroplasia of pulmonary and hepatic fibrosis (62,63). All of these biological functions are relevant to chronic rejection, yet TNF-α levels in BALF from patients with BOS were not found to be significantly elevated, suggesting no significant role for endogenous TNF-α during BOS (57). Similarly, results were found in patients with chronic liver and renal rejection (64,65). In contrast, a study involving 2298 first and 1901 repeat cadaver kidney transplant recipients demonstrated that the TNF-α single-nucleotide polymorphism homozygous for the high TNF-α producer (genotype-308) was associated with decreased kidney survival (66). However, this effect was only found in retransplants and not in primary grafts. This suggests that recipients with TNF-α high responsiveness may require preimmunization/immune priming by rejection of a previous graft in order to exert a true detrimental effect (66). Others have demonstrated in an animal model of BOS that increased expression of TNF-α was associated with tracheal fibro-obliteration (67). Moreover, when TNFR:Fc, an inhibitor of TNF-α, or neutralizing antibodies to TNF-α were administered to recipients of allografts, there was significant attenuation of BOS, suggesting TNF-α may indeed play a role in the pathogenesis of BOS (28,67). Future human and animal studies will be required to determine the exact role of TNF-α during the pathogenesis of BOS.

## THE ROLE OF IL-12 DURING THE PATHOGENESIS OF BOS

IL-12 exists as a p70 heterodimer consisting of p35 and p40 subunits (68,69). These subunits individually interact with distinct components of the IL-12R (70,71). IL-12 is a pivotal cytokine for the promotion of cell mediated (type 1) immune response and has been shown to induce IFN-γ during an allogeneic response (72–84). However, its exact role during allograft rejection remains controversial. In a type 1 immune mediated model of graft versus host disease (GVHD), neutralizing IL-12 or using p40−/−mice (cells from BALB/c p40−/− donors transferred into C57BL/6 p40−/− recipients) was associated with recipient cells having enhanced IL-5 and IL-10, and reduced IFN-γ production (driving a type 1→type 2 response) and attenuated acute GVHD (85–87). Conversely, administration of IL-12 in this model exacerbated acute GVHD and was able to convert a chronic (type 2) GVHD to an acute (type 1) GVHD (77,88). Alternatively, neutralization of IL-12 (either with polyclonal antibodies to IL12 or by IL-12 receptor blockade using a p40 homdimer) in a murine model of cardiac transplantation led to an increased intragraft expression of IL-4 and IL-10 (type 2 response) and accelerated rejection (89). Moreover, the administration of IL-12 in this same model system markedly increased IFN-γ levels without augmentation of the rejection response (72,73,83,84). These studies suggest that high levels of IL-12 can induce superphysiologic levels of IFN-γ, leading an inhibition of the immune response as a result of IFN-γ antiproliferative effects on emerging Th2 cells (IFN-γ receptors are expressed only on Th2 cells) (90,91). Interestingly, a novel heterodimer cytokine IL-23, which is composed of the same p40 subunit of IL-12, but a different p19 subunit, has activity on memory T cells and mononuclear phagocyte function (91–94). Recent studies of autoimmune inflammation demonstrate that IL-23 acts more broadly than IL-12 as an end-stage–effector cytokine through direct action on mononuclear cells (95). To date, there are no know studies that have analyzed IL-23 during BOS, indicating a future need to study this cytokine in the context of lung rejection.

## THE ROLE OF IFN-γ IN THE PATHOGENESIS OF BOS

IFN-γ is a type 1 pleiotropic cytokine that can be induced by IL-12 and inhibited by IL-10 (96–98). With regard to transplantation, IFN-γ can induce classes I and II expression and inhibit T cell proliferation (99–102). In human studies, elevated expression of IFN-γ from BALF was associated with acute and refractory lung allograft rejection, both risk factors for the development of BOS (103,104). In addition, a significant correlation was detected between the presence of a high-expressing human polymorphism at position +874 of the *IFN-γ* gene and BOS (105). Furthermore, in a rat heterotopic tracheal transplantation model of BOS, IFN-γ was found to be persistently elevated during fibro-obliterative events (106). However, other animal models of acute and chronic rejection have demonstrated a few unanticipated results with regard to IFN-γ and rejection. Using an immunosuppressed, murine cardiac transplantation model, IFN-γ−/− recipients demonstrated decreased graft integrin and MHC class II expression, yet accelerated acute parenchymal rejection (107–109). Interestingly, these allografts demonstrated decreased chronic transplantation coronary artery rejection (i.e., graft arterial/vascular disease, which involves intimal lesions containing smooth muscle cells, leukocytes, and ECM deposition) (107–109). Collectively, these studies suggest a role for IFN-γ, in part, limiting acute allograft rejection, due to its antiproliferative effects on T cells and its ability to downregulate the cytotoxic T-lymphocyte (CTL) lytic activity against allogeneic targets. In contrast, IFN-γ secretion by activated infiltrating cells may, in part, worsen chronic rejection by upregulating integrin and MHC class II on the surface of allograft endothelial cells, culminating in the accumulation of activated macrophages secreting profibrotic mediators.

## THE ROLE OF IL-10 DURING THE PATHOGENESIS OF BOS

IL-10 is a pleiotropic type 2 cytokine with immunomodulatory bioactivity including the inhibition of cytotoxicity, MHC class II antigens, and proinflammatory cytokine production (98,110–123). The role of IL-10 in modulating the response to allograft rejection has been controversial. Elevated expression of IL-10 in allografts undergoing rejection and tolerance suggests IL-10 can promote or inhibit alloimmune destruction (124–126). Animal experiments have demonstrated that in vivo IL-10 administration or overexpression accelerated or had no effect on graft failure in islet cell allografts (127,128). Similarly, systemic administration of superphysiologic doses of IL-10 was found to exacerbate murine cardiac allograft rejection while immunosupressed IL-10$-/-$ mice rejected cardiac allografts twice as rapidly as controls (108,129). In addition, the polymorphism in the *IL-10* gene promoter (position $-1082$) (high–IL-10 producers) were associated with acute renal allograft rejection (130). In contrast, the administration of IL-10 at physiologic doses or by liposome-mediated ex-vivo intracoronary *IL-10* gene transfer in animal models of cardiac rejection prolonged survival by attenuating intragraft mononuclear cell recruitment and increasing cytotoxic T cell apoptosis secondary to the Fas/FasL pathway (131,132). Furthermore, either retro- or adenoviral vector delivery of viral IL-10 (vIL-10), not cellular IL-10 (cIL-10), caused prolonged cardiac allograft survival through similar mechanisms (133,134). Moreover, a polymorphism causing high IL-10 production has been shown to be protective in heart and kidney transplantation and associated with the tolerant state in pediatric liver transplantation recipients not receiving immunosuppression therapy (135–139).

With regard to human lung transplantation recipients, the increased IL-10 production genotype (GCC/GCC) protected recipients against acute persistent rejection (a major risk factor for the development of BOS) when compared with the intermediate or decreased IL-10 production genotypes (140). In contrast, IL-10 levels in BALF from patients with BOS did not demonstrate differences when compared with non-BOS controls (57). However, neutralization of IL-10 in a rat heterotopic tracheal transplantation model accelerated airway obliteration, whereas the administration of physiologic doses of IL-10 or local Sedai virus (SeV)–mediated *IL-10* gene transfer targeted to the airway or autologous hematopoetic progenitostem cell–enriched mouse bone marrow transduced with retrovirus encoding vIL-10 attenuated airway fibroplasia (141–144).

The discrepancy in the effect of IL-10 may be related to dose (physiologic vs. superphysiologic), type (vIL-10 vs. cIL-10), timing of the dose, and compartment (systemic or local administration) at which IL-10 is delivered. The effects of systemic IL-10 appear to depend on dosing and timing (i.e., superphysiologic doses augment rejection and physiologic doses given at the right time attenuate rejection) and suggest superphysiologic doses of IL-10 may reflect desensitization of IL-10 biology by unabated proinflammatory effects. With regard to vIL-10 versus cIL-10, vIL-10 does not possess the T cell costimulation activities of cIL-10 and vIL-10 has a 100-fold lower affinity than cIL-10 for binding to the IL-10 receptor (129,133,134,145). Therefore, when vIL-10 or cIL-10 are delivered in equivalent concentrations they will not have the same biological effects (129,133). Last, direct transfer of IL-10 into the transplanted organ may precede local intragraft levels of

IL-10 from systemic administration, making the timing of the administration of IL-10 another variable to be considered (146). Hence, the efficacy of IL-10 manipulation coupled with differences in the type of IL-10 and transplantation microenvironment may explain the inconsistent effects seen in graft survival to date (146). Further investigations of timing, dose, and type of IL-10 in animal models may clarify these controversies.

## THE ROLE OF IL-6 DURING THE PATHOGENESIS OF BOS

IL-6 is a cytokine with both proinflammatory and anti-inflammatory properties and has been associated with a type 2 profile and fibrogenesis (147–151). With respect to an allogeneic response, in vitro studies have demonstrated that allogeneic CD2+ lymphocytes are capable of activating airway-derived epithelial cells to produce high levels of IL-6, possibly promoting airway fibrosis (152). Alternatively, other studies have suggested that IL-6 plays a significant role at different stages of the inflammatory process during the pathogenesis of BOS (153). For instance, in a rat lung transplantation model, IL-6 had a bimodal distribution with early expression during ischemia–reperfusion and then later at maximal rejection (154). In addition, a prospective cohort study of human BALF, analyzed within two months post–lung transplantation, demonstrated that increased levels of IL-6 were predictive of the development of BOS (155). Furthermore, ex vivo data demonstrated that the alveolar macrophages (AM) during acute rejection secrete high levels of IL-6 while TGF-β1 secretion remained normal. Subsequently, at the time of BOS onset, AM production of IL-6 was normal and TGF-β1 production increased. This suggests IL-6 activity is involved in the development of BOS, perhaps by priming resident AM to upregulate their production of the profibrotic cytokine TGF-β. Last, the presence of high-expression polymorphism IL-6 at position −174 significantly increased the risk for the development of BOS, underscoring its possible role during the pathogenesis of BOS (105).

## THE ROLE OF TGF-β DURING THE PATHOGENESIS OF BOS

While TGF-β has a strong history of immunosuppressive activity, it is the most potent inducer of collagen synthesis, fibroblast proliferation, and fibroblast chemotaxis (156,157). Studies involving solid organ transplantation have demonstrated that TGF-β has beneficial effects on acute allograft rejection (158,159). Overexpression of the TGF-β transgene led to a reduction in acute rejection and prolonged graft survival in experimental heart and lung transplantation (158,159). In addition, elevated serum levels of TGF-β have been associated with tolerance induction in an experimental model of lung transplantation. Importantly, the animals' alloimmune responses were restored with the administration of neutralizing antibodies to TGF-β (160). Alternatively, TGF-β has been implicated during the pathogenesis of chronic rejection involving liver, kidney, and heart transplantation (161–163). Similar studies involving lung transplantation have shown augmented expression of TGF-β to be an early marker of BOS and directly correlate with the severity of luminal fibrosis (164–166). In contrast, other studies have demonstrated no difference in BALF protein levels or cellular expression of TGF-β between BOS and non-BOS groups (57,164). However, animal studies have found TGF-β to be localized to infiltrating mononuclear cells and fibrotic tissue in a rodent model of BOS (167). The administration of adenoviral mediated soluble TGF-βIIIR, a functional TGF-β antagonist, topically on day five posttransplantation attenuated rodent BOS (167). However, if soluble TGF-βIIIR was given on day 0 or 10, or intramuscularly posttransplantation, no significant effect on BOS was distinguished (167). These studies demonstrate that compartmentalization and timing of TGF-β augmentation may be important factors with regard to its fibro-obliterative effects during BOS.

Smad3 is a member of the highly conserved Smad family of intracellular signaling proteins, which mediate many of the effects of TGF-β1. Smad3 is directly phosphorylated by the ligand activated TGF-β type I receptor (TβRI) (168). After joining with a common mediator SMAD4, the heteromeric complex translocates into the nucleus and regulates gene transcription of such molecules as PDGF, connective tissue growth factor (CTGF), MMPs, fibronectin, and collagen (169–172). Ramirez and associates, using a murine model of BOS, demonstrated early expression of TGF-β and CTGF localized to inflammatory cells, then later during fibro-obliteration both were predominately localized to fibroblast (173). In addition, the TGF-β intracellular signal transducer, Smad3, was detected in these fibroblasts throughout the fibrous tissue. Importantly, Smad activation was confirmed by demonstrating phosphorylated Smad2/3 in these fibroblasts. Using Smad3−/− recipient mice, these investigators demonstrated a reduction in fibronectin and collagen and BOS, thus establishing Smad3, and possibly other downstream mediators of TGF-β1 may provide possible therapeutic options in the prevention and treatment of BOS.

## THE ROLE OF GROWTH FACTORS DURING THE PATHOGENESIS OF BOS

IGF-1 is a potent profibrogenic mediator acting as a mitogen/stimulator of collagen synthesis by fibroblasts (174–177). The local bioactivity of IGF-1 in the lung is regulated by a system of multiple high-affinity IGF binding proteins (IGFBP) (178), some of which act as inhibitors while others can potentate IGF-1 cellular response (178). In a human study of sequential BALs from lung transplantation recipients, IGF-1 expression was found to be increased prior to the development of BOS and was not affected by acute rejection episodes or CMV infection (179). Similarly, IGFBP-3 was markedly increased from patients who later developed BOS as compared to those who did not, suggesting IGF-1 and IGFBP-3 interaction could have a critical role in the pathogenesis of BOS through potentiation of IGF-1 profibrotic activities (179). Moreover, IGF-1 has been found to be associated with murine BOS and future studies on the inhibition of IGF-1 and the manipulation of its multiple IFGBP may add insight to the role of IGF-1/IFGBP during BOS.

PDGF is another mitogen for mesenchymal cells including fibroblasts and smooth muscle cells. PDGF ligands consist of two polypeptides, the PDGF-A and PDGF-B chains, which can be expressed as homodimers (PDGF-AA and PDGF-BB) or as a heterodimer PDGF-AB (180). The isoforms of PDGF have different affinity to their related receptors, PDGF-Rα and PDGF-Rβ (181,182). PDGF-Rβ binds the PDGF-B chain and PDGF-Rα binds both PDGF-A and PDGF-B chains (181,182). In humans, elevated levels of biologically active PDGF from BALF are associated with BOS (183). Furthermore, the expression of PDGF-AA and were found to be elevated in an animal model of BOS (184). Treatment with a protein tyrosine kinase inhibitor specific for PDGF receptor significantly reduced the myofibroproliferation associated with BOS without effecting inflammation or immune activation (184). These studies suggest a regulatory role for PDGF on fibroplasia during the development of BOS.

Hepatocyte growth factor (HGF) has been found to be highly expressed in the lung and serum during injurious conditions and has been found to help stimulate epithelial cell proliferation and prevent aberrant wound repair (185,186). Aharinejad and associates demonstrated in human lung transplantation recipients that elevated serum HGF concentration was a significant predictor of rejection (187). In contrast, serum HGF concentration was not a predictor for infection, allowing the authors to discriminate between patients with rejection from infection. Thus, elevated serum levels of HGF may be a marker for acute lung allograft rejection. Further studies will be required to find its role in predicting BOS.

## THE ROLE OF CHEMOKINE RECEPTOR/CHEMOKINES DURING THE PATHOGENESIS OF BOS

The persistent elicitation of mononuclear cells within and around the allograft airways eventually leading to fibro-obliteration during the pathogenesis of BOS requires intercellular communication between infiltrating leukocytes, endothelium, parenchymal cells, and components of the ECM. These events are mediated via the generation of adhesion molecules, cytokines, and chemokines. The chemokines, by virtue of their specific cell surface receptor expression, can selectively mediate the local recruitment/activation of distinct leukocytes, allowing for migration across the endothelium and beyond the vascular compartment along established chemotactic gradients.

The chemokine superfamily is divided into four subfamilies (C, CC, CXC, and CX₃C) based on the presence of a conserved cysteine residue at the $NH_2$-terminus (188–190). CXC chemokines have been further subdivided on the basis of the presence or absence of the sequence glutamic acid–leucine–arginine (ELR) near the $NH_2$-terminal. $ELR^+$ chemokines are neutrophil chemoattractants with angiogenic properties. IFN-inducible $ELR^-$ CXC chemokines are chemoattractants of lymphocytes with angiostatic properties (191–195). CC chemokines predominantly recruit mononuclear cells (188,196). The C subfamily consists of lymphotactin-α/XCL1 and lymphotactin-β/XCL2, which attract lymphocytes, while fractalkine/CX3CL1 is the only member of the CX₃C subfamily, and its chemokine domain sits on a mucin stalk allowing for cellular adhesion (197–200). All chemokine action is mediated through seven transmembrane spanning G protein–coupled receptors (201–203).

## THE ROLE OF RECEPTOR/CC CHEMOKINES DURING THE PATHOGENESIS OF BOS

In both human and animal models of BOS, inflammatory and immune responses have been shown to be a requirement for fibro-obliteration (204–214). CC chemokines are potent chemoattractants of leukocytes [CCL5 and CCL3 recruit mononuclear cells expressing CCR1 and CCR5, CCL2 recruits mononuclear cells expressing CCR2, and the ligands (CCL17 and CCL22) recruit mononuclear cells and dendritic cells (DC) expressing CCR4]. CCL5 was found to be elevated during human and animal BOS (106,215,216). Neutralization of endogenous CCL5 in an animal model of BOS reduced the numbers of infiltrating graft CD4+ T-cells, preserved lumen patency, and attenuated early epithelial injury (215,217). Similarly, in a murine model of chronic cardiac rejection CCR1−/− recipient mice completely ablated chronic rejection (218). Collectively, these studies suggest multiple CC chemokines are important in the pathogenesis of chronic rejection. Unfortunately, to date there are no studies that demonstrate whether specific chemokine/chemokine receptor polymorphisms are associated with lung rejection. However, there are studies in humans of chemokine receptor polymorphisms that impact on renal allograft survival (219,220). CCR5Δ32 is a nonfunctional mutant allele of CCR5 (221–223) and in a multicenter study was found to be associated with prolonged renal allograft survival (219). These studies suggest CC chemokines may be a potential target for inflammatory/fibroproliferative disorders such as transplantation rejection.

CCL2 levels in BALF from patients with acute rejection and BOS were found to be markedly elevated, biologically active, and localized to airway epithelium and mononuclear cells (216). Similar results were seen in human renal transplantation recipients (224). This suggests CCL2 is important in

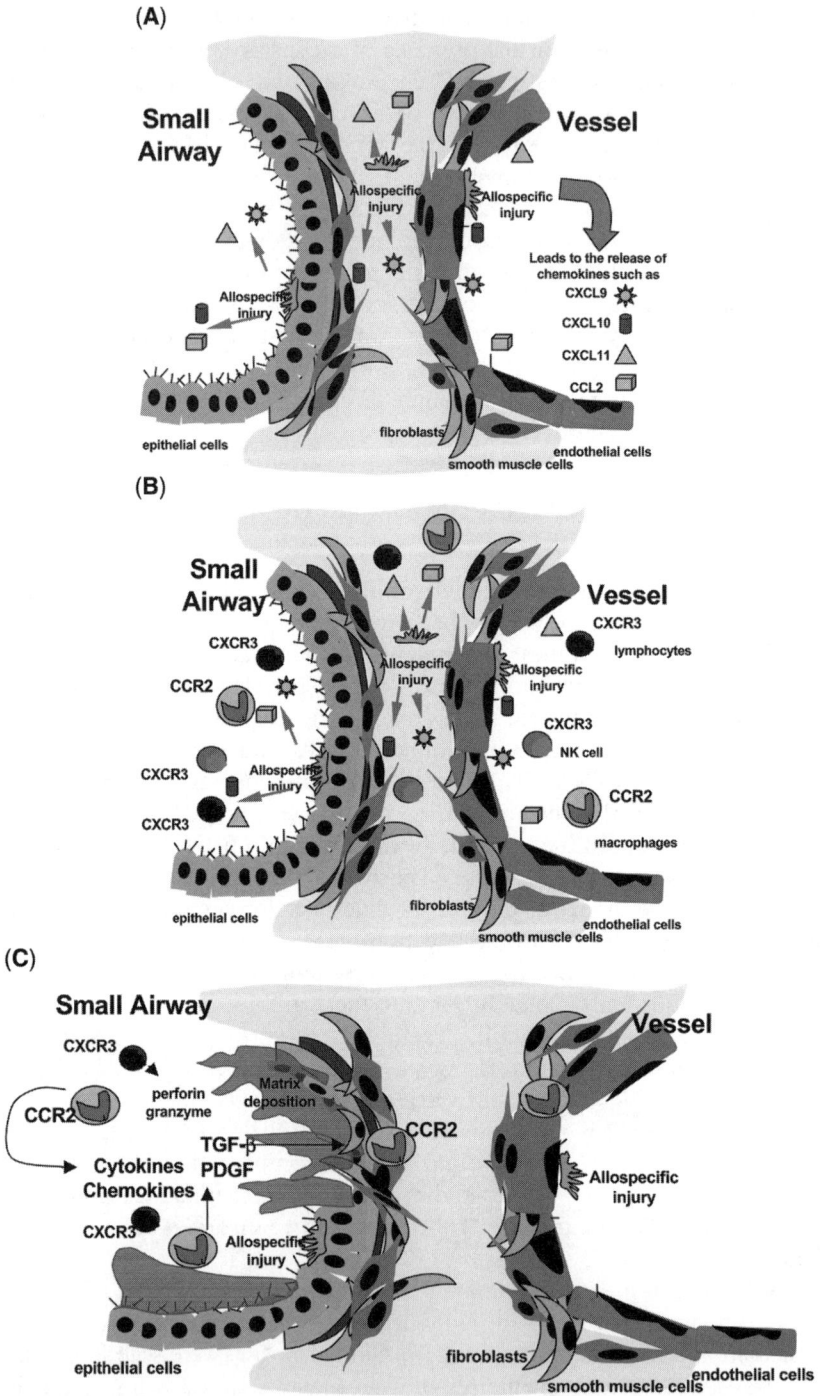

**Figure 2**  (*Caption on facing page*)

the continuum from human acute to chronic allograft rejection by causing persistent accumulation of peribronchiolar leukocytes. Translational studies using rodent models of BOS were consistent with human data demonstrating CCL2 localized to airway columnar epithelium and infiltrating mononuclear cells (216,217). Furthermore, CCL2 levels paralleled the recruitment of mononuclear cells and cellular expression of its receptor, CCR2. A genetic approach was used to determine the effects of inhibiting CCR2 biology on BOS. Allografts from CCR2$-/-$ mice demonstrated significant reductions in mononuclear phagocytes that were not accompanied by significant reductions in lymphocytes as well as significantly less matrix deposition, airway obliteration, and epithelial injury (216). This suggests that a phenotypically distinct mononuclear phagocyte expressing CCR2 (i.e., producing more TGF-β and PDGF) is pivotal during the pathogenesis of BOS (Fig. 2).

CCL17 and CCL22 bind to CCR4, a highly expressed receptor on type 2 cells and used for homing memory T cells (225–227). This receptor has also been identified on monocytes, Langerhans DC cells, monocytes, NK cells, and platelets. While no studies have been performed with regard to transplantation BOS, Alferink and colleagues demonstrated a significant prolongation of cardiac allograft survival when fully mismatched hearts were transplanted into immunosuppressed CCL17$-/-$ recipients (228). This marked enhancement of cardiac survival is presumably due to (i) the absence of expression of CCL17 from recipient DC, suggesting that the expression of CCL17 from recipient DC is indeed important for the recruitment of activated and memory T cells expressing CCR4 and the DC–T cell interactions, and (ii) the expression of CCL17 from recipient cells, which is important for the additional recruitment of CCR4 expressing monocytes, NK cells, and the induction of a type 2 response polarizing inflammation and adaptive immunity to cause chronic rejection. These findings may be pertinent to BOS and will need to be further evaluated in models relevant to BOS.

**Figure 2** (*Facing page*) The role of multiple chemokines during the pathogenesis of BOS. (**A**) Allospecific injury to the lung allograft endothelium, stromal cells, and epithelial cells leads to the release of specific chemokines such as CCL2 and the interferon-inducible ELR$^-$ CXC chemokines (CXCL9, CXCL10, and CXCL11). (**B**) CCL2 recruits a phenotypically distinct population of CCR2-expressing macrophages while the interferon-inducible ELR$^-$ CXC chemokines recruit mononuclear cells expressing CXCR3. (**C**) The interactions of the CXCR3-expressing mononuclear cells with the phenotypically distinct population of CCR2-expressing macrophages leads to the production of cytokines and growth factors, which cause matrix deposition, ultimately ending in fibro-obliteration of the allograft airway. *Abbreviations*: BOS, bronchiolitis obliterans syndrome; CCL, chemoattractant of leukocyte.

## THE ROLE OF RECEPTOR/CXC CHEMOKINES DURING THE PATHOGENESIS OF BOS

Concentrating on airway inflammation, multiple studies have demonstrated that the $ELR^+$ CXC chemokine, CXCL8, in BALF from patients with BOS correlates with airway wall neutrophilia (209–214,229). In addition, CXCL8 localized to α smooth actin positive cells of BOS (214). Interestingly, increased levels of CXCL8 were associated with human ischemia–reperfusion, a risk factor for BOS, and high levels of CXCL8 in human donor lungs were associated with poor graft function and early mortality posttransplantation (230,231). This implies an important role for CXCL8 during the pathogenesis of BOS.

Elevated levels of IFN-inducible $ELR^-$ CXC chemokines CXCL9, CXCL10, and CXCL11 in human BALF were found to be associated with the continuum from acute to chronic rejection (232,233). Translational studies using a murine model of BOS demonstrated increased expression of IFN-inducible $ELR^-$ CXC chemokines paralleling the recruitment of CXCR3 expressing mononuclear cells. In vivo neutralization of CXCR3 or its ligands CXCL9 and CXCL10 decreased intragraft recruitment of CXCR3 expressing mononuclear cells and attenuated BOS. Similar results were seen using murine models of cardiac allograft rejection (234–240). Moreover, elevated levels of human plasma CXCL11 were associated with severe transplantation coronary artery disease (TCAD) as compared to long-term survivors of cardiac transplantation without TCAD (241). Immunohistochemical localization confirmed the presence of infiltrating CXCR3 expressing mononuclear cells within TCAD lesion and the presence of CXCL11, which was found on the surface of endothelial cells within rejected areas of the allograft (241). Collectively, the above chemokine studies demonstrate that chemokines (IFN-inducible $ELR^-$ CXC chemokine ligands/CXCR3 specific for lymphocytes and CCL2/CCR2 specific for mononuclear phagocytes) are acting in parallel during the pathogenesis of acute and chronic (BOS) lung rejection (Fig. 2). Future studies will determine whether combined inhibitors of both chemokine pathways will ultimately lead to additive or syngeneic reductions in the pathogenesis of BOS.

## CONCLUSION

In summary, the above human and preclinical studies in animal models have demonstrated the importance of immune (i.e., HLA matching/mismatching and cytokine expression) and nonimmune (i.e., GERD) mechanisms of allograft injury leading to BOS. Furthermore, the proof of concept studies in humans and animal models of rejection have demonstrated that HLA matching, GERD, and cytokine biology play a pivotal role in mediating the leukocyte infiltration that contributes to chronic (BOS) lung allograft rejection. Furthermore, the finding of these studies should pave the way for the development of pharmaceutical agents and surgical techniques that will target (HLA matching/mismatching, GERD, and cytokines) and provide a novel means to ultimately enhance long-term lung allograft survival.

## ACKNOWLEDGMENT

This work was supported in part by grants from the NIH (HL04493 and HL080206–01 to JAB and HL69978 to SMP).

## REFERENCES

1. Trulock EP. Lung transplantation. Am J Respir Crit Care Med 1997; 155(3):789–818.
2. Arcasoy SM, Kotloff RM. Lung transplantation. N Engl J Med 1999; 340(14):1081–1091.
3. Kelly K, Hertz MI. Obliterative bronchiolitis. Clin Chest Med 1997; 18(2):319–338.
4. Paradis I, Yousem S, Griffith B. Airway obstruction and bronchiolitis obliterans after lung transplantation. Clin Chest Med 1993; 14(4):751–763.
5. Heng D, Sharples LD, McNeil K, Stewart S, Wreghitt T, Wallwork J. Bronchiolitis obliterans syndrome: incidence, natural history, prognosis, and risk factors. J Heart Lung Transplant 1998; 17(12):1255–1263.
6. Valentine VG, Robbins RC, Berry GJ, et al. Actuarial survival of heart-lung and bilateral sequential lung transplant recipients with obliterative bronchiolitis. J Heart Lung Transplant 1996; 15(4):371–383.
7. Wisser W, Wekerle T, Zlabinger G, et al. Influence of human leukocyte antigen matching on long-term outcome after lung transplantation. J Heart Lung Transplant 1996; 15(12):1209–1216.
8. Iwaki Y, Yoshida Y, Griffith B. The HLA matching effect in lung transplantation. Transplantation 1993; 56(6):1528–1529.
9. Quantz MA, Bennett LE, Meyer DM, Novick RJ. Does human leukocyte antigen matching influence the outcome of lung transplantation? An analysis of 3549 lung transplantations. J Heart Lung Transplant 2000; 19(5):473–479.
10. Bando K, Paradis IL, Komatsu K, et al. Analysis of time-dependent risks for infection, rejection, and death after pulmonary transplantation. J Thorac Cardiovasc Surg 1995; 109(1):49–57; discussion 57–59.
11. Schulman LL, Weinberg AD, McGregor CC, Suciu-Foca NM, Itescu S. Influence of donor and recipient HLA locus mismatching on development of obliterative bronchiolitis after lung transplantation. Am J Respir Crit Care Med 2001; 163(2):437–442.
12. Keogh A, Kaan A, Doran T, Macdonald P, Bryant D, Spratt P. HLA mismatching and outcome in heart, heart-lung, and single lung transplantation. J Heart Lung Transplant 1995; 14(3):444–451.
13. Schulman LL, Weinberg AD, McGregor C, Galantowicz ME, Suciu-Foca NM, Itescu S. Mismatches at the HLA-DR and HLA-B loci are risk factors

for acute rejection after lung transplantation. Am J Respir Crit Care Med 1998; 157(6, Pt 1):1833–1837.

14. Sundaresan S, Mohanakumar T, Smith MA, et al. HLA-A locus mismatches and development of antibodies to HLA after lung transplantation correlate with the development of bronchiolitis obliterans syndrome. Transplantation 1998; 65(5):648–653.

15. Kroshus TJ, Kshettry VR, Savik K, John R, Hertz MI, Bolman RM III. Risk factors for the development of bronchiolitis obliterans syndrome after lung transplantation. J Thorac Cardiovasc Surg 1997; 114(2):195–202.

16. Bando K, Paradis IL, Similo S, et al. Obliterative bronchiolitis after lung and heart-lung transplantation. An analysis of risk factors and management. J Thorac Cardiovasc Surg 1995; 110(1):4–13; discussion 13–14.

17. Husain AN, Siddiqui MT, Holmes EW, et al. Analysis of risk factors for the development of bronchiolitis obliterans syndrome. Am J Respir Crit Care Med 1999; 159(3):829–833.

18. Estenne M, Maurer JR, Boehler A, et al. Bronchiolitis obliterans syndrome 2001: an update of the diagnostic criteria. J Heart Lung Transplant 2002; 21(3):297–310.

19. Chalermskulrat W, Neuringer IP, Schmitz JL, et al. Human leukocyte antigen mismatches predispose to the severity of bronchiolitis obliterans syndrome after lung transplantation. Chest 2003; 123(6):1825–1831.

20. SivaSai KS, Smith MA, Poindexter NJ, et al. Indirect recognition of donor HLA class I peptides in lung transplant recipients with bronchiolitis obliterans syndrome. Transplantation 1999; 67(8):1094–1098.

21. Girnita AL, Duquesnoy R, Yousem SA, et al. HLA-specific antibodies are risk factors for lymphocytic bronchiolitis and chronic lung allograft dysfunction. Am J Transplant 2005; 5(1):131–138.

22. Palmer SM, Davis RD, Hadjiliadis D, et al. Development of an antibody specific to major histocompatibility antigens detectable by flow cytometry after lung transplant is associated with bronchiolitis obliterans syndrome. Transplantation 2002; 74(6):799–804.

23. Reznik SI, Jaramillo A, SivaSai KS, et al. Indirect allorecognition of mismatched donor HLA class II peptides in lung transplant recipients with bronchiolitis obliterans syndrome. Am J Transplant 2001; 1(3):228–235.

24. Jaramillo A, Naziruddin B, Zhang L, et al. Activation of human airway epithelial cells by non-HLA antibodies developed after lung transplantation: a potential etiological factor for bronchiolitis obliterans syndrome. Transplantation 2001; 71(7):966–976.

25. Jaramillo A, Zhang L, Mohanakumar T. Binding of anti-HLA class I antibodies to airway epithelial cells induces activation and growth factor production and indirectly upregulates lung fibroblast proliferation. J Heart Lung Transplant 2001; 20(2):166.

26. Jaramillo A, Smith CR, Maruyama T, Zhang L, Patterson GA, Mohanakumar T. Anti-HLA class I antibody binding to airway epithelial cells induces production of fibrogenic growth factors and apoptotic cell death: a possible mechanism for bronchiolitis obliterans syndrome. Hum Immunol 2003; 64(5):521–529.

27. Kelly KE, Hertz MI, Mueller DL. T-cell and major histocompatibility complex requirements for obliterative airway disease in heterotopically transplanted murine tracheas. Transplantation 1998; 66(6):764–771.

28. Smith CR, Jaramillo A, Lu KC, Higuchi T, Kaleem Z, Mohanakumar T. Prevention of obliterative airway disease in HLA-A2-transgenic tracheal allografts by neutralization of tumor necrosis factor. Transplantation 2001; 72(9):1512–1518.

29. Chalermskulrat W, Neuringer IP, Brickey WJ, et al. Hierarchical contributions of allorecognition pathways in chronic lung rejection. Am J Respir Crit Care Med 2003; 167(7):999–1007.

30. Richards DM, Dalheimer SL, Hertz MI, Mueller DL. Trachea allograft class I molecules directly activate and retain CD8+ T cells that cause obliterative airways disease. J Immunol 2003; 171(12):6919–6928.

31. Richards DM, Dalheimer SL, Ehst BD, et al. Indirect minor histocompatibility antigen presentation by allograft recipient cells in the draining lymph node leads to the activation and clonal expansion of CD4+ T cells that cause obliterative airways disease. J Immunol 2004; 172(6):3469–3479.

32. Higuchi T, Maruyama T, Jaramillo A, Mohanakumar T. Induction of obliterative airway disease in murine tracheal allografts by CD8+ CTLs recognizing a single minor histocompatibility antigen. J Immunol 2005; 174(4):1871–1878.

33. Kesten S, Rajagopalan N, Maurer J. Cytolytic therapy for the treatment of bronchiolitis obliterans syndrome following lung transplantation. Transplantation 1996; 61(3):427–430.

34. Kesten S, Chaparro C, Scavuzzo M, Gutierrez C. Tacrolimus as rescue therapy for bronchiolitis obliterans syndrome. J Heart Lung Transplant 1997; 16(9):905–912.

35. Sharples LD, McNeil K, Stewart S, Wallwork J. Risk factors for bronchiolitis obliterans: a systematic review of recent publications. J Heart Lung Transplant 2002; 21(2):271–281 (review; 28 references).

36. Harding SM, Richter JE. The role of gastroesophageal reflux in chronic cough and asthma. Chest 1997; 111(5):1389–1402.

37. Feigelson J, Girault F, Pecau Y. Gastro-oesophageal reflux and esophagitis in cystic fibrosis. Acta Paediatr Scand 1987; 76(6):989–990.

38. Tobin RW, Pope CE II, Pellegrini CA, Emond MJ, Sillery J, Raghu G. Increased prevalence of gastroesophageal reflux in patients with idiopathic pulmonary fibrosis. Am J Respir Crit Care Med 1998; 158(6):1804–1808.

39. Teramoto S, Matsuse T, Ouchi Y. Clinical significance of cough as a defense mechanism or a symptom in elderly patients with aspiration and diffuse aspiration bronchiolitis. Chest 1999; 115(2):602–603.

40. Veale D, Glasper PN, Gascoigne A, Dark JH, Gibson GJ, Corris PA. Ciliary beat frequency in transplanted lungs. Thorax 1993; 48(6):629–631.

41. Lubetkin EI, Lipson DA, Palevsky HI, et al. GI complications after orthotopic lung transplantation. Am J Gastroenterol 1996; 91(11):2382–2390.

42. Reid KR, McKenzie FN, Menkis AH, et al. Importance of chronic aspiration in recipients of heart-lung transplants. Lancet 1990; 336(8709):206–208 (see comment).

43. Abernathy EC, Hruban RH, Baumgartner WA, Reitz BA, Hutchins GM. The two forms of bronchiolitis obliterans in heart-lung transplant recipients. Hum Pathol 1991; 22(11):1102–1110.

44. Young LR, Hadjiliadis D, Davis RD, Palmer SM. Lung transplantation exacerbates gastroesophageal reflux disease. Chest 2003; 124(5):1689–1693.

45. Hadjiliadis D, Duane Davis R, Steele MP, et al. Gastroesophageal reflux disease in lung transplant recipients. Clin Transpl 2003; 17(4):363–368.

46. Davis RD Jr, Lau CL, Eubanks S, et al. Improved lung allograft function after fundoplication in patients with gastroesophageal reflux disease undergoing lung transplantation. J Thorac Cardiovasc Surg 2003; 125(3):533–542.

47. Lau CL, Palmer SM, Howell DN, et al. Laparoscopic antireflux surgery in the lung transplant population. Surg Endosc 2002; 16(12):1674–1678.

48. Cantu I, Edward, Appel I, et al. Early fundoplication prevents chronic allograft dysfunction in patients with gastroesophageal reflux disease. Ann Thorac Surg 2004; 78(4):1142–1151.

49. Zhai Y, Kupiec-Weglinski JW. What is the role of regulatory T cells in transplantation tolerance? Curr Opin Immunol 1999; 11(5):497–503.

50. Mosmann TR, Cherwinski H, Bond MW, Giedlin MA, Coffman RL. Two types of murine helper T cell clone. I. Definition according to profiles of lymphokine activities and secreted proteins. J Immunol 1986; 136(7):2348–2357.

51. Kunzendorf U, Tran TH, Bulfone-Paus S. The Th1-Th2 paradigm in 1998: law of nature or rule with exceptions. Nephrol Dial Transplant 1998; 13(10):2445–2448.

52. Ruth JH, Bienkowski M, Warmington KS, Lincoln PM, Kunkel SL, Chensue SW. IL-1 receptor antagonist (IL-1ra) expression, function, and cytokine- mediated regulation during mycobacterial and schistosomal antigen-elicited granuloma formation. J Immunol 1996; 156(7):2503–2509.

53. Dinarello CA. Biologic basis for interleukin-1 in disease. Blood 1996; 87(6):2095–2147.

54. Arend WP, Welgus HG, Thompson RC, Eisenberg SP. Biological properties of recombinant human monocyte-derived interleukin 1 receptor antagonist. J Clin Invest 1990; 85(5):1694–1697.

55. Wilborn J, Crofford LJ, Burdick MD, Kunkel SL, Strieter RM, Peters-Golden M. Cultured lung fibroblasts isolated from patients with idiopathic pulmonary fibrosis have a diminished capacity to synthesize prostaglandin E2 and to express cyclooxygenase-2. J Clin Invest 1995; 95(4):1861–1868.

56. Naruse K, Shimizu K, Muramatsu M, et al. Long-term inhibition of NO synthesis promotes atherosclerosis in the hypercholesterolemic rabbit thoracic aorta. PGH2 does not contribute to impaired endothelium-dependent relaxation. Arterioscler Thromb 1994; 14(5):746–752 (see comments).

57. Belperio JA, DiGiovine B, Keane MP, et al. Interleukin-1 receptor antagonist as a biomarker for bronchiolitis obliterans syndrome in lung transplant recipients. Transplantation 2002; 73(4):591–599.

58. Vamvakopoulos J, Green C, Metcalfe S. Genetic control of IL-1beta bioactivity through differential regulation of the IL-1 receptor antagonist. Eur J Immunol 2002; 32(10):2988–2996.

59. Vamvakopoulos JE, Taylor CJ, Green C, et al. Interleukin 1 and chronic rejection: possible genetic links in human heart allografts. Am J Transplant 2002; 2(1):76–83.
60. Beutler BA. The role of tumor necrosis factor in health and disease. J Rheumatol 1999; 26(Suppl 57):16–21.
61. Ostensen ME, Thiele DL, Lipsky PE. Tumor necrosis factor-alpha enhances cytolytic activity of human natural killer cells. J Immunol 1987; 138(12):4185–4191.
62. Piguet PF, Collart MA, Grau GE, Kapanci Y, Vassalli P. Tumor necrosis factor/cachectin plays a key role in bleomycin-induced pneumopathy and fibrosis. J Exp Med 1989; 170(3):655–663.
63. He Y, Liu W. The preliminary research on the relationship between TNF- and egg-induced granuloma and hepatic fibrosis of schistosomiasis japonica. J Tongji Med Univ 1996; 16(4):205–208.
64. Hayashi M, Martinez OM, Garcia-Kennedy R, So S, Esquivel CO, Krams SM. Expression of cytokines and immune mediators during chronic liver allograft rejection. Transplantation 1995; 60(12):1533–1538.
65. Noronha IL, Eberlein-Gonska M, Hartley B, Stephens S, Cameron JS, Waldherr R. In situ expression of tumor necrosis factor-alpha, interferon-gamma, and interleukin-2 receptors in renal allograft biopsies. Transplantation 1992; 54(6):1017–1024.
66. Mytilineos J, Laux G, Opelz G. Relevance of IL10, TGFbeta1, TNFalpha, and IL4Ralpha gene polymorphisms in kidney transplantation: a collaborative transplant study report. Am J Transplant 2004; 4(10):1684–1690.
67. Aris RM, Walsh S, Chalermskulrat W, Hathwar V, Neuringer IP. Growth factor upregulation during obliterative bronchiolitis in the mouse model. Am J Respir Crit Care Med 2002; 166(3):417–422.
68. Kobayashi M, Fitz L, Ryan M, et al. Identification and purification of natural killer cell stimulatory factor (NKSF), a cytokine with multiple biologic effects on human lymphocytes. J Exp Med 1989; 170(3):827–845.
69. Stern AS, Podlaski FJ, Hulmes JD, et al. Purification to homogeneity and partial characterization of cytotoxic lymphocyte maturation factor from human B-lymphoblastoid cells. Proc Natl Acad Sci USA 1990; 87(17):6808–6812.
70. Presky DH, Yang H, Minetti LJ, et al. A functional interleukin 12 receptor complex is composed of two beta-type cytokine receptor subunits. Proc Natl Acad Sci USA 1996; 93(24):14002–14007.
71. Presky DH, Minetti LJ, Gillessen S, et al. Evidence for multiple sites of interaction between IL-12 and its receptor. Ann N Y Acad Sci 1996; 795: 390–393.
72. Gately MK, Renzetti LM, Magram J, et al. The interleukin-12/interleukin-12-receptor system: role in normal and pathologic immune responses. Annu Rev Immunol 1998; 16:495–521.
73. Trinchieri G. Interleukin-12: a proinflammatory cytokine with immunoregulatory functions that bridge innate resistance and antigen-specific adaptive immunity. Annu Rev Immunol 1995; 13:251–276.
74. Seder RA, Gazzinelli R, Sher A, Paul WE. Interleukin 12 acts directly on CD4+ T cells to enhance priming for interferon gamma production and

diminishes interleukin 4 inhibition of such priming. Proc Natl Acad Sci USA 1993; 90(21):10188–10192.

75. McKnight AJ, Zimmer GJ, Fogelman I, Wolf SF, Abbas AK. Effects of IL-12 on helper T cell-dependent immune responses in vivo. J Immunol 1994; 152(5):2172–2179.

76. Marshall JD, Secrist H, DeKruyff RH, Wolf SF, Umetsu DT. IL-12 inhibits the production of IL-4 and IL-10 in allergen-specific human CD4+ T lymphocytes. J Immunol 1995; 155(1):111–117.

77. Via CS, Rus V, Gately MK, Finkelman FD. IL-12 stimulates the development of acute graft-versus-host disease in mice that normally would develop chronic, autoimmune graft-versus-host disease. J Immunol 1994; 153(9): 4040–4047.

78. Hsieh CS, Macatonia SE, Tripp CS, Wolf SF, O'Garra A, Murphy KM. Development of TH1 CD4+ T cells through IL-12 produced by Listeria-induced macrophages. Science 1993; 260(5107):547–549.

79. Oswald IP, Caspar P, Jankovic D, Wynn TA, Pearce EJ, Sher A. IL-12 inhibits Th2 cytokine responses induced by eggs of Schistosoma mansoni. J Immunol 1994; 153(4):1707–1713.

80. Pearlman E, Heinzel FP, Hazlett FE Jr, Kazura JW. IL-12 modulation of T helper responses to the filarial helminth, Brugia malayi. J Immunol 1995; 154(9):4658–4664.

81. Gazzinelli RT, Giese NA, Morse HC III. In vivo treatment with interleukin 12 protects mice from immune abnormalities observed during murine acquired immunodeficiency syndrome (MAIDS). J Exp Med 1994; 180(6):2199–2208.

82. Zhou P, Sieve MC, Bennett J, et al. IL-12 prevents mortality in mice infected with Histoplasma capsulatum through induction of IFN-gamma. J Immunol 1995; 155(2):785–795.

83. Rosenberg AS, Singer A. Cellular basis of skin allograft rejection: an in vivo model of immune-mediated tissue destruction. Annu Rev Immunol 1992; 10:333–358.

84. Piccotti JR, Li K, Chan SY, Eichwald EJ, Bishop DK. Interleukin-12 (IL-12)-driven alloimmune responses in vitro and in vivo: requirement for beta1 subunit of the IL-12 receptor. Transplantation 1999; 67(11):1453–1460.

85. Williamson E, Garside P, Bradley JA, More IA, Mowat AM. Neutralizing IL-12 during induction of murine acute graft-versus-host disease polarizes the cytokine profile toward a Th2-type alloimmune response and confers long term protection from disease. J Immunol 1997; 159(3):1208–1215.

86. Orr DJ, Bolton EM, Bradley JA. Neutralising IL-12 activity as a strategy for prolonging allograft survival and preventing graft-versus-host disease. Scott Med J 1998; 43(4):109–111.

87. Welniak LA, Blazar BR, Wiltrout RH, Anver MR, Murphy WJ. Role of interleukin-12 in acute graft-versus-host disease (1). Transplant Proc 2001; 33(1–2): 1752–1753.

88. Williamson E, Garside P, Bradley JA, Mowat AM. IL-12 is a central mediator of acute graft-versus-host disease in mice. J Immunol 1996; 157(2):689–699.

89. Piccotti JR, Chan SY, Goodman RE, Magram J, Eichwald EJ, Bishop DK. IL-12 antagonism induces T helper 2 responses, yet exacerbates cardiac

allograft rejection. Evidence against a dominant protective role for T helper 2 cytokines in alloimmunity. J Immunol 1996; 157(5):1951–1957.

90. Konieczny BT, Dai Z, Elwood ET, et al. IFN-gamma is critical for long-term allograft survival induced by blocking the CD28 and CD40 ligand T cell costimulation pathways. J Immunol 1998; 160(5):2059–2064.

91. Tau GZ, von der Weid T, Lu B, et al. Interferon gamma signaling alters the function of T helper type 1 cells. J Exp Med 2000; 192(7):977–986.

92. Wiekowski MT, Leach MW, Evans EW, et al. Ubiquitous transgenic expression of the IL-23 subunit p19 induces multiorgan inflammation, runting, infertility, and premature death. J Immunol 2001; 166(12):7563–7570.

93. Parham C, Chirica M, Timans J, et al. A receptor for the heterodimeric cytokine IL-23 is composed of IL-12Rbeta1 and a novel cytokine receptor subunit, IL-23R. J Immunol 2002; 168(11):5699–5708.

94. Oppmann B, Lesley R, Blom B, et al. Novel p19 protein engages IL-12p40 to form a cytokine, IL-23, with biological activities similar as well as distinct from IL-12. Immunity 2000; 13(5):715–725.

95. Cua DJ, Sherlock J, Chen Y, et al. Interleukin-23 rather than interleukin-12 is the critical cytokine for autoimmune inflammation of the brain. Nature 2003; 421(6924):744–748.

96. Farrar MA, Schreiber RD. The molecular cell biology of interferon-gamma and its receptor. Annu Rev Immunol 1993; 11:571–611.

97. Thierfelder WE, van Deursen JM, Yamamoto K, et al. Requirement for Stat4 in interleukin-12-mediated responses of natural killer and T cells. Nature 1996; 382(6587):171–174.

98. Fiorentino DF, Zlotnik A, Mosmann TR, Howard M, O'Garra A. IL-10 inhibits cytokine production by activated macrophages. J Immunol 1991; 147(11):3815–3822.

99. Hobart M, Ramassar V, Goes N, Urmson J, Halloran PF. The induction of class I and II major histocompatibility complex by allogeneic stimulation is dependent on the transcription factor interferon regulatory factor 1 (IRF-1): observations in IRF-1 knockout mice. Transplantation 1996; 62(12):1895–1901.

100. Hobart M, Ramassar V, Goes N, Urmson J, Halloran PF. IFN regulatory factor-1 plays a central role in the regulation of the expression of class I and II MHC genes in vivo. J Immunol 1997; 158(9):4260–4269.

101. Hassan AT, Dai Z, Konieczny BT, et al. Regulation of alloantigen-mediated T-cell proliferation by endogenous interferon-gamma: implications for long-term allograft acceptance. Transplantation 1999; 68(1):124–129.

102. Hidalgo LG, Halloran PF. Role of IFN-gamma in allograft rejection. Crit Rev Immunol 2002; 22(4):317–349.

103. Moudgil A, Bagga A, Toyoda M, Nicolaidou E, Jordan SC, Ross D. Expression of gamma-IFN mRNA in bronchoalveolar lavage fluid correlates with early acute allograft rejection in lung transplant recipients. Clin Transpl 1999; 13(2):201–207.

104. Iacono A, Dauber J, Keenan R, et al. Interleukin 6 and interferon-gamma gene expression in lung transplant recipients with refractory acute cellular rejection: implications for monitoring and inhibition by treatment with aerosolized cyclosporine. Transplantation 1997; 64(2):263–269.

105. Lu KC, Jaramillo A, Lecha RL, et al. Interleukin-6 and interferon-gamma gene polymorphisms in the development of bronchiolitis obliterans syndrome after lung transplantation. Transplantation 2002; 74(9):1297–1302.

106. Boehler A, Bai XH, Liu M, et al. Upregulation of T-helper 1 cytokines and chemokine expression in post-transplant airway obliteration. Am J Respir Crit Care Med 1999; 159(6):1910–1917.

107. Nagano H, Mitchell RN, Taylor MK, Hasegawa S, Tilney NL, Libby P. Interferon-gamma deficiency prevents coronary arteriosclerosis but not myocardial rejection in transplanted mouse hearts. J Clin Invest 1997; 100(3):550–557.

108. Raisanen-Sokolowski A, Mottram PL, Glysing-Jensen T, Satoskar A, Russell ME. Heart transplants in interferon-gamma, interleukin 4, and interleukin 10 knockout mice. Recipient environment alters graft rejection. J Clin Invest 1997; 100(10):2449–2456.

109. Raisanen-Sokolowski A, Glysing-Jensen T, Russell ME. Leukocyte-suppressing influences of interleukin (IL)-10 in cardiac allografts: insights from IL-10 knockout mice. Am J Pathol 1998; 153(5):1491–1500.

110. de Waal Malefyt R, Abrams J, Bennett B, Figdor CG, de Vries JE. Interleukin 10(IL-10) inhibits cytokine synthesis by human monocytes: an autoregulatory role of IL-10 produced by monocytes. J Exp Med 1991; 174(5):1209–1220.

111. de Waal Malefyt R, Haanen J, Spits H, et al. Interleukin 10 (IL-10) and viral IL-10 strongly reduce antigen-specific human T cell proliferation by diminishing the antigen-presenting capacity of monocytes via downregulation of class II major histocompatibility complex expression. J Exp Med 1991; 174(4):915–924.

112. de Waal Malefyt R, Yssel H, Roncarolo MG, Spits H, de Vries JE. Interleukin-10. Curr Opin Immunol 1992; 4(3):314–320.

113. de Waal Malefyt R, Yssel H, de Vries JE. Direct effects of IL-10 on subsets of human CD4+ T cell clones and resting T cells. Specific inhibition of IL-2 production and proliferation. J Immunol 1993; 150(11):4754–4765.

114. te Velde AA, de Waal Malefijt R, Huijbens RJ, de Vries JE, Figdor CG. IL-10 stimulates monocyte Fc gamma R surface expression and cytotoxic activity. Distinct regulation of antibody-dependent cellular cytotoxicity by IFN-gamma, IL-4, and IL-10. J Immunol 1992; 149(12):4048–4052.

115. Fiorentino DF, Zlotnik A, Vieira P, et al. IL-10 acts on the antigen-presenting cell to inhibit cytokine production by Th1 cells. J Immunol 1991; 146(10):3444–3451.

116. Bogdan C, Vodovotz Y, Nathan C. Macrophage deactivation by interleukin 10. J Exp Med 1991; 174(6):1549–1555.

117. Ralph P, Nakoinz I, Sampson-Johannes A, et al. IL-10, T lymphocyte inhibitor of human blood cell production of IL-1 and tumor necrosis factor. J Immunol 1992; 148(3):808–814.

118. Hsu DH, de Waal Malefyt R, Fiorentino DF, et al. Expression of interleukin-10 activity by Epstein–Barr virus protein BCRF1. Science 1990; 250(4982):830–832.

119. Hsu DH, Moore KW, Spits H. Differential effects of IL-4 and IL-10 on IL-2-induced IFN-gamma synthesis and lymphokine-activated killer activity. Int Immunol 1992; 4(5):563–569.

120. Chen WF, Zlotnik A. IL-10: a novel cytotoxic T cell differentiation factor. J Immunol 1991; 147(2):528–534.

121. MacNeil IA, Suda T, Moore KW, Mosmann TR, Zlotnik A. IL-10, a novel growth cofactor for mature and immature T cells. J Immunol 1990; 145(12): 4167–4173.

122. Hu S, Chao CC, Ehrlich LC, et al. Inhibition of microglial cell RANTES production by IL-10 and TGF-beta. J Leukoc Biol 1999; 65(6):815–821.

123. Bejarano MT, de Waal Malefyt R, Abrams JS, et al. Interleukin 10 inhibits allogeneic proliferative and cytotoxic T cell responses generated in primary mixed lymphocyte cultures. Int Immunol 1992; 4(12):1389–1397.

124. Bromberg JS. IL-10 immunosuppression in transplantation. Curr Opin Immunol 1995; 7(5):639–643.

125. Zuo XJ, Matsumura Y, Prehn J, et al. Cytokine gene expression in rejecting and tolerant rat lung allograft models: analysis by RT-PCR. Transpl Immunol 1995; 3(2):151–161.

126. Maeda H, Takata M, Takahashi S, Ogoshi S, Fujimoto S. Adoptive transfer of a Th2-like cell line prolongs MHC class II antigen disparate skin allograft survival in the mouse. Int Immunol 1994; 6(6):855–862.

127. Zheng XX, Steele AW, Nickerson PW, Steurer W, Steiger J, Strom TB. Administration of noncytolytic IL-10/Fc in murine models of lipopolysaccharide-induced septic shock and allogeneic islet transplantation. J Immunol 1995; 154(10):5590–5600.

128. Lee MS, Wogensen L, Shizuru J, Oldstone MB, Sarvetnick N. Pancreatic islet production of murine interleukin-10 does not inhibit immune-mediated tissue destruction. J Clin Invest 1994; 93(3):1332–1338.

129. Qian S, Li W, Li Y, et al. Systemic administration of cellular interleukin-10 can exacerbate cardiac allograft rejection in mice. Transplantation 1996; 62(12):1709–1714.

130. Sankaran D, Asderakis A, Ashraf S, et al. Cytokine gene polymorphisms predict acute graft rejection following renal transplantation. Kidney Int 1999; 56(1):281–288.

131. Mulligan MS, Warner RL, McDuffie JE, Bolling SF, Sarma JV, Ward PA. Regulatory role of Th-2 cytokines, IL-10 and IL-4, in cardiac allograft rejection. Exp Mol Pathol 2000; 69(1):1–9.

132. Oshima K, Sen L, Cui G, et al. Localized interleukin-10 gene transfer induces apoptosis of alloreactive T cells via FAS/FASL pathway, improves function, and prolongs survival of cardiac allograft. Transplantation 2002; 73(7):1019–1026.

133. Qin L, Chavin KD, Ding Y, et al. Retrovirus-mediated transfer of viral IL-10 gene prolongs murine cardiac allograft survival. J Immunol 1996; 156(6):2316–2323.

134. Qin L, Ding Y, Pahud DR, Robson ND, Shaked A, Bromberg JS. Adenovirus-mediated gene transfer of viral interleukin-10 inhibits the immune response to both alloantigen and adenoviral antigen. Hum Gene Ther 1997; 8(11):1365–1374.

135. Awad MR, Webber S, Boyle G, et al. The effect of cytokine gene polymorphisms on pediatric heart allograft outcome. J Heart Lung Transplant 2001; 20(6):625–630.

136. Hutchinson IV, Turner D, Sankaran D, Awad M, Pravica V, Sinnott P. Cytokine genotypes in allograft rejection: guidelines for immunosuppression. Transplant Proc 1998; 30(8):3991–3992.

137. Mazariegos GV, Reyes J, Webber SA, et al. Cytokine gene polymorphisms in children successfully withdrawn from immunosuppression after liver transplantation. Transplantation 2002; 73(8):1342–1345.

138. Turner D, Grant SC, Yonan N, et al. Cytokine gene polymorphism and heart transplant rejection. Transplantation 1997; 64(5):776–779.

139. Uboldi de Capei M, Dametto E, Fasano ME, et al. Cytokines and chronic rejection: a study in kidney transplant long-term survivors. Transplantation 2004; 77(4):548–552.

140. Zheng HX, Burckart GJ, McCurry K, et al. Interleukin-10 production genotype protects against acute persistent rejection after lung transplantation. J Heart Lung Transplant 2004; 23(5):541–546.

141. Naidu B, Krishnadasan B, Whyte RI, Warner RL, Ward PA, Mulligan MS. Regulatory role of IL-10 in experimental obliterative bronchiolitis in rats. Exp Mol Pathol 2002; 73(3):164–170.

142. Yonemitsu Y, Kitson C, Ferrari S, et al. Efficient gene transfer to airway epithelium using recombinant Sendai virus. Nat Biotechnol 2000; 18(9):970–973.

143. Shoji F, Yonemitsu Y, Okano S, et al. Airway-directed gene transfer of interleukin-10 using recombinant Sendai virus effectively prevents post-transplant fibrous airway obliteration in mice. Gene Ther 2003; 10(3):213–218.

144. Salgar SK, Yang D, Ruiz P, Miller J, Tzakis AG. Viral interleukin-10-engineered autologous hematopoietic stem cell therapy: a novel gene therapy approach to prevent graft rejection. Hum Gene Ther 2004; 15(2):131–144.

145. Berman RM, Suzuki T, Tahara H, Robbins PD, Narula SK, Lotze MT. Systemic administration of cellular IL-10 induces an effective, specific, and long-lived immune response against established tumors in mice. J Immunol 1996; 157(1):231–238.

146. Lowry RP, Konieczny B, Alexander D, et al. Interleukin-10 eliminates anti-CD3 monoclonal antibody-induced mortality and prolongs heart allograft survival in inbred mice. Transplant Proc 1995; 27(1):392–394.

147. Kishimoto T. Interleukin-6 and its receptor in autoimmunity. J Autoimmun 1992; 5(Suppl A):123–132.

148. Hirano T, Matsuda T, Turner M, et al. Excessive production of interleukin 6/B cell stimulatory factor-2 in rheumatoid arthritis. Eur J Immunol 1988; 18(11):1797–1801.

149. Taga T, Kishimoto T. Gp130 and the interleukin-6 family of cytokines. Annu Rev Immunol 1997; 15:797–819.

150. Shahar I, Fireman E, Topilsky M, et al. Effect of IL-6 on alveolar fibroblast proliferation in interstitial lung diseases. Clin Immunol Immunopathol 1996; 79(3):244–251.

151. Horii Y, Muraguchi A, Iwano M, et al. Involvement of IL-6 in mesangial proliferative glomerulonephritis. J Immunol 1989; 143(12):3949–3955.

152. Borger P, Kauffman HF, Scholma J, Timmerman JA, Koeter GH. Human allogeneic CD2+ lymphocytes activate airway-derived epithelial cells to produce interleukin-6 and interleukin-8. Possible role for the epithelium in chronic allograft rejection. J Heart Lung Transplant 2002; 21(5):567–575.

153. Magnan A, Mege JL, Escallier JC, et al. Balance between alveolar macrophage IL-6 and TGF-beta in lung-transplant recipients. Marseille and Montreal

Lung Transplantation Group. Am J Respir Crit Care Med 1996; 153(4, Pt 1):1431–1436.

154. Rolfe MW, Kunkel S, Lincoln P, Deeb M, Lupinetti F, Strieter R. Lung allograft rejection: role of tumor necrosis factor-alpha and interleukin-6. Chest 1993; 103(2, Suppl):133S.

155. Scholma J, Slebos DJ, Boezen HM, et al. Eosinophilic granulocytes and interleukin-6 level in bronchoalveolar lavage fluid are associated with the development of obliterative bronchiolitis after lung transplantation. Am J Respir Crit Care Med 2000; 162(6):2221–2225.

156. Penttinen RP, Kobayashi S, Bornstein P. Transforming growth factor beta increases mRNA for matrix proteins both in the presence and in the absence of changes in mRNA stability. Proc Natl Acad Sci USA 1988; 85(4):1105–1108.

157. Roberts AB, Sporn MB, Assoian RK, et al. Transforming growth factor type beta: rapid induction of fibrosis and angiogenesis in vivo and stimulation of collagen formation in vitro. Proc Natl Acad Sci USA 1986; 83(12):4167–4171.

158. Mora BN, Boasquevisque CH, Boglione M, et al. Transforming growth factor-beta1 gene transfer ameliorates acute lung allograft rejection. J Thorac Cardiovasc Surg 2000; 119(5):913–920.

159. Qin L, Chavin KD, Ding Y, et al. Gene transfer for transplantation. Prolongation of allograft survival with transforming growth factor-beta 1. Ann Surg 1994; 220(4):508–518; discussion 18–19.

160. Yasufuku K, Heidler KM, O'Donnell PW, et al. Oral tolerance induction by type V collagen downregulates lung allograft rejection. Am J Respir Cell Mol Biol 2001; 25(1):26–34.

161. Demirci G, Nashan B, Pichlmayr R. Fibrosis in chronic rejection of human liver allografts: expression patterns of transforming growth factor-TGFbeta1 and TGF-beta3. Transplantation 1996; 62(12):1776–1783.

162. Shihab FS, Yamamoto T, Nast CC, et al. Transforming growth factor-beta and matrix protein expression in acute and chronic rejection of human renal allografts. J Am Soc Nephrol 1995; 6(2):286–294.

163. Aziz T, Hasleton P, Hann AW, Yonan N, Deiraniya A, Hutchinson IV. Transforming growth factor beta in relation to cardiac allograft vasculopathy after heart transplantation. J Thorac Cardiovasc Surg 2000; 119(4, Pt 1):700–708.

164. Elssner A, Jaumann F, Dobmann S, et al. Elevated levels of interleukin-8 and transforming growth factor-beta in bronchoalveolar lavage fluid from patients with bronchiolitis obliterans syndrome: proinflammatory role of bronchial epithelial cells. Munich Lung Transplant Group. Transplantation 2000; 70(2):362–367.

165. El-Gamel A, Sim E, Hasleton P, et al. Transforming growth factor beta (TGF-beta) and obliterative bronchiolitis following pulmonary transplantation. J Heart Lung Transplant 1999; 18(9):828–837.

166. Charpin JM, Valcke J, Kettaneh L, Epardeau B, Stern M, Israel-Biet D. Peaks of transforming growth factor-beta mRNA in alveolar cells of lung transplant recipients as an early marker of chronic rejection. Transplantation 1998; 65(5):752–755.

167. Liu M, Suga M, Maclean AA, St George JA, Souza DW, Keshavjee S. Soluble transforming growth factor-beta type III receptor gene transfection inhibits

fibrous airway obliteration in a rat model of Bronchiolitis obliterans. Am J Respir Crit Care Med 2002; 165(3):419–423.

168. Massague J, Wotton D. Transcriptional control by the TGF-beta/Smad signaling system. EMBO J 2000; 19(8):1745–1754.

169. Taylor LM, Khachigian LM. Induction of platelet-derived growth factor B-chain expression by transforming growth factor-beta involves transactivation by Smads. J Biol Chem 2000; 275(22):16709–16716.

170. Holmes A, Abraham DJ, Sa S, Shiwen X, Black CM, Leask A. CTGF and SMADs, maintenance of scleroderma phenotype is independent of SMAD signaling. J Biol Chem 2001; 276(14):10594–10601.

171. Isono M, Chen S, Hong SW, Iglesias-de la Cruz MC, Ziyadeh FN. Smad pathway is activated in the diabetic mouse kidney and Smad3 mediates TGF-beta-induced fibronectin in mesangial cells. Biochem Biophys Res Commun 2002; 296(5):1356–1365.

172. Yuan W, Varga J. Transforming growth factor-beta repression of matrix metalloproteinase-1 in dermal fibroblasts involves Smad3. J Biol Chem 2001; 276(42):38502–38510.

173. Ramirez AM, Takagawa S, Sekosan M, Jaffe HA, Varga J, Roman J. Smad3 deficiency ameliorates experimental obliterative bronchiolitis in a heterotopic tracheal transplantation model. Am J Pathol 2004; 165(4):1223–1232.

174. Cambrey AD, Kwon OJ, Gray AJ, et al. Insulin-like growth factor I is a major fibroblast mitogen produced by primary cultures of human airway epithelial cells. Clin Sci (Lond) 1995; 89(6):611–617.

175. Goldstein RH, Poliks CF, Pilch PF, Smith BD, Fine A. Stimulation of collagen formation by insulin and insulin-like growth factor I in cultures of human lung fibroblasts. Endocrinology 1989; 124(2):964–970.

176. Rom WN, Basset P, Fells GA, Nukiwa T, Trapnell BC, Crysal RG. Alveolar macrophages release an insulin-like growth factor I-type molecule. J Clin Invest 1988; 82(5):1685–1693.

177. Homma S, Nagaoka I, Abe H, et al. Localization of platelet-derived growth factor and insulin-like growth factor I in the fibrotic lung. Am J Respir Crit Care Med 1995; 152(6, Pt 1):2084–2089.

178. Jones JI, Clemmons DR. Insulin-like growth factors and their binding proteins: biological actions. Endocrinol Rev 1995; 16(1):3–34.

179. Charpin JM, Stern M, Grenet D, Israel-Biet D. Insulinlike growth factor-1 in lung transplants with obliterative bronchiolitis. Am J Respir Crit Care Med 2000; 161(6):1991–1998.

180. Ross R, Raines EW, Bowen-Pope DF. The biology of platelet-derived growth factor. Cell 1986; 46(2):155–169.

181. Williams LT. Signal transduction by the platelet-derived growth factor receptor. Science 1989; 243(4898):1564–1570.

182. Heldin CH, Westermark B. Platelet-derived growth factor: three isoforms and two receptor types. Trends Genet 1989; 5(4):108–111.

183. Hertz MI, Henke CA, Nakhleh RE, et al. Obliterative bronchiolitis after lung transplantation: a fibroproliferative disorder associated with platelet-derived growth factor. Proc Natl Acad Sci USA 1992; 89(21):10385–10389.

184. Kallio EA, Koskinen PK, Aavik E, Buchdunger E, Lemstrom KB. Role of platelet-derived growth factor in obliterative bronchiolitis (chronic rejection) in the rat. Am J Respir Crit Care Med 1999; 160(4):1324–1332.
185. Defrances MC, Wolf HK, Michalopoulos GK, Zarnegar R. The presence of hepatocyte growth factor in the developing rat. Development 1992; 116(2):387–395.
186. Matsumoto K, Tajima H, Hamanoue M, Kohno S, Kinoshita T, Nakamura T. Identification and characterization of "injurin," an inducer of expression of the gene for hepatocyte growth factor. Proc Natl Acad Sci USA 1992; 89(9):3800–3804.
187. Aharinejad S, Taghavi S, Klepetko W, Abraham D. Prediction of lung-transplant rejection by hepatocyte growth factor. Lancet 2004; 363(9420): 1503–1508.
188. Rollins BJ. Chemokines. Blood 1997; 90(3):909–928.
189. Luster AD. Review articles: mechanisms of disease: chemokines—chemotactic cytokines that mediate inflammation. N Engl J Med 1998; 338(7):436–445.
190. Strieter RM, Kunkel SL. Chemokines and the lung. In: Crystal R, West J, Weibel E, Barnes PJ, eds. Lung: Scientific Foundations. 2nd. New York: Raven Press, 1977:155–186.
191. Bleul CC, Fuhlbrigge RC, Casasnovas JM, Aiuti A, Springer TA. A highly efficacious lymphocyte chemoattractant, stromal cell-derived factor 1 (SDF-1). J Exp Med 1996; 184(3):1101–1109 (see comments).
192. Loetscher M, Gerber B, Loetscher P, et al. Chemokine receptor specific for IP10 and mig: structure, function, and expression in activated T-lymphocytes. J Exp Med 1996; 184(3):963–969 (see comments).
193. Keane MP, Belperio JA, Arenberg DA, et al. IFN-gamma-inducible protein-10 attenuates bleomycin-induced pulmonary fibrosis via inhibition of angiogenesis. J Immunol 1999; 163(10):5686–5692 (in process citation).
194. Keane MP, Belperio JA, Moore TA, et al. Neutralization of the CXC chemokine, macrophage inflammatory protein-2, attenuates bleomycin-induced pulmonary fibrosis. J Immunol 1999; 162(9):5511–5518.
195. Moore BB, Arenberg DA, Addison CL, Keane MP, Strieter RM. Tumor angiogenesis is regulated by CXC chemokines. J Lab Clin Med 1998; 132(2):97–103.
196. Baggiolini M, Dewald B, Moser B. Human chemokines: an update. Annu Rev Immunol 1997; 15:675–705.
197. Robinson LA, Nataraj C, Thomas DW, et al. A role for fractalkine and its receptor (CX3CR1) in cardiac allograft rejection. J Immunol 2000; 165(11):6067–6072.
198. Fong AM, Robinson LA, Steeber DA, et al. Fractalkine and CX3CR1 mediate a novel mechanism of leukocyte capture, firm adhesion, and activation under physiologic flow. J Exp Med 1998; 188(8):1413–1419.
199. Pan Y, Lloyd C, Zhou H, et al. Neurotactin, a membrane-anchored chemokine upregulated in brain inflammation. Nature 1997; 387(6633):611–617. [Published erratum appears in Nature 1997; 389(6646):100.].
200. Bazan JF, Bacon KB, Hardiman G, et al. A new class of membrane-bound chemokine with a CX3C motif. Nature 1997; 385(6617):640–644.

201. Zlotnik A, Yoshie O. Chemokines: a new classification system and their role in immunity. Immunity 2000; 12(2):121–127.
202. Murphy PM, Baggiolini M, Charo IF, et al. International union of pharmacology. XXII. Nomenclature for chemokine receptors. Pharmacol Rev 2000; 52(1):145–176.
203. Segerer S, Nelson PJ, Schlondorff D. Chemokines, chemokine receptors, and renal disease: from basic science to pathophysiologic and therapeutic studies. J Am Soc Nephrol 2000; 11(1):152–176.
204. Uvama T, Winter JB, Groen G, Wildevuur CRH, Monden Y, Prop J. Late airway changes caused by chronic rejection in rat lung allografts. Transplantation 1992; 54:809–812.
205. Uyama T, Sakiyama S, Fukumoto T, et al. Graft-infiltrating cells in rat lung allograft with late airway damage. Transplant Proc 1995; 27(3):2118–2119.
206. Matsumura Y, Marchevsky A, Zuo XJ, Kass RM, Matloff JM, Jordan SC. Assessment of pathological changes associated with chronic allograft rejection and tolerance in two experimental models of rat lung transplantation. Transplantation 1995; 59(11):1509–1517.
207. Tazelaar HD, Prop J, Nieuwenhuis P, Billingham ME, Wildevuur CR. Airway pathology in the transplanted rat lung. Transplantation 1988; 45(5):864–869.
208. Hertz MI, Jessurun J, King MB, Savik SK, Murray JJ. Reproduction of the obliterative bronchiolitis lesion after heterotopic transplantation of mouse airways. Am J Pathol 1993; 142(6):1945–1951.
209. Riise GC, Williams A, Kjellstrom C, Schersten H, Andersson BA, Kelly FJ. Bronchiolitis obliterans syndrome in lung transplant recipients is associated with increased neutrophil activity and decreased antioxidant status in the lung. Eur Respir J 1998; 12(1):82–88.
210. Riise GC, Andersson BA, Kjellstrom C, et al. Persistent high BAL fluid granulocyte activation marker levels as early indicators of bronchiolitis obliterans after lung transplant. Eur Respir J 1999; 14(5):1123–1130.
211. Zheng L, Walters EH, Ward C, et al. Airway neutrophilia in stable and bronchiolitis obliterans syndrome patients following lung transplantation. Thorax 2000; 55(1):53–59.
212. Elssner A, Jaumann F, Dobmann S, et al. Elevated levels of interleukin-8 and transforming growth factor-beta in bronchoalveolar lavage fluid from patients with bronchiolitis obliterans syndrome: proinflammatory role of bronchial epithelial cells. Munich Lung Transplant Group. Transplantation 2000; 70(2):362–367.
213. Elssner A, Vogelmeier C. The role of neutrophils in the pathogenesis of obliterative bronchiolitis after lung transplantation. Transpl Infect Dis 2001; 3(3):168–176.
214. DiGiovine B, Lynch JP III, Martinez FJ, et al. Bronchoalveolar lavage neutrophilia is associated with obliterative bronchiolitis after lung transplantation: role of IL-8. J Immunol 1996; 157(9):4194–4202.
215. Suga M, Maclean AA, Keshavjee S, Fischer S, Moreira JM, Liu M. RANTES plays an important role in the evolution of allograft transplant-induced fibrous airway obliteration. Am J Respir Crit Care Med 2000; 162(5):1940–1948.

216. Belperio JA, Keane MP, Burdick MD, et al. Critical role for the chemokine MCP-1/CCR2 in the pathogenesis of bronchiolitis obliterans syndrome. J Clin Invest 2001; 108(4):547–556.

217. Farivar AS, Krishnadasan B, Naidu BV, Woolley SM, Mulligan MS. The role of the beta chemokines in experimental obliterative bronchiolitis. Exp Mol Pathol 2003; 75(3):210–216.

218. Gao W, Topham PS, King JA, et al. Targeting of the chemokine receptor CCR1 suppresses development of acute and chronic cardiac allograft rejection. J Clin Invest 2000; 105(1):35–44.

219. Fischereder M, Luckow B, Hocher B, et al. CC chemokine receptor 5 and renal-transplant survival. Lancet 2001; 357(9270):1758–1761.

220. Abdi R, Tran TB, Sahagun-Ruiz A, et al. Chemokine receptor polymorphism and risk of acute rejection in human renal transplantation. J Am Soc Nephrol 2002; 13(3):754–758.

221. Martinson JJ, Chapman NH, Rees DC, Liu YT, Clegg JB. Global distribution of the CCR5 gene 32-basepair deletion. Nat Genet 1997; 16(1):100–103.

222. Libert F, Cochaux P, Beckman G, et al. The deltaccr5 mutation conferring protection against HIV-1 in Caucasian populations has a single and recent origin in northeastern Europe. Hum Mol Genet 1998; 7(3):399–406.

223. Stephens JC, Reich DE, Goldstein DB, et al. Dating the origin of the CCR5-Delta32 AIDS-resistance allele by the coalescence of haplotypes. Am J Hum Genet 1998; 62(6):1507–1515.

224. Ruster M, Sperschneider H, Funfstuck R, Stein G, Grone HJ. Differential expression of beta-chemokines MCP-1 and RANTES and their receptors CCR1, CCR2, CCR5 in acute rejection and chronic allograft nephropathy of human renal allografts. Clin Nephrol 2004; 61(1):30–39.

225. Imai T, Baba M, Nishimura M, Kakizaki M, Takagi S, Yoshie O. The T cell-directed CC chemokine TARC is a highly specific biological ligand for CC chemokine receptor 4. J Biol Chem 1997; 272(23):15036–15042.

226. Campbell JJ, Haraldsen G, Pan J, et al. The chemokine receptor CCR4 in vascular recognition by cutaneous but not intestinal memory T cells. Nature 1999; 400(6746):776–780.

227. Luther SA, Cyster JG. Chemokines as regulators of T cell differentiation. Nat Immunol 2001; 2(2):102–107.

228. Alferink J, Lieberam I, Reindl W, et al. Compartmentalized production of CCL17 in vivo: strong inducibility in peripheral dendritic cells contrasts selective absence from the spleen. J Exp Med 2003; 197(5):585–599.

229. Slebos DJ, Postma DS, Koeter GH, Van Der Bij W, Boezen M, Kauffman HF. Bronchoalveolar lavage fluid characteristics in acute and chronic lung transplant rejection. J Heart Lung Transplant 2004; 23(5):532–540.

230. Fisher AJ, Donnelly SC, Hirani N, et al. Elevated levels of interleukin-8 in donor lungs is associated with early graft failure after lung transplantation. Am J Respir Crit Care Med 2001; 163(1):259–265.

231. De Perrot M, Sekine Y, Fischer S, et al. Interleukin-8 release during early reperfusion predicts graft function in human lung transplantation. Am J Respir Crit Care Med 2002; 165(2):211–215.

232. Belperio JA, Keane MP, Burdick MD, et al. Critical role for CXCR3 chemokine biology in the pathogenesis of Bronchiolitis obliterans syndrome. J Immunol 2002; 169(2):1037–1049.

233. Agostini C, Calabrese F, Rea F, et al. Cxcr3 and its ligand CXCL10 are expressed by inflammatory cells infiltrating lung allografts and mediate chemotaxis of T cells at sites of rejection. Am J Pathol 2001; 158(5):1703–1711.

234. Yun JJ, Fischbein MP, Whiting D, et al. The role of MIG/CXCL9 in cardiac allograft vasculopathy. Am J Pathol 2002; 161(4):1307–1313.

235. Whiting D, Hsieh G, Yun JJ, et al. Chemokine monokine induced by IFN-gamma/CXC chemokine ligand 9 stimulates T lymphocyte proliferation and effector cytokine production. J Immunol 2004; 172(12):7417–7424.

236. Miura M, Morita K, Kobayashi H, et al. Monokine induced by IFN-gamma is a dominant factor directing T cells into murine cardiac allografts during acute rejection. J Immunol 2001; 167(6):3494–3504.

237. Kapoor A, Morita K, Engeman TM, et al. Early expression of interferon-gamma inducible protein 10 and monokine induced by interferon-gamma in cardiac allografts is mediated by CD8+ T cells. Transplantation 2000; 69(6):1147–1155.

238. Koga S, Auerbach MB, Engeman TM, Novick AC, Toma H, Fairchild RL. T cell infiltration into class II MHC-disparate allografts and acute rejection is dependent on the IFN-gamma-induced chemokine Mig. J Immunol 1999; 163(9):4878–4885.

239. Hancock WW, Gao W, Csizmadia V, Faia KL, Shemmeri N, Luster AD. Donor-derived IP-10 initiates development of acute allograft rejection. J Exp Med 2001; 193(8):975–980.

240. Hancock WW, Lu B, Gao W, et al. Requirement of the chemokine receptor CXCR3 for acute allograft rejection. J Exp Med 2000; 192(10):1515–1520.

241. Kao J, Kobashigawa J, Fishbein MC, et al. Elevated serum levels of the CXCR3 chemokine ITAC are associated with the development of transplant coronary artery disease. Circulation 2003; 107(15):1958–1961.

# 33

# Pulmonary Physiology Posttransplant

**Marc Estenne**

*Chest Service and Thoracic Transplantation Unit, Erasme University Hospital,
Brussels School of Medicine, Brussels, Belgium*

## INTRODUCTION

Lung transplantation is now accepted as an appropriate treatment for selected patients with end-stage pulmonary disease. Over the last two decades, there has been growing evidence that several aspects of respiratory and exercise physiology present unique changes after lung transplantation. Many of these changes do not affect the clinical status of the patients, but some do; a typical example is the prominent limb muscle dysfunction that impairs the exercise capacity and does not allow the patients to fully benefit from the improvements in pulmonary function and gas exchange. This chapter presents an overview of a large number of studies on posttransplant respiratory and exercise physiology. It deals primarily with human studies because in most areas, physiological changes seen in experimental conditions differ from those occurring after human transplantation; in addition, it focuses on studies done in patients with well-functioning grafts and does not address alterations in physiology associated with specific complications [e.g., broncheolitis obliterans (BO)]. It should be emphasized that most of the studies discussed in this chapter require careful interpretation due to one or more of the following methodological limitations. The studies were frequently retrospective in design, involving a small number of patients with different types of transplants and a variety of pretransplant diseases. The rationale behind the selection of the control group (e.g., healthy subjects vs.

heart transplant recipients) was not always appropriately discussed. Most studies were primarily descriptive. Finally, very few studies provided long-itudinal data obtained pre- and posttransplant, which made it difficult to interpret posttransplant abnormalities.

## EFFECTS OF PULMONARY DENERVATION

Lung transplantation severs both the efferent and the afferent neural con-nections between the lung and the central nervous system, transmitted through the vagus and sympathetic nerves, which both enter the lung at the hilum. Lung transplant recipients may therefore represent a unique model to study the physiological effects of chronic loss of afferent neural information from the lung in humans. However, the validity of this model depends on the assumption that human lungs, unlike canine (1,2) and rodent (3,4) lungs, do not undergo afferent reinnervation after surgery. This assumption is supported by histologic studies of human transplanted lungs (5) and by the following observations made in lung transplant recipients: (i) the classic Hering–Breuer reflex is lost (6), (ii) there is a marked decrease in the cough response to various stimuli (discussed later), (iii) the inhibition of muscle sympathetic nerve activity (MSNA) that follows resumption of breathing after breath-holding (and is mediated, in part, by vagal afferent input from the lung) is decreased (7), (iv) there is a marked attenuation of respiratory sinus arrhythmia (7,8), and (v) intravenous injection of lobeline, which is a potent stimulus of C fibers, does not evoke noxious sensations (9). In the latter study, three patients who were studied 12 months or more after surgery reported some noxious sensations, suggesting that reinnervation of pulmonary receptors may occur in some long-term transplant recipients. However, when present, this reinnervation seems only partial because the sensations reported by the three patients were of less intensity than those experienced by normal controls (9).

### Control of Breathing at Rest

Despite vagal interruption, the resting breathing pattern of lung transplant recipients is no different from that of normal subjects (provided there are no concurrent restrictive or obstructive ventilatory defects) (10,11). The stabi-lity of tidal volume during postural changes is maintained (12). The duration of voluntary breath-holding is not substantially altered (13). There are no disturbances in sleep architecture and oxyhemoglobin saturation, and sleep-disordered events are no more frequent than in normal subjects (10,11). The only significant alteration that was reported in the patients was a less effective than normal coupling between mechanical inflation and neural inspiratory activity during non–rapid eye movement (NREM) sleep (14). Altogether, these studies thus indicate that in humans neural afferent information from the lung does not contribute significantly to the regulation of resting breathing during wakefulness and sleep.

## Control of Breathing During Exercise

Several studies (15–21) have shown that the slope of the relationships between ventilation and oxygen uptake (the ventilatory equivalent for oxygen) or carbon dioxide output (the ventilatory equivalent for carbon dioxide) is greater in lung transplant recipients than in normal subjects. This increased ventilatory response has been attributed to lung denervation causing loss of negative feedback from either vagal (15) or sympathetic afferents (16). However, an increased ventilation in relation to oxygen uptake or carbon dioxide output has also been reported in cardiac transplant recipients who have intact pulmonary innervation (18,19,22,23). In these patients, the increased ventilation has been attributed to peripheral muscle dysfunction and early onset of anaerobic metabolism. As discussed in the section on limb muscle function, such peripheral factors are also present in lung transplant recipients and may contribute to exercise hyperventilation. Data regarding the pattern of breathing during exercise are conflicting. Sciurba and colleagues (23) reported that compared to heart transplant recipients, heart–lung transplantation (HLT) recipients have a slower respiratory rate and a deeper tidal volume response during increasing levels of exercise. This abnormal pattern of breathing was attributed to disruption of pulmonary vagal afferents. Subsequent studies found, however, that respiratory rate and tidal volume in HLT recipients were either similar to, or greater than, those of normal subjects (15,16). Methodological limitations likely explain these discrepancies between studies (described earlier).

## Response to Hypoxia and Hypercapnia

Early studies of HLT recipients suggested that disruption of vagal pathways blunted the ventilatory response to hypercapnia (in particular the breathing frequency response) (24–26), whereas the ventilatory response to hypoxia was maintained (25). These patients, however, had restricted lung volumes, and subsequent studies of recipients with near-normal lung volumes showed normal ventilatory responses (27,28) and normal shortening of inspiratory time during hypercapnia (29).

## Response to Loading

The finding by Duncan et al. (28) that transplant recipients with restricted lung volumes exhibited a reduced response of tidal volume to hypercapnia suggested that, under loaded conditions, afferent information from pulmonary vagal receptors is needed for a normal regulation of inspiratory timing and an appropriate ventilatory response. This is consistent with the observation of Pellegrino et al. (30) that when an expiratory threshold load is imposed during exercise, healthy subjects defend inspiratory duration, but lung transplant recipients prolong inspiration and decrease breathing frequency.

On the other hand, Sciurba and colleagues (31) have reported that transplant recipients with airflow obstruction due to BO have a greater increase in respiratory rate and a slower increment in tidal volume during exercise than transplant recipients without BO. Because this response is similar to that of nontransplanted patients with chronic respiratory impairment, it was suggested that mechanisms outside pulmonary vagal afferents are responsible for the development of a rapid shallow breathing pattern in response to loading (31). The apparent discrepancy between these studies may be related to the different experimental conditions (hypercapnia vs. exercise) and to the different types of respiratory load: four of the six patients studied by Duncan et al. (28) had evidence of extraparenchymal restriction, Pellegrino et al. (30) used an externally applied expiratory load, and all four patients studied by Sciurba et al. (31) had airflow obstruction.

## Other Reflex Responses

Additional studies in lung transplant recipients have demonstrated the integrity of several respiratory reflex responses. These include (i) the neuro-mechanical inhibitory effect of mechanical ventilation on respiratory muscle activity (32), (ii) the inhibition of inspiratory muscle activity during inspiratory occlusion (33), (iii) the generation of respiratory-related evoked potentials by inspiratory occlusion (34), (iv) the tachycardiac response to hypoxia (35) and adenosine infusion (36), (v) the excitatory effect of inspiratory flow rate on breathing frequency during mechanical ventilation (37), and (vi) the influence of respiratory phase (38) and apnea (7) on MSNA. These observations may be interpreted as indicating that these reflex responses depend more on afferent information originating in the chest wall and the respiratory muscles than on pulmonary vagal afferent information. However, unless stretch receptors in the airways above the anastomosis are blocked with airway anesthesia (12,32), a role played by vagal information originating from these receptors cannot be totally excluded.

## Cough and Mucociliary Clearance

A more clinically relevant consequence of afferent vagal denervation is impairment of the cough response to airway irritants. During fiber-optic bronchoscopy, mechanical probing of the bronchi distal to the anastomosis induces less coughing than in nontransplanted patients. Similarly, the cough response to ultrasonically nebulized distilled water or to extract of red pepper (Capsaicin) is strikingly diminished compared to that of normal subjects (39,40). Afferent denervation also diminishes the chronic cough associated with gastroesophageal reflux (41). Transplant recipients may thus be insensitive to microaspiration, which may contribute to the high incidence of bacterial infections, and may be a risk factor for BO (42–44).

There is evidence that mucociliary clearance is impaired after lung transplantation (45,46). In one study, the clearance time of a technetium-labeled aerosol was nearly doubled compared to the clearance rate in normal controls (45). Of course, loss of cough reflex itself will delay clearance of an aerosol. Moreover, passage across the tracheal or bronchial anastomosis is delayed because of interruption of the ciliary carpet. Even well-healed anastomoses are often covered by a layer of white fibrous tissue replacing normal, pink respiratory mucosa. Ciliary function itself (e.g., ciliary beat frequency) may be impaired (47,48), but the mechanism of this alteration is unclear. In one study (47), epithelial abnormalities including ciliary dysfunction were observed both proximal and distal to the anastomosis, whereas in another study (48), reduced ciliary beat frequency was found in the transplanted, but not in the native, bronchi.

A unique phenomenon in airway function is observed in patients with cystic fibrosis (CF). In these individuals, the bioelectric and pharmacological characteristics of the bronchial mucosa below the anastomosis are similar to those found in normal individuals and in non-CF lung transplant recipients, whereas above the anastomosis, bronchial epithelial abnormalities persist (49).

### Respiratory Sensations

Very few data on respiratory sensation after lung transplantation are available. Studies have reported unaltered perception of breathlessness during exercise (15,16,50), and during methacholine-induced bronchoconstriction (51). The detection of an inspiratory resistive load is similar in HLT recipients and normal subjects (52), but one study suggested that the intensity of respiratory sensations was decreased (53). The sensation of breathlessness/ air hunger evoked by injections of lobeline (9) and elicited by voluntary breath-holding (13) is similar in transplant recipients and normal subjects.

## PULMONARY FUNCTION AND GAS EXCHANGE

### Response to Infection and Rejection

Shortly after the introduction of lung transplantation in clinical practice in the early 1980s, it was recognized that pulmonary function is sensitive to complications affecting the allograft. Several studies reported that both acute infection and rejection can produce an obstructive ventilatory defect (Fig. 1) (54–58), and progressive airflow obstruction was identified as the functional hallmark of BO, which is the manifestation of chronic allograft rejection (59,60). As a result, regular measurements of spirometry were proposed as a noninvasive tool to monitor the function of the transplanted lung (61,62).

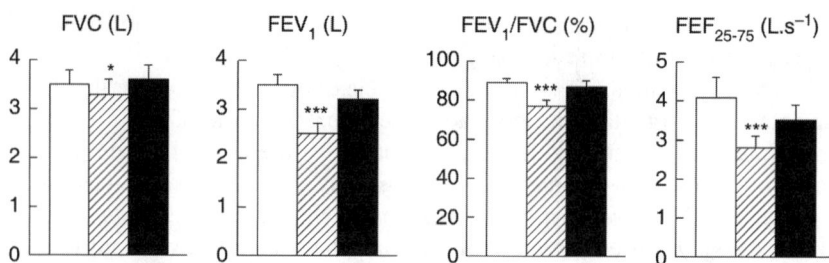

**Figure 1**   Average values (±SE) for FVC, FEV$_1$, FEV$_1$/FVC, and FEF$_{25-75}$ during 16 acute episodes of infection or rejection of the allograft in 13 HLT recipients. Values before (*open bars*), at the time of diagnosis (*shaded bars*), and 25 ± 5 days after (*closed bars*) the episodes are shown. *$P < 0.05$, ***$P < 0.001$ at the time of diagnosis versus before the episodes. *Abbreviations*: FVC, forced vital capacity; FEV$_1$, forced expiratory volume in one second, FEF$_{25-75}$, forced midexpiratory flow rate; HLT, heart–lung transplantation. *Source*: From Ref. 58.

However, the value of such functional monitoring for the detection of acute complications is limited by at least two factors. First, the definition of a significant change in forced expiratory volume in one second (FEV$_1$) from baseline is calculated from the intrasubject variability of the measurement, which is influenced by the time elapsed since surgery, the type of surgical procedure, and the frequency of the measurement. For example, a retrospective review of sequential spirometry measurements after lung transplantation revealed a high degree of variability during the first postoperative year, due to increasing values for forced vital capacity (FVC) and FEV$_1$ (63). After the first year, the value for significant change in FEV$_1$ was 8.9% after bilateral lung transplantation (BLT) and HLT and 13.4% after single-lung transplantation (SLT). These figures, however, may not apply to patients who measure their spirometry on a daily basis. In a study using home monitoring of spirometry by an internet-based telemonitoring system in HLT and BLT recipients (64), the intrasubject variability of FEV$_1$ measurements was much decreased, resulting in a value for significant change of only 6%; this suggests that by performing spirometry on a daily basis, patients may become very reproducible in their spirometric measurements.

The second factor that limits the value of spirometry to monitor the function of the graft is the relatively low sensitivity of pulmonary function for the detection of acute infection and/or rejection. In patients with HLT and BLT, a 10% drop in FEV$_1$ was reported to have an ~75% sensitivity for the detection of these complications (57,61), and this value was not improved by using an Internet-based home telemonitoring system (64). In patients with SLT, the sensitivity of a 10% drop in FEV$_1$ was even smaller, ranging between 31% and 62% according to the preoperative diagnosis (65).

In terms of specificity, lung function is not helpful to distinguish between infection and rejection.

## Stable Lung Transplant Recipients

### Bilateral and Heart–Lung Transplantation

Most BLT and HLT recipients achieve normal static lung volumes, although FVC and total lung capacity (TLC) may not completely normalize (66,67). This mild restrictive defect is partly related to the effects of sternotomy and thoracotomy, since lung volumes tend to improve during the first year after surgery (68–73). The persistent restriction observed in some patients thereafter is not related to an increased lung elastic recoil since the lung pressure–volume curve is normal (74,75). A contribution of inspiratory muscle weakness has been suggested (74) (see section on chest wall and respiratory muscles).

The postoperative TLC is unaffected by the disease of the recipient and by the size of the donor lung. By one year after surgery, recipients have TLC values within the predicted range, even if there are large disparities between the donor predicted TLC and the recipient preoperative or predicted TLC (69,75). Thus, it is most appropriate to use the recipients' predicted lung volumes as the normal values after transplantation, and the best method of matching donor and recipient volumes is to use their respective predicted TLC values (69,76).

In contrast to TLC, functional residual capacity (FRC) and residual volume (RV) values achieved after BLT or HLT may be influenced by the preoperative disease (69,75,77). Whereas patients transplanted for primary pulmonary hypertension (PPH) have normal or near-normal FRC and RV values (69,77), patients transplanted for diseases that produce chronic hyperinflation (e.g., CF or emphysema) show a persistent increase in FRC (range 130–141% of predicted) and RV (range 151–164% of predicted) (Fig. 2) (77,78). This alteration is not seen in all patients, but when present, it does not improve with time (78). The increase in FRC is not related to a decrease in lung elastic recoil, but it appears to relate to persistent hyperinflation of the chest wall (i.e., corresponding to a leftward shift of the chest wall pressure–volume curve).

Measurements of the anteroposterior diameter of the rib cage at FRC averaged 12.1 cm in transplant recipients with CF as compared with only 9.5 cm in patients with PPH (77). Thus, some patients with emphysema and CF may have preoperative changes in rib cage shape that persist in part after transplantation and lead to persistent increases in FRC and RV.

Apart from static lung volumes, other parameters of respiratory function are remarkably intact after BLT or HLT. There is no evidence of airflow obstruction; in fact, the $FEV_1/FVC$ ratio may be higher and airway resistance may be lower than in nontransplanted subjects, reflecting

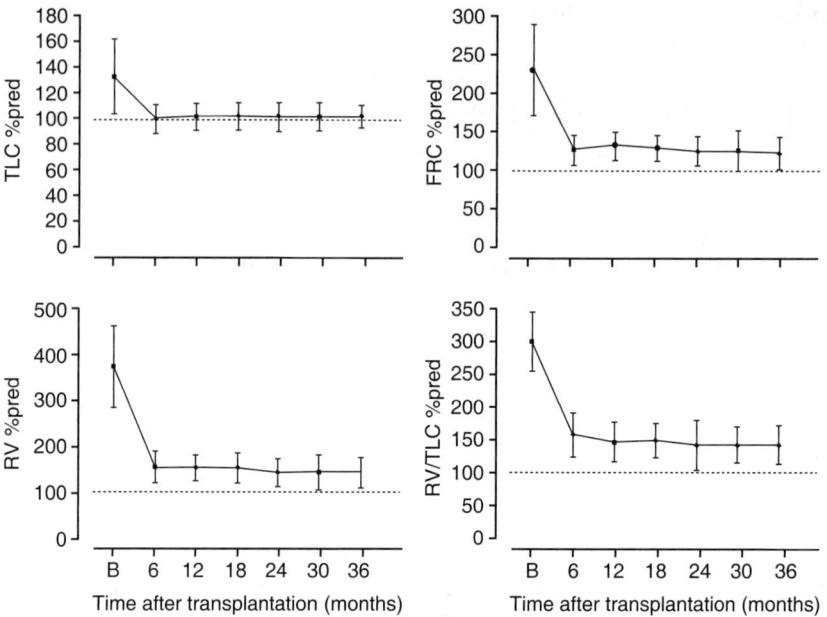

**Figure 2**  Average values (±SE) for TLC, FRC, RV, and RV/TLC before (*B*) and at six-month intervals after HLT or BLT. Predicted values are those of the recipient. Note that FRC, RV, and RV/TLC remain greater than predicted after surgery. *Abbreviations*: TLC, total lung capacity; FRC, functional residual capacity; RV, residual volume; HLT, heart–lung transplantation; BLT, bilateral lung transplantation. *Source*: From Ref. 78.

denervation of the airways with loss of resting vagal bronchomotor tone (79,80). Gas exchange is normal (66).

A few studies in HLT and BLT recipients have assessed the distribution of ventilation using single-breath washouts. Two groups have reported that the slope of the alveolar plateau for nitrogen was normal (58,81), but one study found an increased slope in 82% of the patients (67). This alteration could represent an early sign of BO (58,81,82), but the cross-sectional design of the study (67) did not allow the authors to determine what percentage of their patients eventually developed this complication.

### Single-Lung Transplantation

Pulmonary function in SLT recipients is highly dependent on physiologic interactions with the diseased native lung. For example, in SLT performed for emphysema, mediastinal shift secondary to overdistention of the native emphysematous lung may impair gas exchange and hemodynamics after surgery (83–85). In a single-center study (86), risk factors for early graft failure associated with native lung hyperinflation included a higher preoperative pulmonary artery pressure, a higher transpulmonary gradient, a higher RV, and a lower $FEV_1$, but this observation was not confirmed in a subsequent report (87). When early graft failure or reperfusion injury occurs, mechanical ventilation with positive and expiratory pressure (PEEP) via a single-lumen endotracheal tube can also accentuate the native lung hyperinflation and the mediastinal shift. Several approaches have been proposed to manage acute native lung hyperinflation including differential lung ventilation (88,89), lung volume reduction surgery (LVRS) (86,90–92), lobectomy (86) or pneumonectomy of the native lung (93), and retransplantation (86).

The thorax remains mildly hyperinflated after SLT for emphysema, with TLC ranging from 110% to 126% predicted, FRC ranging from 100% to 161% predicted, and RV ranging from 90% to 170% predicted (76,94,95). The transplant lung invariably appears radiographically "smaller" than the native hyperinflated lung, with the mediastinum shifted toward the graft (Fig. 3); in two previous studies, the angle of mediastinal shift measured by computed tomography (CT) scan averaged 20–25° at FRC (95,97). Although the degree of mediastinal shift is generally stable over time (95), a small subset of patients may show progressive worsening of native lung hyperinflation, leading to clinical and functional changes similar to those produced by BO (98); in this context, LVRS may temporarily improve airflow obstruction, 6-min walking distance, and dyspnea (99).

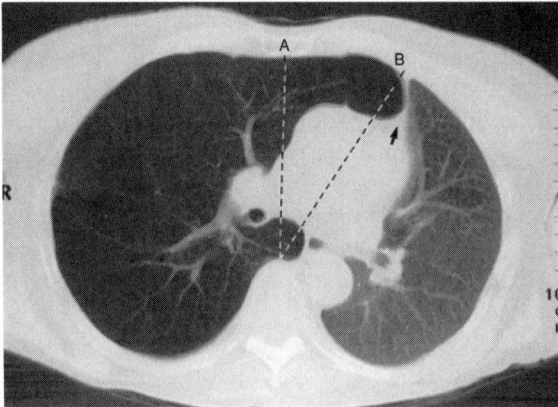

**Figure 3** Representative axial computed tomography slice in an emphysematous patient with a left transplant. The arrow indicates location of the anterior mediastinal line. Note the shift of the mediastinum toward the graft. Line A is the midsagittal line, and line B was drawn from the vertebral body to the anterior mediastinal line. *Source*: From Ref. 96.

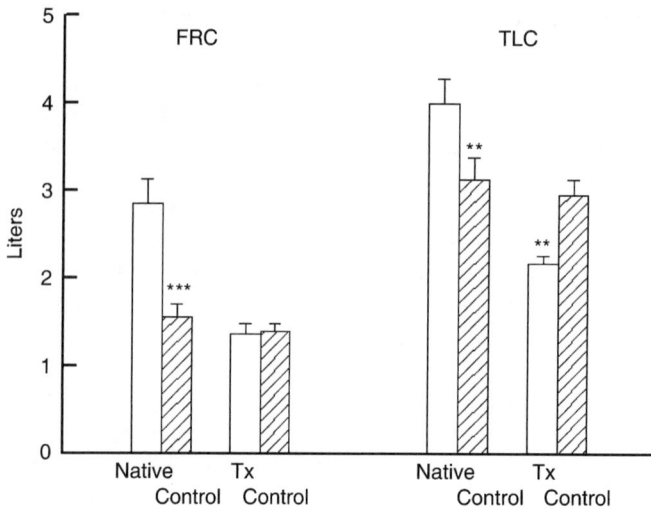

**Figure 4** Average (±SE) values of TLC and FRC of the native lung and of the graft (Tx) in 10 patients who underwent SLT for emphysema (*open bars*). Values are compared with those obtained on the ipsilateral side in 10 matched normal control subjects (*hatched bars*). Statistical differences are shown only for adjacent bars. $^{**}P < 0.005$; $^{***}P < 0.001$. *Abbreviations*: TLC, total lung capacity; FRC, functional residual capacity; SLT, single-lung transplantation. *Source*: From Ref. 95.

Three studies have used standard chest radiograph (94) or CT scan (95,97) to assess the TLC of the graft and the native lung. On average, the graft and native lung had TLC values corresponding to 33% to 39% and 55 % to 75% of predicted TLC, respectively, and the TLC of the graft was decreased by ~20% when compared to the TLC of the ipsilateral lung of normal controls (95). These observations indicate that the presence of the hyperinflated native lung may cause functional restriction of the transplant (Fig. 4) (100). In a recent study using optoelectronic plethysmography, De Groote et al. (97) showed that these unequal lung volumes on the transplanted versus the native side do not translate into differences in the volumes of the two hemithoraces, i.e., differences in the static volumes of the graft and the native lung are accommodated primarily by the shift of the mediastinum.

In contrast to TLC, the FRC of the graft is similar to the FRC of the ipsilateral lung of normal controls (Fig. 4) (95). This observation is best explained by overexpansion of the rib cage at end-expiration on the transplanted side, resulting from the interdependence between the two sides of the cage. This overexpansion likely offsets the restrictive effect of the mediastinal shift on the graft FRC (95).

Despite these volume discrepancies, there is marked clinical improvement, without significant differences in physiologic parameters in patients

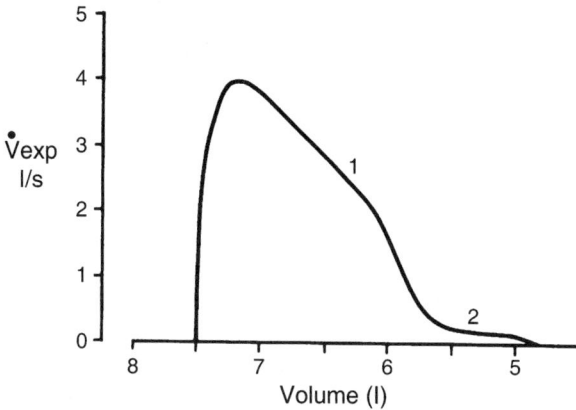

**Figure 5** MEFV curve obtained in one typical patient with SLT for emphysema. Note the biphasic pattern of expiratory flow with an initial high flow phase coming from the graft (*line 1*) followed by a low flow phase coming from the native lung (*line 2*). *Abbreviations*: MEFV, maximum expiratory flow volume, Vexp, expiratory flow; SLT, single-lung transplantation.

undergoing right versus left SLT (68). Spirometry and arterial partial pressure for oxygen ($PaO_2$) improve considerably. Typically, for patients with pulmonary emphysema, $FEV_1$ is multiplied by two to three times and $FEV_1/FVC$ and diffusion capacity for carbon monoxide (DLCO) double (68,72,101,102). Mean $PaO_2$ at rest is close to normal and patients no longer require supplemental oxygen at rest or during exercise. These improvements are sustained in the first few years after transplantation (68,101). A biphasic pattern of expiratory flow is often observed in the flow–volume curve (Fig. 5) (103–105). The initial high flow phase derives from the transplanted lung, and the terminal low flow phase from the native, emphysematous lung. In the absence of anastomotic stenosis, the flow-limiting segment is located in the native bronchus, immediately proximal to the anastomosis (103). Using the conventional approach of superimposing tidal and maximal flow–volume curves, Martinez et al. (50) demonstrated flow limitation at rest in some patients; however, using the more aocurate negative inspiratory pressure method, Murciano et al. (104) found evidence of flow limitation in only one of 13 SLT recipients who were studied at rest in the seated and supine postures.

In SLT performed for pulmonary fibrosis, there are fewer adverse physiologic interactions with the diseased native lung, since the increased elastic recoil of the latter makes the mediastinum move away from the graft. In one study, at one year after transplantation, FVC was 69%, $FEV_1$ 79%, and DLCO 62% of predicted (106). $PaO_2$ was 87 mmHg, and supplemental oxygen was no longer needed by any patient after transplantation. In another study, patients showed normal TLC, but mildly reduced FRC and RV (76). Lung compliance expressed as *K* was mildly reduced (73% predicted); DLCO was also reduced (60% predicted), but transfer coefficient was normal (94%) (76).

## FUNCTIONAL IMAGING OF THE GRAFT

In patients with bilateral grafts who are clinically stable, ventilation ($V_A$) and perfusion (Q) scans show a homogenous pattern and a symmetrical distribution between the two lungs (107). In addition, single-photon emission computerized tomography (SPECT) studies in SLT recipients have shown normal regional distribution of $V_A/Q$ relationships in the graft (108,109). In these patients, most (~70%) of the perfusion is distributed to the transplanted side, whatever the disease affecting the native lung (68,76,101,108, 110,111) and irrespective of the presence or absence of pulmonary hypertension before surgery (110). Ventilation is also predominantly distributed to the graft in patients with parenchymal lung diseases (68,76,102), but it is equally divided between the native and transplanted lung in patients undergoing transplantation for PPH, which results in substantial $V_A/Q$ mismatching (112). The preferential ventilation of the graft in patients with emphysema results from tidal displacement of the mediastinum toward the native lung during inspiration (i.e., from a decrease in the degree of mediastinal shift during inspiration), and not from asymmetrical changes in chest wall volume (Fig. 6) (97). The use of SPECT (113) and [201]Thallium scintigraphy (114) has been advocated for the diagnosis of infection and/or acute rejection, and two studies have suggested that perfusion (115) or ventilation (116) scintigraphy may be a useful adjunct in the early diagnosis of BO.

Recently, several studies using [3]He-magnetic resonance imaging ([3]He-MRI) in lung transplant recipients have been published by the group of Kauczor et al. (117–120). This innovative technique allows separate measurements of lung volumes and regional ventilation in the graft and the native lung, and visualization of ventilatory defects. It has been suggested that it might contribute to the early detection of BO (117), but the complex and expensive nature of the technique makes it ill-suited for wide clinical use.

## CHEST WALL AND RESPIRATORY MUSCLES

Phrenic nerve injury producing partial or complete paralysis of one or both hemidiaphragms can occur during the transplant procedure. The incidence varies widely from 3% to 43%, which is explained by differences in the techniques used to diagnose phrenic nerve injury and/or diaphragm paralysis (121–124). The complication seems to be more frequent after HLT, than BLT or SLT (124), and it results in prolonged postoperative mechanical ventilation, increased need for tracheostomy, and persistent lung volume restriction in the long term (122,124).

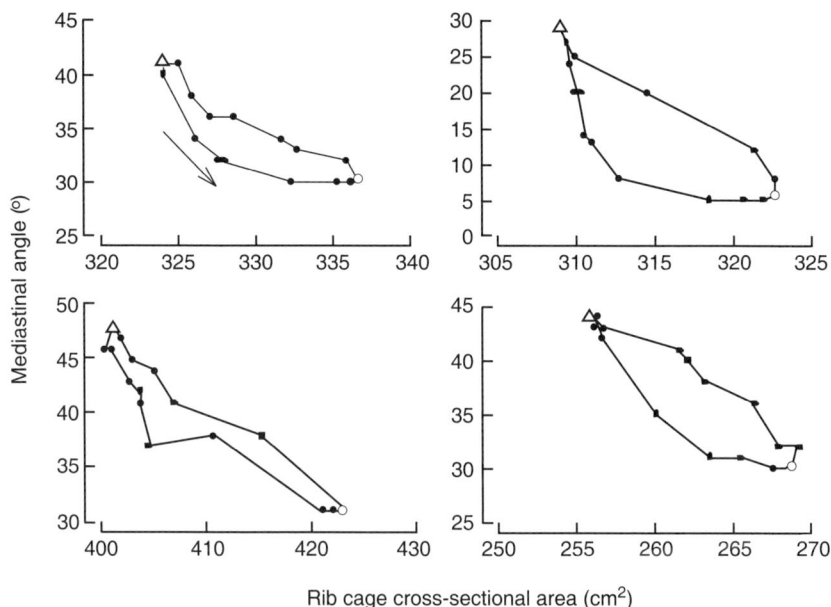

**Figure 6** Changes in the angle of mediastinal shift toward the graft (*y-axis*) and in rib cage cross-sectional area (*x-axis*) during a tidal breath in four representative patients with SLT for emphysema. The open triangle corresponds to end-expiration and the open circle to end-inspiration; the arrow indicates the inspiratory phase of the loop. Note that inspiration is accompanied by a reduction in mediastinal angle, i.e., by displacement of the mediastinum toward the native lung. *Abbreviation*: SLT, single-lung transplantation. *Source*: From Ref. 97.

In patients without phrenic nerve injury, inspiratory muscle strength assessed by measuring either mouth [maximal inspiratory mouth pressure (MIP)] or esophageal pressure during maximal static inspiratory efforts has been reported to be markedly decreased in one study in HLT recipients (23), but other studies in HLT, BLT, or SLT recipients found either normal (77,125) or only mildly decreased (20,66) inspiratory muscle strength. In keeping with these observations, Pinet et al. (126) recently reported normal values of twitch transdiaphragmatic pressure and diaphragm mass in a group of patients with HLT or BLT for CF (Fig. 7). In these patients, as in patients with emphysema, the decrease in the degree of hyperinflation after transplantation produces an increase in the pressure-generating capacity of the diaphragm (126–128), which may contribute to the reduction in neural drive to the muscle during inspiratory threshold loading (129).

Measurement of diaphragm dimensions using CT demonstrated that after SLT for emphysema, the surface areas of the whole diaphragm and of the dome are smaller on the transplanted side than on the native side,

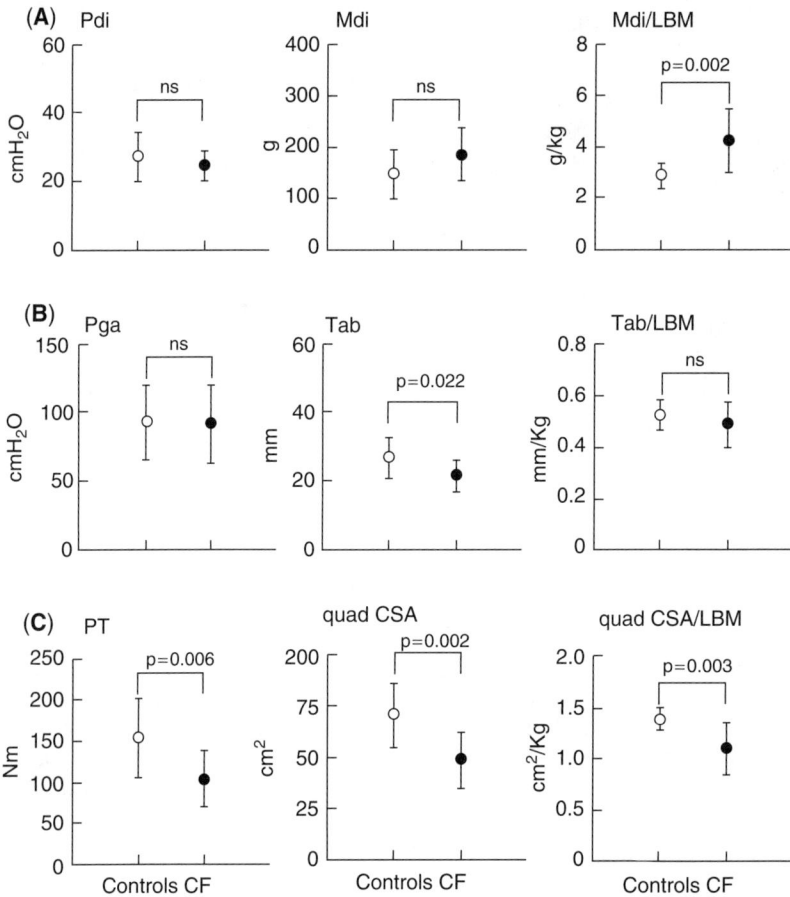

**Figure 7**  (**A**) Average values of transdiaphragmatic pressure (Pdi) elicited by twitch stimulation of the phrenic nerves in 11 transplanted CF patients and 12 controls, and of diaphragm mass (Mdi) in 12 CF patients and 12 controls. (**B**) Average changes in gastric pressure (Pga) elicited by stimulation of the abdominal muscles in 11 transplanted CF patients and 12 controls, and average values of cumulated thickness of the abdominal muscles (Tab) in 12 CF patients and 12 controls. (**C**) Average values of quadriceps peak torque (PT) and cross-sectional area (quad CSA) in 12 transplanted CF patients and 12 controls. *Abbreviations*: CF, cystic fibrosis; LBM, lean body mass. *Source*: From Ref. 127.

reflecting the shift of the mediastinum, and that the curvature of the diaphragm on the transplanted side returns to normal (Fig. 8) (96).

The observation that inspiratory muscle strength measured at RV or FRC is normal or only mildly decreased does not imply that patients are able

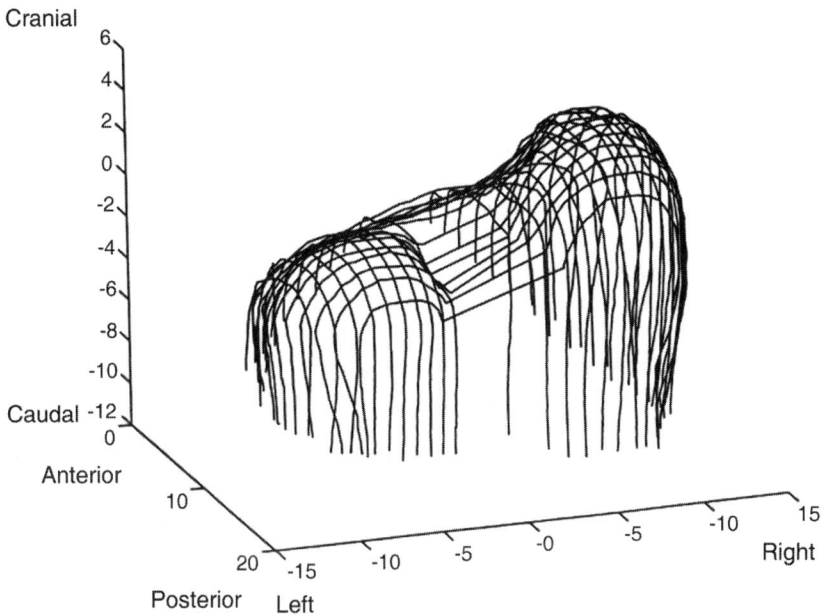

**Figure 8** Three-dimensional reconstruction of the diaphragm at FRC in a patient with a right SLT for emphysema. *Abbreviations*: FRC, functional residual capacity; SLT, single-lung transplantation. *Source*: From Ref. 96.

to generate normal inspiratory pressures at TLC. In this regard, the linear correlation found by Glanville et al. (74) in HLT recipients between MIP and TLC (% predicted) suggested that inspiratory muscle weakness may contribute to the inability of some patients to achieve a normal TLC. After SLT for emphysema, esophageal pressure at TLC is less negative than normal (94), which may contribute to decreasing the volume of the transplanted lung at full inflation (95). Because of the interdependence between the two sides of the chest wall, the hyperinflation on the side of the native lung might make the inspiratory muscles on the side of the graft operate at shorter than optimal lengths, and hence reduce their pressure-generating capacity.

Fewer data are available on expiratory muscle strength after lung transplantation. Three studies showed a reduction in maximal expiratory mouth pressure (MEP) (20,23,125), but a recent study in patients who had undergone HLT or BLT for CF reported normal values of abdominal muscle strength (Fig. 7) (127). Because this study used a nonvolitional technique (magnetic stimulation of the lower thoracic nerve roots), the low values of MEP reported earlier may be related to the inability of the patients to perform the required task. In any case, the results of Pinet et al.

(127) suggest that expiratory muscle weakness, if present, would be due to loss of function in the intercostal muscles and not in the abdominal muscles.

## BRONCHIAL HYPERREACTIVITY

Several studies have reported nonspecific bronchial hyperreactivity (NSBHR) to methacholine or histamine in SLT, BLT, and HLT recipients (40,51,79,130–135). In general, NSBHR was unrelated to the level of $FEV_1$, the time after transplantation, the presence of acute allograft rejection, or a history of asthma in the donor (131), but it tended to be less marked in SLT than in BLT or HLT recipients (130). One study suggested that NSBHR develops only when there is inflammation in the airways (136), but subsequent studies failed to demonstrate any association between NSBHR and airway inflammation (40,134). NSBHR is not a clinical problem after lung transplantation, and diurnal variation in $FEV_1$ is similar to that seen in normal subjects (137). It is remarkable that the presence and degree of NSBHR are highly variable between subjects and within subjects over time (131,135). In one study of four serial methacholine challenges during the first year after transplantation, 62% of patients had exclusively negative challenges, 19% had only one positive challenge, 10% had two positive challenges, 10% had three positive challenges, and no patient had a positive challenge on all occasions (135).

Among possible explanations for posttransplant NSBHR, the mechanism to which most attention has been paid is the suggestion that loss of vagal stimulation to the bronchi results in hypersensitivity of muscarinic receptors. However, an in vitro study of bronchial tissue from HLT recipients revealed normal cholinergic responsiveness, no change in receptors, and normal function of postganglionic cholinergic nerves (138). Furthermore, if NSBHR resulted from denervation hypersensitivity, it is not clear why it should be present in some patients and not in others, and why it should vary in intensity in a given patient from one testing to the next. Other local mechanisms may be involved, such as the peptidergic neurotransmitters of the nonadrenergic, noncholinergic system. Support for this derives from an animal model of lung transplantation demonstrating expression of "sensory neuropeptide" genes despite denervation, including substance P and its main receptor neurokinin-1 (139). In addition, patients with lung denervation may still develop cough in response to angiotensin-converting enzyme inhibitors, supporting local tachykinins as potential mediators (140).

In HLT recipients, methacholine-induced bronchoconstriction makes the distribution of ventilation more heterogenous in the peripheral airways (79). This involvement of peripheral airways may explain why assessing NSBHR in these patients may provide information on the presence of a pathologic process affecting the bronchioles, and hence on the risk of progression to BO.

## EXERCISE PHYSIOLOGY

Although improvements in exercise tolerance and level of physical activity occur after lung transplantation, results of formal exercise testing have shown that these improvements are relatively modest. Despite satisfactory allograft function, the vast majority of transplant recipients have a persistent exercise impairment as defined by lower than normal values of $VO_{2 peak}$ and maximum achievable work rate (15–17,20,21,23,127,141–152). The degree of exercise tolerance is remarkably similar, regardless of the underlying disease (145) and type of transplant procedure (17,66,141). Typically, recipients of HLT, SLT, and BLT have values of $VO_{2 peak}$ decreased to 40% to 60% of predicted during the first year after surgery, with no significant improvement over time. There is a trend for aerobic performance to be slightly higher in HLT and BLT than in SLT recipients, but in most studies the difference did not reach statistical significance. The reduced $VO_{2 peak}$ is accompanied by low peak cardiac frequency, low $O_2$ pulse at peak exercise, high respiratory exchange ratio, and early lactic acidosis (149).

There is no significant ventilatory limitation to exercise in most patients (17,149), but recipients of SLT tend to use a greater percentage of their ventilatory reserve at peak exercise and may have evidence of expiratory flow limitation and dynamic hyperinflation (50,150). Gas exchange is well preserved, although some SLT recipients (in particular those operated for pulmonary fibrosis and pulmonary vascular disease) may show slight increases in alveolar–arterial pressure gradient for $O_2$ and decreases in $O_2$ saturation at peak exercise (17,141,142,149). The ratio of dead space to tidal volume is often elevated at rest and does not decrease toward normal values during exercise due to abnormal ventilation/perfusion matching related to the presence of the native lung (143).

HLT recipients have prominent abnormalities in cardiac performance during exercise, characterized by a blunted chronotropic response due to denervation, an insufficient rise in stroke volume and cardiac output, and an abnormal rise in pulmonary filling pressures (Fig. 9) (21,153); very similar alterations are observed in heart transplant recipients (154). In contrast, most SLT and BLT recipients have normal cardiac and hemodynamic responses to exercise (147,148), though an abnormal rise in mean pulmonary artery pressure and capillary wedge pressure may occasionally be seen in the former (144). The blunted chronotropic response reported by Systrom et al. (147) and others (66,141,142) after SLT and BLT may be related, at least in part, to the reduction in exercising muscle mass (discussed later).

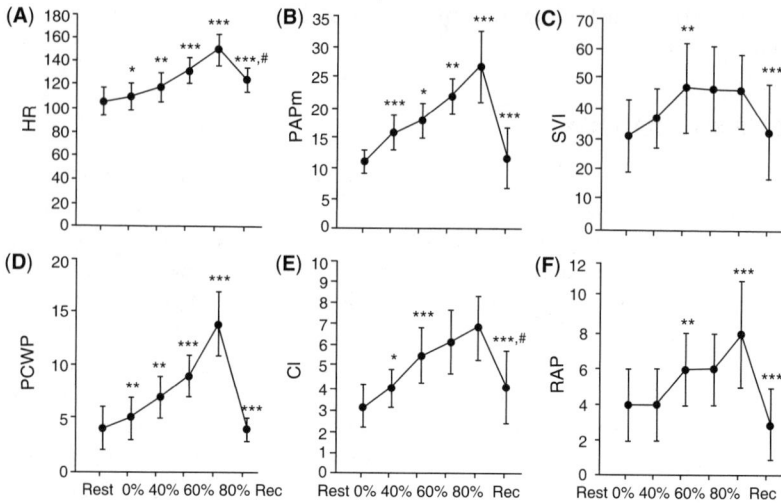

**Figure 9** Results of hemodynamic measurements during exercise in 11 HLT recipients: (**A**) heart rate; (**B**) mean pulmonary artery pressure (PAPm); (**C**) stroke volume index (SVI); (**D**) pulmonary artery wedge pressure (PCWP); (**E**) cardiac index (CI); (**F**) right atrial pressure (RAP), at rest, during exercise (at 0%, 40%, 60%, and 80% of predetermined maximal workload), and during recovery (Rec). $^*P < 0.05$, $^{**}P < 0.01$, $^{***}P < 0.001$ compared to preceding stage; $^{#}P < 0.05$ between rest and recovery. *Source*: From Ref. 21.

Anemia is frequently present in lung transplant recipients, which could contribute to the reduction in $VO_{2\,peak}$. This factor, however, is likely to play only a limited role because the degree of anemia is generally mild.

Altogether these studies indicate that neither the ventilatory nor the hemodynamic abnormalities seen after lung transplantation are sufficient to account for the persistence of a substantial limitation to exercise performance. In fact, the low peak cardiac frequency, low $O_2$ pulse, and high respiratory exchange ratio at peak exercise, and the early lactic acidosis are all consistent with a defect originating in the peripheral muscles (155).

## LIMB MUSCLE FUNCTION

### Muscle Strength and Mass

Four studies have reported a 30% to 40% decrease in quadriceps and/or leg strength in patients studied one year or more after lung transplantation (20,125,127,148). In the study by Pinet et al. (127), which included exclusively patients transplanted for CF, quadriceps cross-sectional area measured by CT was proportionately decreased such that values of quadriceps strength per unit cross-sectional area were similar in the patients and in the control subjects (Fig. 7); this indicates that quadriceps weakness was entirely accounted for by atrophy (as opposed to myopathy). On the other hand, values of quadriceps cross-sectional area normalized by lean body mass were significantly decreased in patients compared with controls, suggesting that generalized muscle wasting did not fully account for atrophy (i.e., there was a disproportionate loss of quadriceps bulk) (Fig. 7) (127).

Because these studies did not include measurements performed before and after transplantation, it is difficult to assess to what extent the reduction in quadriceps strength and bulk seen after surgery was a reflection of changes already present in the pretransplant condition. It is worth emphasizing, however, that the alterations reported by Pinet et al. (127) after transplantation are very similar to those reported by the same authors in a group of non-transplanted CF patients (126). In a longitudinal study in recipients of cardiac transplantation, quadriceps weakness and atrophy were both present before surgery and did not significantly improve after transplantation (156).

## Muscle Metabolism and Histology

The leg muscle weakness observed after lung transplantation probably accounts for part of the reduction in exercise capacity, but several observations indicate that a reduction in endurance and muscle oxidative capacity has a key role. Transplant recipients invariably report leg fatigue and pain as the reason for stopping the exercise test, and the patient's maximal workload is better correlated with measures of leg muscle endurance than strength (148). Lung transplant recipients have a shorter time to exhaustion during knee-extension exercise than age- and sex-matched control subjects (152). Finally, the observation that values of $VO_{2\,peak}$ per unit quadriceps strength are lower in lung transplant recipients than in controls indicates that quadriceps atrophy alone cannot account for all of the impairment in $VO_{2\,peak}$ (Fig. 10) (127).

Skeletal muscle metabolism has been examined in lung transplant recipients with a nuclear imaging technique, [31]P-magnetic resonance spectroscopy. Using this technique, Evans et al. (152) demonstrated that the quadriceps had a reduced intracellular pH at rest, and that incremental lower-extremity exercise produced a greater increase in muscle lactate concentration, a greater decline in phosphocreatine/inorganic phosphate ratio, and a drop in intracellular pH at a lower metabolic rate than in control subjects. The early drop in pH was associated with a shorter exercise endurance time and a lower $VO_{2\,peak}$. These findings indicate a greater reliance on anaerobic metabolism and may be the result of poor $O_2$ uptake or utilization by the muscle, an alteration that was subsequently demonstrated using optical near-infrared spectroscopy in the quadriceps of patients with SLT and BLT (157). This defect in $O_2$ metabolism is in keeping with the finding that

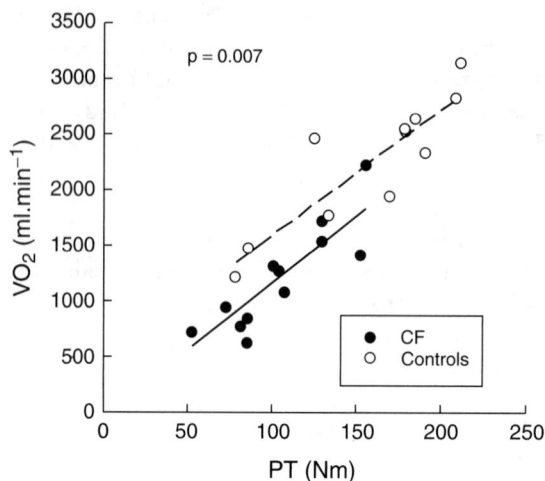

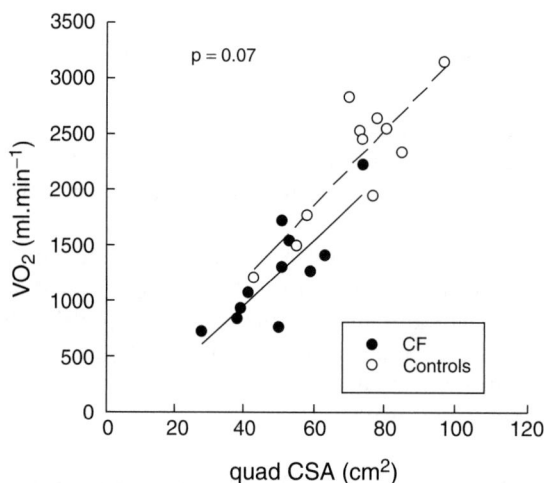

**Figure 10**  Relationships between peak VO$_2$ and quadriceps strength (PT) (*upper panel*) or quad CSA (*lower panel*) in 11 transplanted CF patients and 11 control subjects. The *P* value refers to the significance of the difference in vertical distance between the two regression lines as tested by covariance analysis. *Abbreviations*: VO$_2$, oxygen uptake; PT, peak torque; CSA, cross-sectional area; CF, cystic fibrosis. *Source*: From Ref. 127.

systemic extraction of O$_2$ during exercise (measured from the arterial–venous O$_2$ content) is reduced in both SLT and BLT recipients (147,158).

Two studies have examined biopsies from the vastus lateralis muscle in lung transplant recipients (159,160). Compared to matched controls, the muscle from the patients had a lower proportion of type I (oxidative fatigue-resistant) fibers, a lower oxidative enzyme activity, a decrease in mitochondrial mass and volume, and an impairment of mitochondrial metabolism. In addition to this abnormal muscle oxidative function, lung transplant recipients have impaired muscle $Ca^{2+}$ and $K^+$ regulation. In two elegant studies (151,160), the group of Williams et al. showed that these patients have markedly abnormal sarcoplasmic reticulum (SR) $Ca^{2+}$ regulation with lower $Ca^{2+}$ release and $Ca^{2+}$ uptake rates, as well as lower $Ca^{2+}$–ATPase activity. In addition, $K^+$ regulation was abnormal with an excessive increase in plasma $K^+$ during incremental exercise and a slower rate of decline during recovery; this was observed despite an increased maximal $Na^+$–$K^+$–ATPase activity. Several correlations were found between SR function or $K^+$ variables and $VO_{2\ peak}$ (Fig. 11), suggesting that the impaired muscle $Ca^{2+}$ and $K^+$ regulation contributes to the poor exercise performance that persists after lung transplantation.

Several mechanisms may account for these alterations in muscle metabolism and histology, including muscle disuse and atrophy, immobilization, physical deconditioning, factors related to the pretransplant condition, and use of immune suppressive agents. Morton et al. (161) showed that the reduction in the proportion of type I fibers and oxidative enzymes of the quadriceps was already present in patients before transplantation [pretransplant diagnosis was chronic obstructive pulmonary disease (COPD), CF, bronchiectasis, pulmonary fibrosis, or Eisenmenger syndrome]; a second biopsy taken three months after surgery showed no significant change compared to the pretransplant condition. Similarly, Oelberg et al. (158) showed that the ability of peripheral exercising muscles to extract $O_2$ is similarly impaired before and after transplantation. So, there is no doubt that the skeletal muscle dysfunction seen in lung transplant recipients reflects, at least in part, an ongoing process that started with the pretransplant disease. These alterations in muscle metabolism are likely to result primarily from chronic disuse, but a genetic abnormality in muscle $O_2$ metabolism might also contribute in patients with CF (127,162).

Pretransplant abnormalities in muscle function may be accentuated by the immune suppressive agents taken by the patients after transplantation, in particular the corticosteroids and cyclosporine. Treatment with high doses of methylprednisolone for acute rejection produces a transient decrease in limb and inspiratory muscle strength in ~50% of the patients (163), and long-term corticosteroid therapy may produce proximal limb muscle weakness and atrophy (involving primarily type IIb muscle fibers) (164). In the study by Pinet et al. (127), the cumulative dose of methylprednisolone received by the patients between transplantation and study was predictive of quadriceps bulk by multivariate analysis.

Cyclosporine may impair skeletal muscle metabolism; cyclosporine inhibits skeletal muscle mitochondrial respiration in vitro (165,166), and this effect may be amplified by prednisolone and azathioprine (167).

**(A)**

**(B)**

$$VO_{2\,peak}\ (ml.Kg^{-1}.min^{-1})$$

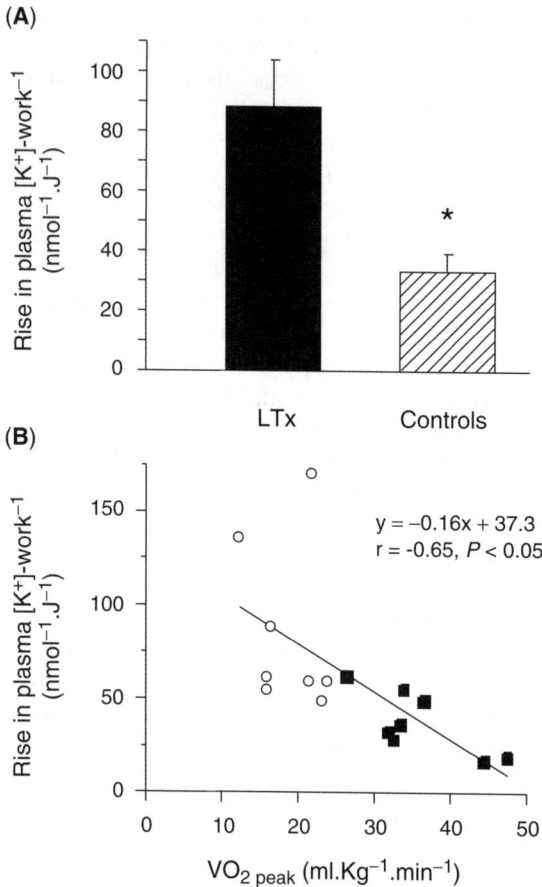

**Figure 11** (A) Rise in plasma $[K^+]$-to-work ratio for lung transplant recipients (LTx) and healthy, matched controls. Values are means $\pm$ SE; $n = 8$ for both groups. $^*P < 0.05$. (B) Relationship between $VO_{2\,peak}$ and rise in plasma $[K^+]$-to-work ratio for LTx (*open circles*) and controls (*filled squares*). Regression line (*solid line*) and equation are shown for pooled LTx and control data; $n = 16$. *Source*: From Ref. 160.

Cyclosporine, which inhibits calcineurin-activated pathways, also leads to a slow-to-fast muscle fiber phenotype conversion and hence may contribute to increase the proportion of type II fibers (168). In addition, cyclosporine causes vasoconstriction, which could contribute to disrupting the matching of perfusion and metabolic demand in exercising peripheral muscles. Studies in heart transplant recipients taking cyclosporine have shown a reduction in quadriceps muscle capillary density, but whether this alteration was entirely due to the pretransplant condition or also reflected cyclosporine toxicity is unclear (169,170). Although no data are available on the potential toxicity of tacrolimus on muscle metabolism, there does not appear to be any difference in exercise performance between patients taking cyclosporine and those on tacrolimus (149).

## Impact of Revalidation

Aerobic exercise training after transplantation increases $VO_{2\,peak}$ and leg muscle strength. In one study in nine lung transplant recipients, a 6-week exercise training program improved peak work (66 vs. 81 W) and $VO_{2\,peak}$ (1.1 vs. 1.3 L/min) (171). In another study in 10 HLT recipients, 41 days of exercise training increased $VO_{2\,peak}$ from 14.2 to 18.2 mL/kg/min and quadriceps strength from 48 to 55 N m (20). Yet, values of $VO_{2\,peak}$ after revalidation remained markedly abnormal in both studies. These preliminary results thus indicate that exercise training has only limited effects in lung transplant recipients. This observation is in keeping with studies in heart transplant recipients that showed that recovery of abnormalities in limb muscle morphology and biochemistry after surgery is incomplete (170). Yet, on rare occasions, extraordinarily high levels of $VO_{2\,peak}$ may be achieved by highly competitive recipients of lung transplants (172).

The relatively mild impact of revalidation may be related to the toxicity of immune suppressive agents (discussed earlier), and to the fact that some alterations (e.g., the reduction in $Ca^{2+}$–ATPase muscle content) do not respond to training (173). It is possible that adding strategies aimed at increasing muscle bulk, such as strength training or anabolic drugs, to endurance training alone may produce greater gains in exercise tolerance (127).

## CONCLUSION

This chapter summarizes a large number of studies that have been devoted to respiratory and exercise physiology after human lung transplantation. They showed that (i) chronic lung denervation does not result in clinically significant alterations in the control of breathing; (ii) lung and chest wall physiology undergo unique changes, in particular after SLT for emphysema; and (iii) the posttransplant exercise tolerance remains substantially impaired due primarily to limb muscle dysfunction related to a combination of factors including pretransplant abnormalities and toxicity of immune suppressive agents.

## REFERENCES

1. Edmunds LH Jr, Nadel JA, Graf PD. Reinnervation of the reimplanted canine lung. J Appl Physiol 1971; 31(5):722–727.
2. Clifford PS, Bell LB, Hopp FA, et al. Reinnervation of pulmonary stretch receptors. J Appl Physiol 1987; 62(5):1912–1916.

3.  Kawaguchi AT, Shirai M, Yamano M, et al. Afferent reinnervation after lung transplantation in the rat. J Heart Lung Transplant 1998; 17(4):341–348.
4.  Buvry A, Yang YR, Tavakoli R, et al. Calcitonin gene-related peptide-immunoreactive nerves and neuroendocrine cells after lung transplantation in the rat. Am J Respir Cell Mol Biol 1999; 20(6):1268–1273.
5.  Springall DR, Polak JM, Howard L, et al. Persistence of intrinsic neurones and possible phenotypic changes after extrinsic denervation of human respiratory tract by heart–lung transplantation. Am Rev Respir Dis 1990; 141(6): 1538–1546.
6.  Iber C, Simon P, Skatrud JB, et al. The Breuer–Hering reflex in humans. Effects of pulmonary denervation and hypocapnia. Am J Respir Crit Care Med 1995; 152(1):217–224.
7.  Khayat RN, Przybylowski T, Meyer KC, et al. Role of sensory input from the lungs in control of muscle sympathetic nerve activity during and after apnea in humans. J Appl Physiol 2004; 97(2):635–640.
8.  Taha BH, Simon PM, Dempsey JA, et al. C. Respiratory sinus arrhythmia in humans: an obligatory role for vagal feedback from the lungs. J Appl Physiol 1995; 78(2):638–645.
9.  Butler JE, Anand A, Crawford MR, et al. Changes in respiratory sensations induced by lobeline after human bilateral lung transplantation. J Physiol 2001; 534(2):583–593.
10. Shea SA, Horner RL, Banner NR, et al. The effect of human heart–lung transplantation upon breathing at rest and during sleep. Respir Physiol 1988; 72(2):131–149.
11. Sanders MH, Costantino JP, Owens GR, et al. Breathing during wakefulness and sleep after human heart–lung transplantation. Am Rev Respir Dis 1989; 140(1):45–51.
12. Kinnear W, Higenbottam T, Shaw D, et al. Ventilatory compensation for changes in posture after human heart–lung transplantation. Respir Physiol 1989; 77(1):75–88.
13. Ninane V, Estenne M. Regulation of breathholding time and sensation after heart–lung transplantation. Am J Respir Crit Care Med 1995; 152(3): 1010–1015.
14. Simon PM, Habel AM, Daubenspeck JA, et al. Vagal feedback in the entrainment of respiration to mechanical ventilation in sleeping humans. J Appl Physiol 2000; 89(2):760–769.
15. Banner NR, Lloyd MH, Hamilton RD, et al. Cardiopulmonary response to dynamic exercise after heart and combined heart–lung transplantation. Br Heart J 1989; 61(3):215–223.
16. Kimoff RJ, Cheong TH, Cosio MG, et al. Pulmonary denervation in humans. Effects on dyspnea and ventilatory pattern during exercise. Am Rev Respir Dis 1990; 142(5):1034–1040.
17. Levy RD, Ernst P, Levine SM, et al. Exercise performance after lung transplantation. J Heart Lung Transplant. 1993; 12(1):27–33.
18. Grassi B, Ferretti G, Xi L, et al. Ventilatory response to exercise after heart and lung denervation in humans. Respir Physiol 1993; 92(3):289–304.

19. Nixon PA, Flicker FJ, Noyes BE, et al. Exercise testing in pediatric heart, heart–lung, and lung transplant recipients. Chest 1995; 107(5):1328–1335.

20. Ambrosino N, Bruschi C, Callegari G, et al. Time course of exercise capacity, skeletal and respiratory muscle performance after heart–lung transplantation. Eur Respir J 1996; 9(7):1508–1514.

21. Vachiery JL, Niset G, Antoine M, et al. Haemodynamic response to dynamic exercise after heart–lung transplantation. Eur Respir J 1999; 14(5):1131–1135.

22. Savin WM, Haskell WL, Schroeder JS, et al. Cardiorespiratory responses of cardiac transplant patients to graded, symptom-limited exercise. Circulation 1980; 62(1):55–60.

23. Sciurba FC, Owens GR, Sanders MH, et al. Evidence of an altered pattern of breathing during exercise in recipients of heart-lung transplants. N Engl J Med 1988; 319(18):1186–1192.

24. Trachiotis GD, Knight SR, Pohl MS, et al. Tidal volume and respiratory rate changes during $CO_2$ rebreathing after lung transplantation. Ann Thorac Surg 1994; 58(6):1718–1720.

25. Sanders MH, Owens GR, Sciurba FC, et al. Ventilation and breathing pattern during progressive hypercapnia and hypoxia after human heart–lung transplantation. Am Rev Respir Dis 1989; 40(1):38–44.

26. Frost AE, Zamel N, McClean P, et al. Hypercapnic ventilatory response in recipients of double-lung transplants. Am Rev Respir Dis 1992; 146(6): 1610–1612.

27. Duncan SR, Kagawa FT, Kramer MR, et al. Effects of pulmonary restriction on hypercapnic responses of heart-lung transplant recipients. J Appl Physiol 1991; 71(1):322–327.

28. Duncan SR, Kagawa FT, Starnes VA, et al. Hypercarbic ventilatory responses of human heart–lung transplant recipients. Am Rev Respir Dis 1991; 144(1): 126–130.

29. Kagawa FT, Duncan SR, Theodore J. Inspiratory timing of heart–lung transplant recipients during progressive hypercapnia. J Appl Physiol 1991; 71(3): 945–950.

30. Pellegrino R, Rodarte JR, Frost AE, et al. Breathing by double-lung recipients during exercise: response to expiratory threshold loading. Am Respir Crit Care Med 1998; 157(1):106–110.

31. Sciurba FC, Owens GR, Sanders MH, et al. The effect of obliterative bronchiolitis on breathing pattern during exercise in recipients of heart–lung transplants. Am Rev Respir Dis 1991; 144(1):131–135.

32. Simon PM, Skatrud JB, Badr MS, et al. Role of airway mechanoreceptors in the inhibition of inspiration during mechanical ventilation in humans. Am Rev Respir Dis 1991; 144(5):1033–1041.

33. Butler JE, McKenzie DK, Glanville AR, et al. Pulmonary afferents are not necessary for the reflex inhibition of human inspiratory muscles produced by airway occlusion. J Neurophysiol 1997; 78(1):170–176.

34. Zhao W, Martin AD, Davenport PW. Respiratory-related evoked potentials elicited by inspiratory occlusions in double-lung transplant recipients. J Appl Physiol 2002; 93(3):894–902.

35. Simon PM, Taha BH, Dempsey JA, et al. Role of vagal feedback from the lung in hypoxic-induced tachycardia in humans. J Appl Physiol 1995; 78(4): 1522–1530.
36. Morgan-Hughes NJ, Corri PA, Healey MD, et al. Cardiovascular and respiratory effects of adenosine in humans after pulmonary denervation. J Appl Physiol 1994; 76(2):756–759.
37. Mitrouska I, Bshouty Z, Younes M, et al. Effects of pulmonary and intercostal denervation on the response of breathing frequency to varying inspiratory flow. Eur Respir J 1998; 11(4):895–900.
38. Seals DR, Suwarno NO, Joyner MJ, et al. Respiratory modulation of muscle sympathetic nerve activity in intact and lung denervated humans. Circ Res 1993; 72(2):440–454.
39. Higenbottam T, Jackson M, Woolman P, et al. The cough response to ultrasonically nebulized distilled water in heart–lung transplantation patients. Am Rev Respir Dis 1989; 140(1):58–61.
40. Hathaway TJ, Higenbottam TW, Morrison JF, et al. Effects of inhaled capsaicin in heart–lung transplant patients and asthmatic subjects. Am Rev Respir Dis 1993; 148(5):1233–1237.
41. Ing AJ, Ngu MC, Breslin AB. Pathogenesis of chronic persistent cough associated with gastroesophageal reflux. Am J Respir Crit Care Med 1994; 149(1):160–167.
42. Reid KR, McKenzie FN, Menkis AH, et al. Importance of chronic aspiration in recipients of heart–lung transplants. Lancet 1990; 336(8709):206–208.
43. Berkowitz N, Schulman LL, McGregor C, et al. Gastroparesis after lung transplantation. Potential role in postoperative respiratory complications. Chest 1995; 108(6):1602–1607.
44. Palmer SM, Miralles AP, Howell DN, et al. Gastroesophageal reflux as a reversible cause of allograft dysfunction after lung transplantation. Chest 2000; 118(4):1214–1217.
45. Herve P, Silbert D, Cerrina J, et al. Impairment of bronchial mucociliary clearance in long-term survivors of heart/lung and double-lung transplantation. The Paris-Sud Lung Transplant Group. Chest 1993; 103(1):59–63.
46. Tomkiewicz RP, App EM, Shennib H, et al. Airway mucus and epithelial function in a canine model of single lung autotransplantation. Chest 1995; 107(1):261–265.
47. Read RC, Shankar S, Rutman A, et al. Ciliary beat frequency and structure of recipient and donor epithelia following lung transplantation. Eur Respir J 1991; 4(7):796–801.
48. Veale D, Glasper PN, Gascoigne A, et al. Ciliary beat frequency in transplanted lungs. Thorax 1993; 48(6):629–631.
49. Tsang VT, Alton EW, Hodson ME, et al. In vitro bioelectric properties of bronchial epithelium from transplanted lungs in recipients with cystic fibrosis. Thorax 1993; 48(10):1006–1011.
50. Martinez FJ, Orens JB, Whyte RI, et al. Lung mechanics and dyspnea after lung transplantation for chronic airflow obstruction. Am J Respir Crit Care Med 1996; 153(5):1536–1543.

51. Banner NR, Heaton R, Hollingshead L, et al. Bronchial reactivity to methacholine after combined heart–lung transplantation. Thorax 1988; 43(12): 955–959.

52. Tapper DP, Duncan SR, Kraft S, et al. Detection of inspiratory resistive loads by heart–lung transplant recipients. Am Rev Respir Dis 1992; 145(2):458–460.

53. Peiffer C, Silbert D, Cerrina J, et al. Respiratory sensation related to resistive loads in lung transplant recipients. Am J Respir Crit Care Med 1996; 154(4): 924–930.

54. Higenbottam T, Stewart S, Penketh A, et al. Transbronchial lung biopsy for the diagnosis of rejection in heart–lung transplant patients. Transplantation 1988; 46(4):532–539.

55. Hoeper MM, Hamm M, Schäfers HJ, et al. Evaluation of lung function during pulmonary rejection and infection in heart–lung transplant patients. Chest 1992; 102(3):864–870.

56. Otulana BA, Higenbottam TW, Scott JP, et al. Lung function associated with histologically diagnosed acute lung rejection and pulmonary infection in heart–lung transplant patients. Am Rev Respir Dis 1990; 142(2):329–332.

57. Van Muylem A, Melot C, Antoine M, et al. Role of pulmonary function in the detection of allograft dysfunction after heart–lung transplantation. Thorax 1997; 52(7):643–647.

58. Van Muylem A, Antoine M, Yernault JC, et al. Inert gas single-breath washout after heart-lung transplantation. Am J Respir Crit Care Med 1995; 152(3):947–952.

59. Estenne M, Hertz MI. Bronchiolitis obliterans after human lung transplantation. Am J Respir Crit Care Med 2002; 166(4):440–444.

60. Estenne M, Maurer JR, Boehler A, et al. Bronchiolitis obliterans syndrome 2001: An update of the diagnostic criteria. J Heart Lung Transplant 2002; 21(3):297–310.

61. Otulana BA, Higenbottam TW, Ferrari L, et al. The use of home spirometry in detecting acute lung rejection and infection following heart–lung transplantation. Chest 1990; 97(2):353–357.

62. Bjortuft O, Johansen B, Boe J, et al. Daily home spirometry facilitates early detection of rejection in single lung transplant recipients with emphysema. Eur Respir J 1993; 6(5):705–708.

63. Martinez JA, Paradis IL, Dauber JH et al. Spirometry values in stable lung transplant recipients. Am J Respir Crit Care Med 1997; 155(1):285–290.

64. Morlion B, Knoop C, Paiva M, et al. Internet-based home monitoring of pulmonary function after lung transplantation. Am J Respir Crit Care Med 2002; 165(5):694–697.

65. Becker FS, Martinez FJ, Brunsting LA, et al. Limitations of spirometry in detecting rejection after single-lung transplantation. Am J Respir Crit Care Med 1994; 150(1):159–166.

66. Williams TJ, Patterson GA, McClean PA, et al. Maximal exercise testing in single and double lung transplant recipients. Am Rev Respir Dis 1992; 145(1):101–105.

67. Arens R, McDonough JM, Zhao H, et al. Altered lung mechanics after double-lung transplantation. Am J Respir Crit Care Med 1998; 158(1):1403–1409.

68. Levine SM, Anzueto A, Peters JI, et al. Medium term functional results of single-lung transplantation for endstage obstructive lung disease. Am J Respir Crit Care Med 1994; 150(2):398–402.

69. Tamm M, Higenbottam TW, Dennis CM, et al. Donor and recipient predicted lung volume and lung size after heart–lung transplantation. Am J Respir Crit Care Med 1994; 150(2):403–407.

70. Sundaresan RS, Shiraishi Y, Trulock EP, et al. Single or bilateral lung transplantation for emphysema? J Thorac Cardiovasc Surg 1996; 112(6):1485–1494; discussion 1494–1495.

71. Bavaria JE, Kotloff R, Palevsky H, et al. Bilateral versus single lung transplantation for chronic obstructive pulmonary disease. J Thorac Cardiovasc Surg 1997; 113(3):520–527; discussion 528.

72. Pochettino A, Kotloff RM, Rosengard BR, et al. Bilateral versus single lung transplantation for chronic obstructive pulmonary disease: intermediate-term results. Ann Thorac Surg 2000; 70(6):1813–1818; discussion 1818–1819.

73. Ueno T, Smith JA, Snell GI, et al. Bilateral sequential single lung transplantation for pulmonary hypertension and Eisenmenger's syndrome. Ann Thorac Surg 2000; 69(2):381–387.

74. Glanville AR, Theodore J, Harvey J, et al. Elastic behavior of the transplanted lung. Exponential analysis of static pressure–volume relationships. Am Rev Respir Dis 1988; 137(2):308–312.

75. Chacon RA, Corris PA, Dark JH, et al. Respiratory mechanics after heart–lung and bilateral lung transplantation. Thorax 1997; 52(8):718–722.

76. Chacon RA, Corris PA, Dark JH, et al. Comparison of the functional results of single lung transplantation for pulmonary fibrosis and chronic airway obstruction. Thorax 1998; 53(1):43–49.

77. Guignon I, Cassart M, Gevenois PA, et al. Persistent hyperinflation after heart–lung transplantation for cystic fibrosis. Am J Respir Crit Care Med 1995; 151(2):534–540.

78. Pinet C, Estenne M. Effect of preoperative hyperinflation on static lung volumes after lung transplantation. Eur Respir J 2000; 16(3):482–485.

79. Van Muylem A, Paiva M, Estenne, M. Involvement of peripheral airways during methacholine-induced bronchoconstriction after lung transplantation. Am J Respir Crit Care Med 2001; 164(7):1200–1203.

80. Estenne M, Ketelbant P, Primo G, et al. Human heart–lung transplantation: physiologic aspects of the denervated lung and post-transplant obliterative bronchiolitis. Am Rev Respir Dis 1987; 135(4):976–978.

81. Reynaud-Gaubert M, Thomas P, Badier M, et al. Early detection of airway involvement in obliterative bronchiolitis after lung transplantation. Functional and bronchoalveolar lavage cell findings. Am J Respir Crit Care Med 2000; 161(6):1924–1929.

82. Estenne M, Van Muylem A, Knoop C, et al. Detection of obliterative bronchiolitis after lung transplantation by indexes of ventilation distribution. Am J Respir Crit Care Med 2000; 162(3, Pt 1):1047–1051.

83. Smiley RM, Navedo AT, Kirby T, et al. Postoperative independent lung ventilation in a single-lung transplant recipient. Anesthesiology 1991; 74(6):1144–1148.

84. Officer TM, Wheeler DR, Frost AE, et al. Respiratory control during independent lung ventilation. Chest 2001; 120(2):678–681.
85. Malchow SC, McAdams HP, Palmer SM, et al. Does hyperexpansion of the native lung adversely affect outcome after single lung transplantation for emphysema? Preliminary findings. Acad Radiol 1998; 5(10):688–693.
86. Yonan NA, el-Gamel A, Egan J, et al. Single lung transplantation for emphysema: predictors for native lung hyperinflation. J Heart Lung Transplant 1998; 17(2):192–201.
87. Weill D, Torres F, Hodges TN, et al. Acute native lung hyperinflation is not associated with poor outcomes after single lung transplant for emphysema. J Heart Lung Transplant 1999; 18(11):1080–1087.
88. Harwood RJ, Graham TR, Kendall SW, et al. Use of a double-lumen tracheostomy tube after single lung transplantation. J Thorac Cardiovasc Surg 1992; 103(6):1224–1226.
89. Popple C, Higgins TL, McCarthy P, et al. Unilateral auto-PEEP in the recipient of a single lung transplant. Chest 1993; 103(1):297–299.
90. Kapelanski DP, Anderson MB, Kriett JM, et al. Volume reduction of the native lung after single-lung transplantation for emphysema. J Thorac Cardiovasc Surg 1996; 111(4):898–899.
91. Kroshus TJ, Bolman RM III, Kshettry VR. Unilateral volume reduction after single-lung transplantation for emphysema. Ann Thorac Surg 1996; 62(2): 363–368.
92. Anderson MB, Kriett JM, Kapelanski DP, et al. Volume reduction surgery in the native lung after single lung transplantation for emphysema. J Heart Lung Transplant 1997; 16(7):752–757.
93. Novick RJ, Menkis AH, Sandler D, et al. Contralateral pneumonectomy after single-lung transplantation for emphysema. Ann Thorac Surg 1991; 2(6): 1317–1319.
94. Cheriyan AF, Garrity ER Jr, Pifarre R, et al. Reduced transplant lung volumes after single lung transplantation for chronic obstructive pulmonary disease. Am J Respir Crit Care Med 1995; 151(3):851–853.
95. Estenne M, Cassart M, Poncelet P, et al. Volume of graft and native lung after single-lung transplantation for emphysema. Am J Respir Crit Care Med 1999; 159(2):641–645.
96. Cassart M, Verbandt Y, de Francquen P, et al. Diaphragm dimensions after single-lung transplantation for emphysema. Am J Respir Crit Care Med 1999; 159(6):1992–1997.
97. De Groote A, Van Muylem A, Scillia P, et al. Ventilation asymmetry after transplantation for emphysema: role of chest wall and mediastinum. Am J Respir Crit Care Med 2004; 170(11):1233–1238.
98. Moy ML, Loring SH, Ingenito EP, et al. Causes of allograft dysfunction after single lung transplantation for emphysema: extrinsic restriction versus intrinsic obstruction. Brigham and Women's Hospital Lung Transplantation Group. J Heart Lung Transplant 1999; 18(10):986–993.
99. Schulman LL, O'Hair DP, Cantu E, et al. Salvage by volume reduction of chronic allograft rejection in emphysema. J Heart Lung Transplant 1999; 18(2): 107–112.

100. Loring SH, Leith DE, Connolly MJ, et al. Model of functional restriction in chronic obstructive pulmonary disease, transplantation, and lung reduction surgery. Am J Respir Crit Care Med 1999; 160(3):821–828.

101. Low DE, Trulock EP, Kaiser LR, et al. Morbidity, mortality, and early results of single versus bilateral lung transplantation for emphysema. J Thorac Cardiovasa Surg 1992; 103(6):1119–1126.

102. Mal H, Sleiman C, Jebrak G, et al. Functional results of single-lung transplantation for chronic obstructive lung disease. Am J Respir Crit Care Med 1994; 149(6):1476–1481.

103. Herlihy JP, Venegas JG, Systrom DM, et al. Expiratory flow pattern following single-lung transplantation in emphysema. Am J Respir Crit Care Med 1994; 150(6):1684–1689.

104. Murciano D, Pichot MH, Boczkowski J, et al. Expiratory flow limitation in COPD patients after single lung transplantation. Am J Respir Crit Care Med 1997; 155(3):1036–1041.

105. Villaran Y, Sekela ME, Burki NK. Maximal expiratory flow patterns after single-lung transplantation in patients with and without chronic airways obstruction. Chest 2001; 119(1):163–168.

106. Grossman RF, Frost A, Zamel N, et al. Results of single-lung transplantation for bilateral pulmonary fibrosis. The Toronto Lung Transplant Group. N Engl J Med 1990; 322(11):727–733.

107. Lisbona R, Hakim TS, Dean GW, et al. Regional pulmonary perfusion following human heart–lung transplantation. J Nucl Med 1989; 30(8): 1297–1301.

108. Ross DJ, Koerner SK, Elashoff J, et al. Isogravitational heterogeneity of perfusion after unilateral lung transplantation. Clin Sci (Lond) 1995; 89(3): 285–291.

109. Ross DJ, Kass RM, Mohsenifar Z. Assessment of regional VA/Q relationships by SPECT after single lung transplantation. Transplant Proc 1998; 30(1):180–186.

110. Bjortuft O, Simonsen S, Geiran OR, et al. Pulmonary haemodynamics after single-lung transplantation for end-stage pulmonary parenchymal disease. Eur Respir J 1996; 9(10):2007–2011.

111. Berthezene Y, Croisille P, Bertocchi M, et al. Lung perfusion demonstrated by contrast-enhanced dynamic magnetic resonance imaging. Application to unilateral lung transplantation. Invest Radiol 1997; 32(6):351–356.

112. Levine SM, Gibbons WJ, Bryan CL, et al. Single lung transplantation for primary pulmonary hypertension. Chest 1990; 98(5):1107–1115.

113. Colt HG, Cammilleri S, Khelifa F, et al. Comparison of SPECT lung perfusion with transbronchial lung biopsy after lung transplantation. Am J Respir Crit Care Med 1994; 150(2):515–520.

114. Karetzky MS, Jasani RR, Zubair MA. Thallium-201 scintigraphy in the evaluation of graft dysfunction in lung transplantation. Newark Beth Israel Medical Center Lung Transplant Group. Eur Respir J 1996; 9(12):2553–2559.

115. Hardoff R, Steinmetz AP, Krausz Y, et al. The prognostic value of perfusion lung scintigraphy in patients who underwent single-lung transplantation for emphysema and pulmonary fibrosis. J Nucl Med 2000; 41(11):1771–1776.

116. Ouwens JP, van der Bij W, van der Mark TW, et al. The value of ventilation scintigraphy after single lung transplantation. J Heart Lung Transplant 2004; 23(1):115–121.

117. Gast KK, Viallon M, Eberle B, et al. MRI in lung transplant recipients using hyperpolarized ³He: comparison with CT. J Magn Reson Imaging 2002; 15(3):268–274.

118. Markstaller K, Kauczor HU, Puderbach M, et al. ³He-MRI-based vs. conventional determination of lung volumes in patients after unilateral lung transplantation: a new approach to regional spirometry. Acta Anaesthesiol Scand 2002; 46(7):845–852.

119. Gast KK, Puderbach MU, Rodriguez I, et al. Distribution of ventilation in lung transplant recipients: evaluation by dynamic ³He-MRI with lung motion correction. Invest Radiol 2003; 38(6):341–348.

120. Zaporozhan J, Ley S, Gast KK, et al. Functional analysis in single-lung transplant recipients: a comparative study of high-resolution CT, ³He-MRI, and pulmonary function tests. Chest 2004; 125(1):173–181.

121. Sheridan PH Jr, Cheriyan A, Doud J, et al. Incidence of phrenic neuropathy after isolated lung transplantation. The Loyola University Lung Transplant Group. J Heart Lung Transplant 1995; 14(4):684–691.

122. Maziak DE, Maurer JR, Kesten S. Diaphragmatic paralysis: a complication of lung transplantation. Ann Thorac Surg 1996; 61(1):170–173.

123. Dorffner R, Eibenberger K, Youssefzadeh S, et al. Diaphragmatic dysfunction after heart or lung transplantation. J Heart Lung Transplant 1997; 16(5): 566–569.

124. Ferdinande P, Bruyninckx F, Van Raemdonck D, et al. Phrenic nerve dysfunction after heart–lung and lung transplantation. J Heart Lung Transplant 2004; 23(1):105–109.

125. Pantoja JG, Andrade FH, Stoki DS, et al. Respiratory and limb muscle function in lung allograft recipients. Am J Respir Crit Care Med 1999; 160(4): 1205–1211.

126. Pinet C, Cassart M, Scillia P, et al. Function and bulk of respiratory and limb muscles in patients with cystic fibrosis. Am J Respir Crit Care Med 2003; 168(8):89–94.

127. Pinet C, Scillia P, Cassart M, et al. Preferential reduction of quadriceps over respiratory muscle strength and bulk after lung transplantation for cystic fibrosis. Thorax 2004; 59(9):783–789.

128. Wanke T, Merkle M, Formanek D, et al. Effect of lung transplantation on diaphragmatic function in patients with chronic obstructive pulmonary disease. Thorax 1994; 49(5):459–464.

129. Brath H, Lahrmann H, Wanke T, et al. The effect of lung transplantation on the neural drive to the diaphragm in patients with severe COPD. Eur Respir J 1997; 10(2):424–429.

130. Maurer JR, McLean PA, Cooper JD, et al. Airway hyperreactivity in patients undergoing lung and heart/lung transplantation. Am Rev Respir Dis 1989; 139(4):1038–1041.

131. Higenbottam T, Jackson M, Rashdi T, et al. Lung rejection and bronchial hyperresponsiveness to methacholine and ultrasonically nebulized distilled

water in heart–lung transplantation patients. Am Rev Respir Dis 1989; 140(1):52–57.

132. Glanville AR, Gabb GM, Theodore J, Robin ED. Bronchial responsiveness to exercise after human cardiopulmonary transplantation. Chest 1989; 96(2): 281–286.

133. Glanville AR, Theodore J, Baldwin JC, et al. Bronchial responsiveness after human heart–lung transplantation. Chest 1990; 97(6):1360–1366.

134. Liakakos P, Snell GI, Ward C, et al. Bronchial hyperresponsiveness in lung transplant recipients: lack of correlation with airway inflammation. Thorax 1997; 52(6):551–556.

135. Stanbrook MB, Kesten S. Bronchial hyperreactivity after lung transplantation predicts early bronchiolitis obliterans. Am J Respir Crit Care Med 1999; 160(6):2034–2039.

136. Herve P, Heard N, Le Roy Ladurie M, et al. Lack of bronchial hyperresponsiveness to methacholine and to isocapnic dry air hyperventilation in heart/ lung and double-lung transplant recipients with normal lung histology. The Paris-Sud Lung Transplant Group. Am Rev Respir Dis 1992; 145(6): 1503–1505.

137. Morrison JF, Higenbottam TW, Hathaway TJ, et al. Diurnal variation in $FEV_1$ after heart–lung transplantation. Eur Respir J 1992; 5(7):834–840.

138. Stretton CD, Mak JC, Belvisi MG, et al. Cholinergic control of human airways in vitro following extrinsic denervation of the human respiratory tract by heart–lung transplantation. Am Rev Respir Dis 1990; 142(5):1030–1033.

139. Fontan JJ, Cortright DN, Krause JE, et al. Substance P and neurokinin-1 receptor expression by intrinsic airway neurons in the rat. Am J Physiol Lung Cell Mol Physiol 2000; 278(2):L344–L355.

140. Gabbay E, Small T, Corris PA. Angiotensin converting enzyme inhibitor cough: lessons from heart–lung transplantation. Respirology 1998; 3(1):39–40.

141. Miyoshi S, Trulock EP, Schaefers HJ, et al. Cardiopulmonary exercise testing after single and double lung transplantation. Chest 1990; 97(5):1130–1136.

142. Gibbons WJ, Levine SM, Bryan CL, et al. Cardiopulmonary exercise responses after single lung transplantation for severe obstructive lung disease. Chest 1991; 100(1):106–111.

143. Ross DJ, Waters PF, Waxman AD, et al. Regional distribution of lung perfusion and ventilation at rest and during steady-state exercise after unilateral lung transplantation. Chest 1993; 104(1):130–135.

144. Ross DJ, Waters PF, Mohsenifar Z, et al. Hemodynamic responses to exercise after lung transplantation. Chest 1993; 103(1):46–53.

145. Orens JB, Becker FS, Lynch JP, et al. Cardiopulmonary exercise testing following allogeneic lung transplantation for different underlying disease states. Chest 1995; 107(1):144–149.

146. Gaissert HA, Trulock EP, Cooper JD, et al. Comparison of early functional results after volume reduction or lung transplantation for chronic obstructive pulmonary disease. J Thorac Cardiovasc Surg 1996; 111(2):296–306; discussion 306–307.

147. Systrom DM, Pappagianopoulos P, Fishman RS, et al. Determinants of abnormal maximum oxygen uptake after lung transplantation for chronic

obstructive pulmonary disease. J Heart Lung Transplant 1998; 17(12): 1220–1230.

148. Lands LC, Smountas AA, Mesiano G, et al. Maximal exercise capacity and peripheral skeletal muscle function following lung transplantation. J Heart Lung Transplant 1999; 18(2):113–120.

149. Schwaiblmair M, Reichenspurner H, Muller C, et al. Cardiopulmonary exercise testing before and after lung and heart–lung transplantation. Am J Respir Crit Care Med 1999; 159(4):1277–1283.

150. Murciano D, Ferretti A, Boczkowski J, et al. Flow limitation and dynamic hyperinflation during exercise in COPD patients after single lung transplantation. Chest 2000; 118(5):1248–1254.

151. Hall MJ, Snell GI, Side EA, et al. Exercise, potassium, and muscle deconditioning post-thoracic organ transplantation. J Appl Physiol 1994; 77(6):2784–2790.

152. Evans AB, Al-Himyary AJ, Hrovat MI, et al. Abnormal skeletal muscle oxidative capacity after lung transplantation by $^{31}$P-MRS. Am J Respir Crit Care Med 1997; 155(2):615–621.

153. Scott JP, Otulana BA, Mullins PA, et al. Late pulmonary haemodynamic changes in heart–lung transplantation. Eur Heart J 1992; 13(4):503–507.

154. Pflugfelder PW, McKenzie FN, Kostuk WJ. Hemodynamic profiles at rest and during supine exercise after orthotopic cardiac transplantation. Am J Cardiol 1988; 61(15):1328–1333.

155. Krieger AC, Szidon P, Kesten S. Skeletal muscle dysfunction in lung transplantation. J Heart Lung Transplant 2000; 19(4):392–400.

156. Schaufelberger M, Eriksson BO, Lonn L, et al. Skeletal muscle characteristics, muscle strength and thigh muscle area in patients before and after cardiac transplantation. Eur J Heart Fail 2001; 3(1):59–67.

157. Tirdel GB, Girgis R, Fishman RS, et al. Metabolic myopathy as a cause of the exercise limitation in lung transplant recipients. J Heart Lung Transplant 1998; 17(12):1231–1237.

158. Oelberg DA, Systrom DM, Markowitz DH, et al. Exercise performance in cystic fibrosis before and after bilateral lung transplantation. J Heart Lung Transplant 1998; 17(11):1104–1112.

159. Wang XN, Williams TJ, McKenna MJ, et al. Skeletal muscle oxidative capacity, fiber type, and metabolites after lung transplantation. Am J Respir Crit Care Med 1999; 160(1):57–63.

160. McKenna MJ, Fraser SF, Li JL, et al. Impaired muscle $Ca^{2+}$ and $K^+$ regulation contribute to poor exercise performance post-lung transplantation. J Appl Physiol 2003; 95(4):1606–1616.

161. Morton JM, McKenna MJ, Fraser SF, et al. Reductions in type I fibre proportions and oxidative enzyme activity in skeletal muscle exist pre and post lung transplantation (abstract). J Heart Lung Transplant 1999; 18(2):52.

162. de Meer K, Jeneson JA, Gulmans VA, et al. Efficiency of oxidative work performance of skeletal muscle in patients with cystic fibrosis. Thorax 1995; 50(9):980–983.

163. Nava S, Fracchia G, Callegari G, et al. Weakness of respiratory and skeletal muscles after a short course of steroids in patients with acute lung rejection. Eur Respir J 2002; 20(2):497–499.

164. Gayan-Ramirez G, Decramer M. Corticosteroids and muscle function in stable COPD. In: Lenfant C, ed. Clinical Management of Stable COPD. New York: Marcel Dekker Inc., 2002:639–658.

165. Hokanson JF, Mercier JG, Brooks GA. Cyclosporine A decreases rat skeletal muscle mitochondrial respiration in vitro. Am J Respir Crit Care Med 1995; 151(6):1848–1851.

166. Mercier JG, Hokanson JF, Brooks GA. Effects of cyclosporine A on skeletal muscle mitochondrial respiration and endurance time in rats. Am J Respir Crit Care Med 1995; 151(5):1532–1536.

167. Simon N, Zini R, Morin G, et al. Prednisolone and azathioprine worsen the cyclosporine A-induced oxidative phosphorylation decrease of kidney mitochondria. Life Sci 1997; 61(6):659–666.

168. Bigard X, Sanchez H, Zoll J, et al. Calcineurin co-regulates contractile and metabolic components of slow muscle phenotype. J Biol Chem 2000; 275(26): 19653–19660.

169. Lampert E, Mettauer B, Hoppeler H, et al. Structure of skeletal muscle in heart transplant recipients. J Am Coll Cardiol 1996; 28(4):980–984.

170. Bussieres LM, Pflugfelder PW, Taylor AW, et al. Changes in skeletal muscle morphology and biochemistry after cardiac transplantation. Am J Cardiol 1997; 79(5):630–634.

171. Stiebellehner L, Quittan M, End A, et al. Aerobic endurance training program improves exercise performance in lung transplant recipients. Chest 1998; 113(4):906–912.

172. Fink G, Lebzelter J, Blau C, et al. The sky is the limit: exercise capacity 10 years post- heart–lung transplantation. Transplant Proc 2000; 32(4):733–734.

173. Madsen K, Franch J, Clausen T. Effects of intensified endurance training on the concentration of Na,K-ATPase and Ca-ATPase in human skeletal muscle. Acta Physiol Scand 1994; 150(3):251–258.

# 34

# Imaging of the Posttransplant Lung

Robert D. Suh, Tikvah Myers, and Jonathan G. Goldin

*Department of Radiological Sciences, David Geffen School of Medicine at UCLA, Los Angeles, California, U.S.A.*

## INTRODUCTION

Adult lung transplantation, an established technique in the treatment of end-stage pulmonary disease, has reported survival rates of 73% at one year, 45% at five years, and 23% at 10 years (1). The overall lung transplantation operative mortality rate is less than 10% (2). Common indications for single lung and double lung transplantation are listed in Table 1. The risk of infection, rejection, and death is greatest in the first 100 days following lung transplantation (3). Early recognition and treatment of complications that present within the postoperative period can be instrumental in improving long-term outcome. However, a broad spectrum of nonspecific, and sometimes confusing, clinical and radiographic findings complicates the immediate postoperative period and beyond. By linking the clinical and radiological findings to their time of onset relative to transplantation, postoperative complications can be easily and usefully organized to aid in narrowing the clinician's differential diagnosis (Table 2). Within this chapter, post lung transplant complications are organized based upon a time continuum: immediate (within 24 hours), early (24 hours to 1 week), intermediate (first 2 months), primary late (2–4 months), and secondary late (> 4 months). Within each time frame, the radiological features of the complications on plain radiography, computed tomography (CT), and high-resolution computed tomography (HRCT) are accordingly described (Table 3). In addition, the

**Table 1**   Common Indications for Adult Lung Transplantation

---
COPD/emphysema
Idiopathic pulmonary fibrosis
Cystic fibrosis
Alpha-1-antitrypsin deficiency
Primary pulmonary hypertension
Sarcoidosis
Bronchiectasis
Lymphangioleiomyomatosis
Retransplantation 2° bronchiolitis obliterans
Bronchiolitis obliterans (non-retransplantation)
Retransplantation: non-bronchiolitis obliterans
Connective tissue disorder
Cancer
Histiocytosis
Other

---

*Note*: Indications are based upon data reported by the Registry of the International Society for Heart and Lung Transplantation for adult lung transplants performed between January 1995 and June 2002.
*Abbreviation*: COPD, chronic obstructive pulmonary disease.
*Source*: From Ref. 1.

potential future applications of modalities, such as ventilation scintigraphy, $^3$helium magnetic resonance imaging [$^3$He MRI], $^{18}$F-fluorodeoxyglucose positron emission tomography (FDG-PET), and multidetector CT with computerized reformations are discussed.

## IMMEDIATE (WITHIN 24 HOURS)

### Postoperative Monitoring

Several perioperative lines and tubes are in place in the transplant recipient patient. Portable chest radiography remains the primary modality to evaluate proper placement of central lines (intravenous catheters, Swan-Ganz catheters), endotracheal, nasogastric and thoracostomy tubes, and if malpositioned, their associated complications (Table 4). On frontal chest radiographs, the tip of a central venous catheter should terminate within the mid superior vena cava, proximal to the right atrium. Swan-Ganz catheters should terminate within the main, lobar, or proximal interlobar pulmonary artery. Associated complications with placement of central venous catheters include pneumothorax or hemothorax, intra- and extrathoracic hematomas, perforation of the mediastinal vasculature, and cardiac arrhythmias (4). On chest radiographs, a region of radiolucency with absent vascular markings and a sharp pleural edge could signify the presence of a pneumothorax. An apical cap or widened mediastinum suggests hemomediastinum, often

**Table 2** Post–Lung Transplant Complications and Time Period of Occurrence

| Complications | Immediate (within 24 hr) | Early (24 hr to 1 wk) | Intermediate (within 2 mo) | 1° late (2–4 mo) | 2° late (>4 mo) |
|---|---|---|---|---|---|
| Size mismatch | +++++ | | | | |
| Acute pleural complications | +++ | +++++ | | | |
| Hyperacute rejection | +++++ | ++ | | | |
| Ischemic–reperfusion injury | ++++ | +++++ | | | |
| Acute rejection | | | +++++ | +++ | ++ |
| Bronchial anastomotic complications | | ++ | +++++ | ++ | |
| Bacterial infection | | + | +++++ | +++ | +++ |
| CMV | | | ++ | +++++ | +++ |
| RSV | | | | +++++ | +++ |
| *Aspergillus* | | | | +++++ | +++ |
| Candida pneumonia | | | ++++ | +++ | |
| *Mycobacterium* | | | ++ | +++ | ++++ |
| Bronchiolitis obliterans | | | | +++ | +++++ |
| PTLD | | | | ++ | +++++ |
| Upper lobe fibrosis | | | | | +++++ |
| TBB complications | +++ | +++ | +++ | +++ | +++ |
| Recurrence 1° disease | | | ++ | +++ | +++++ |
| PE and infarction | | | ++++ | +++ | |
| Bronchogenic carcinoma | | | | ++ | +++++ |
| Native lung complications | | | | ++++ | +++ |

*Key*: +++++, occurs predominantly; ++++, occurs frequently; +++, may occur at times; ++, may occur but infrequently; +, uncommon.
*Abbreviations*: CMV, cytomegalovirus; RSV, respiratory synctial virus; PTLD, posttransplantation lymphoproliferative disorder; TBB, transbronchial biopsy; PE, pulmonary embolism.

as a result of a perforated mediastinal vein or artery (4). Fluid accumulation, presenting as hazy opacification of the affected hemithorax and/or blunting of the costophrenic angle or diaphragmatic margins, may be seen in varying degrees of severity with pleural perforation (4). Finally, cardiac arrhythmias that result from central venous catheter placement can often be attributed to

**Table 3**  Computed Tomography Abnormalities and Time Continuum of Lung Transplant Complications

| CT abnormality | Complication/time frame | | |
| --- | --- | --- | --- |
|  | <2 mo | 2–4 mo | >4 mo |
| Pleural effusion | Acute rejection | CMV | *Mycobacterium* |
|  | Bacterial infection | PE with infarction | PTLD |
|  | Acute pleural complication | *Aspergillus* |  |
| GGO | Acute rejection | CMV | PTLD |
|  | Bacterial infection | Parainfluenza | Upper lobe fibrosis |
|  | Ischemic– reperfusion | RSV | TBB complication |
|  |  | *Aspergillus* |  |
|  |  | PE with infarction |  |
| Parenchymal densities | Acute rejection | CMV | *Mycobacterium* |
|  | Bacterial infection | *Aspergillus* | PTLD |
|  | Candida pneumonia | PE with infarction[a] | Bronchiolitis obliterans |
|  | Hemothorax | Adenovirus | Upper lobe fibrosis |
|  | Ischemic– reperfusion | RSV |  |
| Bronchial wall thickening |  | CMV | Bronchiolitis obliterans |
|  |  | Adenovirus | Recurrent panbronchiolitis |
|  |  | RSV |  |
|  |  | *Aspergillus*[b] |  |
| Septal lines/ thickening | Acute rejection | CMV | *Mycobacterium* |
|  | Bacterial infection | *Aspergillus* | Bronchiolitis obliterans |
|  |  |  | PTLD |
|  |  |  | Bronchogenic carcinoma |
|  |  |  | Upper lobe fibrosis |
| Bronchial narrowing | Bronchial dehiscence | *Aspergillus*[b] |  |
|  | Bronchial stenosis |  |  |
| Tree-in-bud appearance | Bacterial infection | CMV | Bronchiolitis obliterans |
|  |  |  | *Aspergillus* |
|  |  |  | Recurrent panbronchiolitis |

(*Continued*)

**Table 3** Computed Tomography Abnormalities and Time Continuum of Lung Transplant Complications (*Continued*)

| CT abnormality | Complication/time frame | | |
|---|---|---|---|
| | <2 mo | 2–4 mo | >4 mo |
| Mediastinal LAD | Bacterial infection | Viral infections[c] | *Mycobacterium* PTLD Bronchogenic carcinoma Recurrent LAM |
| Nodules (single/ multiple) | Bacterial infection TBB complication Candida pneumonia | CMV Parainfluenza *Aspergillus* TBB complication | *Mycobacterium* PTLD Bronchogenic carcinoma TBB complication Recurrent sarcoidosis Recurrent LCH |
| Cavitary lesions | Empyema TBB complication | *Aspergillus* TBB complication | *Mycobacterium* TBB complication |
| Atelectasis | | PE with infarction | Bronchogenic carcinoma |
| Volume contraction | Acute rejection Mechanical complications | | Bronchiolitis obliterans Upper lobe fibrosis |

[a]Wedged shape.
[b]It involves the bronchial anastomotic site.
[c]Includes CMV, adenovirus, parainfluenza, RSV, and influenza.
*Abbreviations*: CT, computed tomography; CMV, cytomegalovirus; PE, pulmonary embolism; PTLD, posttransplantation lymphoproliferative disorder; GGO, ground glass opacity; RSV, respiratory synctial virus; LAD, lymphadenopathy; TBB, transbronchial biopsy.

an improperly placed catheter or a catheter curled or kinked within the right atrium, right ventricle, or both (4).

Although most lung transplant patients are extubated within the first 24 to 48 hours, accurate assessment of endotracheal tube placement is critical. The endotracheal tube tip ideally should terminate within the mid-trachea, approximately 50–70 mm above the carina (5). If the carina cannot be adequately visualized, its location can be estimated by comparing current and ear lier images. Alternatively, anatomical knowledge of the carina can allow adequate approximation of endotracheal tube placement (4,5). Complications associated with poor endotracheal tube placement include mainstem bronchial intubation with improper lung aeration, extrathoracic

**Table 4**  Chest Radiograph Abnormalities and Time Continuum of Lung
Transplant Complications

| Radiographic abnormality | Complication/time frame | | |
|---|---|---|---|
| | <2 mo | 2–4 mo | 4 mo and beyond |
| Parenchymal densities | Ischemic–reperfusion | CMV | Adenovirus |
| | Bacterial infection | Adenovirus | *Mycobacterium* |
| | Candida pneumonia | *Aspergillus* | PTLD |
| | Hyperacute rejection | Parainfluenza | Parainfluenza |
| | Acute rejection | RSV | RSV |
| | TBB complication | Influenza | Influenza |
| | Acute pleural complication | PE with infarction TBB complication | TBB complication |
| Air-fluid levels | Empyema Hemothorax Complicated pneumothorax | | |
| Mediastinal shift | Mechanical complications Empyema (+/−) Pneumothorax (+/−) | Native lung hyperinflation | |
| Septal lines/ thickening | Acute rejection Ischemic–reperfusion Hydrostatic edema | | *Mycobacterium* |
| Pleural effusion | Acute pleural complication | Adenovirus | Adenovirus |
| | Acute rejection | PE | *Mycobacterium* |
| | Bacterial infection | | Bronchogenic carcinoma |
| | Empyema | | |
| Atelectasis | Mechanical complications | PE | Bronchiolitis obliterans |
| | Bacterial infection | | |
| Cavitary lesions | Empyema | *Aspergillus* | *Mycobacterium* |
| Nodules (single/ multiple) | Candida pneumonia | *Aspergillus* | *Mycobacterium* PTLD Bronchogenic carcinoma TBB complication |
| Mediastinal LAD | Bacterial infection | Viral infections[a] | PTLD *Mycobacterium* Bronchogenic carcinoma |

[a]Viral infections include CMV, adenovirus, parainfluenza, RSV, and influenza.
*Abbreviations*: CMV, cytomegalovirus; PE, pulmonary embolism; PTLD, posttransplantation
lymphoproliferative disorder; TBB, transbronchial biopsy; RSV, respiratory synctial virus;
LAD, lymphadenopathy.

tracheal intubation, and tracheal or pharyngeal perforation. Mainstem bronchial intubation can result in hyperinflation of the intubated lung with ipsilateral diaphragmatic flattening, rapid collapse of the contralateral lung, and pneumomediastinum or pneumothorax secondary to barotrauma from mechanical ventilation. Shallow intubation with the endotracheal tube terminating in the region of the vocal cords can lead to vocal cord damage, aspiration, and regurgitation and retraction of the tube into the pharynx causing loss of airway continuity (4).

Thoracostomy tubes are commonly placed in the apical and basal regions of the chest to drain fluid or air after lung transplantation (4,6). Following extubation, apical chest tubes are typically removed in the absence of an air leak, while basal chest tubes remain in place until postoperative day five or seven (6). Thoracostomy tube placement, including kinked tubing and proximity to great vessels and proper drainage of both air and fluid from within the pleural space, should be documented (4).

## Mechanical Complications Related to Donor–Recipient Mismatch

A mismatch between the size of the donor lung and the recipient thorax can quickly lead to potential mechanical complications. The best approach to determining appropriate donor to recipient size matching remains unclear in the literature (7–10). More recently, established equations based upon donor and recipient normal predicted lung values (total lung capacity, vital capacity) have been better able to accurately gauge lung size (7,8). Alternate methods to provide better measures of size and match prediction include use of the submammary thoracic perimeter (9) and inspiratory chest radiography to measure the height of the lung at the midclavicular line and width of the thorax at the level of the dome of the diaphragm (10). Acceptable size differences of 10% to 25% between donor lung and recipient thorax have been reported (7,9,10).

Atelectasis and impaired ventilation occur as a consequence of implanting a large donor lung into a comparatively smaller recipient thorax (7,11). In patients undergoing single lung transplant for emphysema, implantation of a small donor lung into a large recipient hemithorax leads to allograft compression by the remaining hyperexpanded, emphysematous, and relatively compliant native lung (7,12). As a result, in rare instances, altered hemodynamic and ventilatory lung patterns may emerge (12–14).

## Hyperacute Rejection

Hyperacute rejection in post lung transplantation is a rare occurrence with a high associated mortality rate (15–17). The mechanism is not entirely clear, but the presence of preformed antibodies to donor organ specific HLA or ABO antigens is thought to play a major role (15,16,18). Documented case reports describe hyperacute rejection in lung transplant patients as a rapid and aggressive clinical syndrome, which occurs within hours of transplantation. The clinical syndrome includes a sudden increase in airway pressure, abundant frothy, pink fluid out-flowing from the orifice of the endotracheal tubing, cardiovascular collapse, oxygen desaturation, coagulopathy, and thrombocytopenia, in conjunction with diffuse edema of the transplanted lung (15,16,18). On chest radiographs, hyperacute rejection appears as diffuse, homogenous infiltration of the entire transplanted lung (15). Diagnosis is based upon the rapid and severe development of the clinical symptoms described earlier and clinical suspicion. Treatment has focused on regimens used in other solid organ transplantation populations and includes immediate alteration in immunosuppressive therapy, induction of plasmaphoresis, administration of antithymocyte globulin, and cyclophosphamide therapy aimed at reduction of the presence and production of preformed antibodies thought to be the cause of the rejection (15,16).

## EARLY (24 HOURS TO 1 WEEK)

### Ischemic–Reperfusion Injury

Ischemic–reperfusion injury, also known as reimplantation response or reperfusion edema, is a type of non-cardiogenic or permeability pulmonary edema associated with lung transplantation. Its etiology may be due to surgical trauma, ischemia, lymphatic interruption, and denervation in the donor lung (19). Radiographic signs of ischemic-reperfusion injury can be seen as early as 3 to 12 hours, peak at approximately 48 to 72 hours, and dissipate by postoperative day five or seven (13,20,21). Although reperfusion edema occurs in nearly all lung transplants, it is only clinically significant in 15% to 35% and is a diagnosis of exclusion (22). Clinically, patients exhibit signs of volume overload, impaired oxygenation, and decreased lung compliance. Findings in the transplanted lung on chest radiograph are non-specific and include perihilar, basal or diffuse interstitial and alveolar consolidation, peribronchial and perivascular thickening, and reticular interstitial or air-space opacities (Fig. 1) (13,19,20,23,24). The middle and lower lung zones are often more involved (20). Similar radiographic findings can be seen in patients with left ventricular failure, volume overload, atelectasis, mucous plugging, acute rejection, and infection (13,20). In some instances, CT imaging can be helpful, but more often, it discloses similar findings as on plain radiography of ground-glass, interstitial, and air-space opacities. In general, poor correlation exists between the severity of radiographic findings and physiologic pulmonary function (20). As a result, a diagnosis of ischemic-reperfusion injury must be consistent with the timing of radiographic findings and is made only after alternate diagnoses have been excluded.

**(A)**

**(B)**

**(C)**

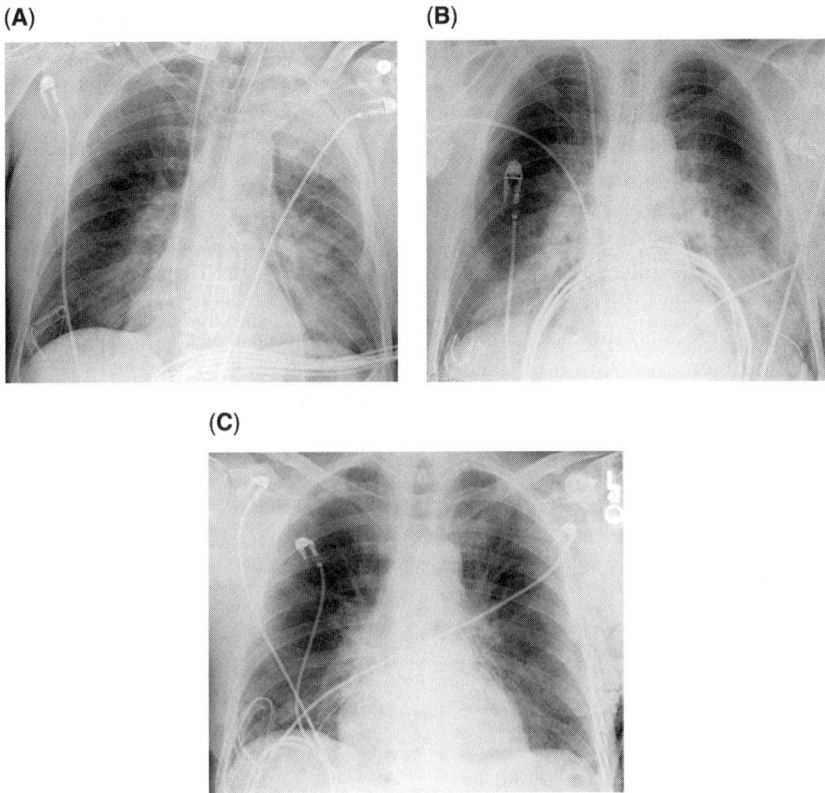

**Figure 1** (A–C) Ischemic–reperfusion injury. (A) A single radiograph obtained 24 hours post bilateral lung transplantation shows bilateral lower lobe heterogeneous air-space opacities. (B) Chest radiograph taken one day later demonstrates worsening of bilateral air-space opacities. (C) An additional chest radiograph taken 48 hours later demonstrates improvement of the air-space opacities identified on (A) and (B). Clinical and radiographic findings are consistent with ischemic–reperfusion injury.

## Acute Pleural Complications

Postoperative acute pleural complications for lung transplant patients include pleural effusion, hemothorax, and pneumothorax, which have been shown to occur as early as 24 hours posttransplantation (25). Empyema, an additional postoperative pleural complication, has been documented to occur as early as postoperative day 14 (26). Clinically, a patient with a pleural effusion, hemothorax, or pneumothorax may exhibit nonspecific symptoms of dyspnea and chest pain (localized and/or pleuritic), signs of progressive hypoxemia and hemodynamic instability. Empyemas are often due to infectious organisms, such as aerobic and anaerobic gram negative bacilli, Mycobacterium, fungi, or

*Staphylococcus aureus* (27). As a result, patients can exhibit signs of infection, such as fever, chills, malaise, dyspnea, chest pain, and productive cough (27,28).

Hazy opacification of the affected hemithorax, obscuration of the diaphragmatic margins, and blunting of the costophrenic angle can indicate a pleural effusion on chest radiograph (Fig. 2). Loculated or coagulated blood due to a hemothorax is often indistinguishable from other types of pleural fluid. Regions of radiolucency with the absence of vascular markings on chest radiographs are concerning for pneumothorax. Often in the supine patient, the air collects within the least dependent aspect of the hemithorax causing the pneumothorax to be anteriorly located (medially or basally) (4,29). If there is doubt and the patient's condition allows, expiratory maneuvers improve visualization of pneumothoraces. Persistent air leaks (air leakage that continues beyond seven days) present as a continued pneumothorax,

(A)                                                    (B)

(C)                                                    (D)

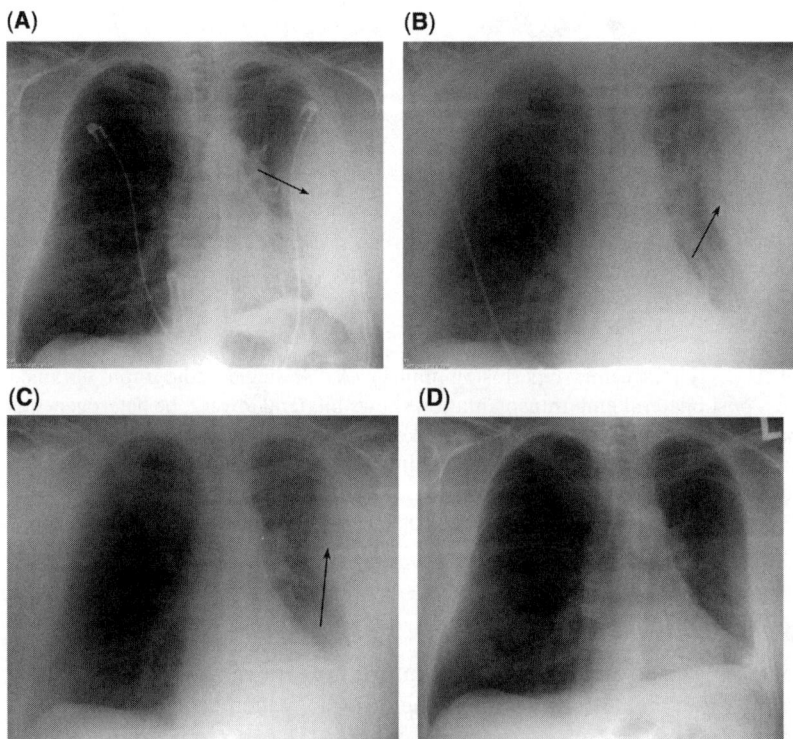

**Figure 2** (A–D) Persistent pleural effusion. (A) A series of frontal chest radiographs show a large, loculated pleural effusion (*black arrow*) in a single left lung transplant patient. (B) Post-thoracostomy tube placement and drainage, the left pleural effusion (*black arrow*) is evident with only mild resolution 48 hours later. (C) Following five days of minimal drainage, the thoracostomy tube is removed. (D) Follow-up chest radiograph one month later finally shows complete resolution of the left pleural effusion.

pneumomediastinum, or subcutaneous emphysema on chest radiographs (28). Loculated pleural effusions with or without air fluid levels, often causing mass effect on the transplant lung and mediastinum, suggest the presence of an empyema on chest radiograph (28,30,31).

In the setting of a normal or indeterminate chest radiograph, CT has been shown to be a sensitive modality in differentiating pleural fluid from peripheral lung infiltrates or pleural thickening. Additionally, CT scanning can detect the presence of loculated air and/or effusion and can characterize abnormal pleural surfaces (27). For simple postoperative pleural effusions, CT demonstrates dependent lenticular or sickle-shaped hypodensities within the expected pleural, including fissural spaces. For hemothorax, CT reveals heterogenous collections, due to blood products, within the pleural, including fissural spaces (Fig. 3). On occasion, a fluid-hematocrit level can be seen (28). CT findings for empyema include elongated regions with thin uniform walls which conform to the shape of the chest wall and compress the adjacent lung parenchyma (27). In addition, when intravenous contrast is administered, the inflamed pleural surfaces become enhanced and appear separated by the intermediary empyema fluid, known as the "split pleura sign" (27). Transient or persistent air leak findings on CT are similar to the findings observed on chest radiograph and include pneumothorax, pneumomediastinum, and subcutaneous emphysema (28).

**(A)**          **(B)**

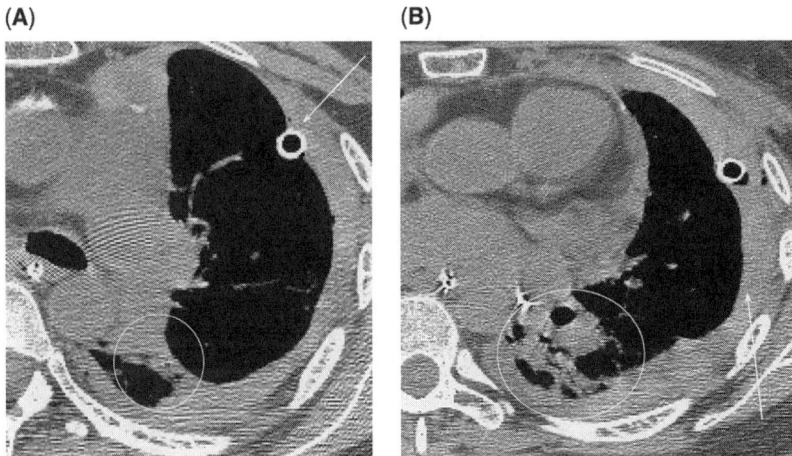

**Figure 3** (**A** and **B**) Left lung posttransplant hemothorax. (**A**) A moderately large collection of blood is visualized with extension into the major fissure (*encircled region*) on soft tissue window. A single thoracostomy tube is visualized (*thin white arrow*). (**B**) On a more caudal image, the collection of blood is again seen (*encircled region*) showing characteristic increased attenuation consistent with organized fresh blood. This is better appreciated within the costal pleural space (*white arrow*).

## INTERMEDIATE (FIRST 2 MONTHS)

### Acute Rejection

Acute rejection is characterized histologically by perivascular and subendothelial mononuclear cell infiltrates (32). It occurs in approximately 50% of all lung transplant patients (23), rarely resulting in death (3). In the literature, repeated episodes of acute rejection have been linked to the development of bronchiolitis obliterans, or chronic rejection, the major obstacle to long-term survival post lung transplantation (33). The development of acute rejection may occur at any point during the postoperative course, with peak incidence in the second postoperative week and most episodes occurring within two months of lung transplantation (34,35). Clinically, patients with acute allograft rejection complain of new onset tachypnea, nonproductive cough, low-grade fever, and malaise, accompanied by a decline in pulmonary function (13,35). As with reperfusion edema, findings on chest radiographs are relatively nonspecific and include perihilar and lower lobe opacities, interlobular septal thickening or lines, and pleural effusions in the absence of clinical signs of volume overload (Figs 4 and 5) (13,35). Chest radiograph findings cannot be heavily relied upon in patients suspected of acute rejection because a reported 24% of patients clinically diagnosed with acute rejection have normal findings on chest radiographs (13).

CT improves detection of acute rejection, especially when the chest radiograph is apparently normal. Findings reported on HRCT include focal, multifocal, or diffuse ground-glass opacities, often with basal distribution, peribronchial cuffing, interlobular septal thickening, volume loss, and new or increased pleural effusions (Fig. 6) (36,37). However, these observations are relatively nonspecific, with reported variations in sensitivity for diagnosing acute rejection being overall poor (35–65%) (36,37). Further, the CT can appear normal, even when pathology demonstrates rejection on transbronchial biopsy (TBB) specimens. Histopathologic evidence for rejection on TBB is currently regarded as the gold standard for making the diagnosis despite its own documented limitations (38). In the absence of invasive procedures like TBB, a CT diagnosis of acute rejection is supported by improvement of clinical and radiological abnormalities 24 to 48 hours after administration of intravenous methylprednisone (13,39).

### Bronchial Anastomotic Complications

With improvements in anastomotic techniques, the prevalence of airway-related complications currently ranges between 10% and 20% (40–42). Ischemia of the donor bronchus due to disruption of the native bronchial circulation is a key factor adversely influencing airway anastomosis healing (43,44). Bronchial anastomotic complications following lung transplantation include bronchial dehiscence, bronchomalacia, bronchial stenosis, and

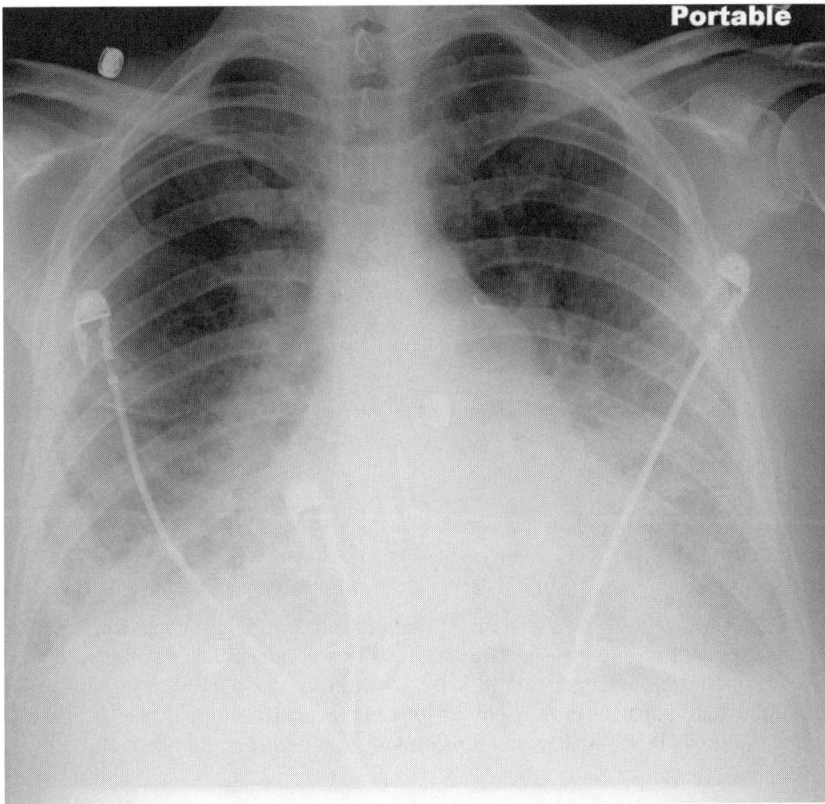

**Figure 4** Acute rejection. Bilateral pulmonary opacities in the middle and lower lung on frontal chest radiograph in a patient complaining of shortness of breath three weeks after bilateral lung transplantation. Transbronchial biopsy revealed perivascular and interstitial mononuclear infiltrates consistent with minimal acute rejection (Grade A1).

anastomotic infection (43,44). Anastomotic complications, reported in 5% to 18% of cases, occur within the first weeks to months following transplantation with dehiscence usually presenting within the first 30 days and stenosis presenting later, usually within four months (28,43–45). Interestingly, in one study of 127 consecutive lung transplants, actuarial survival was not different for patients with airway complications compared to those without (44).

Depending on the type of postoperative bronchial complication, clinical presentation is variable; some patients are asymptomatic while others exhibit a progressive decline in respiratory function with or without pleuritic chest pain, cough, wheezing, and stridor. In the presence of an anastomotic infection, patients may exhibit signs of fever, chills, tachycardia, and malaise.

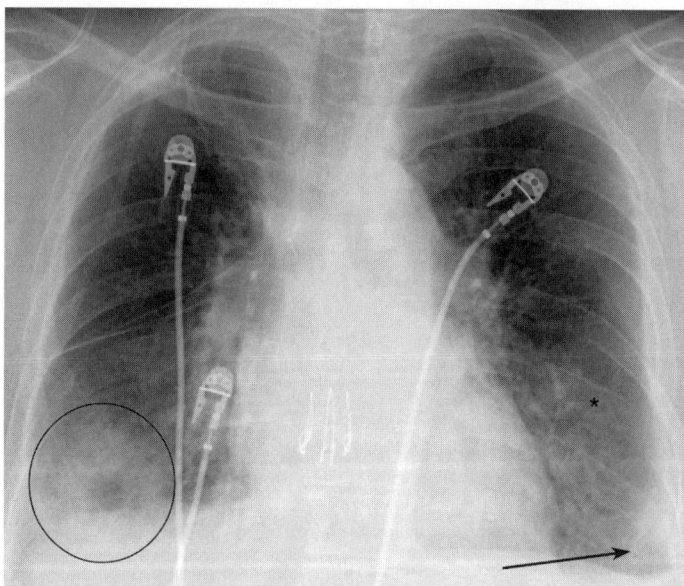

**Figure 5** Acute rejection. Several manifestations of acute rejection can be present at the same time, including pleural effusion (*black arrow*), air-space opacities (*encircled region*), and interlobular septal thickening (*asterisk*), on plain chest radiograph. Transbronchial biopsy of the right lower lobe in this bilateral lung transplant patient revealed findings highly suspicious for Grade A3 moderate acute rejection.

Chest radiography is relatively poor in detecting anastomotic complications (19). Defects in the bronchial wall, accumulation of extraluminal air surrounding the anastomotic site or some distance from it, bronchial irregularity, and bronchial narrowing are direct features of dehiscence observed on CT (Fig. 7) (28). Indirect features suggestive of bronchial dehiscence include intrathoracic air collections, such as pneumomediastinum, pneumopericardium, pneumothorax, and on occasion, pulmonary interstitial emphysema (Fig. 8). Several studies evaluating CT detection of dehiscence have demonstrated high sensitivity and specificity, both in the presence and in the absence of extraluminal air (46). Direct bronchoscopy should be used in CT negative cases when the diagnosis is suspected (43).

Fixed bronchial narrowing is classically described on CT in the setting of bronchial stenosis or stricture (28), with significant obstruction defined as greater than 50% diameter narrowing (47). Excessive airway collapse observed with bronchomalacia is best detected with direct bronchoscopic visualization during spontaneous breathing. However, transient airway narrowing can be readily detected with paired inspiratory and expiratory CT imaging of the anastomosis or airway segment in question, or by dynamic CT scanning during exhalation (48–50).

**(A)**

**(B)**

**(C)**

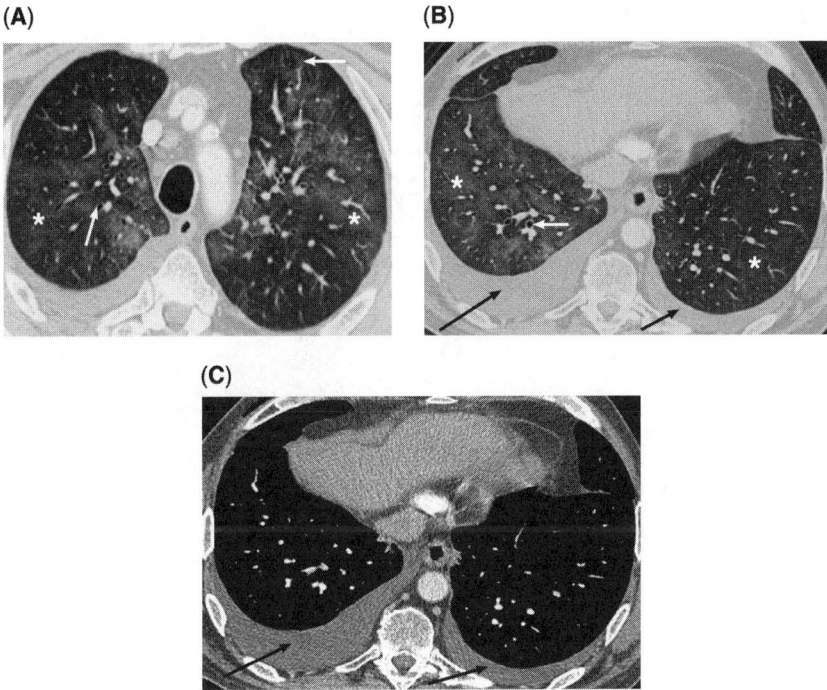

**Figure 6** (A–C) Acute rejection. (A) A single image through the upper lobes demonstrates diffuse, bilateral ground-glass opacities (*asterisks*), peribronchial thickening (*solid white arrow*), and septal thickening (*dashed white arrow*) in a bilateral lung transplant patient with acute rejection. (B) A single axial high-resolution computed tomography slice at the base of the lungs, of the same patient, also demonstrates bilateral ground-glass opacities (*asterisks*) and peribronchial thickening (*white arrow*). Bilateral pleural effusions are also evident (*black arrows*). (C) Soft tissue windows at the lung bases confirm bilateral pleural effusions (*black arrows*).

## Bacterial Infections

Bacterial infections usually occur within the first 6 months and are the most common type of acute infection in the post lung transplant patient (6,19,24). Pneumonia is the most common manifestation, occurring in up to 75%, and catheter-related bacteremia or overt sepsis are less common presentations, occurring in up to 30% of patients (6,24). The most frequent organisms cultured include gram negative organisms (*Pseudomonas aeruginosa, Klebsiella* species, *Enterobacteriaceae*), gram positive organisms (*Staphylococcus aureus, Streptococcus pneumoniae, Hemophilus influenza*), and *Actinomyces* (6,51,52). Pulmonary infections tend to occur as a result of aspiration of gastric secretions, bacterial colonization of an atelectatic lobe (28), impaired mucociliary transport in the denervated lung, altered phagocytosis in the

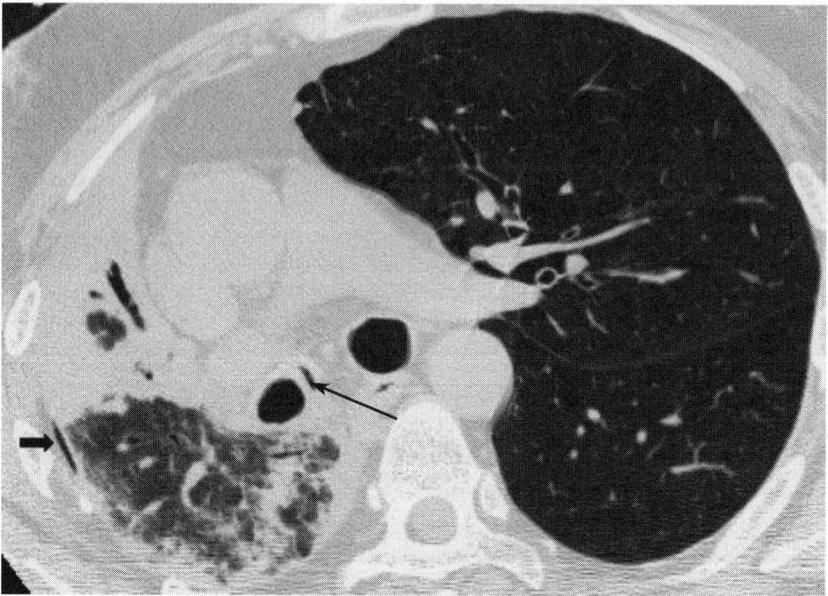

**Figure 7** Dehiscence. On high-resolution computed tomography, medial to the right mainstem bronchus, an irregular pocket of air is outside of the airway (*thin black arrow*). A small pneumothorax (*thick black arrow*) related to the anastomic leak is also present.

alveolar macrophages, direct communication of the donor lung with the atmosphere, loss of the cough reflex, and interruption of the lymphatic drainage (19,24). Risk factors for early infection include longer donor ischemic time (>76 hours), lower donor arterial oxygen tension (<350 mmHg) before harvest, older recipient age (>40 years), positive donor sputum culture, prolonged ventilatory support, and difficulty clearing tracheal–bronchial secretions (3,28). Overall, the risk of developing an infection (bacterial, viral, or fungal) is extremely high within the first 100 days post lung transplantation (3,52). Patients are at the greatest risk from bacterial infections within the first month following lung transplantation and remain at risk throughout their lifetime (6,52). Patients with bacterial infections clinically present with fevers, chills, malaise, pleuritic chest pain, tachypnea, and cough with or without sputum production.

Chest X ray findings include atelectasis, patchy and confluent bronchopneumonic opacities, lobar air-space consolidation, and pleural effusions (Figs. 9 and 10) (28). Findings observed on chest radiographs related to bacterial infections usually occur within the transplant lung and tend to lag behind the development of clinical symptoms. As a result, a negative chest radiograph does not exclude a diagnosis of postoperative pneumonia (28).

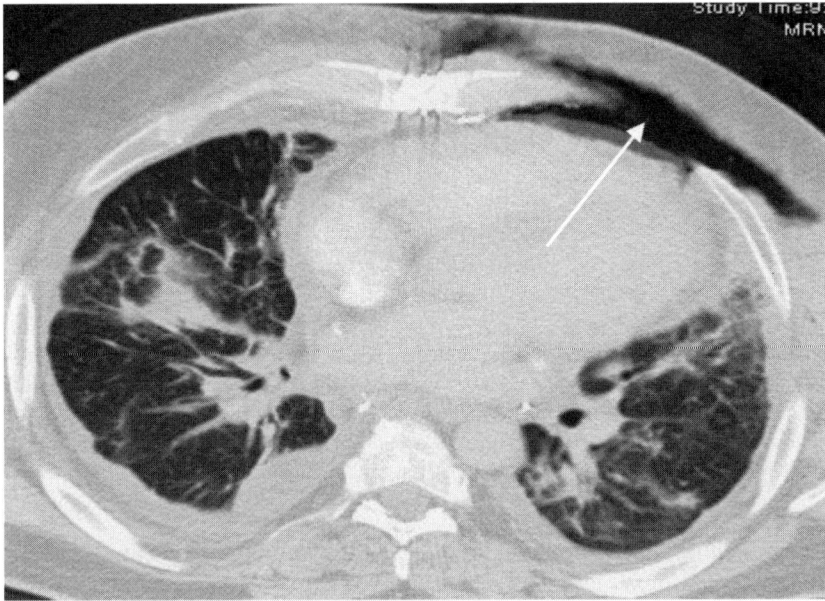

**Figure 8** Dehiscence. A one-month postoperative high-resolution computed tomography scan demonstrates a large collection of subcutaneous air extending along the left anterior chest wall (*white arrow*) in a transplant patient complaining of leakage from the operative site.

In fact, the chest X ray has been reported to be apparently negative in 50% of cases, making it neither a very sensitive or specific test (53,54). CT is more sensitive for the detection of abnormalities but remains nonspecific with respect to the causative organism (51,52). CT appearances have a spectrum of features, including nodules with smooth or irregular margins and ground-glass components, branching nodular or linear opacities often described as a "tree-in-bud" appearance, air-space consolidation (unilateral or bilateral with asymmetry), ground-glass opacification, interlobular septal thickening, pleural effusions, and enlarged hilar or mediastinal lymph nodes (Fig. 11) (52). For the most part, the role of CT involves subjectively quantifying the presence and extent of infiltrates, localizing ideal regions of the lung for biopsy, and determining the response to specific antimicrobial treatment (51,55). Overall, the role of antibiotic prophylaxis has dramatically reduced the morbidity and morality related to posttransplant lung infections (19,24).

### Candida Infections

*Candida* and *Aspergillus* account for the majority of fungal infections that affect lung transplant patients (6,56–58). *Candida* infections can manifest

(A)                                    (B)

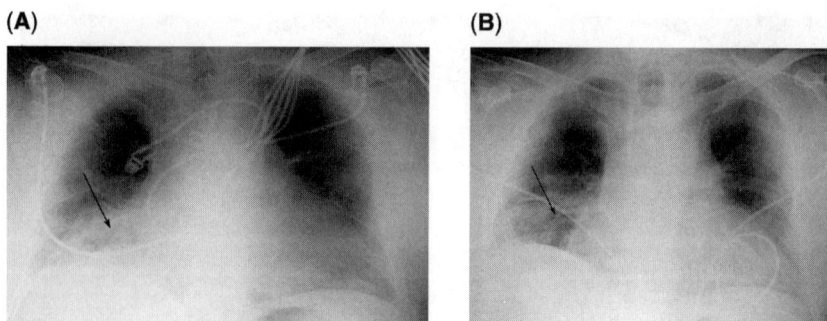

**Figure 9**   (A and B) Bacterial pneumonia. (A) Single frontal chest radiograph demonstrates air-space opacities and consolidation in the right lower lobe (*black arrow*). Fiberoptic bronchoscopy with biopsy performed the same day yielded cultures positive for *Streptococcus viridians*. (B) Chest radiograph taken five days later following antibiotic treatment shows improvement in the right lower lobe pneumonia (*black arrow*).

as candidemia, mucocutaneous infections, pneumonia, mediastinitis, bronchial anastomotic infections, catheter-associated candidiasis, or esophagitis (56–60). Infection due to *Candida* is thought to be directly related to the intricate technique of lung transplantation surgery (56), colonization of the bronchial segment in the donor lung (43,56) and/or pretransplant fungal colonization of the transplant patient (56). *Candida* infections occur earlier as compared to aspergillus infections, typically within the first 3 months post lung transplantation (55,56,60,61). In a study of 73 post lung and heart–lung transplant patients, 26% of the patients were shown to have *Candida* species isolated from either blood or bodily secretions. Of these identified patients, about half were shown to be colonized (11/19) and half were ultimately diagnosed with invasive disease (8/19) (62). Clinically, patients may present with progressive dyspnea, respiratory failure, fever, and hypotension (62).

*Candida* pneumonia rarely occurs, although it is more common among lung transplant patients as compared to other solid organ transplant patients (61,63). Chest radiograph findings range from normal to nonspecific and include local or diffuse infiltrates and slowly enlarging nodules, which occasionally occur in a miliary pattern (59,62–65). CT findings include patchy and confluent infiltrates, nodular and mass-like or air-space consolidation and interstitial lung patterns (Fig. 12) (66). *Candida* has been shown to be a common isolate of respiratory secretions from immunocompromised patients in general and usually represents colonization rather than infection (6,63). Diagnosis of *Candida* species infection can be performed by bronchoscopy with bronchoalveolar lavage (BAL) or TBB. In addition, blood, sputum, and urine cultures are also helpful (62). As has been shown previously, definitive diagnosis is often difficult without histologic and pathologic evidence (62). As a result, in addition to bronchoscopy, fine needle

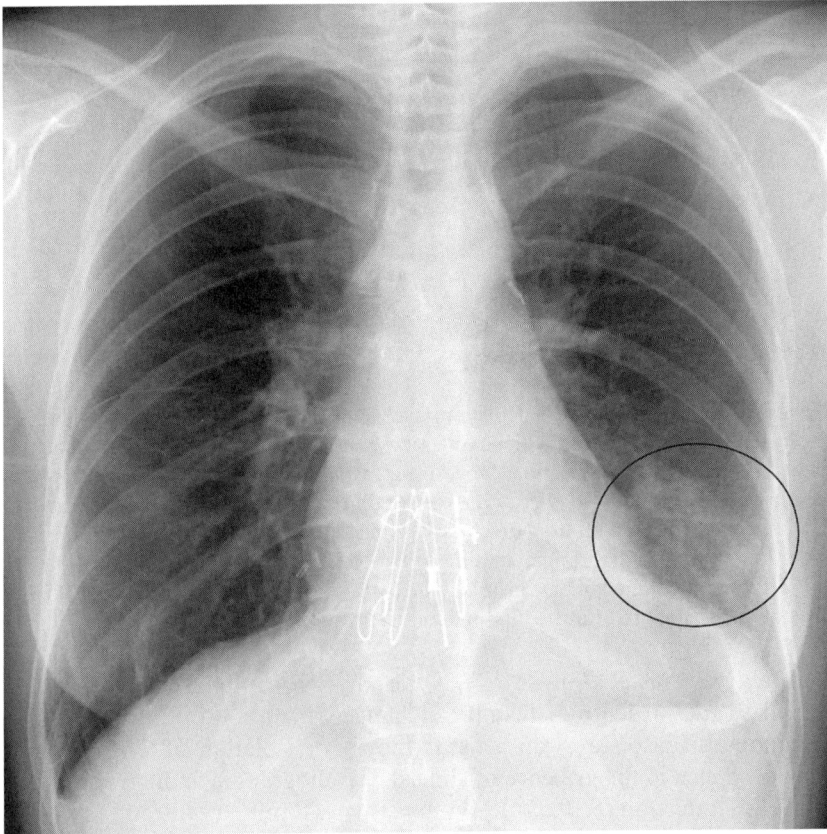

**Figure 10** Bacterial pneumonia. Single frontal chest radiograph in a double lung transplant patient demonstrates patchy and confluent air-space consolidation with air bronchograms (*encircled region*) within the lingula; cultures identified *Pseudomonas aeruginosa*.

aspiration or open lung biopsy may be needed (62). More recently, focus has been on the development of rapid antigen detection measures to facilitate early diagnosis prior to the development of invasive fungal disease (57,59).

## PRIMARY LATE (2–4 MONTHS)

### Cytomegalovirus Infections

Cytomegalovirus (CMV) is a common opportunistic infection observed in solid organ transplant patients and is the second most common infection in lung transplant recipients (55). CMV infection is defined as detection of the virus in serum or in BAL obtained specimens by culture, polymerase

**(A)**                              **(B)**

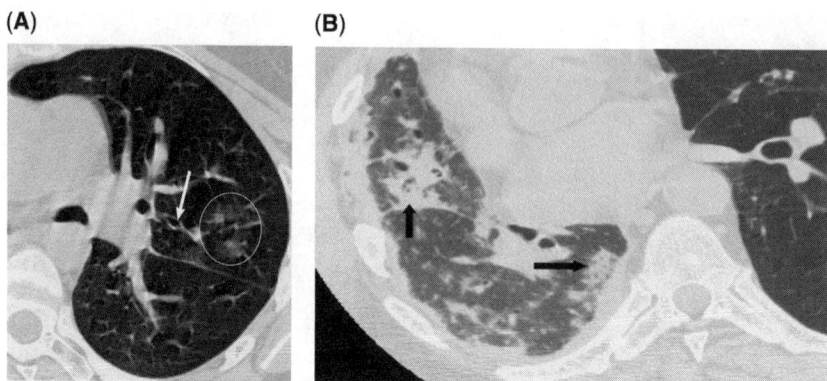

**Figure 11**  (**A** and **B**) Bacterial pneumonia. (**A**) High-resolution computed tomography shows peribronchial thickening (*white arrow*) and centrilobular opacities (*encircled region*) in the left upper lobe of a transplanted lung. The patient was treated empirically with a 14-day course of levaquin for presumed bacterial pneumonia and improved with resolution of clinical symptoms. Subsequent scans confirmed resolution of the radiographic findings. (**B**) Axial computed tomography image demonstrates focal consolidation (*black arrows*) within the right middle and lower lobes of a transplanted lung, a finding consistent with bacterial pneumonia.

chain reaction (PCR), or CMV DNA by hybrid capture. CMV disease is defined as the presence of histologic changes (inclusion bodies or positive immunoperoxidase stain) on a tissue biopsy or isolation of CMV from a tissue specimen in the presence of clinical or radiographic findings consistent with CMV infection (6,19,55). CMV presents as a primary infection (when a seronegative recipient receives a seropositive donor lung (D+/R−) and develops CMV disease) or secondary infection (CMV disease as a result of viral reactivation or reinfection from a donor lung) (24). D+/R− patients have been shown to have the highest risk of infection (19) with the incidence of CMV disease overall in lung or heart–lung transplant patients reported to be at least 50% (55,60).

Pneumonia is the most common manifestation of CMV disease (19). The clinical and radiographic findings associated with CMV rarely occur before two weeks posttransplant (19). Typically, between one and six months post lung transplantation, patients show signs of CMV disease (60). Presenting symptoms are nonspecific and include fever, chills, malaise, and nonproductive cough (55). Findings on chest radiographs include reticulonodular, reticular or ground glass opacities, and consolidation (24). CT findings of CMV pneumonia include nodules (can be multiple and of varying sizes), nodular and branching linear opacities (tree-in-bud appearance), consolidation (unilateral or bilateral with asymmetry), ground-glass opacification, interlobular septal thickening, pleural effusions, thickened and/or enhancing pleura, bronchiectatic airways, and bronchial thickening (Fig. 13) (51,52). CMV

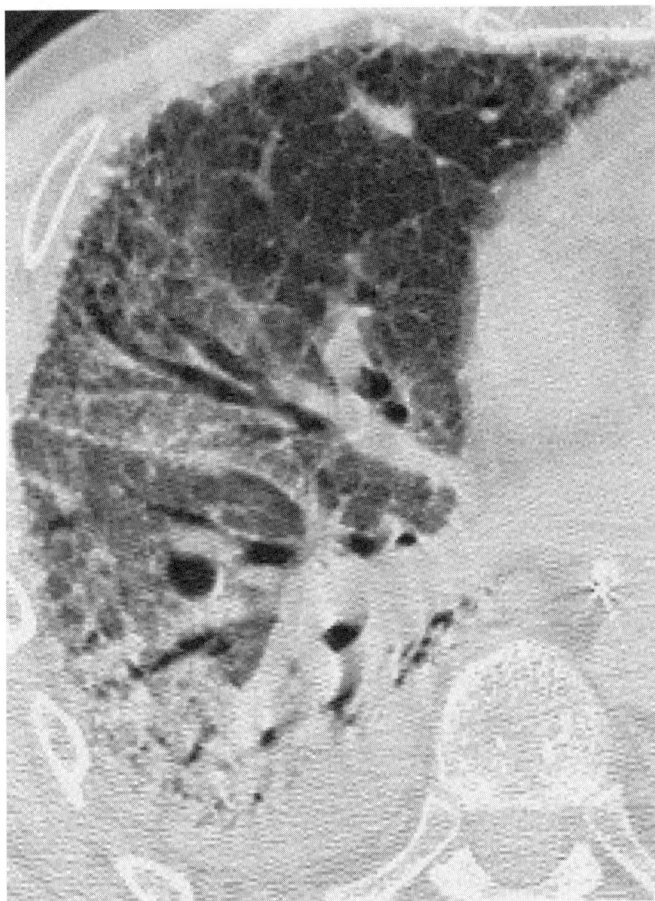

**Figure 12** Aspiration pneumonia. High-resolution computed tomography image demonstrates extensive multifocal ground glass and air-space opacities within the right middle and lower lobes of the native lung. Sputum cultures later yielded *Candida lusitanae*. The findings noted in the native right lung were thought clinically to be attributed to an aspiration pneumonitis.

pneumonia can involve any region within the transplanted lung, native lung, or both (52). As in the setting of bacterial infections, CT findings for CMV infection are nonspecific and are used to characterize extent of disease, determine optimal locations for biopsy, and determine response to treatment (52).

**Respiratory Viral Infections**

Community acquired respiratory viral infections, such as respiratory syncytial (RSV), parainfluenza (PIV), adenovirus, and influenza virus also affect

(A)                                    (B)

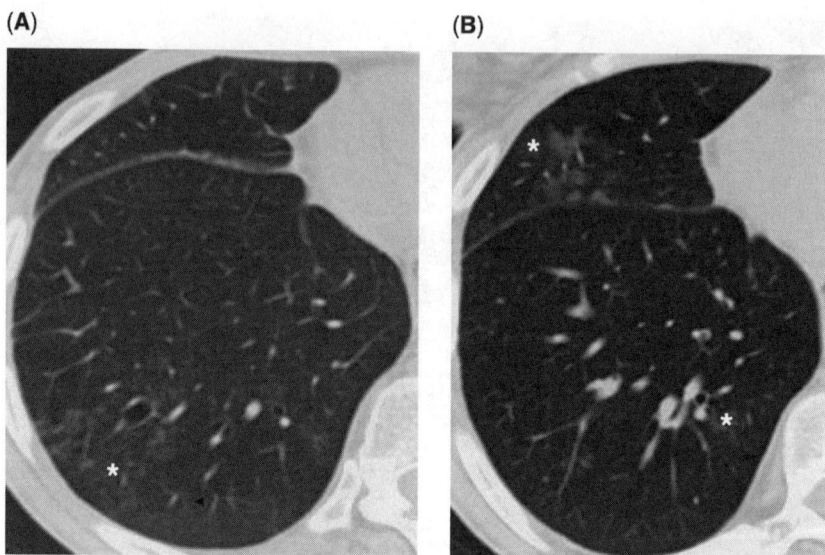

**Figure 13**   (**A** and **B**) Cytomegalovirus (CMV) pneumonitis. Axial image (**A** and **B**) of the right lung of a bilateral transplant patient shows patchy and confluent ground glass nodularities (*asterisks*) in the right middle and lower lobes. Transbronchial biopsy later found inclusion bodies consistent with CMV.

the post lung transplant patient (19,67). The incidence of viral infection is reported to be between 8% and 14% (67–70). The timetable for the development of clinical symptoms and/or radiographic findings is wide, ranging from two weeks to two years posttransplantation (67,69). Early viral infections may be secondary to nosocomial infections or reactivation of latent virus, while late infections may be primarily related to community-acquired infections (67,69). In addition, seasonal viral infections, such as RSV and influenza, tend to occur in the winter and spring months, while PIV and adenovirus tend to occur year round (67–69). Clinically, patient presentation is highly variable with some patients asymptomatic and other patients with mild or severe disease. Symptoms and signs include fever, dry cough, wheezing, dyspnea, progressive loss of lung function, and hypoxemia (67,69,71). Community-acquired respiratory viral infections have been shown to be a significant risk factor for the development of bronchiolitis obliterans after lung transplantation (70). As a consequence, early detection and antiviral treatment are important clinical strategies to prevent or modify the posttransplant course complicated by viral infection (69,70).

In PIV and RSV infections, chest radiograph findings include perihilar and heterogenous opacities (Fig. 14) (67,71). In adenovirus infections, the radiographic findings are usually more extensive and include heterogenous,

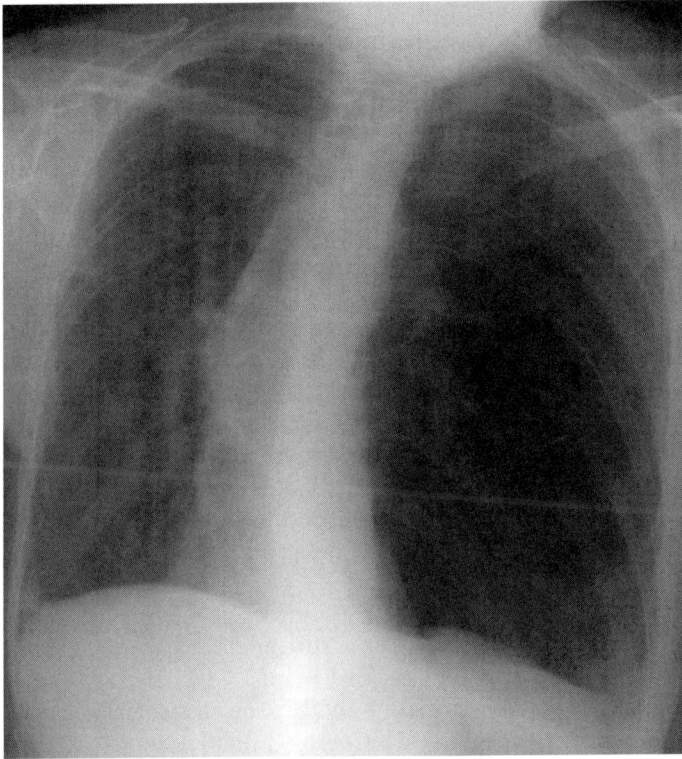

**Figure 14** Respiratory synctial virus (RSV) pneumonitis. Following a two-week history of increasing cough and shortness of breath, chest radiograph shows diffuse ground-glass and patchy air-space consolidation of the right single lung transplant. Respiratory cultures were positive for RSV antigen.

homogenous or peribronchial opacities, focal mass-like consolidations, and pleural effusions (67). In influenza, reported findings on chest radiographs include heterogenous opacities and bronchial wall thickening (67). CT findings of the community-acquired respiratory viral infections are nonspecific with diffuse or multifocal patterns located peripherally or centrally in the native lung, transplanted lung, or both (67,68). Findings include centrilobular nodules (parainfluenza), ground-glass opacities (parainfluenza, RSV), bronchial wall thickening (adenovirus, RSV), air-space opacities (adenovirus, RSV), and bronchial dilation (RSV) (67,68).

## Aspergillus

Infection due to *Aspergillus* can result in tracheobronchitis, bronchial anastomotic infection, an aspergilloma, necrotizing pneumonia, invasive pulmonary disease, empyema, or disseminated infection (6,24,43,52,56, 58,72). The donor lung's direct exposure to the external environment and airborne fungal spores, denervation of the lung leading to impaired mucociliary function and loss of the cough reflex, altered alveolar phagocytic function, and postoperative immunosuppression all potentially can cause patients to become susceptible to colonization and invasive fungal disease (56,61,73). Infection due to aspergillus has been shown to occur between one and six months post lung transplantation, with the highest incidence within the first 3 months posttransplant (6,52,55,56,60,73). The incidence of aspergillus is reported between 6% and 20% in the literature, (73–75) with high mortality rates estimated around 50% (61,73) for the lung transplant population. In elderly patients who received single lung transplants secondary to chronic obstructive pulmonary disease, aspergillus infection tends to occur later and present as an invasive infection with a higher associated mortality rate as compared to other lung transplant patients (73). Clinically, similar to other postoperative infections affecting lung transplant patients, nonspecific symptoms include fever, chills, malaise, hemoptysis, pleuritic chest pain, recurrent wheezing, and dyspnea (72).

Findings on chest radiograph are again nonspecific and include focal, nodular infiltrates with well-defined borders surrounded by aerated lungs (55,74,76), consolidation (55,72,73,76), cavitary lesions (72,73), nodules (multiple or solitary) (72,76,77), mass-like lesions with associated soft tissue opacities (72,73), and pleural thickening (72). Common findings on CT include nodules which are often multiple of differing sizes, with irregular or smooth margins (19,72,76) and associated cavitations (52,76). The nodules have been described as having an associated decreased surrounding density referred to as a "halo sign" (Fig. 15A) (72,74,76). Other radiologic manifestations of aspergillus infection on CT include consolidation (19,52), ground-glass opacification (19,52), interlobular septal thickening (52), and pleural effusions (Fig. 15B) (52). If the fungal infection involves the bronchial anastomotic site, circumferential bronchial wall thickening and bronchial obstruction can be seen on CT (72). Aspergillus has been shown to affect any region of the lung (52).

Similar to its use in the setting of suspected bacterial and viral infections, CT can isolate parenchymal abnormalities and highlight an optimal site for BAL or TBB (76). Diagnosis of an infection due to aspergillus can be established by several methods, including culture of BAL fluid or sputum, histologic diagnosis by TBB or open lung biopsy and/or serologic testing (6,43,74,76). In the literature, extensive research has focused on the prophylaxis and treatment of aspergillus through intravenous and aerosolized formulations. However, wide variabilities in dosage, length of prophylaxis, and route of administration have been reported across institutional sites (6,73,74).

**(A)**

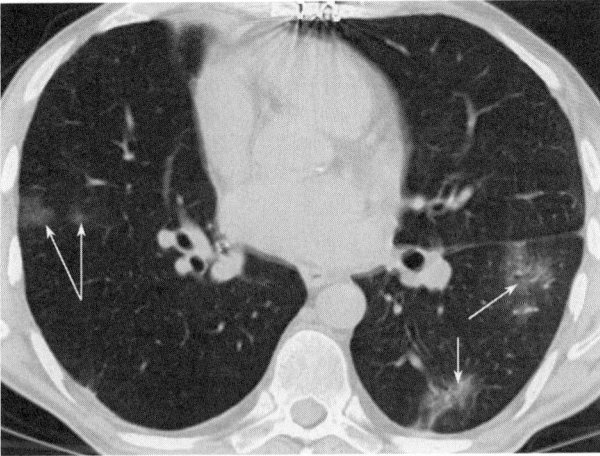

**(B)**

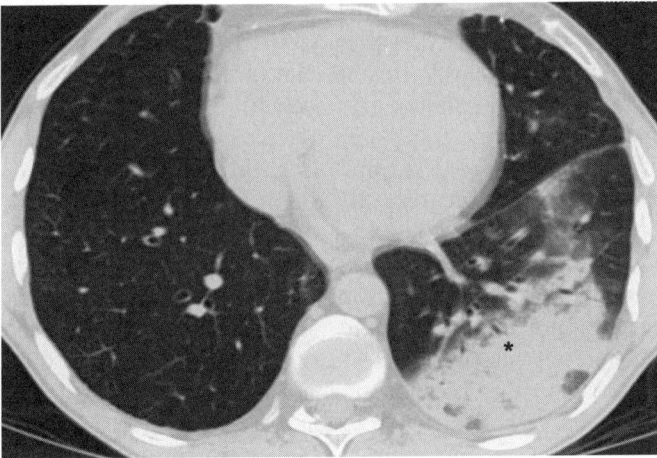

**Figure 15** (**A** and **B**) *Aspergillus* pneumonia. (**A**) In a patient culture positive for *Aspergillus*, ground-glass nodules (*white arrows*) with surrounding decreased density, often called "halo sign," are scattered throughout both lungs on high-resolution computed tomography. (**B**) A single axial slice through the left lower lobe demonstrates dense air-space consolidation (*asterisk*), another radiographic feature of *Aspergillus* infection.

## Pulmonary Embolism and Infarction

Pulmonary embolism (PE) and pulmonary infarction may be an underdiagnosed complication in lung transplant patients (78). In a study of 126 adult single lung, double lung, and heart–lung transplant patients at autopsy, the reported incidence of PE was 27% (79). Risk factors accounting for increased incidence of clinically silent PE included single and double lung transplantation versus heart–lung transplantation and prolonged mechanical ventilation >48 hours within the early posttransplant period (78,79). One postulated mechanism suggested is increased perfusion occurring within the allograft and the arterial anastomotic site, which acts as a thrombogenic surface. PE occurs both early and late in the post lung transplant period, with 75% of patients affected <4 months posttransplant (79). Pulmonary infarction occurring as a result of a PE is reported in up to 37.5% of patients, of which some were receiving anticoagulant prophylaxis therapy (78). It is thought that infarction occurs within the early postoperative period secondary to poorly developed collateral circulation (79). Clinically, patients may be asymptomatic or present with progressive dyspnea, tachypnea, chest pain, and hypoxemia. Overall the mortality rate associated with PE is 7% early in the postoperative period (<30 days) and 5% late in the postoperative period (>30 days) (79).

Radiographic findings of PE are relatively nonspecific and indirect, in that only secondary signs are observed. These include ill defined linear opacities, regions of parenchymal hyperlucency, atelectasis, hyperinflation, wedge-shaped consolidation, pleural effusion, elevation of the hemidiaphragm, enlargement of the central pulmonary vasculature, and cardiomegaly (80). CT pulmonary angiography (CTPA) clearly offers a superior method for diagnosing suspected pulmonary thromboembolic disease. Direct findings of acute PE on CTPA include central arterial filling defects, arterial occlusion, and localized arterial distension. Indirect or secondary findings for acute PE on CTPA include wedge-shaped consolidation with or without ground-glass opacity within the context of pulmonary infarction, differential parenchymal attenuation due to differences in regional perfusion termed "mosaic hypoperfusion" or oligemia, atelectasis, and pleural effusion (80). In addition, CTPA may further provide evidence of acutely elevated pulmonary arterial pressures, right ventricular strain, and secondary pericardial effusion. PE has been shown to preferentially affect the transplanted side with the majority occurring within the allograft (78).

## Conditions of the Native Lung Complicating Lung Transplantation

In patients undergoing single lung transplantation, the native lung is not only susceptible to the infections that occur within the allograft, namely bacterial, viral, fungal, and mycobacterial pathogens, but also situations unique to the remaining diseased lung. Within the context of single lung transplantation for end stage emphysema, hyperinflation of the native lung is a common finding but has been shown to be rarely associated with any significant morbidity or mortality (12,81). Other conditions arising from the native lung post transplantation include pneumothorax, primary lung malignancy, and less commonly, PE and pulmonary infarction (79,82). Native lung complications can occur from one month to five years posttransplantation (25,52,82). Excluding hyperinflation, the literature shows the incidence of complications involving the native lung as 11% (82). The associated mortality with native lung complications appears to be significant. In a small study of 111 transplants, 5 of 17 (29%) documented native lung complications (excluding hyperinflation) resulted in death (82).

In the presence of infection, patient symptoms include cough, dyspnea, pleuritic chest pain, fever, and hemoptysis (82). In the presence of pulmonary malignancy, patient presentation is variable with most patients asymptomatic and others with cough, progressive dyspnea, shoulder pain, chest pain, fatigue, and weakness (82,83). In the presence of native lung hyperinflation, patients are usually asymptomatic but may present with hemodynamic and ventilatory abnormalities (12,81).

Findings on chest radiographs or CT for native lung occurrences as a result of infection and malignancy are nonspecific and include new homogenous, heterogenous, lobar or segmental opacities, nodules (solitary or multiple), and atelectasis (Fig. 16) (82). PE, but more specifically, pulmonary infarction, as described earlier is associated with homogenous and/or heterogenous opacification within the native lung on chest radiograph or CT. Native lung hyperinflation presents as volume asymmetry between the native lung and transplanted lung with the native lung exerting cardiomediastinal shift and ipsilateral diaphragmatic flattening on chest radiographs and CT (12,81).

## SECONDARY LATE (>4 MONTHS)

### Mycobacterial Infection

Mycobacterial infections occurring post lung transplantation are relatively uncommon (0.8–3.8% of cases) and can manifest as both pulmonary and extrapulmonary infections (55,84–86). Development of infection in the transplanted patient is thought to be a result of donor lung colonization (52,84–86), native lung colonization (84), and transmission from the external environment (86). Typically, infection due to nontuberculosis and tuberculosis mycobacterial organisms occurs late in the post lung transplantation time continuum with most documented cases occurring at least four months after surgery (52,63,84,86). Clinically, patients may be asymptomatic or present with cough, increased sputum, dyspnea, fever, and weight loss (84,86).

Chest radiograph findings include clusters of multiple small nodules, nodular opacities or infiltrates, consolidation, cavitation, interlobular septal thickening, pleural thickening, unilateral or bilateral pleural effusions, and mediastinal lymphadenopathy (19,52,55,63,84–86). Findings on CT include multiple nodules, consolidation, interlobular septal lines or thickening,

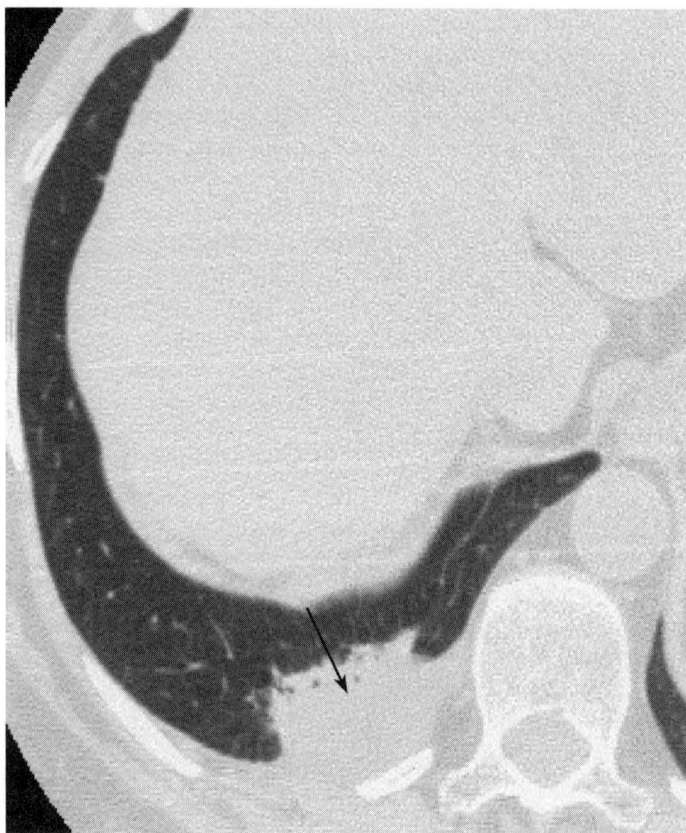

**Figure 16** Native lung infection. An axial image demonstrates mass-like consolidation (*black arrow*) within the right lower lobe posterior basal segment in the native lung of a single lung transplant patient. Bronchoalveolar lavage washings were positive for *Scedosporium apiospermum*.

cavitation, pleural effusions, and lymphadenopathy (Fig. 17) (19,52). On both methods of evaluation, the pattern of involvement is variable with infiltrative patterns described as focal, miliary, nodular, or cavitary affecting the native or transplanted lung (63).

Diagnosis can be obtained from several sources such as sputum, pleural fluid, and bronchial washings obtained from bronchoscopy with BAL or TBB (84,86). Although treatment is similar to nontransplant patient populations (84), limitations exist in the lung transplant patient population due to immunosuppression, enhanced drug toxicity, and drug interactions that have been described between rifampicin and cyclosporine or prednisone (86). Overall, treatment response to antimycobacterial medications has been, at best, variable and may be due to other opportunistic lung infections

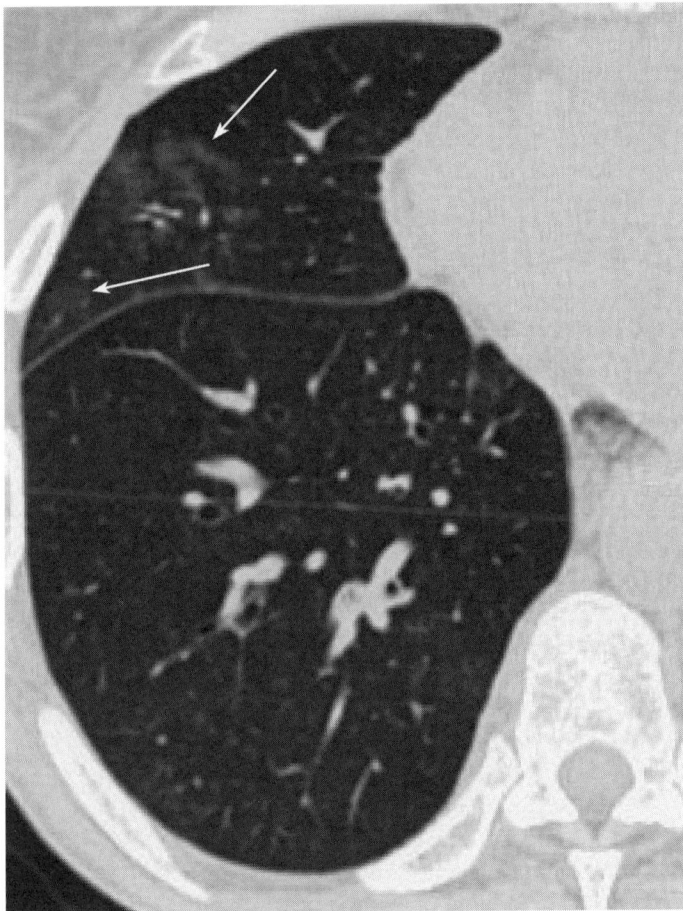

**Figure 17** Nontuberculous *Mycobacterium*. A single axial image demonstrates nodular ground glass (*white arrow*) within the right middle and lower lobe in a bilateral lung transplant patient. Bronchoalveolar lavage cultures later were positive for nontuberculous *Mycobacterium*.

and/or coexistent native lung disease that contribute to the irreversible airway damage and loss of lung function observed in the post lung transplant patient (84,86).

## Chronic Lung Rejection

Chronic allograft rejection is defined as the clinicopathologic syndrome characterized histopathologically by bronchiolitis obliterans (BO). Bronchiolitis obliterans syndrome (BOS) is used to describe less specific graft dysfunction with physiologic airflow obstruction (32,87). Histologically, BO is characterized by the development of dense, eosinophilic fibrous scarring within the small airways (32). Clinically, BOS is characterized by a decrease in forced expiratory volume in one second ($FEV_1$) from a baseline value obtained after lung transplantation (87). Chronic allograft rejection remains the major late complication of lung transplantation with at least 50% of patients affected by five years posttransplantation, regardless of age, gender, or underlying disease (1,33). Immunologic as well as nonimmunologic factors, such as infection, may play a primary role, although the etiology of chronic rejection remains unclear (87). Accepted risk factors include acute rejection and lymphocytic bronchitis, while potential risk factors include CMV pneumonitis, non-CMV pulmonary infections, and HLA-mismatching (3,19,33). Development of pathological or clinical symptoms of chronic rejection usually do not begin to occur until approximately one year post lung transplantation (19,32,88), but have been reported as early as three months posttransplant. Clinically, patients may be asymptomatic or present with slow, progressive dyspnea, cough with or without sputum, fever, atypical chest pain, malaise, recurrent lower respiratory tract infections, and a decline in conventional pulmonary function measures (3,19,21,89).

Findings associated with chronic rejection and BO/BOS on chest radiographs include absence of abnormal findings, hyperinflation, decreased peripheral vascular markings, regional volume contraction, subsegmental atelectasis, increased linear opacities, and bronchiectasis (21,90,91). Conventional and thin-section CT have both been employed to characterize the early and late associated findings of BO/BOS. Despite various approaches, reported CT findings of chronic rejection remain similar to those seen on chest radiographs and include bronchiectasis, bronchial wall thickening, nodular and linear branching opacities, air trapping, regional volume expansion/contraction, mosaic lung attenuation (defined as heterogenous areas of lung attenuation), decreased or distorted peripheral arteries, interlobular septal thickening, and peribronchovascular infiltrates (Figs. 18–20) (19,51,88–90,92–94).

Air trapping as detected on expiratory CT as mosaic pattern of lung attenuation, bronchiectasis, and bronchial wall thickening have all been suggested to be predictive of BO/BOS (Fig. 21) (89,92,95–97). TBB is used in addition to imaging to diagnose patients with a clinical suspicion of BO (91,98). Diagnosis by tissue sample is not without its complications and can often lead to over and under-diagnosis of BO (19,87,91,98). Inadequate tissue sampling, coexisting infection or pathology seen on biopsy, and the unequal pattern distribution with which BO affects the lung all potentially contribute to the poor sensitivity of TBB to detect BO (87,91). The observed decline in $FEV_1$ may in part be due to other posttransplantation complications, including infection, airway complications, and underlying

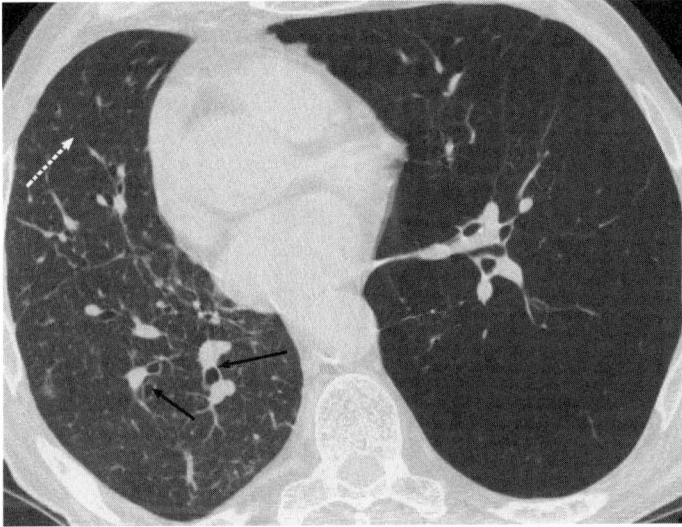

**Figure 18** Chronic lung rejection. A 62-year-old male patient status post right lung transplant secondary to end-stage, tobacco-induced emphysema shows evidence of rightward mediastinal shift, peribronchial thickening (*solid arrows*), and interlobular septal thickening (*white dashed arrow*) on inspiratory high-resolution computed tomography. The native left lung shows evidence of severe emphysema and marked lung destruction with multiple avascular regions of decreased attenuation.

disease (3,87). Overall, as a result, BO/BOS is a diagnosis usually made following exclusion of other causes.

Goals for treatment of BO/BOS include halting or retarding the progressive loss of respiratory function. Without definitive standard of care, limited available treatment options include alteration of immunosuppressive therapy (33) and retransplantation (99).

## Bronchiolitis Obliterans Organizing Pneumonia

Bronchiolitis obliterans organizing pneumonia (BOOP), also sometimes referred to as cryptogenic organizing pneumonia, is characterized histologically by the presence of inflammation and fibromyxomatous granulation tissue within the alveoli, alveolar ducts, and small airways (100–103). The incidence of BOOP in lung transplant patients ranges from 10% to 28% in the published literature (104,105). BOOP is most commonly associated with acute rejection (104,105). However, CMV pneumonitis, bacterial infection, and chronic rejection have also been observed to occur in conjunction with BOOP in lung transplant patients (104,105). On average, eight to nine months postoperatively, clinical and radiographic evidence of BOOP can be

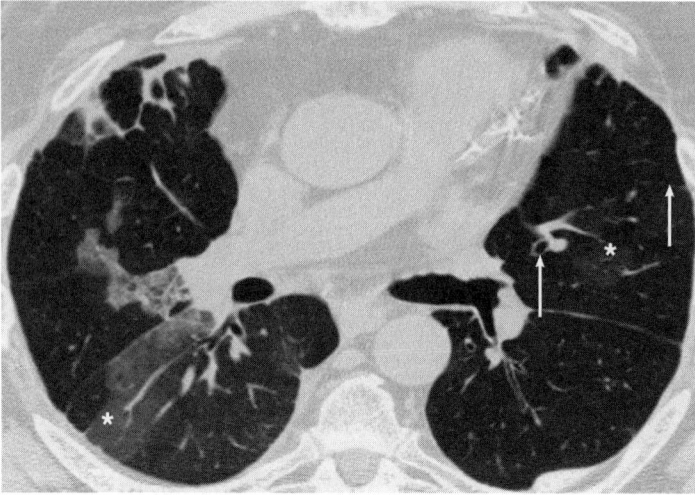

**Figure 19** Chronic lung rejection. Air trapping, a hallmark feature of chronic lung rejection, is characterized by the black or hypo-attenuated regions of the lung. Overall, on the axial high-resolution computed tomography image, mosaic attenuation with both hyper- and hypo-attenuated regions is evident. Bilateral, patchy ground-glass opacities (*asterisks*), interlobular septal thickening (*solid arrows*), and peribronchial thickening (*dashed arrow*) are also demonstrated.

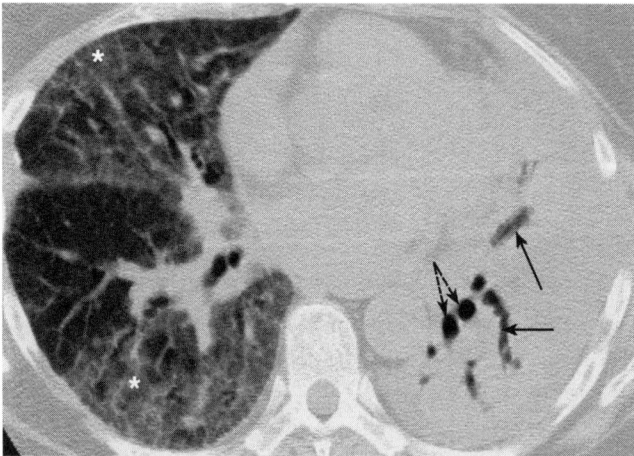

**Figure 20** Chronic lung rejection. Opacification of a single left lung transplant secondary to complete atelectasis is shown. Air bronchograms (*solid arrows*) with dilated bronchi (*dashed arrows*) are present. There are severe changes of idiopathic pulmonary fibrosis (*asterisks*) involving the right native lung. At autopsy, the cause of death for this patient was determined to be respiratory failure due to severe chronic rejection.

**(A)**

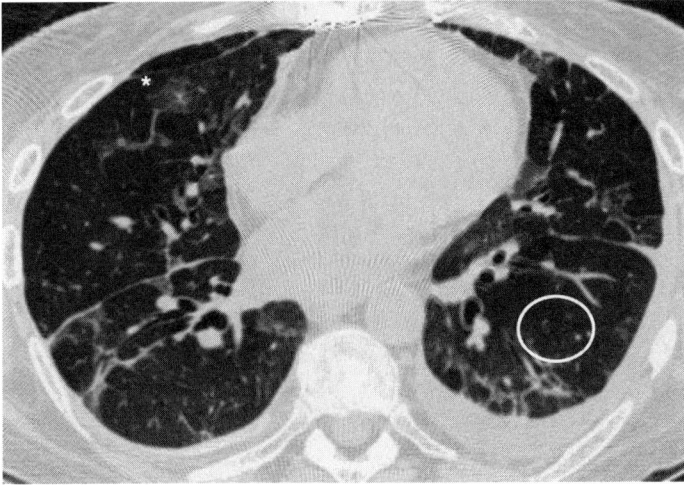

**(B)**

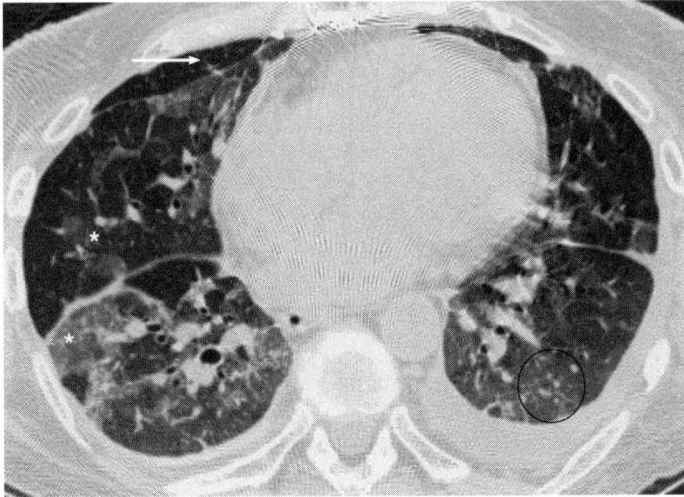

**Figure 21** (**A** and **B**) Chronic lung rejection. (**A**) A single, axial inspiratory high-resolution computed tomography (HRCT) image demonstrates regions of heterogenous opacities (*asterisk*), mosaic attenuation, and centrilobular nodularity (*encircled region*). (**B**) The expiratory HRCT image at the same level as (**A**) demonstrates air trapping characterized by bilateral hypo-attenuated regions, nodularity (*encircled region*), interlobular septal thickening (*black arrow*), and patchy regions of ground-glass opacities (*asterisks*). Right lung biopsy was positive for active bronchiolitis obliterans with associated mononunclear cellular infiltrates and epithelial damage.

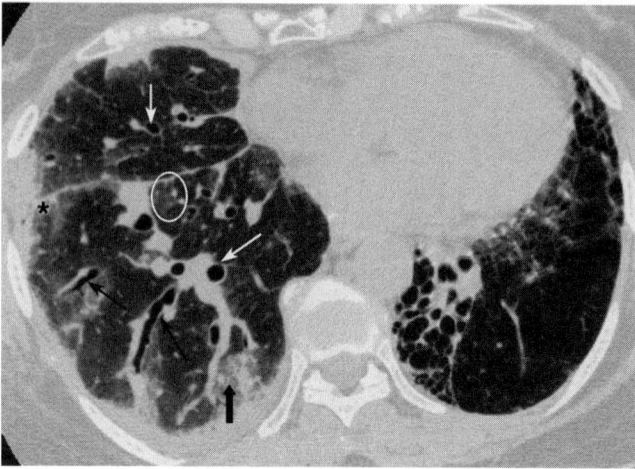

**Figure 22** Bronchiolitis obliterans organizing pneumonia. Single axial high-resolution computed tomography in a right lung transplant patient demonstrates patchy regions of consolidation (*thick black arrow*), multifocal ground glass (*asterisk*), airspace opacities (*encircled region*), scattered bronchiectasia (*thin black arrows*), and peribronchial thickening (*white arrows*) in the right lung. Right lobe transbronchial biopsy revealed an organizing pneumonia.

observed (104,105). Clinically, patients may show no evidence of acute disease and/or present with fever, cough, sputum production, and dyspnea (104,105).

Radiographically, bilateral, patchy, diffuse, or localized infiltrates can be seen on plain films of the chest (104,105). HRCT often shows evidence of air-space consolidation, ground-glass opacities, nodules or masses, and linear or reticular opacities. Additional CT findings include bronchial dilation, bronchial wall thickening, fibrosis, lung volume loss, and air trapping (Fig. 22) (104,106,107).

A diagnosis of BOOP can be obtained clinically, radiographically, and/or by open lung biopsy, TBB, and analysis of BAL fluid (104–107). Both the radiographic and clinical findings of BOOP have been shown to be reversible with supportive measures and administration of high dose corticosteroids (104).

## Posttransplantation Lymphoproliferative Disorder

Posttransplantation lymphoproliferative disorder (PTLD) can be characterized by a spectrum of lymphoid neoplasms (primarily B-cell) (1,108). Epstein–Barr virus (EBV) seronegative status is thought to be the major risk factor for development of PTLD (109). The incidence of PTLD reported in post lung transplant patients varies between 2.8% and 6.1% at one year posttransplant (110–113). The majority of PTLD presents within the first posttransplant year, but late disease can develop beyond one year posttransplantation (19,51,111). Early disease tends to have a benign course and is associated with intrathoracic manifestations which commonly affect the transplanted lung (109,111). Cases of early abdominal–pelvic lymphoproliferative disease have also been described post lung transplantation (114). Late disease rarely affects the transplanted lung and is associated with gastrointestinal involvement including gastric, colonic, and small bowel ulcerations (109,111). Involvement of the liver, spleen, kidneys, mesentery, and adrenal glands has also been described (108,114,115). For either early or late disease, patients may be asymptomatic or complain of nonspecific flu-like symptoms, including cough, fever, chills, and general malaise (24). Specific to abdominal–pelvic manifestations, patients may present with diffuse or localized abdominal or pelvic pain of varying severity, upper or lower gastrointestinal tract bleeding, and/or hematuria (114,115).

Intrathoracic chest radiograph findings include solitary or multiple pulmonary nodules, multifocal alveolar infiltrates, and mediastinal lymphadenopathy (Fig. 23A) (113). Intrathoracic CT findings include multiple, well-circumscribed pulmonary nodules, nodules with associated ground-glass opacities (halo sign), consolidation, interlobular septal thickening, pleural effusion, and mediastinal lymphadenopathy (Fig. 23B and C) (51,108,110,116–118). Abdominal–pelvic CT findings of PTLD are highly variable depending on the affected organ and can include homogenously enlarged peritoneal or retroperitoneal lymph nodes, enlarged focal or nodular low-attenuating lesions within the liver or spleen, and round, solid, hypoattenuated lesions within the kidneys (108,115,119). Gastrointestinal tract manifestations on CT include circumferential wall thickening, ulcerations, eccentric mass(es), dilatation or narrowing of bowel lumen, perforation, and intussusception (Fig. 24) (108,115,119).

Diagnosis of intrathoracic PTLD can be obtained by fine needle aspiration or core needle biopsy, TBB, or surgical excision (111). Diagnosis of abdominal–pelvic PTLD can also be obtained by tissue biopsy and surgical excision or resection (114). Immediate antiviral therapy following transplantation with lifetime maintenance therapy has been shown to lower the incidence of PTLD in lung transplant patients (112). Other treatment options include reduction in immunosuppressive therapy, conventional chemotherapy, surgical resection, interferon-alpha therapy, and anti-CD20 monoclonal antibody therapy (19,108,111).

## Upper Lobe Fibrosis

More recently, findings of progressive upper lobe fibrosis on HRCT were described as a potential late complication in post lung transplant patients. In a study of 391 post lung transplant patients, seven were described as having similar clinical, radiological, and pathological findings without a clear etiology

**(A)**

**(B)**

**(C)**

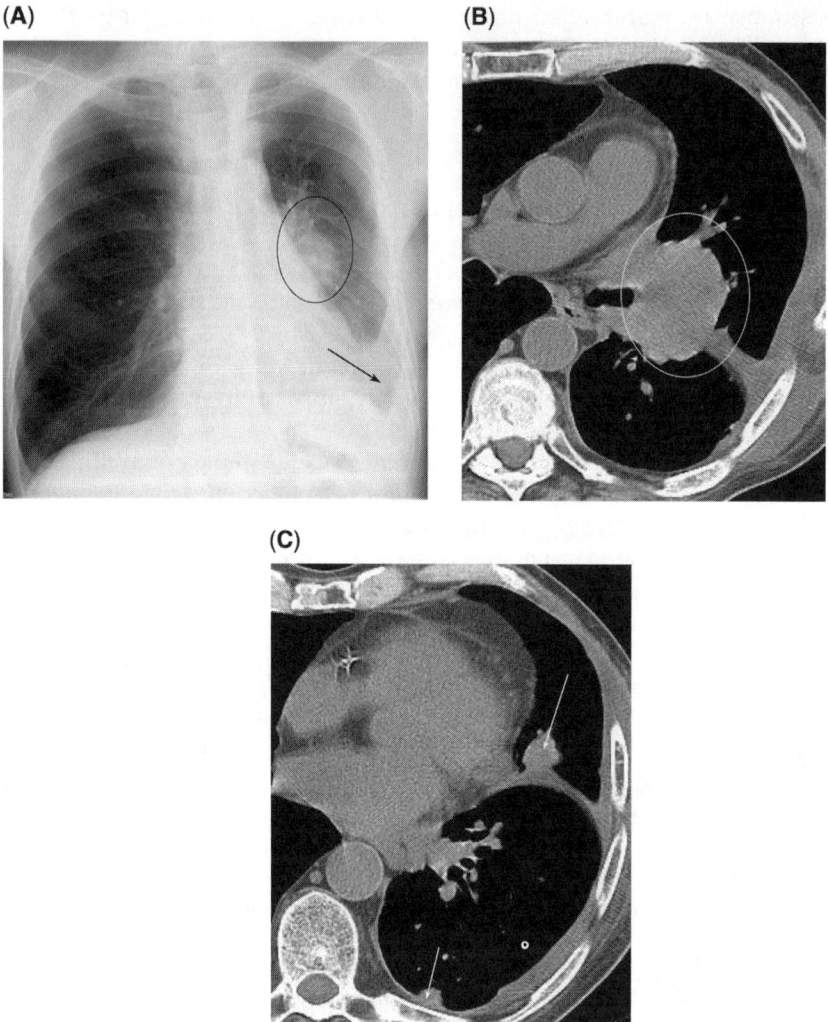

**Figure 23**  (A–C) Posttransplantation lymphoproliferative disorder. (A) A frontal chest radiograph demonstrates a large left hilar mass (*encircled region*) within the left transplant lung in a single allograft recipient and a small accompanying left pleural effusion (*black arrow*). (B and C) Mid- and lower axial images further demonstrate the left hilar mass (*encircled region*) seen on chest radiograph and two additional nodules within the lingula and left lower lobe (*white arrows*).

that could explain the observed similarities. HRCT findings when studied retro-spectively were observed rarely prior to the first postoperative year and occurred commonly between one and four years posttransplantation. Clinically, patients present with progressive dyspnea, declining exercise tolerance, and a worsening

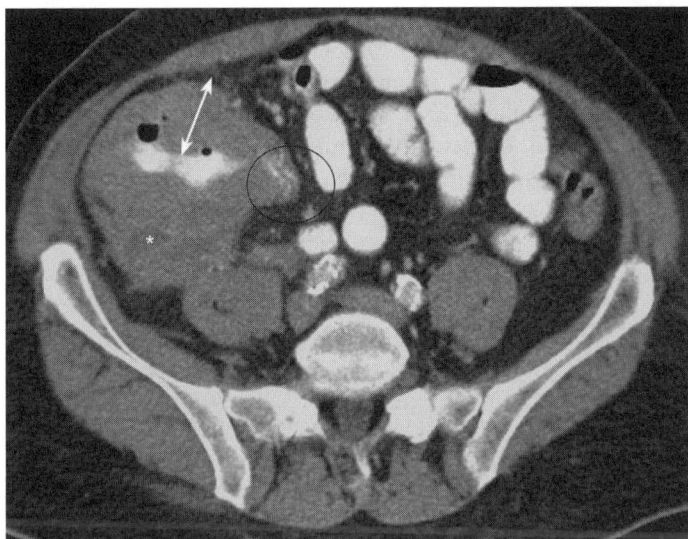

**Figure 24** Abdominal posttransplant lymphoproliferative disorder (PTLD). Axial computed tomography slice of the abdomen demonstrates a large soft tissue mass (*asterisk*) encasing the bowel, marked thickening of the cecal wall (*double-sided arrow*), and narrowing of the contrast filled bowel lumen. The terminal ileum is also seen (*encircled*). Biopsy findings were consistent with PTLD.

combination of restrictive and obstructive lung patterns as opposed to post-operative baseline conventional pulmonary function tests (120).

Initially, nonspecific interstitial lung disease findings were observed on CT. These findings included interlobular septal thickening and reticular or ground glass opacities. With time, findings of pulmonary fibrosis developed and included traction bronchiectasis, honeycombing, architectural distortion within the lung parenchyma, and loss of lung volume observed primarily in the upper lobes. All observed CT findings followed a gradual pattern of development and were very similar from patient to patient (120).

Pathologic findings (TBB or open lung biopsy) were inconclusive showing nonspecific inflammatory and fibrotic changes in all affected patients. With exclusion of mycobacterial infection and exposure to pulmonary cytotoxic medications as potential causes, the HRCT findings of upper lobe fibrosis were hypothesized to perhaps be part of the spectrum associated with chronic lung rejection. However, this hypothesis remains to be proven definitively in the published literature (120).

### Recurrence of Primary Disease

Recurrence of primary diseases such as sarcoidosis, lymphangioleiomyomatosis (LAM), langerhans cell histiocytosis (LCH), talc granulomatosis, diffuse panbronchiolitis, and pulmonary alveolar proteinosis have been reported in the literature (19,51,121,122). Observation of the radiologic findings and/or clinical presentation of recurrent disease has ranged from two weeks to two years posttransplant (121). Most often, the diagnosis of recurrent disease occurs as a result of incidental findings seen on CT or at biopsy with patients often being asymptomatic (121).

Sarcoidosis, the most likely primary pulmonary disease to recur at a frequency of approximately 35%, is often seen as a solitary pulmonary nodule or as numerous perilymphatic or miliary pulmonary nodules on HRCT (Fig. 25) (121,122). An enlarged retrocural lymph node observed on CT or the lack of radiologic abnormalities has been reported with recurrent LAM (121). Similar to sarcoidosis, a solitary pulmonary nodule was observed on CT in one case of recurrent LCH (121). Additionally, findings on CT for recurrent panbronchiolitis include bronchiectasis, bronchiolectasis, bronchial wall thickening, and tree-in-bud opacities (121).

Typically, recurrence of primary disease is diagnosed by fine needle aspiration, TBB, open lung biopsy, or autopsy (121). Overall, of the reported disease types that recur, none include the common indications

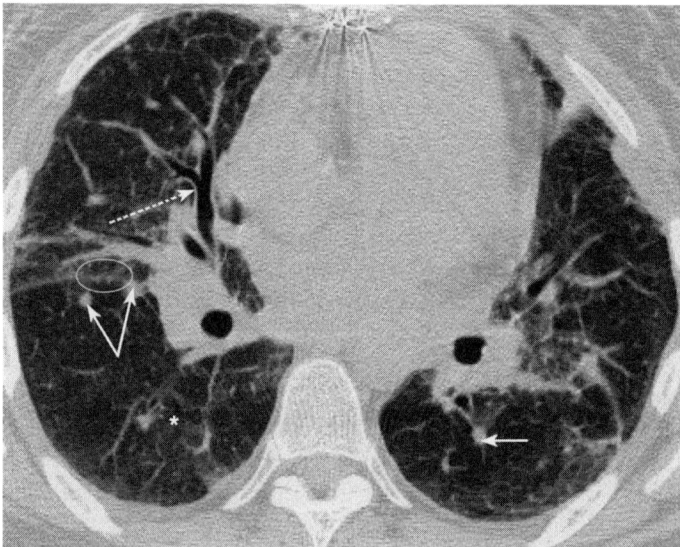

**Figure 25** Recurrent sarcoidosis. High-resolution computed tomography scan shows multiple subcentimeter pulmonary nodules (*solid white arrows*), nodularity along the right major fissure (*encircled region*), subtle peribronchial thickening (*dashed white arrow*), ground-glass opacities (*asterisk*), and peripheral scarring of the lung parenchyma. Biopsies of the right middle and lower lobes reveal noncaseating granulomas with airway inflammation consistent with sarcoidosis. Two months earlier, this patient received a double lung transplant due to sarcoidosis.

for lung transplantation such as emphysema, cystic fibrosis, and idiopathic pulmonary fibrosis (1).

## Bronchogenic Carcinoma

In addition to PTLD, post lung transplant patients are at increased risk for developing bronchogenic carcinoma (83). Frequency of development has been reported between 0.2% and 1.1% in the general lung transplant population and 2% to 4% in patients receiving lung transplantation secondary to emphysema or pulmonary fibrosis (83,85,123–125). Time from transplantation to development of radiological features typically occurs after the first postoperative year (83,124,125). Patients often complain of a combination of symptoms, including cough, hemoptysis, wheezing, dyspnea, fever, night sweats, shoulder pain, chest pain, fatigue, weakness, anorexia, and weight loss (83,125).

The most common radiographic findings include a solitary pulmonary nodule or mass with irregular margins (83,85,124,125). Other findings described on chest radiography include multiple nodules or masses with well circumscribed margins, lymphadenopathy, and pleural effusions (83). Findings on CT include single or multiple nodules or masses of varying sizes with irregular or well-circumscribed margins, air bronchograms, distal atelectasis, interlobular septal thickening, lymphadenopathy, and local tumor invasion into adjacent anatomical structures (carina, mediastinum, chest wall) (83). The majority of the observed nodules on chest radiograph or CT are noncalcified and more commonly affect the native lung (83,85,125).

The majority of bronchogenic carcinomas develop in post lung transplant patients with a history of heavy tobacco use (83,85,124). Additional risk factors include advancing age, impaired immunosuppression, and a pretransplantation diagnosis of pulmonary fibrosis or emphysema (83). The overall risk of developing a pulmonary malignancy appears low (123). However, when bronchogenic carcinoma is diagnosed in the post lung transplant patient, it is associated with a poor prognosis (83). Focus remains on early detection with annual radiographic screening and when clinically indicated, the use of necessary follow-up imaging and invasive screening tools, such as bronchoscopy with TBB (83).

## ANY STAGE

### Transbronchial Biopsy–Associated Complications

Bronchoscopy with TBB may be performed at any stage posttransplant, as a screening tool, a follow-up tool, and certainly, a diagnostic tool in any post lung transplant patient presenting with new clinical symptoms (126). It has been shown to aid in the diagnosis and differentiation of acute rejection and infection (51,126). TBB is well tolerated, but several potential complications do exist (51). Alveolar hemorrhage (blood loss > 100 mL), pulmonary hematomas, pulmonary lacerations, intrapulmonary cavitations or air cysts, pneumothoraces, and infection have been described as a result of transbronchial lung biopsies (38,51,126–129). Overall, the complication rate is reported between 6% and 12% (38,126). Chest radiographic findings are variable, dependent on the complication incurred. Apart from air leaks, pulmonary parenchymal injuries are the most common and can result in edematous and hemorrhagic contusions, lacerations, hematomas, and pneumatoceles. Findings on chest radiography include focal nodular or nonspecific alveolar opacities which are thought to be pulmonary lacerations, focal hemorrhage, and/or hematomas at the biopsy sites (128,129). Findings of TBB-associated complications may not always be easily discernable on chest radiographs and may appear one to two weeks post bronchoscopy (127,129). In such cases, CT has been shown to be superior (127,129). CT findings include small round or ovoid nodules, ranging in size from 2 to 15 mm, usually located within 2 cm of the pleura corresponding to the biopsy sites (51,127). These nodules can be solid or cavitary, can often exhibit a surrounding halo of ground glass and can persist up to one month following TBB (Fig. 26) (127). The mortality rate associated with the procedure is 0% (38,126). Overall, although associated risks of morbidity exist, TBB is a sensitive screening tool for the diagnosis of acute or chronic rejection and infection in symptomatic patients (126).

## Extrathoracic Complications

In addition to abdominal pelvic PTLD, extrathoracic complications occurring within the post lung transplant period include central nervous system (CNS) neurotoxicities and complications involving the gastrointestinal tract unrelated to PTLD.

In organ transplantation, cyclosporine A and tacrolimus are a routine part of immunosuppressive therapy. In several case reports, CNS neurotoxicities, as a result of both pharmacological agents, have been described (130–134) along with numerous other side effects. The potential to develop CNS neurotoxicity is well known (135); however, the frequency at which the post lung transplant population is affected remains largely unknown. From the available case reports, neurotoxicity secondary to cyclosporine or tacrolimus occurs in the lung transplant patient anywhere from days to years following transplantation (130–134,136). Patient symptoms are very similar, with headache, seizures, lethargy, disorientation, visual disturbances, and hypertension described in both drug-induced neurotoxicities (130–134,137).

CT and primarily MRI are the imaging modalities thought best to characterize the abnormal neuropathology associated with cyclosporine and tacrolimus toxicity. Findings on head CT with contrast due to cyclosporine toxicity include edema and bilateral symmetric nonenhancing or

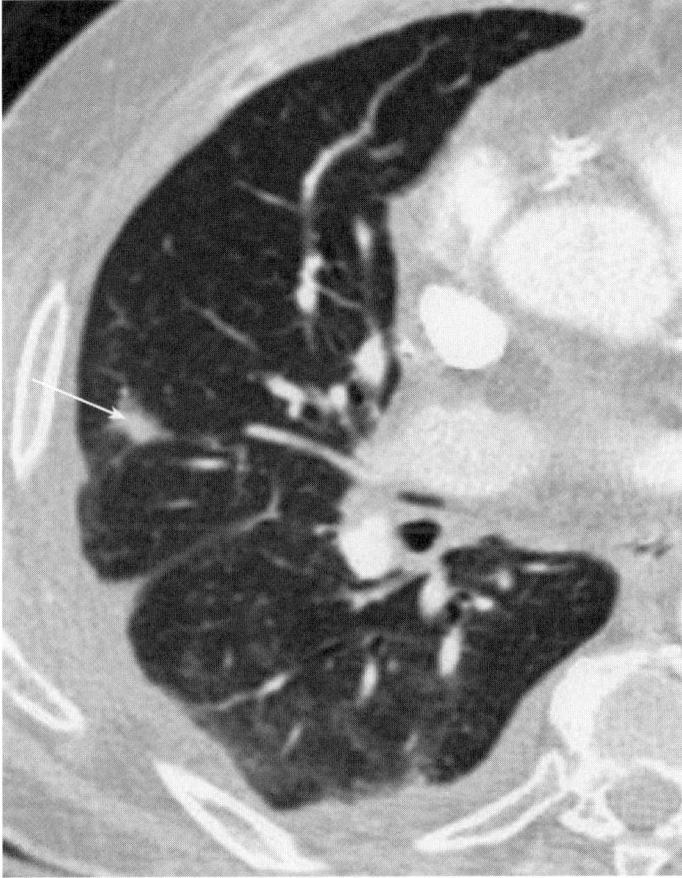

**Figure 26** Transbronchial biopsy–associated hematoma. A single axial high-resolution computed tomography scan two days post-transbronchial biopsy demonstrates the appearance of a new solitary nodule (*white arrow*), which resolved spontaneously on subsequent scans.

hypodense regions within the subcortical white matter (131,137). Similarly, multiple, bilateral hypodense, or enhancing regions within the subcortical white matter and cerebellar hemispheres, reduction in ventricle size, and diffuse edema have been observed on head CT in association with tacrolimus toxicity (Fig. 27A and B) (132–134). MRI using fluid attenuated inversion recovery $T_2$ weighted images (FLAIR) in both cyclosporine and tacrolimus toxicity shows multiple, bilateral, and symmetric hyperintensity involving the white matter with cortical and subcortical changes (Fig. 28A and B). Involvement of the cerebellum and brainstem have also been described (130–133,136,137).

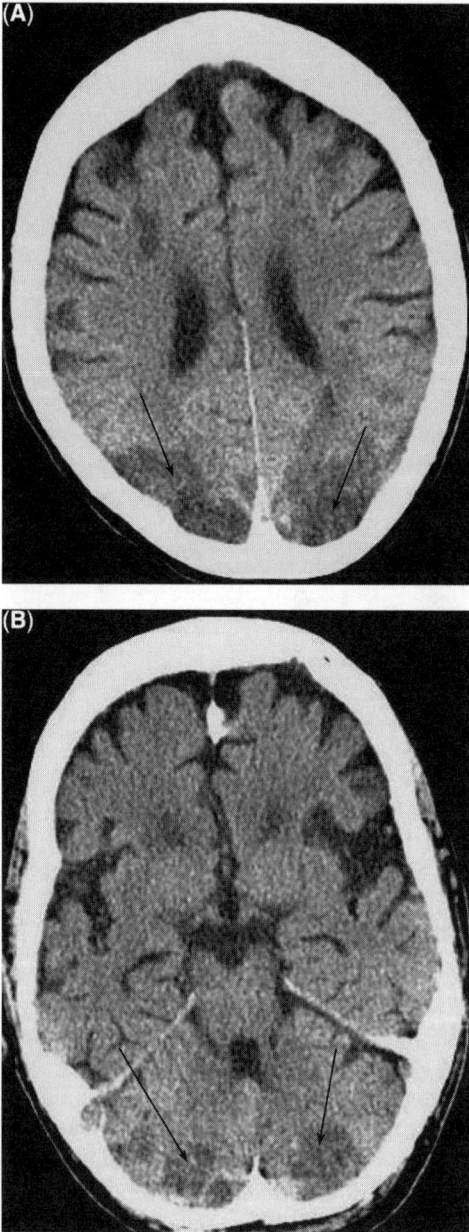

**Figure 27** (**A** and **B**) Tacrolimus-induced neurotoxicity. Axial computed tomography image with contrast (both **A** and **B**) demonstrates bilateral, symmetric hypodense regions (*black arrows*) within the subcortical white matter in a liver transplant patient receiving tacrolimus. Similar radiological findings have been described in lung transplant patients.

The pathogenesis leading to CNS neurotoxicity in the setting of cyclosporine or tacrolimus immunosuppression is unknown. The majority of what is observed on CT and MRI is reversible with reduction or cessation of the offending drug (Fig. 28C and D) (130–134). In addition, treatment is often aimed at controlling associated symptomatic hypertension and correcting electrolyte imbalances if present (130,136). Interestingly, several case reports show development of neurotoxicity is not related to dosage of either cyclosporine or tacrolimus, and findings of neurotoxicity have been reported in lung transplant patients, both with therapeutic and elevated drug levels (130,132–134,136).

Post lung transplantation, reports of several gastrointestinal complications, including prolonged adynamic ileus, colonic perforation (most commonly secondary to diverticulitis), colitis, esophagitis, gastrointestinal bleeding, and gall bladder disease, have been described (138–142). Overall, the incidence of abdominal complications following lung transplantation ranges from 6% to 18% (139–142). Complications tend to occur both within the first 30 days following transplantation (140,141) and thereafter (140). Patient presentation, based upon the severity and type of gastrointestinal complication, may vary from being asymptomatic to having anorexia, nausea, vomiting, progressive, crampy abdominal or epigastric pain, diarrhea, fever, and abdominal distention or tenderness (141,142).

Findings of free air in the abdomen on plain radiograph and collections of retroperitoneal air on CT have been described in the setting of colonic or gastric perforation (Fig. 29) (140–142). Large amounts of free intraperitoneal fluid, left lower quadrant mass or phlegmon, and/or thickening of the sigmoid colon with associated fat stranding has been described on CT in patients with diverticulitis or perforation secondary to diverticulitis (Fig. 30) (142,143). In the setting of colitis, lung transplant patients may show evidence of thickened loops of bowel in the large and small intestine on CT of the abdomen and pelvis (144). For complications involving the gall bladder, ultrasound may reveal thickening of the gall bladder wall, sludge within the organ itself, and/or cholelithiasis (138).

Following lung transplantation, development of gastrointestinal complications is a significant risk of mortality (20–50%) (140–142). Overall, consensus exists in the literature that among lung transplant patients complaining of abdominal symptoms, a high index of suspicion with aggressive management including appropriate diagnostic studies and surgical intervention to exclude life-threatening abdominal complications is necessary (140–143).

## FUTURE DIRECTIONS IN IMAGING

Ventilation scintigraphy, FDG-PET, $^3$He-MRI, and multi-detector CT with computerized reformations are potential future techniques that may aid in

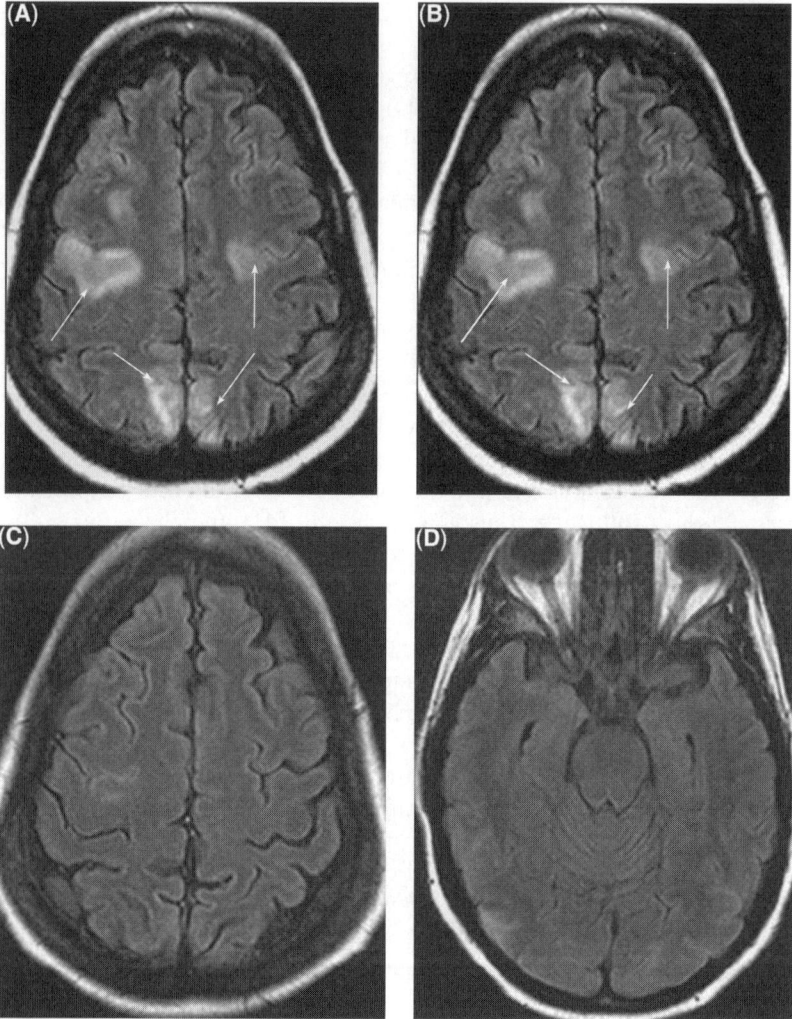

**Figure 28** (A–D) Tacrolimus-induced neurotoxicity. Fluid attenuation inversion recovery (FLAIR) images (both **A** and **B**) demonstrate multiple bilateral, symmetric hyperintense regions (*white arrows*) involving the white matter. This patient, a renal transplant recipient receiving tacrolimus, presented initially with new onset seizures. Images (**C**) and (**D**) (taken at the same level as **A** and **B**, one month later) show no evidence of the multiple hyperintense regions seen previously on FLAIR. Tacrolimus therapy had been terminated one month earlier following acquisition of images (**A**) and (**B**).

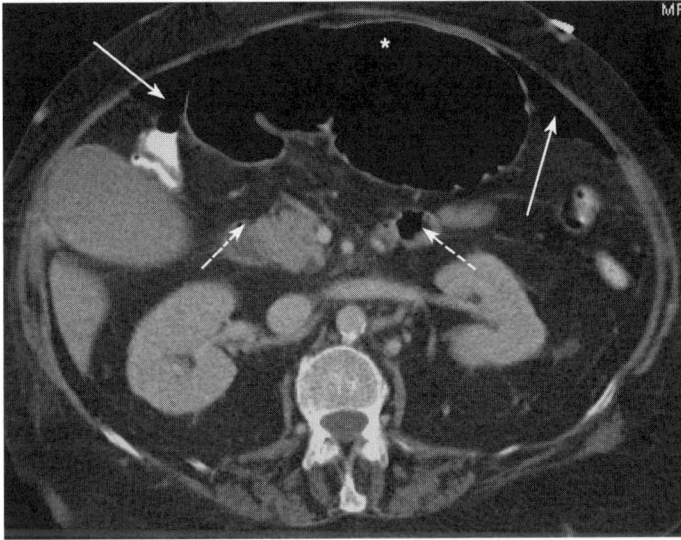

**Figure 29** Bowel perforation. Abdominal computed tomography demonstrates a large collection of free intraperitoneal air (*solid arrows*) and dilatation of the bowel lumen (*asterisk*). Intramural air is also present within the second and fourth portions of the duodenum (*dashed arrows*). At laparotomy, the patient was found to have perforation of the ileum with segments of necrotic bowel extending to portions of the right colon.

the description of complications that occur within the post lung transplantation period.

Ventilation scintigraphy, commonly used in the setting of PE, has been applied to the post lung transplant patient to detect native and transplanted lung function by quantifying their contribution to $FEV_1$ (145). This technique may play a potential role in the detection of early BO in single lung transplant patients with vascular or restrictive lung disease (145). Ventilation scintigraphy is a noninvasive and potentially repeatable imaging modality, offering a safe alternative to bronchoscopy with TBB (145). However, with radiation exposure and only small clinical studies examining the viability of ventilation scintigraphy to quantify pulmonary dysfunction in lung transplant patients, further investigation is needed.

As an additional modality under investigation, FDG-PET can detect neutrophil activation in regions of inflammation or infection in the post lung transplant patient (146). Infection is associated with enhanced neutrophil activation and a corresponding increased FDG-PET signal, and acute rejection is associated with limited neutrophil activation and minimal FDG-PET signal uptake (146). One major potential application is the use of FDG-PET to discriminate between infection and rejection. Other

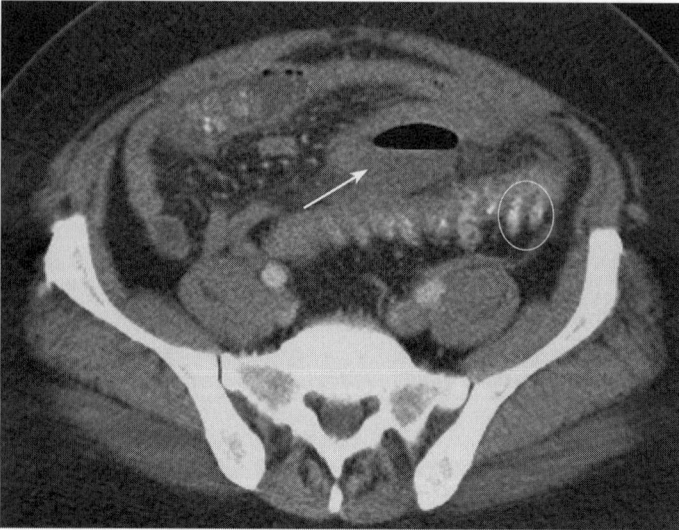

**Figure 30** Diverticulitis. Axial computed tomography of the abdomen demonstrates diverticulosis of the sigmoid colon with multiple contrast filled diverticula
(*encircled*). Within the mesentery, a large abscess containing both air and fluid is seen
(*arrow*).

applications include staging of PTLD and the characterization of extrathoracic PTLD sites missed by conventional CT imaging (147). FDG-
PET, like ventilation scintigraphy, is noninvasive and safe, thus having
the potential to be used multiple times in the same patient with minimal risk
of injury (146). In the future, this may lead to an overall reduction in the
number of transbronchial biopsies needed to screen, diagnose and follow
patients with acute or chronic lung rejection (146). FDG-PET also carries
a risk of exposure to radiation, which may potentially limit its use as a follow-up tool (148).

$^3$He-MRI has both static and dynamic potential to characterize the
ventilated regions of native and transplanted lungs (149–151). In comparison studies to conventional CT imaging, $^3$He-MRI is superior in detecting
the ventilated region of the lung participating in gas exchange in patients
with emphysema (148). As a consequence, $^3$He-MRI may play a role, as a
noninvasive follow-up tool to monitor transplanted lung outcome over
time, in characterizing regional ventilatory defects during dynamic breathing maneuvers and in detecting early BO (148–150,152,153). Static lung
volume $^3$He-MRI images have the advantage of better spatial and temporal
resolution, as compared to ventilation scintigraphy and PET (148). However, in comparison, dynamic $^3$He-MRI images still need improvement in
temporal resolution (150). Particular advantages of $^3$He-MRI, compared

to scintigraphy, PET, and multi-detector CT, are the lack of radiation exposure and its application as both a dynamic and a static imaging modality (148–150). Disadvantages of the technique include lack of standard methods for inspiration of $^3$He gas and the low availability and high cost of $^3$He (149,150).

Multidetector CT allows rapid acquisition of thin-section data of the entire thorax in a single breath hold. This allows for detailed review of the lung parenchyma as well as for advanced computerized aided reformations and three-dimensional visual images of the tracheobronchial tree and its associated vasculature (154). This modality may be particularly useful in characterizing the extent and location of bronchial anastomic complications, such as bronchial stenosis or bronchomalacia (154,155). The advantage of the technique lies in its ability to characterize an abnormality in three dimensions with multiple viewing planes (154). Disadvantages include radiation exposure and potential for motion artifacts and misregistration. Compared to bronchoscopy with TBB, other disadvantages of multidetector CT include its inability to biopsy regions of interest and its lack of adequate evaluation of color, vascularity, and structure of the mucous membrane, all of which are easily obtained when bronchoscopy is performed (154).

Computer-assisted density and texture feature analysis has been successfully used in the detection of a variety of parenchymal and airway abnormalities (50,156–158). With the ability to distinguish between such lung parenchymal patterns as honeycombing, ground glass, nodularity, and emphysema (157), and assess split lung function in the native versus the transplanted lung (50,158), these techniques may have a future, applicable role in improving the CT detection and quantitation of various transplant-related complications, particularly BO.

## CONCLUSION

With lung transplantation, as discussed, a myriad of complications can occur within the posttransplant period, often with nonspecific, sometimes overlapping clinical presentations, imaging findings, and at times, lack of accurate diagnostic testing. By gaining an understanding of the clinical and radiological findings and their relationships relative to transplantation, the postoperative complications of lung transplantation can be easily and usefully organized to aid in narrowing the clinician's differential diagnosis.

## REFERENCES

1. Trulock EP, Edwards LB, Taylor DO, et al. The Registry of the International Society for Heart and Lung Transplantation: Twentieth Official Adult Lung and Heart–Lung Transplant Report—2003. J Heart Lung Transplant 2003; 22:625–635.

2. Davis RD Jr, Pasque MK. Pulmonary transplantation. Ann Surg 1995; 221:14–28.
3. Bando K, Paradis IL, Komatsu K, et al. Analysis of time-dependent risks for infection, rejection, and death after pulmonary transplantation. J Thorac Cardiovasc Surg 1995; 109:49–57; discussion 57–59.
4. Wechsler RJ, Steiner RM, Kinori I. Monitoring the monitors: the radiology of thoracic catheters, wires, and tubes. Semin Roentgenol 1988; 23:61–84.
5. Goodman LR, Conrardy PA, Laing F, Singer MM. Radiographic evaluation of endotracheal tube position. Am J Roentgenol 1976; 127:433–434.
6. Lau CL, Patterson GA, Palmer SM. Critical care aspects of lung transplantation. J Intensive Care Med 2004; 19:83–104.
7. Frost AE. Donor criteria and evaluation. Clin Chest Med 1997; 18:231–237.
8. Ouwens JP, van der Mark TW, van der Bij W, Geertsma A, de Boer WJ, Koeter GH. Size matching in lung transplantation using predicted total lung capacity. Eur Respir J 2002; 20:1419–1422.
9. Massard G, Badier M, Guillot C, et al. Lung size matching for double lung transplantation based on the submammary thoracic perimeter. Accuracy and functional results. The Joint Marseille–Montreal Lung Transplant Program. J Thorac Cardiovasc Surg 1993; 105:9–14.
10. Winton TL. Lung transplantation: donor selection. Semin Thorac Cardiovasc Surg 1992; 4:79–82.
11. Egan TM, Thompson JT, Detterbeck FC, et al. Effect of size (mis)matching in clinical double-lung transplantation. Transplantation 1995; 59:707–713.
12. Weill D, Torres F, Hodges TN, Olmos JJ, Zamora MR. Acute native lung hyperinflation is not associated with poor outcomes after single lung transplant for emphysema. J Heart Lung Transplant 1999; 18:1080–1087.
13. Anderson DC, Glazer HS, Semenkovich JW, et al. Lung transplant edema: chest radiography after lung transplantation—the first 10 days. Radiology 1995; 195:275–281.
14. Kuno R, Kanter KR, Torres WE, Lawrence EC. Single lung transplantation followed by contralateral bullectomy for bullous emphysema. J Heart Lung Transplant 1996; 15:389–394.
15. Bittner HB, Dunitz J, Hertz M, Bolman MR III, Park SJ. Hyperacute rejection in single lung transplantation—case report of successful management by means of plasmapheresis and antithymocyte globulin treatment. Transplantation 2001; 71:649–651.
16. Frost AE, Jammal CT, Cagle PT. Hyperacute rejection following lung transplantation. Chest 1996; 110:559–562.
17. Zander DS, Baz MA, Visner GA, et al. Analysis of early deaths after isolated lung transplantation. Chest 2001; 120:225–232.
18. Choi JK, Kearns J, Palevsky HI, et al. Hyperacute rejection of a pulmonary allograft. Immediate clinical and pathologic findings. Am J Respir Crit Care Med 1999; 160:1015–1018.
19. Collins J. Imaging of the chest after lung transplantation. J Thorac Imaging 2002; 17:102–112.
20. Kundu S, Herman SJ, Winton TL. Reperfusion edema after lung transplantation: radiographic manifestations. Radiology 1998; 206:75–80.

21. Stewart KC, Patterson GA. Current trends in lung transplantation. Am J Transplant 2001; 1:204–210.
22. Siegleman SS, Sinha SB, Veith FJ. Pulmonary reimplantation response. Ann Surg 1973; 177:30–36.
23. Thabut G, Vinatier I, Stern JB, et al. Primary graft failure following lung transplantation: predictive factors of mortality. Chest 2002; 121:1876–1882.
24. Ward S, Muller NL. Pulmonary complications following lung transplantation. Clin Radiol 2000; 55:332–339.
25. Ferrer J, Roldan J, Roman A, et al. Acute and chronic pleural complications in lung transplantation. J Heart Lung Transplant 2003; 22:1217–1225.
26. Nunley DR, Grgurich WF, Keenan RJ, Dauber JH. Empyema complicating successful lung transplantation. Chest 1999; 115:1312–1315.
27. de Hoyos A, Sundaresan S. Thoracic empyema. Surg Clin North Am 2002; 82:643–671, viii.
28. Kim EA, Lee KS, Shim YM, et al. Radiographic and CT findings in complications following pulmonary resection. Radiographics 2002; 22:67–86.
29. Tocino IM, Miller MH, Fairfax WR. Distribution of pneumothorax in the supine and semirecumbent critically ill adult. Am J Roentgenol 1985; 144:901–905.
30. Murray JF, Nadel JA, eds. Textbook of Respiratory Medicine. 3rd ed. Philadelphia, PA: WB Saunders, 2000.
31. Spirn PW, Gross GW, Wechsler RJ, Steiner RM. Radiology of the chest after thoracic surgery. Semin Roentgenol 1988; 23:9–31.
32. Yousem SA, Berry GJ, Cagle PT, et al. Revision of the 1990 working formulation for the classification of pulmonary allograft rejection: Lung Rejection Study Group. J Heart Lung Transplant 1996; 15:1–15.
33. Sharples LD, McNeil K, Stewart S, Wallwork J. Risk factors for bronchiolitis obliterans: a systematic review of recent publications. J Heart Lung Transplant 2002; 21:271–281.
34. Herman SJ, Rappaport DC, Weisbrod GL, Olscamp GC, Patterson GA, Cooper JD. Single-lung transplantation: imaging features. Radiology 1989; 170:89–93.
35. King-Biggs MB. Acute pulmonary allograft rejection. Mechanisms, diagnosis, and management. Clin Chest Med 1997; 18:301–310.
36. Loubeyre P, Revel D, Delignette A, Loire R, Mornex JF. High-resolution computed tomographic findings associated with histologically diagnosed acute lung rejection in heart–lung transplant recipients. Chest 1995; 107:132–138.
37. Gotway MB, Dawn SK, Sellami D, et al. Acute rejection following lung transplantation: limitations in accuracy of thin-section CT for diagnosis. Radiology 2001; 221:207–212.
38. Hopkins PM, Aboyoun CL, Chhajed PN, et al. Prospective analysis of 1,235 transbronchial lung biopsies in lung transplant recipients. J Heart Lung Transplant 2002; 21:1062–1067.
39. Lawrence EC. Diagnosis and management of lung allograft rejection. Clin Chest Med 1990; 11:269–278.
40. Schmid RA, Boehler A, Speich R, Frey HR, Russi EW, Weder W. Bronchial anastomotic complications following lung transplantation: still a major cause of morbidity? Eur Respir J 1997; 10:2872–2875.

41. Schafers HJ, Haydock DA, Cooper JD. The prevalence and management of bronchial anastomotic complications in lung transplantation. J Thorac Cardiovasc Surg 1991; 101:1044–1052.

42. Date H, Trulock EP, Arcidi JM, Sundaresan S, Cooper JD, Patterson GA. Improved airway healing after lung transplantation. An analysis of 348 bronchial anastomoses. J Thorac Cardiovasc Surg 1995; 110:1424–1432; discussion 1432–1433.

43. Nunley DR, Gal AA, Vega JD, Perlino C, Smith P, Lawrence EC. Saprophytic fungal infections and complications involving the bronchial anastomosis following human lung transplantation. Chest 2002; 122:1185–1191.

44. Kshettry VR, Kroshus TJ, Hertz MI, Hunter DW, Shumway SJ, Bolman RM III. Early and late airway complications after lung transplantation: incidence and management. Ann Thorac Surg 1997; 63:1576–1583.

45. Alvarez A, Algar J, Santos F, et al. Airway complications after lung transplantation: a review of 151 anastomoses. Eur J Cardiothorac Surg 2001; 19:381–387.

46. Semenkovich JW, Glazer HS, Anderson DC, Arcidi JM Jr, Cooper JD, Patterson GA. Bronchial dehiscence in lung transplantation: CT evaluation. Radiology 1995; 194:205–208.

47. Trulock EP. Lung transplantation. Am J Respir Crit Care Med 1997; 155: 789–818.

48. Boiselle PM. Multislice helical CT of the central airways. Radiol Clin North Am 2003; 41:561–574.

49. Boiselle PM, Feller-Kopman D, Ashiku S, Weeks D, Ernst A. Tracheobronchomalacia: evolving role of dynamic multislice helical CT. Radiol Clin North Am 2003; 41:627–636.

50. Szold O, Levine M, Goldin JG. Late expiratory plateau patients in post-single lung transplant patients with emphysema. Am J Respir Crit Care Med 1995; 151:A85.

51. Soyer P, Devine N, Frachon I, et al. Computed tomography of complications of lung transplantation. Eur Radiol 1997; 7:847–853.

52. Collins J, Muller NL, Kazerooni EA, Paciocco G. CT findings of pneumonia after lung transplantation. Am J Roentgenol 2000; 175:811–818.

53. Tew J, Calenoff L, Berlin BS. Bacterial or nonbacterial pneumonia: accuracy of radiographic diagnosis. Radiology 1977; 124:607–612.

54. Franquet T. Imaging of pneumonia: trends and algorithms. Eur Respir J 2001; 18:196–208.

55. Fishman JA, Rubin RH. Infection in organ-transplant recipients. N Engl J Med 1998; 338:1741–1751.

56. Dharnidharka VR, Stablein DM, Harmon WE. Fungal infections. Am J Transplant 2004; 4:110–134.

57. Grossi P, Farina C, Fiocchi R, Dalla Gasperina D. Prevalence and outcome of invasive fungal infections in 1,963 thoracic organ transplant recipients: a multicenter retrospective study. Italian Study Group of Fungal Infections in Thoracic Organ Transplant Recipients. Transplantation 2000; 70:112–116.

58. Singh N. Fungal infections in the recipients of solid organ transplantation. Infect Dis Clin North Am 2003; 17:113–134, viii.

59. Patterson TF. Approaches to fungal diagnosis in transplantation. Transpl Infect Dis 1999; 1:262–272.
60. Syndman DR. Infection in solid organ transplantation. Transpl Infect Dis 1999; 1:21–28.
61. Patterson JE. Epidemiology of fungal infections in solid organ transplant patients. Transpl Infect Dis 1999; 1:229–236.
62. Kanj SS, Welty-Wolf K, Madden J, et al. Fungal infections in lung and heart-lung transplant recipients. Report of 9 cases and review of the literature. Medicine (Baltimore) 1996; 75:142–156.
63. Shorr AF, Susla GM, O'Grady NP. Pulmonary infiltrates in the non-HIV-infected immunocompromised patient: etiologies, diagnostic strategies, and outcomes. Chest 2004; 125:260–271.
64. McAdams HP, Rosado-de-Christenson ML, Templeton PA, Lesar M, Moran CA. Thoracic mycoses from opportunistic fungi: radiologic–pathologic correlation. Radiographics 1995; 15:271–286.
65. Buff SJ, McLelland R, Gallis HA, Matthay R, Putman CE. *Candida albicans* pneumonia: radiographic appearance. Am J Roentgenol 1982; 138: 645–648.
66. Potente G. CT findings in fungal opportunistic pneumonias: body and brain involvement. Comput Med Imaging Graph 1989; 13:423–428.
67. Matar LD, McAdams HP, Palmer SM, et al. Respiratory viral infections in lung transplant recipients: radiologic findings with clinical correlation. Radiology 1999; 213:735–742.
68. Ko JP, Shepard JA, Sproule MW, et al. CT manifestations of respiratory syncytial virus infection in lung transplant recipients. J Comput Assist Tomogr 2000; 24:235–241.
69. Palmer SM Jr, Henshaw NG, Howell DN, Miller SE, Davis RD, Tapson VF. Community respiratory viral infection in adult lung transplant recipients. Chest 1998; 113:944–950.
70. Khalifah AP, Hachem RR, Chakinala MM, et al. Respiratory viral infections are a distinct risk for bronchiolitis obliterans syndrome and death. Am J Respir Crit Care Med 2004; 170:181–187.
71. Billings JL, Hertz MI, Wendt CH. Community respiratory virus infections following lung transplantation. Transpl Infect Dis 2001; 3:138–148.
72. Franquet T, Muller NL, Oikonomou A, Flint JD. Aspergillus infection of the airways: computed tomography and pathologic findings. J Comput Assist Tomogr 2004; 28:10–16.
73. Singh N, Husain S. Aspergillus infections after lung transplantation: clinical differences in type of transplant and implications for management. J Heart Lung Transplant 2003; 22:258–266.
74. Minari A, Husni R, Avery RK, et al. The incidence of invasive aspergillosis among solid organ transplant recipients and implications for prophylaxis in lung transplants. Transpl Infect Dis 2002; 4:195–200.
75. Mehrad B, Paciocco G, Martinez FJ, Ojo TC, Iannettoni MD, Lynch JP III. Spectrum of aspergillus infection in lung transplant recipients: case series and review of the literature. Chest 2001; 119:169–175.

76. Diederich S, Scadeng M, Dennis C, Stewart S, Flower CD. Aspergillus infection of the respiratory tract after lung transplantation: chest radiographic and CT findings. Eur Radiol 1998; 8:306–312.
77. Husain S, Singh N. Bronchiolitis obliterans and lung transplantation: evidence for an infectious etiology. Semin Respir Infect 2002; 17:310–314.
78. Burns KE, Iacono AT. Incidence of clinically unsuspected pulmonary embolism in mechanically ventilated lung transplant recipients. Transplantation 2003; 76:964–968.
79. Burns KE, Iacono AT. Pulmonary embolism on postmortem examination: an under-recognized complication in lung-transplant recipients? Transplantation 2004; 77:692–698.
80. Coche E, Verschuren F, Hainaut P, Goncette L. Pulmonary embolism findings on chest radiographs and multislice spiral CT. Eur Radiol 2004; 14: 1241–1248.
81. Mal H, Brugiere O, Sleiman C, et al. Morbidity and mortality related to the native lung in single lung transplantation for emphysema. J Heart Lung Transplant 2000; 19:220–223.
82. McAdams HP, Erasmus JJ, Palmer SM. Complications (excluding hyperinflation) involving the native lung after single-lung transplantation: incidence, radiologic features, and clinical importance. Radiology 2001; 218:233–241.
83. Collins J, Kazerooni EA, Lacomis J, et al. Bronchogenic carcinoma after lung transplantation: frequency, clinical characteristics, and imaging findings. Radiology 2002; 224:131–138.
84. Kesten S, Chaparro C. Mycobacterial infections in lung transplant recipients. Chest 1999; 115:741–745.
85. Schulman LL, Htun T, Staniloae C, McGregor CC, Austin JH. Pulmonary nodules and masses after lung and heart–lung transplantation. J Thorac Imaging 2000; 15:173–179.
86. Malouf MA, Glanville AR. The spectrum of mycobacterial infection after lung transplantation. Am J Respir Crit Care Med 1999; 160:1611–1616.
87. Cooper JD, Billingham M, Egan T, et al. A working formulation for the standardization of nomenclature and for clinical staging of chronic dysfunction in lung allografts. International Society for Heart and Lung Transplantation. J Heart Lung Transplant 1993; 12:713–716.
88. Ikonen T, Kivisaari L, Taskinen E, Piilonen A, Harjula AL. High-resolution CT in long-term follow-up after lung transplantation. Chest 1997; 111:370–376.
89. Miller WT Jr, Kotloff RM, Blumenthal NP, Aronchick JM, Gefter WB, Miller WT. Utility of high resolution computed tomography in predicting bronchiolitis obliterans syndrome following lung transplantation: preliminary findings. J Thorac Imaging 2001; 16:76–80.
90. Morrish WF, Herman SJ, Weisbrod GL, Chamberlain DW. Bronchiolitis obliterans after lung transplantation: findings at chest radiography and high-resolution CT. The Toronto Lung Transplant Group. Radiology 1991; 179:487–490.
91. Kramer MR, Stoehr C, Whang JL, et al. The diagnosis of obliterative bronchiolitis after heart–lung and lung transplantation: low yield of transbronchial lung biopsy. J Heart Lung Transplant 1993; 12:675–681.

92. Leung AN, Fisher K, Valentine V, et al. Bronchiolitis obliterans after lung transplantation: detection using expiratory HRCT. Chest 1998; 113: 365–370.
93. Lee ES, Gotway MB, Reddy GP, Golden JA, Keith FM, Webb WR. Early bronchiolitis obliterans following lung transplantation: accuracy of expiratory thin-section CT for diagnosis. Radiology 2000; 216:472–477.
94. Choi YW, Rossi SE, Palmer SM, DeLong D, Erasmus JJ, McAdams HP. Bronchiolitis obliterans syndrome in lung transplant recipients: correlation of computed tomography findings with bronchiolitis obliterans syndrome stage. J Thorac Imaging 2003; 18:72–79.
95. Knollmann FD, Ewert R, Wundrich T, Hetzer R, Felix R. Bronchiolitis obliterans syndrome in lung transplant recipients: use of spirometrically gated CT. Radiology 2002; 225:655–662.
96. Siegel MJ, Bhalla S, Gutierrez FR, Hildebolt C, Sweet S. Post-lung transplantation bronchiolitis obliterans syndrome: usefulness of expiratory thin-section CT for diagnosis. Radiology 2001; 220:455–462.
97. Konen E, Gutierrez C, Chaparro C, et al. Bronchiolitis obliterans syndrome in lung transplant recipients: can thin-section CT findings predict disease before its clinical appearance? Radiology 2004; 231:467–473.
98. Chamberlain D, Maurer J, Chaparro C, Idolor L. Evaluation of transbronchial lung biopsy specimens in the diagnosis of bronchiolitis obliterans after lung transplantation. J Heart Lung Transplant 1994; 13:963–971.
99. Novick RJ, Stitt L. Pulmonary retransplantation. Semin Thorac Cardiovasc Surg 1998; 10:227–236.
100. Colby TV. Pathologic aspects of bronchiolitis obliterans organizing pneumonia. Chest 1992; 102:38S–43S.
101. Abernathy EC, Hruban RH, Baumgartner WA, Reitz BA, Hutchins GM. The two forms of bronchiolitis obliterans in heart–lung transplant recipients. Hum Pathol 1991; 22:1102–1110.
102. Yousem SA, Duncan SR, Griffith BP. Interstitial and airspace granulation tissue reactions in lung transplant recipients. Am J Surg Pathol 1992; 16: 877–884.
103. Epler GR, Colby TV, McLoud TC, Carrington CB, Gaensler EA. Bronchiolitis obliterans organizing pneumonia. N Engl J Med 1985; 312:152–158.
104. Siddiqui MT, Garrity ER, Husain AN. Bronchiolitis obliterans organizing pneumonia-like reactions: a nonspecific response or an atypical form of rejection or infection in lung allograft recipients? Hum Pathol 1996; 27:714–719.
105. Chaparro C, Chamberlain D, Maurer J, Winton T, Dehoyos A, Kesten S. Bronchiolitis obliterans organizing pneumonia (BOOP) in lung transplant recipients. Chest 1996; 110:1150–1154.
106. Arakawa H, Kurihara Y, Niimi H, Nakajima Y, Johkoh T, Nakamura H. Bronchiolitis obliterans with organizing pneumonia versus chronic eosinophilic pneumonia: high-resolution CT findings in 81 patients. Am J Roentgenol 2001; 176:1053–1058.
107. Ujita M, Renzoni EA, Veeraraghavan S, Wells AU, Hansell DM. Organizing pneumonia: perilobular pattern at thin-section CT. Radiology 2004; 232: 757–761.

108. Scarsbrook AF, Warakaulle DR, Dattani M, Traill Z. Post-transplantation lymphoproliferative disorder: the spectrum of imaging appearances. Clin Radiol 2005; 60:47–55.

109. Verschuuren E, van der Bij W, de Boer W, Timens W, Middeldorp J, The TH. Quantitative Epstein–Barr virus (EBV) serology in lung transplant recipients with primary EBV infection and/or post-transplant lymphoproliferative disease. J Med Virol 2003; 69:258–266.

110. Rappaport DC, Chamberlain DW, Shepherd FA, Hutcheon MA. Lymphoproliferative disorders after lung transplantation: imaging features. Radiology 1998; 206:519–524.

111. Paranjothi S, Yusen RD, Kraus MD, Lynch JP, Patterson GA, Trulock EP. Lymphoproliferative disease after lung transplantation: comparison of presentation and outcome of early and late cases. J Heart Lung Transplant 2001; 20:1054–1063.

112. Malouf MA, Chhajed PN, Hopkins P, Plit M, Turner J, Glanville AR. Antiviral prophylaxis reduces the incidence of lymphoproliferative disease in lung transplant recipients. J Heart Lung Transplant 2002; 21:547–554.

113. Pickhardt PJ, Siegel MJ, Anderson DC, Hayashi R, DeBaun MR. Chest radiography as a predictor of outcome in posttransplantation lymphoproliferative disorder in lung allograft recipients. Am J Roentgenol 1998; 171:375–382.

114. Hachem RR, Chakinala MM, Yusen RD, et al. Abdominal–pelvic lymphoproliferative disease after lung transplantation: presentation and outcome. Transplantation 2004; 77:431–437.

115. Pickhardt PJ, Siegel MJ. Posttransplantation lymphoproliferative disorder of the abdomen: CT evaluation in 51 patients. Radiology 1999; 213:73–78.

116. Collins J, Muller NL, Leung AN, et al. Epstein-Barr-virus-associated lymphoproliferative disease of the lung: CT and histologic findings. Radiology 1998; 208:749–759.

117. Carignan S, Staples CA, Muller NL. Intrathoracic lymphoproliferative disorders in the immunocompromised patient: CT findings. Radiology 1995; 197:53–58.

118. Dodd GD III, Ledesma-Medina J, Baron RL, Fuhrman CR. Posttransplant lymphoproliferative disorder: intrathoracic manifestations. Radiology 1992; 184:65–69.

119. Pickhardt PJ, Siegel MJ. Abdominal manifestations of posttransplantation lymphoproliferative disorder. Am J Roentgenol 1998; 171:1007–1013.

120. Konen E, Weisbrod GL, Pakhale S, Chung T, Paul NS, Hutcheon MA. Fibrosis of the upper lobes: a newly identified late-onset complication after lung transplantation? Am J Roentgenol 2003; 181:1539–1543.

121. Collins J, Hartman MJ, Warner TF, et al. Frequency and CT findings of recurrent disease after lung transplantation. Radiology 2001; 219:503–509.

122. Kazerooni EA, Jackson C, Cascade PN. Sarcoidosis: recurrence of primary disease in transplanted lungs. Radiology 1994; 192:461–464.

123. de Perrot M, Wigle DA, Pierre AF, et al. Bronchogenic carcinoma after solid organ transplantation. Ann Thorac Surg 2003; 75:367–371.

124. Choi YH, Leung AN, Miro S, Poirier C, Hunt S, Theodore J. Primary bronchogenic carcinoma after heart or lung transplantation: radiologic and clinical findings. J Thorac Imaging 2000; 15:36–40.
125. Lee P, Minai OA, Mehta AC, DeCamp MM, Murthy S. Pulmonary nodules in lung transplant recipients: etiology and outcome. Chest 2004; 125: 165–172.
126. Boehler A, Vogt P, Zollinger A, Weder W, Speich R. Prospective study of the value of transbronchial lung biopsy after lung transplantation. Eur Respir J 1996; 9:658–662.
127. Kazerooni EA, Cascade PN, Gross BH. Transplanted lungs: nodules following transbronchial biopsy. Radiology 1995; 194:209–212.
128. Root JD, Molina PL, Anderson DJ, Sagel SS. Pulmonary nodular opacities after transbronchial biopsy in patients with lung transplants. Radiology 1992; 184:435–436.
129. Daly BD, Martinez FJ, Brunsting LA III, Deeb GM, Cascade PN, Lynch JP III. High-resolution CT detection of lacerations in the transplanted lung after transbronchial biopsy. J Thorac Imaging 1994; 9:160–165.
130. Lischke R, Simonek J, Stolz AJ, et al. Cyclosporine-related neurotoxicity in a patient after bilateral lung transplantation for cystic fibrosis. Transplant Proc 2004; 36:2837–2839.
131. Goodman JM, Kuzma B. Encephalopathy following heart–lung transplantation. Surg Neurol 1996; 46:157.
132. Thyagarajan GK, Cobanoglu A, Johnston W. FK506-induced fulminant leukoencephalopathy after single-lung transplantation. Ann Thorac Surg 1997; 64:1461–1464.
133. Kiemeneij IM, de Leeuw FE, Ramos LM, van Gijn J. Acute headache as a presenting symptom of tacrolimus encephalopathy. J Neurol Neurosurg Psychiatry 2003; 74:1126–1127.
134. Small SL, Fukui MB, Bramblett GT, Eidelman BH. Immunosuppression-induced leukoencephalopathy from tacrolimus (FK506). Ann Neurol 1996; 40:575–580.
135. Scott LJ, McKeage K, Keam SJ, Plosker GL. Tacrolimus: a further update of its use in the management of organ transplantation. Drugs 2003; 63: 1247–1297.
136. Goldstein LS, Haug MT III, Perl J II, et al. Central nervous system complications after lung transplantation. J Heart Lung Transplant 1998; 17:185–191.
137. Casey SO, Sampaio RC, Michel E, Truwit CL. Posterior reversible encephalopathy syndrome: utility of fluid-attenuated inversion recovery MR imaging in the detection of cortical and subcortical lesions. Am J Neuroradiol 2000; 21:1199–1206.
138. Gupta D, Sakorafas GH, McGregor CG, Harmsen WS, Farnell MB. Management of biliary tract disease in heart and lung transplant patients. Surgery 2000; 128:641–649.
139. Hoekstra HJ, Hawkins K, de Boer WJ, Rottier K, van der Bij W. Gastrointestinal complications in lung transplant survivors that require surgical intervention. Br J Surg 2001; 88:433–438.

140. Smith PC, Slaughter MS, Petty MG, Shumway SJ, Kshettry VR, Bolman RM III. Abdominal complications after lung transplantation. J Heart Lung Transplant 1995; 14:44–51.

141. Lubetkin EI, Lipson DA, Palevsky HI, et al. GI complications after orthotopic lung transplantation. Am J Gastroenterol 1996; 91:2382–2390.

142. Beaver TM, Fullerton DA, Zamora MR, et al. Colon perforation after lung transplantation. Ann Thorac Surg 1996; 62:839–843.

143. Khan S, Eppstein AC, Anderson GK, et al. Acute diverticulitis in heart- and lung transplant patients. Transpl Int 2001; 14:12–15.

144. Nichols L, Strollo DC, Kusne S. Legionellosis in a lung transplant recipient obscured by cytomegalovirus infection and *Clostridium difficile* colitis. Transpl Infect Dis 2002; 4:41–45.

145. Ouwens JP, van der Bij W, van der Mark TW, et al. The value of ventilation scintigraphy after single lung transplantation. J Heart Lung Transplant 2004; 23:115–121.

146. Jones HA, Donovan T, Goddard MJ, et al. Use of 18FDG-pet to discriminate between infection and rejection in lung transplant recipients. Transplantation 2004; 77:1462–1464.

147. Marom EM, McAdams HP, Butnor KJ, Coleman RE. Positron emission tomography with fluoro-2-deoxy-d-glucose (FDG-PET) in the staging of post transplant lymphoproliferative disorder in lung transplant recipients. J Thorac Imaging 2004; 19:74–78.

148. Gast KK, Viallon M, Eberle B, et al. MRI in lung transplant recipients using hyperpolarized $^3$He: comparison with CT. J Magn Reson Imaging 2002; 15:268–274.

149. Salerno M, Altes TA, Mugler JP III, Nakatsu M, Hatabu H, de Lange EE. Hyperpolarized noble gas MR imaging of the lung: potential clinical applications. Eur J Radiol 2001; 40:33–44.

150. Gast KK, Puderbach MU, Rodriguez I, et al. Distribution of ventilation in lung transplant recipients: evaluation by dynamic $^3$He-MRI with lung motion correction. Invest Radiol 2003; 38:341–348.

151. Zaporozhan J, Ley S, Gast KK, et al. Functional analysis in single-lung transplant recipients: a comparative study of high-resolution CT, $^3$He-MRI, and pulmonary function tests. Chest 2004; 125:173–181.

152. Gast KK, Zaporozhan J, Ley S, et al. (3)He-MRI in follow-up of lung transplant recipients. Eur Radiol 2004; 14:78–85.

153. Markstaller K, Kauczor HU, Puderbach M, et al. $^3$He-MRI-based versus conventional determination of lung volumes in patients after unilateral lung transplantation: a new approach to regional spirometry. Acta Anaesthesiol Scand 2002; 46:845–852.

154. Konen E, Yellin A, Greenberg I, et al. Complications of tracheal and thoracic surgery: the role of multisection helical CT and computerized reformations. Clin Radiol 2003; 58:341–350.

155. McAdams HP, Palmer SM, Erasmus JJ, et al. Bronchial anastomotic complications in lung transplant recipients: virtual bronchoscopy for noninvasive assessment. Radiology 1998; 209:689–695.

156. Uppaluri R, Mitsa T, Sonka M, Hoffman EA, McLennan G. Quantification of pulmonary emphysema from lung computed tomography images. Am J Respir Crit Care Med 1997; 156:248–254.
157. Uppaluri R, Hoffman EA, Sonka M, Hartley PG, Hunninghake GW, McLennan G. Computer recognition of regional lung disease patterns. Am J Respir Crit Care Med 1999; 160:648–654.
158. Levine M, Shpiner R, Martin K. Clinical evaluation of stent placement in patients with persistent dyspnea in post single lung transplants (SLT). Am J Respir Crit Care Med 1997; 155:A275.

# 35

# Cardiac, Lipid, and Atherosclerotic Complications Among Lung and Heart–Lung Recipients

Jignesh K. Patel, Jon A. Kobashigawa, and Michele Hamilton

*Division of Cardiology, David Geffen School of Medicine at UCLA, Center for Health Sciences, Los Angeles, California, U.S.A.*

## INTRODUCTION

Cardiovascular disease as a determinant of long-term outcome becomes more important as allograft survival continues to improve and the median age of transplant recipients increases. The posttransplant state is characterized by a number of endocrine and metabolic abnormalities, which may contribute to the development or progression of cardiovascular disease. Lung and combined heart–lung transplantation is associated with a proatherogenic milieu and transplant patients are more prone to develop atherosclerotic cardiovascular disease for a variety of reasons. Immunosuppressive agents have a number of atherogenic effects. These agents contribute to the development of hypertension, hyperlipidemia, diabetes mellitus, and post-transplant obesity. Infectious agents, particularly cytomegalovirus, have been implicated in the pathogenesis of atherosclerosis and the development of transplant coronary artery disease in heart transplant recipients. Increased risk of infection following transplantation also places them at risk for developing infective endocarditis or inflammatory myocarditis.

Cardiovascular management of the lung or heart–lung recipient focuses first on the determination of preexisting cardiac disease prior to

transplantation. Following transplantation, the emphasis is more on prevention and addressing risk factors, which were frequently not present prior to
transplantation. If cardiovascular disease does develop following transplantation, detection, evaluation, and treatment become essential for minimizing
cardiovascular morbidity and mortality.

Despite improvements in immunosuppression and general posttransplant management, long-term outcomes in lung and heart–lung transplantation remain chiefly limited by the development of bronchiolitis and graft
failure. However, as survival rates continue to improve, cardiovascular complications also become more prominent. Five-year mortality from cardiovascular disease for lung transplant recipients was 4.6% by the latest
International Society of Heart and Lung Transplantation (ISHLT) registry
data and 8.5% for heart–lung recipients (Tables 1 and 2).

## PREOPERATIVE CARDIOVASCULAR EVALUATION

The prevalence of coronary artery disease in potential lung transplant recipients has not been extensively studied. In the Duke cohort of 345 lung
transplant recipients, the prevalence of significant coronary artery disease
was 5% (1). Fibrotic lung diseases have been associated with an increased
risk of coronary artery disease (2).

Determination of preexisting cardiovascular disease prior to transplantation is important in minimizing perioperative risk. Approximately
10% of all deaths within 30 days of lung or heart–lung transplantation are
attributed to a cardiovascular cause (Tables 1 and 2). One of the major

**Table 1**  Early and Late Cause of Death Among Adult Lung Transplant Recipients

| Cause of death | 0–30 days (N = 937) | 31 days to 1 yr (N = 1,345) | >1–3 yr (N = 1,096) | >3–5 yr (N = 572) | >5 yr (N = 456) |
|---|---|---|---|---|---|
| Bronchiolitis | 5 (0.5%) | 74 (5.5%) | 313 (28.6%) | 185 (32.3%) | 142 (31.1%) |
| Acute rejection | 46 (4.9%) | 27 (2.0%) | 21 (1.9%) | 4 (0.7%) | 2 (0.4%) |
| Lymphoma | 1 (0.1%) | 44 (3.3%) | 23 (2.1%) | 9 (1.6%) | 18 (3.9%) |
| Malignancy, other | | 27 (2.0%) | 52 (4.7%) | 43 (7.5%) | 40 (8.8%) |
| CMV | 1 (0.1%) | 56 (4.2%) | 17 (1.6%) | 4 (0.7%) | 2 (0.4%) |
| Infection, non-CMV | 220 (23.5%) | 521 (38.7%) | 284 (25.9%) | 113 (19.8%) | 79 (17.3%) |
| Graft failure | 286 (30.5%) | 236 (17.5%) | 175 (16.0%) | 99 (17.3%) | 58 (12.7%) |
| Cardiovascular | 108 (11.5%) | 58 (4.3%) | 36 (3.3%) | 24 (4.2%) | 21 (4.6%) |
| Technical | 78 (8.3%) | 37 (2.8%) | 12 (1.1%) | 1 (0.2%) | 2 (0.4%) |
| Other | 192 (20.5%) | 265 (19.7%) | 163 (14.9%) | 90 (15.7%) | 92 (20.2%) |

*Source*: From Ref. 9.

**Table 2**  Early and Late Cause of Death Among Adult Heart–Lung
Transplant Recipients

| Cause of death | 0–30 days ($N=181$) | 31 days to 1 yr ($N=117$) | >1–3 yr ($N=96$) | >3–5 yr ($N=56$) | >5 yr ($N=82$) |
|---|---|---|---|---|---|
| Bronchiolitis | | 4 (3.4%) | 25 (26.0%) | 21 (37.5%) | 17 (20.7%) |
| Acute rejection | 3 (1.7%) | 3 (2.6%) | 1 (1.0%) | 1 (1.8%) | 1 (1.2%) |
| Lymphoma | | 3 (2.6%) | 4 (4.2%) | 3 (5.4%) | 1 (1.2%) |
| Malignancy, other | | 1 (0.9%) | 6 (6.3%) | 2 (3.6%) | 5 (6.1%) |
| CMV | | 1 (0.9%) | | 1 (1.8%) | |
| Infection, non-CMV | 37 (20.4%) | 52 (44.4%) | 31 (32.3%) | 3 (5.4%) | 11 (13.4%) |
| Graft failure | 57 (31.5%) | 23 (19.7%) | 17 (17.7%) | 8 (14.3%) | 20 (24.4%) |
| Cardiovascular | 17 (9.4%) | 7 (6.0%) | 5 (5.2%) | 8 (14.3%) | 7 (8.5%) |
| Technical | 35 (19.3%) | 2 (1.7%) | 1 (1.0%) | | |
| Other | 32 (17.7%) | 21 (17.9%) | 6 (6.3%) | 9 (16.1%) | 20 (24.4%) |

*Source*: From Ref. 9.

cardiac problems posttransplant is coronary ischemia. Since the most
common etiology for which lung transplantation is carried out is chronic
obstructive pulmonary disease, these patients invariably have an extensive
smoking history and may also have additional contributing cardiovascular
risk factors. Coronary artery disease has in general been considered to be
a contraindication to lung transplantation (3), but is no longer an absolute
contraindication in some centers. An initial detailed history and physical
evaluation will determine overall risk of cardiovascular disease for patients
being considered for lung transplantation. Symptoms may be more difficult
to interpret as lung disease may mask the extent of cardiovascular disease.
Pulmonary disease may also limit significant patient activity, which may
prevent the manifestation of cardiovascular symptoms. Particular note
should be made of chest pain syndromes, palpitations, dizziness, or history
of syncope. Careful clinical examination should reveal signs of significant
left or right ventricular dysfunction and pulmonary hypertension.

A variety of diagnostic studies are generally required for comprehensive pretransplant cardiovascular evaluation. The aim is to determine the
presence, etiology, and severity of cardiovascular disease. An electrocardiogram is important to rule out arrhythmias, assess right or left ventricular
hypertrophy, and determine the presence of possible prior myocardial
infarction. A chest X ray will show evidence of pulmonary vascular congestion and cardiomegaly. Echocardiography is very useful for determining left
and right ventricular size and systolic function, diastolic dysfunction,

valvular disease, prior myocardial infarction, and pulmonary hypertension. The determination of the latter is particularly important in patients being considered for lung transplantation as this may determine the need for bilateral versus single-lung transplant or combined heart–lung transplantation. Patients with significant chronic pulmonary hypertension may have right ventricular enlargement and dysfunction. Generally, invasive evaluation of cardiac hemodynamics is the optimal approach. Echocardiographic bubble-contrast study is useful for identifying patients with a patent foramen ovale, which may warrant closure at the time of lung transplantation. The rationale behind closing a patent foremaen ovale at the time of transplant relates to concern about ischemia–reperfusion injury–related pulmonary vascular resistance and elevated right heart pressures, which may lead to a right-to-left shunt and worsening hypoxemia.

Graded exercise stress testing is the most common form of preoperative evaluation for suspected coronary artery disease. Patients for lung transplant, however, usually have limited exercise capacity due to the extent of pulmonary disease. Pharmacologic stress testing in conjunction with echocardiography or radionuclide imaging may provide important clues to the physiologic importance of coronary lesions. Adenosine and persantine need to be avoided in patients with significant bronchospasm, in which case dobutamine would be the pharmacologic stress agent of choice. Diminished ejection fraction at rest, but particularly with stress, coupled with wall motion abnormalities denote a substantive adverse prognosis. Large areas of myocardial hypoperfusion documented by radionuclide imaging, particularly when associated with left ventricular dilatation and depressed ejection fraction, portend the highest cardiovascular risk. However, in one study comparing results of preoperative dobutamine thallium-201 stress testing with those of coronary angiography, specificity of radionuclide imaging was low with a large number of false-positive results (4).

Given that significant coronary disease affects perioperative outcomes and may be amenable to treatment with bypass grafting at the time of lung transplantation or by preoperative percutaneous coronary intervention, coronary angiography is generally the preferred method for detecting coronary atherosclerosis due to its high sensitivity and specificity. Due to the limited donor supply, a high degree of sensitivity for detecting occult disease is essential. It is unclear, however, whether all patients need to undergo invasive coronary angiography. In a retrospective study, Thaik et al. (5) studied both the clinical indications for coronary angiography and the extent of coronary arteriosclerotic disease in 105 consecutive potential lung transplant candidates. Forty-nine percent of patients underwent angiography to either exclude asymptomatic atherosclerosis ($n = 46$) or define the extent of known symptomatic ischemic heart disease ($n = 5$). The perceived risk of occult disease according to a semiquantitative coronary risk assessment score that included hypertension, hyperlipidemia, diabetes, smoking, a family history of coronary artery disease, and electrocardiographic or echocardiographic abnormalities influenced the decision to perform angiography: 4 of 44 patients (9%) with two or fewer risk factors underwent angiography versus 42 of 56 patients (75%) with more than two risk factors ($P \leq 0.05$). A higher risk factor score also correlated with angiographic evidence of coronary artery disease. In the 46 patients without symptoms who were studied, two hemodynamically significant but unsuspected coronary lesions were identified. Six other patients without symptoms had noncritical (<50%) lesions. Among the five patients with angina or a prior myocardial infarction, coronary angiography showed either minimal atherosclerosis ($n = 2$) or non–life-threatening anatomy ($n = 3$). In this study, angiographic findings did not exclude any patient from transplant listing. The authors concluded that coronary angiography appears most useful in patients without symptoms with multiple coronary risk factors and in a subset of patients who might otherwise be excluded from lung transplantation because of a history of symptomatic cardiovascular disease. In another study (6), when coronary angiography was performed in patients >50 years old with at least one cardiovascular risk factor, 39% of patients were identified with coronary artery disease and half of these cases had significant stenoses. Five patients subsequently underwent preoperative percutaneous coronary intervention or coronary bypass surgery at the time of transplant. One of these patients died within 90 days of transplant. The authors concluded that significant coronary artery disease is a common finding in older patients who are presenting for lung transplantation and coronary revascularization for severe large vessel stenoses can allow acceptable posttransplant survival. Furthermore, coronary artery disease risk factors may predict who should undergo coronary angiography. Other centers have subsequently also reported favorable outcomes following coronary revascularization and lung transplantation (1,3). At our center, though coronary atherosclerosis is considered a relative contraindication for lung transplantation, patients who have discreet, single-vessel coronary artery disease amenable to either percutaneous angioplasty and stenting prior to transplant or single-vessel bypass at the time of transplant have been successfully treated. In patients undergoing stenting, transplant listing is delayed until it is felt to be safe to discontinue clopidegrel to reduce operative bleeding risk. Patients with known coronary artery disease must of course be carefully screened for other evidence of atherosclerosis (i.e., with carotid duplex scanning and peripheral arterial Doppler analysis).

Some forms of valvular heart disease, such as primary mitral regurgitation or secondary tricuspid regurgitation, may not be absolute contraindications to lung transplantation and may be able to be addressed surgically at the time of transplant. As mentioned later, tricuspid regurgitation may improve spontaneously post lung transplantation once pulmonary hypertension resolves.

## EARLY POSTTRANSPLANT CARDIOVASCULAR COMPLICATIONS

Despite aggressive preoperative screening for cardiovascular disease, cardiac complications following lung and heart–lung transplantation are particularly prominent in the early posttransplant period (Tables 1 and 2). According to the ISHLT registry, 11.4% of deaths within the first 30 days of lung transplant were attributed to a cardiovascular event between January 1992 and June 2003. The figure was similar for heart–lung transplants (9.4%). Other major cardiac adverse events such as myocardial infarction and heart failure are more difficult to quantify. The increased perioperative cardiovascular morbidity and mortality may be related to the high catecholamine stress and at times persistent pulmonary hypertension.

Management of acute coronary syndromes early post-transplant can be particularly problematic. Percutaneous coronary intervention invariably requires systemic anticoagulation and antiplatelet therapy, carrying with it significant risk of perioperative bleeding. Congestive heart failure may complicate early posttransplant management as it may compound effects of ischemia–reperfusion injury, which in itself can lead to pulmonary edema and hypoxemia.

Atrial fibrillation is a frequent complication after lung transplant. In a recent retrospective study at Duke University (7), several factors were identified by multivariate analysis as contributing to the development of atrial fibrillation, which occurred in 39% of patients. Advanced age, idiopathic pulmonary fibrosis as a cause for transplant, known coronary disease, enlarged left atrium, and use of postoperative vasopressors increased the risk for developing atrial fibrillation. The development of posttransplant atrial fibrillation was associated with significantly prolonged hospital stay and increased mortality. Atrial flutter may occur secondary to macro-reentry at the anastomotic site between the pulmonary veins and the left atrium and may be treated with radiofrequency ablation (8). Though there are few data, postoperative betablockade may be helpful in reducing the risk of atrial fibrillation and flutter as long as there is no major concern of bronchospasm in the nontransplanted lung.

### LUNG TRANSPLANT VS. HEART–LUNG TRANSPLANT

Cardiac dysfunction, either primary or as a result of pulmonary disease, may determine the type of procedure being considered. Patients with severe left ventricular dysfunction or major congenital abnormalities may require heart–lung transplantation. Those with cardiac issues limited to right ventricular dysfunction secondary to pulmonary hypertension, however, are now usually felt to be candidates for double-lung transplantation. Severe chronic pulmonary hypertension leads to right ventricular pressure overload.

Adverse cardiac remodeling will then cause right ventricular dysfunction, right ventricular enlargement, severe tricuspid regurgitation, and a leftward shift and flattening of the interventricular septum. Clinically, this causes symptomatic right heart failure with severe ascites, renal impairment, malnutrition, and immobility. Many of these patients have traditionally been considered for combined heart–lung transplantation. However, while outcomes with combined heart–lung transplantation are comparable to those for lung transplantation alone (9) the availability of organs for combined heart and lung transplantation is limited and doubles the waiting time for transplantation when compared to isolated lung transplantation. Latest registry data show that less than 75 combined heart–lung transplants were performed worldwide in 2002 due to limited organ availability. Recent experience, however, suggests that many of these patients may undergo isolated bilateral lung transplantation with acceptable outcomes and significant reverse remodeling of the right ventricle can occur following lung transplantation. Of course, maximal optimization of right ventricular failure to reduce hepatic congestion preoperatively is warranted to try to decrease operative bleeding risk. Kasimir (10) reported on 17 patients at the University of Vienna who underwent bilateral lung transplantation between 2000 and 2002 for severe primary pulmonary hypertension associated with severe alterations in cardiac structure. All patients were in heart failure New York Heart Association (NYHA) class III or IV, most of them with intractable ascites, established renal impairment, malnutrition, and immobility, continuously deteriorating despite various forms of pharmacological treatment including intravenous and inhalative prostacyclin, diuretics, calcium channel antagonists, bosentan, and catecholamines. Echocardiography and Doppler echocardiography measurements were performed before and three months after lung transplantation. Left and right ventricular diameters and function were assessed and tricuspid valve regurgitation was determined. The authors reported comparable short-term mortality to combined heart–lung transplantation. At three months after lung transplantation surviving patients were in NYHA I or II. Echocardiography showed normal left ventricular function and markedly improved right ventricular function with normal size of the right ventricle. The leftward shifted flattened interventricular septum had returned in its physiological position and the high-grade tricuspid insufficiency had disappeared in all patients. The authors concluded that advanced alterations of cardiac morphology and function normalize completely and preexisting tricuspid insufficiency disappears in primary pulmonary hypertension patients after isolated bilateral lung transplant. Quality of life is excellent and bilateral lung transplantation is therefore preferred and safe in patients with advanced primary pulmonary hypertension even with severe right ventricular dysfunction.

## HYPERLIPIDEMIA

Lipid levels have been shown to be widely elevated following cardiac transplantation (11). A number of factors are thought to contribute to post-transplant hyperlipidemia. Steroids contribute to increased apolipoprotein B production and also to post-transplant obesity. Cyclosporine may enhance this effect and also independently increase hepatic lipase activity and decrease lipoprotein lipase activity (12). This results in impaired very low-density lipoprotein (VLDL) and low-density lipoprotein (LDL) clearance.

Hyperlipidemia is a well-established risk factor for nontransplant atherosclerosis and should be aggressively treated post lung transplant. Heart–lung transplant patients have the additional risk of developing transplant vasculopathy, an accelerated form of coronary atherosclerosis felt to be related to chronic rejection in the transplanted heart. Both clinical and experimental observations in heart transplant recipients suggest that hyperlipidemia may be important in the development of transplant vasculopathy (13,14).

In a small retrospective study in heart transplant recipients, elevated lipid values six months following transplantation had a strong predictive value for the development of transplant vasculopathy at three years (13). In a more recent study, post-transplant elevation of LDL at one year was the only predictor for the development or progression of transplant vasculopathy by intravascular ultrasound (15). The allogeneic state following heart–lung transplantation also leads to endothelial activation, which may further augment the vascular response to hyperlipidemia. In this respect, greater intimal thickening, more intimal angiogenesis, and a greater accumulation of T cells is seen in transplanted vasculature compared to native vessels in animals exposed to the same level of hyperlipidemia (16,17).

Interestingly, treatment following cardiac transplantation with an inhibitor of the rate-limiting enzyme in the cholesterol biosynthetic pathway, 3-hydroxyl-3-methylglutryl coenzyme A (HMG Co-A) reductase, is associated not only with decreased development of coronary intimal thickening, but also a lower frequency of hemodynamically compromising rejection episodes and improved survival in heart transplant recipients (18,19). These agents likely have an immunosuppressive effect in addition to their lipid-lowering activity. The mechanism for this apparent immunosuppressive benefit of statins has recently been determined (20). Statins effectively repress the induction of major histocompatibility complex (MHC-II) expression by interferon-$\gamma$ and thereby inhibit T-cell proliferation. The specific molecular mechanism of inhibition by statins on MHC-II induction is a selective repressive effect on the induction of expression of promoter IV of the MHC-II transactivator CIITA gene. Given these beneficial effects, statin therapy has now become an integral part of the immunosuppressive

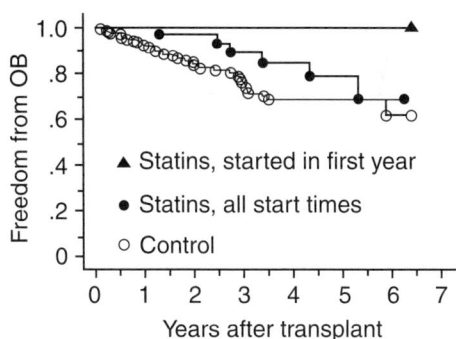

**Figure 1** Freedom from obliterative bronchiolitis (OB). Cumulative incidence of OB among all recipients who received statins at any time after lung transplantation (*solid circles, >N = 39*) tends to be less than that of control subjects (*open circles, N = 161*) (*P = 0.06*). Recipients receiving statins within the first year after transplantation (*solid triangles, N = 15*) remain entirely free of OB (*P = 0.02*). *Source*: From Ref. 21.

regimen in cardiac transplantation. Their use in lung transplantation has also been associated with improved allograft function and survival. In a nonrandomized study, Johnson et al. (21) evaluated possible effects of these agents after lung transplantation by comparing outcomes of 39 allograft recipients, who were prescribed statins for hyperlipidemia, with those of 161 contemporaneous control recipients who did not receive these drugs. Acute rejection was significantly less frequent in the statin group. The cumulative incidence of obliterative bronchiolitis among recipients who received statins at any time after lung transplantation tended to be less than that of control subjects (Fig. 1). Interestingly, recipients who received statins within the first year after transplantation remained entirely free of obliterative bronchiolitis up to six years after transplantation. Total cellularity in bronchoalveolar lavages, as well as proportions of inflammatory neutrophils and lymphocytes, were significantly lower in statin recipients. Among double-lung recipients, those taking statins had significantly better spirometry. The six-year survival of recipients taking statins (91%) was much greater than that of control subjects (54%) (*P < 0.01*) (Fig. 2). These data suggest statin use may have substantial clinical benefits after pulmonary transplantation and, therefore, all lung and heart–lung transplant recipients should receive HMG Co-A reductase inhibitors when tolerated.

## HYPERTENSION

There is a clear link between hypertension and conventional coronary atherosclerosis and stroke. Hypertension is a common problem following transplantation, related in part to the use of corticosteroids, frequent

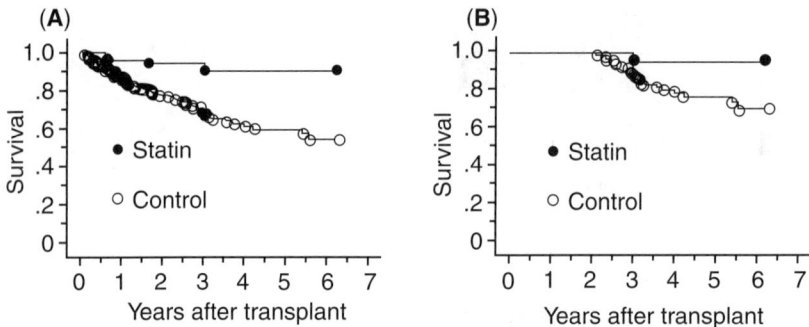

**Figure 2** Survival of control and patients on statins after lung transplantation. Kaplan–Meier analysis for survival for control subjects (*open circles*) and statin recipients (*solid circles*). (**A**) Kaplan–Meier analysis that includes all control subjects and all patients who received statins at any time after lung transplantation. The proportion of patients surviving six years after transplantation in this study was 0.91 for statin patients and 0.54 for control subjects ($P = 0.02$). (**B**) Analysis limited to recipients who survived at least two years after transplantation. The proportion surviving six years after transplantation was 0.96 for statin recipients and 0.70 for control subjects ($P = 0.03$). *Source*: From Ref. 21.

associated weight gain, and use of calcineurin inhibitors. Although no studies have specifically addressed the issue of whether hypertension is a risk factor for the development of coronary disease after transplantation, it seems likely that it is based on risk factors for native coronary atherosclerosis. Traditional antihypertensive medications should be tailored individually for tight blood pressure control.

## DRUGS AND TRANSPLANT VASCULOPATHY

The impact of immunosuppressive agents on transplant vasculopathy in heart or heart–lung recipients is not well defined. The indirect effects of long-term steroid therapy on lipid metabolism has already been described. This effect is enhanced by the use of cyclosporine although there is some evidence that substitution of cyclosporine for the newer calcineurin inhibitor tacrolimus may abrogate the rise in serum lipids (22). The number and severity of episodes of acute rejection may contribute to the subsequent development of transplant vasculopathy (23,24). More effective immunosuppressive regimens may therefore have a beneficial impact on the development of allograft vasculopathy.

Tacrolimus, a calcineurin inhibitor with actions similar to cyclosporine, has been studied extensively in liver transplantation and shown to be superior to cyclosporine in preventing chronic rejection (25). In cardiac transplantation, while it has been demonstrated to cause less hypertension and hyperlipidemia than cyclosporine (22), data on preventing transplant vasculopathy have been less conclusive. In one study, treatment with tacrolimus has been associated with the lower incidence of antiendothelial antibodies (26).

Mycophenolate mofetil (MMF), an inhibitor of the de novo pathway for purine biosynthesis, has been shown to be more effective at reducing cardiac allograft rejection and post-transplant mortality (27). More recent studies suggest that it may also be more effective at reducing allograft vasculopathy (28,29). This effect may be related at least in part to the ability of mycophenolate to reduce B cell responses as patients treated with this agent developed lower antivimentin titers and this was correlated with the lower incidence of transplant vasculopathy by intravascular ultrasound. The improved immunosuppression profile seen with MMF may therefore also translate into a lower incidence of cardiac allograft vasculopathy, although clinical benefit in this regard has yet to be demonstrated. There have been no convincing trials, however, demonstrating the superiority of MMF over azathioprine in lung transplantation in terms of survival or reduction in acute rejection episodes (30,31).

Sirolimus (rapamycin), a macrolide antibiotic with potent immunosuppressive effects, has been shown to have antiproliferative effects on smooth muscle cells in vitro and in experimental animal models of vascular injury. It has also been shown to reduce the process of in-stent restenosis following angioplasty and tent placement in native coronary artery disease (32–34). Sirolimus and the related agent everolimus block activation of T cells following autocrine stimulation by interleukin-2. Their action is therefore complementary to the calcineurin inhibitors. Sirolimus has been shown to effectively prevent acute graft rejection and inhibit refractory acute graft rejection in heart transplant recipients (35). Though sirolimus is associated with increased risks of hypertension and hyperlipidemia, it is also known to have antiproliferative effects on smooth muscle cells and was shown to decrease the development of cardiac allograft vasculopathy as assessed by intravascular ultrasound at six months (36). This benefit was maintained at two years (37). In another angiographic study of cardiac transplant patients with established transplant vasculopathy, sirolimus was also shown to slow down the disease progression (38).

Similarly, a related agent, everolimus has been shown to significantly reduce markers for allograft vasculopathy relative to azathiopine through 24 months in cardiac transplantation (39). Use of sirolimus in lung transplantation early following surgery, however, has been limited by airway anastomotic dehiscence (40). However, sirolimus may be useful in the treatment of chronic lung rejection which manifests as bronchiolitis obliterans syndrome, a condition characterized by fibro-intimal proliferation of small airways, analogous to transplant vasculopathy seen in chronic cardiac allograft rejection (41).

## SUMMARY

Cardiac complications are major contributors to morbidity and mortality following lung and heart–lung transplantation. Patients should be carefully screened for antecedent cardiovascular disease. Select cardiac problems including limited coronary artery disease and secondary right ventricular dysfunction may not prohibit successful lung transplantation. Risk factors for atherosclerosis, common posttransplant, should be aggressively treated. Patients undergoing heart–lung transplant face the additional risk of transplant vasculopathy. In addition to agents used in the treatment and prevention of conventional atherosclerosis, including aspirin and HMG Co-A reductase inhibitors, newer immunosuppressive agents such as MMF and sirolimus appear to have additional benefits.

## REFERENCES

1. Patel VS, Palmer SM, Messier RH, Davis RD. Clinical outcome after coronary artery revascularization and lung transplantation. Ann Thorac Surg 2003; 75(2):372–377; discussion 377.
2. Kizer JR, Zisman DA, Blumenthal NP, et al. Association between pulmonary fibrosis and coronary artery disease. Arch Intern Med 2004; 164(5):551–556.
3. Lee R, Meyers BF, Sundt TM, Trulock EP, Patterson GA. Concomitant coronary artery revascularization to allow successful lung transplantation in selected patients with coronary artery disease. J Thorac Cardiovasc Surg 2002; 124(6):1250–1251.
4. Henzlova MJ, Padilla ML, Freilich A, et al. Dobutamine thallium 201 perfusion imaging in candidates for lung transplantation. J Heart Lung Transplant 1995; 14(2):251–256.
5. Thaik CM, Semigran MJ, Ginns L, Wain JC, Dec GW. Evaluation of ischemic heart disease in potential lung transplant recipients. J Heart Lung Transplant 1995; 14(2):257–266.
6. Snell GI, Richardson M, Griffiths AP, Williams TJ, Esmore DS. Coronary artery disease in potential lung transplant recipients >50 years old: the role of coronary intervention. Chest 1999; 116(4):874–879.
7. Nielsen TD, Bahnson T, Davis RD, Palmer SM. Atrial fibrillation after pulmonary transplant. Chest 2004; 126(2):496–500.
8. Lazaro MUP, Merimo J. Atrial fibrillation, atrial flutter, or both after pulmonary transplantation. Chest 2005; 127:1461–1462.
9. Trulock EP, Edwards LB, Taylor DO, Boucek MM, Keck BM, Hertz MI. The Registry of the International Society for Heart and Lung Transplantation: twenty-first official adult heart transplant report—2004. J Heart Lung Transplant 2004; 23(7):804–815.
10. Kasimir MT, Seebacher G, Jaksch P, et al. Reverse cardiac remodelling in patients with primary pulmonary hypertension after isolated lung transplantation. Eur J Cardiothorac Surg 2004; 26(4):776–781.
11. Stamler JS, Vaughan DE, Rudd MA, et al. Frequency of hypercholesterolemia after cardiac transplantation. Am J Cardiol 1988; 62(17):1268–1272.

12. Superko HR, Haskell WL, Di Ricco CD. Lipoprotein and hepatic lipase activity and high-density lipoprotein subclasses after cardiac transplantation. Am J Cardiol 1990; 66(15):1131–1134.

13. Eich D, Thompson JA, Ko DJ, et al. Hypercholesterolemia in long-term survivors of heart transplantation: an early marker of accelerated coronary artery disease. J Heart Lung Transplant 1991; 10(1, Pt 1):45–49.

14. Esper E, Glagov S, Karp RB, et al. Role of hypercholesterolemia in accelerated transplant coronary vasculopathy: results of surgical therapy with partial ileal bypass in rabbits undergoing heterotopic heart transplantation. J Heart Lung Transplant 1997; 16(4):420–435.

15. Kapadia SR, Nissen SE, Ziada KM, et al. Impact of lipid abnormalities in development and progression of transplant coronary disease: a serial intravascular ultrasound study. J Am Coll Cardiol 2001; 38(1):206–213.

16. Tanaka H, Sukhova GK, Libby P. Interaction of the allogeneic state and hypercholesterolemia in arterial lesion formation in experimental cardiac allografts. Arterioscler Thromb 1994; 14(5):734–745.

17. Raisanen-Sokolowski A, Tilly-Kiesi M, Ustinov J, et al. Hyperlipidemia accelerates allograft arteriosclerosis (chronic rejection) in the rat. Arterioscler Thromb 1994; 14(12):2032–2042.

18. Kobashigawa JA, Katznelson S, Laks H, et al. Effect of pravastatin on outcomes after cardiac transplantation. N Engl J Med 1995; 333(10):621–627.

19. Wenke K, Meiser B, Thiery J, et al. Simvastatin initiated early after heart transplantation: 8-year prospective experience. Circulation 2003; 107(1):93–97.

20. Kwak B, Mulhaupt F, Myit S, Mach F. Statins as a newly recognized type of immunomodulator. Nat Med 2000; 6(12):1399–1402.

21. Johnson BA, Iacono AT, Zeevi A, McCurry KR, Duncan SR. Statin use is associated with improved function and survival of lung allografts. Am J Respir Crit Care Med 2003; 167(9):1271–1278.

22. Taylor DO, Barr ML, Radovancevic B, et al. A randomized, multicenter comparison of tacrolimus and cyclosporine immunosuppressive regimens in cardiac transplantation: decreased hyperlipidemia and hypertension with tacrolimus. J Heart Lung Transplant 1999; 18(4):336–345.

23. Kobashigawa JA, Miller L, Yeung A, et al. Does acute rejection correlate with the development of transplant coronary artery disease? A multicenter study using intravascular ultrasound. Sandoz/CVIS Investigators. J Heart Lung Transplant 1995; 14(6, Pt 2):S221–S226.

24. Hornick P, Smith J, Pomerance A, et al. Influence of acute rejection episodes, HLA matching, and donor/recipient phenotype on the development of 'early' transplant-associated coronary artery disease. Circulation 1997; 96(9, Suppl II): 148–153.

25. Williams R, Neuhaus P, Bismuth H, et al. Two-year data from the European multicentre tacrolimus (FK506) liver study. Transplant Int 1996; (9, Suppl I): S144–S150.

26. Jurcevic S, Dunn MJ, Crisp S, et al. A new enzyme-linked immunosorbent assay to measure anti-endothelial antibodies after cardiac transplantation demonstrates greater inhibition of antibody formation by tacrolimus compared with cyclosporine. Transplantation 1998; 65(9):1197–1202.

27. Kobashigawa J, Miller L, Renlund D, et al. A randomized active-controlled trial of mycophenolate mofetil in heart transplant recipients. Mycophenolate Mofetil Investigators. Transplantation 1998; 66(4):507–515.

28. Kobashigawa J, Tobis J, Mentzer R, et al. Further analysis of the intravascular ultrasound data from the randomized mycopenolate mofetil (MMF) trial in heart transplant recipients (abstract). J Heart Lung Transplant 2004; 23(2, Suppl 0):S42.

29. Rose MLDA, Smith JD, Keogh AM, Dureau G, Kobashigawa JA, Dunn MJ. Mycophenolate mofetil (MMF) depresses antibody production after cardiac transplantation. Circulation 2000; 102(18S):II.490.

30. Corri P, Glanville A, McNeil K, et al. One year analysis of an ongoing international randomized study of mycophenolate mofetil (MMF) vs azathioprine (AZA) in lung transplantation. J Heart Lung Transplant 2001; 20(2):149–150.

31. Palmer SM, Baz MA, Sanders L, et al. Results of a randomized, prospective, multicenter trial of mycophenolate mofetil versus azathioprine in the prevention of acute lung allograft rejection. Transplantation 2001; 71(12):1772–1776.

32. Rensing BVJ, Smits P, Foley D, et al. Coronary restenosis prevention with a rapamycin coated stent. J Am Coll Cardiol 2001; 37(2, Suppl A):47A.

33. Morice M-C, Serruys PW, Sousa JE, et al. A randomized comparison of a sirolimus-eluting stent with a standard stent for coronary revascularization. New Engl J Med 2002; 346(23):1773–1780.

34. Moses JW, Leon MB, Popma JJ, et al. Sirolimus-eluting stents versus standard stents in patients with stenosis in a native coronary artery. New Engl J Med 2003; 349(14):1315–1323.

35. Radovancevic B, Vrtovec B. Sirolimus therapy in cardiac transplantation. Transplant Proc 2003; 35(3, Suppl):171S–176S.

36. Keogh A, Group TSCTT. Sirolimus immunotherapy reduces the rates of cardiac allograft rejection: 6-month results from a phase 2, open label study. Am J Transplant 2002; 2(Suppl 3):246.

37. Keogh A, Muller DW, Faddy S, Ruygrok PN, Richardson M, Galbaith A. Sirolimus from the time of heart transplantation-persistent protection from graft vasculopathy at 2 years (abstract). J Heart Lung Transplant 2004; 23(2, Suppl 0):S106–S107.

38. Mancini D, Pinney S, Burkhoff D, et al. Use of rapamycin slows progression of cardiac transplantation vasculopathy. Circulation 2003; 108(l):48–53.

39. Tuzcu EM, Kobashigawa J, Eisen H, et al. Favorable effect of everolimus on cardiac allograft vasculopathy is maintained through 24 months (abstract). J Heart Lung Transplant 2004; 24(2, Suppl 0):S51.

40. King-Biggs MB, Dunitz JM, Park SJ, Kay Savik S, Hertz MI. Airway anastomotic dehiscence associated with use of sirolimus immediately after lung transplantation. Transplantation 2003; 75(9):1437–1443.

41. Cahill BC, Somerville KT, Crompton JA, et al. Early experience with sirolimus in lung transplant recipients with chronic allograft rejection. J Heart Lung Transplant 2003; 22(2):169–176.

# Metabolic Bone Disease in Lung Transplant Recipients

Janet R. Maurer

*Health Dialog Services Corporation, Phoenix, Arizona, U.S.A.*

## INTRODUCTION

Osteopenia and osteoporosis are common medical problems in both patients with end-stage lung disease (1) and in posttransplant patients (2). Metabolic bone disease is a complication not only in lung transplant candidates, but also in patients who are candidates for other solid organs and in the recipients of those organs (3). Metabolic bone disease has also been identified as a complication of stem cell transplant recipients (4).

The World Health Organization classified bone mineral loss in 1994 as a comparison to normal young healthy adult values by the use of T-scores. According to this classification, a T-score that is 1 to 2.5 standard deviations below the mean represents osteopenia; a T-score that is greater than 2.5 standard deviations below the mean represents osteoporosis. Z-scores, another type of classification, differ from T-scores in that they reflect a normalization of the bone mineral density to age to take account of the normal bone loss healthy adults experience as they get older. A Z-score deviation of two standard deviations below normal is consistent with osteoporosis in this classification (5).

## RISK FACTORS

Steroids have long been implicated in the metabolic bone disease of patients with advanced lung disease; however, significant bone mineral loss is also seen in patients who have never used steroids (6). Most often the cause is multifactorial. Contributing factors include vitamin D deficiency and other nutritional deficits (e.g., cystic fibrosis), inactivity, and reduced levels of hormones particularly in older patients (7–10). An increased rate of bone mineral loss has been documented in lung and other solid organ recipients in the early posttransplant period. This has been attributed to the use of both steroids and calcineurin inhibitors; however, the mechanism by which calcineurin inhibitors might cause bone mineral loss remains unclear (11).

The impact of osteoporosis was first observed and reported in lung transplant recipients in the mid-1990s. Aris et al. conducted a cross-sectional study of 100 lung transplant recipients, 55 of whom were pretransplant and 45 of whom were posttransplant. Spine and femoral neck bone mineral density was measured. Using Z-scores, the authors found that 45% of pretransplant and 73% of posttransplant patients were below the fracture threshold (2). More than half of the patients in each group had either chronic obstructive pulmonary disease (COPD) or cystic fibrosis (CF). CF patients had the lowest scores, followed by COPD. Patients with pulmonary fibrosis and pulmonary vascular disease appear to have a lower risk of metabolic bone disease (2,12). Fifteen fractures were recorded in the study group, 80% of them posttransplant. Subsequent studies in candidates for lung transplant have confirmed a prevalence of osteoporosis varying from 35% to greater than 50% in the lumbar spine and femoral neck (6,12–15). In addition, these studies document an association with vitamin D deficiency (6,7) and low body mass index (7,9) in the pretransplant population.

Ferrari et al. prospectively assessed the bone mineral density in 21 candidates for lung transplant. In this study, 35% of patients had preoperative osteoporosis. Despite treatment with vitamin D and calcium, within six months of surgery, 8 of 12 patients reassessed had a significant increase in bone mineral loss and two had new vertebral fractures (13).

In a second prospective study, Spira et al. measured bone mineral density in 28 patients pretransplant and again within one year posttransplant. Patients were treated with vitamin D and calcium posttransplant. Patients experienced a mean fall in bone mineral density of approximately 5% in both lumbar spine and femoral neck in spite of the treatment. In addition, five posttransplant fractures were documented (12).

Metabolic bone disease in lung transplant recipients has been associated with some unusual complications. A patient with multiple vertebral compression fractures was reported to experience fat embolism with a fatal outcome (16). Another report noted four insufficiency fractures of the sacrum in a population of 71 posttransplant patients. These fractures were heralded by back pain and were detected by radionuclide bone scans (17).

## MANAGEMENT

While osteopenia and osteoporosis have been well-documented as significant medical problems in both pre- and posttransplant lung transplant patients for the past decade, approaches to management are not yet well established.

### Vitamin D/Calcium

At least four published series of transplant recipients received treatment for their metabolic bone disease with calcium and vitamin D but continued to have significant bone mineral loss and fracture. Thus, while this supplementation is important, it does not appear sufficient to address the bone loss in these patients (12,13,15,18,19).

### Hormone Replacement

Estrogen and testosterone deficiency have known relationships to bone mineral loss. Hormone replacement has been tried in some patients but has not been shown to improve or significantly reduce the loss of bone mineral. Hormone replacement may be contraindicated in postmenopausal females because of the potential impact on breast cancer and cardiovascular risk.

### Bisphosphonates

Bisphosphonates have received the most attention as treatment for osteopenia/osteoporosis in this population. Two small, randomized controlled trials (total 65 patients) have been conducted in pre- and posttransplant CF patients using intravenous pamidronate every three months. Axial bone density was increased, but the posttransplant fracture rate did not change in treated patients relative to controls (20). In addition, patients not taking corticosteroids experienced significant bone pain.

Trombetti et al. studied 29 patients determined on preoperative evaluation to have either osteopenia or osteoporosis. Pamidronate was given to 14 patients, hormone replacement to 5, and calcium/vitamin D to 10. The patients receiving antiresorptive therapy had significantly less bone loss of the spine at six months and actually an increase in bone mineral density at one year compared to the other groups (21). In a pilot study by Cahill et al., pre- and posttransplant patients were treated prospectively with calcium/vitamin D, hormone replacement (if indicated), and pamidronate. At 12 months posttransplant the fracture rate and bone densities were compared to those of a historical control group. The regimen appeared to be most effective in preserving bone in patients who started treatment before transplant. Overall, the treated patients had improved bone mineral density and reduced fracture rate compared to controls (22).

In another small study of patients recruited within a week of transplant with varying diagnoses, patients were randomized to either calcitriol or two cycles of etidronate followed by calcium carbonate. Patients were followed for 18 months and were compared to a historical control group. Despite treatment, both calcitriol and etidronate groups had significant posttransplant bone loss and some fractures; the loss, however, was less than that observed in historical, nontreated controls. Treatment was carried out for six months with an additional follow-up of six months. Patients were observed to have ongoing bone loss in the six months of follow-up, leading the authors to suggest therapy at least for a year posttransplant (22).

It is of interest that bisphosphonate studies have primarily used pamidronate, an expensive, parenteral drug. It is easier and cheaper to use oral bisphosphonates like alendronate (Fosamax), risedronate (Actonel), etidronate (Didronel), or ibandronate (BONIVA). Probably, the lack of studies using these drugs is due to the extended time period required to reach a large enough absorption to reach therapeutic quantities of the drugs.

Other potential approaches include the use of calcitonin or teriparatide. The use of either of these drugs has not yet been reported in lung transplant recipients. Teriparatide, which is parathyroid hormone (rh-PTH) (1–34) and acts as endogenous PTH, actually increases bone mineral density, whereas the primary impact of most other treatments is a decrease in resorption, which prevents further mineral loss. Thus, this drug may have a role in some of the highest risk patients; however, that remains unproven.

All potential lung transplant candidates should undergo assessment of bone mineral density via DEXA scan at the time of evaluation. Any patient with bone mineral density at least one standard deviation below normal should begin appropriate treatment, usually including an antiresorptive, during the pretransplant period. Following transplant, the treatment should be continued. A repeat DEXA scan six months to one year posttransplant will assist in guiding ongoing treatment. A goal of posttransplant management should be to prevent fractures, which not only can cause a lower quality of life, but can also impact graft function if fracture pain impairs the ability to cough.

## REFERENCES

1. Gluck O, Colice G. Recognizing and treating glucocorticoid-induced osteoporosis in patients with pulmonary disease. Chest 2004; 125:1859–1876.
2. Aris RM, Neuringer IP, Weiner MA, et al. Severe osteoporosis before and after lung transplantation. Chest 1996; 109:1176–1183.
3. Maalouf NM, Shane E. Osteoporosis after solid organ transplantation. J Clin Endocrinol Metab 2004.
4. Schulte C, Beelen DW, Schaefer UW, Mann K. Bone loss in long-term survivors after transplantation of hematopoietic stem cells: a prospective study. Osteoporos Int 2000; 11:344–353.

5. Prevention and management of osteoporosis. World Health Organ Tech Rep Ser 2003; 921:1–164.

6. Shane E, Silverberg SJ, Donovan D, et al. Osteoporosis in lung transplantation candidates with end-stage pulmonary disease. Am J Med 1996; 101:262–269.

7. Forli L, Halse J, Haug E, et al. Vitamin D deficiency, bone mineral density and weight in patients with advanced pulmonary disease. J Intern Med 2004; 256:56–62.

8. Aringer M, Kiener HP, Koeller MD, et al. High turnover bone disease following lung transplantation. Bone 1998; 23:485–488.

9. Tschopp O, Boehler A, Speich R, et al. Osteoporosis before lung transplantation: association with low body mass index, but not with underlying disease. Am J Transplant 2002; 2:167–172.

10. Aris RM, Renner JB, Winders AD, et al. Increased rate of fractures and severe kyphosis: sequelae of living into adulthood with cystic fibrosis. Ann Int Med 1998; 128:186–193.

11. Sprague SM. Mechanism of transplantation-associated bone loss. Pediatr Nephrol 2000; 14:650–653.

12. Spira A, Gutierrez C, Chaparro C, et al. Osteoporosis and lung transplantation: a prospective study. Chest 2000; 117:476–481.

13. Ferrari SL, Nicod LP, Hamacher J, et al. Osteoporosis in patients undergoing lung transplantation. Eur Respir J 1996; 9:2378–2382.

14. Haworth CS, Webb AK, Egan JJ, et al. Bone histomorphometry in adult patients with cystic fibrosis. Chest 2000; 118:434–439.

15. Shane E, Papadopoulos A, Staron RB, et al. Bone loss and fracture after lung transplantation. Transplantation 1999; 68:220–227.

16. Day JD, Walden SM, Stuart SR, et al. Fatal fat embolism syndrome after numerous vertebral body compression fractures in a lung transplant recipient. J Heart Lung Transplant 1994; 13:785–790.

17. Schulman LL, Addesso V, Staron BB, et al. Insufficiency fractures of sacrum: a cause of low back pain after lung transplantation. J Heart Lung Transplant 1997; 16:181–185.

18. Henderson K, Eisman J, Keogh A, et al. Protective effect of short-term calcitriol or cyclical etidronate on bone loss after cardiac or lung transplantation. J Bone Miner Res 2001; 16:565–571.

19. Hecker TM, Aris RM. Management of osteoporosis in adults with cystic fibrosis. Drugs 2004; 64:133–147.

20. Brenckmann C, Papaioannou A. Bisphosphonates for osteoporosis in people with cystic fibrosis. Cochrane Database Syst Rev 2001; 4:CD002010.

21. Trombetti A, Gerbase MW, Spiliopoulos A, et al. Bone mineral density in lung-transplant recipients before and after graft: prevention of lumbar spine posttransplantation-accelerated bone loss by pamidronate. J Heart Lung Transplant 2000; 19:736–743.

22. Cahill BC, O'Rourke MK, Parker S, et al. Prevention of bone loss and fracture after lung transplantation: a pilot study. Transplantation 2001; 72:1251–1255.

# Lymphoproliferative Disorders Complicating Solid Organ Transplantation

**S. Samuel Weigt and Joseph P. Lynch III**

*Division of Pulmonary and Critical Care Medicine and Hospitalists, Department of Internal Medicine, David Geffen School of Medicine at UCLA, Los Angeles, California, U.S.A.*

**Lucy R. Langer**

*Division of Hematology and Oncology, Department of Internal Medicine, David Geffen School of Medicine at UCLA, Los Angeles, California, U.S.A.*

**Michael C. Fishbein**

*Department of Pathology and Laboratory Medicine, David Geffen School of Medicine at UCLA, Los Angeles, California, U.S.A.*

## INTRODUCTION

Posttransplant lymphoproliferative disorder (PTLD) is an infrequent but potentially lethal complication of solid-organ transplantation (1,2). The designation PTLD refers to a spectrum of lymphoid proliferations with varying histological features, clinical presentation, and prognosis (2–4). Histological features of PTLD are heterogenous, ranging from cytologically benign polyclonal lymphoid proliferation to overtly malignant lymphomas (3,5,6). Lymphoproliferative disorders (including lymphomas) may also complicate various forms of inherited and acquired immunosuppressive (IMS) disorders [e.g., ataxia telangiectasia (7), autoimmune diseases (8), and acquired human immunodeficiency virus syndrome (AIDS) (9)], but in this manuscript we limit our discussion to PTLDs. As early as 1969, immunosuppressed solid organ transplant (SOT) recipients were noted to have an increased incidence of lymphomas (10). Lymphoproliferative disorders account for 21% of all malignancies posttransplant, compared to only 5% in the general population (11). Posttransplant lymphomas have increased extranodal involvement, a more aggresssive clinical course, a poorer response to conventional therapies, and poorer outcomes in general than lymphomas in the general population (12).

Data regarding PTLD among lung transplant recipients (LTRs) are limited, so much of the evidence is extrapolated from the experience in non–lung SOT recipients (discussed in this chapter).

## CLASSIFICATION OF PTLD

The vast majority ($\geq$76–95%) of PTLDs are associated with Epstein–Barr virus (EBV) and are of B-cell origin (13–16). T-cell proliferations comprise up to 14% of PTLDs (17–19); natural killer (NK) cells comprise 1% (20).

### Histopathology

Subclassification of PTLD is standarized according to morphologic criteria set forth by the World Health Organization (17). Four major categories include (i) early lesions (i.e., reactive plasma cell hyperplasia and infectious mononucleosis-like proliferations); (ii) polymorphic proliferation; (iii) monomorphic proliferation corresponding to typical lymphomas (e.g., B- or T-cell lymphomas and their subtypes); and (iv) Hodgkin's or Hodgkin-like lymphoma (Table 1, Fig. 1) (5,14,17,21). However, morphologic classification of PTLD does not reliably predict disease behavior (23,24).

### Immunohistochemistry

Analysis of histogenetic and clonal patterns of PTLD may prove to be more important for prognosis and treatment than morphology alone. T-cell lymphomas usually express CD3 and may exhibit T-cell gene rearrangement (25). CD20 is a B-cell surface marker and is expressed in >85% of PTLD (26). In some CD20 negative PTLDs, a B-cell origin can be affirmed by reactivity with a panel of other B-cell lymphoid markers or by gene rearrangement studies (26).

Markers can also identify the stage of development in the cell lineage. Bcl-6 is a well-defined histogenetic marker present only while the B-cell is in the germinal center (GC) stage (27). MUM1/IRF4 expression occurs in the final step of differentiation in the GC and is maintained afterward (27). CD138 is acquired after exit from the GC late in the B-cell's differentiation into plasma/memory cells (27). SHP-1 expression is another marker acquired

**Table 1**  Classification of Posttransplant Lymphoproliferative Disorders

Early lesions
   Reactive plasmacytic hyperplasia
   Infectious mononucleosis–like lesions
Polymorphic PTLD
Monomorphic PTLD (classified by type of lymphoma)
   B-cell lymphoma
      Diffuse large cell——centroblastic and immunoblastic variants
      Burkitt/Burkitt-like lymphoma
      Plasma cell myeloma
      Plasmacytoma-like lesions
      Maltoma
   T-cell lymphomas
      Peripheral T-cell lymphomas
      Anaplastic large cell lymphoma (T cell or null cell)
      $\gamma-\delta$ T-cell lymphoma
      T-NK cell
Hodgkin's and Hodgkin-like lymphoma

*Abbreviations*: PTLD, posttransplant lymphoproliferative disorder; NK, natural killer.
*Source*: Adapted from Refs. 2, 3, and 22.

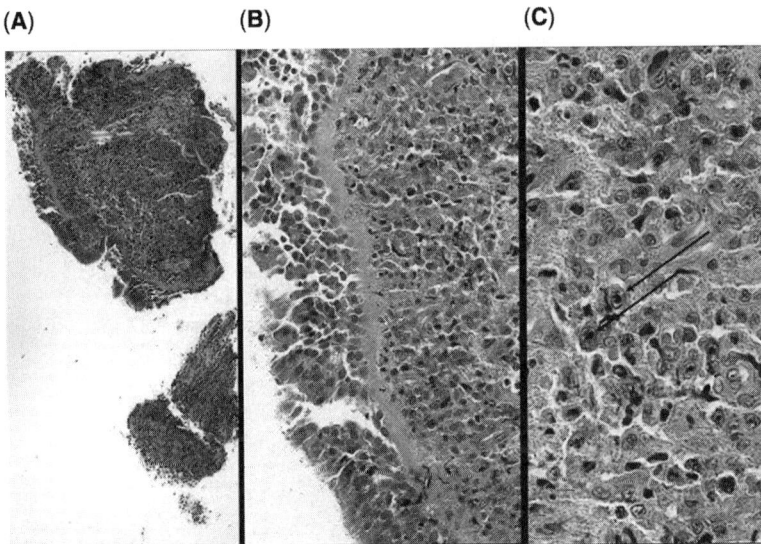

**Figure 1**  Lung biopsy five months S/P lung transplant: low (**A**, ×40), medium (**B**, ×100), and high (**C**, ×400) power photomicrographs of bronchial wall with marked infiltration by pleomorphic, atypical, plasmacytoid-appearing lymphoid cells (*arrows*), characteristic of posttransplant lymphoma, diffuse large-cell immunoblastic variant (all H&E stain).

early after the exit from the GC (28). VS38c is a plasma cell antigen and identifies the plasmacytoid types (14). Staining for κ and λ light chains may indicate whether the plasma cell proliferation is monoclonal or polyclonal (Fig. 2). Additional studies are needed to determine what prognostic and treatment implications these markers may have.

In the majority of cases of PTLD associated with EBV infection, EBV can be identified in tissues by in situ hybridization of EBV-encoded RNA (EBER) (Fig. 3) (29,30), or by immunochemical analysis of EBV antigens latent membrane protein (LMP)-1 and Epstein–Barr nuclear antigen (EBNA)-2 (26,31). Certain EBV-related malignancies express EBER but not LMP-1 (15,32). Further, the pattern of staining differs according to histologic subtype. Monomorphic PTLDs express LMP-1 diffusely in virtually all tumor cells, whereas polymorphic PTLD express LMP-1 in < 5% of lesional cells (26).

Hodgkin's disease (HD) (33,34) or lymphomas resembling HD (35) account for fewer than 3% of PTLD (36). Classic Reed–Sternberg (RS) cells stain positive for CD15, CD30, and EBV RNA (33). Other cases with atypical RS-like cells may fail to express CD15 or EBV RNA but retain CD30 and are LMP-1 positive (37).

**(A)**                                        **(B)**

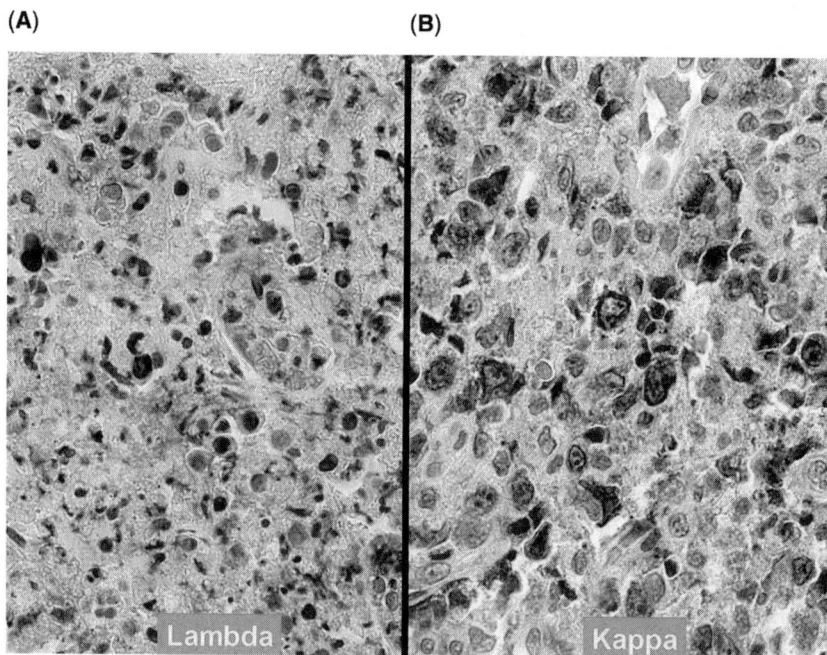

**Figure 2**  Immunohistochemical stains for Lambda (**A**) and Kappa (**B**) light chains showing that the proliferation is monoclonal for κ light chains (**A** and **B**, ×400, peroxidase stain).

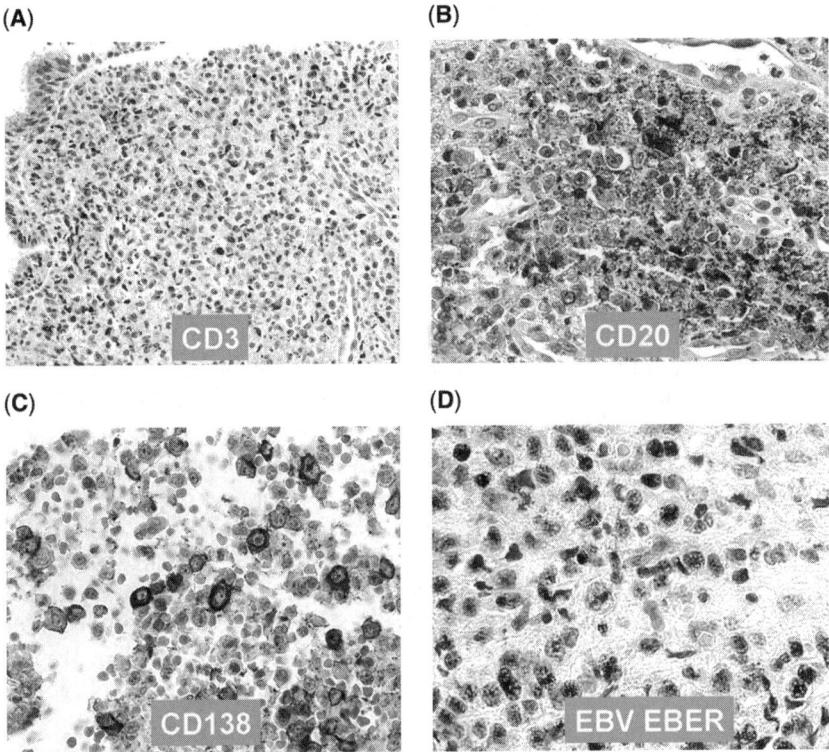

**Figure 3** Immunohistochemical staining of lymphoid infiltrate shows only rare T cells (**A**), numerous B cells (**B**), numerous plasma cells (**C**), and positive staining for Epstein–Barr virus (**D**, showing positive nuclei) (**A**, ×200; **B–D**, ×400; **A–C**, peroxidase stains).

Synchronous and metachronous lesions of PTLD may arise from distinct clones of proliferating lymphocytes. Multiple pathologic subtypes of PTLD have been noted in different locations in the same patient simultaneously (38,39). Further, recurrent disease may represent a new subtype of PTLD and not reactivation of the previous clone (39).

## PATHOGENESIS

Reactivation of EBV and the resultant unchecked virus-driven lymphocytic proliferation in the setting of immunosuppression are responsible for the vast majority of PTLDs (15,40–42). The cellular source of EBV (principally B-cells) is derived from the recipient in >90% of PTLDs complicating SOT (26,40,43), whereas PTLDs among bone marrow or stem cell transplant (SCT) recipients arise predominantly from the donor (26). EBV is ubiquitous, and 85% of adults >35 years of age are seropositive (41,42,44).

The primary target of EBV in the immunocompetent host is the B-cell (45). During the course of naive B-cell infection, EBV-coded proteins mimic pathways followed when naive B-cells encounter antigen and thereby establish EBV latency in memory B-cells (2,15). In this state, the virus is "invisible" to the immune system (2). Further, differentiation of EBV-infected B-cells to memory cells downregulates latent EBV gene expression (2). When B-cells differentiate into plasma cells, the lytic EBV cycle is triggered and infectious virus is produced (2). Long-lasting EBV-specific memory cytotoxic T-lymphocytes (CTL) are critical for controlling EBV (46–48). These virus-specific CD8 positive lymphocytes lyse EBV-infected B-cells if viral proteins are presented to the cell surface (49). In the immunocompetent host, an equilibrium between virus and host is established (2). In immunocompromised hosts, this equilibrium is disrupted and rates of proliferation exceed rates of clearance and differentiation.

Immunosuppressive drugs used in SOT recipients suppress the function of EBV-specific CTL, allowing uncontrolled proliferation of EBV-infected B-cells (50,51). Development of PTLD is associated with elevated EBV DNA levels and a deficiency of EBV-specific CTL (52). The load of EBV-infected lymphocytes in peripheral blood correlates with the risk of PTLD (53). Typically, uncontrolled proliferation of B-cells results in polyclonal proliferation. However, the local microenvironment (cytokine milieu) may provide specific clones a growth advantage, resulting in oligoclonal or monoclonal proliferation (2). Certain cytokines may play a role in induction of PTLD as well as tolerance and tumor regression. For example, interleukin (IL)-10 enhances B-cell proliferation, immunoglobulin G (IgG) secretion, and maintenance of B-cells in culture, and may facilitate EBV-associated PTLD (54,55). In one study, elevated serum IL-10 was a better predictor of PTLD than EBV viral load (56). In contrast, IL-18 induces T-lymphocyte synthesis of interferon-$\gamma$, and may contribute to PTLD tumor regression (54).

Lymphocytes infected with EBV in vitro are often transformed to immortalized EBV-infected lymphoblastoid cell lines (2). This transformation process is the primary basis for the oncogenic potential of the virus. In some cases, unchecked lymphoid proliferation activates oncogenes (57) and evolves to malignant lymphoma (58). Mutations occuring during the lymphoproliferative process dictate the cellular phenotype. For example, c-myc activation may elicit Burkitt's lymphoma (58), whereas mutations at the GC stage may result in HD (2). Most PTLD cases occurring early after transplantation are derived from naive B-cells, whereas PTLD occurring late after transplantation are derived from GC or post-GC cells (2).

## RISK FACTORS FOR PTLD

Pretransplant seronegative EBV status is the primary risk factor for PTLD (41,42,59,60). The intensity of immunosuppression is the other major

**Table 2**   Risk Factors for Posttransplant Lymphoproliferative Disorder in Lung Transplantation

| |
|---|
| Independent risk factors |
|   Recipient EBV seronegative immune status |
|   Intense immunosuppression |
|     Monoclonal and polyclonal T-cell antibody induction |
|     Monoclonal and polyclonal T-cell antibody anti-rejection therapy |
|     High-dose maintenance |
| Other possible risk factors |
|   Organ transplanted |
|     Heart–lung > lung > heart > liver > kidney |
|   Age of recipient |
|     Pediatric recipients |
|     Adult recipients > 55 years old |
|   Higher acute rejection frequency |
|   CMV and other viral infections |

*Abbreviations:* EBV, Epstein–Barr virus; CMV, cytomegalovirus.

determinant of risk. Other factors, including IMS agent, donor EBV status, and recipient cytomegalovirus (CMV) status have also been evaluated as risk factors for the development of PTLD but studies have not demonstrated conclusive independent correlations (Table 2).

**EBV Serological Status**

Healthy individuals who develop primary EBV infection rapidly develop antibodies to EBV viral capsid antigen (VCA) (61). However, the protective role of EBV humoral antibodies is unclear. Nonetheless, pretransplant EBV seronegative status in the recipient is the primary risk factor for the development of PTLD. In a cohort of 40 EBV seronegative adult liver transplant recipients, 95% developed primary EBV infection posttransplant; 13 (33%) developed PTLD (42). Among LTRs, PTLD developed in 5 of 15 (33%) patients who were seronegative for EBV prior to transplantation compared to 1 of 60 (2%) who were seropositive for EBV pretransplant (60). Similarly, data from Australia identified PTLD in 5 of 16 (31%) EBV-mismatched (D+/R−) LTRs but in only 2 of 187 (1%) non-EBV mismatched LTRs (62). Multiple studies have shown children are at increased risk for PTLD owing to a higher proportion of EBV-naive individuals (42,63–67).

The EBV viral load in peripheral blood is elevated in patients with PTLD, and the elevated viral load has been shown to preceed the development of PTLD (68), and therefore may be a good marker for risk of developing PTLD. EBV viral loads decrease with antiviral treatment (68), and there is some evidence that preemptive use of antiviral medications may reduce the risk of PTLD (2,69).

## Effect of Immunosuppression

The intensity of immunosuppression appears to be strongly associated with risk of PTLD (12). However, evidence for which IMS medications confer a greater risk has been conflicting. Some studies suggest the incidence of PTLD is increased among SOT recipients receiving cyclosporine-based IMS therapy (70,71). Others have questioned such associations and attribute the increased incidence to the inclusion of recipients of nonrenal transplants that require a greater degree of immune suppression (12,15,72,73).

Some studies indicate that the incidence of PTLD is lower among renal transplant recipients receiving mycophenolate mofetil (MMF) (15,65,74). This apparent protective effect of MMF may reflect potentiation of antiviral activity by MMF (75) or reduced risk of rejection episodes requiring intensification of IMS therapy (65). In a study by Ciancio et al. the use of MMF in combination with tacrolimus was associated with an increased incidence of PTLD in renal transplant recipients (76). Other studies note an association between the use of tacrolimus and the increased risk of PTLD among pediatric renal and liver transplant recipients (77–80), but data from >6700 pediatric renal transplant recipients found no increased risk with the use of tacrolimus, MMF, or the combination of both agents (81).

The Collaborative Transplant Study database includes approximately 200,000 SOT recipients from 42 countries followed over a 10-year period (12). In this database, MMF conferred no protective effect; tacrolimus was associated with a twofold increased risk of PTLD among kidney but not hepatic transplant recipients, and cyclosporine had no effect compared to azathioprine/steroid treatment (12).

PTLD was also linked to the use of the monoclonal antibody OKT3 (82,83), and polyclonal antibodies antilymphocyte globulin (ALG) (83) and antithymocyte globulin (ATG) in some (84–86) but not all studies (15). In a cohort of >38,000 renal transplant recipients, the incidence of PTLD was slightly increased with the receipt of monoclonal (0.85%) or polyclonal (0.81%) antibodies compared to IL-2 receptor antibody (0.50%) or no induction therapy (0.51%) (65). In one retrospective study of renal transplant recipients, all four of the patients who developed PTLD (of a total of 162 studied) had received ALG induction therapy. Of the four PTLD patients, three also received OKT3 as treatment for steroid-resistant rejection (87). Use of OKT3 induction therapy was associated with an increased incidence of PTLD in heart transplant recipients at one center (82) but others found no such association (63).

In the Collaborative Transplant Study, induction therapy with either OKT3 or ATG increased the risk of lymphoma during the first year. Anti-rejection therapy with either OKT3 or ATG also increased the risk (12). The use of IL-2 receptor monoclonal antibodies was not associated with an increased risk of PTLD (12).

In general, it appears that the degree of immunosuppression is a crucial factor in the early posttransplant period. Risk of acute rejection in SOT necessitates early intense immunosupression. The incidence of PTLD correlates with this early period of heightened immunosuppression and appears to level off after the first two years posttransplant (12). It is likely that degree of immunosuppression, rather than the individual agent, is the key determinant of risk for PTLD.

### Effect of Organ Transplanted

Multiple studies have demonstrated that lung, heart, and heart–lung transplants are associated with a greater risk for PTLD than kidney or liver transplants (2,12,63,88,89). The degree of immunosuppression probably explains the variability in the incidence of PTLD by organ transplanted. For example, in the Collaborative Transplant Study database, 61% of heart transplant recipients received antibody induction therapy, compared to only 27% of kidney recipients (12).

However, local immune reaction against the graft may be a factor in malignant transformation. Among SOT recipients, PTLD frequently involves the graft and other proximal organs (12,90,91). In this context, chronic antigenic stimulation by the allograft may play a role in PTLD pathogenesis (15).

### CMV, Hepatitis C Virus, and Other Viral Infections

CMV inhibits the tumor-suppression gene p53 (63), and may play a permissive role in the development of PTLD. Several studies implicated CMV as a possible cofactor in the development of PTLD among renal, hepatic, and cardiac allograft recipients (42,65,92–94). Evaluation of a small series of LTRs demonstrated that all three patients seronegative for EBV had CMV viremia at the time of PTLD diagnosis (95). Although CMV infection may also be a marker for overall degree of immunosuppression, CMV mismatching (donor seropositive and recipient seronegative) was an independent risk factor for PTLD among liver transplant recipients (92). Among renal transplant recipients, pretransplant CMV negative status was associated with an increased risk of PTLD (65), but in a separate study of renal allograft recipients, CMV mismatch was not a risk factor for PTLD (96). Further, CMV may precipitate allograft rejection (97), which triggers escalation of the IMS regimen.

Additional viruses may act as cofactors in the pathogenesis of PTLD. Liver transplantation for hepatitis C virus (HCV) cirrhosis is a risk factor for PTLD (86,98), probably via HCV-induced clonal B-cell expansion in the posttransplant setting. Rare cases of adult T-cell leukemia (ATL) due to human T-cell lymphotropic virus 1 (HTLV-1) have been described among SOT recipients (25). The association between PTLD and HCV, CMV, and other viruses is complex, and merits further epidemiologic and prospective prevention studies.

## Human Leukocyte Antigen Mismatch

Human leukocyte antigen (HLA) matching did not correlate with the incidence of PTLD in a large cohort (>38,000 patients) of renal transplant recipients (65). No significant associations between HLA-A or HLA-DR mismatching were noted among heart, heart–lung, or LTRs, but a trend toward increased risk of PTLD was observed with increased HLA-B mismatching (99). In a small cohort of 16 EBV-mismatched (D+/R−) LTRs, two or more HLA mismatches were present in four of five patients with PTLD but in none of 11 without PTLD (62).

## INCIDENCE OF PTLD

The incidence of PTLD varies according to the organ transplanted (2,12,63,88,89). In one review (89), incidence rates according to the organ transplanted were as follows: renal (≤1%), liver (2.2%), heart (3.4%), lung (1.8–7.9%), heart–lung (9.4%), and intestinal (7–11%). In the Collaborative Transplant Study, the incidence was highest in combined heart–lung and LTRs (12).

### Renal

The incidence of PTLD following renal transplantation is low, ranging from 0.3% to 2% (13,65,81,100). The incidence is higher (1–10%) in pediatric renal transplant recipients (101).

### Bone Marrow

The reported incidence of PTLD among bone marrow transplant recipients ranges from 0.6% to 1.6% (102–104). In a series reported from the Fred Hutchison Cancer Research Center in Seattle, Washington, 13 out of 13 cases tested positive for EBV genomic sequences by Southern blot and 77% (10 of 13) were of donor cell origin (102).

### Liver

PTLD occurs in 2% to 4% of adult liver transplant recipients (13,16,86,105–108) and 4% to 12% of pediatric recipients (66,109–111). The main risk factors for PTLD among liver transplant recipients are EBV infection (88,109) and the use of antilymphocyte antibodies (ATG or OKT3) (86,105,106). The incidence is highest (31%) among EBV-naive recipients of EBV seropositive grafts (42,109).

### Heart Transplant Recipients

The reported incidence of PTLD among cardiac transplant recipients ranges from 0.3% to 6.8% (4,13,25,63,82,91,112–115), with higher rates (14%)

among pediatric patients (25). Cumulative experience of 274 cases of PTLD in cardiac transplant recipients cited one- and three-year survival rates of 45% and 30%, respectively (113). Cardiomyopathy as the indication for transplant was associated with increased incidence of PTLD in at least two studies (113,116). The use of OKT3 in cardiac transplant recipients was associated with an increased risk of PTLD in one study (82) but others found no such association (115).

## Lung Transplant Recipients

The reported incidence of PTLD in lung transplants at different centers ranges from very low (1.3%) (117), to alarmingly high (20%) (118). Typically however, most centers report an incidence around 2% to 8% (12,13,40,41, 60,63,64,91,95,99,117–122). This is higher than usually reported for other SOTs other than heart, and may be attributable to the higher level of immunosuppression required to prevent both acute and chronic rejection of the lung allograft.

As would be predicted, recipient EBV seronegative immune status at the time of transplant is the major risk factor for development of PTLD. PTLD develops in 30% to 40% of EBV seronegative LTRs who receive EBV seropositive lungs, compared with less than 5% in EBV seropositive recipients (62). An analysis of reported literature in which EBV serostatus of LTRs was examined prior to transplant shows the EBV seronegative recipients always have a much higher incidence of PTLD (40,41,60,62,123,124). Generally, the EBV seronegative status results in a five- to sevenfold increased incidence of PTLD (Table 3).

There appears to be a bimodal distribution of PTLD incidence by age among LTRs. Several studies have noted an increased risk among pediatric LTRs (63–65). This is attributable to a lower prevalence of exposure to EBV in children, and thus a higher likelihood of an EBV seronegative host receiving seropositive lungs. In another study, PTLD was found to be more common in patients >55 years old (117). This probably reflects the impact of immunosuppression on the senescent immune system.

Interestingly, the incidence of PTLD among heart–lung transplant recipients is higher than either heart or lung transplants alone, ranging from 5.3% to 19% (12,63,64,125,126). The explanation for this finding remains unclear.

## CLINICAL MANIFESTATIONS OF PTLD
## IN LUNG TRANSPLANTATION

The spectrum of PTLD is highly diverse (2). The disease may be nodal or extranodal, localized or widely disseminated (2). Among LTRs, 69% to 89% of PTLD involves the thorax (91,122); the next most commonly

**Table 3** Incidence of Posttransplant Lymphoproliferative Disorder in Lung Transplant Patients

| | No. of LTRs | Incidence of PTLD in LTRs (%) | Incidence of PTLD in EBV (−) LTRs (%) | Incidence of PTLD in EBV (+) LTRs (%) |
|---|---|---|---|---|
| Armitage et al. (91) | 63 | 5 (7.9) | N/A | N/A |
| Montone et al. (118) | 45 | 9 (20) <br> 7 polymorphous <br> 2 B-cell monoclonal | N/A | N/A |
| Aris et al. (60) | 94 | 6 (6.4) | 5/15 (33) | 1/60 (1.7) |
| Angel et al. (123) | 129 (survived >1 mo) | 2 (1.8) | 1/5 (2) | 1/104 (1) |
| Wigle et al. (40) | 300 (total) 242 (>12 mos) | 12 (4-5) <br> 4 B-cell unspecified <br> 7 monomorphic B-cell <br> 1 Hodgkin's lymphoma | 4/13 (30.8) | 6/133 (4.5) |
| Ramalingam et al. (13) | 244 | 8 (3.3) <br> 3 polymorphic B-cell <br> 5 monomorphic B-cell | N/A | N/A |
| Malouf et al. (124) | Pre-1996: 167 <br> Post-1996: 149 | 7 (4.2) <br> 2 (1.3) | N/A <br> 1/18 (5.6) | N/A <br> 1/131 (0.8) |
| Reams et al. (117) | 400 | 10 (2.5) <br> 4 polymorphic B-cell <br> 3 monomorphic B-cell <br> 2 B-cell unspecified <br> 1 anaplastic T-cell | N/A | N/A |
| Verschuuren et al. (41) | 118 | 11 (9.3) | 4/12 (33) | 7/103 (7) |
| Wong et al. (62) | 237, 218 (>1 mo) | 7 (3) | 5/16 (31) | 2/221 (0.9) |
| Lee et al. (120) | 234 | 9 (3.9) | N/A | N/A |

*Abbreviations:* EBV, Epstein–Barr virus; LTRs, lung transplant recipients.

involved site is the abdomen (20–34% of PTLDs) (13,95,122,126,127). Primary central nervous system involvement with PTLD is an uncommon but highly refractory variant (128).

In LTRs, PTLD typically presents early (within the first year posttransplant) (60). Early-onset PTLD appears to be more common in LTRs compared to other SOTs (126). Early PTLD among LTRs has a predilection for the allograft (Fig. 4) (13,40,60,117,121,129). In one series, 80% of PTLD among LTRs occurred in the lung allograft(s) but only 2 of 15 PTLD in heart transplant recipients developed within the cardiac allograft (91). Similarly, investigators from the Cleveland Clinic noted that PTLD involved the allograft in five of eight LTRs; in striking contrast, the allograft was never involved in 20 non–lung SOTs with PTLD (13). At Duke University, 7 of 10 cases of PTLD involved the lung allograft (117). In another series, 10 of 12 cases of PTLD among LTRs presented with lung or mediastinal involvement (40). Further, survival was better among PTLD involving the lung allograft (121). The proclivity for the lung allograft may reflect the relatively large amount of lymphoid tissue present in the transplanted lung.

Late-onset PTLD in lung transplantation is less likely to involve the graft and carries a worse prognosis. Investigators from Washington

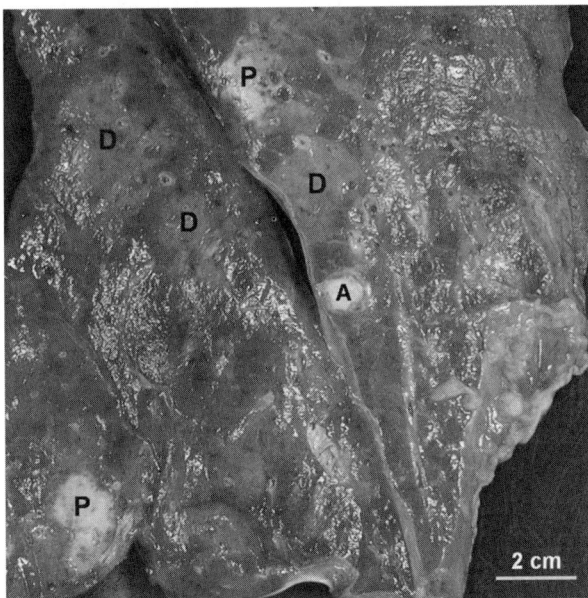

**Figure 4**   Autopsy photograph of patient who died with posttransplant lymphoproliferative disorder (PTLD). The lung showed diffuse alveolar damage (*D*), aspergillosis (*A*), and nodules of PTLD (*P*).

University noted that late-onset PTLD involved the lung allograft in only 2 of 16 (12%) cases (121). In a subsequent study from Washington University, abdominal–pelvic PTLD was found in 19 of 603 (3%) adult lung or heart–lung transplant recipients (95). Three cases presented early (< 1 year) post-transplantation; 16 presented late. Gastrointestinal tract involvement was noted in 12 patients; bleeding, nonhealing ulcers, or bowel perforation were often the presenting features. Liver involvement was noted in three patients. Despite aggressive therapy, 16 died (14 as a direct result of PTLD) (95). EBV seronegative non-Hodgkin's lymphomas (NHL) (99,130), T-cell lymphomas (18,19), and HD (15) typically develop late (>1–4 years after transplantation) and are more aggressive than early lesions (25,26,130–134). Similarly, EBV seropositive Burkitt's lymphoma occurs late post SOT (mean >4 years) (58).

## RADIOGRAPHIC IMAGING

Computed tomographic (CT) scanning is invaluable to stage the nature and extent of intrathoracic PTLD (127,129,135). Typical features include multiple parenchymal nodules (46–85% of patients)(Fig. 5, panels A–C) and hilar or mediastinal adenopathy (10–25%)(Fig. 5, panel D) (40,90,122,126,136–138). The nodules are generally well circumscribed, ranging in size from 3 mm to >5 cm (90,126). Central low attenuation (consistent with necrosis) may be observed in some cases (122,126). Patchy or diffuse alveolar infiltrates may also be observed (126,129). Pleural effusion as an isolated finding is uncommon, but may be found in the setting of parenchymal manifestations of PTLD (126).

Abdominal–pelvic CT features of PTLD are variable, and include enlarged focal or nodular low-attenuation lesions in liver, spleen, or kidneys. Additional gastrointestinal tract manifestations of PTLD include ulcerations, masses, circumferential wall thickening, dilatation or stenosis of bowel lumen, and perforation (127,135,139).

## DIAGNOSIS

In the appropriate clinical setting, radiographic findings can be strongly suggestive of the diagnosis of PTLD. Positron emission tomography with fluoro-2-deoyx-d-glucose (FDG-PET) may supplement CT. In one series of PTLD complicating LTR, all pulmonary nodules larger than 5 mm in diameter were FDG-PET positive (138).

Peripheral blood semiquantitative EBV polymerase chain reaction (140,141) may identify patients at increased risk for PTLD, and may be a surrogate marker for disease burden (41). By contrast, serologies (i.e., EBV-specific antibodies) are of limited value (41,47). Antibody responses to three EBV viral antigens have been developed and include EBNA-1,

**(A)**

**(B)**

**(C)**

**(D)**

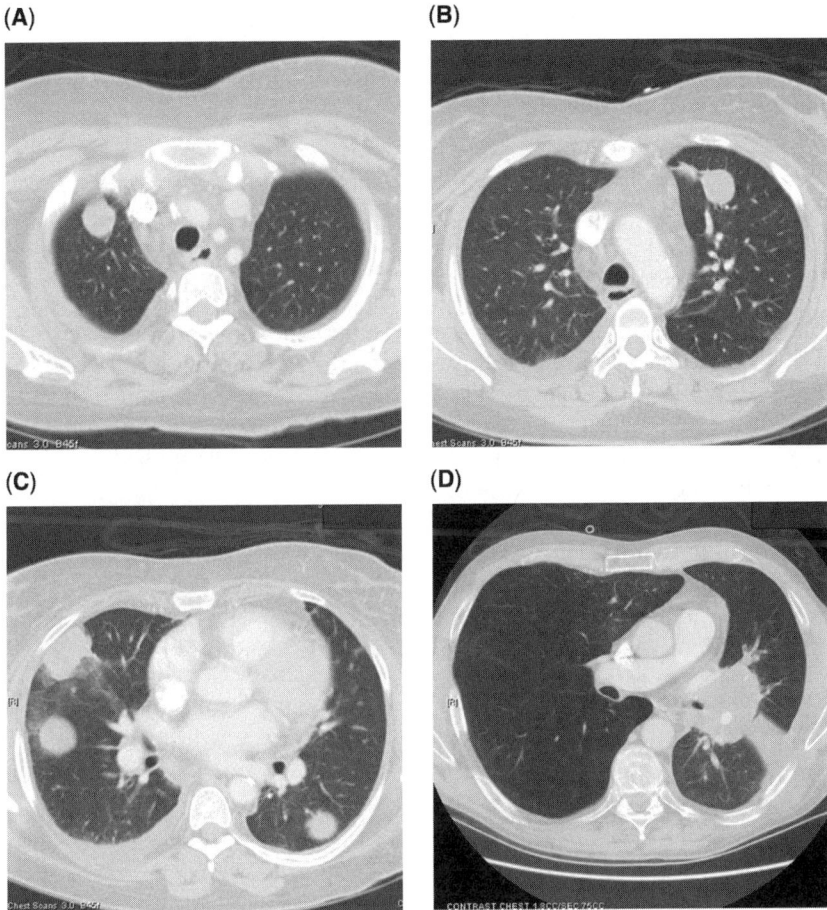

**Figure 5** Computed tomography chest of renal transplant recipient with posttransplant lymphoproliferative disorder (PTLD) and multiple pulmonary parenchymal nodules (**A–C**), and of patient with emphysema after single-lung transplant with PTLD manifest as hilar mass in left allograft (**D**).

diffuse early antigen [EA(D)], and VCA (41). In one study of LTRs who developed PTLD, an increase in EBV antibodies was noted in only two of seven patients with preexisting EBV(+) and increased EA(D) was noted in only two of four previously seronegative patients (41). Generation of EBV-specific CTL and elevated EBV DNA levels are more sensitive, and were present in four patients who developed PTLD despite *persistently negative* EBV antibody levels (47). Immunosuppressive agents such as MMF suppress humoral antibody responses (142) and may contribute to absent or blunted EBV antibody responses in organ transplant recipients.

While clinical presentation, radiographic findings, and high EBV viral load can strongly suggest PTLD, the specific diagnosis requires tissue sampling with biopsy. When possible, an excisional biopsy with intact architecture is preferred to fully characterize the lesion (88). The biopsy not only confirms the suspected clinical diagnosis of PTLD, but identifies the histopathological subtype of disease, which cannot be predicted by noninvasive methods (135).

## RISK REDUCTION OR PREVENTION OF PTLD

Because of the important role of immunosuppression in the pathogenesis of PTLD, the degree of immunosuppression should be limited when possible. In one study, the incidence of PTLD in pediatric renal transplant recipients was reduced by the institution of a protocol for aggressive tapering of tacrolimus and a lower target trough level (143). This approach applied generally may reduce the overall incidence of PTLD.

Although randomized, controlled studies are lacking, the "preemptive" use of antiviral agents reduced the incidence of PTLD in some transplant centers (2,69,109,144,145). In addition to direct effects on EBV, antiviral agents may indirectly reduce the incidence of PTLD by preventing CMV infection, which acts as a cofactor in PTLD pathogenesis (2).

One retrospective review evaluated the use of prophylactic antiviral agents in lung or heart–lung transplants between November 1986 and December 2000 at a single center (124). After 1996, patients in this study were routinely evaluated for EBV serotype prior to transplant. EBV seronegative patients then received routine antiviral prophylaxis with either acyclovir or valacyclovir. Ganciclovir was substituted in patients who were also CMV seronegative and received a CMV seropositive transplant. The incidence of PTLD in all transplanted patients prior to 1996 was 4.2% and dropped to 1.3% after 1996. Among EBV seronegative recipients after 1996, the incidence of PTLD was only 5.6% (1/18) (124), much lower than the 30% to 40% historically reported for this at-risk population (62).

## TREATMENT OF PTLD

Optimal management of PTLD is controversial (88) and requires close collaboration among transplant physicians, pathologists, and oncologists (146,147). No randomized controlled trials of PTLD management have been performed (2). Therapy for PTLD needs to be tailored according to the histopathology, extent of disease, and host factors (Fig. 6) (148).

The first-line of treatment in all cases of PTLD should be reduction or elimination of immunosuppression (66,149). However, this approach is associated with a risk of graft loss (113). Although successful retransplantation of renal and liver grafts following curative treatment of PTLD has been

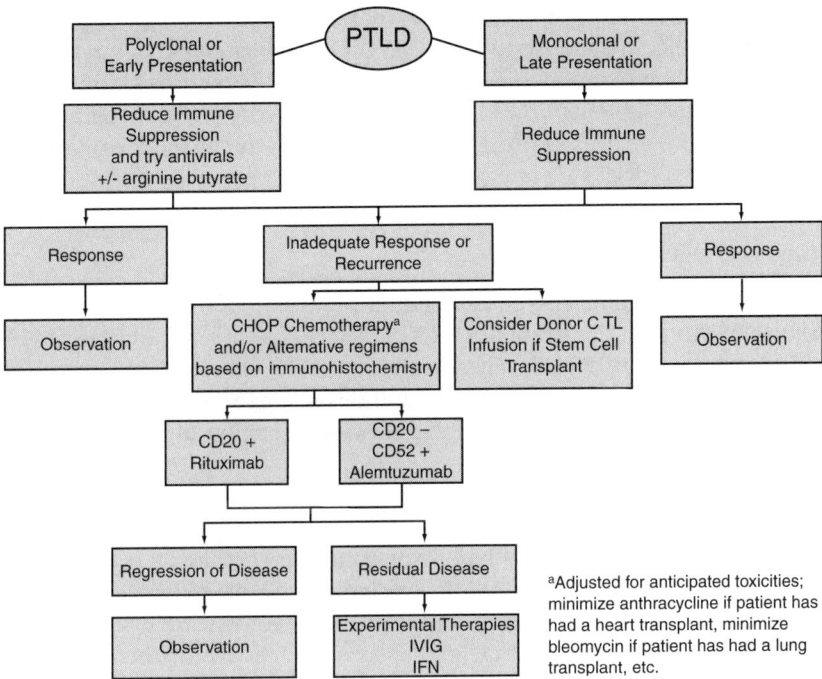

**Figure 6** Treatment algorithm for posttransplant lymphoproliferative disorder.

accomplished (54), the loss of heart or lung allografts can be fatal. Careful consideration of the risks and benefits must form the foundation for treatment of PTLD among SOT recipients.

Treatment of PTLD must be individualized, taking into account the extent and nature of PTLD, histology (or immunohistochemical markers), clonality (polyclonal vs. monoclonal), and type of organ transplant. For early, polyclonal PTLD, reducing the level of immunosuppression and initiating antiviral therapy (e.g., acyclovir, valacyclovir, ganciclovir, or foscarnet) may be adequate (2,40,42,88,150,151). Response rates of 23% to 86% were cited for treatment of polyclonal PTLD occurring within the first year of transplantation (5,14,66,91,152). Although reducing immunosuppression enhances the risk of allograft rejection (113), patients with PTLD are typically profoundly immunosuppressed, and IMS drugs can be tapered or withdrawn in many cases, provided careful monitoring is ensured (2). In a cohort of cardiac transplant recipients with PTLD, minimization of IMS therapy was associated with improved survival, whereas chemotherapy had no benefit (113). Similarly, immunosuppression was withdrawn in a cohort of 38 pediatric liver transplant recipients, with no graft loss (66). Episodes of rejection were successfully treated with standard therapy (66). Reduction (but not elimination) of immunosuppression has been employed among LTRs with PTLD, with inconsistent results (95,117). Unfortunately, this strategy is usually ineffective for monomorphic proliferations, lymphomas, non–B-cell or EBV negative lesions, or PTLD occurring >1 year posttransplantation (2,38,42,69,153). In this context, cytotoxic therapy or novel therapies are warranted (154) (discussed later).

### Intravenous IgG

Several reports documented an association between loss or absence of antibody against at least one of the EBNAs in the organ recipients and the subsequent development of PTLD. There is thus a theoretical role for intravenous IgG as antibody replacement in PTLD and this is supported by evidence that rising antibodies to EBNAs are associated with regression of PTLD (155).

### Antiviral Treatment

Antiviral agents that target the lytic virus cycle (e.g., acyclovir, valacyclovir, ganciclovir, or foscarnet) are routinely employed both to prevent and to treat PTLD, but their efficacy has not been convincingly established (2,113). The efficacy of these agents depends on the role of the lytic cycle in the pathogenesis of PTLD. The majority of EBV DNA in peripheral blood is in transcriptionally silent memory B-cells, and will not be affected by lytic agents (2). Although EBV-driven lymphoproliferation is largely independent of the lytic virus cycle, lytic infection may play a contributory role during the early stages of infection (156,157). During the acute phase of infection, the cytotoxic T-cell response is dominated by a response to EBV lytic antigens, but later (during recovery or with persistent infection) switches to a response directed to latent antigens (156,157). A phase I/II trial suggests that arginine butyrate can cause latent virus to enter the lytic phase and may make the PTLD more susceptible to antivirals (158).

### Cytotoxic Drug Therapy (Chemotherapy)

Monomorphic lymphoproliferative lesions or frank lymphomas require more aggressive treatment with multiagent chemotherapy, surgery, or radiation therapy (54,117,159). *Localized* lesions may be treated with surgery and/or radiotherapy, with reported cures (95,117,133). Responses to radiation therapy have been cited in anecdotal case reports (117,160,161) and small series (102,103,162). Low-dose radiation was efficacious in three children with PTLD recalcitrant to treatment with anti-CD20 antibody (103). Endobronchial photodynamic therapy, combined with anti-CD20 antibody, was curative in a patient with endobronchial PTLD (163). However, most experts believe that PTLD should be treated as a systemic disease.

Cyclophosphamide, hydroxydaunomycin (doxorubicin), oncovin (vincristine), and prednisone (CHOP) chemotherapy, the standard treatment for NHL, is frequently used for PTLD, but is associated with moderate toxicity and a risk of septic complications (40). Alternate chemotherapy regimens such as PRO-MACE-CytaBOM are also used but toxicities and complications remain high (38–40,133,164,165). Initial experience with multiagent chemotherapy for PTLD was disappointing. Remissions were achieved in a minority of patients, and toxicities were frequent (117,162,166). Chemotherapy-associated toxicities included cardiotoxicity (anthracyclines), pulmonary fibrosis (bleomycin), hepatic toxicity (anthracyclines and antimetabolites), and renal toxicity (cyclophosphamide) (39). However, some studies cited high durable response rates (>70%) with traditional chemotherapeutic regimens (38,153,164,165). "Tailored" (individualized) chemotherapy aims to minimize toxicity (39). In one series, the dose of doxorubicin was reduced in cardiac allograft recipients; bleomycin was avoided in LTRs (39). This approach achieved durable remissions in six of seven children with PTLD (39). Chemotherapy was stopped after known active disease was eradicated (usually two to four cycles). Thereafter, IMS medications were resumed; no patient had recurrent PTLD (39).

Only 16 cases of PTLD-myeloma have been reported in the literature (15 adult, one pediatric) (167). This form of PTLD has not been definitively associated with EBV seropositivity, and tailored treatment of multiple myeloma with thalidomide or melphalan with steroids (168) may be warranted.

The BCL-6 oncogene has prognostic value in PTLD (38,57). This oncogene is expressed in large-cell lymphomas, AIDS-associated NHL, and some PTLDs (38). In one series of 36 patients with PTLD, all BCL-6 negative cases but none of the BCL-6 positive cases resolved with reduction in immunosuppression (38). Importantly, some of the BCL-6 exhibited polymorphic histology and not malignant lymphoma morphology. Thus, the presence of BCL-6 identifies patients in need of adjuvant chemotherapy.

### γ-Interferon

γ-Interferon has both antiviral and antiproliferative effects and anecdotal responses were noted with conventional lymphomas (169) and EBV-associated PTLD (55,170,171). Its effect is thought to counteract the production by EBV-infected B-cells of an IL-10 homolog that interferes with endogenous synthesis of γ-interferon. Phase I–II clinical trials using an anti-IL-6 monoclonal antibody reported response rates of 41% to 75% for early PTLD (172,173); this drug is not commercially available.

### Monoclonal Antibodies Against B-Cells

Monoclonal antibodies against B-cells have been used to treat PTLD in solid organ (174,175), heart (176), lung (117,159,177), bone marrow (178), and SCT recipients (179), with promising results (180,181). In early seminal studies, excellent responses were achieved among polymorphic PTLDs treated with humanized monoclonal antibodies against CD21 and CD24 (175,178). These agents are not commercially available. Rituximab, a murine/human chimeric monoclonal antibody specific for CD20, a cell-surface molecule expressed on B-cells, is considered by some experts to be first-line therapy for PTLD expressing CD20 (159,182). Rituximab has been associated with response rates as high as 61% to 76% for PTLD (2,180,183). Efficacy of rituximab requires expression of CD20 by neoplastic cells (26,184). In a retrospective review of 30 cases of PTLD (15 received rituximab; 15 other therapies), treatment with rituximab was associated with improved survival (33% vs. 17%) (183). Reams et al. cited favorable responses in all four LTRs treated with rituximab (three were cured) (117). In one small series, remissions were achieved with rituximab (combined with chemotherapy and reduction of immunosuppression) in three of three SOT recipients with Burkitt's lymphoma (58). Relapses may occur after initial remissions with rituximab (159,180,185). In addition, outgrowth of CD20 negative subclones may occur (159,186). Preemptive therapy with rituximab prevented PTLD in high-risk patients following allogeneic SCT (187) but data are limited among SOTs. In some patients, rituximab may result in severe, prolonged depletion of B-cells (6–16 months) (159,188). Prolonged hypogammaglobulinemia, opportunistic infections, and reactivation of viral infections (particularly CMV and hepatitis B and C) may complicate its use (2,159). Coadministration of IMS medications (especially MMF) may inhibit restoration of the peripheral B-cell pool (159). Serum IgG levels should be monitored following rituximab (159).

### Alemtuzumab (Campath-1H)

Alemtuzumab (Campath-1H), which targets the CD52 membrane protein, may be considered for PTLD lacking the CD20 antigen, but its value is unproven. Futher, the use of alemtuzumab conditioning in SCTs may contribute to the development of PTLD (189).

### Hydroxyurea

Hydroxurea inhibits ribonucleotide reductase and eradicated latent EBV in Burkitt's lymphoma cell lines (190). Anecdotal responses to low-dose hydroxyurea were noted in central nervous system lymphomas in two patients with human immunodeficiency virus infection (191) and one patient with PTLD (192).

### Everolimus (RAD)

Everolimus (RAD, Novartis Pharma AG, Basel, Switzerland), a derivative of rapamycin, inhibited the growth of EBV positive B-lymphoblastoid cell lines in vitro (193,194) and in a murine model (194). The role of everolimus or rapamycin in patients with PTLD has not been established.

## Adoptive Cellular Immunotherapy

Adoptive cellular immunotherapy using EBV-specific CTLs has been tried to both treat and prevent PTLD (54,156,195–198). This approach involves in vitro expansion of EBV-specific recipient T-cells by stimulating them with viral antigens and cytokines that promote T-cell growth (196). The resulting polyclonal mixture of T-cells is then infused into the patient, where tumor-specific cytotoxicity relies on recognition of EBV peptides bound to HLA molecules on the surface of tumor cells (195). Adoptive immunotherapy requires matching HLA molecules on CTL to those on the tumor cells (197). Since the vast majority (>90%) of PTLD among SOT recipients are of recipient origin, EBV-specific T-cells must be matched to the recipient's major histocomptibility complex type (26). In contrast, among bone marrow or SCT recipients, PTLD cells are of donor origin (2,197). In this context, expansion of donor-derived EBV CTLs is required. Expansion of EBV-specific CTLs is expensive and labor-intensive, requires several weeks, and is available in selected research centers.

## REFERENCES

1. Boubenider S, Hiesse C, Goupy C, Kriaa F, Marchand S, Charpentier B. Incidence and consequences of post-transplantation lymphoproliferative disorders. J Nephrol 1997; 10(3):136–145.
2. Preiksaitis JK. New developments in the diagnosis and management of posttransplantation lymphoproliferative disorders in solid organ transplant recipients. Clin Infect Dis 2004; 39(7):1016–1023.
3. Nalesnik MA. The diverse pathology of post-transplant lymphoproliferative disorders: the importance of a standardized approach. Transpl Infect Dis 2001; 3(2):88–96.
4. Nalesnik MA. Clinicopathologic characteristics of post-transplant lymphoproliferative disorders. Recent Results Cancer Res 2002; 159:9–18.
5. Chadburn A, Cesarman E, Knowles DM. Molecular pathology of posttransplantation lymphoproliferative disorders. Semin Diagn Pathol 1997; 14(1):15–26.
6. Nalesnik MA, Starzl TE. Epstein–Barr virus, infectious mononucleosis, and posttransplant lymphoproliferative disorders. Transplant Sci 1994; 4(1):61–79.
7. Elenitoba-Johnson KS, Jaffe ES. Lymphoproliferative disorders associated with congenital immunodeficiencies. Semin Diagn Pathol 1997; 14(1):35–47.
8. Mellemkjaer L, Andersen V, Linet MS, Gridley G, Hoover R, Olsen JH. Non-Hodgkin's lymphoma and other cancers among a cohort of patients with systemic lupus erythematosus. Arthritis Rheum 1997; 40(4):761–768.
9. Goedert JJ, Cote TR, Virgo P, et al. Spectrum of AIDS-associated malignant disorders. Lancet 1998; 351(9119):1833–1839.
10. Penn I, Hammond W, Brettschneider L, Starzl TE. Malignant lymphomas in transplantation patients. Transplant Proc 1969; 1(1):106–112.

11. Penn I. Cancers complicating organ transplantation. N Engl J Med 1990; 323(25):1767–1769.
12. Opelz G, Dohler B. Lymphomas after solid organ transplantation: a collaborative transplant study report. Am J Transplant 2004; 4(2):222–230.
13. Ramalingam P, Rybicki L, Smith MD, et al. Posttransplant lymphoproliferative disorders in lung transplant patients: the Cleveland Clinic experience. Mod Pathol 2002; 15(6):647–656.
14. Ziarkiewicz-Wroblewska B, Gornicka B, Oldakowska U, et al. Plasmacytic hyperplasia—the early form of posttransplant lymphoproliferative disorder—with atypical morphology and clinical course in patient after liver transplantation: a case report. Transplant Proc 2003; 35(6):2320–2322.
15. Birkeland SA, Hamilton-Dutoit S. Is posttransplant lymphoproliferative disorder (PTLD) caused by any specific immunosuppressive drug or by the transplantation per se? Transplantation 2003; 76(6):984–988.
16. Leblond V, Choquet S. Lymphoproliferative disorders after liver transplantation. J Hepatol 2004; 40(5):728–735.
17. Jaffe E, Harris NL, Stein H, et al. Tumors of hematopoietic and lymphoid tissues. In: Jaffe ES, Harris NL, Stein H, Vardiman JW, eds. World Health Organization Classification of Tumors. Lyon, France: IARC Press, 2001.
18. Lundell R, Elenitoba-Johnson KS, Lim MS. T-cell posttransplant lymphoproliferative disorder occurring in a pediatric solid-organ transplant patient. Am J Surg Pathol 2004; 28(7):967–973.
19. Sebire NJ, Malone M, Ramsay AD. Posttransplant lymphoproliferative disorder presenting as CD30+, ALK+, anaplastic large cell lymphoma in a child. Pediatr Dev Pathol 2004; 7(3):290–293.
20. Bustillo M, Perez Melon C, Otero Glz A, et al. High grade lymphoma in a post-renal transplant patient. Description of a case and literature review. Nephron 2000; 84(2):189–191.
21. Harris NL, Ferry JA, Swerdlow SH. Posttransplant lymphoproliferative disorders: summary of society for hematopathology workshop. Semin Diagn Pathol 1997; 14(1):8–14.
22. Harris N, Swerdlow SH, Frizzera G, et al. Posttransplant lymphoproliferative disorders (PTLD) pathology and genetics: tumours of haematopoietic and lymphoid tissues. In: Jaffe ES, Harris NL, Stein H, Vardiman JW, eds. WHO Classification of Tumors. Lyons, France: IARC Press, 2001:264–269.
23. Nalesnik MA, Jaffe R, Starzl TE, et al. The pathology of posttransplant lymphoproliferative disorders occurring in the setting of cyclosporine A-prednisone immunosuppression. Am J Pathol 1988; 133(1):173–192.
24. Knowles DM, Cesarman E, Chadburn A, et al. Correlative morphologic and molecular genetic analysis demonstrates three distinct categories of posttransplantation lymphoproliferative disorders. Blood 1995; 85(2):552–565.
25. Draoua HY, Tsao L, Mancini DM, Addonizio LJ, Bhagat G, Alobeid B. T-cell post-transplantation lymphoproliferative disorders after cardiac transplantation: a single institutional experience. Br J Haematol 2004; 127(4): 429–432.
26. Gulley ML, Swinnen LJ, Plaisance KT Jr, Schnell C, Grogan TM, Schneider BG. Tumor origin and CD20 expression in posttransplant lymphoproliferative

disorder occurring in solid organ transplant recipients: implications for immune-based therapy. Transplantation 2003; 76(6):959–964.

27. Abed N, Casper JT, Camitta BM, et al. Evaluation of histogenesis of B-lymphocytes in pediatric EBV-related post-transplant lymphoproliferative disorders. Bone Marrow Transplant 2004; 33(3):321–327.

28. Paessler M, Kossev P, Tsai D, et al. Expression of SHP-1 phosphatase indicates post-germinal center cell derivation of B-cell posttransplant lymphoproliferative disorders. Lab Invest 2002; 82(11):1599–1606.

29. Fan H, Gulley ML. In situ hybridization to Epstein–Barr virus encoded RNA (EBER) transcripts. In: Killeen A, ed. Molecular Pathology Protocols. Totowa, NJ: Humana Press, 2001.

30. Hamilton-Dutoit SJ, Pallesen G. Detection of Epstein–Barr virus small RNAs in routine paraffin sections using non-isotopic RNA/RNA in situ hybridization. Histopathology 1994; 25(2):101–111.

31. Pallesen G, Hamilton-Dutoit SJ, Rowe M, Young LS. Expression of Epstein–Barr virus latent gene products in tumour cells of Hodgkin's disease. Lancet 1991; 337(8737):320–322.

32. Gulley ML. Molecular diagnosis of Epstein–Barr virus-related diseases. J Mol Diagn 2001; 3(1):1–10.

33. Dharnidharka VR, Douglas VK, Hunger SP, Fennell RS. Hodgkin's lymphoma after post-transplant lymphoproliferative disease in a renal transplant recipient. Pediatr Transplant 2004; 8(1):87–90.

34. Bierman PJ, Vose JM, Langnas AN, et al. Hodgkin's disease following solid organ transplantation. Ann Oncol 1996; 7(3):265–270.

35. Nalesnik MA, Randhawa P, Demetris AJ, Casavilla A, Fung JJ, Locker J. Lymphoma resembling Hodgkin disease after posttransplant lymphoproliferative disorder in a liver transplant recipient. Cancer 1993; 72(9):2568–2573.

36. Penn I. Neoplastic complications of transplantation. Semin Respir Infect 1993; 8(3):233–239.

37. Chetty R, Biddolph S, Gatter K. An immunohistochemical analysis of Reed-Sternberg-like cells in posttransplantation lymphoproliferative disorders: the possible pathogenetic relationship to Reed-Sternberg cells in Hodgkin's disease and Reed-Sternberg-like cells in non-Hodgkin's lymphomas and reactive conditions. Hum Pathol 1997; 28(4):493–498.

38. Swinnen LJ, Mullen GM, Carr TJ, Costanzo MR, Fisher RI. Aggressive treatment for postcardiac transplant lymphoproliferation. Blood 1995; 86(9): 3333–3340.

39. Watts RG, Hilliard LM, Berkow RL. Tailored chemotherapy for malignant lymphoma arising in the setting of posttransplant lymphoproliferative disorder after solid organ transplantation. J Pediatr Hematol Oncol 2002; 24(8):622–626.

40. Wigle DA, Chaparro C, Humar A, Hutcheon MA, Chan CK, Keshavjee S. Epstein–Barr virus serology and posttransplant lymphoproliferative disease in lung transplantation. Transplantation 2001; 72(11):1783–1786.

41. Verschuuren E, van der Bij W, de Boer W, Timens W, Middeldorp J, The TH. Quantitative Epstein–Barr virus (EBV) serology in lung transplant recipients with primary EBV infection and/or post-transplant lymphoproliferative disease. J Med Virol 2003; 69(2):258–266.

42. Manez R, Breinig MC, Linden P, et al. Posttransplant lymphoproliferative disease in primary Epstein–Barr virus infection after liver transplantation: the role of cytomegalovirus disease. J Infect Dis 1997; 176(6):1462–1467.
43. Weissmann DJ, Ferry JA, Harris NL, Louis DN, Delmonico F, Spiro I. Post-transplantation lymphoproliferative disorders in solid organ recipients are predominantly aggressive tumors of host origin. Am J Clin Pathol 1995; 103(6):748–755.
44. Gray J, Wreghitt TG, Pavel P, et al. Epstein–Barr virus infection in heart and heart–lung transplant recipients: incidence and clinical impact. J Heart Lung Transplant 1995; 14(4):640–646.
45. Thorley-Lawson DA, Gross A. Persistence of the Epstein–Barr virus and the origins of associated lymphomas. N Engl J Med 2004; 350(13):1328–1337.
46. Murray RJ, Kurilla MG, Brooks JM, et al. Identification of target antigens for the human cytotoxic T cell response to Epstein–Barr virus (EBV): implications for the immune control of EBV-positive malignancies. J Exp Med 1992; 176(1):157–168.
47. Davis JE, Sherritt MA, Bharadwaj M, et al. Determining virological, serological and immunological parameters of EBV infection in the development of PTLD. Int Immunol 2004; 16(7):983–989.
48. Savoldo B, Cubbage ML, Durett AG, et al. Generation of EBV-specific CD4+ cytotoxic T cells from virus naive individuals. J Immunol 2002; 168(2): 909–918.
49. Rickinson AB, Moss DJ. Human cytotoxic T lymphocyte responses to Epstein–Barr virus infection. Annu Rev Immunol 1997; 15:405–431.
50. Ho M. Risk factors and pathogenesis of posttransplant lymphoproliferative disorders. Transplant Proc 1995;27(5, Suppl 1):38–40.
51. Tosato G, Teruya-Feldstein J, Setsuda J, Pike SE, Jones KD, Jaffe ES. Post-transplant lymphoproliferative disease (PTLD): lymphokine production and PTLD. Springer Semin Immunopathol 1998;20(3–4):405–423.
52. Smets F, Latinne D, Bazin H, et al. Ratio between Epstein–Barr viral load and anti-Epstein–Barr virus specific T-cell response as a predictive marker of posttransplant lymphoproliferative disease. Transplantation 2002; 73(10): 1603–1610.
53. Savoie A, Perpete C, Carpentier L, Joncas J, Alfieri C. Direct correlation between the load of Epstein–Barr virus-infected lymphocytes in the peripheral blood of pediatric transplant patients and risk of lymphoproliferative disease. Blood 1994; 83(9):2715–2722.
54. Birkeland SA, Hamilton-Dutoit S, Bendtzen K. Long-term follow-up of kidney transplant patients with posttransplant lymphoproliferative disorder: duration of posttransplant lymphoproliferative disorder-induced operational graft tolerance, interleukin-18 course, and results of retransplantation. Transplantation 2003; 76(1):153–158.
55. Setsuda J, Teruya-Feldstein J, Harris NL, et al. Interleukin-18, interferon-gamma, IP-10, and Mig expression in Epstein–Barr virus-induced infectious mononucleosis and posttransplant lymphoproliferative disease. Am J Pathol 1999; 155(1):257–265.

56. Muti G, Klersy C, Baldanti F, et al. Epstein–Barr virus (EBV) load and interleukin-10 in EBV-positive and EBV-negative post-transplant lymphoproliferative disorders. Br J Haematol 2003; 122(6):927–933.

57. Cesarman E, Chadburn A, Liu YF, Migliazza A, Dalla-Favera R, Knowles DM. BCL-6 gene mutations in posttransplantation lymphoproliferative disorders predict response to therapy and clinical outcome. Blood 1998; 92(7): 2294–2302.

58. Gong JZ, Stenzel TT, Bennett ER, et al. Burkitt lymphoma arising in organ transplant recipients: a clinicopathologic study of five cases. Am J Surg Pathol 2003; 27(6):818–827.

59. Walker RC, Paya CV, Marshall WF, et al. Pretransplantation seronegative Epstein–Barr virus status is the primary risk factor for posttransplantation lymphoproliferative disorder in adult heart, lung, and other solid organ transplantations. J Heart Lung Transplant 1995; 14(2):214–221.

60. Aris RM, Maia DM, Neuringer IP, et al. Post-transplantation lymphoproliferative disorder in the Epstein–Barr virus-naive lung transplant recipient. Am J Respir Crit Care Med 1996; 154(6, Pt 1):1712–1717.

61. Bailey RE. Diagnosis and treatment of infectious mononucleosis. Am Fam Physician 1994; 49(4):879–888.

62. Wong JY, Tait B, Levvey B, et al. Epstein–Barr virus primary mismatching and HLA matching: key risk factors for post lung transplant lymphoproliferative disease. Transplantation 2004; 78(2):205–210.

63. Gao SZ, Chaparro SV, Perlroth M, et al. Post-transplantation lymphoproliferative disease in heart and heart–lung transplant recipients: 30-year experience at Stanford University. J Heart Lung Transplant 2003; 22(5):505–514.

64. Boyle GJ, Michaels MG, Webber SA, et al. Post-transplantation lymphoproliferative disorders in pediatric thoracic organ recipients. J Pediatr 1997; 131(2):309–313.

65. Cherikh WS, Kauffman HM, McBride MA, Maghirang J, Swinnen LJ, Hanto DW. Association of the type of induction immunosuppression with posttransplant lymphoproliferative disorder, graft survival, and patient survival after primary kidney transplantation. Transplantation 2003; 76(9):1289–1293.

66. Hurwitz M, Desai DM, Cox KL, Berquist WE, Esquivel CO, Millan MT. Complete immunosuppressive withdrawal as a uniform approach to post-transplant lymphoproliferative disease in pediatric liver transplantation. Pediatr Transplant 2004; 8(3):267–272.

67. Schwab M, Boswald M, Korn K, Ruder H. Epstein–Barr virus in pediatric patients after renal transplantation. Clin Nephrol 2000; 53(2):132–139.

68. Kenagy DN, Schlesinger Y, Weck K, Ritter JH, Gaudreault-Keener MM, Storch GA. Epstein–Barr virus DNA in peripheral blood leukocytes of patients with post-transplant lymphoproliferative disease. Transplantation 1995; 60(6):547–554.

69. Green M. Management of Epstein–Barr virus-induced post-transplant lymphoproliferative disease in recipients of solid organ transplantation. Am J Transplant 2001; 1(2):103–108.

70. Dantal J, Hourmant M, Cantarovich D, et al. Effect of long-term immunosuppression in kidney-graft recipients on cancer incidence: randomised comparison of two cyclosporin regimens. Lancet 1998; 351(9103):623–628.

71. Hojo M, Morimoto T, Maluccio M, et al. Cyclosporine induces cancer progression by a cell-autonomous mechanism. Nature 1999; 397(6719):530–534.

72. Landewe RB, van den Borne BE, Breedveld FC, Dijkmans BA. Does cyclosporin A cause cancer? Nat Med 1999; 5(7):714.

73. Persson C. Clinical research or classical clinical research? Nat Med 1999; 5(7):714–715.

74. Birkeland SA, Andersen HK, Hamilton-Dutoit SJ. Preventing acute rejection, Epstein–Barr virus infection, and posttransplant lymphoproliferative disorders after kidney transplantation: use of aciclovir and mycophenolate mofetil in a steroid-free immunosuppressive protocol. Transplantation 1999; 67(9): 1209–1214.

75. Neyts J, Andrei G, De Clercq E. The novel immunosuppressive agent mycophenolate mofetil markedly potentiates the antiherpesvirus activities of acyclovir, ganciclovir, and penciclovir in vitro and in vivo. Antimicrob Agents Chemother 1998; 42(2):216–222.

76. Ciancio G, Siquijor AP, Burke GW, et al. Post-transplant lymphoproliferative disease in kidney transplant patients in the new immunosuppressive era. Clin Transpl 1997; 11(3):243–249.

77. Ellis D, Jaffe R, Green M, et al. Epstein–Barr virus-related disorders in children undergoing renal transplantation with tacrolimus-based immunosuppression. Transplantation 1999; 68(7):997–1003.

78. Sokal EM, Antunes H, Beguin C, et al. Early signs and risk factors for the increased incidence of Epstein–Barr virus-related posttransplant lymphoproliferative diseases in pediatric liver transplant recipients treated with tacrolimus. Transplantation 1997; 64(10):1438–1442.

79. Cox KL, Lawrence-Miyasaki LS, Garcia-Kennedy R, et al. An increased incidence of Epstein–Barr virus infection and lymphoproliferative disorder in young children on FK506 after liver transplantation. Transplantation 1995; 59(4):524–529.

80. Younes BS, McDiarmid SV, Martin MG, et al. The effect of immunosuppression on posttransplant lymphoproliferative disease in pediatric liver transplant patients. Transplantation 2000; 70(1):94–99.

81. Dharnidharka VR, Ho PL, Stablein DM, Harmon WE, Tejani AH. Mycophenolate, tacrolimus and post-transplant lymphoproliferative disorder: a report of the North American Pediatric Renal Transplant Cooperative Study. Pediatr Transplant 2002; 6(5):396–399.

82. Swinnen LJ, Costanzo-Nordin MR, Fisher SG, et al. Increased incidence of lymphoproliferative disorder after immunosuppression with the monoclonal antibody OKT3 in cardiac-transplant recipients. N Engl J Med 1990; 323(25):1723–1728.

83. Cockfield SM, Preiksaitis J, Harvey E, et al. Is sequential use of ALG and OKT3 in renal transplants associated with an increased incidence of fulminant posttransplant lymphoproliferative disorder? Transplant Proc 1991; 23(1, Pt 2):1106–1107.

84. Hibberd AD, Trevillian PR, Wlodarzcyk JH, et al. Cancer risk associated with ATG/OKT3 in renal transplantation. Transplant Proc 1999; 31(1–2): 1271–1272.

85. Jamil B, Nicholls K, Becker GJ, Walker RG. Impact of acute rejection therapy on infections and malignancies in renal transplant recipients. Transplantation 1999; 68(10):1597–1603.

86. Duvoux C, Pageaux GP, Vanlemmens C, et al. Risk factors for lymphoproliferative disorders after liver transplantation in adults: an analysis of 480 patients. Transplantation 2002; 74(8):1103–1109.

87. Cockfield SM, Preiksaitis JK, Jewell LD, Parfrey NA. Post-transplant lymphoproliferative disorder in renal allograft recipients. Clinical experience and risk factor analysis in a single center. Transplantation 1993; 56(1):88–96.

88. Paya CV, Fung JJ, Nalesnik MA, et al. Epstein–Barr virus-induced posttransplant lymphoproliferative disorders. ASTS/ASTP EBV-PTLD Task Force and The Mayo Clinic Organized International Consensus Development Meeting. Transplantation 1999; 68(10):1517–1525.

89. Cockfield SM. Identifying the patient at risk for post-transplant lymphoproliferative disorder. Transpl Infect Dis 2001; 3(2):70–78.

90. Rappaport DC, Chamberlain DW, Shepherd FA, Hutcheon MA. Lymphoproliferative disorders after lung transplantation: imaging features. Radiology 1998; 206(2):519–524.

91. Armitage JM, Kormos RL, Stuart RS, et al. Posttransplant lymphoproliferative disease in thoracic organ transplant patients: ten years of cyclosporine-based immunosuppression. J Heart Lung Transplant 1991; 10(6):877–886; discussion 86–87.

92. Walker RC, Marshall WF, Strickler JG, et al. Pretransplantation assessment of the risk of lymphoproliferative disorder. Clin Infect Dis 1995; 20(5): 1346–1353.

93. Manez R, Breinig MK, Linden P, et al. Factors associated with the development of post-transplant lymphoproliferative disease (PTLD) in Epstein–Barr virus (EBV)-seronegative adult liver transplant recipients. Transplant Int 1994; 7(Suppl 1):S235–S237.

94. Mattila PS, Aalto SM, Heikkila L, et al. Malignancies after heart transplantation: presence of Epstein–Barr virus and cytomegalovirus. Clin Transpl 2001; 15(5):337–342.

95. Hachem RR, Chakinala MM, Yusen RD, et al. Abdominal-pelvic lymphoproliferative disease after lung transplantation: presentation and outcome. Transplantation 2004; 77(3):431–437.

96. Shahinian VB, Muirhead N, Jevnikar AM, et al. Epstein–Barr virus seronegativity is a risk factor for late-onset posttransplant lymphoroliferative disorder in adult renal allograft recipients. Transplantation 2003; 75(6):851–856.

97. Duncan SR, Paradis IL, Yousem SA, et al. Sequelae of cytomegalovirus pulmonary infections in lung allograft recipients. Am Rev Respir Dis 1992; 146(6):1419–1425.

98. Hezode C, Duvoux C, Germanidis G, et al. Role of hepatitis C virus in lymphoproliferative disorders after liver transplantation. Hepatology 1999; 30(3): 775–778.

99. Higgins CD, Swerdlow AJ, Smith JD, et al. Risk of lymphoid neoplasia after cardiothoracic transplantation: the influence of underlying disease and human leukocyte antigen type and matching. Transplantation 2003; 75(10): 1698–1703.

100. Soler MJ, Puig JM, Mir M, et al. Posttransplant lymphoproliferative disease: treatment and outcome in renal transplant recipients. Transplant Proc 2003; 35(5):1709–1713.

101. Shroff R, Rees L. The post-transplant lymphoproliferative disorder-a literature review. Pediatr Nephrol 2004; 19(4):369–377.

102. Zutter MM, Martin PJ, Sale GE, et al. Epstein–Barr virus lymphoproliferation after bone marrow transplantation. Blood 1988; 72(2):520–529.

103. Kang SK, Kirkpatrick JP, Halperin EC. Low-dose radiation for posttransplant lymphoproliferative disorder. Am J Clin Oncol 2003; 26(2):210–214.

104. Swinnen LJ. Treatment of organ transplant-related lymphoma. Hematol Oncol Clin North Am 1997; 11(5):963–973.

105. Levy M, Backman L, Husberg B, et al. De novo malignancy following liver transplantation: a single-center study. Transplant Proc 1993; 25(1, Pt 2): 1397–1399.

106. McAlister V, Grant D, Roy A, Yilmaz Z, Ghent C, Wall W. Post-transplant lymphoproliferative disorders in liver recipients treated with OKT3 or ALG induction immunosuppression. Transplant Proc 1993; 25(1, Pt 2):1400–1401.

107. Penn I. Posttransplantation de novo tumors in liver allograft recipients. Liver Transpl Surg 1996; 2(1):52–59.

108. McCarthy M, Ramage J, McNair A, et al. The clinical diversity and role of chemotherapy in lymphoproliferative disorder in liver transplant recipients. J Hepatol 1997; 27(6):1015–1021.

109. Heo JS, Park JW, Lee KW, et al. Posttransplantation lymphoproliferative disorder in pediatric liver transplantation. Transplant Proc 2004; 36(8): 2307–2308.

110. Cacciarelli TV, Reyes J, Jaffe R, et al. Primary tacrolimus (FK506) therapy and the long-term risk of post-transplant lymphoproliferative disease in pediatric liver transplant recipients. Pediatr Transplant 2001; 5(5):359–364.

111. Wagner HJ, Wessel M, Jabs W, et al. Patients at risk for development of posttransplant lymphoproliferative disorder: plasma versus peripheral blood mononuclear cells as material for quantification of Epstein–Barr viral load by using real-time quantitative polymerase chain reaction. Transplantation 2001; 72(6):1012–1019.

112. Haldas J, Wang W, Lazarchick J. Post-transplant lymphoproliferative disorders: T-cell lymphoma following cardiac transplant. Leukoc Lymphoma 2002; 43(2): 447–450.

113. Aull MJ, Buell JF, Trofe J, et al. Experience with 274 cardiac transplant recipients with posttransplant lymphoproliferative disorder: a report from the Israel Penn International Transplant Tumor Registry. Transplantation 2004; 78(11):1676–1682.

114. Chen JM, Barr ML, Chadburn A, et al. Management of lymphoproliferative disorders after cardiac transplantation. Ann Thorac Surg 1993; 56(3):527–538.

115. Mihalov ML, Gattuso P, Abraham K, Holmes EW, Reddy V. Incidence of post-transplant malignancy among 674 solid-organ-transplant recipients at a single center. Clin Transpl 1996; 10(3):248–255.
116. Weintraub J, Warnke RA. Lymphoma in cardiac allotransplant recipients. Clinical and histological features and immunological phenotype. Transplantation 1982; 33(4):347–351.
117. Reams BD, McAdams HP, Howell DN, Steele MP, Davis RD, Palmer SM. Posttransplant lymphoproliferative disorder: incidence, presentation, and response to treatment in lung transplant recipients. Chest 2003; 124(4):1242–1249.
118. Montone KT, Litzky LA, Wurster A, et al. Analysis of Epstein–Barr virus-associated post-transplantation lymphoproliferative disorder after lung transplantation. Surgery 1996; 119(5):544–551.
119. Levine SM, Angel L, Anzueto A, et al. A low incidence of posttransplant lymphoproliferative disorder in 109 lung transplant recipients. Chest 1999; 116(5):1273–1277.
120. Lee P, Minai OA, Mehta AC, DeCamp MM, Murthy S. Pulmonary nodules in lung transplant recipients: etiology and outcome. Chest 2004; 125(1):165–172.
121. Paranjothi S, Yusen RD, Kraus MD, Lynch JP, Patterson GA, Trulock EP. Lymphoproliferative disease after lung transplantation: comparison of presentation and outcome of early and late cases. J Heart Lung Transplant 2001; 20(10):1054–1063.
122. Siegel MJ, Lee EY, Sweet SC, Hildebolt C. CT of posttransplantation lymphoproliferative disorder in pediatric recipients of lung allograft. AJR Am J Roentgenol 2003; 181(4):1125–1131.
123. Angel LF, Cai TH, Sako EY, Levine SM. Posttransplant lymphoproliferative disorders in lung transplant recipients: clinical experience at a single center. Ann Transplant 2000; 5(3):26–30.
124. Malouf MA, Chhajed PN, Hopkins P, Plit M, Turner J, Glanville AR. Antiviral prophylaxis reduces the incidence of lymphoproliferative disease in lung transplant recipients. J Heart Lung Transplant 2002; 21(5):547–554.
125. Yousem SA, Randhawa P, Locker J, et al. Posttransplant lymphoproliferative disorders in heart–lung transplant recipients: primary presentation in the allograft. Hum Pathol 1989; 20(4):361–369.
126. Lim GY, Newman B, Kurland G, Webber SA. Posttransplantation lymphoproliferative disorder: manifestations in pediatric thoracic organ recipients. Radiology 2002; 222(3):699–708.
127. Pickhardt PJ, Siegel MJ. Posttransplantation lymphoproliferative disorder of the abdomen: CT evaluation in 51 patients. Radiology 1999; 213(1):73–78.
128. Castellano-Sanchez AA, Li S, Qian J, Lagoo A, Weir E, Brat DJ. Primary central nervous system posttransplant lymphoproliferative disorders. Am J Clin Pathol 2004; 121(2):246–253.
129. Pickhardt PJ, Siegel MJ, Anderson DC, Hayashi R, DeBaun MR. Chest radiography as a predictor of outcome in posttransplantation lymphoproliferative disorder in lung allograft recipients. AJR Am J Roentgenol 1998; 171(2):375–382.

130. Leblond V, Davi F, Charlotte F, et al. Posttransplant lymphoproliferative disorders not associated with Epstein–Barr virus: a distinct entity? J Clin Oncol 1998; 16(6):2052–2059.

131. Swerdlow AJ, Higgins CD, Hunt BJ, et al. Risk of lymphoid neoplasia after cardiothoracic transplantation. A cohort study of the relation to Epstein–Barr virus. Transplantation 2000; 69(5):897–904.

132. Nelson BP, Nalesnik MA, Bahler DW, Locker J, Fung JJ, Swerdlow SH. Epstein–Barr virus-negative post-transplant lymphoproliferative disorders: a distinct entity? Am J Surg Pathol 2000; 24(3):375–385.

133. Dotti G, Fiocchi R, Motta T, et al. Lymphomas occurring late after solid-organ transplantation: influence of treatment on the clinical outcome. Transplantation 2002; 74(8):1095–1102.

134. Dotti G, Fiocchi R, Motta T, et al. Epstein–Barr virus-negative lymphoproliferate disorders in long-term survivors after heart, kidney, and liver transplant. Transplantation 2000; 69(5):827–833.

135. Scarsbrook AF, Warakaulle DR, Dattani M, Traill Z. Post-transplantation lymphoproliferative disorder: the spectrum of imaging appearances. Clin Radiol 2005; 60(1):47–55.

136. Dodd GD III, Ledesma-Medina J, Baron RL, Fuhrman CR. Posttransplant lymphoproliferative disorder: intrathoracic manifestations. Radiology 1992; 184(1):65–69.

137. Collins J, Muller NL, Leung AN, et al. Epstein–Barr-virus-associated lymphoproliferative disease of the lung: CT and histologic findings. Radiology 1998; 208(3):749–759.

138. Marom EM, McAdams HP, Butnor KJ, Coleman RE. Positron emission tomography with fluoro-2-deoxy-d-glucose (FDG-PET) in the staging of post transplant lymphoproliferative disorder in lung transplant recipients. J Thorac Imaging 2004; 19(2):74–78.

139. Pickhardt PJ, Siegel MJ. Abdominal manifestations of posttransplantation lymphoproliferative disorder. Am J Roentgenol 1998; 171(4):1007–1013.

140. Stevens SJ, Verschuuren EA, Pronk I, et al. Frequent monitoring of Epstein–Barr virus DNA load in unfractionated whole blood is essential for early detection of posttransplant lymphoproliferative disease in high-risk patients. Blood 2001; 97(5):1165–1171.

141. Verschuuren EA, Stevens S, Pronk I, et al. Frequent monitoring of Epstein–Barr virus DNA load in unfractionated whole blood is essential for early detection of post-transplant lymphoproliferative disease in lung transplant patients. J Heart Lung Transplant 2001; 20(2):199–200.

142. Smith KG, Isbel NM, Catton MG, Leydon JA, Becker GJ, Walker RG. Suppression of the humoral immune response by mycophenolate mofetil. Nephrol Dial Transplant 1998; 13(1):160–164.

143. Shapiro R, Scantlebury VP, Jordan ML, et al. Pediatric renal transplantation under tacrolimus-based immunosuppression. Transplantation 1999; 67(2): 299–303.

144. McDiarmid SV, Jordan S, Kim GS, et al. Prevention and preemptive therapy of posttransplant lymphoproliferative disease in pediatric liver recipients. Transplantation 1998; 66(12):1604–1611.

145. Darenkov IA, Marcarelli MA, Basadonna GP, et al. Reduced incidence of Epstein–Barr virus-associated posttransplant lymphoproliferative disorder using preemptive antiviral therapy. Transplantation 1997; 64(6):848–852.

146. Gross TG. Treatment of Epstein–Barr virus-associated posttransplant lymphoproliferative disorders. J Pediatr Hematol Oncol 2001; 23(1):7–9.

147. Meijer E, Dekker AW, Weersink AJ, Rozenberg-Arska M, Verdonck LF. Prevention and treatment of Epstein–Barr virus-associated lymphoproliferative disorders in recipients of bone marrow and solid organ transplants. Br J Haematol 2002; 119(3):596–607.

148. Chadburn A, Chen JM, Hsu DT, et al. The morphologic and molecular genetic categories of posttransplantation lymphoproliferative disorders are clinically relevant. Cancer 1998; 82(10):1978–1987.

149. Mazariegos GV, Reyes J, Marino IR, et al. Weaning of immunosuppression in liver transplant recipients. Transplantation 1997; 63(2):243–249.

150. Starzl TE, Nalesnik MA, Porter KA, et al. Reversibility of lymphomas and lymphoproliferative lesions developing under cyclosporin-steroid therapy. Lancet 1984; 1(8377):583–587.

151. Oertel SH, Ruhnke MS, Anagnostopoulos I, et al. Treatment of Epstein–Barr virus-induced posttransplantation lymphoproliferative disorder with foscarnet alone in an adult after simultaneous heart and renal transplantation. Transplantation 1999; 67(5):765–767.

152. Rondinara GF, Muti G, De Carlis L, et al. Posttransplant lymphoproliferative diseases: report from a single center. Transplant Proc 2001; 33(1–2):1832–1833.

153. Hayashi RJ, Kraus MD, Patel AL, et al. Posttransplant lymphoproliferative disease in children: correlation of histology to clinical behavior. J Pediatr Hematol Oncol 2001; 23(1):14–18.

154. Gross TG. Low-dose chemotherapy for children with post-transplant lymphoproliferative disease. Recent Results Cancer Res 2002; 159:96–103.

155. Riddler SA, Breinig MC, McKnight JL. Increased levels of circulating Epstein–Barr virus (EBV)-infected lymphocytes and decreased EBV nuclear antigen antibody responses are associated with the development of posttransplant lymphoproliferative disease in solid-organ transplant recipients. Blood 1994; 84(3):972–984.

156. Sherritt MA, Bharadwaj M, Burrows JM, et al. Reconstitution of the latent T-lymphocyte response to Epstein–Barr virus is coincident with long-term recovery from posttransplant lymphoma after adoptive immunotherapy. Transplantation 2003; 75(9):1556–1560.

157. Khanna R, Moss DJ, Burrows SR. Vaccine strategies against Epstein–Barr virus-associated diseases: lessons from studies on cytotoxic T-cell-mediated immune regulation. Immunol Rev 1999; 170:49–64.

158. Mentzer SJ, Perrine SP, Faller DV. Epstein—Barr virus post-transplant lymphoproliferative disease and virus-specific therapy: pharmacological re-activation of viral target genes with arginine butyrate. Transpl Infect Dis 2001; 3(3):177–185.

159. Verschuuren EA, Stevens SJ, van Imhoff GW, et al. Treatment of posttransplant lymphoproliferative disease with rituximab: the remission, the relapse, and the complication. Transplantation 2002; 73(1):100–104.

160. Tsai DE, Stadtmauer EA, Canaday DJ, Vaughn DJ. Combined radiation and chemotherapy in posttransplant lymphoproliferative disorder. Med Oncol 1998; 15(4):279–281.

161. Koffman BH, Kennedy AS, Heyman M, Colonna J, Howell C. Use of radiation therapy in posttransplant lymphoproliferative disorder (PTLD) after liver transplantation. Int J Cancer 2000; 90(2):104–109.

162. Morrison VA, Dunn DL, Manivel JC, Gajl-Peczalska KJ, Peterson BA. Clinical characteristics of post-transplant lymphoproliferative disorders. Am J Med 1994; 97(1):14–24.

163. Legere BM, Saad CP, Mehta AC. Endobronchial post-transplant lymphoproliferative disorder and its management with photodynamic therapy: a case report. J Heart Lung Transplant 2003; 22(4):474–477.

164. Mamzer-Bruneel MF, Lome C, Morelon E, et al. Durable remission after aggressive chemotherapy for very late post-kidney transplant lymphoproliferation: a report of 16 cases observed in a single center. J Clin Oncol 2000; 18(21):3622–3632.

165. Haas RJ, Schmid I, Schon C, Soballa-Stehr E, Stachel D. Non-Hodgkin lymphoma after heart-lung transplantation: response to chemotherapy. Med Pediatr Oncol 1999; 32(3):229–230.

166. Dror Y, Greenberg M, Taylor G, et al. Lymphoproliferative disorders after organ transplantation in children. Transplantation 1999; 67(7):990–998.

167. Tcheng WY, Said J, Hall T, Al-Akash S, Malogolowkin M, Feig SA. Posttransplant multiple myeloma in a pediatric renal transplant patient. Pediatr Blood Cancer 2005 (Epub ahead of print).

168. Jagannath S. Treatment of myeloma in patients not eligible for transplantation. Curr Treat Options Oncol 2005; 6(3):241–253.

169. Street SE, Trapani JA, MacGregor D, Smyth MJ. Suppression of lymphoma and epithelial malignancies effected by interferon gamma. J Exp Med 2002; 196(1):129–134.

170. Davis CL, Wood BL, Sabath DE, Joseph JS, Stehman-Breen C, Broudy VC. Interferon-alpha treatment of posttransplant lymphoproliferative disorder in recipients of solid organ transplants. Transplantation 1998; 66(12):1770–1779.

171. Faro A, Kurland G, Michaels MG, et al. Interferon-alpha affects the immune response in post-transplant lymphoproliferative disorder. Am J Respir Crit Care Med 1996; 153(4, Pt 1):1442–1447.

172. Durandy A. Anti-B cell and anti-cytokine therapy for the treatment of posttransplant lymphoproliferative disorder: past, present, and future. Transpl Infect Dis 2001; 3(2):104–107.

173. Haddad E, Paczesny S, Leblond V, et al. Treatment of B-lymphoproliferative disorder with a monoclonal anti-interleukin-6 antibody in 12 patients: a multicenter phase 1–2 clinical trial. Blood 2001; 97(6):1590–1597.

174. Leblond V, Sutton L, Dorent R, et al. Lymphoproliferative disorders after organ transplantation: a report of 24 cases observed in a single center. J Clin Oncol 1995; 13(4):961–968.

175. Benkerrou M, Jais JP, Leblond V, et al. Anti-B-cell monoclonal antibody treatment of severe posttransplant B-lymphoproliferative disorder: prognostic factors and long-term outcome. Blood 1998; 92(9):3137–3147.

176. Zilz ND, Olson LJ, McGregor CG. Treatment of post-transplant lymphoproliferative disorder with monoclonal CD20 antibody (rituximab) after heart transplantation. J Heart Lung Transplant 2001; 20(7):770–772.
177. Cook RC, Connors JM, Gascoyne RD, Fradet G, Levy RD. Treatment of post-transplant lymphoproliferative disease with rituximab monoclonal antibody after lung transplantation. Lancet 1999; 354(9191):1698–1699.
178. Fischer A, Blanche S, Le Bidois J, et al. Anti-B-cell monoclonal antibodies in the treatment of severe B-cell lymphoproliferative syndrome following bone marrow and organ transplantation. N Engl J Med 1991; 324(21):1451–1456.
179. Kuehnle I, Huls MH, Liu Z, et al. CD20 monoclonal antibody (rituximab) for therapy of Epstein–Barr virus lymphoma after hemopoietic stem-cell transplantation. Blood 2000; 95(4):1502–1505.
180. Milpied N, Vasseur B, Parquet N, et al. Humanized anti-CD20 monoclonal antibody (Rituximab) in post transplant B-lymphoproliferative disorder: a retrospective analysis on 32 patients. Ann Oncol 2000; 11(Suppl 1):113–116.
181. Zompi S, Tulliez M, Conti F, et al. Rituximab (anti-CD20 monoclonal antibody) for the treatment of patients with clonal lymphoproliferative disorders after orthotopic liver transplantation: a report of three cases. J Hepatol 2000; 32(3):521–527.
182. Faye A, Van Den Abeele T, Peuchmaur M, Mathieu-Boue A, Vilmer E. Anti-CD20 monoclonal antibody for post-transplant lymphoproliferative disorders. Lancet 1998; 352(9136):1285.
183. Ghobrial I, Habermann T, Ristow K, et al. Prognostic factors in patients with post-transplant lymphoproliferative disorders (PTLD) in the rituximab era. Leukoc Lymphoma 2005; 46(2):191–196.
184. Yang J, Tao Q, Flinn IW, et al. Characterization of Epstein–Barr virus-infected B cells in patients with posttransplantation lymphoproliferative disease: disappearance after rituximab therapy does not predict clinical response. Blood 2000; 96(13):4055–4063.
185. Kinoshita T, Nagai H, Murate T, Saito H. CD20-negative relapse in B-cell lymphoma after treatment with rituximab. J Clin Oncol 1998; 16(12):3916.
186. Davis TA, Czerwinski DK, Levy R. Therapy of B-cell lymphoma with anti-CD20 antibodies can result in the loss of CD20 antigen expression. Clin Cancer Res 1999; 5(3):611–615.
187. van Esser JW, Niesters HG, van der Holt B, et al. Prevention of Epstein–Barr virus-lymphoproliferative disease by molecular monitoring and preemptive rituximab in high-risk patients after allogeneic stem cell transplantation. Blood 2002; 99(12):4364–4369.
188. Maloney DG, Grillo-Lopez AJ, White CA, et al. IDEC-C2B8 (rituximab) anti-CD20 monoclonal antibody therapy in patients with relapsed low-grade non-Hodgkin's lymphoma. Blood 1997; 90(6):2188–2195.
189. Snyder MJ, Stenzel TT, Buckley PJ, et al. Posttransplant lymphoproliferative disorder following nonmyeloablative allogeneic stem cell transplantation. Am J Surg Pathol 2004; 28(6):794–800.
190. Chodosh J, Holder VP, Gan YJ, Belgaumi A, Sample J, Sixbey JW. Eradication of latent Epstein–Barr virus by hydroxyurea alters the growth-transformed cell phenotype. J Infect Dis 1998; 177(5):1194–1201.

191. Slobod KS, Taylor GH, Sandlund JT, Furth P, Helton KJ, Sixbey JW. Epstein–Barr virus-targeted therapy for AIDS-related primary lymphoma of the central nervous system. Lancet 2000; 356(9240):1493–1494.

192. Pakakasama S, Eames GM, Morriss MC, et al. Treatment of Epstein–Barr virus lymphoproliferative disease after hematopoietic stem-cell transplantation with hydroxyurea and cytotoxic T-cell lymphocytes. Transplantation 2004; 78(5):755–757.

193. Majewski M, Korecka M, Joergensen J, et al. Immunosuppressive TOR kinase inhibitor everolimus (RAD) suppresses growth of cells derived from posttransplant lymphoproliferative disorder at allograft-protecting doses. Transplantation 2003; 75(10):1710–1717.

194. Majewski M, Korecka M, Kossev P, et al. The immunosuppressive macrolide RAD inhibits growth of human Epstein–Barr virus-transformed B lymphocytes in vitro and in vivo: a potential approach to prevention and treatment of posttransplant lymphoproliferative disorders. Proc Natl Acad Sci USA 2000; 97(8):4285–4290.

195. Liu Z, Savoldo B, Huls H, et al. Epstein–Barr virus (EBV)-specific cytotoxic T lymphocytes for the prevention and treatment of EBV-associated posttransplant lymphomas. Recent Results Cancer Res 2002; 159:123–133.

196. Khanna R, Bell S, Sherritt M, et al. Activation and adoptive transfer of Epstein–Barr virus-specific cytotoxic T cells in solid organ transplant patients with posttransplant lymphoproliferative disease. Proc Natl Acad Sci USA 1999; 96(18):10391–10396.

197. Straathof KC, Savoldo B, Heslop HE, Rooney CM. Immunotherapy for posttransplant lymphoproliferative disease. Br J Haematol 2002; 118(3):728–740.

198. Rooney CM, Smith CA, Ng CY, et al. Infusion of cytotoxic T cells for the prevention and treatment of Epstein–Barr virus-induced lymphoma in allogeneic transplant recipients. Blood 1998; 92(5):1549–1555.

# Index

Abdominal infections, 596–597
Acid-fast bacilli (AFB), 627
Acquired immunodeficiency syndrome
   (AIDS), 597, 609, 632
ACR. *See* Acute cellular rejection
*Actinomyces odontolyticus*, 599
Activator protein one (AP-1), 443
Acute cellular rejection (ACR), 698
   clinical presentation, 662
   diagnosis of, 668–669
   incidence of, 662
   noninvasive markers of, 669
   pathogenesis of, 670–672
   pathology of, 670
   treatment of, 675–676
Acute humoral rejection (AHR), 662,
   673–674, 697
Acute interstitial pneumonia (AIP), 167
Acute respiratory distress syndrome
   (ARDS), 437, 450
Acyclovir, 245
Adhesion molecules, 441–442
AHR. *See* Acute humoral rejection
AIDS. *See* Acquired immunodeficiency
   syndrome
Airway
   complications, 380, 468–469
   ischemia, 729
   obstruction, 471

[Airway]
   tissue remodeling, 760
   wound repair, 760
Alemtuzumab (campath-1H), 920
Allergic bronchopulmonary aspergillosis
   (ABPA), 560
Alloantigens, 755
Allograft
   assessment prior to procurement,
   352
   implantation, 257–258
   rejection, 3, 52, 245, 704
   survival, 54
Alloimmune responses, 754
Allorecognition pathways, 49
Alpha-1 antitrypsin deficiency
   ($\alpha$1-ATD), 65, 98
Altered peptide ligands (APLs), 25
Alveolar macrophage
   (AM), 439, 442, 766
AM. *See* Alveolar macrophage
American Society of Transplant
   Physicians, 62
American Thoracic Society, 62
Amphotericin B, 541, 560
Anaerobic glycolysis, 327
Anastomosis, vascular, 404
Anastomotic dehiscence, 468–469
Angiomyolipomas, 213

Anti-CD25 antibodies, 409
Anticholinergics, 74–75
Antiestrogen, 220
Antigen-presenting cells (APCs),
    48, 52
Anti-inflammatory cytokine, 339
Antilymphocyte globulin (ALG), 497,
    908
Antilymphocyte serum (ALS), first form
    of lympholytic therapy, 402
Antimetabolites, 373–379
Antithymocyte globulins (ATG), 431,
    908
ANZODR. *See* Australian and
    New Zealand Organ Donor
    Registry
APCs. *See* Antigen-presenting cells
Apoptosis, 444
    inducing, 382
ARDS. *See* Adult respiratory distress
    syndrome
Area-under-the-curve monitoring
    (AUC), 366
Aspergillus, 119, 476, 845
    clinical presentation, 560
    diagnosis, 561
        culture, 562
        DNA-based methods, 565
        histopathology, 563
        radiology, 562
    incidence, 558
    pathogenesis, 557
    risk factors, 558
    treatment, 555, 568
*Aspergillus hyphae*, 564
ATG. *See* Antithymocyte globulins
Atovaquone, 601
Atrial fibrillation, 886
Atrial flutter, 886
Atrial septostomy, 126, 273
Australian and New Zealand Organ
    Donor Registry (ANZODR),
    309, 314
Australian Human Tissue
    Act 1982, 309
AZA. *See* Azathioprine
Azathioprine (AZA), 168, 374, 739

BALF. *See* Bronchoalveolar lavage fluid
Bacterial pneumonia, 690–691
BAL. *See* Bronchoalveolar lavage
Basiliximab, 410
β-Adrenergic agonists, 76, 78
Bilateral and heart–lung
    transplantation, 795
Bilateral hilar lymphadenopathy (BHL),
    184
Bilateral infiltrate, 358
Bilateral lung transplantation (BLT),
    93
Bilateral sequential lung transplants
    (BSLT), 166
Bisphosphonates, 897
*Blastomyces dermatitidis*, 552
Blastomycosis, 552–553
BLT. *See* Bilateral lung transplantation
BMT. *See* Bone marrow transplant
Bolus steroids, 445, 895
Bone disease, 109
Bone marrow transplant (BMT), 600,
    611, 624–625, 637
Bone mass density (BMD), 109
BOOP. *See* Bronchiolitis obliterans
    organizing pneumonia
BOS. *See* Bronchiolitis obliterans
    syndrome
Brain death, 22, 445
Brain natriuretic peptide (BNP), 176
Bronchial anastomosis in lung
    transplantation, 466
    complications, 836
    dehiscence, 468–470
    healing grade classification, 468
    hyperreactivity, 802
    stenosis, 471
Bronchiectasis, 112
Bronchiolitis obliterans organizing
    pneumonia (BOOP), 691,
    705, 853
Bronchiolitis obliterans syndrome
    (BOS), 13, 22, 122, 127, 245, 350,
    371, 404, 455–456, 489, 661
    causes of, 51
    chemokines in, 768–742
    cytokines in, 760–761

[Bronchiolitis obliterans syndrome
(BOS)]
gastroesophageal reflux in, 758–760
growth factor in, 767–768
HLA in, 754–758
IFN-γ in, 764
IL-12 in, 763–764
IL-10 in, 764–766
IL-6 in, 766
incidence and prevalence of, 723–724
TGF-β in, 766–767
TNF-α in, 761–763
treatment of, 734–735, 737–741
Bronchioloalveolar carcinoma (BAC),
681
Bronchoalveolar lavage (BAL),
169, 441, 508, 564, 591, 626,
669, 696
Bronchoalveolar lavage fluid (BALF),
94, 760
Bronchodilators, 62, 71, 80, 84
Bronchogenic carcinoma, 97
Bronchomalacia, 469
Bronchoscopic lung volume reduction,
89
Bronchoscopy, 275, 354, 477
Bronchus-associated lymphoid tissue
(BALT), 702
*Burkoldheria*, 594
*Burkholderia cepacia*, 238
*Burkholderia* species, 118

CAL. *See* Chronic airflow limitation
Calcineurin inhibitors (CNIs), 49, 54,
363, 628, 891
effects of, 444
Calcium channel blocker therapy, 273
Campath-1H, 405–406, 427–429
*Candida* infections, 841–843
Carcinoid tumorlets, 712
Cardiac dysfunction, 886
Cardiomyopathy, 910
Cardiopulmonary bypass (CPB), 127,
241, 449–450
Cardiopulmonary exercise testing
(CPET), 173, 208

Cardiovascular complications,
posttransplant, 886
CARV. *See* Community-acquired
respiratory viruses
Caspofungin, 542
Cavitary lung disease, 612
CD4 antibodies, 24
CD4+/CD25+ regulatory cells, 53
Cell cycle proteins, 379
Cell injury, endothelial, 328
Cell–cell communication, 442
Cellular immunotherapy, adoptive, 921
Cepacia syndrome, 593
Cerebral vascular accident (CVA),
310
CF. *See* Cystic fibrosis
CF-related diabetes (CFRD), 124–125
CF transmembrane conductance
regulator (CFTR) protein, 112
Charcoal yeast extract, 609
Chemokine subfamilies, 739
Chronic airflow limitation (CAL), 64
Chronic obstructive pulmonary disease
(COPD), 22, 287, 448, 698, 896
definition, 61
natural history/predictive indices, 62
Chronic pulmonary sarcoidosis, 183
Chronic respiratory disease
questionnaire (CRDQ), 73
Chylothorax, 215
Chylous effusions, management
of, 222–223
*Clostridium difficile*, 596
CMV. *See* Cytomegalovirus
Coccidioidomycosis, 527
clinical disease, 527–529
diagnosis, 536
epidemiology and geographic
occurrence, 530
immunology, 532
incidence, 530
mycology, 528
pretransplant evaluation, 532–534
prevention, 543
skin tests, 539
treatment, 539
Cold flushing, 329

Collagen vascular disease–associated
  pulmonary fibrosis (CVD-PF),
  165
Collagen, type V, 23
Community-acquired pneumonia
  (CAP), 608
Community-acquired respiratory viruses
  (CARV), 485
  clinical syndromes, 507
  diagnosis, 507–508
  epidemiology, 506–507
  treatment, 508–510
Complement antagonist, 339
Connective tissue growth factor
  (CTGF), 767
COPD. *See* Chronic obstructive
  pulmonary disease
Coreceptor blockade, 28–30
Corticosteroids, combination
  of inhaled, 84
Costimulatory molecules, 754
Costimulatory receptors, 51
Cowdry A or owl's eye, 695
CPB. *See* Cardiopulmonary bypass
*Cryptococcal meningitis*, 571
*Cryptococcus*, 560, 570, 572
*Cryptococcus neoformans*, 570
Cryptogenic fibrosing alveolitis
  (CFA), 166
Cryptogenic organizing pneumonia
  (COP), 167
CsA. *See* Cyclosporine A
CSF. *See* Cerebrospinal fluid
CTGF. *See* Connective tissue growth
  factor
CTL. *See* Cytotoxic T-lymphocytes
CT pulmonary angiography
  (CTPA), 848
Cushing's syndrome, 384
Cyclophilins, 364
Cyclosphosphamide (CP), 168, 181
Cyclosporine, 3, 6, 250, 423–425, 810
Cyclosporine A (CsA), 364, 366
Cystic fibrosis (CF), 22, 112, 271, 287,
  588, 592–594, 793
Cytochrome P450 enzyme 3A4
  (CYP3A4), 364, 383

Cytokines, 440–441
Cytokine-induced neutrophil
  chemoattractant
  (CINC), 440, 442
Cytokine release syndrome, 409
Cytolytic T lymphocyte (CTL), 500
Cytomegalovirus (CMV), 275,
  279, 485–487
  antiviral resistance, 495
  clinical syndromes, 487–488
  infection, 50, 843
  monitoring techniques, 490–491
  prevention, 489–490
  treatment, 494–495
Cytotoxic drug therapy
  (chemotherapy), 918–919
Cytotoxic T-lymphocytes
  (CTL), 425, 906

Daclizumab, 410, 736
Dapsone, 600
Dematiaceous molds, 572
Dendritic cells, 22, 32
Dermatomyositis (DM), 182
Desquamative interstitial pneumonia
  (DIP), 167
Diffuse alveolar damage (DAD),
  688
Directed observed therapy (DOT),
  628
Domino heart transplantation, 270–272
Donor core cooling. *See* Lung
  preservation, techniques for
Donor lobectomy, 257–258
Donor lungs, 49
  allocation, 116
  criteria for, 314, 353–355
  selection, 256
Donor tracheal cultures (DTC), 590
Donor–recipient mismatch, mechanical
  complications related to, 829
Donor-related risk factors, 444–447
Double-lung transplantation, 7
Drug pharmacokinetics, 120–121
Drug safety profiles, 407
Dyspnea, 220

Early growth response one (EGR-1), 443

EBNA. *See* Epstein–Barr nuclear antigen

EBV. *See* Epstein–Barr virus

EBV-encoded RNA (EBER), 904

ECMO. *See* Extracorporeal membrane oxygenation

Eisenmenger's syndrome, 15, 149, 270, 274, 280

Empyema, 594–595

Endogenous nitric oxide (eNOS), 336

Endothelin receptor, 126

Enzyme immunoassays (EIA), 508

Enzyme-linked immunosorbent assay (ELISA), 564

Eosinophils, 23, 208

Eepithelioid histiocytes, 692

Epstein–Barr nuclear antigen (EBNA), 681, 904

Epstein–Barr virus (EBV), 276, 485, 500–502, 709, 856
clinical presentations, 501–502
risk factors, 501
serological status, 907
treatment, 503–504
viral load determination, 503

Ethambutol (EMB), 628

European Respiratory Society, 62

Eurotransplant, 303–305

Everolimus, 892, 921

Extracellular matrix deposition (ECM), 754

Extracorporeal membrane oxygenation (ECMO), 156, 238, 439, 454, 688

Extracorporeal photochemotherapy (ECP), 737

Fiber-optic bronchoscopy (FOB), 590

Fibroblast proliferation, 376

Fluconazole, 551

Fluoroquinolones, 629

Food and Drug Administration (FDA), 471, 630

FoxP3 gene, 27

Fractional concentration of exhaled nitric oxide (FENO), 734

Fungal infections, 475–477

Fusarium, 564

Galactomannan (GM), 564

Gameable factors, 293

γ-Interferon, 919

Ganciclovir
monotherapy, 491
prophylaxis, 275

Gastroesophageal reflux (GER), 729

Gastroesophageal reflux disease (GERD), 121–122, 246, 708, 754

Gastrointestinal colonization, 632
complications, 755
function, 249

Gastroparesis, 249

GER. *See* Gastroesophageal reflux

Gingival hyperplasia, 369

Glucocorticoids, 382

Gonadotropin-releasing hormone (GrRH), 220

Graft dysfunction, quantified grades of, 326

Graft, functional imaging of, 800

Graft rejection, 12, 127

Graft reperfusion, mode of, 451

Graft versus host disease (GVHD), 625, 761

Granzyme B (GB), 425–426

GVHD. *See* Graft versus host disease

Health-related quality of life (HRQOL), 67

Heart failure, congestive, 886

Heart transplant recipients, 625, 637–638, 910–911

Heart–lung transplantation (HLT), 147, 269, 723
economic evaluation of, 276
indications for, 270–272
medical alternatives to, 273
patients awaiting transplantation, 272–273

[Heart–lung transplantation
(HLT)]
    postoperative complications,
        275–276
    recipient selection criteria, 272
    results of, 276–277
Hematopoietic stem cell transplants
    (HSCTs), 624
Hematoxylin and eosin (HE) stains,
    686, 694
Hemodynamic donor, 445
Hemolytic uremic syndrome, 373, 381
Hepatic transplant recipients, 625, 638
Hepatitis C virus (HCV), 909
Hepatobiliary disease, 123
Hepatocyte growth factor (HGF),
    768
Hepatotoxicity, 628, 631
Hereditary hemorrhagic telangiectasia
    (HHT), 149
Herpes simplex virus (HSV), 485
Herpesvirus infection syndrome, 498
High-resolution computed tomography
    (HRCT), 216–217, 627,
    732–733
    in sarcoidosis, 184
*Histoplasma capsulatum*, 549
Histoplasmosis, 549–552
HIV. *See* Human immunodeficiency
    virus
HLA. *See* Human leukocyte antigen
HLT. *See* Heart–lung transplantation
HMG-CoA reductase inhibitors, 371
HMPV. *See* Human metapneumovirus
Hodgkin's disease (HD), 904
Hormone replacement, 897
HRCT. *See* High-resolution computed
    tomography
HRQOL. *See* Health-related quality of
    life
HSV-1, 2 and VZV, 504–506
Human antimouse antibodies (HAMA),
    408
Human herpesviridae (HHVs), 486
Human herpesvirus, 498–500
Human immunodeficiency virus (HIV),
    597, 628

Human leukocyte antigen (HLA), 48,
    128, 257, 673, 909
    role of, 754
    mismatches, 22, 754
Human metapneumovirus (hMPV), 485,
    512–513
Human T-cell lymphotropic virus 1
    (HTLV-1),
Humoral allograft rejection, 697
Humoral rejection, 50, 697
Hyalohyphomycetes, 694
Hydroxurea, 920
3-Hydroxyl-3-methylglutryl coenzyme A
    (HMG Co-A) reductase, 888
Hyperacute rejection, 697–698,
    829–830
Hyperinflation, 331
Hyperlipidemia, 279, 888–890
Hypothermia, 328
Hypoxemia, 173


ICAM. *See* Intracellular adhesion
    molecule
Idiopathic interstitial pneumonias (IIPs),
    167
Idiopathic pulmonary arterial
    hypertension (IPAH), 147, 151
Idiopathic pulmonary fibrosis (IPF),
    114, 165–166, 286
    clinical features, 167
    definition, 167
    epidemiology of, 167
    histopathology, 167–168
    treatment of, 168–169
IDO. *See* Indolamine 2,3-dioxygenase
IGF. *See* Insulin-like growth factor
IGF binding proteins (IGFBP),
    767
IL. *See* Interleukin
Immune globulin monotherapy, 493
Immune reprogramming, 24
Immune response type I and II,
    development of, 732
Immunodiffusion tube precipitins
    (IDTP), 539
Immunoperoxidase stains, 686

Immunosuppression, 121, 243, 275, 406, 907–909
Immunosuppressive drugs, 363, 402, 906
Indolamine 2,3-dioxygenase (IDO), 33
Infectious complications, 356
INH. *See* Isoniazid
Inherited and acquired immunosuppressive (IMS) disorders, 901
Inosine monophosphate dehydrogenase, inhibition of, 376
Insulin-like growth factor 1 (IGF-1), 757
bioactivity of, 767
Intercellular adhesion molecule one (ICAM-1), 441
Interferon gamma (IFN-Ð), 761
Interleukin-2 (IL-2) synthesis, inhibition of. *See* Cyclosporine A (CsA), mechanism of action
Interleukin beta (IL-β), 440
Intermittent Positive Pressure Breathing Trial (IPPB), 62
International Society for Heart and Lung Transplantation (ISHLT), 62, 127, 165, 235, 670, 724, 755
Interstitial lung disease (ILD), 165
Intestinal dysmotility, 121–122
Intracellular adhesion molecule (ICAM), 489
IPAH. *See* Idiopathic pulmonary arterial hypertension
IPAH/secondary PAH, 154–155
morbidity and mortality, 156–157
IPF. *See* Idiopathic pulmonary fibrosis
Ischemia–reperfusion injury, 49, 326, 334, 437, 687, 830
ISHLT. *See* International Society of Heart and Lung Transplantation
Isoniazid (INH), 628, 631
Itraconazole, 567

Kaplan–Meier analysis, 219
Kaposi's sarcoma (KS), 486
Kidney transplant recipients, 625, 638
Kinyoun's carbol fuchsin stain, 686

KS. *See* Kaposi's sarcoma
KS herpesvirus (KSHV), 486

LAM. *See* Lymphangioleiomyomatosis
Langerhans cells (LCs), 208–209
Langerhans cell histiocytosis (LCH), 205, 859
Late acute chronic rejection, 724
Latent membrane protein (LMP), 681, 904
Latent tuberculous infection (LTBI), 630–631
LCH. *See* langerhans cell histiocytosis
Legionella, in solid organ transplantation
epidemiology, 610
microbiology and pathogenesis, 609–610
treatment, 613–614
virulence factors for, 609
*Legionella pneumophila*, 597
Legionellosis, nosocomial, 612
Legionnaires' disease, 608
diagnosis of, 612–613
incidence of, 610
incubation period for, 611
Leukocyte activation, 439
Leukopenia, Aza-induced, 375
LHRH. *See* Luteinizing hormone–releasing hormone
Limb muscle function, 807
Lipid peroxidation, 328
Lipid-formulations of amphotericin B (LFAB), 541
Living donor lung transplantation (LDLT), 242
Living lobar lung transplantation, 9, 350
LMP. *See* Latent membrane protein
Lobar lung transplantation
indications for, 256
operative technique, 257–259
Lobar torsion, diagnosis of, 450
Lofgren's syndrome, 184
Long-term oxygen therapy (LTOT), 63
Low-density lipoprotein (LDL), 888
Low-potassium dextran (LPD), 446

Low-potassium dextran (LPD)–glucose
solution, 328
LT. *See* Lung transplantation
LTRs. *See* Lung transplant recipients
Lung allocation score
definition, 294
determining, 297–298
Lung allograft
dysfunction, 356
rejection, preventing, 54
Lung function testing, 249–250
Lung hyperinflation, native, 96
Lung ischemia reperfusion injury
(LIRI), 440
Lung perfusion scans, 667
Lung preservation techniques, 326, 448
Lung transplant biopsies, examination
of, 686
Lung transplant recipients (LTRs), 625,
638–639, 723, 902, 911
Lung transplant vs. heart–lung
transplant, 886–887
Lung transplantation (LT)
anatomic considerations and surgical
techniques, 153–154, 465–468
in Australia, 311, 316–317
for CVD-PF, 180
in CF patients, 127–129
for IPAH, 126
for IPF, results of, 166–167
for LAM, 223
for PLCH, 212
and pulmonary vascular disease, 157
referral criteria for, 114–116
for sarcoidosis, results of, 183,
186–188
Lung volume reduction surgery (LVRS),
70, 85
impact on subsequent transplantation,
87
Lupus erythematosus, 53
Luteinizing hormone–releasing hormone
(LHRH), 220
Lymphangioleiomyomatosis (LAM),
213, 859
clinical manifestations of, 215
course and prognosis of, 219

[Lymphangioleiomyomatosis (LAM)]
pathogenesis, 210
pulmonary function tests, 218
radiographic features, 215
treatment, 218–210
Lymphocytic bronchiolitis, 727
Lymphocyte depletion, 431
Lymphocytic interstitial pneumonia
(LIP), 167
Lympholytic therapy, 402


Maastricht categories, 332
Macrophage inflammatory protein one
alpha (MIP-1 $\alpha$), 440, 442
Major histocompatibility complex
(MHC), 489, 672, 677, 754
Masson's trichrome, 686
MCP. *See* Monocyte chemoattractant
protein
Mean pulmonary-artery pressure
(mPAP), 150–151
Mediastinitis, 595
Medroxyprogesterone acetate (MPA),
220
6-Mercaptopurine (6-MP), 373
Metalloproteinase (MMP), 761
Methylxanthines, 81, 82
MHC. *See* Major histocompatibility
complex
Mixed connective tissue disease
(MCTD), 182–183
Mofetil mycophenolate (MMF), 735
Monoclonal antibodies against
B-cells, 920
Monocyte chemoattractant protein one
(MCP-1), 440, 442, 510
Mononuclear inflammatory
cells, 703
Mosaic hypoperfusion, 848
Multidrug-resistant (MDR) TB, 628
Multiorgan donors in Australia, 310
Multiply antibiotic-resistant
(MAR), 118
Muscarinic receptors, 74
Muscle sympathetic nerve activity
(MSNA), 790

Mycobacerium avium complex (MAC), 633
Mycobacterial infections (MBIs), 692
incidence of, 623
Mycobacterium avium-intracellulare complex, treatment of, 640
*Mycobacterium gordonae*, 634
*Mycobacterium haemophilum*, 634
treatment of, 641
*Mycobacterium kansasii*, 634
treatment of, 640
*Mycobacterium malmoense*, 635
*Mycobacterium marinum*, 635
*Mycobacterium scrofulaceum*, 635
*Mycobacterium simiae*, 635–636
*Mycobacterium szulgai*, 636
*Mycobacterium tuberculosis*, 624
clinical manifestations of, 626–627
diagnosis, 627
risk factors for, 624
treatment, 627–629
*Mycobacterium ulcerans*, 636
*Mycobacterium xenopi*, 636–637
Mycophenolate mofetil (MMF), 243, 375–378, 891, 908
*Mycoplasma hominis*, 594

*N*-acetyl cysteine (NAC), 169
Natural killer (NK) cells, 760
Natural killer T (NKT) cells, 28
Neoplastic disease, 315
Neoplastic disorders, 134–135
Neutrophils, 703
New York Heart Association (NYHA), 273
NHBDs. *See* Non–heart-beating donors
*Nocardia farcinica*, 598
Nocturnal Oxygen Therapy Trial (NOTT), 64
Non–heart-beating donors (NHBDs), 10, 332
Nonalloimmune responses, 754
Noncytomegalovirus infections (non-CMV), 13
Non-hodgkin's lymphomas (NHL), 914

Non–rapid eye movement (NREM) sleep, 790
Nonspecific bronchial hyperreactivity (NSBHR), 802
Nonspecific interstitial pneumonia (NSIP), 167, 177–178
Nontuberculous mycobacteria (NTM), 96, 118–119, 623, 631–632
clinical features of, 639
diagnostic testing, 639–640
epidemiology, 632–633
NTM. *See* Nontuberculous mycobacteria
Nuclear factor kappa B (NFkB), 442–443
Nystatin, oral, 245

OB. *See* Obliterative bronchiolitis
Obliterative bronchiolitis (OB), 157, 704, 723, 726
clinical presentation, 724
diagnosis of, 731
histopathologic features, 754
incidence and prevalence of, 723–724
treatment of, 734–735, 737–741
OKT3, 407
Omental wrap, 6, 8
Oophorectomy, 220
Opsonization, 407
Organ donation, 302, 309–310
Organ harvest, 49
Organ preservation, principles, 326
Organ procurement agencies (OPAs), 309
Organ Procurement and Transplant Network (OPTN), 286
Organ transplant recipients (OTRs), 624
Osteopenia, 895
Osteoporosis, 384, 895
Overlap syndrome, 182
Oxygen therapy, long-term, 82
Oxygenation, 173

PAEC. *See* Pulmonary artery endothelial cells
PAH. *See* Pulmonary arterial hypertension
Panel reactive antibodies (PRA), 697
PAP. *See* Pulmonary arterial pressure
Para influenza virus (PIV), 485, 843
Parameters, clinicopathologic, 697
Parvovirus B19 (PVB19), 511, 686
PCR. *See* Polymerase chain reaction
PDGF. *See* Platelet-derived growth factor
Pentoxifylline administration, 337
Perfadex®, 353. *See also* Low-potassium dextran (LPD)–glucose solution
Periodic Acid-Schiff (PAS), 686
Peripheral tolerance, 54
PET. *See* Positron emission tomography
PFT. *See* Pulmonary function test
Phrenic nerve injury, 801
PIV. *See* Para influenza virus
Plasmapheresis, 404
Platelet activating factor antagonist, 338
Platelet aggregation, 406
Platelet-derived growth factor (PDGF), 757
Platelia®, 564
PLCH. *See* Pulmonary Langerhans cell histiocytosis
Pleiotropic cytokine, 764
PMNs. *See* Polymorphonuclear leukocytes
*Pneumocystis carinii*, 259, 694
*Pneumocystic carnii* pneumonia (PCP), 275
*Pneumocystis jiroveci*, 245, 599
Pneumonectomy, recipient, 257–258
Pneumonia, 588, 589
Polymerase chain reaction (PCR), 488, 490, 627, 843
Polymorphonuclear chemotaxis, 328
Polymorphonuclear leukocytes (PMNs), 609
Polymyositis (PM), 182
Posaconazole, 541

Positron emission tomography (PET), 627
Postmortem functional assessment, 352
Posttransplant lung, imaging of, 861
  imaging of, early (24 hours to 1 week), 830
  immediate (within 24 hours), 794
  intermediate (first 2 months), 833
  primary late (2–4 months), 843
  secondary late (>4 months), 849
Posttransplant lymphoproliferative disorder (PTLD), 248–249, 404, 486
  classification of, 902–903
  clinical manifestations of, 911
  diagnosis of, 914
  histological features of, 901
  incidence of, 910, 912
  risk factors for, 906–907
  treatment of, 916–918
Posttransplant malignancy, 276
PPH. *See* Primary pulmonary hypertension
PRA. *See* Panel reactive antibodies
Prednisone, 382–384
Pretransplant panel reactivity testing, 50
Primary graft dysfunction (PGD), 355, 437
  definition and diagnosis, 437–439
  grading system, 439
  management of, 452–453
  outcomes of, 455
  retransplantation, 455
Primary graft failure (PGF), 154, 687
Primary pulmonary hypertension (PPH), 114, 270, 448
Profibrotic factors, 757
Progressive systemic sclerosis (PSSc), 180
Prostacylin in pulmonary hypertension, 273
Prostaglandins, 453
Prostaglandin E1 (PGE1), 337, 446
*Pseudomonas aeruginosa*, 118
PTLD. *See* Posttransplant lymphoproliferative disorder

Pulmonary arterial hypertension (PAH), 148, 175
  diagnosis and classification systems, 148
  medical management of, 150
  natural history of, 150–152
  pathology of, 149
Pulmonary arterial pressure (PAP), 66, 148, 289
Pulmonary arterial stenosis, 450
Pulmonary artery endothelial cells (PAEC), 442
Pulmonary artery hypertension, surgical treatments, 273–275
Pulmonary cryptococcosis, symptoms of, 571
Pulmonary denervation, effects, 790–793
Pulmonary edema, 409
Pulmonary embolism (PE), 847–848
Pulmonary eosinophilic granuloma, 210
Pulmonary function, 62
  analysis of, 261–262
  and gas exchange, 793–795
  parameters as predictors of mortality, 171
  postoperative, 261
Pulmonary function test (PFT), 662, 665–667
Pulmonary hypertension, 66
Pulmonary infarction, 847–848
Pulmonary Langerhans cell histiocytosis (PLCH), 205
  clinical features, 206
  course and prognosis, 210
  pathogenesis of, 210
  pathology, 208
  pulmonary function tests (PFTs), 208
  radiographic features, 206–208
  therapy, 211–212
Pulmonary rehabilitation, 64
Pulmonary thromboendarterectomy, 274
Pulmonary vascular disease, biology of, 149–150
Pulmonary vascular disorders, 278
Pulmonary vascular resistance (PVR), 151, 449

Pulmonary vasodilators, 272, 280
Pulmonary vein, donor, 258
Purified protein derivative (PPD), 630
Purine biosynthesis, 376
Puriritic skin rashes, 405
Purulent secretions, 358
PVB. *See* Parvovirus B
PVR. *See* Pulmonary vascular resistance
Pyrazinamide (PZA), 628–629, 631
PZA. *See* Pyrazinamide

Rabbit antithymocyte globulin (RATG), 674, 736
RANTES, 425–426
Rapamycin, 221, 470, 739
Rapamycin-related airway complications, 470–471
Rapid growing mycobacteria (RGM), 633, 641
RATG. *See* Rabbit antithymocyte globulin
Recipient hepatic dysfunction, 452
Recurrent acute rejection (RAR), 735
Reed–Sternberg (RS) cells, 904
Regulatory T (Treg) cells, 21
Regulatory T lymphocytes, 53
Rejection episodes, in nonstandard donors, 357, 405
Renal impairment (chronic), principal cause of, 380
Renal insufficiency, 124
Renal toxicity, 367, 409
Respiratory bronchiolitis interstitial lung disease (RB-ILD), 167
Respiratory failure and mechanical ventilation, 120
Respiratory reflex responses, 792
Respiratory syncytial virus (RSV), 485, 508, 708, 843
Reticuloendothelial system (RES), 404
RGM. *See* Rapid growing mycobacteria
Rhabdomyolysis, 372
Rheumatoid arthritis (RA), 181
Rhinosinusoidal disease, 123–124
*Rhodococcus equi*, 597

Rifampin (RIF), 628
  role of, 629
RSV. *See* Respiratory syncytial virus

Salmeterol, 72
Saprophytic fungal organisms, 475
Sarcoidosis, 183, 860
  clinical features and prognosis of, 184
  mortality, 186
  treatment of, 183
Scedosporium, 574
Scientific Registry of Transplant
      Recipients (SRTR), 290
Sedai virus (SeV), 765
Seizures, 247–248
Severe acute respiratory syndrome
      coronavirus (SARS-CoV), 485,
      514
Single flush perfusion. *See* Lung
      preservation, techniques used for
Single-lung transplantation (SLT), 9, 93,
      127, 667
Sirolimus (SRL), 379–382, 892
Sjogren's syndrome (SS), 183
Skin malignancies, 276
SLT. *See* Single lung transplantation
Smoker's macrophages, 714
Solid organ transplant
      (SOT), 406, 611, 626, 902
Solid organ transplant recipients
      (SOTRs), 527
SOT. *See* Solid organ transplant
Spirometry, 62
Stable lung transplant recipients, 795
Steroids, 895
Streptomycin (SM), 628
Sulfobutyl ether β-cyclodextrin
      (SBECD), 566
Surface recognition receptors, 48
Surfactant dysfunction, 334
Surveillance bronchoscopy, 669–670
Systemic hypertension, 279
Systemic lupus erythematosus
      (SLE), 182
Systolic pulmonary artery pressure
      (sPAP), 149

Tacrolimus, 369–373, 891
TB. *See* Tuberculosis
TBB. *See* Transbronchial biopsies
TCAD. *See* Transplantation coronary
      artery disease
T-cell activation cascade, 365
T-cell depletion strategies, 23
T-cell subsets, 402
Teriparatide, 109
TGF. *See* Transforming growthfactor
Theophylline, 81
Thoracic donor organs, 311
Thoracic simulated allocation model
      (TSAM), 297
Thoracosternotomy incision, 8
Thoracostomy tubes, 221, 829
Thrombocytopenia, 406
Tiotropium, 74, 76
T-lymphocyte activation. *See*
      Cyclosporine A (CsA),
      mechanism of action
TMP-SMX. *See* Trimethoprim–
      sulfamethoxazole
Total lymphoid irradiation
      (TLI), 736
TNF. *See* Tumor necrosis factor
Tracheobronchitis, 559
Transbronchial biopsies
      (TBB), 668–669, 731
Transcription factor activation, 443
Transesophageal echocardiography
      (TEE), 450
Transforming growthfactor beta
      (TGF- β), 27, 53, 364, 757
Transplantation coronary artery disease
      (TCAD), 772
Treg cells, types, 26. *See also* Regulatory
      T cells
Treprostinil, 126
Trimethoprim–sulfamethoxazole
      (TMP-SMX), 245, 275, 598
Trough level monitoring, 366
Tryptophan depletion, 33
TSAM. *See* Thoracic simulated
      allocation model
Tuberculin skin testing (TST), 630
Tuberculosis (TB), incidence of, 624

Tuberous sclerosis complex (TSC), 213
Tumor necrosis factor alpha (TNF-α),
    440, 487, 761


UIP. *See* Usual interstitial pneumonia
United Network for Organ Sharing
    (UNOS), 233, 280
Upper lobe fibrosis, 857
Upper respiratory tract infections
    (URTI), 507
URTI. *See* Upper respiratory tract
    infections
Usual interstitial pneumonia
    (UIP), 166, 171


Valganciclovir (VGCV), 492
Valvular heart disease, 885
Varicella–Zoster virus (VZV), 485
Vascular cell adhesion molecule
    (VCAM), 489
VATS. *See* Videoassisted thoracoscopic
    surgery
VCA. *See* Viral capsid antigen

VCAM. *See* Vascular cell adhesion
    molecule
Ventilation indexes, 733
Ventilation–perfusion mismatch, 336
Very low-density lipoprotein
    (VLDL), 888
VGCV. *See* Valganciclovir
Video-assisted thoracoscopic surgery
    (VATS), 85, 217, 685
Viral capsid antigen (VCA), 907
Viral infections, 248
    community-acquired, 695–696
    opportunistic, 694–695
Vitamin D/calcium, 897
VLDL. *See* Very low-density
    lipoprotein
Voriconazole, 566
VZV. *See* Varicella–Zoster virus


West Nile virus (WNV), 485, 513–514
Williams–Campbell syndrome, 713


Zygomycetes, 567